THIRD EDITION

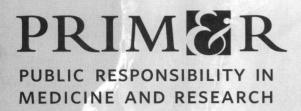

PRIM&R

PUBLIC RESPONSIBILITY IN
MEDICINE AND RESEARCH

Institutional
Review Board

Management and Function

THIRD EDITION

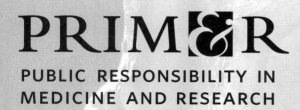

PUBLIC RESPONSIBILITY IN MEDICINE AND RESEARCH

Institutional Review Board

Management and Function

Elizabeth A. Bankert, MA

Director Emerita
Office of the Committee for
the Protection of Human
Subjects
Dartmouth College

Bruce G. Gordon, MD

Assistant Vice-Chancellor
for Regulatory Affairs
Professor of Pediatric
Hematology/Oncology
University of Nebraska
Medical Center

Elisa A. Hurley, PhD

Executive Director
Public Responsibility
in Medicine and
Research (PRIM&R)

Sharon P. Shriver, PhD

Director of Programs
Public Responsibility in
Medicine and Research
(PRIM&R)

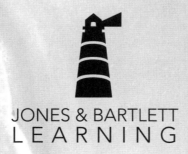

JONES & BARTLETT
LEARNING

World Headquarters
Jones & Bartlett Learning
5 Wall Street
Burlington, MA 01803
978-443-5000
info@jblearning.com
www.jblearning.com

Jones & Bartlett Learning books and products are available through most bookstores and online booksellers. To contact Jones & Bartlett Learning directly, call 800-832-0034, fax 978-443-8000, or visit our website, www.jblearning.com.

Substantial discounts on bulk quantities of Jones & Bartlett Learning publications are available to corporations, professional associations, and other qualified organizations. For details and specific discount information, contact the special sales department at Jones & Bartlett Learning via the above contact information or send an email to specialsales@jblearning.com.

Production Credits
VP, Product Development: Christine Emerton
Director of Product Management: Matt Kane
Product Manager: Tina Chen
Content Strategist: Melina Leon-Haley
Project Manager: Kristen Rogers
Senior Project Specialist: Alex Schab
Senior Digital Project Specialist: Angela Dooley
Senior Marketing Manager: Lindsay White
Content Services Manager: Colleen Lamy

Product Fulfillment Manager: Wendy Kilborn
Composition: S4Carlisle Publishing Services
Cover Design: Michael O'Donnell
Text Design: Michael O'Donnell
Senior Media Development Editor: Troy Liston
Rights Specialist: Rebecca Damon
Cover Image (Title Page, Part Opener, Chapter Opener):
 © Santiago Urquijo/Getty Images.
Printing and Binding: McNaughton & Gunn

Library of Congress Cataloging-in-Publication Data
Names: Bankert, Elizabeth A., editor. | Gordon, Bruce G., editor. | Hurley,
 Elisa A., editor. | Shriver, Sharon P., editor. | Public Responsibility
 in Medicine and Research (Association), issuing body.
Title: Institutional review board : management and function / [edited by]
 Elizabeth A. Bankert, Bruce G. Gordon, Elisa A. Hurley, Sharon P.
 Shriver, Public Responsibility in Medicine & Research (PRIM&R).
Other titles: Institutional review board (Amdur)
Description: Third edition. | Burlington, Massachusetts : Jones & Bartlett
 Learning, [2021] | Includes bibliographical references and index. |
 Summary: "The National Institutes of Health (NIH) invests over $37
 billion per year in support of research to improve human health. All
 research funded by NIH that involves human subjects is subject to
 regulatory oversight, requiring institutions to staff and manage
 Institutional Review Boards (IRBs). IRB members, chairs, and the many
 associated human subjects protections oversight professionals who
 support the work of the IRB must navigate complex federal regulations
 issued by multiple agencies. This book is the industry standard
 reference work for the research oversight community, providing
 comprehensive, understandable interpretations of the regulations, clear
 descriptions of the ethical principles on which the regulations are
 based, and practical best-practices guidelines for effectively
 implementing regulatory oversight"-- Provided by publisher.
Identifiers: LCCN 2020044754 | ISBN 9781284181159 (paperback)
Subjects: MESH: Ethics Committees, Research--organization & administration
Classification: LCC R725.3 | NLM W 20.5 | DDC 174.2--dc23
LC record available at https://lccn.loc.gov/2020044754

6048

Printed in the United States of America
25 24 23 22 21   10 9 8 7 6 5 4 3 2 1

Contents

Foreword

Reflections on *Belmont* at Forty

Suzanne M. Rivera

The *Belmont Report* turned 40 in 2019, and, just as adults ask themselves existential questions as they age, so, too, was there much handwringing about the relevance, vitality, and staying power of the *Belmont Report* on the occasion of its milestone birthday.

Like adults facing a midlife crisis, the academic fields of bioethics and public policy—among others—took the opportunity to question where we are, how we got here, and whether we should have made different choices. This generated a flurry of scholarly think pieces about the *Belmont Report*, exploring the impact of the document and ruminating about its applicability as it heads into its fifth decade.* Although a good number of the commentaries were complimentary about *Belmont*'s staying power, others called for a reexamination of the principles (and even of principlism as an approach to ethical decision making). Perhaps not unsurprisingly, common themes emerged in the *Belmont*-at-40 literature oeuvre.

First, it seems there is a general (although not universal) consensus that the ethical principles of respect for persons, beneficence, and justice have provided a valuable framework for moral decision making regarding human research and the protection of research subjects' rights and welfare. Indeed, these principles have become downright canonical in research ethics scholarship, while at the same time serving as a mantra for legions of IRB members and staff, who do the hard work each day of trying to operationalize their meaning and intent.

Second (and somewhat paradoxically), there is both a reverence for the historical significance of the document and a willingness to question the process of its creation and the outcomes of the exercise to produce it. Each of these impulses merits further consideration.

With regard to process, it is worth recalling the circumstances under which the commission that wrote the report was established. In the wake of concerns in 1972 about the now notorious Public Health Service–funded study of syphilis in the "negro" male, the U.S. government set about designing a new ethical, legal, and regulatory landscape for the protection of human research subjects. In a visionary attempt to avoid putting the cart before the horse, this redesign process began, not with a rush to produce regulations, but with an effort to establish the fundamental principles that could provide a foundation for the policies, rules, and practices that would follow.

Because the commission's first meeting took place at the Belmont Conference Center in Elkridge, Maryland, the final report was given the name of that

---

*One of these was co-authored by Kyle Brothers, Aaron Goldenberg, and me. The drafting of that article heavily influenced my thinking about this essay.

center: "Belmont Report: Ethical Principles and Guidelines for the Protection of Human Subjects of Research, Report of the National Commission for the Protection of Human Subjects of Biomedical and Behavioral Research."

By today's standards, the group charged with writing the report was exceedingly homogeneous and therefore did not reflect the diversity of the U.S. population or the various constituencies we currently would expect to be given a seat at the table for such an undertaking. Indeed, if such a commission were chartered today, we would expect to see a very different roster. That said, we in the field of research ethics owe a debt of gratitude to the architects of the *Belmont Report*, who wrestled valiantly with some of the thorniest conflicts, challenges, and dilemmas of that time—many of which continue to characterize the enterprise of human research today.

Nevertheless, there has been much questioning of and reflection on the report's drafting and ultimate conclusions. Was the process sound? Were the "right" voices in the room? Might we need additional principles today? These have not so much constituted a critique of the *Belmont* principles *per se* but rather are evidence of the ways in which the public's perspectives and values have changed since the report was first published in 1979.

Numerous societal changes have influenced the myriad ways we think differently today about human research protections than we did 40 years ago. These include skepticism of authority, the imperative to "do it yourself," a more sophisticated appreciation for human diversity and intersecting forms of oppression and inequality, and evolving notions of ownership (both with regard to data and biological specimens). There also have been changes in the research enterprise itself.

Some of these changes may be attributable to the development of new technologies. The rapid expansion of multisite research, which brought with it new challenges related to data sharing and storing of specimens, has been made possible in large part due to the opportunities for collaboration created by the internet. However, societal changes cannot be explained by the availability of new technologies alone. Consider, for example, emerging practices like the inclusion of community members in research oversight, expanded efforts to make research data publicly available, and the participation of patient advocacy groups in collecting and sharing data. To some extent, new technologies made these activities possible, but they also reflect a change in cultural values.

Patients are now far less likely to accept a "doctor knows best" approach and instead expect that healthcare providers will welcome shared decision making. This trend toward leveling the power differential between professionals and their clients is not limited to medicine. To varying degrees, professionals in many fields—lawyers, accountants, realtors, bankers, etc.—have begun to shift toward playing an advisory role to their clients. Given this shift, it should not be surprising that researchers have begun to adopt—and research participants have begun to expect—approaches to research that encourage study participants to take a more active role in the research process.

As times have changed, IRBs have had to (and will continue to) navigate an ever-evolving landscape of new technologies and shifting cultural values. And, like the middle-aged parent of a teenager who must adjust to the sounds of unfamiliar musical artists and a later curfew, those of us responsible for protecting human subjects' rights and welfare must learn to apply the *Belmont* principles in the context of today's world.

The enduring relevance of *Belmont* speaks volumes about the elegance of the principles and their applicability despite changing norms. However, the weight given to each of the principles has shifted over time. For many years, respect for persons was treated like the primary principle to be observed by IRBs and researchers, with beneficence and justice playing supporting roles. In today's context, it is more common to think about the three principles as points on a triangular plane, resting precariously on a fulcrum. As the IRB or researcher attempts to maximize one principle, it becomes elevated over the other two. Thus, an emphasis on beneficence can reduce justice. Under the best circumstances, IRBs and researchers can strive for something closer to balance by attending to all three principles.

Our understanding of the principles also has shifted over time. The evolving interpretation of the justice principle provides a keen example. The commissioners who framed the *Belmont Report*, responding to legitimate and urgent concerns about the exploitation of vulnerable populations, such as those enrolled in the aforementioned PHS-funded syphilis study, focused on the aspect of justice that has to do with avoiding exploitation of vulnerable populations. Accordingly, the report's discussion of the justice principle asserted that, "the selection of research subjects needs to be scrutinized in order to determine whether some classes (e.g., welfare patients, particular racial and ethnic minorities, or persons confined to institutions) are being systematically selected simply because of their easy availability, their compromised position, or their manipulability, rather than for reasons directly related to the problem being studied."

Although the principle of justice still requires fairness, modern IRBs do not and should not focus exclusively on the aspects of justice that have to do with avoiding exploitation; indeed, most research ethicists now emphasize the importance of avoiding the unjustified and unfair *exclusion* of certain populations from research. We recognize now that the paternalistic "protection" from research that for many years kept children, so-called "women of child-bearing potential," and members of minoritized groups out of studies resulted in research findings that often were not broadly applicable and that neglected the specific and unique health needs of large segments of the population.

A close reading of the *Belmont Report* reveals that its framers understood the complexity of the justice principle, evidenced by that fact that they encouraged us to think about fairness in a variety of ways: "injustice arises from social, racial, sexual and cultural biases institutionalized in society. Thus, even if individual researchers are treating their research subjects fairly, and even if IRBs are taking care to assure that subjects are selected fairly within a particular institution, unjust social patterns may nevertheless appear in the overall distribution of the burdens and benefits of research." It would be hard to argue that these words are any less relevant in today's world.

We can thank members of patients' rights, civil rights, and various liberation movements for drawing attention to the aspects of justice that require intentional and deliberate inclusion of diverse populations in research to achieve fairness. We also should applaud the many IRB members and staff who, over the years, have worked tirelessly to honor the spirit of the *Belmont* principles while applying them in the context of changing cultural norms.

This is no easy feat. To serve on an IRB is a great responsibility. Doing it well requires intellectual curiosity, good judgment, and a genuine desire to promote high-quality research for the benefit of society. IRB members must deftly execute their duty to protect subjects' rights and welfare and a concurrent obligation to avoid unnecessary impediments to important research that sometimes are created by excessive institutional risk aversion. An openness to learning is essential, which is why books like this one are so helpful—not only for "onboarding" of new IRB members and staff but also as a reference manual to help guide decision making when ethically challenging questions arise in the review and oversight of human research studies.

The regulations that eventually were written after the publication of the *Belmont Report* promulgated the belief that a group of thoughtful people, working together to think about and resolve moral questions and ethical dilemmas, could arrive at more sound and appropriate decisions than a simple bureaucratic form or administrative procedure. And, for the most part, this belief has borne fruit. Communities of researchers, scholars, public policy experts, research subjects, and others have, over the years, built a community concerned with advancing best practices for IRBs and promoting the highest ethical standards for the conduct of research. By publishing and periodically updating this book, PRIM&R contributes to those efforts.

But continuous improvement is never done. So, having been subjected to reexamination at its 40th birthday, the *Belmont Report* now stands firmly in mature adulthood—older, wiser, and more comfortable with the ambiguities of life, ready for the inevitable challenges ahead, and open to the potential for reflection, change, and reinvention.

Preface

It is hard to believe it has been 15 years since the publication of the last edition of *Institutional Review Board: Management and Function*. We know the community has been eagerly awaiting this new edition, as the research environment has changed significantly since 2005. The ascendance of "big data," patient-engaged research, centralized IRB review, data transparency and sharing, and research conducted in "real-world" settings, among other developments, means that the methods used to collect and share research data, the types and quantities of information available for study, and who counts as a subject and stakeholder in research have all evolved in significant ways over the past decade and a half. These changes have brought new challenges for those who oversee research, raising questions about how to apply ethical principles and research regulations in a variety of new contexts. In addition, this period has seen the first major revisions to the core federal regulations governing human research since 1991, as well as increasing specialization and professionalization of the research oversight field.

Given these developments, when creating this edition, we carefully considered both content and structure. While all of the topics covered in previous editions are represented here, the content has been rewritten to reflect new regulations and evolving best practices. Many new chapters have been added to address newer research areas, methodologies, and challenges. Finally, an overall reorganization and refreshing of the presentation, including highlighting when topics cross over between chapters, the use of sidebars to call out background material, and the inclusion of case studies, have resulted in a book that is easy to use both as a thorough orientation to the field and as a quick, on-the-ground reference. We thank the contributors of prior editions for providing such a firm foundation on which to build.

While human subjects research has continued to evolve, the dedication of the human research oversight community to their work, to the ethical principles of research, and to each other has remained constant. This generosity of spirit is reflected in this volume, to which a total of 180 professionals contributed. We are extremely grateful to the chapter authors for sharing their wisdom, insights, and practical experience on all aspects of human subjects research oversight. We also appreciate those who reviewed the work in progress and the team at Jones & Bartlett Learning who led us through the production process. *Institutional Review Board: Management and Function* is a book written for research oversight professionals by research oversight professionals, and we hope the support and dedication of your colleagues is evident in its pages.

This edition was produced at a particular moment in time—when we are facing unprecedented challenges, including the COVID-19 global pandemic, rising recognition of the need to address racial injustice and inequity as they manifest in research, and increasing public distrust of science and demand for transparency. These are the issues that demand our attention now. It is certain that in the future, IRB professionals will face similarly unprecedented circumstances and be called on to address their impacts on research. Historically, this field has met challenges as they arise by returning to foundational ethical principles and applying them anew. Our hope is that this book provides the background, resources, and tools needed to continue this tradition of excellence, in whatever moment it is being used.

Liz Bankert
Bruce Gordon
Elisa Hurley
Sharon Shriver
October 2020

A Few Notes on Terminology

"Subject" vs. "participant": Throughout this book, we use the term research "subject" to refer to the people who donate their time, bodies, information, or biological specimens to make research possible. We recognize that many people prefer the term "participant" to refer to research volunteers. This may be especially true for some domains and types of research, for instance, research that makes a point of engaging patients as partners in some aspect of the research conduct or design, or research in the social sciences that involves the careful cultivation of long-term trusting relationships with those who are being studied and with whom the resulting knowledge is "co-created." In cases like these, in which the individual in question is engaged in an active and ongoing way in some sort of shared endeavor, the term research "participant" may well be more fitting.

While acknowledging these points, we thought it important to use one term consistently across the book, for clarity, and we have chosen "subject" for two reasons. First, "subject" is used in the federal regulations that provide the framework for the IRB's work. The second, more substantive reason is that we believe that the term "subject" more accurately reflects the unavoidable power and knowledge asymmetries between researchers and those upon whom research procedures are done, or about whom information is being collected, that are endemic to most types of research. Using the term "subject" makes clear an individual's position of relative vulnerability when enrolled in a research study, as well as the need for independent mechanisms to ensure that the rights, welfare, and interests of those who volunteer for research are adequately protected.

2018 revisions to the Common Rule: This volume was put together shortly after the revisions to the Federal Policy for the Protection of Human Subjects, or Common Rule, went into effect in 2018. Unless otherwise noted, references to "the Common Rule" are to this current rule. When the context calls for distinguishing between the Common Rule that was revised in 2018 and the earlier version of the regulations, we use "2018 Common Rule" and the "pre-2018 Common Rule" to make clear which set of regulations are being referred to. We recognize that some ongoing research may still be reviewed under the pre-2018 Common Rule and that not all federal agencies have signed on to adopt the revised regulations. While most of the guidance provided by this book will be applicable to such research, readers are advised to consult the text of the earlier version of the rule when appropriate.

How to Use This Book

Regulatory References

The regulations governing various aspects of research with human subjects are codified in the U.S. Code of Federal Regulations, or CFR. We use standard regulatory notation to refer to or cite specific regulations, which involves referencing the Title, Part, Section, and Subpart of the Code of Federal Regulation where the regulations appear. For example, the FDA regulations that deal with IRBs comprise Title 21, Part 56, of the Code of Federal Regulations, so the shorthand to refer to these regulations is 21 CFR 56. The criteria for IRB approval of FDA-regulated research, more specifically, can be found in Section 111 of these regulations: 21 CFR 56.111. Within each section, subsections and paragraphs are indicated with additional letters and numbers, and these designations follow the section number in parentheses. For example, 21 CFR 56.111(a)(2) refers to the specific IRB criterion for approval that says risks to subjects are reasonable in relation to anticipated benefits.

Because the Common Rule and the FDA human subjects regulations are referred to in the text of nearly every chapter of the book, they are not included in the reference lists at the end of each chapter. 45 CFR 46, 21 CFR 50, and 21 CFR 56 (as they appear at the time of publication of this book) have been reproduced in full in Part 13, along with full references and links to the sources. For regulations that are less commonly cited, for instance, the HIPAA Privacy Rule, we use regulatory notation in the body of the text, but also include a full citation in the reference list at the end of the chapter.

As of this writing, 19 federal departments and agencies are either signatories to the Revised Common Rule, or follow the rule by executive order. Each agency that is a signatory to the Common Rule includes in its respective title and part of the CFR section numbers and language that are identical to Department of Health and Human Services (DHHS) regulations at 45 CFR 46 subpart A. This information is reproduced in Part 13, "Adoption of the Common Rule by Participating Agencies." Given this harmonization, and for ease of reading, we use 45 CFR 46 to cite or refer to the Common Rule, although other agencies may use a different regulatory designation for the same language.

Symbols and Conventions Used in This Book

Introduction: The Concept of Vulnerability

The Common Rule requires that "when some or all of the subjects are likely to be vulnerable … additional safeguards have been included in the study to protect the rights and welfare of these subjects" [45 CFR 46.111(b)]. This requirement is based, in part, on the *Belmont Report* principle of respect for persons. *Belmont* states that "persons with diminished autonomy are entitled to protection" (National Commission, 1979).

⊘ 1-1

Regulatory citations are indicated with **bold, shaded text**.

Regulatory excerpts (quotes) are shaded.

A crosslink symbol (⊘) in the margin indicates where information related to the corresponding underlined text may be found in another chapter.

Boxes are used to highlight key points or brief summaries.

RESOURCES TO ASSIST IRBS WITH DEVELOPMENT OF AI/AN COMMUNITY ENGAGEMENT PROCEDURES

- **Collaborative Research Center for American Indian Health (CRCAIH)**, especially its IRB Toolkit and Data Management Toolkit
- **Indigenous Wellness Research Institute (IWRI)**, especially its Research Ethics Training for Health in Indigenous Communities (rETHICS) curriculum, a culturally adapted version of Collaborative Institutional Training Initiative's (CITI's) human subjects training
- **National Congress of American Indians (NCAI) Policy Research Center**, especially its *Research That Benefits Native Peoples: A Guide for Tribal Leaders* curriculum
- **Native American Cancer Prevention Center—Outreach Core Resources**, especially researcher guidelines and *How to* resources in the publications library
- **Public Responsibility in Medicine and Research (PRIM&R)**. See resources developed with the NCAI Policy Research Center, Northwest Indian College, and others, especially several free webinars (search for "Tribal" and "Indian" within past and archived webinars)
- **Urban Indian Health Institute (UIHI)**, especially support and materials for Urban Indian Programs.

VOLUNTARY INFORMED CONSENT CAPACITY

In exploring whether subjects might have difficulty providing voluntary informed consent, the IRB might consider asking the following questions:

- Are there decisional issues or communication issues that might interfere with the ability of the prospective subject to understand the research or their rights, to process that information and make a reasoned choice based on their own goals and values, or to communicate their wishes?
- Are there social conditions that limit the subject's options?
- Does the subject's hope for medical benefit influence their judgment?
- Are the conditions for informed consent satisfied? That is, is information presented in an understandable manner, do the subjects comprehend the details of the research and their rights as research subjects, and is the process of consent conducive to true voluntariness?

adults. In early 1982, however, it was recognized that infusion of IV medications containing benzyl alcohol to low birth weight premature infants caused severe metabolic acidosis, encephalopathy, and respiratory depression with gasping, leading to the death of 16 infants. Benzyl alcohol is metabolized to benzoic acid and then conjugated in the liver and excreted as hippuric acid. This latter metabolic pathway is less functional in premature infants, allowing accumulation of benzoic acid with resulting toxicity. Removal of benzyl alcohol from IV medications in one NICU was associated with a decrease of mortality rate for very small infants from 81% to 46% (Hiller et al., 1986). Similar pediatric therapeutic disasters have occurred, reflecting the danger of extrapolating safety and dosage from adult studies to children (Christensen et al., 1999). These episodes clearly demonstrate the necessity of controlled testing of drugs in children before the use of these drugs, approved in adults, becomes standard practice.

Sidebars are used for additional background or explanatory material.

☻ *Federal Ethics Panel Review*

In 2017, FDA conducted the first review under 21 CFR 50.54 for a commercially sponsored pediatric protocol. The IRB referral asked whether placement of a central venous catheter was acceptable for study-drug infusion (including for subjects receiving placebo) during the 96-week study period. Children in this study were having significant difficulty with peripheral venous access due to their disease. The review was completed within 10 weeks, highlighting that the 21 CFR 50.54 process can be completed in an efficient and timely manner. Transparency was promoted throughout the process, although some documents were redacted for public comment to protect commercial confidential information. Parent and patient community input were instrumental in contributing to the outcome (FDA, 2017a; Snyder et al., 2018; Snyder & Nelson, 2018).

Case studies are presented in special boxes with a case study symbol (☻).

Reviewers

Susan Ahlf, CIP
Children's Wisconsin
Milwaukee, WI

Laura Bezler, MSRC, CCRC
Children's Wisconsin
Milwaukee, WI

Mina Busch, MS, CCRP, CIP
Cincinnati Children's Hospital
Cincinnati, OH

Benjamin "Rocky" Byington, CIP
Cincinnati Children's Hospital
Cincinnati, OH

Nichelle Cobb, PhD
University of Wisconsin
Madison, WI

Rebecca Dahl, PhD, CIP
Stony Brook University
Stony Brook, NY

Dianne Ferris, MS, CIP
Stanford University
Palo Alto, CA

Martha Jones, MA, CIP
Mass General Brigham
Boston, MA

Michelle Martin, BA, MSW, MILS, JD, CIP
Children's Wisconsin
Milwaukee, WI

Melissa McGee, JD
University of New Hampshire
Durham, NH

Sara Meeder
Maimonides Medical Center
Brooklyn, NY

Jonathan Miller, MPPA, CIP
University of Alabama at Birmingham
Birmingham, AL

Nancy Olson, JD
University of Mississippi Medical Center (retired)
Jackson, MS

Nancy Ondrusek, PhD
Public Health Ontario; University of Toronto
Toronto, Ontario

Annette Rid, MD, PhD
National Institutes of Health
Bethesda, MD

Michele Russell-Einhorn, JD
Advarra, Inc.
Columbia, MD

Julie Simpson, PhD
University of New Hampshire
Durham, NH

Amy Waltz, JD, CIP
Indiana University
Indianapolis, IN

Alexa Williams, RN
Children's Wisconsin
Milwaukee, WI

Chris Witwer, CIP
Stanford University
Palo Alto, CA

Brandon Woodruff
Children's Wisconsin
Milwaukee, WI

Laura Youngblood, MPH, CIP
Centers for Disease Control and Prevention
Atlanta, GA

Contributors

Melissa Abraham, PhD, MS
Harvard Medical School
Boston, MA

Emily E. Anderson, PhD, MPH
Loyola University Chicago
Maywood, IL

Deana Around Him, DrPH, ScM*
Child Trends, Inc.
Bethesda, MD

Elizabeth A. Bankert, MA
Dartmouth College
Hanover, NH

Deborah Barnard, MS
University of Colorado
Denver, CO

Mark Barnes, JD, LLM
Ropes & Gray, LLP
Boston, MA

John R. Baumann, PhD
Indiana University
Indianapolis, IN

Jill Beck, MD
University of Nebraska Medical Center
Omaha, NE

Amy Ben-Arieh, JD, MPH
The Fenway Institute at Fenway Health
Boston, MA

Stacey Berg, MD
Baylor College of Medicine
Houston, TX

Rachel Bibeault, CIP
Dartmouth College
Hanover, NH

Barbara E. Bierer, MD
Brigham and Women's Hospital
Harvard Medical School
Boston, MA

Marianna Bledsoe, MA
Colorado Springs, CO

David Borasky, MPH, CIP
WIRB – Copernicus Group
Cary, NC

Kristina Borror, PhD*
Veterans Health Administration
Washington, DC

Joseph S. Brown, PhD
University of Nebraska–Omaha
Omaha, NE

Stephanie Bruce
Department of Defense
Office of Human Research Protections
Alexandria, VA

Elizabeth Buchanan, PhD
Marshfield Clinic Research Institute
Marshfield, WI

Mina Busch, MS, CCRP, CIP
Cincinnati Children's Hospital Medical Center
Cincinnati, OH

Judith Carrithers, JD, MPA
Advarra, Inc.
Columbia, MD

Cecilia Brooke Cholka, PhD, CIP
University of Nevada, Reno
Reno, NV

Delia Wolf Christiani, MD, JD, MSCI
Harvard T.H. Chan School of Public Health
Boston, MA

Karen Christianson, RN, BSN
HRP Consulting Group
Lake Success, NY

Paul Christopher, MD
Brown University
Providence, RI

---

*The views expressed by this contributor are the author's own and do not necessarily represent those of their institution or organization.

Nichelle Cobb, PhD
University of Wisconsin
Madison, WI

Linda M. Coleman, JD, CIP, CHC, CHRC, CCEP-I
Yale University
New Haven, CT

Charlotte Coley, MACT, CIP
University of North Carolina
Chapel Hill, NC

Kindra Cooper, JD, MPA, MA
Advarra, Inc.
Seattle, WA

Jacqueline Corrigan-Curay, JD, MD*
U.S. Food and Drug Administration
Silver Spring, MD

Jeremy Corsmo, MPH
Cincinnati Children's Hospital
Cincinnati, OH

Tracey Craddock, CCRP
University of Alabama
Birmingham, AL

Kristi DeHaai, MS, CIP
University of Virginia
Charlottesville, VA

Lisa Denney, CIP, MPH
Stanford University
Palo Alto, CA

Neal W. Dickert, MD
Emory University School of Medicine
Atlanta, GA

Francis J. DiMario Jr., MD, MA, CIP
Connecticut Children's Medical Center
Hartford, CT

Megan Doerr, MS, LGC
Sage Bionetworks
Seattle, WA

Anastasia Doherty, BS, CIP
Stanford University
Palo Alto, CA

Teresa Doksum, PhD, MPH
Abt Associates Inc.
Cambridge, MA

Stacey Donnelly, MPH, MS
Broad Institute of MIT and Harvard
Cambridge, MA

James M. DuBois, PhD, DSc
Washington University in St. Louis
St. Louis, MO

Emily Eldh, BA, CIP
Advarra, Inc.
Columbia, MD

Melissa A. Epstein, PhD, MBE, CIP
Albert Einstein College of Medicine
Bronx, NY

Laverne Estanol, MS, CIP
University of California, Santa Cruz
Santa Cruz, CA

Helena Estes-Johnson, AAS, CIP
University of Virginia
Charlottesville, VA

Nir Eyal, DPhil Politics
Center for Population-Level Bioethics
Rutgers University
New Brunswick, NJ

Joshua Fedewa, MS, CIP*
University of Texas Southwestern Medical Center
Dallas, TX

Michelle Feige, MSW, LCSW-C
AAHRPP
Washington, DC

Susan S. Fish, PharmD, MPH
Boston University
Boston, MA

Faith E. Fletcher, PhD, MA
University of Alabama
Birmingham, AL

David Forster, JD, MA, CIP
WIRB – Copernicus Group
Puyallup, WA

William L. Freeman, MD, MPH, CIP
Northwest Indian College
Bellingham, WA

Francine Gachupin, PhD, MPH
University of Arizona
Tucson, AZ

Dean Gallant, AB
HRP Consulting Group
Lake Success, NY

*The views expressed by this contributor are the author's own and do not necessarily represent those of their institution or organization.

Aaron Goldenberg, PhD, MPH
Case Western Reserve University
Cleveland, OH

Sara Goldkind, MD, MA
Goldkind Consulting, LLC
Potomac, MD

Bruce G. Gordon, MD
University of Nebraska Medical Center
Omaha, NE

Julia G. Gorey, JD*
Office for Human Research Protections
U.S. Department of Health and Human Services
Rockville, MD

Christine Grady, RN, PhD
NIH Clinical Center
Bethesda, MD

Jennifer A. Graf, BA*
Takeda Pharmaceuticals International Co.
Cambridge, MA

Jonathan Green, MD, MBA
National Institutes of Health
Bethesda, MD

William E. Grizzle, MD, PhD*
University of Alabama, Birmingham
Birmingham, AL

Marielle S. Gross, MD, MBE
Johns Hopkins Berman Institute of Bioethics
Baltimore, MD

John A. Guidry, PhD, MA
TRX Development Solutions, LLC
Brooklyn, NY

Karen Hale, RPh, MPH
The Ohio State University (retired)
Columbus, OH

Charles B. Hall, PhD
Albert Einstein College of Medicine
Bronx, NY

Lauren Hartsmith, JD*
Office for Human Research Protections
U.S. Department of Health and Human Services
Rockville, MD

Erica Heath, MBA, CIP
Independent Review Consulting, Inc.
San Anselmo, CA

John Heldens, CIP, RAC
University of Colorado Denver
Anschutz Medical Campus
Aurora, CO

Ross Hickey, CIP, CPIA, JD
University of Southern Maine
Portland, ME

Susie Hoffman, BSN, CIP
University of Virginia
Charlottesville, VA

Fariba Houman, PhD
Boston Children's Hospital
Boston, MA

Leslie M. Howes, MPH, CIP
Harvard T.H. Chan School of Public Health
Boston, MA

Sara Chandros Hull, PhD*
National Institutes of Health
Bethesda, MD

Elisa A. Hurley, PhD
Public Responsibility in Medicine & Research
Boston, MA

Peter R. Iafrate, PharmD
University of Florida
Gainesville, FL

Courtney Jarboe, MS, MA, CIP
University of Minnesota
Minneapolis, MN

Karen Jeans, PhD, CCRW*
Veterans Health Administration
Washington, DC

Ann Johnson, PhD, MPH, CIP
University of Utah
Salt Lake City, UT

Bethany Johnson, JD, CIP
Indiana University
Indianapolis, IN

Martha F. Jones, MA, CIP
Mass General Brigham
Boston, MA

Stefanie E. Juell, MA, CIP
Albert Einstein College of Medicine
Bronx, NY

*The views expressed by this contributor are the author's own and do not necessarily represent those of their institution or organization.

Joy Jurnack, RN, CCRC, CIP, FACRP
Northwell Health
Manhasset, NY

Julie Kaneshiro, MA*
Office for Human Research Protections
U.S. Department of Health and Human Services
Rockville, MD

Elizabeth Kipp-Campbell, MS, PhD, CIP
Maine Health System
Portland, ME

Richard Klein
GE2P2 Global Foundation
Philadelphia, PA

Molly Klote, MD, CIP*
Veterans Health Administration
Washington, DC

Susan Kornetsky, MPH
Boston Children's Hospital
Boston, MA

Christopher J. Kratochvil, MD
University of Nebraska Medical Center/
   Nebraska Medicine
Omaha, NE

Helene Lake-Bullock, PhD, JD
University of Kentucky
Lexington, KY

Emily A. Largent, JD, PhD, RN
University of Pennsylvania
Philadelphia, PA

Lisa Leventhal, MSS, CIP*
Oregon State University
Corvallis, Oregon

Maggie Little, PhD
Georgetown University
Washington, DC

Sue Logsdon, MS, CIP
University of Nebraska Medical Center
Omaha, NE

Abbey Lowe, MA
University of Nebraska Medical Center
Omaha, NE

Bryan Ludwig, BA, CIP
University of Nebraska Medical Center
Omaha, NE

Anne Drapkin Lyerly, MD, MA
University of North Carolina
Chapel Hill, NC

Kimberly A. Lyford, BA, CIP
Dartmouth College CPHS
Hanover, NH

Monica Magalhaes, PhD
Center for Population-Level Bioethics
Rutgers University
New Brunswick, NJ

Monika Markowitz, PhD, MA, MSN, RN
Virginia Commonwealth University
Richmond, VA

Peter J. Marshall, CIP
Air Force Research Oversight and Compliance Office
Falls Church, VA

Judy Matuk, MS
HRP Consulting Group
Lake Success, NY

Linda (Petree) Mayo, BA, CIP
University of New Mexico
Albuquerque, NM

Kathy McClelland, BS
Stanford University
Palo Alto, CA

Tristan McIntosh, PhD
Washington University in St. Louis
St. Louis, MO

Ross McKinney, MD
Association of American Medical Colleges
Washington, DC

Lindsay McNair, MD, MPH, MSB
WIRB – Copernicus Group
Princeton, NJ

Sara Meeder
Maimonides Medical Center
Brooklyn, NY

Jonathan E. Miller, MPPA, CIP
University of Alabama at Birmingham
Birmingham, AL

Lauren Milner, PhD*
U.S. Food and Drug Administration
Silver Spring, MD

*The views expressed by this contributor are the author's own and do not necessarily represent those of their institution or organization.

Stephanie Morain, PhD, MPH
Baylor College of Medicine
Houston, TX

Lawrence H. Muhlbaier, PhD
Duke University
Durham, NC

Kathleen E. Murphy, MSW, PhD, MLIS, CIP
Retired
Glenview, IL

Daniel K. Nelson, MS
University of North Carolina (Emeritus)
U.S. Environmental Protection Agency (Emeritus)
Chapel Hill, NC

Robert M. Nelson, MD, PhD*
Johnson & Johnson
Spring House, PA

Eunice Yim Newbert, MPH
Boston Children's Hospital
Boston, MA

Robert Nobles, DrPH, MPH
Emory University
Atlanta, GA

Kelley A. O'Donoghue, MPH, CIP
University of Rochester
Rochester, NY

Ann O'Hara, BS, CIP
Dartmouth College
Hanover, NH

Kelly O'Keefe, MPH
Population Services International
Washington, DC

Laura Odwazny, JD, MA*
U.S. Department of Health and Human Services
Rockville, MD

Nancy Olson, JD
University of Mississippi Medical Center (retired)
Jackson, MS

David Peloquin, JD
Ropes & Gray, LLP
Boston, MA

Heather Pierce, JD, MPH
Association of American Medical Colleges
Washington, DC

Ernest D. Prentice, PhD
University of Nebraska Medical Center
Omaha, NE

Ivor Pritchard, PhD*
Office for Human Research Protections
U.S. Department of Health and Human Services
Rockville, MD

Josiah Rich, MD, MPH
Brown University
Providence, RI

Jessica Ripton, MPH, CIP
Partners Healthcare System, Inc.
Somerville, MA

Suzanne M. Rivera, PhD, MSW*
Macalester College
St. Paul, MN

Laura Lyman Rodriguez, PhD*
Geisinger Research
North Bethesda, MD

Lori Roesch, CIM, CIP*
Children's Wisconsin
Milwaukee, WI

Stephen Rosenfeld, MD, MBA
Freeport Research Systems
Freeport, ME

Brenda Ruotolo, CIP, BA*
Columbia University
New York, NY

Michele Russell-Einhorn, JD
Advarra, Inc.
Columbia, MD

Victor M. Santana, MD
St. Jude Children's Research Hospital
Memphis, TN

Cheryl Savini
HRP Consulting Group
Lake Success, NY

Toby Schonfeld, PhD*
Department of Veterans Affairs
Washington, DC

Meghan Scott, BA
Fred Hutchinson Cancer Research Center
Seattle, WA

*The views expressed by this contributor are the author's own and do not necessarily represent those of their institution or organization.

Ada Sue Selwitz, MA
University of Kentucky
Lexington, KY

Shannon Sewards, MA, CIP
Harvard University
Cambridge, MA

J. Jina Shah, MD, MPH
Kite Pharmaceuticals
Santa Monica, CA

J. Graham Sharp, PhD
University of Nebraska Medical Center
Omaha, NE

Sharon P. Shriver, PhD
Public Responsibility in Medicine & Research
Boston, MA

Robert Silbergleit, MD
University of Michigan
Ann Arbor, MI

Julie Simpson, PhD
University of New Hampshire
Durham, NH

Megan Kasimatis Singleton, JD, MBE, CIP
Johns Hopkins University School of Medicine
Baltimore, MD

Julia Slutsman, PhD
Children's National Hospital
George Washington University School of Medicine
    and Health Sciences
Washington, DC

Belinda Smith, MS, RD, CCRC
University of Kentucky
Lexington, KY

Lynn Smith, JD
Tampa General Hospital
Tampa, FL

Donna L. Snyder, MD*
U.S. Food and Drug Administration
Silver Spring, MD

Marjorie Speers, PhD
Clinical Research Pathways
Atlanta, GA

Ryan Spellecy, PhD
Medical College of Wisconsin
Milwaukee, WI

Matthew Stafford, MPH
Boston Children's Hospital
Boston, MA

Irene Stith-Coleman, PhD*
Office for Human Research Protections
U.S. Department of Health and Human Services
Rockville, MD

David Strauss, MD
Columbia University
New York, NY

Walter Straus, MD, MPH*
Merck & Co., Inc.
Kenilworth, NJ

Elyse I. Summers, JD
AAHRPP
Washington, DC

Catherine Sutherland
University of Colorado
Aurora, CO

Kelly Tanguay, CIP
Dartmouth College
Hanover, NH

Erica Tauriello, BA, CIP
Wentworth-Douglass Hospital
Dover, NH

Amy Waltz, JD, CIP
Indiana University
Indianapolis, IN

Cheryl Crawford Watson, JD, MPA, MBE*
National Institute of Justice
Office of Justice Programs
US Department of Justice
Washington, DC

Meaghann Weaver, MD, MPH, FAAP
University of Nebraska Medical Center
Omaha, NE

Carol J. Weil, JD*
National Cancer Institute
Rockville, MD

Gabriella Weston, MS, CIP
Albert Einstein College of Medicine
Bronx, NY

Lorri Wettemann, BS, CIP, MA
Dartmouth College CPHS
Hanover, NH

*The views expressed by this contributor are the author's own and do not necessarily represent those of their institution or organization.

Libby White, CIP, MBA, MPH
U.S. Department of Energy
Washington, DC

Chris Witwer, CIP
Stanford University
Palo Alto, CA

Laura Youngblood, MPH, CIP*
Centers for Disease Control and Prevention
Atlanta, GA

Sharon Zack, MS*
Westat
Rockville, MD

---

*The views expressed by this contributor are the author's own and do not necessarily represent those of their institution or organization.

Ethical and Historical Background

Ethical Foundations of Human Research Protections

Elisa A. Hurley
Sharon P. Shriver

Abstract

The Common Rule and other regulations governing human research oversight are built on a foundation of ethical principles. Familiarity with some of the core concepts of ethics and an understanding of ethical reasoning will provide context for the day-to-day work of the IRB, help IRB administrators effectively apply the rules and regulations, and provide guidance and resources for navigating novel or complex situations or those not covered by the regulations. This chapter provides an outline of the core principles of ethics and ethical reasoning and a framework for their application in effective research oversight.

Introduction

The responsibility to protect the rights and welfare of human research subjects is codified in the Common Rule and other human research subject regulations, but it is ultimately a matter of ethics: what sort of conduct is right or wrong, good or bad, acceptable or unacceptable. Historical narratives describing the development of the field of human subjects research regulation and oversight often quote bioethicist Carol Levine who, in 1998, wrote "[T]he basic approach to the ethical conduct of research and approval of investigational drugs was born in scandal and reared in protectionism" (Levine, 1988). While it is true that the current codification of research regulations was stimulated by 20th-century revelations of gross mistreatment of human research subjects, the principles of ethics that guide how we ought to act and treat others have been around for centuries and inform much of how we live together.

While it is not essential to have a deep understanding of the philosophical underpinnings of human subjects protections in order to interpret and apply the regulations, a familiarity with ethical concepts will provide important context for the day-to-day work of the IRB. IRBs are in the business of ethical reasoning, whether they are explicitly aware of it or not. Ethical reasoning involves (1) identifying that there is a moral question or problem at hand, a question of what we ought or ought not to do; (2) accurately understanding the facts and circumstances of the situation; (3) drawing on ethical frameworks and principles to identify the ethical dimensions and morally relevant features of the situation; (4) weighing the various moral considerations against each other; (5) making a considered moral judgment about what to do, how to act, and being able to articulate the reasons in favor of that judgment. While the IRB's process rarely involves this kind of step-by-step moral reasoning, knowledge of ethical principles and reasoning processes can be key in navigating novel or complex situations or those not covered by the regulations. As the research landscape, technology, and society change, an understanding of the principles and history of ethics in human subjects protections will provide a solid foundation for adapting to such changes.

Ethics

Definitions vary, but most generally, *ethics* can be thought of as a system of moral principles that define right and wrong for individuals and society. The term *ethics* also refers to the branch of philosophy that deals with right vs. wrong, good vs. evil, and the actions or motivations that correspond to those values. Some of the earliest recorded writings concern ethics and ethical conduct, and the fundamental principles on which our current ethical consensus is based can trace their origins to this early philosophical work.

There are different theories of ethics, such as consequentialism, deontology, and virtue ethics, which differ in terms of whether they put the consequences of our actions, duties and obligations, or character at the center of their conception of morality (see sidebar: Examples of Ethical Theories). All of the ethical frameworks that have been developed attempt to provide answers to important questions of morality, including, What is the right or best way to act? Even the most skilled philosopher, however, may encounter situations in which there is no clear moral path, and where reasonable people might disagree about the morally best thing to do. In fact, given the complexity of human life, some problems may not have a "correct" answer. In these cases, taking any action will require making ethical trade-offs.

Furthermore, different approaches to ethics may be appropriate for different situations. For example, in some situations, focusing on the *consequences* of actions might be appropriate—dislocating someone's arm to remove them from a car wreck is likely the right thing to do, even though intentionally hurting someone is typically a bad thing to do. On the other hand, there are some things we just should not do, even if the consequences of doing them would be good.

Although a doctor might wish to spare a patient the painful news of a poor prognosis, it is generally considered morally unacceptable to withhold the truth from competent adults, regardless of how difficult it might be to hear. A focus on maximizing well-being might be the appropriate guiding framework for a domain like public health, where we agree that considerations about what will bring about the greatest good for the greatest number of people should override duties to respect individuals' wishes. The clinician–patient relationship, on the other hand, seems more appropriately governed by concepts of a doctor's fiduciary duties to their patients and their wishes.

Ethical theories also highlight what we should pay attention to in the situations we face. Being familiar with ethical theories and principles can help us know what to look for when we are not sure what we should do. For example, ethics tells us that we should look at the consequences of each of our possible courses of action, but we should also think about whether the people in the situation, including us, might have duties to act in certain ways (or to refrain from acting in certain ways). Identifying what might be ethically relevant to the situation helps us to focus on the features that we should consider in decision making and to ignore the features that are morally irrelevant.

Now that we have a general sense of what ethics is and the role that ethical reasoning plays in moral decision making, let us look more closely at how these principles and theories play a role in effective oversight of human subjects research.

> **EXAMPLES OF ETHICAL THEORIES**
>
> *Consequentialism:* A type of ethical theory that says whether an action or policy is right or wrong depends on the consequences that action or policy brings about. This approach is sometimes associated with the idea that "the ends justify the means." The most well-known form of consequentialism, Utilitarianism, says that actions are right to the extent that they maximize happiness or well-being.
>
> *Deontology:* A type of ethical theory that is centered on the idea of duties. Some actions are right or wrong in and of themselves, regardless of their consequences, and we have a duty to either do those things or refrain from doing them. A deontologist would disagree that ends justify the means; they would argue that the means *themselves* matter.
>
> *Virtue ethics:* A type of ethical theory that focuses on the idea of character rather than on the consequences of actions or on duties. Good actions are those that flow from a good and virtuous character.

Applied Ethics

Applied ethics refers to the use of ethical reasoning, principles, or theories in practical day-to-day contexts and decision making. Anyone living in society makes ethical decisions many times every day, from choosing which products to purchase, to deciding whether to tell the truth, to calculating how much to tip the coffee shop barista. When we make these decisions, we are "doing" applied ethics. Applied ethics is also an umbrella term for approaches to ethics in various practical domains, such as law, business, the environment, and medicine.

Biomedical ethics, or *bioethics*, is concerned with ethical decisions and ethical conduct in the domain of medicine and health care. Bioethics touches on a wide range of questions: When is it justifiable for physicians to aid patients in dying? What is the best way to allocate scarce healthcare resources? What is the moral view of paid surrogacy? What sort of post-trial obligations do research sponsors have to research subjects and their communities?

Bioethics encompasses clinical ethics, which is sometimes referred to as "ethics at the bedside," as well as research ethics. *Research ethics* is a broad category concerned with ethical issues that arise in the conduct of research and includes a more focused area known as the Responsible Conduct of Research (RCR), which applies to the professional activities of scholars and researchers. RCR principles have implications for all aspects, stages, and personnel involved in the research process and cover a broad range of issues, including the proper conduct of research with animals and human beings, publication and authorship, teaching and mentoring, and the creation, integrity, and sharing of research data (**Figure 1.1-1**). Research involving human subjects is a key research integrity issue, and it often overlaps with other areas of RCR, such as financial management of grants or authorship of research articles. In the United

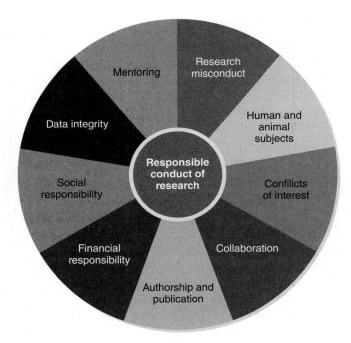

Figure 1.1-1 Principles of RCR

States, the National Science Foundation and the National Institutes of Health (NIH) require education in RCR topics for certain funding recipients (National Science Foundation, n.d.). IRB personnel will benefit from a general understanding of RCR and the place that human subjects oversight has in the larger context of research ethics.

Ethical Foundations of Human Subjects Protections

Research with human subjects has at its core a central ethical dilemma or tension: *while the goal of research is to develop generalizable knowledge that can improve human health and well-being for all, it is individuals who are asked to take on the burdens and possible risks of research, often without the potential of direct benefit to them.* Although people who participate in research may, in fact, benefit—perhaps from receiving an effective experimental therapy, or in the form of enhanced care or post-trial benefits—the *aim* of research, by definition and design, is to benefit society, not the individual. The core principles of research ethics recognize this basic fact and seek to provide guidance on how to balance the obligation to protect individuals from harm with the desire to maximize the benefits to human well-being that research may provide.

These core principles have been articulated and further specified in a number of national and international ethics codes, which together form a rough "framework" for the protection of the rights and welfare of human subjects of research. These codes have emerged at different points in time, in some cases (as noted later), in response to specific events. The revelation of research scandals or atrocities, the advent of new research technologies and practices, and changing social norms continue to drive changes to the codes themselves or, in some cases, to the ways they are interpreted and applied. We can think of these events as "inflection points" for research ethics—episodes or circumstances that prompt new thinking about particular aspects of ethical research. For example, the 1999 death of <u>Jesse Gelsinger</u> in a clinical trial led to increased precautions around investigator and institutional conflicts of interest and prompted a re-conceptualization of the IRB as just one part of a broader <u>human research protections program</u> (HRPP). The 2013 revelation that cells from <u>Henrietta Lacks</u> had been used for years without her consent informed the process of revising the Common Rule and, to some extent, the shape of the final rule. These inflection points and their effects are highlighted at relevant points throughout the book and are listed in the historical timeline that follows this chapter.

🔗 1-2

🔗 2-1

🔗 1-2

Research Ethics Codes

Existing research ethics codes do not have the force of regulations or law but are instead widely accepted as offering guiding principles for both the creation of national laws and regulations and for the conduct of research. The most influential of these codes are the *Belmont Report,* the *Nuremberg Code*, and the *Declaration of Helsinki* (National Commission for the Protection of Human Subjects of Biomedical and Behavioral Research, 1979; Nuremberg Code, 1949; World Medical Association, 2013).

The Nuremberg Code is the oldest of the modern research ethics codes. It was drafted in 1947, following World War II, at the close of the "Doctors' trial" at Nuremberg, Germany, during which Nazi doctors who had conducted a series of horrific experiments on prisoners were tried for war crimes and other offenses. At the conclusion of the trial, the Nuremberg judges articulated a set of 10 guiding principles for research, beginning with an absolute requirement to seek and obtain the voluntary consent of every human research subject (Nuremberg Code, 1949). This was one of the first times that the obligation to seek informed consent was articulated in the context of human experimentation (Shuster, 1997).

In 1964, the World Medical Association, an international organization representing physicians, formally adopted the Declaration of Helsinki, a set of ethical principles for medical research involving human subjects that was heavily influenced by the Nuremberg Code (Carlson, Boyd, & Webb, 2004). The Declaration of Helsinki has been amended several times, most recently in 2013, to reflect both evolving norms and changing research practices (World Medical Association, 2013). While the Declaration was originally addressed to physicians, later versions explicitly encourage other stakeholders in the human subjects research enterprise to adopt its principles. The most recent Declaration includes 37 short provisions arranged within 10 general topic areas: risks, burdens, and benefits; vulnerable groups and individuals; scientific requirements and research protocols; research ethics committees; privacy and confidentiality; informed consent; use of placebo; post-trial provisions; research registration and publication and dissemination of results; and unproven interventions in clinical practice.

In 1974, it was revealed that the U.S. government, in collaboration with the Tuskegee Institute, had been conducting a <u>study of untreated syphilis</u> in poor Black men in Macon County, Alabama, for 40 years—and had withheld proven syphilis treatment for 20 of those years. In response, the National Research Act was passed to examine and improve research practices in the United States. Among other things, the National Research Act created the National Commission for the Protection of Human Subjects of Biomedical and Behavioral Research. The National Commission was charged with

🔗 1-2

"identifying the basic ethical principles that should underlie the conduct of biomedical and behavioral research involving human subjects and developing guidelines to assure that such research is conducted in accordance with those principles" (Department of Health and Human Services, 2016). After 4 years of deliberation and discussion, in April 1979, the National Commission published the *Belmont Report*, which identified three basic ethical principles described as "generally accepted in our cultural tradition . . . respect of persons, beneficence, and justice" (National Commission, 1979). *Belmont* outlines the application of these principles in three basic requirements for conducting research: informed consent, risk/benefit assessment, and selection of research subjects (see box: Ethical Codes Guiding Human Subjects Research). The framework provided in the *Belmont Report* serves as the foundation for the Federal Policy for the Protection of Human Subjects, or Common Rule, and remains the foundational document for research ethics and oversight in the United States.

ETHICAL CODES GUIDING HUMAN SUBJECTS RESEARCH

Nuremberg Code: 1947 statement by jurists following the Nuremberg trials of Nazi doctors that lists 10 ethical principles for research with human subjects.

World Medical Association Declaration of Helsinki: First adopted in 1964 and revised multiple times, the most recent version (2013) details 37 provisions in 10 topic areas, largely based on the Nuremberg Code principles.

Belmont Report: The 1979 report of the U.S. National Commission for the Protection of Human Subjects of Biomedical and Behavioral Research describing respect for persons, beneficence, and justice as three overarching principles for human subjects research.

Singapore Statement on Research Integrity: Drafted following the Second World Congress on Research Integrity, this internationally created statement published in 2010 lists four principles (honesty, accountability, professional courtesy and fairness, good stewardship) and 14 related professional responsibilities to support integrity in research.

Council for International Organizations of Medical Sciences (CIOMS) International Ethical Guidelines for Health-Related Research Involving Humans: Written in collaboration with the World Health Organization (WHO), and most recently updated in 2016, this publication lists 25 guidelines to protect humans in research.

The *Belmont* Principles

Respect for persons: As elaborated in *Belmont*, respect for persons breaks down into two parts. First is the idea that individuals should be treated as autonomous agents. An autonomous agent is someone who is capable of deliberating about their personal goals, and who is then able to act on those deliberations. Thus to respect persons is to acknowledge and "give weight" to their considered judgments and choices, and to refrain from interfering with their acting on those judgments and choices, unless there is some good reason to do so. The idea that individuals possess autonomy is central to the *deontological* approach to ethics mentioned earlier—it is because people are autonomous that we have certain duties and obligations to them.

The second part of respect for persons is the conviction that people with diminished autonomy are entitled to protection. While some people are capable of self-determination, others—perhaps because they are not yet mature enough, are temporarily incapacitated by illness, or permanently lack the capacity due to disability—are not as capable, and those individuals require protection. They need someone else to look out for their interests, either permanently or temporarily.

> *Application*: The principle of respect for persons gives rise to the practical requirement to seek potential research subjects' informed consent, thereby giving them the opportunity to choose what will or will not happen to them. *Belmont* breaks down informed consent into three components—the *information* provided, the subject's *comprehension* of that information, and the *voluntariness* of the subject's decision that results. Special provisions to facilitate consent will be needed in cases where (1) the validity of the research requires incomplete disclosure of information (e.g., deception research), (2) subjects are limited in their ability to comprehend information, either temporarily or permanently, and (3) subjects are being asked to consent in conditions that may involve (perceived) coercion or undue influence.

🔗 Section 6

Beneficence: The second principle outlined in *Belmont* is beneficence: the idea of securing someone's well-being. Beneficence incorporates two requirements: to do no harm (nonmaleficence) and to maximize possible benefits and minimize possible harm (the maximizing principle). *Belmont* is clear that beneficence encompasses both individual benefits as well as potential benefits to society, including the benefits of knowledge that is expected to be gained from research. Beneficence, and in particular the maximizing principle, are *consequentialist* ideas—they appeal to the consequences that our actions will bring about, and they call on us to maximize the good consequences and minimize the bad.

> *Application*: The principle of beneficence gives rise to the practical requirement to assess the risks and the benefits of research and to the requirement that research must be justified on the basis of a "favorable" risk/benefit assessment. This means that in order for a research project to be ethically justified, the risks of research must be *reasonable* in relation to the anticipated benefits of the research (to the individual and/or to society).

Justice: The third principle outlined in *Belmont* is justice. The sense of justice that *Belmont* appeals to is known as "distributive justice"; it is concerned with the fair distribution of the benefits and burdens of research. *Belmont* does not explicitly define what would count as a "fair" distribution but points out that injustice occurs when a benefit to which someone is otherwise entitled is denied them without a good reason or when a burden is "unduly" imposed on someone (or on a particular group of people).

> *Application*: The principle of justice gives rise to the practical requirement that there be "fair procedures and outcomes in the selection of research subjects." It is unethical, for instance, to involve in research groups who are not likely to benefit from the applications of that research. According to *Belmont*, justice also requires being especially careful not to add research burdens to groups who are already burdened by socioeconomic conditions, illness, institutionalization, or bias, especially if that research does not offer the prospect of direct benefit.

The *Belmont Report* does not suggest that any of the principles takes priority over the other. There is relatively wide consensus that the three principles will often be in tension with each other and that, when they are, treating research subjects ethically requires attending to all three principles and doing our best to balance them. *Belmont* recognizes this tension when introducing the principle of beneficence, noting that "Persons are treated in an ethical manner not only by respecting their decisions and protecting them from harm, but also by making efforts to secure their well-being" (National Commission, 1979). Here, *Belmont* makes clear that both principles (autonomy and beneficence) are relevant for treating subjects ethically, but does not suggest one be considered before the other or be weighed more heavily than the other. *Belmont* does acknowledge that the application of each principle might give rise to competing claims. Respect for persons, for instance, might, on the one hand, demand providing prisoners the opportunity to volunteer for research but, on the other, seem to require that—as individuals whose autonomy may be compromised—prisoners be protected from the burdens of research. Indeed, the introduction to *Belmont* states explicitly, "These principles cannot always be applied so as to resolve beyond dispute particular ethical problems. The objective is to provide an analytical framework that will guide the resolution of ethical problems arising from research involving human subjects" (National Commission, 1979). The implementation of the principles takes ethical judgment and reasoning.

Belmont and Its Critics

While the *Belmont Report* continues to provide the core ethical foundation for research oversight in the United States, some have suggested that its principles are outdated and should be revised, replaced, or supplemented by additional principles. As noted previously, the *Belmont Report* was created following revelations about the <u>Tuskegee Study</u> of Untreated Syphilis in the Negro Male. The first two-thirds of the 20th century had seen a number of other egregious examples of research on vulnerable and relatively powerless populations, including sick children, residents of psychiatric hospitals, and prisoners. *Belmont*'s principle of justice is, as a result, primarily concerned with ensuring that those who are asked to take on the burdens of research should also be in a position to enjoy its benefits and that some should not be unfairly burdened for others' benefit. But beginning as early as the 1980s, when acquired immunodeficiency syndrome (AIDS) activists advocated for access to clinical trials, some began to see the framework codified in *Belmont* as overly protectionist. Today, many agree that the justice principle requires thinking just as carefully about how to ensure broad and equitable access to research and its potential benefits as about how to protect people from its burdens and harms. Others suggest that justice considerations call for more than the fair distribution of the benefits and burdens of research. Rather, attending to the principle of justice demands looking at which communities have a voice in setting the research agenda in the first place and thinking critically about whether, in certain circumstances, people might have an obligation to participate in research (Saghai, 2018).

Still others have suggested that since *Belmont* was created in response to specific research scandals, its scope is too narrowly focused on particular transgressions. In an influential 2000 paper, Emanuel and colleagues provide a novel ethical framework for biomedical research that seeks to improve what they see as deficiencies in existing research ethics guidelines, including *Belmont*. Emmanuel et al. (2000) identify and specify seven principles of ethical research: social value, scientific validity, fair participant selection, favorable risk–benefit ratio, independent review, informed consent, and respect for persons. They provide benchmarks that provide practical interpretations of each principle, and later added an eighth principle, collaborative partnership (Emanuel, Wendler, & Grady, 2000, 2008).

More recently, given how dramatically the research enterprise and public attitudes about research have changed in the 40 years since *Belmont* was published, some have suggested that it is time to entirely rethink the ethics framework underlying our regulatory and research system (Faden et al., 2013; Friesen, Kearns, Redman, & Caplan, 2017; Kass et al., 2013; National Academies of Science, Engineering, and Medicine, 2016; Parasidis, Pike, & McGraw, 2019; Raymond, 2019). Those who make these arguments point to the rise of technologies and methodologies that were not part of the research landscape when *Belmont* was written, such as comparative effectiveness research and the learning healthcare system, research involving deidentified biospecimens, cluster randomized trials, research involving large data sets, gene editing technologies, internet research, and mHealth research. There are also long-standing questions about the applicability of rules written for the biomedical research context to social and behavioral research (National Research Council, 2013). In addition, patients and the public are now engaged in research, as participants and partners, in ways that were not imaginable 40 years ago, as evidenced by the rise of patient-centered research. Current research ethics literature often refers to values and principles that were not part of the research ethical landscape at the time *Belmont* was written: transparency and trust; reciprocity (the idea that subjects' contributions to research should be acknowledged by providing some sort of benefit or recognition); stewardship and governance (of biospecimens and data, for example); obligations to participate; and patient or community engagement. A revision or updating of the *Belmont Report* was not part of the 2011–2018 process of revising the Common Rule, but an awareness of these changes and their implications is vital to the effective application of the *Belmont* principles by IRBs today.

🖉 10-8
🖉 10-10 🖉 10-11
🖉 12-4 🖉 10-13 🖉 10-14
🖉 10-5 🖉 12-5

🖉 12-9

Applying Principles of Research Ethics for the IRB

The regulations require IRBs to fulfill certain requirements for protecting the rights and welfare of research subjects. However, it is important to note that making ethical decisions is usually more than just following the requirements. We often talk about the distinction between *compliance* and *ethics*. Compliance is a matter of doing something simply because it is required by some set of rules or requirements. Ethics involves doing things because they are the right or best things to do. There are three types of reasons why IRBs should understand themselves to be *doing ethics*, beyond merely complying with rules, when they do their day-to-day work.

1. **The regulations require interpretation.**
   The regulations do not apply themselves; they require interpretation. Anyone who has witnessed an IRB discussion will have heard questions like, "Is this study minimal risk?" or "Is this proposed procedure a 'benign behavioral intervention' under exemption category 3?" and likely heard a range of different answers. Some have cited this kind of variability as a flaw in the IRB system, because it indicates a kind of arbitrariness in IRB judgments and decision making (Friesen, Yusof, & Sheehan, 2019). There may be some merit to that argument, but the variability also reveals a truth about rules, which is that it takes judgment to interpret and apply them and that reasonable people might come to different conclusions.

Consider, for example, the concept of "minimal risk," which is defined in the regulations to "mean that the probability and magnitude of harm or discomfort anticipated in the research are not greater in and of themselves than those ordinarily encountered in daily life or during the performance of routine physical or psychological examinations or tests" [45 CFR 46.102(j)]. This definition of "minimal risk" is open to different interpretations. For example, it is not clear whose "daily life" should be the standard: should it be based on the risk faced by an average person in the general population, or should the level of daily risk reflect that of a member of the particular study population? While the latter option may seem more appropriate to a particular study, it can unjustly distribute research risks, if the daily life of the study population just happens to expose those individuals to greater risk. There is no official guidance on the interpretation of the phrase "daily life," and similar conundrums are raised when trying to interpret phrases such as "routine . . . examinations" or determine what constitutes "harm or discomfort."

2. **The regulations themselves call for the use of ethical judgment and reasoning.**

Consider the requirement that "risks to subjects are reasonable in relation to anticipated benefits, if any, to subjects, and the importance of the knowledge that may reasonably be expected to result" [45 CFR 46.111(a)(2)]. Notice that this requires the IRB to make judgments regarding what is a "reasonable" balance of risks and benefits, and what constitutes "important" knowledge, because these terms are not defined in the regulations. Making such judgments involves identifying the potential harms of the research—including physical, psychological, social, informational, and economic harms—and their probability and magnitude. It also involves identifying and understanding what might reasonably be expected in terms of individual benefit, whether from access to the study therapy itself or from ancillary benefits such as additional monitoring. The IRB must also evaluate the importance to society of the knowledge that might be gained from the research and then determine whether those individual and social benefits together *justify* asking a potential subject to take on the risks identified. There is no formula for this evaluation, and because the two things (risks and benefits) being "balanced" are incommensurate—that is, they are not the same kind of thing—the decision is unavoidably a matter of judgment and reasoning.

🔗 12-2

There are other examples of concepts invoked in the regulations whose application specifically calls for ethical judgment. One is "undue" inducement, which the regulations do not define, and we discuss further later. The regulations also call for the IRB to determine whether the selection of subjects is "equitable," without providing a definition of equity or even offering much in the way of considerations that should go into such a determination. It is up to the IRB to consider factors such as features of the target population(s); the risk/benefit profile of the research; the available risk mitigation strategies; whether and how much compensation is offered; recruitment strategies; and the adequacy of justification offered for excluding any groups. The IRB must assign various weights to these factors and, ultimately, determine whether the proposed subject selection approach seems equitable.

3. **The regulations are incomplete and require supplementation.**

The regulations reflect knowledge and practice at a single point in time, and they must be general enough to be applicable to a range of different kinds of studies. There are, therefore, topics and areas that are not addressed in the Common Rule or not covered in much detail. By its nature, the research enterprise is constantly evolving, as discoveries are made, advances in technology permit global collaborations, and society changes. Therefore, it is inevitable that those charged with the ethical oversight of research will encounter research studies that present novel or unclear situations with respect to the regulations. See sidebar: Research Scenarios Not Addressed by the Regulations for examples of some current challenges where IRBs need to use ethical reasoning in order to practically and effectively assess research and situations that are not well characterized in the regulations.

RESEARCH SCENARIOS NOT ADDRESSED BY THE REGULATIONS

Voluntariness: Although this is a cornerstone concept of ethical research, the Common Rule provides little explanation of the concept of voluntariness or guidance for ensuring that research participation is voluntary. In fact, the only places where voluntariness is explicitly mentioned in the regulations is in the context of the requirements for informed consent. The second general requirement for informed consent is that researchers should seek informed consent only under circumstances "that minimize the possibility of coercion or undue influence" **[45 CFR 46.116(a)(2)]**. Further on, the regulation states that a basic required element of informed consent is "a statement that participation is voluntary" **[45 CFR 46.116(b)(8)]**. Consequently, informed consent forms often include a statement like, "Taking part in this study is voluntary . . . you may withdraw from the study at any time."

Whether research subjects are approached, recruited, or treated as volunteers is hardly captured by these brief mentions of voluntariness in the context of consent or by the corresponding statements in consent forms. *Belmont* contains a helpful discussion of the meaning of "voluntariness," summarizing some of the conditions that can undermine voluntariness. For instance, *Belmont* points out that undue influence occurs through an "excessive, unwarranted, inappropriate, or improper reward or other overture in order to obtain compliance," and that "unjustifiable pressures" occur when persons in position of authority . . . urge a course of action for the subject" (National Commission, 1979). *Belmont*'s discussion calls ethical reasoning and judgment into play because "it is impossible to state precisely where justifiable persuasion ends and undue influence begins" (National Commission, 1979). IRBs should be prepared to use ethical reasoning to determine how undue influence and coercion can be avoided when they review protocols, including by looking at recruitment strategies and materials and offers of compensation for research participation.

Return of research results and incidental findings: The Common Rule is relatively silent on the issue of how to handle situations where research procedures produce important or useful information about research subjects, other than requiring a statement in the informed consent about whether and in what conditions clinically relevant research results will be returned to subjects. This information may comprise research results, or it may involve "incidental findings" (findings that do not relate to the aims of the research). The chance of incidental findings comes up most often in genetics research, where, for instance, information about one subject may inadvertently provide information about family members; and in imaging research, where, for example, a study aimed at improving brain scan technology might reveal a brain tumor. The question of whether, when, and how to return such information to subjects implicates questions of respect

🔗 12-1

🔗 12-1

for people's autonomy, questions about risk and benefit, and questions of justice and fairness. IRBs need to be able to both identify the potential for these situations to arise during research they are reviewing in order to ensure research protocols adequately plan for such findings and utilize their knowledge of general ethical principles and reasoning to determine what constitutes an appropriate plan for returning results and incidental findings (or not) to research subjects (Wolf, 2013).

🔗 10-8

Comparative effectiveness research: A growing area of research concerns the comparison of two existing treatments or healthcare interventions. Often, each of the treatments was tested and developed against a placebo or the prior "standard of care," and little information exists directly comparing the two treatments, both of which may be commonly and widely used. Comparative effectiveness research (CER) involves randomizing patients to one standard treatment or the other, typically in "real world" settings, in order to compare and evaluate their outcomes, risks, and benefits. There is disagreement about how the Common Rule is best applied to CER, and IRBs will need to use their judgment to think about the intent of the regulations and how they fit the CER context (Joffe & Wertheimer, 2014; O'Neil, 2014).

Much of the difficulty rests on whether CER qualifies as minimal risk research. Some suggest that CER is almost always minimal risk, because the subjects will not incur any additional risk over and above what they would experience as patients receiving one of the standard treatments outside of the context of the trial. After all, the Common Rule states, "In evaluating risks and benefits, the IRB should consider only those risks and benefits that may result from the research (as distinguished from risks and benefits of therapies subjects would receive even if not participating in the research)" **[45 CFR 46.111(a)(2)]**. Thus, many IRBs choose to identify and evaluate only "incremental risks"—the risk added by participating in the study, above and beyond the risk of receiving a standard of care therapy. Other IRBs consider *all* of the risks involved as research risks, so that CER studies can only be designated minimal risk if they are comparing treatments that are themselves minimal risk (Lantos et al., 2015).

Another challenge in oversight of CER research concerns disclosure: some believe that regardless of the level of research risk involved, subjects (out of respect for their autonomy) should be told that in CER, the treatment they receive will be determined by a randomization procedure and not by clinician judgment, as it would if they were not enrolled in the research. Those who agree on this principle of disclosure, however, may disagree on whether that requires traditional informed consent or can allow for something less formal.

Post-trial obligations: Once a clinical trial has concluded, do the researchers or study sponsors have any ongoing obligations to the research subjects? The Common Rule and other research regulations are silent on this issue, though some international guidelines outline post-trial obligations. The Declaration of Helsinki, for example, states that sponsors and researchers have a responsibility to make provisions for individual research subjects and host communities to receive post-trial access to "interventions identified as beneficial in the trial" (World Medical Association, 2013). Another international guideline, produced by the Council for International Organizations of Medical Sciences (CIOMS), goes further, stating that "As part of their obligation, sponsors, and researchers must also make every effort. . . to make available . . . any intervention or product developed, and knowledge generated, for the population or community in which the research is carried out, and to assist in building local research capacity. In some cases, in order to ensure an overall fair distribution of the benefits and burdens of the research, additional benefits such as investments in the local health infrastructure should be provided to the population or community" (CIOMS, 2016; Cho, Danis, & Grady, 2018; Doval, Shirili, & Sinha, 2015).

There is ongoing debate about the scope of post-trial obligations, including questions such as who should get access, what the post-trial support should include, how long it should last, and who should bear the costs. At the close of a drug trial, for example, if the trial drug proved beneficial, a subject may wish to continue the treatment post trial. If the trial conditions were not beneficial to the subject, some argue that the researcher has a moral imperative to offer a more effective treatment to the subject. Regardless of the effectiveness of the intervention, researchers may have an obligation to provide support to subjects as they transition off the trial (post-trial care), perhaps by providing access to other medical care or social services. Although there is currently little consensus around these issues, many agree that doing nothing for research subjects after their trial participation is over may exploit research subjects and is therefore unethical (Cho et al., 2018). IRBs may be asked to review post-trial access and care plans, which may be described in research protocols and for prospective subjects in the informed consent documents, and determine if they are ethical. They will have to think about what is fair and equitable, given particulars of the study population and the trial, and consider what is a reasonable use of limited research resources.

Creating a Culture of Ethics

In this chapter, we have discussed the benefit to IRBs of understanding ethical principles and engaging in ethical reasoning. However, an understanding of and commitment to ethics is not only the purview of the IRB. Institutions have a shared responsibility for creating an institutional culture of ethical research, rather than a culture of mere compliance. Institutional policies, procedures, and practices that emphasize ethical principles will encourage well-conceived and properly executed research and may help mitigate the view of IRBs as the "ethics police." Institutional leaders can help foster such a culture by communicating in their words and actions that the institution's commitment to ethical research is not separate from its commitment to excellent research but rather is integral to it.

References

Carlson, R. V., Boyd, K., & Webb, D. J. (2004). The revision of the Declaration of Helsinki: Past, present and future. www.ncbi.nlm.nih.gov/pmc/articles/PMC1884510/#app1

Cho, H. L., Danis, M., & Grady, C. (2018). Post-trial responsibilities beyond post-trial access. *The Lancet, 391*(10129), 1478–1479. https://doi.org/10.1016/S0140-6736(18)30761-X

Council for International Organizations of Medical Sciences (CIOMS). (2016). *International ethical guidelines for health-related research involving humans.* CIOMS.

Doval, D. C., Shirali, R., & Sinha, R. (2015). Post-trial access to treatment for patients participating in clinical trials. *Perspectives in Clinical Research, 6*(2), 82–85. doi:10.4103/2229-3485.154003

Department of Health and Human Services (2016) The Belmont Report. www.hhs.gov/ohrp/regulations-and-policy/belmont-report/index.html

Emanuel, E. J., Wendler, D., & Grady, C. (2000). What makes clinical research ethical? *JAMA, 283*(20), 2701–2711.

Emanuel, E. J., Wender, D., & Grady, C. (2008). An ethical framework for biomedical research. In E. J. Emanuel et al. (Eds.), *The Oxford textbook of clinical research ethics.* Oxford University Press.

Faden, R. R., Kass, N. E., Goodman, S. N., Provonost, P., Tunis, S., & Beauchamp, T. L. (2013). An ethics framework for a learning health care system: A departure from traditional research ethics and clinical ethics. *Hastings Center Special Report, 43*(1), S16–S27.

Friesen, P., Kearns, L., Redman, B., & Caplan, A. L. (2017). Rethinking the Belmont Report? *American Journal of Bioethics, 17*(7), 15–21.

Friesen, P., Yusof, A. N. M., & Sheehan, M. (2019). Should the decisions of institutional review boards be consistent? *Ethics and Human Research, 41*(4), 2–14. doi:10.1002/eahr.500022

Joffe, S., & Wertheimer, A. (2014). Determining minimal risk for comparative effectiveness research. *The Hastings Center, 36*(3). www.thehastingscenter.org/irb_article/determining-minimal-risk-for-comparative-effectiveness-research/

Kass, N. E., Faden, R. R., Goodman, S. N., Provonost, P., Tunis, S., & Beauchamp, T. L. (2013). The research–treatment distinction: A problematic approach for determining which activities should have ethical oversight. *Hastings Center Special Report, 43*(1): S4–S15. doi:10.1002/hast.133

Lantos, J. D., Wendler, D., Septimus, E., Wahba, S., Madigan, R., and Bliss, G. (2015) Considerations in the evaluation and determination of minimal risk in pragmatic clinical trials. *Clinical Trials, 12*(5): 485–493.

Levine, C. (1988). Has AIDS changed the ethics of human subjects research? *Journal of Law, Medicine and Health Care, 16*(3–4):167–173. doi:10.1111/j.1748-720x.1988.tb01942.x

National Academies of Science, Engineering, and Medicine. (2016). Optimizing the nation's investment in academic research: A new regulatory framework for the 21st century. Washington, DC: National Academies Press. doi:1017226/21824

National Commission for the Protection of Human Subjects of Biomedical and Behavioral Research. (1979). *The Belmont Report: Ethical principles and guidelines for the protection of human subjects in biomedical and behavioral research.* www.hhs.gov/ohrp/regulations-and-policy/belmont-report/index.html

National Research Council. (2013). Proposed revisions to the Common Rule: Perspectives of social and behavioral scientists: Workshop summary. Washington, DC: National Academies Press. https://doi.org/10.17226/18383

National Science Foundation. (n.d.). America COMPETES Act RECR training requirements. www.nsf.gov/bfa/dias/policy/rcr.jsp

Nuremberg Code. (1949). Originally published in "Permissible medical experiments." In *Trials of war criminals before the Nuremberg Military Tribunals under Control Council Law, 10*(2), 181–182. Washington, DC: U.S. Government Printing Office. https://history.nih.gov/research/downloads/nuremberg.pdf

O'Neil, C. (2014). Consent and rights in comparative effectiveness trials. *Virtual Mentor, 16*(4), 289–294. doi:10.1001/virtualmentor.2014.16.4.msoc1-1404

Parasidis, E., Pike, E., & McGraw, D. (2019). A *Belmont Report* for health data. *New England Journal of Medicine, 380,* 1493–1495. doi:10.1056/NEJMp1816373

Raymond, N. (2019). Safeguards for human studies can't cope with big data. *Nature, 568,* 277. doi:10.1038/d41586-019-01164-z

Saghai, Y. (2008). Theorizing justice in health research. In J. P. Kahn, A. C. Mastroianni, & J. Sugarman (Eds.), *Beyond consent: Seeking justice in research* (p. 187). Oxford University Press.

Shuster, E. (1997). The significance of the Nuremberg Code. *New England Journal of Medicine, 337,* 1436.

Wolf, S. M. (2013). Return of individual research results and incidental findings: Facing the challenges of translational science. *Annual Review of Genomics and Human Genetics, 14,* 557–577. doi:10.1146/annurev-genom-091212-153506

World Medical Association. (2013). World Medical Association Declaration of Helsinki: Ethical principles for medical research involving human subjects. *JAMA, 310*(20), 2191–2194.

Historical Timeline

Bruce G. Gordon
Sharon P. Shriver

Key events in the history of human subjects protection can be traced to ancient times, such as the creation of the Hippocratic Oath in the 4th century BCE (physicians should do no harm); the Adab al-Tabib (Conduct of a Physician), a 9th-century treatise on medical ethics by Ishaq bin Ali Rahawi; and the 1752 introduction of peer review for papers submitted to the Philosophical Transactions of the Royal Society of London. Although the entire history of medicine and research ethics has contributed to the regulatory framework of today, this timeline will focus on summarizing key events from 1900 to 2020. The framework for human research ethics has evolved over this time period in response to medical advances, new technologies, globalization, and revelations of past missteps. Many of the events listed here were pivotal points in shaping the current research ethics oversight environment.

Date	Detailed Description	Event
1900	Walter Reed was a major in the U.S. Army appointed to study tropical diseases in Cuba. His research on yellow fever confirmed the theory of the Cuban doctor Carlos Finlay that yellow fever is transmitted by a particular mosquito species, rather than by direct contact. The research was conducted with human subjects who were deliberately infected with the disease; three of the subjects died as a result of the yellow fever infection. Unprecedented for his era, Reed drew up a written contract in English and in Spanish informing subjects of the risk of death from yellow fever and obtained written consent. The research was responsible for identifying the mosquito as the vector of disease transmission and led to a significant decrease in mortality rates from yellow fever. Reed and the Yellow Fever Commission were regarded as the first research group to use consent forms in their research.	Walter Reed Yellow Fever Study

Date	Detailed Description	Event
1939	This social science experiment set out to prove that stuttering is a learned behavior that can be induced in children through psychological pressure. Over a 6-month period, Dr. Wendell Johnson, a nationally renowned pioneer in the field of speech pathology, and his staff tested his theory on 22 children who were in the care of the state-run Iowa Soldiers' Orphans' Home. This particular study group was chosen because they formed a convenient sample to abuse and berate. Some were subjected to steady harassment, badgering, and other negative therapy in an attempt to get them to stutter; the rest served as a control group.	Stuttering Study
1946	The Nazi "Doctors' trial" began in 1946 following World War II. Criminal proceedings were brought against 23 German doctors for participating in war crimes and crimes against humanity. Sixteen were found guilty, and seven were sentenced to death because of their participation in experiments on prisoners held by the Nazis that involved painful and frequently fatal procedures.	Nazi Doctors' Trial
1947	As part of their judgment in the Nazi Doctors' trial, the judges articulated "certain basic principles must be observed in order to satisfy moral, ethical and legal concepts" (Nuremberg Code, 1949). These 10 principles form the Nuremberg Code. Though never officially accepted as law by any nation or as official ethics guidelines by any association, the Code nonetheless has had a profound influence, forming the basis of the Declaration of Helsinki and influencing the *Belmont Report*. Key provisions of the Code include: ■ The voluntary consent of the human subject is absolutely essential; ■ Human research should be founded on preliminary results from animal studies; ■ Unnecessary physical and mental suffering should be avoided; ■ Degree of risk to subjects should never exceed the humanitarian importance of the problem to be solved by the experiment; ■ Only sufficiently qualified persons should be allowed to conduct the research; ■ The researcher must stop the experiment if it becomes apparent that injury, disability, or death is a likely result of continuation.	Nuremberg Code
1953	American medical researchers were generally unconcerned by the precepts of the Code; many did not perceive specific personal implications in the medical trial. Joseph Gardella, Dean of the Harvard Medical School in 1953, stated, "The Nuremberg Code was conceived in reference to Nazi atrocities and was written for the specific purpose of preventing brutal excesses from being committed or excused in the name of science. The code . . . is in our opinion not necessarily pertinent to or adequate for the conduct of medical research in the United States" (ACHRE, n.d. a). Physician–researchers felt they were adequately governed by the Hippocratic ideal, reframed in the Declaration of Geneva in 1948: "The health of my patient will be my first consideration."	American medical community response to the Nuremberg Code
1950s	Between 1946 and 1953, researchers fed radioactive cereal to more than 70 children at the Fernald School, a state home for mentally disabled children in Massachusetts. Small amounts of radioactive calcium and iron were put in the children's cereal, allowing researchers to track the absorption of those nutrients as the oatmeal was digested. Although permission of the parents and children was sought, the information provided was incomplete and inaccurate. Furthermore, to entice their participation, the children were told they were part of a science club.	Radioactive Cereal Experiments at Fernald

Date	Detailed Description	Event
1950s	Researchers at the Willowbrook State School in New York, an institution for mentally disabled children, deliberately infected children with a mild form of hepatitis during a series of studies of the progression, prevention, and treatment of viral hepatitis that extended from 1956 to 1972. The results eventually contributed to the development of a successful hepatitis vaccine. However, the ethics of the studies has been challenged; questions have been raised about the quality and content of parental consent, including evidence that studies were incompletely and inaccurately described. In addition, many have condemned the deliberate infection of these institutionalized children.	Willowbrook Experiment
1956–1972	In the late 1950s, thalidomide was approved as a sedative in Europe. Although thalidomide was not FDA approved for use in the United States, at that time manufacturers were permitted to give samples to U.S. physicians and pay them to study the safety and efficacy of their drugs. By 1961 it became clear that thalidomide caused significant damage if a fetus was exposed during the first trimester of pregnancy, causing children to be born severely deformed. Although this case did not involve research, it prompted the 1962 amendments to the Food, Drug, and Cosmetics Act, which required drug manufacturers to establish a drug's effectiveness prior to marketing.	Thalidomide Effects
1961–1962	Stanley Milgram conducted a social science study in an attempt to understand the role of obedience to authority. The research design was to have an authority figure instruct subjects to do something that they would not do under ordinary circumstances. In the study, Milgram told the subjects that another research subject (actually a research associate) would be completing a memory task. The associate was connected to a device that appeared to deliver an electrical charge, and the subjects were told to administer a shock if the associate answered incorrectly on the memory task. The associate responded as if an actual shock had been received. The researcher instructed the subjects to increase the "electrical charge" each time the associate answered incorrectly. The research subjects had no idea that the associates were not actually being shocked, and some of them suffered emotional distress after witnessing the responses they thought they had inflicted.	Milgram Study
1963	Researchers at Sloan-Kettering Cancer Research Institute, funded by the National Institutes of Health (NIH), injected live cancer cells into indigent, chronically ill elderly patients at Brooklyn's Jewish Chronic Disease Hospital. Consent of the subjects was at best incomplete and in some cases completely absent. The experiment was intended to measure the patients' ability to reject the cells and was not related to their treatment.	Jewish Chronic Disease Hospital
1964	The Declaration of Helsinki was developed in 1964 by the World Medical Association as an international statement of ethical principles to guide medical professionals conducting research involving human subjects. Notably, the Declaration described two separate categories of clinical research (therapeutic and nontherapeutic), with distinct guidelines for consent.	The Declaration of Helsinki
1965	In 1965, Humphreys began what became a controversial study involving deception, in which he covertly observed men having sex with men in a public bathroom. Humphreys subsequently interviewed the subjects to obtain background information about them, having used their car license numbers to identify them, and then posed as a health services surveyor to obtain their cooperation for the interviews (Humphreys, 1970).	Tearoom Trade Study

Date	Detailed Description	Event
1966	Surgeon General William H. Stewart issued a policy statement requiring Public Health Service (PHS) grantee institutions to address three topics by committee review prior to all proposed research involving human subjects: "This review should assure an independent determination (1) of the rights and welfare of the individual or individuals involved, (2) of the appropriateness of the methods used to secure informed consent, and (3) of the risks and potential medical benefits of the investigation (US Congress, 1966)." The policy was especially significant for the recognition that patient-subjects (like healthy subjects) should be included in the consent provisions.	PHS Policy: Clinical investigations using human subjects.
1966	Dr. Henry Beecher published an article in the *New England Journal of Medicine* that cited 22 published studies with serious ethical flaws. Examples included one study in which researchers assigned some patients with acute streptococcal infections to a "control group" and did not allow them to receive effective treatment. More than 70 of these patients developed rheumatic fever. In another study of immune response, researchers injected live cancer cells into subjects without their informed consent. Many of them died.	Beecher article in the *New England Journal of Medicine*
1971	In 1971, Stanford University researcher Philip Zimbardo conducted a study of the psychology of imprisonment by setting up a mock prison using volunteer college student subjects to assume the roles of prisoners and guards. The student "guards" brutalized the student "prisoners." Ethical concerns about the research include underestimation of the likelihood and severity of psychological harm to the subjects and that the researcher himself played a role (prison director) in the research rather than safeguarding the welfare of the research subjects.	Stanford Prison Experiment
1972	The U.S. Public Health Service Tuskegee Study of Untreated Syphilis in the Negro Male (the Tuskegee Study) began in 1932. Six hundred poor Black men, sharecroppers from Alabama, were recruited—400 test subjects who had syphilis and 200 controls who did not. The subjects were not informed of their diagnosis or possible treatments, and spinal taps to assess for neurosyphilis were described as "special free treatment." While study subjects were provided some subadequate treatment, none was offered treatment with penicillin, even though the antibiotic was proven to be effective against syphilis and was offered to nonstudy patients by the PHS after 1943. In 1969, the CDC convened a Blue Ribbon Panel, composed almost entirely of physicians and scientists participating in the Tuskegee Study, which voted, with one dissension, to continue the project. In 1972, the story of the Tuskegee Study was published in several major newspapers. This was followed by a review by the Tuskegee Syphilis Study Ad Hoc Advisory Panel, convened by the Department of Health, Education, and Welfare, which called the study ethically unjustified, recommended treatment of all surviving subjects, and found existing protections for human subjects not effective. In 1973, partly in response to this finding, Senator Edward Kennedy convened hearings on human experimentation, which ultimately led to the National Research Act. The Tuskegee Study formally ended in 1973 when the surviving subjects finally received penicillin.	US PHS Tuskegee Study
1972	The Office for Protection from Research Risks (OPRR) was created in 1972 as part of the National Institutes of Health (NIH). (OPRR was later replaced by the Office for Human Research Protections [OHRP].)	OPRR created

Date	Detailed Description	Event
1974	The National Research Act of 1974 established the National Commission for the Protection of Human Subjects of Biomedical and Behavioral Research, which met from 1974 to 1978. In accord with its charge, the Commission produced reports and recommendations regarding independent review of research by institutional review boards, as well as research involving "children, prisoners, and the institutionalized mentally infirm."	National Research Act
1974	U.S. Department of Health, Education, and Welfare published 45 CFR 46 subpart A (Basic Policy for the Protection of Human Research Subjects) in accordance with requirements of the National Research Act. The 1974 regulations established IRB review procedures.	45 CFR 46 subpart A
1978	FDA Guidance: General Considerations for the Clinical Evaluation of Drugs. This guidance recommended that women of childbearing potential be excluded from participation in Phase I and early Phase II clinical trials. Even though it was later reversed, this policy (and similar practices in non-FDA clinical research) led to the widespread exclusion of women from clinical and scientific trials, resulting in a lack of information about the effects of many therapies and drugs on women.	FDA guidance excluding women of childbearing potential from clinical trials
1978	The National Commission published "Report and Recommendations: Institutional Review Boards," evaluating the performance of institutional review boards and recommending steps to improve the ethical review process.	National Commission report on IRBs
1979	The National Commission released "The Ethical Principles and Guidelines for the Protection of Human Subjects of Research" (called the *Belmont Report* after the conference center where discussions were held in 1976). It defined three fundamental ethical principles that should underlie research involving human subjects: 1. *Respect for persons*: Protecting the autonomy of all people and requiring informed consent 2. *Beneficence*: Maximizing benefits of the research while minimizing risks of harm to the research subjects 3. *Justice*: Ensuring fair recruitment of subjects and fair distribution of both the burdens and benefits of research These principles form the ethical foundation for federal regulations designed to protect human subjects of research.	*Belmont Report*
1980	The Department of Health, Education, and Welfare (DHEW) became the Department of Health and Human Services (DHHS) on May 4, 1980.	DHEW becomes DHHS
1981	DHHS published a revision of 45 CFR 46, responding to recommendations of the National Commission and incorporating the *Belmont* principles. The revision set out in greater specificity IRB responsibilities and the procedures IRBs were to follow.	Revision of 45 CFR 46 subpart A in response to National Commission
1981	President's Commission for the Study of Ethical Problems in Medicine and Biomedical and Behavioral Research recommended the adoption of DHHS regulations by all federal agencies.	President's Commission
1980, 1981	FDA issued 21 CFR 50 (Protection of Human Subjects, 1980) and 21 CFR 56 (Institutional Review Boards, 1981), establishing requirements for IRB review and informed consent for FDA-regulated clinical trials. This extended protections to any research study involving drugs or devices regulated by the FDA (in contrast to DHHS regulations, which only apply to federally funded programs).	FDA requires IRB review of clinical trials

Date	Detailed Description	Event
1991	The Federal Policy for the Protection of Human Subjects was published by DHHS and adopted as the "Common Rule" by other federal agencies and departments. The 1991, the DHHS human subjects regulations at 45 CFR 46 included four subparts: subpart A, Basic HHS Policy for Protection of Human Subjects (Common Rule); subpart B, additional protections for pregnant women, human fetuses, and neonates; subpart C, additional protections for prisoners; and subpart D, additional protections for children. Subpart A was codified in the regulations of 15 federal agencies or departments, which include in their chapters of the Code of Federal Regulations section numbers and language that are identical to those of the DHHS codification at 45 CFR part 46, subpart A. In addition, four departments or agencies follow this "Common Rule" by statutory mandate (Department of Homeland Security, Social Security Administration, Office of the Director of National Intelligence, and Central Intelligence Agency). Prior to 1991, different federal agencies used a variety of policies and procedures to protect human research subjects.	Common Rule published and adopted by various federal agencies
1993	FDA issued Guideline for the Study and Evaluation of Gender Differences in the Clinical Evaluation of Drugs. The guideline was developed amid growing concerns that the drug development process did not provide adequate information about the effects of drugs or biological products in women and a general consensus that women should be allowed to determine for themselves the appropriateness of participating in early clinical trials. The Guideline lifted a restriction on participation by most women with childbearing potential from entering Phase 1 and early Phase 2 trials, and now encouraged their participation. The Guideline also stated that sponsors should collect gender-related data during research and development and should analyze the data for gender effects.	FDA Guideline for the Study and Evaluation of Gender Differences in the Clinical Evaluation of Drugs
1993	In response to the NIH Revitalization Act of 1993 (PL 103-43), NIH published Policy and Guidelines on the Inclusion of Women and Minorities as Subjects in Clinical Research. The policy stated that women and members of minority groups must be included in all NIH-funded clinical research, unless a clear and compelling rationale and justification establishes that inclusion is inappropriate with respect to the health of the subjects or the purpose of the research.	NIH Policy on Inclusion of Women and Minorities as Subjects in Clinical Research
1995	The U.S. government published a report entitled "Human Radiation Experiments: The Department of Energy Roadmap to the Story and Records." It discusses human radiation experiments that were conducted on thousands of U.S. citizens during and after World War II, including the injection of plutonium into hospital patients without their consent and the intentional release of radiation into the environment. The ethical issues raised by these experiments include lack of informed consent, lack of fairness in the selection of subjects, failure to report the existence or results of the experiments, and failure to maintain proper records of the experiments.	U.S. Radiation Experiments
1995	Nicole Wan, a healthy 19-year-old nursing student, died after volunteering for a medical research study in which University of Rochester researchers performed a bronchoscopy. An investigation revealed that researchers exceeded the maximum dosage of lidocaine established by the research protocol.	University of Rochester Bronchoscopy Case

Date	Detailed Description	Event
1998	Jesse Gelsinger, an 18-year-old research subject, died while taking part in a clinical experiment using gene transfer to treat ornithine transcarbamylase (OTC) deficiency, a genetic disease that disrupts metabolism. Jesse's OTC deficiency was not severe, and he was able to live a relatively normal life. During the experiment conducted at the University of Pennsylvania in 1998, Gelsinger developed a massive immune response after being injected with the study substance. He died 4 days later. An FDA investigation concluded that the informed consent provided to Gelsinger was inadequate for a number of reasons, including failures to fully describe the risks of the research study and to reveal financial conflicts of interest on the part of the researcher.	Jesse Gelsinger
1998–2001	OPRR, on behalf of the federal government, suspended federally funded human subjects research at 15 institutions due to various lapses in human subjects research oversight. In many cases, the violations involved failure to obtain adequate informed consent from research subjects.	Research suspensions
1999	The Office for Human Research Protections (OHRP) was established in the Office of the Assistant Secretary for Health, within the DHHS, to elevate its stature and effectiveness. OHRP replaced the NIH's Office for Protection from Research Risks (OPRR).	OHRP established
2000	The National Human Research Protections Advisory Committee (NHRPAC) was established to advise DHHS on human subject protection. The NHRPAC was later replaced by the Secretary's Advisory Committee on Human Research Protections (SACHRP).	NHRPAC established
2001	Ellen Roche, a healthy 24-year-old lab technician at the Johns Hopkins Asthma Center, died after participating in an experiment designed to understand the natural defenses of healthy people against asthma. Roche had received inhaled hexamethonium, a drug that induced a mild asthma attack. Within 24 hours of inhaling the drug, Roche developed worsening respiratory failure; she died within a month. The consent form she signed warned of coughing, dizziness, and tightness in the chest, but not death. The informed consent document referred to hexamethonium as a "medication" and did not mention the fact that hexamethonium used by inhalation was experimental (hexamethonium was withdrawn from human use by the FDA in the 1970s and had never been approved for administration via inhalation). In its evaluation of the human subjects protection system at the Johns Hopkins Hospital and School of Medicine, OHRP found, among other deficiencies, that Hopkins was failing to perform "substantive and meaningful IRB review." On July 19, OHRP suspended nearly all federally funded medical research involving human subjects.	Ellen Roche
2000	The Health Insurance Portability and Accountability Act (HIPAA) Privacy Rule was issued. The rule addresses the uses and disclosures of private health information (PHI) for research purposes.	HIPAA Privacy Rule
2002	The Secretary's Advisory Committee on Human Research Protections (SACHRP) replaced the NHRPAC. SACHRP is charged with providing advice to the Secretary of DHHS on matters relating to the responsible conduct of research involving human subjects. This includes research issues involving special populations, such as children, neonates, prisoners, and the decisionally impaired; pregnant women, embryos, and fetuses; individuals and populations in international studies; populations in which there are individually identifiable samples, data, or information; and investigator conflicts of interest.	SACHRP

Date	Detailed Description	Event
2003	The Surfactant, Positive Pressure, and Oxygenation Randomized Trial (SUPPORT) was an early example of comparative effectiveness research (CER) to determine the optimum oxygen therapy protocol for premature infants. The NIH-sponsored multicenter trial randomly assigned approximately 1,300 premature infants to either a low or high oxygen treatment protocol. Considerable controversy about this study has been raised, focusing on several issues. OHRP found that the parents in the study were insufficiently informed of the risks involved, a conclusion that has been disputed by some in the medical research and bioethics communities. Other controversial issues include the random assignment of infants to treatment groups, rather than assignment by a physician based on the infants' best interests, and whether there was already sufficient medical knowledge at the time, making a randomized trial inappropriate.	SUPPORT
2005–2009	The Havasupai tribe settled with Arizona State University (ASU) concerning their claim that blood collected in the 1990s by ASU researchers to study the genetic origins of diabetes among tribe members was used for unrelated projects, including studies of schizophrenia, inbreeding, and theories of the tribe's geographical origins that contradict their traditional stories. The Havasupai had consented to the diabetes study, but the other studies were performed without their knowledge or consent.	Havasupai settlement
2010	Dr. Susan Reverby, a medical historian, announced her discovery of a syphilis study conducted in Guatemala from 1946 to 1948. In the study, funded by the U.S. government, nearly 700 Guatemalans were deliberately infected with sexually transmitted disease organisms in an effort to test the effectiveness of penicillin. In 2010, U.S. President Barack Obama apologized to the government of Guatemala and the survivors and descendants of those infected, calling the experiments "clearly unethical."	Guatemala syphilis study exposed
2010	Rebecca Skloot published *The Immortal Life of Henrietta Lacks*, a book that describes the short life and long legacy of Henrietta Lacks, who died in 1951 from cervical cancer at age 31. Her cancer cells were the originators of the HeLa cell line, an incredibly robust line that has contributed to countless scientific advances over the years. Her descendants' realization of their mother's "immortality" (for which she received no compensation or recognition) is the focus of the book. The book sparked a national dialogue about the ethics of collection and subsequent use of biological tissue for research purposes and the exploitation of communities of color in research.	*The Immortal Life of Henrietta Lacks*
2011–2019	In 2011, DHHS announced an Advance Notice of Proposed Rulemaking (ANPRM), signaling that the government was considering revising the regulations overseeing research on human subjects. In 2015, DHHS and fifteen other federal departments and agencies announced proposed revisions to the Common Rule. The Notice of Proposed Rulemaking (NPRM) sought comment on proposals to better protect human subjects involved in research, while facilitating valuable research and reducing burden, delay, and ambiguity for investigators. The revised Common Rule (designated the "2018 Requirements" to distinguish it from previous language) was published in the Federal Register on January 19, 2017. Following a number of delays, the 2018 Requirements (or revised Common Rule) went fully into effect on January 21, 2019.	Process to revise the Common Rule
2014–2016	An outbreak of the Ebola virus in West Africa killed over 11,000 people across six countries in just under 2 years. The urgent need to treat the disease led to rapid approval of clinical trials in affected areas, raising novel ethical questions about researching unproven therapies during public health emergencies.	Ebola outbreak in West Africa

Date	Detailed Description	Event
2014	The social media platform Facebook conducted a massive experiment in which the news feeds of over 600,000 Facebook users were manipulated without their knowledge or consent. The study, published by the Proceedings of the National Academy of Sciences in 2014, purported to show that emotional contagion, a well-characterized phenomenon in offline environments, also occurs online. News of the experiment raised widespread ethical concerns around the ideas of privacy, industry–academic partnerships, and the nature of informed consent.	Facebook Emotional Contagion Study
2016	The 21st Century Cures Act was signed into law, providing broad support for biomedical research and implementing measures to reduce administrative burden. Impacts to human research protections included allowances for waiver or alteration of informed consent for FDA-regulated minimal risk studies, and for use of a single IRB for multisite medical device studies, as well as a call for harmonization of FDA regulations and the Common Rule. Provisions to support increased diversity among clinical research subjects, protect vulnerable populations in research, and enhance privacy protections for subjects' sensitive data, were also included.	21st Century Cures Act
2016	NIH mandated that all multisite cooperative research funded by it must rely upon ethical review and approval conducted by a single IRB of record. The rule was proposed in 2016 and, after some delays, was implemented in January 2018. The revised Common Rule followed suit and included a requirement for single IRB review of cooperative research to take effect in 2020.	Single IRB mandates
2018	He Jiankui, a scientist from Shenzhen, China, announced the birth of twin babies who had undergone genome editing as embryos. He claimed to have used CRISPR-Cas 9 technology to modify the CCR5 gene in human embryos, to make the resulting babies resistant to human immunodeficiency virus (HIV) infection. Questions regarding the ethics of He's experiments, including whether there had been institutional review and approval for this work, led many scientists and policymakers to call for a ban on genome editing in the human germline.	CRISPR Babies
2019	The U.S. National Academy of Medicine, the U.S. National Academy of Sciences, and the Royal Society of the UK formed the International Commission on the Clinical Use of Human Germline Genome Editing to develop an ethical framework to guide clinicians, scientists, and policymakers in assessing potential clinical applications of human germline genome editing.	International Commission on the Clinical Use of Human Germline Genome Editing
2019	Originating in Wuhan City of Hubei Province, China, the Severe Acute Respiratory Syndrome Coronavirus 2 (SARS-CoV-2) rapidly spread internationally. The resulting illness, COVID-19, prompted the World Health Organization to declare a pandemic in March 2020, and sickened at least 70 million worldwide as of December 2020. Overload of healthcare systems, quarantines, social distancing requirements, and financial uncertainty forced HRPPs and IRBs to consider a host of ethical and regulatory issues, including emergency use of new drugs and therapies, remote consent and monitoring of subjects in research, fair distribution of investigational drugs, and human vaccine challenge studies.	SARS-CoV-2 pandemic

References and Resources

Advisory Committee on Human Radiation Experiments (ACHRE). (n.d. a). *ACHRE Final Report. Chapter 2: new times, new codes.* bioethicsarchive.georgetown.edu/achre/final/chap2_6.html

Advisory Committee on Human Radiation Experiments (ACHRE). (n.d. b). *ACHRE Final Report. Chapter 14: The federal policy for human subject protections (the Common Rule).* bioethicsarchive. georgetown.edu/achre/final/chap14_2.html

Breault, J. L. (2006). Protecting human research subjects: The past defines the future. *The Ochsner Journal,* 2006, 15–20.

Congressional Research Service Report for Congress. (2005). *Federal protection for human research subjects: An analysis of the Common Rule and its interactions with FDA regulations and the HIPAA Privacy Rule.* fas.org/sgp/crs/misc/RL32909.pdf

Humphreys, L. (1970). Tearoom trade: Impersonal sex in public places. Aldine Transaction.

Jones, J. H. (1981). *Bad blood: The Tuskegee syphilis experiment.* Free Press.

National Academies of Sciences, Engineering, and Medicine. (2019, May 22). *New international commission launched on clinical use of heritable human genome editing.* [Press release]. www .nationalacademies.org/news/2019/05/new-international-commission-launched-on-clinical -use-of-heritable-human-genome-editing

Nuremberg Code. (1949). Originally published in "Permissible medical experiments." In *Trials of war criminals before the Nuremberg Military Tribunals under Control Council Law, 10*(2): 181–182. U.S. Government Printing Office. https://history.nih.gov/research/downloads /nuremberg.pdf

Oxtoby, K. (2016). Is the Hippocratic oath still relevant to practising doctors today? *BMJ, 355,* i6629. https://doi.org/10.1136/bmj.i6629

Rahim, A. B. A. (2013). Understanding Islamic ethics and its significance on the character building. *International Journal of Social Science and Humanity, 3*(6), 508–513.

Resnik, D. B. (2020). *Research ethics timeline.* National Institute of Environmental Health Sciences. www.niehs.nih.gov/research/resources/bioethics/timeline/index.cfm

Reverby, S. (Ed.). (2000). *Tuskegee's truths: Rethinking the Tuskegee syphilis study.* University of North Carolina Press.

Sparks, J. (2002). *Timeline of laws related to the protection of human subjects.* Office of History, National Institutes of Health. history.nih.gov/about/timelines_laws_human.html

United States Congress (1966) Investigation of HEW, Hearings Before the Special Subcommittee on Investigation of the Department of Health, Education, and Welfare of . . ., 89-2 . . ., April 18, 19, 20, 21, 22; May 27; June 20, 1966. https://books.google.com /books?id=CaAXDyl0Y0sC&source=gbs_navlinks_s

Organizing the IRB Office

Overview of the Human Research Protection Program

Charlotte H. Coley

Judy Matuk

Abstract

The concept of a human research protection program (HRPP) captures the idea that all components of an institution that are involved in human subjects research are responsible for the protection of the rights and welfare of those subjects, not just the IRB. When it recognizes the multiple systems and processes needed to conduct responsible human subjects research, an institution can better tie the components together into a cohesive unit with a shared mission and goal, and is in a better position to clarify the respective roles and responsibilities of, and improve communication among, those components. This chapter provides the history and rationale of the idea of an HRPP and a description of the HRPP components.

Background

For decades after the 1974 National Research Act became the first law to "provide for the protection of human subjects involved in biomedical and behavioral research," it was widely believed that the IRB was the only entity that needed to be put into place to provide those protections (National Research Service Act, 1974). In June 1998, a Department of Health and Human Services (DHHS) Inspector General's Report was released, with clear conclusions that IRBs were overworked and understaffed (DHHS-OIG, 1998). As a result, the National Institutes of Health (NIH) Office for the Protection from Research Risks (OPRR) and the Food and Drug Administration (FDA) audited, and then suspended, human subjects research at several major universities due to noncompliance with federal regulations and/or failure to adequately protect research volunteers. Events such as the 1999 research-related death of Jesse Gelsinger at the University of Pennsylvania, as well as the increasing complexity

🖉 1-2

🖉 1-2

of research moving away from the single-researcher/single-site model, made it abundantly clear that the processes believed to be in place to protect subjects were inadequate, and were not providing the protections intended under the National Research Act. Eventually it became apparent (see, e.g., the Institute of Medicine's 2001 publication, "Preserving Public Trust") that it would take a co-ordinated, dedicated effort of multiple entities at an organization to form an integrated system to maximize oversight and create a culture of compliance that would ensure the protection of human subjects in research (IOM, 2001). With that, the concept of the human research protection program (HRPP) was born.

Picture a car that is disassembled with all the parts laid out next to each other. Some of the parts make the car move, while others keep the passenger safe while the car is moving. Which of those parts are not needed? Are there any connections between those parts that are unnecessary? Would you get into a car and attempt to drive it, knowing that some of the parts or connections were missing? Now consider research involving human subjects. Would you want to volunteer, or have a loved one volunteer, in research where the system that should be in place to protect them and keep them safe throughout their participation does not have all its necessary parts connected properly? It is the identification and cooperation of all necessary "parts," along with the coordination of effort and synchronized communication among them, that creates the harmonized system known as HRPP.

With an HRPP, we leave behind the concept of a single entity (the IRB) with responsibility for the welfare of subjects in research, and turn our attention to a shared responsibility of multiple components, filling in the myriad gaps surrounding the jurisdiction of the IRB. With all such components interconnected properly, a "safety net" is formed to help ensure the optimal protection of the rights and welfare of the subjects.

The identification of all relevant HRPP components, followed by the creation, promulgation, execution, and maintenance of policies and procedures that describe a fully functioning HRPP, is hard work. The culture at an institution must be such that the importance of the HRPP is fully appreciated and supported. The individual(s) assigned the task of bringing together previously "siloed" processes must have appropriate working knowledge (or access to it) of all the steps in the life of a human subjects research activity (funded or not), along with the (potentially multiple) regulatory requirements to be met before proceeding to a next step. If planned and documented appropriately, with education provided throughout the process, the result becomes a set of step-by-step directions describing how to conduct compliant and safe research involving human subjects.

Even though the field has moved from an IRB-only to an HRPP model for the protection of subjects, it is important to distinguish the roles and responsibilities of the IRB from those of the HRPP, particularly in the context of the

✐ Section 4

federal mandate to use a <u>single IRB</u> in multisite studies (NIH, 2016). It would be unfortunate for an organization to assume that its oversight responsibilities for a study are removed when the IRB of record is outside of that organization. That study is still being conducted at the organization; it is part of the organization's active research, with implications for researcher education, conflict of interest oversight, proper handling of study funds, proper conduct of the study, and so on. In other words, even when one component of the HRPP—namely, regulatory human subjects review—is outsourced, the rest of the components of the HRPP must continue their respective functions and communicate as they always do.

Components of an HRPP

HRPPs are as varied in size and complexity as the research institutions they support. HRPPs need to be designed and resourced to match the needs of the research portfolio, supporting a compliant and safe research program that functions in an efficient and facilitative way. An HRPP that supports 100 active studies will require a different structure from one supporting 5,000 studies. In addition, other variables factor into institutional support requirements, such as the type of research (social/behavioral vs. biomedical studies), requirements for single-IRB reliance, review levels, etc.

Some of the various components that may be found within an HRPP are listed next. Not every HRPP will have (or require) all of these functions. Some HRPPs may have distinct offices that are responsible for each role, whereas others will have a centralized office that handles the majority of them (see section "Structure of the HRPP"). The number of staff and specific responsibilities in those distinct or centralized offices can vary greatly as well, and in a way that does not necessarily correlate with size of the institution or research portfolio. It is for this reason that there needs to be a regularly scheduled process for evaluating these variables that is coordinated via the institutional official (see later), to assess efficiencies, effectiveness, and compliance of the programs, with improvements made and resources allocated accordingly.

Institutional Review Boards

There is no question that IRBs play an integral role in protecting the rights and welfare of human research subjects by approving only those research proposals that meet rigorous ethical and regulatory standards. The federal regulations governing human research grant IRBs a narrow, albeit very important, charge. Guidance from OHRP (DHHS, 2018) states:

> Both the HHS regulations at **45 CFR 46.108(a)(3)** and **(4)** the FDA regulations at **21 CFR 56.108(a)** and **(b)** state that IRBs must follow written <u>procedures</u> for the following functions and operations:
>
> - Conducting initial and <u>continuing review</u> of research and reporting findings and actions to the researcher and the institution;
> - Determining which projects require review more often than annually and determining which projects need verification from sources other than the researcher that no material changes have occurred since previous IRB review;
> - Ensuring prompt reporting to the IRB of proposed <u>changes</u> in a research activity and ensuring that changes in approved research, during the period for which IRB approval has already been given, may not be initiated without IRB review and approval except where necessary to eliminate apparent immediate hazards to the human subjects;
> - Ensuring prompt reporting to the IRB, appropriate institutional officials, and the department or agency head (i.e., OHRP) for research conducted or supported by HHS, and FDA for FDA-regulated research of any:
>   - <u>Unanticipated problems</u> involving risks to human subjects or others;

🖉 2-3
🖉 7-2

🖉 7-1

🖉 7-3

🔗 7-6

- Instance of serious or continuing <u>noncompliance</u> with the applicable HHS and FDA regulations or the requirements or determinations of the IRB;
- Suspension or termination of IRB approval.

From a regulatory standpoint, both the Common Rule **[45 CFR 46.107]** and FDA **[21 CFR 56.107]** require that IRBs "... shall be able to ascertain the acceptability of proposed research in terms of institutional commitments (including policies and resources) and regulations, applicable law, and standards of professional conduct and practice. The IRB shall therefore include persons knowledgeable in these areas." In assuring that research risks to subjects are minimized, IRBs must be confident that researchers have the necessary expertise not only in the field of study but also in their ability to conduct the research safely and in accordance with federal, state, and local institutional requirements for the protection of human subjects.

🔗 Section 6

While federally funded human subjects research requires the approval of the IRB, the execution of that research requires the involvement of others in the organization. The IRB is not responsible for obtaining <u>consent</u> from potential study subjects; conducting study procedures; managing the processes for securing and disbursement of external funding for the research; making sure that the HRPP is properly resourced to ensure compliant research is being conducted; coordinating other federally mandated reviews to which the research might be subject, such as Public Health Service-required review of researcher

🔗 12-6

financial disclosures to identify potential <u>conflicts of interest</u>, or the NIH Office of Science Policy-required review of the use of vaccines or antibodies that may have been created using recombinant techniques.

Institutional Official

🔗 8-1

The institutional official (IO) is the signatory official on the <u>Federalwide Assurance</u> (FWA), which assures an institution's compliance with the Federal Policy for the Protection of Human Subjects (the Common Rule). Authority over, and responsibility for, the institution's HRPP rests with this individual. Federal regulators (e.g., OHRP, FDA) will address questions that may arise regarding an institution's HRPP to the IO. These questions may come from complaints or concerns made to the federal agency or from results of inspections or audits conducted by that agency. It is essential that the IO be knowledgeable about the regulatory requirements for the protection of human subjects, as well as the federal regulatory expectations of the IO's role (even if some of their responsibilities have been transferred to designees, such as a deputy or the head of the HRPP office).

The IO, or their designee, is responsible for allocating necessary resources to support the HRPP components, including appropriate staffing, funds for training and space, appointment of IRB members and chairs, and determining the component offices that make up the HRPP. The IO, or designee, can disapprove an IRB-approved study, but cannot approve research disapproved by the IRB. Along with the IRB, the IO can suspend a study or researcher and can terminate a study or prevent a researcher from doing research at the institution.

IRB Administration Staff

🔗 2-2

IRB administration <u>staff</u> are responsible for facilitating the process of moving submissions through the IRB review pipeline. They are key contacts, coordinators, and liaisons among the researcher, IRB, and other HRPP components (e.g., pharmacy, conflicts of interest, institutional biosafety committee, etc.) that are responsible for assessing aspects of the proposed research that fall within their expertise area.

Education

Researchers cannot conduct compliant research if they do not know the ethical standards, regulations, policies, and procedures that impact compliance. Maintaining organizational standards that are required for certification within the various HRPP roles, ensuring compliance with these organizational standards, and providing <u>education</u> about human research protection issues are often the responsibility of central HRPP staff. These staff must maintain, or have access to, a current database of certified researchers. The communication pathway between these staff and those who review IRB submissions must be clear, so that approval of submissions can be withheld if all study researchers do not meet the institutional training requirements.

    8-5

    Effective education is not a "one and done" event. It is a continuing process, not only to maintain acquired knowledge, but also to enable adaptation when processes need to change to increase efficiencies or meet new federal or institutional mandates. The research world is not static; knowledge and technology are constantly evolving, posing new challenges and risks. This, in turn, generates new regulatory requirements that require guidance and additional training. The HRPP staff responsible for researcher education may also contribute to ongoing <u>educational efforts for IRB members</u>.

    8-4

    Additional educational needs of the research organization can be handled by this group or split among other components of the HRPP. These educational efforts may include orientation for new IRB staff; continuing IRB member and staff education and workshops; noncompliant researcher reeducation; training on new or updated operational processes, forms, and documents; electronic submission system training; research staff training; and more.

Post-Approval Monitoring; Quality Assurance/Quality Improvement

Another function required within an HRPP is the monitoring of compliance, not only for active research studies, but for other components of the HRPP. This may fall into the category of <u>post-approval monitoring</u> (PAM) or quality assurance/quality improvement (QA/QI) efforts. Although the research enterprise at an institution is necessarily dependent on the assumption that research will be conducted ethically and compliantly, monitoring and auditing by HRPP staff provide an important check on the system. This monitoring could be required by the IRB or by other offices when concerns arise about a study, researcher, or research team. It can also be effective when done randomly within the institution's research portfolio, to find and correct issues early and prevent them from becoming serious or continuing <u>noncompliance</u>. PAM or QA/QI staff can also assist in preparation when a researcher has been notified that a federal or sponsor <u>audit</u> is being scheduled.

    7-4

    7-6

    8-6

    <u>Monitoring</u> of the compliance of the IRB and other offices of the HRPP can also be part of this component's charge; for example, monitoring IRB minutes to check with federally required compliance, assessing whether contracts and consent forms are aligned in terms of injury payment provisions, etc.

    2-7

Researchers

Scientific questions developed by researchers in the biomedical and social/behavioral fields become the proposals that IRBs review and approve so that the research can be conducted and knowledge advanced. One of the most important roles of researchers is their face-to-face interaction with research subjects (or their identifiable data or biospecimens). Researchers are literally on the front line of human research protections. They are entrusted with ensuring that consent is obtained from subjects in an informed and noncoercive way, following the research study as approved by the IRB, and treating each subject with respect at all times.

⊘ Section 6

It is important to remember that IRBs review and approve research proposals. At the point of initial proposal submission to the IRB, the researcher thinks they know the subject population, the number of subjects, the procedures, the frequency of visits, etc. needed to answer the research question. Once the research is approved, the study shifts from a theoretical plan to one being conducted in real time. The importance of communication between the IRB and the researcher becomes significant, going well beyond continuing review or progress reports. It is the responsibility of the researcher to assess whether any aspect of the study must be amended, and to not do so without IRB approval, with very limited exceptions [45 CFR 46.108 (a)(3)(iii)].

⊘ 7-2

⊘ 7-1
⊘ 7-5
⊘ 8-5
⊘ 7-3
⊘ 7-6

The organization must ensure proper education of the researcher so that any unanticipated problems involving risks to subjects or others or noncompliance associated with the conduct of the study will be reported in a timely manner. Unintentional mistakes in following the study protocol or unexpected issues may occur. Notification of the IRB via the IRB or HRPP office regarding these types of events constitutes a critical signal that the protections in place for the research subjects may be in jeopardy 45 CFR 46.108(a)(4)(i).

The Grants or Sponsored Programs Office

Researchers seeking funding for their research must write requests (grant applications or responses to requests for proposals [RFPs]) or partner with industry to obtain the resources needed to carry out research. The proper submission of grant applications, execution of contracts, and compliant disbursement and expenditure of resulting funds often requires involvement of the organization's Grants Office/Office of Sponsored Programs (although the process to apply for internal funding within the organization may occur via a different process). With respect to its role in the HRPP, this office is a necessary gatekeeper to ensure that funds are not spent on activities involving human subjects without a valid IRB approval, thus requiring a solid communication path to the IRB office.

⊘ 12-2

Although a grant-protocol congruency review is no longer required by the regulations, the grants office might be charged by the institution with reviewing the grant proposal to ensure congruency with the associated IRB approval. If a submission to the IRB proposes compensation to subjects, the grants office must ensure that the amount and scheduling of those payments are consistent with what the IRB approves.

⊘ Section 6

Industry contracts need to address who will pay in case of subject injury, and that provision in the contract must match what the subject agrees to in the informed consent document they sign. The HRPP policies and procedures must clearly state who will make this assessment, and confirm that the two documents are consistent in this regard, before the contract is signed and/or IRB approval is issued (the timing between the two will vary among institutions, but must be clearly defined; e.g., the contract is signed before IRB approval, or the contract signing is held until IRB approval).

Industry studies are often conducted across many research centers, and in this case the associated contract should have provisions for timely dissemination of safety information across all sites. This allows individual study sites to assess whether the study's risk profile is still acceptable to permit the study to continue at that site. If the study can continue, do subjects need to be informed of the new information so they may decide if they wish to continue to participate or withdraw from the study? If the safety information from the industry sponsor is sent to the researcher, the researcher must know, through proper education, to forward it to the IRB office for triaging within the time frame required by the institution.

Financial Conflict of Interest

Why must an HRPP be concerned with <u>financial conflicts of interest</u> (FCOIs)? All scientific endeavors require objectivity at all stages, from designing and conducting the research, to interpreting the data, to publishing the results. Researchers who have FCOIs can have a real or perceived bias, however unintentional, at any or all of those stages. The resulting effect is the eroding of critical scientific rigor and, ultimately, public trust, including trust from the communities from which we seek volunteers to participate in research. For transparency's sake, it is important for researchers to disclose FCOIs to appropriate individuals or offices at their institution, to the IRB reviewing their work, and, if a management plan is deemed necessary, to the human subjects they recruit. Disclosed FCOIs must be managed or eliminated, and it is ultimately the IRB that will determine if the management plan allows the research to be approved and move forward.

🖉 12-6

Conflict of interest disclosure and management became a federal mandate shortly after the Office for Human Research Protections (OHRP) and FDA discovery of FCOIs at both the researcher and institutional levels during their investigation into the death of research subject <u>Jesse Gelsinger</u>. As a result, HRPPs must have in place a solid process whereby researchers disclose any potential conflicts to some entity at an organization, and that entity notifies the IRB of potential FCOIs. This may be accompanied by a proposed plan to manage the FCOI, which could include removing the conflict (e.g., the researcher resigns from the pharmaceutical company speaker bureau); disclosure in resulting publications; or having an unbiased researcher monitor the conduct of the study. The IRB can accept or modify the plan (e.g., require disclosure to subjects in the consent process and in the consent document) and approve the research, or it can determine that the FCOI cannot be managed and the study cannot move forward.

🖉 1-2

Pharmacy/Investigational Drug Service

The services and expertise of an investigational drug service (IDS) are essential for the successful implementation of a drug study whose results will be submitted to FDA for review and potential approval for the marketing of a new drug. Researchers investigating new drugs for submission to FDA have requirements for the handling, storage, and compounding of these drugs and/or placebos that need the expertise of a pharmacist to properly manage. This responsibility can be formally delegated to the IDS. The IDS can inventory the drugs received, package them for the study in the dosages needed, store them at the correct temperature, and compound the drug or placebo, as needed.

11-2   Generally, the Investigational New Drug (IND) application from FDA is held by the sponsor of the study. However, there are instances when the IND is held by an institutional researcher. The IDS can assist and provide training for researchers on the application process, reporting requirements, and documentation required by FDA.

Institutional Biosafety Committee

The NIH Guidelines for Research Involving Recombinant or Synthetic Nucleic Acid Molecules (rsNAM) requires institutional biosafety committee (IBC) review of activities involving rsNAM, including research involving human subjects (DHHS, 2019). Such research may involve gene transfer studies or testing of biologics created using rsNAM technology. The IBC and IRB review and approval process must be coordinated so that each is aware of the others' actions (e.g., a required change to a study made by the IRB must be known by the IBC for their review, and vice versa). If not located in the same office, IBC and IRB administrators must ensure that the research in question does not commence without both approvals in place (along with any other approvals that might be necessary).

10-14

Counsel's Office

Institutional legal counsel must be available for consultation to all those involved in the HRPP, as the myriad laws that impact and intersect with human research protections can be complicated, with some having implications at the state level (e.g., wards of the state, age of majority, emancipation, requirements for legally authorized representatives, research with adults with diminished capacity, the Health Insurance Portability and Accountability Act (HIPAA) regulations, European Union data protection laws, international research standards, etc.). The development of policies and procedures for the HRPP must be constructed, and should operate in practice, with legal counsel consultation to ensure that compliance with state and federal laws is assured.

11-6

At many institutions, legal counsel involvement in the HRPP occurs when an allegation of noncompliance also meets the definition of research misconduct. Regulations governing research misconduct for human research funded by the Public Health Service and the National Science Foundation are codified at **42 CFR 50** and **93**, and **45 CFR 689**, respectively. The research integrity officer (RIO) must also become involved in cases of misconduct to ensure that due process occurs during the stages of a misconduct investigation. In confirmed cases of misconduct involving human subjects research, not only is it possible that current subjects were put at risk by the events in question, but the public record may be tainted as well, thus impacting the safety and welfare of subjects who participate in future research based on those (falsified or fabricated) results. The intersection of human research protections and research misconduct is one of the most important connections in the HRPP; for a discussion of handling allegations of noncompliance and research misconduct, see "Research Misconduct Involving Noncompliance in Human Subjects Research Supported by the Public Health Service: Reconciling Separate Regulatory Systems" (Bierer & Barnes, 2014).

7-6
1-1, 8-5

Other Reviews, Other HRPP Components

Depending on an institution's research portfolio and policies, there may be other reviews required within the HRPP, such as the following:

- *Scientific review*: Part of the IRB's mandate is to find that proposed research is of "sound research design," not exposing subjects to unnecessary risk **45 CFR 46.111(a)(1)(i)**. Thus, the IRB must include an assessment of the proposed scientific research design. Regardless of the diversity of expertise on an institution's IRB, it is impossible for that membership to have in-depth knowledge of all subject areas and the soundness of every scientific hypothesis brought forward to them for review. Therefore, there is a need for an individual or group to examine the scientific validity of the proposed research. If the research is being peer-reviewed for funding, the IRB may accept that the activity has scientific merit if funding is approved. Internal reviews at an institution may be conducted by a scientific review board or via a department-level review.

  Often, IRBs depend on specialized reviews by consultants, such as for statistical considerations for a study. It is important to know whether a proposal is sufficiently powered to answer the research question. If too few subjects are proposed, the study will not be able to meet the stated aims. If too many subjects are proposed, then some may be unnecessarily exposed to research risk.

  Whatever the method for scientific review upon which an IRB depends, communication of the outcome of such review to the IRB must be clear. The pathway for such communication is often via the IRB administration staff at central levels of the HRPP. With such a review completed, administration staff can forward the study to the IRB, which in turn can concentrate on their ethical and regulatory review knowing that the scientific merit of the activity has been verified.
- *Radiology*: Radiology departments are often involved in the IRB review process for clinical studies, at least as consultants, to review the amount of radiation exposure to human subjects, as well as to ensure that the description of the radiation is in lay language for ease of the subject's understanding of the associated risk.
- *HIPAA*: Institutions are covered entities under <u>HIPAA</u> regulations if protected health information (PHI) is accessed, used, or disclosed for research purposes. As such, the institution, the privacy board, and the IRB (if not serving as the privacy board) must coordinate efforts to ensure compliance with HIPAA and the human research regulations, as required for a particular study.

  🔗 11-6
- *Material transfer agreements*: Offices at institutions that execute material transfer agreements (MTAs) must communicate with the IRB office to ensure that an MTA was obtained for any human "material" (such as cells or tissues) that is being transferred out of the institution. Oversight must ensure that that material is being used in accordance with federal regulations, institutional policies, and the consent (and authorization, if PHI is included) of the subject from whom the material was obtained.

Structure of the HRPP

The preceding list provides some examples of how broadly the HRPP reaches within an institution, sometimes just for a single study. Following the course of research activities from "cradle to grave" (i.e., from birth of the idea, through funding, obtaining all approvals, monitoring research conduct, and ultimately the disposition of data and biospecimens) helps those charged with developing the HRPP understand all the stakeholders needed to weave together a cooperative system of compliance and subject protection.

Although some HRPPs may have distinct offices that are responsible for each role, others will have a centralized office that handles the majority of them. The HRPP office, or set of offices, is an important hub of the HRPP system, often serving as the support center for coordination of all other HRPP component functions. A director or manager usually heads the operation and is responsible for general oversight of the HRPP. This individual is in regular contact with the IO and other HRPP constituents to ensure they are current on issues, concerns, and regulatory/local policy or procedure updates that might impact their part of the HRPP. The HRPP office director is often the organizational contact for general communications with federal and other external agencies on matters concerning the HRPP. If the HRPP is formed of distinct offices, it is essential that the various office directors of each of the HRPP entities meet on a regular basis. Equally important is for the staff members of each entity to be knowledgeable about the operations of the other entities and how their job complements and fits into the overall HRPP. Communication is key to building a culture of compliance and a strong HRPP.

The responsibility for HRPP transparency and outreach to subjects may also fall to a centralized HRPP office. This includes not only responsibility for compliance with registration requirements for certain studies on the clinicaltrials .gov website and posting of certain Common Rule consent forms on a federally acceptable website (including clinicaltrials.gov), but also maintaining general outreach efforts (e.g., user-friendly websites, etc.) to the surrounding community from which study subjects are derived. Such outreach can explain what type of research is conducted at the institution, what it means to be a volunteer in research, and the importance of doing so for the advancement of science and medicine.

🔗 12-9

Conclusion

Proactive and ongoing assessment of the HRPP helps to ensure that the safety net that protects the rights and welfare of subjects is strong and secure. The challenge for an HRPP is to be a vibrant, active component in the daily life of the research community protecting research subjects by ensuring that research is conducted ethically and responsibly, and not merely an organizational chart that exists only on paper. The following are some suggestions for how to strengthen an HRPP:

- Hold regularly scheduled presentations or workshops hosted by members of the HRPP for others within the program. This provides a forum for transparency and information exchange and an opportunity for exploring ways to improve cooperation, coordination, and synergy within the HRPP.
- Identify opportunities for operational efficiencies. If there is an electronic IRB management system, can other HRPP offices access, review, and if necessary, input information regarding IRB submissions? For example, can members of the sponsored programs office access the proposed consent documents and review them for consistency with indemnification injury language negotiated in the associated contract? Can the IDS input training dates and confirm the IND/IDE number for relevant drug or device studies?
- Set up a shadowing program for different parts of the HRPP. A more in-depth understanding of how other entities operate, especially those that extensively interact, could involve arranging a staff "exchange" for a day. Allowing a colleague from one part of the HRPP to shadow the operations of another department can provide a practical demonstration of operations

and enhance understanding of the host department's role in the HRPP. This also creates an opportunity for identifying and improving efficiencies.

- Hold regular meetings of HRPP components. Regular meetings of the IO, HRPP directors, IRB staff, and IRB chairs are an excellent way to ensure that all parties are aware of issues, potential problems, regulatory changes, and challenges.

Such channels of communication are essential to protecting research subjects and fostering a culture of compliance.

References

Bierer, B. E., & Barnes, M. (2014). Research misconduct involving noncompliance in human subjects research supported by the Public Health Service: Reconciling separate regulatory systems. *Hastings Center, 44*(S3), S2–S26. onlinelibrary.wiley.com/doi/abs/10.1002/hast.336

Department of Health and Human Services (DHHS). (2018). *Institutional review board (IRB), Written procedures: Guidance for institutions and IRBs.* www.fda.gov/media/99271/download

Department of Health and Human Services (DHHS). (2019). *NIH guidelines for research involving recombinant or synthetic nucleic acid molecules.* https://osp.od.nih.gov/wp-content/uploads/NIH_Guidelines.pdf

Department of Health and Human Services, Office of Inspector General (DHHS-OIG). (1998). *Institutional review boards: Their role in reviewing approved research* (Report No. OEI-01-97-00190). https://oig.hhs.gov/oei/reports/oei-01-97-00190.pdf

Institute of Medicine (IOM). (2001). *Preserving public trust: Accreditation and human research participant protection programs.* The National Academies Press. https://doi.org/10.17226/10085

National Institutes of Health (NIH). (2016). *Final NIH policy on the use of a single institutional review board for multi-site research.* (Notice Number: NOT-OD-16-094). https://grants.nih.gov/grants/guide/notice-files/NOT-OD-16-094.html

National Research Service Act. (1974). Public Law 93-348 (42 USC 28g1-1). https://history.nih.gov/research/downloads/PL93-348.pdf

Administrative Reporting Structure for the IRB

Susan Kornetsky

Jessie Ripton

Abstract

The purpose of this chapter is to discuss the reporting structure of the IRB. In this context, "reporting structure" refers to the administrative home of the IRB, the administrative reporting structure for the IRB chair and administrative director, and the position(s) in the institution that controls IRB resources. The reporting structure of the IRB is important because it may have significant influence on the quality and efficiency of IRB function. Support from the highest levels of an institution for the IRB and the administrative staff that support the IRB demonstrates a commitment to the protection of human subjects. This helps contribute to the ability of the IRB to function within a culture of compliance and commitment to human subjects protections.

Where Should the Administrative Office That Supports an IRB Be Positioned?

For an IRB to function effectively, it is essential that it have adequate resources and work in an environment where the IRB can make independent decisions related to the protection of research subjects. Federal regulations do not address the reporting structure of the IRB. The IRB reporting structure must be organized so that no real or perceived <u>conflict of interest</u> compromises IRB function or credibility. In larger institutions, the IRB administrative office often reports to a dean or vice president of research or research administration. This individual may have oversight of other research administration functions; however, they should also be able to advocate for the independence of IRB decisions. In smaller institutions, fewer individuals are assigned responsibilities for institutional oversight of research administration. In these situations it may be tempting to assign administrative oversight of the IRB to the same person who oversees the grants and contracts (sponsored programs) operations. However,

🔗 12-7

IRB offices administratively housed within grants and contracts or the sponsored research office must be able to operate independently, without concern for increasing research volume. Therefore, whenever possible, it is desirable to not have the IRB administrative function reporting to the same individual responsible for the oversight of grants and contracts/sponsored program offices (although this may not be possible in smaller institutions).

⊘ 2-1

In considering where an administrative office for an IRB should be positioned, it is also important to recognize that in some institutions, the IRB administrative office also coordinates interactions with other components of the human research protection program (HRPP) or research infrastructure. For example, if a research protocol involves a drug, the pharmacy may need to review the research protocol; if the research involves radiation exposure, the radiation safety committee may be required to review the protocol. The breadth and scope of these reviews is determined by the institution. If an IRB administrative office is used to help coordinate the components of these reviews, this should be a consideration in the positioning and support of the administrative office.

⊘ 12-7

It is important that the IRB reporting structure be organized so that no real or perceived conflict of interest compromises IRB function or credibility, and there is access to resources and institutional support. In the absence of definitive federal guidance, it is recommended that the IRB be administratively independent from offices that have any direct responsibility for the recruitment of research dollars to the institution.

Institutional Official

Each institution should appoint a high-ranking administrative officer who is legally authorized to act for the institution and assume overall responsibility for compliance with the federal regulations for the protection of human subjects. This individual is designated as the institutional official (IO), who signs the Office for Human Research Protections (OHRP) Federalwide Assurance and obligates the institution to the terms of the assurance. The IO is responsible for ensuring that the HRPP or the research infrastructure functions effectively, and that the institution provides the resources and support necessary to comply with all requirements applicable to research involving human subjects. The IO is usually the president, chancellor, director general, chief executive officer, or chief operating officer for the legal entity. The IO should be at a level of responsibility sufficient to allow authorization of necessary administrative or legal action should that be required. Thus, department chairs, division directors, or other officials who only have authority over one portion of the institution would generally not be an appropriate IO. Further information about the responsibilities of the IO may be found in draft guidance published on the OHRP website (Department of Health and Human Services [DHHS], 2008). Training on the IO's responsibilities and the Assurance of Compliance are available on the OHRP website (DHHS, 2017).

Lines of Authority

IRB Chair

⊘ 3-2

The reporting structure for IRB chairs varies among institutions. There is no one right reporting relationship, and the final choice of reporting structure should be one that allows the IRB chair to work independently with the IRB. In some institutions, the IRB chair may report to the IO, or even to a president or dean. Hospitals and other medical settings often have a physician as the IRB chair, and this person may have dual reporting to their division/departmental chief as well as to the IO or other senior member of the institution. It is important that the IRB chair have support from the highest levels of the institution.

Regardless of to whom the IRB chair reports, it is important to remember that the IRB chair acts on behalf of the IRB, and the IO acts on behalf of the institution. It is, therefore, essential that there be regular communication between these two individuals. In some institutions an IRB may be a standing committee of the medical staff or of the "deans' council," and therefore the IRB chair may have the responsibility for providing periodic reports to these committees. This type of relationship may be acceptable for purposes of information sharing, obtaining feedback for consideration, and allowing ongoing support from the medical staff/faculty; however, these relationships should not be a direct reporting relationship. It is important to preserve the autonomy of the IRB and insulate it from pressure exerted by individuals or groups that are inconsistent with the mission of the IRB. The IRB chair and IRB must be able to act as an independent and objective body.

Chief IRB Administrator

The chief administrator of the IRB is usually the director of the IRB's administrative office. This individual should report to the IO or other high-level officer who can act on behalf of the IO on matters related to the administrative operation and support of the IRB. In general, the director would not report to the IRB chair. However, it is important that the IRB chair and director work closely together. IRB chairs are usually faculty members who serve as the chair on a voluntary and part-time basis. While the IRB chair assumes responsibility for leading the review process for the IRB, the director addresses administrative staffing, personnel issues, budgets, development of electronic review and support systems, and other administrative matters. The director and IRB chair work closely together on policy development, protocol reviews, and other activities of the IRB. The effectiveness of this interaction, however, is not dependent on a direct reporting relationship.

Qualifications for a chief IRB administrator depend on the scope and volume of research reviewed at the institution. In general, there needs to be depth of regulatory knowledge, as well as the ability to manage individuals and complex review processes within an institution. Credentials such as the Certified IRB Professional (CIP) certification help demonstrate both knowledge and experience often needed by the chief IRB administrator.

IRB Staff

The volume and nature of the research conducted at an institution should determine the number of IRB committees and the size of the IRB staff. A small institution may have only one IRB committee with two IRB staff persons, whereas a large institution may have four or more IRB committees and 30 or more IRB staff. The administrative reporting structure and the specific roles of staff within an IRB office vary among institutions; however, it is critical that IRBs are adequately staffed to support a consistent, efficient, and high-quality review process.

IRB staffing and reporting structures adopted by large institutions with multiple IRB committees are usually more complex than the systems employed by smaller institutions. A common model among mid-size to large institutions involves support staff assigned to specific departments within the institution or to functions within the IRB office such as triaging or intake and administrative review of new research applications. This structure is combined with dedicated staff who support the <u>review</u> conducted by the IRB committee, as well as the <u>expedited</u> review process. Typically, each committee of the IRB will have dedicated staff to support the review of research. The lead staff person supporting the IRB committee is usually a senior member of the IRB office, often at level of assistant or associate director, and this person will generally attend all of the meetings to ensure consistency in review. The IRB office may also include protocol analysts or administrators organized to support a specific IRB committee and/or assigned to specific departments within the institutions. Senior members of the IRB with sufficient expertise and education may perform expedited review or <u>exemption</u> determination. Recently, many IRB offices have added staff to focus on supporting <u>reliance arrangements</u> for collaborative research. Midsize to large IRBs may have a dedicated reliance specialist focused on support of IRB review.

Consistency of reviews may be challenging, and it can be helpful for IRB staff, particularly those performing expedited review, to have regular contact with the IRB chair. However, oversight of the IRB staff should be provided by the IRB administrator/director. Reporting structures for IRB staff vary based on size of the office. Many small and mid-size institutions have all staff report directly to the lead IRB administrator/director. Larger institutions may have additional layers, with support staff and protocol analysts or administrators reporting to an assistant or associate director. Regardless of the staffing model, the IRB office must be organized in a way to support consistent and high-quality review.

Conclusion

The IRB should occupy a highly visible and elevated position within the administrative research structure of the institution. A culture of compliance is best established from the top down, and ideally, the chief executive officer or other high-ranking official should serve as the IO and play an active role in fostering the important work of the IRB. When an institution's IRB does not command the respect and support of the highest administrative officials, its effectiveness and credibility are jeopardized. Thus, it is incumbent on the institution to establish an administrative reporting structure for the IRB that will allow it to operate in a highly functional manner that best serves the institution, its investigators, and research subjects.

References

Department of Health and Human Services (DHHS). (2008). *Draft example of guidance to be developed drawing on current OHRP materials, Draft VA guidance, and subpart A subcommittee suggestions.* www.hhs.gov/ohrp/sachrp-committee/recommendations/2008-september-18-letter-attachment/index.html

Department of Health and Human Services (DHHS). (2017). *Assurance training.* www.hhs.gov/ohrp/education-and-outreach/human-research-protection-program-fundamentals/index.html/assurance-training

Documentation, Policies, and Procedures

Deborah Barnard

Michelle M. Feige

Abstract

This chapter emphasizes the importance of written procedures in the administration and operation of a human research protection program (HRPP). Creating and using written procedures entails a systematic and thorough approach to transparent, concise, and thoughtfully presented standard operating procedures for the HRPP and IRB staff, researchers, and the institution.

Introduction

This chapter provides an overview of the creation and implementation of written policies and procedures for institutions, HRPPs, and IRBs, or ethics committees (ECs), as they are commonly known outside the United States. In recognition of the increased use of computer systems, we use the general term "policies and procedures" to refer to all materials in written or electronic form that describe the operation of the HRPP. In addition to policies and procedures, this also includes things such as worksheets and checklists, as well as IRB applications. All of these materials describe the function and operation of the HRPP, and some serve a dual purpose—a worksheet may describe the criteria an IRB member is to use to review research, and, when completed, can also serve as documentation of the review.

    In general, policies are more general statements, and procedures focus on the operational details of implementation. However, whether they are called policies, procedures, standard operating procedures, or something else, ultimately the most important concept is that organizations must clearly describe in writing the operation of the HRPP. For many organizations, having policies and procedures is not just a good idea, it is required by law or regulation (e.g., 45 CFR 46.108(a)(4)). This chapter emphasizes the importance of creating and using written procedures in the administration and operation of an HRPP. This entails a systematic and thorough approach to transparent, concise, and

📎 2-1

thoughtfully presented standard operating procedures for the HRPP and IRB staff, researchers, and the institution. Ultimately, the purpose of policies and procedures is to ensure high-quality, efficient, and effective HRPPs that protect subjects, but it is important to remember that policies and procedures may also be required by law and regulation for those organizations whose research is covered by regulation.

Differentiating Procedures from Policies

Policies and procedures describe how the HRPP operates. Policies tend to be general statements of broad principles, strategies, and philosophical goals. They are guiding principles used to direct an organization and delegate authority. Procedures, on the other hand, are practical, specific, step-by-step tactics and detailed directives about how to *implement* a policy. A procedure is a mechanism for accomplishing the goals set in policies, and it should be designed as a series of steps that can be followed consistently to accomplish those ends. Thus, policies provide overall guidance, and procedures are what an HRPP, the IRB, its administrative staff, and the institution's researchers consult on a regular basis.

	Cooking	IRB
Policy	Creating meringue	Decisions are made at properly constituted meetings
Procedure	Beat 2 egg whites in a bowl with a mixer until stiff. Be sure there is no grease in the bowl. Add 2 tablespoons of sugar slowly when the egg whites have begun to stiffen.	Quorum consists of one-half of the regular membership plus one person. If a quorum is present, including a nonscientist as part of the quorum, a meeting is considered properly constituted.

With the increasing use of computer systems to manage IRB review, it is important to recognize that organizations may choose to describe parts of the operation of the HRPP through checklists and worksheets. In addition, many organizations have their policies and procedures online and accessible, and they do so in a variety of ways. One university, for instance, may have its policies and procedures housed on a single website. In contrast, a medical research center might house its policies on a webpage that is completely discrete from its procedures. Many institutions opt for a hybrid system when communicating their policies and procedures, such as an institution that has one webpage dedicated to discussing the larger goals of its human subjects research program (its policies) and another page that gives information on both policies and the specific procedures used by the staff of the university. The policies typically refer to more complete sets of procedures that are likely to be developed at the office level, rather than at the institutional level. Another format would entail an integrated document, with the policy as the opening paragraph, followed by higher level procedures that implement the policy.

Why Have Written Procedures?

The purpose of having written policies and procedures is to ensure that review of research protects subjects; is consistent and efficient; and complies with any applicable requirements in institutional policy, law and regulations, and ethical principles. For some organizations, having policies and procedures is required by federal regulation and for compliance with the standards of the Association for the Accreditation of Human Research Protection Programs, Inc. (AAHRPP). Although *unwritten* procedures are used to some degree, they are not as effective as written ones for the simple reason that written procedures produce predictable and replicable results. Institutions operating primarily on written procedures are generally organized, transparent, well staffed, knowledgeable, consistent, precise, efficient, and effective.

The Office for Human Research Protections (OHRP), the Food and Drug Administration (FDA), and AAHRPP <u>accreditation</u> standards require that an institution has written procedures for IRB functioning. The regulations describe outcomes and, in some cases, specify steps an organization must take, but do not prescribe how organizations are to operationalize and implement regulatory requirements. Where the regulations are silent, AAHRPP has filled in some of the gaps. This was accomplished with the assistance of a grassroots community effort to require flexible standard operating procedures (SOPs) for areas not covered in the regulations, but which the research community felt were critical to protecting research subjects. For example, AAHRPP has three overarching domains that cover the organization, the IRB, and researchers. Each domain has standards and elements that require written policies to address each area of the HRPP. Subsequent sections refer to a variety of situations for which the institution must have and follow procedures, such as addressing <u>single IRB review</u>, <u>conflict of interest</u>, grants and contracts, and allegations of <u>noncompliance</u>. Finally, when working with sponsors or single IRBs, it is becoming increasingly common for these entities to request copies of certain written procedures.

In summary, institutions should create written procedures to address a variety of audiences: regulatory, accreditation, sponsors, and single IRBs.

✐ 8-7

✐ Section 4
✐ 12-6, 12-7, 12-8 ✐ 7-6

Federal Requirements

Some organizations are covered by federal regulations, based on research funding or the conduct of research regulated by an agency such as the FDA. The federal regulations of all 17 Common Rule agencies require that IRBs establish and follow written procedures. The required procedures outlined in these regulations form the basis of IRB operations. Both the Department of Health and Human Services (DHHS) regulations at **45 CFR 46.103(b)(4)** and **(5)** and the FDA regulations at **21 CFR 56.108(a)** and **(b)** as well as the regulations governing all other Common Rule organizations state that IRBs must follow written procedures for the following functions and operations:

- Conducting initial and <u>continuing review</u> of research and reporting findings and actions to the investigator and the institution;

- Determining which projects require review more often than annually and determining which projects need verification from sources other than the investigator that no material changes have occurred since previous IRB review;

- Ensuring prompt reporting to the IRB of <u>proposed changes</u> in a research activity and ensuring that changes in approved research, during the period for which IRB approval has already been given, may not be initiated without IRB review and approval except where necessary to eliminate apparent immediate hazards to the human subjects;

✐ 7-2

✐ 7-1

- Ensuring prompt reporting to the IRB, appropriate institutional officials, and the department or agency head (i.e., OHRP) for research conducted or supported by DHHS, and FDA for FDA-regulated research of any:

  🔗 7-3
  - Unanticipated problems involving risks to human subjects or others;

  🔗 7-6
  - Instance of serious or continuing noncompliance with the applicable DHHS and FDA regulations or the requirements or determinations of the IRB;
  - Suspension or termination of IRB approval.

The 2018 Common Rule requires additional documentation in certain situations:

Waiver of consent—additional criterion

🔗 6-4

The IRB may waive the requirement or approve an alteration of elements of informed consent if it finds and documents that the research meets certain criteria. The 2018 Common Rule added a waiver criterion that the research could not practicably be carried out without accessing or using information or biospecimens in an identifiable format. Researchers will need to provide justification that all five criteria are met in the study protocol.

Waiver of documentation of consent

🔗 6-5

The IRB may waive the requirement to obtain a signed consent document for some or all the subjects if it finds and documents that the research meets certain criteria. Under the 2018 Common Rule a waiver may be granted for international research where the signature on the consent form is not culturally appropriate. Justification will need to be provided that all five criteria are met in the study protocol.

In 2017 and 2018, OHRP and FDA, respectively, published joint guidance on the topics of "Minutes of Institutional Review Board (IRB) Meetings Guidance for Institutions and IRBs" and "Institutional Review Board Written Procedures: Guidance for Institutions and IRBs" (DHHS, 2017, 2018). In part, the publication of these coordinated guidelines was a response to the passage of the 21st Century Cures Act (Cures Act), which was signed into law on December 13, 2016. Title III, section 3023, of the Cures Act requires the Secretary of DHHS to harmonize differences between DHHS's human subjects regulations and FDA's human subjects regulations. These publications were significant in that they are the first updated guidance from OHRP/FDA on the topic of written procedures since 2011, and the first formal guidance in general about meeting minutes. Although it only reflects OHRP's and FDA's current thinking on the topics, and institutions may use alternate approaches to meet the regulatory requirements, guidance may be useful in ensuring that institutions and IRBs adequately prepare and maintain IRB meeting minutes and written policies and procedures.

However, problems can arise when IRBs develop written procedures that simply restate the regulations at **45 CFR 46.103(b)(4)** and **(5)** and at **21 CFR 56.108(a)** and **(b)**, and do not provide operational details, which may include descriptions of the roles and responsibilities of people involved in the process; time frames for completing the process; references to any worksheets or supporting materials; and references to other related procedures (e.g., a procedure for review of noncompliance might refer to another procedure on reporting to regulatory agencies).

> Developing meaningful content for written procedures involves a comprehensive and critical assessment of the IRB's responsibilities, functions, and operations, and the institution's organizational structure. (DHHS, 2018)

The DHHS regulations were originally written to operationalize ethical principles defined in the _Belmont Report_. While having well-written policies and procedures will improve compliance with regulations, it also helps an organization to protect subjects and live up to the ethical principles that define our field. However, organizations need to follow policies and principles in practice, and they should become an integral, practical description of the various IRB functions. Indeed, solid policies and procedures are clear, transparent, and go beyond basic regulatory requirements. Alongside meeting regulatory standards, successful SOPs will engender many positive outcomes, such as the following:

⌒ 1-1

1. Establishing consistency in how situations are handled. This is especially valuable for instances that may not occur frequently enough for the handling to become a well-learned pattern. Researchers appreciate greater consistency and view IRB decisions more credibly.
2. Reducing errors. It is harder to overlook critical procedural aspects if they are in writing.
3. Clarifying who is responsible for what. The written procedures explicitly address responsibilities, so that tasks are not left undone because neither the chair nor the administrator realizes it is their responsibility.
4. Efficient and effective training for new faculty, IRB members, and IRB staff. New staff members have a reference, and new IRB members have a complete procedural framework on which to structure their review of protocols.

⌒ 8-4, 8-5

5. Defending against complaints, grievances, or lawsuits about inequitable treatment with respect to IRB determinations and functions.

Policies and Procedures for Whom?

Three sets of interlocking procedures need to be developed, including those for the IRB office, researchers, and IRB members.

IRB Administrative Office

These procedures serve as an expanded reference for all staff working with the IRB, including, for example, application intake procedures, schedules, contacts, application routings, procedures for operating and maintaining the electronic IRB system, and a catalog of applicable document files. They can even include procedures for producing procedure manuals, with the frequency and method for revising them. The administrative manual is useful for educating new staff and is critical for maintaining consistency in handling studies.

Researchers

Historically called an _institutional handbook_ or _manual_, policies and procedures inform researchers about the application process, researcher responsibilities, and specific techniques such as obtaining a child's assent for research. It would

1-1   be useful to include the location of core resources such as the _Belmont Report_, the federal regulations, and other institutional procedures (such as for graduate advisors). These documents are typically maintained on an institutional website with pages dedicated to the IRB and its processes.

The IRB

The IRB's procedures must describe how to implement the laws and regulations that govern the IRB. For example, for U.S. organizations that receive funding from the National Institutes of Health (NIH), this means compliance with DHHS regulations. For organizations outside the United States, it means com-

10-9   pliance with that country's laws and regulations. Regardless of location, it may also mean conformity to guidelines, such as the guidelines produced by the

8-2   International Council for Harmonisation (ICH). However, policies and procedures will be expanded to include the institutional and committee interpretations and implementations of those regulations.

How to Produce Written Procedures

Policies and procedures are widely available, and many organizations are willing to share and allow other organizations to use their policies. Many AAHRPP-accredited organizations publish policies, which means there are many examples of organizations that have undergone stringent peer review for completeness and compliance with regulations. Adapting another institution's procedures to make them complete and pertinent to your institution is one expedient way of beginning. Indeed, it is almost always easier to begin with some existing written procedures and modify them for your purposes. Contact IRB administrators at other institutions similar to yours, and ask whether you could receive a copy of their written procedures to adapt. Likewise, consult the web for the procedures of other institutions to see what topics they include. IRB administrators are typically quite generous in allowing use or adaptation of their documents; it is a courtesy to acknowledge the source in your finished product.

Getting Started

One of the largest hurdles faced by an IRB administrator in writing procedures is simply getting started. The task can seem insurmountable, and breaking it down into smaller steps will make the project less intimidating. Suggestions for first steps include involving leadership and stakeholders; assessing your existing policies and procedures by using the OHRP/FDA checklist and AAHRPP self-assessment tool to determine what is there and what is missing; and reviewing existing standards that your organization follows (internal institutional policies, international standards, additional agency requirements, etc.). The following are some overarching tips on how to get started, along with issues to keep in mind:

- Create working groups to tackle specific tasks and areas. Create IRB/executive committees that can focus on specific areas, and assign appropriate staff.
- Decide on your institutional practices and the scope and format in which your SOPs will exist.
- Always be mindful of flexibility. Because regulatory agencies and AAHRPP will hold your organization accountable to what your SOPs say, be sure that

you have "wiggle room" written into your SOPs to provide enough room for updates, changes, and timelines.

- Be careful with the terms "must" and "should." According to OHRP/FDA guidance, "must" means something is required, and "should" is a suggestion or a recommendation but not a requirement. Similar care should be taken with the word "shall," which can mean "must" or "will."
- Do not just restate the regulations. SOPs should contain enough detail so that all staff know what to do and who should be doing it in an efficient, consistent, and effective manner so that the rights and welfare of subjects are protected.
- Get researcher, IRB, and staff input. Are the SOPs realistic? Protective? Doable? Practical?
- Create an approval process that is clear and efficient.
- Ensure high-level "buy-in" by establishing communication and making sure this support trickles down by providing education.
- Collaborate with other organizations to share SOPs, forms, resources, etc.

The OHRP/FDA written procedures self-evaluation checklist, included in the guidance document, offers a helpful start with respect to topics that might be covered (DHHS, 2018). This checklist affords a workable map for comprehensive IRB procedures.

> Written procedures should be sufficiently detailed to help IRB staff understand how to carry out their duties in a consistent and effective way that ensures that the rights and welfare of subjects are protected and that the IRB operates in compliance with the regulations. When preparing written procedures, institutions/IRBs should generally identify who carries out specific duties by reference to position title (e.g., IRB chairperson) rather than by name to avoid the need to update written procedures if duties change, or there are changes in IRB membership. (DHHS, 2018)

DHHS and FDA have stated that they understand that institutions may vary in the way they record their written policies and procedures, both in terms of content and format (DHHS, 2016). Policies and procedures can be kept in paper format or electronically. It is likely, however, that some sections will need to be written from scratch. To get started, consider the following approach:

1. Brainstorm a list of all the topics that need to be covered. Pay no attention to order. Do not worry about including too much; extraneous topics can be weeded out later. Attempt to capture every related aspect.
   Example: Appointing new members. Should not be appointed by researchers. Authorized institutional official (IO) makes final decision. Involve appropriate leadership. New members need to train. Need to represent research areas reviewed by IRB. Pay attention to diversity (gender, ethnicity). Watch representation on IRB (longevity, scientist/nonscientist, physicians, prisoner representative, community membership). Have an order in which various bodies are consulted. Make the appointment in writing from IO. Get current curriculum vitae. The IRB administration team provides instructional materials and basic orientation.
2. Order the topics by grouping them into logical relationships, chronologic sequence, or some other system.
   Example: Selecting → Appointing → Finalizing the appointment

3. Create an outline of the topics that is a further refinement of the grouping.
   Example:
   1.0 Procedure for Appointing New IRB Members
   　　1.1 Selecting candidates
   　　　　1.1.1 Timing
   　　　　1.1.2 IRB starts process
   　　　　1.1.3 Input from leadership
   　　　　1.1.4 Who can propose? Who can select?
   　　　　1.1.5 Prioritizing and getting list to authorized IO
   　　　　1.1.6 The appointment
   　　　　1.1.7 Communicating to new member and IRB committee/panel

4. Then finalize and polish each procedure. Assess the situation needing a written procedure. Think through the variations and exceptions that can occur.
   a. Gather and review background material: existing procedures, laws, and regulations from federal, state, and local sources; previous IRB actions (both those that worked and those that did not).
   b. Draft the procedure. Write rapidly and do not worry about grammatical precision. Get it down in a train of thought. Organize by introductory paragraph containing policy, description of procedure, summary of main points. Depending on the ultimate audience and use of the procedures, you may wish to cite pertinent regulations.
   c. Let the draft procedures rest at least 24 hours. When you return to them, you will see them with new eyes and are likely to see aspects you missed in the first draft.
   d. Test the procedure. "Drop" actual situations through the procedure to see whether it works. You may identify gaps or needed variations or additions, some of which may require IRB or IRB administration action to rectify processes or approve new ones.
   e. Revise procedures as necessary.

Example of Resulting Procedure
1.0 Procedure for Appointing New IRB Members
　　Members shall be appointed to the IRB such that requirements of Common Rule § 107 are met.
　　1.1. Selecting candidates
　　　　1.1.1 The selection process for routine appointments shall begin approximately three months before the appointment date; ad hoc appointments needed to fill unanticipated vacancies shall begin as soon as possible after the announcement is given.
　　　　1.1.2 The IRB shall ascertain what attributes a new member needs to possess (community member, scientist/nonscientist, duration of term, diversity, representation for vulnerable populations, academic standing, research specialty).
　　　　1.1.3 The IRB leadership will communicate these attributes to institutional leadership either by memo or email, asking on behalf of the IRB for suggested candidates. A response date should be stipulated.
　　　　1.1.4 The IRB shall likewise suggest candidates.
　　　　1.1.5 At a convened meeting, the IRB shall prioritize the list of candidates, listing briefly the reasons for the priority ranking. The IRB leadership will communicate the listing to the authorized IO within three working days of receiving the list.

1.1.6 The IO shall appoint the new member. The IO retains this responsibility exclusively; researchers may not appoint new members; the IRB and others may recommend but may not appoint.

1.1.7 The IO shall convey in memo or email his/her appointments to the IRB leadership, who shall:

1.1.7.1 Notify the appropriate IRB chair of the appointment.

1.1.7.2 Prepare the official appointment letter to the new member, using the model retained electronically at [file location] with alterations as needed to fit the circumstances.

5. Have others review the procedures. You may wish to use several reviewers, including a "typical user" as well as a knowledgeable colleague.

6. Determine a workable layout for your procedures: numbering system; format (outline, paragraph, play script); fonts; headings; how to handle graphics and appendices; issue and revision numbers and/or dates; pagination scheme; logo/institutional name; how new material will be inserted; front and back matter such as preface, table of contents, glossary, appendix, index; headers and footers; justification style. Be sure the format accommodates revisions, additions, and withdrawn procedures. Be sure there is a procedure for making these changes as well.

7. Produce final version. Consider whether multiple venues are necessary, though now, avoiding paper documents is strongly encouraged.

8. Promulgate the procedures among the target audience.

9. Follow procedures.

10. Revisit procedures on schedule to ascertain they are current.

11. Revise procedures as needed.

12. Post on intranet or internet as allowed by institutional policy

13. Share with colleagues

Creating Well-Written Procedures

Simply *having* procedures—meeting the letter of the law—is not adequate. Unduly complex or unrealistic procedures are difficult to follow. They may misinform or introduce ambiguity. Precise language and concision are vital; provide enough detail so that individuals unfamiliar with your institution (whether new researchers or federal regulatory staff) can follow your procedures and understand your process. High-quality written procedures will have the following features:

1. Be appropriate to the audience in terms of content, detail, and tone.

2. Be concise, so that users do not get lost in verbiage or unnecessary detail.

3. Be clear; for example, explicitly stating whether "10 days" refers to working days, calendar days, or 10 days from a designated event.

4. Use the active voice; for example, "Mail the approval letter" instead of "The approval letter is mailed." The active voice is more dynamic and readable and reduces ambiguity.

5. Be coherent, with an obvious, complete, and typically sequential organization.

6. Be factual, so that the procedures reflect what is accurate and will be implemented.

7. Avoid vague, superfluous words such as the superlatives *really*, *actually*, and *very*.
8. Explain acronyms, jargon, special terms, and shortcuts to the reader before using them, and perhaps include a glossary or index.
9. Avoid repetition, unless necessary.
10. Use a positive rather than a negative tone (e.g., "Use the provided form," instead of "Do not use forms other than the one provided").
11. Use bullets, numbers, flow charts or special formatting to increase readability, and effectively use embedded links to provide additional details, cross-references, and immediate definitions.
12. Judiciously employ cross-referencing to place the procedures in a broader context and reduce repetition. Overuse of cross-referencing may make the procedures difficult to follow.

Conclusion

Producing, maintaining, and using written procedures for the IRB, its administrative staff, and researchers are necessary to ensure protection of subjects in research. For many organizations, they are also required by law or regulation. Although the task may seem daunting, its alternatives are distinctly unappealing and could culminate in federal sanctions against the institution. A methodological approach is available that, although time consuming, has a high probability of generating workable procedures. After development, the procedures must be followed, revisited on a regular basis, and revised as necessary.

References

Department of Health and Human Services (DHHS). (2016). *Institutional review board (IRB) written procedures: Guidance for institutions and IRBs*. www.hhs.gov/ohrp/regulations-and-policy/requests-for-comments/guidance-for-institutions-and-irbs/index.html

Department of Health and Human Services (DHHS). (2017). *Minutes of institutional review board (IRB) meetings: Guidance for institutions and IRBs*. www.hhs.gov/ohrp/minutes-institutional-review-board-irb-meetings-guidance-institutions-and-irbs.html-0

Department of Health and Human Services (DHHS). (2018). *Institutional review board written procedures: Guidance for institutions and IRBs*. www.hhs.gov/ohrp/regulations-and-policy/guidance/institutional-issues/institutional-review-board-written-procedures/index.html

Administrative Tasks Before Each IRB Meeting

Ann E. O'Hara

Erica W. Tauriello

Abstract

The most efficient and effective IRB meetings require thoughtful and thorough preparation to ensure that the IRB is able to make a definitive determination regarding each agenda item. To accomplish this goal, IRB staff must work with researchers to ensure study materials are complete and contain all of the information required to address regulatory and ethical requirements and that all logistical requirements for an effective meeting are considered and the meeting is well prepared for. The purpose of this chapter is to discuss the administrative tasks to be done in preparation for the full committee meeting.

Introduction

Thorough IRB meeting preparations are respectful of the time constraints of members, researchers, and staff and can assist in the development of goodwill and mutual respect within the research community. The specific internal office processes that each organization adopts will depend on many variables, such as the size of the research portfolio, the number of committees, and the number of office staff. Examples of preparatory tasks in this chapter are from the IRB offices of a small research institution with a single monthly IRB meeting and a larger institution with several committees meeting monthly.

🖉 3-3

Work With Your Researchers/IRB Office Outreach Activities

Whenever possible, it is important to promote a climate within the research community of your institution that welcomes questions and provides educational outreach. Outreach efforts can help to build a camaraderie between IRB staff and researchers and help ensure communication and regulatory compliance throughout the life of a study. Some examples are sending regular newsletters, designating open office hours, and providing regular educational discussion sessions on special topics such as writing consent forms.

IRB Submissions

🔗 5-7

Prior to the assignment of a study to a <u>convened meeting</u>, IRB staff should conduct a prereview process. As a first step, they should provide a checklist for researchers. The materials needed will depend on the type of study, and they may also depend on the type of submission system that an institution uses. Many institutions use electronic submission systems, in which some information is collected in fields in the system, and other information is provided through uploaded documents.

The following list provides an example of required materials for a new submission of a research study:

Materials needed for submission

1. Documentation of local departmental and scientific review or study feasibility review, as applicable. If the principal investigator is not part of the department or institution from which subjects will be drawn, additional documentation of review may be needed.
2. Protocol: Sponsor protocol, or if no sponsor protocol exists, a local template designed for the study type. Dartmouth College IRB forms are publicly available at www.dartmouth.edu/~cphs, and include forms for study types, such as clinical trials, minimal risk nonclinical studies, and studies involving analysis of data only.

🔗 Section 9
🔗 9-7
🔗 Section 6

3. Documents supplemental to the protocol: for example, information about devices needed to determine regulatory status and determinations, and forms specific to <u>special populations</u> such as individuals with <u>impaired decision-making capacity</u>.
4. <u>Consent</u> and assent forms.
5. Recruitment materials.
6. Study instruments, such as surveys and interview scripts.
7. Documentation of ancillary reviews, such as radiation safety.
8. Documentation of drugs or devices used in the study, such as Investigator Brochures and instructions for use.

🔗 8-5

9. Human subjects protections <u>training</u> requirement completion, such as from an online course.
10. IRB review fees as applicable, depending upon your institutional funding source and study sponsor requirements.

🔗 Section 9
🔗 10-3 🔗 6-4
🔗 9-6

The prereview process should involve checking all aspects of the application for completeness, identifying all areas in which additional materials or information may be needed to review the study. For example, edits to study materials may be required in order to thoroughly address potential issues such as enrollment of <u>vulnerable populations</u>. Additional information may be needed to justify the use of <u>deception</u> or requests for <u>waivers</u> of consent or of <u>parental permission</u>. If necessary, IRB staff may refer researchers to other resources within or outside of the organization for assistance, such as an experienced researcher willing to act as mentor or protocol and consent form templates.

🔗 5-7
🔗 5-3 🔗 5-5

As part of the prereview process, applications should be screened to determine whether review at a <u>convened meeting</u> is required or whether the study may be eligible for <u>exemption</u> or <u>expedited</u> review.

IRB staff, along with the <u>IRB chair</u>, may determine that the IRB expertise is appropriate for review of a study or may decide to seek out a consultant to assist with the review and advise the IRB. If a consultant is used, it is important to ensure that appropriate documentation is maintained by the IRB and that any potential <u>conflict of interest</u> has been identified and appropriately addressed.

If time permits, it can be very helpful to invite the researcher to a convened meeting to present a new study and answer questions. For a study that was previously deferred or disapproved at a convened meeting, it can be especially useful to invite researchers to discuss their study at the time of resubmission.

Consideration should be given to the use of a primary reviewer system, in which an IRB member is assigned to provide a verbal summary of the study and any potential issues at the meeting (Department of Health and Human Services [DHHS], 2010). All members are expected to review all studies, and comments of all members are welcomed and encouraged during the discussion.

    3-2

    12-6, 12-7, 12-8

Resubmission of Deferred or Disapproved Study

In spite of communication with researchers and thorough IRB meeting preparation, at times a study may be deferred to a future meeting or disapproved by the full committee. When either of these situations occurs, IRB staff should collaborate with researchers to respond to IRB concerns and help remove barriers to IRB approval, when possible and within the regulatory framework. If the institution has multiple IRB committees, consideration should be given to whether a response would best be reviewed by the same committee as the initial review for consistency. Consistency may also be accomplished by requesting that the initial reviewers review the resubmission prior to a meeting and provide comments for presentation to the members in attendance. It is helpful to require a response memo from the researcher, addressing each issue, in addition to revised materials with changes tracked.

Study Modifications

Study <u>modifications</u> should be reviewed by IRB staff to determine whether review at a convened meeting is needed. Modifications to full committee studies that involve minor changes may be reviewed through an <u>expedited</u> procedure. In determining whether a change is minor, it may be useful to evaluate the change in terms of "purpose, procedure, and population." Changes to any of these aspects of a study will usually not qualify as a "minor" change, and so would not be eligible for expedited review. A change in study procedure that involves increasing the risk to subjects, for example, would require review at a convened meeting. In addition, it is important to consider whether a proposed modification to an expedited study may move the study out of the category or risk level eligible for expedited review. For modifications requiring review at a convened meeting, a description of the modification may be included on the meeting agenda.

    7-1

    5-5

Continuing Review

IRB review must be conducted prior to a study's expiration date in order for the study to continue uninterrupted and to maintain compliance with regulations

7-2

for human research subjects protection. Many institutions have adopted the policy of using a fixed anniversary date for continuing review, as described in OHRP guidance on continuing review (DHHS, 2010). In the anniversary date system, a continuing review conducted within 30 days of the anniversary of the original IRB approval expiration may maintain the same approval date. For all studies, a submission deadline should be assigned, allowing time to preview the submission and permitting several meeting cycles prior to the expiration of approval. IRB staff should develop a standard method to remind researchers to provide applications for renewal. The reminder should include instructions for applying for renewal using the forms and submission system required by the institution. These practices may assist in ensuring there is an IRB determination prior to the study review expiration date, while allowing for unforeseen circumstances that may affect IRB meeting attendance, such as inclement weather.

Special Reports

7-2 7-1
7-3 7-4 7-6
7-7

In addition to new studies, continuing reviews, modifications, reports of unanticipated problems, post-approval monitoring, noncompliance, and study closure may all require review at a convened meeting. A comment added to the IRB meeting agenda can provide guidance to members regarding any potential regulatory determinations that may be needed. IRB policy should describe how these reports are handled within the organization and what is shared during IRB meetings. For example, for expedited studies for which continuing review reporting is not a regulatory requirement, study status reports may be requested from researchers and provided for review at the meeting. These status reports may inform the IRB of study completion or plans for continuation of the study.

Preparing the Agenda

3-1

When inviting members to attend and creating the meeting agenda, it is important to note schedules of guest speakers, consultants, and members, in order to maintain a quorum throughout the meeting and to run the meeting efficiently. The committee roster should be referenced, to be sure that regulatory requirements are met throughout the meeting, including the presence of a nonscientist member.

9-7

The agenda may be used as a guide for IRB members, noting potential regulatory issues for discussion and determinations required for each study. IRB staff may develop a template of commonly used agenda comments as a guide for composing agenda notes for each study. Potential regulatory determinations are added to the agenda with citations. For example, if a study involves individuals with impaired decision making, the agenda might note the need for a determination and may refer to the information provided by the research team to aid in this determination. It may also be helpful to provide specific training or educational resources to guide members on special topics. These may include laminated sheets set out at the meeting table containing regulatory information such as the criteria for approval, and special issues such as inclusion of minors and individuals with impaired decision-making capacity.

Full Committee Review Histories

3-3

When a modification or continuing review is assigned to the agenda of a convened meeting, it is helpful to provide reviewers with a history of all reviews of the study that have occurred at a convened meeting, in one document, with excerpts from the minutes and notes from the IRB office that are appropriate. IRB members appreciate being able to quickly view the IRB review history of a study, and this information is important for ongoing review. Many electronic management systems designed for IRB work provide this type of summary. If members need to be able to obtain their own summary through the electronic system, it is important to ensure that access is easy and intuitive; a high number of "clicks" or a less intuitive pathway to the desired information increases the burden to members (Food and Drug Administration [FDA], 2012).

Distribution of Review Materials to Committee Members

Meeting materials should be made available to members in a timely way, whether distributed electronically or in paper form. For a smaller institution not utilizing an online system, materials may be distributed via a secure file hosting service. Minutes from prior meetings may be provided to IRB members to aid in the review of study modifications or continuing reviews. Dartmouth College prepares a document for each study under review, including the minutes excerpts for each time the study was reviewed.

As described previously, depending on your policy and resources, you may use a "primary reviewer system," in which a primary reviewer assigned to each agenda item presents a verbal overview for all members. Alternatively, all IRB members may be equally responsible for reviews, with the IRB chair providing an overview and leading discussion of all items. In either case, IRB members should arrive at the meeting having reviewed the agenda items, including proposed new studies, study modifications, and continuing review of ongoing studies.

All IRB members should be encouraged to send questions to researchers or to IRB staff to relay to researchers prior to the IRB meeting. An effort to resolve any questions and concerns prior to the IRB meeting helps ensure productive meetings and clear IRB determinations.

Attendance at IRB Meetings

Meeting attendance should be confirmed well in advance of a meeting, to ensure quorum and that regulatory requirements are met. Use of a worksheet is recommended to track planned attendance, including the need to invite alternate members to meet quorum and other review requirements. Maintaining a <u>roster</u> that includes alternates for members of the IRB can assist in these goals. 🔗 3-1 Alternates may attend all meetings, but they may only vote when the full member is unavailable. Or alternates may attend only when the full member is not in attendance; this may vary according to institutional policy.

At the time of invitation to a meeting, members should be reminded to share any scheduling constraints including late arrival or early departure, so that any potential quorum issues can be addressed in advance.

Requests from nonmembers to observe meetings may be approved by the committee chair and announced with a note on the agenda. Consideration should be given to having guests complete nondisclosure agreements, if this is not accomplished by other means at your institution. Reminding the committee of the confidential nature of meeting discussions is always an appropriate practice.

Note Taking and Meeting Minutes

⊘ 3-3

The agenda document may be used to create a template for note taking. IRB staff may find it helpful to include highlighted notes for reference during the <u>meeting</u>, including any special issues for which a prompt to the members may be needed.

⊘ 2-5, 2-6

In addition, notes taken during the meeting can then be used to assist in formulating the communication of meeting proceedings to researchers and the composition of the final <u>meeting minutes</u>. Depending on the size of the agenda and number of IRB staff in attendance, it may be helpful to prepare a spreadsheet for each meeting to record the votes for each item. This allows staff to easily document each vote as it occurs, rather than adding the vote count to the notes document.

At many institutions, minutes for the previous meeting are provided for review by the committee at the next meeting. Although not a regulatory requirement, a vote is then made to approve the minutes. In addition, a listing of expedited reviews and exempt determinations completed outside of the meeting may be communicated to the IRB via electronic means or during the IRB meeting as time allows.

Continuing Education

⊘ 8-4

Continuing <u>education</u> of IRB members may be accomplished in a variety of ways. For each meeting, several articles may be selected and one member assigned to present and lead a discussion. Subscriptions to external resources such as the CITI Program (citiprogram.org), IRB EasyEd (apexethical.com), or Public Responsibility in Medicine and Research (PRIM&R) (primr.org) membership publications may aid in educational discussions or provide case studies for review. Regulatory or other member education items may be shared and presented by IRB staff. It can be useful to leave time for IRB member feedback and contributions, which may lead to lively discussions.

Meeting Environment

⊘ 3-3

Consideration should be given to the time of day for <u>IRB meetings</u> and the length of each meeting. It can be difficult to accommodate members, researchers, guest speakers, and community volunteers. It is ideal for the IRB office to try to create a welcoming and comfortable atmosphere for IRB meetings; refreshments may be provided, depending on the time of day and anticipated length of the meeting. Participants and members may be given the option to teleconference or videoconference as well, as technology allows.

It is worthwhile to consider the use of projection screens or other means to make meeting materials visible to members as a group during the meeting. Dartmouth College has found it best to have a staff member dedicated to navigating the study materials for projection during the meeting. This individual does not have any responsibility for note taking during the meeting but is dedicated only to this important task.

Documentation Storage

Organizing and storing IRB documentation may be viewed as a task needed (or at least initiated) prior to each IRB meeting. Depending on your technology, you may need to create an electronic repository for IRB meeting documents and preparation. This may include IRB meeting notes; agenda; attendance log; prior meeting minutes; study documents; IRB evaluation forms (criteria for review); training materials (and discussion points); outstanding action notes since the last IRB meeting; new business (that did not require an IRB determination at a full convened meeting); documentation of privacy board/officer review and concerns; and documentation of information systems review and concerns, as applicable.

- Create an "inspection-ready" IRB file for each study (electronic, paper, or both). This may be an automated process depending on the technology at your institution. Ensure all IRB study file documents will be deposited into that file and available for audits/inspections at any time.
- In addition, create an auditable IRB file for each IRB meeting to show compliance with regulations for IRB review.

Conclusion

There are a variety of administrative tasks that need to be carefully executed prior to each IRB meeting to ensure the meeting is efficient and effective and to keep researchers and IRB members engaged. Education and engagement of IRB members, and effective communication and meeting preparation with researchers, will result in the most productive meetings and definitive IRB determinations.

References

Department of Health and Human Services (DHHS). (2010). *Continuing review guidance*. www.hhs .gov/ohrp/regulations-and-policy/guidance/guidance-on-continuing-review-2010/index.html

Food and Drug Administration (FDA). (2012). *Guidance for IRBs, clinical investigators, and sponsors: IRB continuing review after clinical investigation approval*. www.fda.gov/media/83121 /download

Administrative Tasks During Each IRB Meeting

Rachel D. Bibeault
Bryan M. Ludwig

Abstract

The purpose of this chapter is to describe the administrative tasks during the convened IRB meeting. The federal regulations and guidance documents do not provide specific details on all the tasks performed during the IRB meeting; rather they focus on attendance requirements, quorum, and meeting minutes documentation. IRBs are free to choose the format of the meeting that works best for their organization, whether this is a standard in-person meeting format or a remote video-based format. Regardless what meeting format is used, administrative support is essential for an effective and efficient meeting. While administrative tasks may vary slightly among organizations, they can be essentially summarized into four main tasks: (1) meeting setup, (2) board education, (3) tracking attendance/quorum and documenting minutes, and (4) documenting IRB determinations, questions, or concerns for each individual study in order to effectively communicate this information to researchers in writing [45 CFR 46.109].

Introduction

Although all administrative tasks discussed here are important, the main administrative task during the meeting is documenting the discussion and determinations in meeting minutes. The regulations at 45 CFR 46.115(2) dictate what is required in the minutes:

> Minutes of the IRB meetings [...] shall be in sufficient detail to show attendance at the meetings; actions taken by the IRB; the vote on these actions including the number of members voting for, against, and abstaining; the basis for requiring changes in or disapproving the research; and a written summary of the discussion of controverted issues and their resolution.

How minutes are recorded will vary among organizations, number of administrative support personnel, and availability of technology. IRB staff can take minutes directly on a computer, making the process more efficient than transcribing an audio recording. Alternatively, some IRB systems have a function allowing the minutes to be entered directly into the electronic system in real time. Many IRBs choose to have administrative staff take notes and prepare the formal minutes <u>after the meeting</u>. With regard to taking minutes, IRBs may find it more efficient to break up the task of taking minutes by having one staff member focus on attendance and the vote counts and another staff member focus on taking accurate notes of the IRB's determinations on individual studies. For the purposes of this chapter, documenting IRB meetings in minutes will be broken down into recording attendance/vote counts, with a separate section for documenting the reasons for the IRB's determination for each individual research study and other documentation as suggested by Office for Human Research Protections (OHRP) and Food and Drug Administration (FDA) guidance documents.

IRB Meeting Setup

Because IRB meetings require substantial commitments of time and resources from both IRB staff and members, preparation <u>prior to the start of the meeting</u> will ensure the meeting commences when scheduled and runs smoothly and efficiently. The meeting facility should be set up with appropriate seating, refreshments (if offered), and the agenda with supporting documentation provided for each member. Reference guides such as the example in **Figure 2.5-1** may be useful. If utilized, media such as telephones, computers, projectors, or televisions should be set up to facilitate support during deliberations or continuing education presentations. Media should be checked prior to the meeting for proper connections, software updates, and internet access to prevent unnecessary delays during the meeting.

As members arrive, the IRB staff should document the number of members in attendance, recording primary members, those alternating for primary members, the presence of a nonscientist, and whether guests are present. Should a member be unable to physically attend a convened meeting but be available by telephone or other real-time electronic media, they should be connected using a speakerphone or other appropriate device, allowing the member participating remotely to discuss the study with the other members in real time and to vote. Once quorum is reached, the IRB staff should notify the <u>IRB chair</u> that the meeting may begin.

IRB Meeting Education

It is worth mentioning that many IRBs conduct continuing <u>education</u> at the beginning of the meeting, as it is a convenient way to provide education to as many IRB members and staff as possible at a single time. Education can either be formal or informal depending on the need and time available. Informal types of education can include providing relevant articles from journals such as *Ethics & Human Research* for members to read on their own time. Another option is to have slides showing in the background before the meeting starts, reminding members of changes to institutional or human research protection program (HRPP) policies or state or federal regulations. Formal education can include an in-depth presentation of changes in policies or regulations, having an IRB member or staff present on a relevant topic, or inviting a researcher to present on a research topic that has resulted in extended discussion at previous IRB meetings.

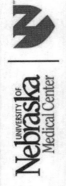

Criteria for IRB Approval of Research
45 CFR 46.111 and 21 CFR 56.111

(1) Risks to subjects are minimized (i) By using procedures that are consistent with sound research design and that do not unnecessarily expose subjects to risk, and (ii) Whenever appropriate, by using procedures already being performed on the subjects for diagnostic or treatment purposes.

(2) Risks to subjects are reasonable in relation to anticipated benefits, if any, to subjects, and the importance of the knowledge that may reasonably be expected to result

(3) Selection of subjects is equitable

(4) Informed consent will be sought from each subject

(5) Informed consent will be documented

(6) Research plan make adequate provision for monitoring the data collected to ensure the safety of subjects.

(7) There are adequate provisions to protect the privacy of subjects and to maintain the confidentiality of data.

(8) Additional safeguards have been included in the study to protect the rights and welfare of vulnerable subjects

Waiver or Alteration of Informed Consent
45 CFR 46.116(f)

- The research involves no more than minimal risk to the subjects; AND
- The research could not practicably be carried out without the waiver or alteration; AND
- If the research involves using identifiable private information or identifiable biospecimens, the research could not practicably be carried out without using such information or biospecimens in an identifiable format; AND
- The waiver or alteration will not adversely affect the rights and welfare of the subjects; AND
- Whenever appropriate, the subjects will be provided with additional pertinent information after participation

Waiver of Documentation of Informed Consent
45 CFR 46.117(c)

- The only record linking the subject and the research would be the informed consent form AND the principal risk would be potential harm resulting from a breach of confidentiality; OR
- The research presents no more than minimal risk AND the research involves no procedures for which written consent is normally required outside of the research context; OR
- The subjects are members of a distinct cultural group or community in which signing forms is not the norm, AND the research presents no more than minimal risk AND there is an appropriate alternative mechanism for documenting that informed consent was obtained

Subpart D Categories
45 CFR 46 and 21 CFR 56

§404 - Research not involving greater than minimal risk

1. Assent of children and permission of parents or guardians

§405 - Research involving greater than minimal risk but presenting the prospect of direct benefit to the individual subjects

1. Risk is justified by the anticipated benefit to subjects; AND

2. Risk/benefit is at least as favorable as that presented by available alternative approaches; AND

3. Assent of children and permission of parents or guardians

§406 - Research involving greater than minimal risk and no prospect of direct benefit to individual subjects

1. Risk represents a minor increase over minimal risk; AND

2. Research presents experiences to subjects that are reasonably commensurate with those inherent in their actual or expected medical, dental, psychological, social, or educational situations; AND

3. Research is likely to yield generalizable knowledge about the subjects' disorder or condition which is of vital importance for the understanding or amelioration of the subjects' disorder or condition; AND

4. Assent of children and permission of parents or guardians

Figure 2.5-1 Example of reference guide

Documentation of Quorum and the Vote

Although responsibility for tracking attendance was covered earlier in the administrative tasks during meeting setup, it also important to track attendance throughout the meeting. Members may leave the room during the meeting for a variety of reasons, and a count of voting members in the room should constantly be tracked to ensure quorum is maintained.

For IRB meeting purposes, quorum is defined as more than half (a majority) of the members assigned to a particular board, not just those present at the meeting. The regulations at 45 CFR 46.108(b), and equivalent FDA regulations, require a quorum for a convened IRB meeting, meaning that a majority of members assigned to that committee must be present. This must include a member who is a nonscientist. This person can have training in a nonscientific discipline, such as an attorney, ethicist, or clergy member. Nonscientist members should not be confused with nonaffiliated members, who must have no connection with the institution in which the IRB is housed. In addition, the regulations state that in order for a research study to be approved, it must receive the approval of the majority of those members present at the meeting.

As noted previously, the regulations require that the vote on the IRB actions be documented to include the number of IRB members voting for or against, abstaining, or recused. IRBs may find it useful to create a form to assist in documenting the vote, that quorum was maintained during the vote, and the members who were absent during the vote (see **Figure 2.5-2** for an example). In the case that quorum is lost, the individual responsible for tracking attendance and quorum should notify the IRB chair that quorum has been lost and that the meeting should be halted until quorum returns.

The individual responsible for tracking attendance and quorum should also prepare for the meeting by determining if any IRB member has a conflict of interest related to research being reviewed at the meeting, in order to remind the chair that that member must be recused before the discussion and vote. According to the regulations at 45 CFR 46.107(e), "No IRB may have a member participate in the IRB's initial or continuing review of any project in which the member has a conflicting interest, except to provide information requested by the IRB." Another consideration for tracking the vote is the presence of guests or consultants. The regulations at 45 CFR 46.107(f) allow IRBs to invite guests or consultants to assist in the review of issues that require expertise beyond, or in addition to, that available on the IRB. However, it must be documented that these individuals did not vote and are not counted toward quorum.

Joint OHRP and FDA guidance documents provide recommendations on other items that IRBs should include in the minutes, such as documenting whether any members not present participated in the meeting via telephone or video conference, and whether they received copies of the review documents in advance of the meeting. It is recommended to record the length of discussion before a motion is made, since some IRBs may limit the length of a discussion before the chair calls for a motion or for a vote on an extended discussion. If review of the research leads to a particularly extended discussion, this should be documented in the minutes, since it may be viewed as a controverted issue. OHRP and FDA do not suggest a verbatim transcript of the meeting but a summary of the relevant information that "contributes to an understanding of the IRB's findings and determinations" (Department of Health and Human Services, 2017).

IRB Full Board Review/Actions

Chair _____   QUORUM: 10

Start Time: _____   Date of **PEDS** IRB Meeting _4-23-2019_   End Time _____

	Commercial	Grants (NIH)	Cooperative	Other	Full Approval	Conditional	Tabled	Declined Rev	Disapproved	Subcommittee	# PRESENT	For	Against	Abstain	Chair Abstain	Absent	Absent/Conflict	Misc. Abstentions i.e. PP; Peer Reviewer	Chair or Vice-Chair Abstention	Members absent from Meeting at Time of Vote	Members Absent Conflict PI, SI's or Faculty Advisor	Additional Comments
IRB # PI NAME New				X		X					15	12	0	0	1	2	0	None	MS	Smith, Davis	None	Department Funds
IRB # PI NAME New				X		X					15	14	0	0	1	0	0	None	MS	-	None	No Funds
IRB # PI NAME RFC					X						15	13	0	1	1	0	0	Smith	MS	-	None	
IRB # PI NAME CR					X						15	13	0	0	1	0	1	None	MS	-	Davis	
IRB # PI NAME CR						X					15	13	0	0	1	1	0	None	MS	Jones	None	

Present: Actual number of members who were at the meeting for any length of time
For, Against, Abstain or Chair Abstain — all count towards quorum

Figure 2.5-2 Sample form to assist in documenting the vote

University of Nebraska Medical Center IRB Office

Documentation of IRB Determination of Individual Studies

One of the most important responsibilities of the IRB staff, and a key to well-conducted research involving human subjects, is appropriate documentation of determinations made during the course of an IRB meeting. Proper documentation will assist the IRB in conveying their decisions and determinations to the researcher in a clear and concise manner [45 CFR 46.109(d)]. The IRB staff must document all findings, determinations, and controverted issues in order to fulfill regulatory requirements [45 CFR 46.109], and this typically includes prior meeting minutes, new individual studies, modifications to existing studies, continuing reviews, and reportable new information.

Meeting minutes are presented to the IRB members for review at a subsequent meeting by a reviewer from the prior meeting, and a vote is taken (and documented) to either accept the minutes as submitted or to indicate if modifications to the prior meeting minutes are needed.

🖉 5-7　Each research study requiring review and approval by a <u>full board IRB</u> is addressed separately at a convened meeting. The primary reviewers present the studies and provide a summary including any significant concerns; determination of risk level; and recommendation for either approval, requiring modifications for approval, deferral, or disapproval of the proposed research. After the reviewers have presented their summaries of the studies and the IRB members have discussed the agenda items, it is time for IRB members to vote. Each item on the agenda is given a separate vote, and it is the responsibility of the IRB staff to document and summarize the discussion, including controverted issues, motions, and voting results. As noted previously, the IRB staff must also record the names of members who abstain from voting or leave the meeting due to a conflicting interest (or any other reason). IRBs handle documentation of the discussion and determinations in different ways. Some IRBs will include a checklist for each individual study, allowing the IRB members to check each determination and to attach documentation supporting the determination. Other IRBs have forms that are included in the initial submission that describe each separate item (e.g., research involving children, prisoners, those with incapacitated decision making, or a nonsignificant risk device), and the discussion is organized around those documents and what determinations will be needed. The IRB may also record whether a study is eligible

🖉 5-5 🖉 7-2　for <u>expedited review</u> in the future and whether <u>continuing review</u> is needed at intervals appropriate to the degree of risk [45 CFR 46.109].

Conclusion

IRB administrative support, which includes efficient preparation of the IRB meeting space, preparing IRB education items to keep members up-to-date on current ethical issues in the research world, keeping accurate record of quorum at the beginning and throughout the meeting, and documenting the discussion and determinations of the IRB for each study accurately and efficiently, ensures the IRB meeting will be as productive and efficient as possible.

Reference

Department of Health and Human Services (DHHS). (2017). *Minutes of institutional review board (IRB) meetings guidance for institutions and IRBs.* www.hhs.gov/ohrp/minutes-institutional-review-board-irb-meetings-guidance-institutions-and-irbs.html-0

Administrative Tasks After Each IRB Meeting

Kristi DeHaai

Helena Estes-Johnson

Kelly Tanguay

Abstract

Administrative tasks following a convened IRB meeting serve to ensure that all regulatory and institutional requirements are appropriately addressed, documented, and communicated with the researchers and board members. This chapter provides guidance on administrative tasks and the types of items that should be included in the documentation following an IRB meeting.

Introduction

The federal regulations require the IRB to inform the researcher and the institution, in writing, of the board's determination to approve or disapprove a proposed research study [45 CFR 46.109(d)]. The reasoning behind the determination and, if applicable, a list of any modifications required to secure approval, should be included in the written correspondence. The regulations also make provisions for the researcher to respond to this communication. While the regulations are written in a manner to address new studies and modifications, it is important to remember that any determination, such as the risk determination of an investigational device or the determination of whether a compliance issue represents continuing or noncontinuing compliance, must be formally documented in the minutes (45 CFR 46.109(d)):

> An IRB shall notify investigators and the institution in writing of its decision to approve or disapprove the proposed research activity, or of modifications required to secure IRB approval of the research activity. If the IRB decides to disapprove a research activity, it shall include in its written notification a statement of the reasons for its decision and give the investigator an opportunity to respond in person or in writing 45 CFR 46.109(d).

Researcher Letters

The following information should be included in formal correspondence to the researchers following IRB review.

For all letters, regardless of IRB determination:

1. The date of the letter and the date of IRB review
2. The name of the researcher
3. The study identification number and study title
4. The IRB determination: approved, approvable with conditions, or disapproved. In the case of risks and noncompliance determinations, the final determination with justification, if the determination is a controverted issue

For items not approved by the IRB (i.e., those approved with conditions, tabled, or disapproved):

1. A statement indicating that the proposed research activity may not begin until all conditions for approval have been met, at which time the IRB will issue a formal approval letter
2. A clear list of the conditions of approval or a detailed justification for tabling/disapproving of the study
3. A deadline for action following determinations requiring further modification or resubmission to the IRB

For items approved by the IRB:

1. Risk determination (minimal or greater than minimal risk).
   a) If minimal risk and the IRB determined the study to be approvable under one of the <u>expedited</u> review categories, the letter should document the applicable expedited category.

   🔗 5-5

2. Any subpart <u>B</u>, <u>C</u>, or D determinations, as applicable. For <u>subpart D</u> determinations it is helpful to the researchers to specify the number of parent signatures, assent requirements, and age of majority re-consent requirements.

   🔗 9-4 🔗 9-5 🔗 9-6

3. Citations of Department of Health and Human Services (DHHS) regulations, Health Insurance Portability and Accountability Act (<u>HIPAA</u>) regulations, as well as any non–Common Rule agency regulations that apply (e.g., Food and Drug Administration [FDA], Department of Justice [DOJ]).

   🔗 11-6

4. Date of expiration and duration of approval.
5. <u>Continuing reviews</u> and <u>modifications</u> of studies approved prior to the implementation of the 2018 Common Rule (January 19, 2019) should indicate which version of the Common Rule is applicable to the study (e.g., pre-2018 Requirements or the revised Common Rule, known as the 2018 Requirements).

   🔗 7-2 🔗 7-1

6. A synopsis of any issues related to the study that involved extended board discussion.
7. A list of study materials reviewed by the board, such as protocol, <u>consent</u> forms, Investigator Brochure, advertisements/recruitment materials, questionnaires, etc. As appropriate, this list should include version control information, such as version number and date.

   🔗 Section 6

Letters to researchers are often used as a notification of other pertinent regulations, IRB policies, and institutional policies. The following are examples of additional notifications:

1. The research must be conducted in accordance with the documents reviewed and approved by the IRB. Any changes in the protocol or other study documents, such as the consent form, must be reviewed and approved by the IRB prior to implementing the changes.

2. Protocol <u>violations</u> and <u>adverse events</u> should be reported to the IRB as soon as possible and in accordance with institutional policy.

🔗 7-5 🔗 7-3

3. Study document retention rules/policies.
4. As applicable, a reminder that subjects are to receive a copy of the consent form.
5. For conditionally approved new studies, it is prudent to reiterate that no research activities, such as recruitment, enrollment, and data collection, are authorized at this time.
6. For conditional approvals of <u>modifications</u> to a previously approved study, the letter should include a statement indicating that the previously approved study activities may continue; however, the proposed modifications may not be implemented until the IRB finds the conditions have been met.

🔗 7-1

Minutes

The regulations require that the minutes document (1) attendance; (2) actions; (3) vote counts; (4) reason for changes required in the research as determined by the board, or for disapproval; and (5) discussion of controverted issues and the resolution thereof **[45 CFR 46.115(a)(2)]**. The <u>minutes</u> should provide sufficient detail to reflect the committee vote, as well as capture the committee's discussion in a way that would be understandable to a person who was not present at the meeting. The IRB staff member responsible for writing the minutes should attend the IRB meeting to take notes. Minutes may be generated retrospectively or in real time during the meeting. Sometimes the working minutes are projected for the IRB to view during the meeting. Because the regulations do not include specific format requirements for minutes, IRBs may use best practices and develop a template. The minutes template is used to facilitate the minute writing process, ensuring required regulatory and institutional information is included. Standardized minutes templates also help to ensure consistency in meeting minutes in offices that involve multiple individuals writing minutes. In many cases, the minutes also serve to document determinations and considerations made by the IRB, as required in other sections of the Common Rule (e.g., <u>criteria</u> for IRB approval **[45 CFR 46.111]**; documentation of <u>informed consent</u> **[45 CFR 46.117]**; and additional protections for vulnerable populations **[subparts B, C, and D]**).

🔗 2-5

🔗 5-4
🔗 Section 6

> **45 CFR 46.115(a)**
> (a) An institution, or when appropriate an IRB, shall prepare and maintain adequate documentation of IRB activities, including the following:

> **45 CFR 46.115(a)(2)**
> Minutes of IRB meetings, which shall be in sufficient detail to show attendance at the meetings; actions taken by the IRB; the vote on these actions including the number of members voting for, against, and abstaining; the basis for requiring changes in or disapproving research; and a written summary of the discussion of controverted issues and their resolution.

Attendance and Vote Count

Although the regulations require that attendance and number of members voting for, against, and abstaining be included in the minutes, it may be beneficial to also include the number of members required to achieve quorum, a list of voting and nonvoting members in attendance, visitors, and any attendees absent at the time of vote. Of note, IRB members participating via telephone or video conference are considered present while they are connected. It is recommended that their mode of attendance be documented in the minutes. When both a primary and alternate IRB member are present, only the primary IRB member counts toward quorum.

Actions Taken by the IRB

The minutes should include the actions taken by the IRB (approved, approvable with conditions, or disapproved). If the IRB votes to approve with conditions, the minutes should detail the required modifications and the specific reasons for the required changes, which will serve to document the committee's concerns and justifications for the requested modifications required in order to secure approval. For studies that are disapproved, the minutes must document the reason for disapproval.

Summary of the Committee Discussion of Controverted Issues and Their Resolution

Any issue requiring extended discussion during the meeting must be summarized within the minutes. The minutes are not intended to be a transcription of the committee discussion, but should succinctly capture the pertinent discussion points and concerns raised. The minutes should be written in a collective voice (e.g., "The committee discussed . . . ," "The IRB finds . . . ," or "The board presumes . . .") in order to avoid identifying individual committee members' specific commentary or opinions. Because the minutes are a document subject to audit, it is best to avoid incomplete statements. Any concerns expressed by the IRB and written in the minutes should include a description of their resolutions.

To ensure accuracy of information and to disseminate results to researchers in a timely manner, administrative tasks following a convened IRB meeting should be a priority. Researchers appreciate being informed of the status of their submissions as soon as possible, which fosters a positive relationship between IRBs and the research communities. IRBs should be aware that submissions are often time sensitive with respect to reporting guidelines for other regulatory, institutional, or funding source deadlines.

Additional Documentation

Although the regulations do not require the minutes to include all determinations and considerations made at a convened meeting, many IRBs include the following:

Administrative documentation:

1. Length of approval. For example, some institutions may require that studies involving controversial issues (e.g., gene transfer, stem cell research) be reviewed every 6 months.
2. Determination of greater than minimal or minimal risk,
   a) If the board determines a study meets the definition of minimal risk and can be approved under an expedited category, the minutes should note the reclassification as an <u>expedited</u> study, all of the applicable expedited categories that apply, and state that continuing review is not applicable.

b) If the board determines a study meets the definition of minimal risk but cannot be approved under an expedited category, the study must remain under full board review. The board, however, may allow for expedited continuations under expedited category 9 (DHHS, 2018c). The minutes should capture whether the <u>continuing review</u> may be conducted by expedited or <u>full board review</u>.

🔗 7-2
🔗 5-7

3. Synopsis of IRB education, if applicable.

Regulatory citations:

The minutes should document the applicable regulations for each given study reviewed by the full board. For example:

- Vulnerable populations [**45 CFR 46 subparts B, C, and D**]
- Investigational and marketed drugs [**21 CFR 50, 56; 21 CFR 312, 314, 812**]; (see FDA/DHHS 2018a–2018e)
- HIPAA Privacy and Security Rules [**45 CFR 160, 164**]; (see DHHS 2018a, 2018b)
- Applicable federal, state, and local laws.
- Citations for other non–Common Rule agencies (e.g., FDA, DOJ).

Minutes should be reviewed by the IRB chair, or designee, for accuracy. A finalized copy of the minutes should be shared (either electronically or as a paper copy) with all IRB members. Finalized minutes should be stored and maintained in the IRB office.

Maintenance of research study materials:

IRBs should maintain study documents in an organized fashion, easily accessible to IRB staff and auditors. Currently, many IRBs have a dual system for maintaining study documents involving both electronic and hard copy documentation. IRBs should keep a record of where the documentation is located (electronically, in a file cabinet, or in a storage facility) so that documents may be easily retrieved.

All study-related records must be stored and maintained for a minimum of 3 years (6 years if HIPAA applies). State laws or institutional policies may require maintaining these records for longer periods.

What to maintain for each study:

1. Protocol
2. IRB application and other IRB required forms (e.g., investigator assurance/agreement, data security plan, reliance agreements)
3. Consent forms (if there is a locked or stamped document [i.e., a stamped consent form as a pdf], one version of the consent that may be edited, such as in Microsoft Word format, should also be saved.)
4. All additional institutional reviews and approvals required for research (e.g., radiation safety, embryonic stem cell research oversight [ESCRO], institutional animal care and use committee [IACUC], grants and contracts, investigational drug pharmacy, cancer center approval, conflict of interest committee, etc.)
5. Recruitment materials
6. Supporting documents (i.e., Investigator Brochures, DSMB charters, FDA correspondence, sponsor's consent template, etc.)
7. Surveys/questionnaires
8. Any item that will be given to the subject, such as instructional information or study card, and documentation of tangible items that subjects may receive (e.g., tote bags, pens, stuffed animals, or other small items that may be given to a subject during their participation in the research)
9. Pertinent correspondence related to the review
10. Letters issued to the researcher on behalf of the IRB
11. Applicable checklists and IRB reviewer comments

Study Tracking

It is commonplace for IRBs to use an electronic tracking system, either commercially available or institutionally developed, to maintain a record of IRB reviews and submissions throughout the life cycle of a research study. Many electronic tracking systems have the ability to notify researchers of IRB determinations regarding their study. The electronic tracking system captures the status and dates of reviews for a study, including when a continuing review is due. These tracking systems often contain version control information and a timeline of IRB-related events for each study. The tracking system is a helpful tool for IRBs and study teams for organizing and maintaining study-related materials and study-related information. Therefore, it is critical that updating the tracking system be a priority.

IRB Fee Invoicing

There is great variability across institutions with respect to charging and invoicing for IRB review. There is no standardization of items such as the amount; the types of IRB reviews that require invoicing; the time point at which the fee is applicable; who initiates the invoicing; or how the fees and invoicing are tracked. Many IRBs currently charge for commercially sponsored full board studies but do not charge for federally funded studies. Recent changes in National Institutes of Health (NIH) policy allow for payment of IRB fees when the fee is not covered in the organization's indirect costs, which will likely result in an increasing number of IRBs charging fees for federally funded research (NIH, 2019). IRBs charging for review must have a process for invoicing IRB fees. Invoicing and tracking may be initiated within the IRB office or designated to a source external to the IRB, such as to accounting, a clinical trials office, or the office responsible for sponsored projects. The invoice may be automatically generated within the IRB's tracking system or may require an altogether separate system and process.

Conclusion

In summary, this chapter provides the framework for administrative tasks required to document a convened IRB meeting according to the federal regulations. Many institutions utilize electronic systems for recording and managing meeting activities, or a combination of hard copy and electronic systems. The most important consideration is to have a well-organized and accurate documentation system to capture the requirements of federal regulations as well as institutional requirements and state and local laws.

References

Department of Health and Human Services (DHHS). (2018a). *Code of Federal Regulations Title 45 Public Welfare Part 160 General administrative requirements.* www.ecfr.gov/cgi-bin/text-idx?SID=04b58098bf25a320be1c59f40f5d3a4d&pitd=20180719&tpl=/ecfrbrowse/Title45/45cfr160_main_02.tpl

Department of Health and Human Services (DHHS). (2018b). *Code of Federal Regulations Title 45 Public Welfare Part 164 Security and privacy.* www.ecfr.gov/cgi-bin/text-idx?SID=04b58098bf25a320be1c59f40f5d3a4d&pitd=20180719&tpl=/ecfrbrowse/Title45/45cfr164_main_02.tpl

Department of Health and Human Services (DHHS). (2018c). *2018 Requirements FAQs: How should IRBs approach the continuing review of research that remains active beyond long-term follow-up or data analysis, but that is eligible for expedited review under categories 8(b) or 9 of the 1998 OHRP Expedited Review List in light of the new provision at §46.109(f)(1)(i) of the 2018 Requirements, which eliminates the requirement for such continuing review unless an IRB determines otherwise?* www.hhs.gov/ohrp/regulations-and-policy/guidance/faq/2018-requirements -faqs/index.html

Food and Drug Administration, Department of Health and Human Services (FDA/DHHS). (2018a). *Code of Federal Regulations Title 21 Food and Drug Part 50 Protection of human subjects.* www.ecfr.gov/cgi-bin/text-idx?SID=46e31711c66a1e29033448fe93990bc8&mc=true &tpl=/ecfrbrowse/Title21/21cfr50_main_02.tpl

Food and Drug Administration, Department of Health and Human Services (FDA/DHHS). (2018b). *Code of Federal Regulations Title 21 Food and Drug Part 56 Institutional review boards.* www.ecfr .gov/cgi-bin/text-idx?SID=46e31711c66a1e29033448fe93990bc8&mc=true&tpl= /ecfrbrowse/Title21/21cfr56_main_02.tpl

Food and Drug Administration, Department of Health and Human Services (FDA/DHHS). (2018c). *Code of Federal Regulations Title 21 Food and Drug Part 312 Investigational new drug application.* www.ecfr.gov/cgi-bin/text-idx?SID=46e31711c66a1e29033448fe93990bc8&mc=true&tpl= /ecfrbrowse/Title21/21cfr312_main_02.tpl

Food and Drug Administration, Department of Health and Human Services (FDA/DHHS). (2018d). *Code of Federal Regulations Title 21 Food and Drug Part 314 Applications for FDA approval to market a new drug.* www.ecfr.gov/cgi-bin/text-idx?SID=46e31711c66a1e29033448fe93990bc8 &mc=true&node=pt21.5.314&rgn=div5

Food and Drug Administration, Department of Health and Human Services (FDA/DHHS). (2018e). *Code of Federal Regulations Title 21 Food and Drug Part 812 Investigational device exemptions.* www.ecfr.gov/cgi-bin/text-idx?SID=46e31711c66a1e29033448fe93990bc8&mc=true&tpl =/ecfrbrowse/Title21/21cfr812_main_02.tpl

National Institutes of Health (NIH). (2019). *7.9 Allowability of costs/activities.* Retrieved from https://grants.nih.gov/grants/policy/nihgps/html5/section_7/7.9_allowability_of_costs _activities.htm

IRB Evaluation, Metrics, and Process Improvement

Jennifer A. Graf

Cheryl A. Savini

Abstract

The IRB office that supports the administration and management of an IRB is an integral component of an institution's human research protection program (HRPP). An IRB office should undergo regular and objective assessment and, as needed, improvement, so that its critical role in an HRPP is assured, especially given the changing domestic and international regulatory landscape and the need to ensure compliance with applicable regulations, laws, and institutional policies. This chapter focuses on evaluation of the IRB office, including metrics for evaluation and their interpretation, as well as resultant process improvements.

Introduction

A robust <u>HRPP</u> consists of four basic components: the IRB; education; quality assurance/quality improvement (QA/QI); and ancillary committees/departments. The IRB office may also serve as the facilitating office and formal communication hub among other components within an HRPP, including the offices for grants and contracts, legal counsel, medical records, environmental health and safety, clinical trials office, finance, pharmacy, etc. An IRB office should undergo regular and objective assessment and, as needed, improvement, so that its critical role in an HRPP is assured, especially given the changing domestic and international regulatory landscape and the need to ensure compliance with applicable regulations, laws, and institutional policies. An HRPP may have models other than the IRB office as the facilitating office. Throughout this chapter, we use the IRB office serving as the facilitating office as our example.

As outsourcing of IRB review increases, it is even more critical to remember that an HRPP includes additional components (e.g., education, QA/QI communication), regardless of which IRB review model is used (i.e., local or outsourced). This ensures organizational oversight for the conduct of the research.

<img> 2-1

Why Evaluate an IRB Office?

The process of evaluating how well an IRB office operates is important to an institution's ongoing efforts to ensure a robust, efficient, and compliant HRPP. Coupled with other institutional assessments, including evaluation of the IRB committee and of other components of the HRPP, such a process can allow an institution to detect, correct, and improve issues before they rise to a level that undermines the institution's research mission, leads to regulatory noncompliance, or worse, endangers the rights and welfare of research subjects.

Conducting ongoing evaluations of the IRB office informs and facilitates real-time process improvement. For example, evaluation of an IRB office can help assess whether the following are needed:

- Staffing adjustments and/or allocation of full-time employee commitment to specific areas within the office
- Process adjustments post review to improve turnaround times for the different types of reviews
- 🔗 8-4   Education of IRB staff to help ensure compliance with federally mandated documentation in IRB records and with required communication with researchers and study personnel, external sponsors, and regulatory agencies

Such an evaluation can also provide insight into needed improvements at many levels of an HRPP:

Institutional level: Is resource allocation appropriate? Is policy revision or development needed? Is the IRB office's location within the institutional structure appropriate? Is there institutional liability?

Researcher level: Are the IRB office's processes and procedures streamlined and compliant to support the researcher and facilitate research?

IRB office level: Are IRB staff levels adequate to support the work of the IRB? Are the number of IRB meetings held appropriate given the institution's research portfolio? If there is a frequent need for consultant reviews, does this indicate that the composition of the IRB requires review and modification?

Leadership will need to determine who will perform the evaluation(s) of the IRB office and how frequently the evaluation(s) will occur. These decisions are predicated (in part) on the volume and type of research conducted under the auspices of the institution (e.g., biomedical, social/behavioral, collaborative) and the number and level of experience of institutional staff and staff within the IRB office. When determining what to evaluate, it is important that 🔗 2-3   the IRB's written policies and procedures themselves are evaluated, not only to confirm compliance with regulatory requirements and whether or not policies and procedures are actually being followed but also to determine whether they are user-friendly and understandable to all stakeholders.

Regardless of what is evaluated, to avoid actual or perceived conflict of interest or bias, and to have validity and credibility, the assessments and the evaluators must be objective. IRB leadership and the local research community need to trust and hold in high regard the person(s) who performs the evaluation(s) to ensure that the results are trusted and respected.

🔗 8-6   IRB offices always need to be prepared for a federal inspection, because the U.S. Food and Drug Administration (FDA) or the Office for Human Research Protections (OHRP) may conduct routine or for-cause (directed) audits of an IRB to ensure compliance with regulations. IRB leadership should refer to the FDA "Institutional Review Board Inspection" document; the OHRP "QA

Self-Assessment Tool;" as well as the Association for the Accreditation of Human Research Protection Programs (AAHRPP) "Evaluation Instrument for Accreditation" as guides and for insight in determining what to monitor.

Because human and financial resources may be limited, careful consideration should be given to evaluating those data and systems that maximize the derivation of actionable information. In all instances, concerted efforts should be made to use objective criteria. Commonly evaluated elements include the following:

- Confirmation of appropriate types of reviews (e.g., convened IRB vs. expedited or designated review of amendments, new studies, exemptions)
- Length of review time for all review types and comparison against a national standard (refer to AAHRPP "Metrics for HRPP Performance")
- Review of IRB meeting minutes to confirm that federally mandated determinations were made and documented according to federal regulation and guidance (e.g., criteria for approval under 45 CFR 46.111 or granting of a waiver of consent or a waiver of documentation of consent under 45 CFR 46.116 or 117), as well as conformity with institutional policies and other requirements
- IRB-associated noncompliance
- IRB office staff and IRB leadership (e.g., chair, vice-chair)

Too frequently, IRB offices are evaluated based solely on administrative efficiency (e.g., volume reviewed in a period of time, length of review time). However, evaluating an IRB office in this way does not necessarily represent an accurate or complete assessment of an IRB office's performance. Study complexity, research team response time, etc., are among the variables that contribute to such measures, but are not often captured or reflected in such standard metrics. IRB leadership should be cautious when considering speed instead of accuracy when evaluating an IRB and IRB office, as such data should not be analyzed in isolation. A careful balance between speed and compliance review is needed to consider an IRB office "efficient."

In addition, evaluation of IRB members, including the IRB chair and vice-chair(s), as well as IRB office staff should be performed. IRB members and office staff should periodically perform self-evaluations as well. IRB office staff and chair/vice-chair(s) should be evaluated to assess knowledge and overall performance on an annual basis. Differences in institutional structure and position titles will dictate who would be appropriate to conduct these assessments. For example, the institutional official is commonly the individual responsible for the evaluation of the IRB chair/vice-chair(s), with input from IRB staff (IRB director/manager/administrator) and IRB members. The research community (e.g., researchers and study team) should also have an opportunity to provide feedback on IRB office performance. The users of the services offer a different perspective and are also in a position to provide constructive feedback.

The frequency with which an IRB office's processes and staff are evaluated may be on a scheduled, periodic basis or on a continuous, ongoing basis.

What Measures (Metrics) Are Important in Evaluating an IRB Office's Performance?

In order to evaluate the IRB office, one must have sufficient information/ data about what is actually being evaluated. The goal is not only to assess the office's compliance with federal regulations, state laws, and local policies, but its efficiency as well. Another goal is to determine whether the institution has provided sufficient resources to ensure a culture of ethics and respect for the protection of human research subjects.

Metrics

1. **Total number of submissions over the past year**
   This will determine volume and workload for staff processing and IRB review. Collect the number of:

   - Not human subjects research and exempt determinations
   - Initial submissions
   - Continuing reviews
   - Modifications/amendments
   - Reportable events (unanticipated problems, deviations, violations)
   - Noncompliance reports
   - Closures

   The significance of these data would be augmented by reviewing the total number of these submission types over a period of time (e.g., months, years). This would help an institution observe trends and determine what may have caused any change in numbers (e.g., faculty hires, a new clinical trials office).

2. **Review path**
   Collect the number of:

   - Not human subject research determinations
   - Exempt determinations
   - Expedited studies
   - Convened IRB review studies

   After the data for #1 and #2 are collected, evaluators should choose random studies within each category and assess whether the review path was correct. This helps assess the division of workload between the IRB members and IRB staff. Evaluators should also determine which individuals are responsible for processing/reviewing the following, along with a check on appropriateness of review type:

   - Not human subject determinations (staff?)
   - Exempt determinations (staff?)
   - Expedited reviews (staff designated as IRB members or all IRB members)
   - Convened IRB
   - Miscellaneous (e.g., amendments, reportable events)

3. **Categories or types of research submitted**
   The following will help determine the expertise needed for IRB membership and the effect on workload for the IRB staff to seek consultants when necessary:

   - *Topic area*: For example, oncology, urology, or other areas, such as research that involves illegal behaviors (e.g., domestic violence, illegal drug use, criminal activities) or sensitive topics (e.g., sexual practices, health status, such as HIV).
   - *Vulnerable or unique populations*: For example, children, elderly, decisionally impaired, prisoners, students, or employees.
   - *Submissions by department/division.*

- *Funding*: Types (e.g., federal, industry, internal, private grants) and volume of each type.

4. **Submission trends**
   Collect the following:

   - Total number of submissions by month
   - Total number of submissions by faculty, students, others

   Submission trends will help determine workload on a cycling basis with respect to staff and IRB member time (e.g., if there is a need for additional IRB meetings, or to shift staff assignments during high submission peaks). Once trends are established, determining the reason for the timing is important (e.g., funding or fiscal deadlines, the start of a new academic year, summer programs), so that resources are appropriately allocated within the IRB office.

5. **Submission turnaround times (the life of a study)**
   - Knowing only the length of time from researcher submission to IRB approval does not necessarily provide information about IRB office efficiency. Details such as the length of time for the researcher to respond to inquiries and the length of IRB review time also offer important insights. Collect the following (for all submission types, including initial review, continuing review, modifications/amendments, reportable events, and closures):
     - Date initially submitted by the researcher.
     - Length of time for office staff to conduct administrative and/or preview.
     - Length of time (if applicable) back with researcher to make changes or provide additional information to complete the submission.
     - Length of time with the IRB or IRB office for review (exempt, expedited, or convened IRB review, reportable events).
     - Length of time (if applicable) between when the researcher received notification from the IRB for required changes to the time the researcher submits those changes.
     - The number of times (and number of days) for the researcher to complete the submission.
     - Final approval date (the time to finalize approval of the research, once researcher has sufficiently responded).
     - Length of time between IRB approval and researcher notification of final approval.

   Lengthy review time could indicate the need for <u>researcher education</u>   🖉 8-5
   on the quality of submissions, IRB staff education on conducting a more robust preview, or improving submission forms to more clearly describe what information the IRB requires to make its required determinations.

   Review of trends regarding the reasons studies are not approved (via the conditions or modifications required in order to secure approval) could also provide insight into the clarity of submission form questions and/or researcher education. For example, are there trends in what researchers are interpreting or submitting inaccurately? Are they not understanding what is expected or how to answer a question, or is there miscommunication (e.g., how the communication is being delivered and how clear is the articulation of the information being requested)?

   Analyzing information provided in continuing review submissions may also offer insights into potential areas of process improvement. For example, a high incidence of self-reported or other discoveries of noncompliance may be indicative of the need for additional education or increased monitoring.

6. **Other metrics to consider for review**
    - The numbers and lengths of IRB meetings (staff workload, such as number of agenda items, as well as IRB member time commitment).
    - The time required to finalize IRB meeting minutes.
    - The numbers and types of educational sessions *conducted for* IRB members, researchers, and their coordinators, by the IRB office staff.
    - The numbers and types of educational sessions *conducted by* IRB members.
    - The numbers and types of educational sessions *attended by* IRB staff and IRB members.
    - The numbers of not-for-cause inspections and for-cause audits *conducted by* the IRB office (QA/QI activities).
    - The types and numbers of post-approval monitoring events conducted by the IRB office staff (QA/QI activities).
    - The numbers of scheduled office visits to work directly with researchers to provide guidance on study submissions (if applicable).
    - The numbers of updates to the research community on regulatory or policy changes in the field. For example, the Common Rule 2018 Requirements or the various NIH requirements/guidance changes, such as the single IRB requirement, clinical trial registration for basic researchers, and the genomic summary results now being classified as unrestricted.
        - A high number of updates provides data to indicate the additional workload and education required to implement those changes. A low number of updates to the community, or no updates at all, may indicate a need for additional communication to strengthen transparency and compliance within the HRPP.
    - The number or which, and for which institutions, your institution is the IRB of record. There is a significant dedication of time and effort for staff to manage additional sites and studies.
    - The numbers and types of IRBs upon which your institution relies (i.e., independent IRB or other collaborative or institutional IRB). The IRB office, in these cases, needs to implement a process for "registering" the study locally as an active study. As stated earlier, whether a study is reviewed by the local IRB or an external IRB of record, the institution and researcher are still responsible for the compliant conduct and oversight of the research. Additional education for researchers may be necessary to ensure they understand their responsibilities to the institution, as well as the IRB of record with respect to the conduct of the research and submission processes and reporting requirements.

The means to collect the data depends upon institutional resources, but can include, for example, use of an electronic system's reporting function, maintaining an electronic spreadsheet, conducting interviews (e.g., IRB chair, researchers, coordinators, ancillary committees), or reviewing past IRB meeting minutes. Tracking metrics over time can help an institution discover emerging issues before they impact IRB office performance.

Reviewing the Previously Referenced Data can Help an Institution Make Informed Decisions Regarding the Following:

- Process improvements or streamlining that may be needed to better facilitate the review and approval of research and ensure compliance with federal regulations, state laws, institutional policies, and best practice.

- Further evaluation of IRB members to ensure diversity of membership, adequate size and expertise for the types of research being reviewed, or to determine the need for consultants in areas where additional expertise is required.
- Whether the current record-keeping system is adequate (i.e., commercial or in-house).
- Educational needs for IRB office staff, researchers, IRB members, and the research community at large.
- Determining whether the institution conducts QA/QI activities and whether the activities are adequate to the research conducted at the institution.
- The need for improvements to maintain community awareness (e.g., website improvements, educational sessions, available informational/guidance documents).
- Improvements that may be needed to current "tools" (e.g., submission forms, reviewer checklists, and any other guidance documents).
- Staffing needs (e.g., the number of staff or additional expertise) as well as possible institutional structure changes that might be indicated.
- Submission cycles: Determining the time(s) of year when ramping up, reworking staff responsibilities, or increasing the number of IRB meetings might be beneficial due to a larger volume of submissions.
- The validation of the institutional culture to support the protection of human subjects.
- Whether or not an institution may be ready to apply for human research protection program <u>accreditation</u>.

✐ 8-7

How Can the Data Collected Be Used to Improve IRB Office Processes and Performances?

It is not enough to merely *assess* quality—improvement is also needed. If, when data are collected as described earlier, it is found that compliance or efficiencies are not at the level the institution expects or are not commensurate with other relevantly similar institutions, the institution must consider quality *improvement* activities.

Perhaps it was determined that an extended length of time between researcher submission and IRB approval was due to submissions that were often incomplete, resulting in days or weeks before the IRB office can move the submission ahead for review. In this example, it might be beneficial to conduct dedicated office hours for researchers who are submitting studies or to send "e-blasts" to the research community on proper submission of IRB documents. Then, in a few months, reassess that metric again. Did the effort work? If there was improvement, but not to the goal originally set, what else can be done? In this example, creation of a "submission completeness checklist" for researcher use prior to submission may further improve the quality of submissions. See the Appendix for a sample checklist.

It is also not enough to report on data, without putting them in perspective. For example, an observed increase in average turnaround times over the past 3 years may be accompanied by metrics showing that the number of new submissions has increased from 100 to 1,000 annually. This increase alone can account for slow turnaround times, impacting efficiencies across the HRPP. The institution might then determine there is a need to increase IRB staffing and/or additional institutional staff to monitor ongoing research, increase the number of IRB meetings, or increase the number of IRBs. Consideration may also be given to implementation of an electronic record-keeping system or improvements to an existing system.

IRB office performance may also be strengthened by ensuring professional growth and development for qualified staff. It is important to organize and structure an IRB office to offer opportunities for growth and promotion (e.g., IRB analyst, senior IRB analyst, IRB director), in order to preserve institutional memory, engender commitment from staff, and ensure continuity of operations in a compliant and efficient manner. It is critical that (at least) senior IRB office staff maintain ongoing education to ensure current knowledge and awareness of national trends, new guidance, etc., and are on the forefront to ensure the IRB office is well equipped and trained to support the research enterprise at the institution.

What Are Possible Outcomes of IRB Office Program Evaluations and Improvements?

When conducted thoughtfully and thoroughly, ongoing evaluations of metrics and process improvements for an IRB office can yield important benefits for the HRPP, including the following:

- Greater safety and protection of study subjects
- Compliance with applicable regulations, laws, and policies based on a culture of ethically conducted research
- Streamlined and compliant processes and procedures throughout an HRPP
- High-quality submission forms and reviewer checklists, as well as other guidance documents
- Appropriate staffing and expertise of IRB office staff and appropriate institutional structure
- Adequate and compliant record keeping
- Adequate education for IRB office staff, researchers, IRB members, and the community at large
- Adequate QA/QI activities for compliant institutional oversight
- Robust communication throughout the institution with respect to human subjects protections
- Better quality of IRB reviews
- Shortened turnaround times
- Preparedness for internal and external inspections
- Preparedness for possible human research accreditation or reaccreditation

Resources

Association for the Accreditation of Human Research Protection Programs, Inc. (2018). *Metrics for HRPP performance.* www.aahrpp.org/apply/resources/metrics-on-hrpp-performance

Association for the Accreditation of Human Research Protection Programs, Inc. (2019a). *AAHRPP accreditation standards.* www.aahrpp.org/apply/process-overview/standards

Association for the Accreditation of Human Research Protection Programs, Inc. (2019b). *Evaluation instrument for accreditation.* www.aahrpp.org/apply/resources/annual-report-documents /evaluation-instrument-for-accreditation

National Institutes of Health. (2016). *Final NIH policy on the use of a single institutional review board for multi-site research.* https://grants.nih.gov/grants/guide/notice-files/NOT-OD-16-094.html

National Institutes of Health. (2017). *Registering with ClinicalTrials.gov.* www.niams.nih.gov/grants-funding/conducting-clinical-research/register-trials-gov

National Institutes of Health. (2018). *Access to genomic summary results: Get up to date on updated policy.* www.niaid.nih.gov/grants-contracts/access-genomic-summary-results

Food and Drug Administration. (2006). *FDA institutional review board inspections.* www.fda.gov/media/75192/download

Food and Drug Administration. (2019). *Information sheet guidance for institutional review boards (IRBs), clinical investigators, and sponsors.* www.fda.gov/science-research/guidance-documents-including-information-sheets-and-notices/information-sheet-guidance-institutional-review-boards-irbs-clinical-investigators-and-sponsors

Office for Human Research Protections. (2002). *QA self-assessment tool.* www.hhs.gov/ohrp/education-and-outreach/human-research-protection-program-fundamentals/ohrp-self-assessment-tool/index.html

Office for Human Research Protections. (2009). *Compliance oversight procedures for evaluating institutions (2009).* www.hhs.gov/ohrp/compliance-and-reporting/evaluating-institutions/index.html

Office for Human Research Protections. (2019). *Guidance.* www.hhs.gov/ohrp/regulations-and-policy/guidance/index.html

Office for Human Research Protections et al. (2018). *Institutional review board (IRB) written procedures: Guidance for institutions and IRBs.* www.fda.gov/media/99271/download

Appendix

Institutional Review Board

Completeness Review

This checklist is designed to ensure that the submission is complete prior to proceeding to prereview.

IRB #:	PI:	
IRB staff conducting completeness review:		
☐	PI signature present?	
☐	☐ NA Ancillary services/committees identified	

☐ Billing analysis	☐ Biosafety
☐ Clinical and translational research unit interest	☐ Conflict of interest
☐ Dual use research of concern	☐ Embryonic stem cell research oversight
☐ MRI safety	☐ Pathology
☐ Pharmacy	☐ Radiation safety
☐ Radioactive drug research committee	☐ Research compliance
☐ Sponsored programs office	☐ Scientific review committee
☐	☐

Have all ancillary approvals been obtained?

(Note: Projects can proceed to the pre-review review without all ancillary approvals. However, approvals should be in place before board review.)

Notes:

☐ | **Other sites engaged in research**:

☐ None
☐ Other site(s):
    ☐ Protocol indicates that sites(s) will obtain local IRB approval.
    ☐ Site(s) are requesting to rely on the **[Institution Name]** IRB.
☐ Multisite study coordinated by the **[Institution Name]** PI.
☐ The **[Institution Name]** PI is conducting the study internationally
    (Note: Consult HRPP director)

Note: *If the research is federally funded and* **[Institution Name]** *is the lead site or coordinating center, verify that the engaged site has an FWA.*

Notes:

☐ | IRB application is present and complete

☐ Submission form

☐ | Supplemental forms identified: NA ☐

Form: Form: Form:
Form: Form: Form:

Supplements present and complete ☐ Yes ☐ No

Notes:

☐ | ☐ Protocol is present

    Protocol version number and/or date:

☐ | Consent document is present ☐ NA – waiver of informed consent is being requested

    Consent version # and date:

    HIPAA authorization is: Included ☐ Separate ☐ NA ☐

☐ | Use this space if additional consent documents have been included (e.g., assent, etc.)

Consent type: Version # and date: HIPAA included ☐
separate ☐   NA ☐

Consent type: Version # and date: HIPAA included ☐
separate ☐   NA ☐

Consent type: Version # and date: HIPAA included ☐
separate ☐   NA ☐

Notes:

| ☐ | All study personnel are listed and human subjects protection training is current. |

Name	Training	Notes
	☐	
	☐	
	☐	
	☐	
	☐	
	☐	
	☐	
	☐	

| ☐ | Any subject materials have been included (e.g., subject diaries)   ☐ NA

Notes: |

| ☐ | Any surveys/questionnaires have been included   ☐ NA

Notes: |

| ☐ | Any recruitment materials have been included   ☐ NA

Notes: |

| ☐ | Investigator brochure/package insert/device instructions for use have been included   ☐ NA

Notes: |

| ☐ | Grant proposal included *(for investigators directly awarded federal grant funds)*   ☐ NA |
| ☐ | Grant congruency completed

Notes: |

FOR TRACKING PURPOSES

| ☐ | **Information requested for completeness**   Date: ☐ NA

Follow-up notes: |

Organizing the IRB Committee

The Composition of the IRB

Cecilia Brooke Cholka
Matthew Stafford

Abstract

IRBs are charged with reviewing proposed research to ensure the protection of the rights and welfare of research subjects. The federal regulations prescribe specific membership requirements for an IRB so that this charge can be met. However, interpreting the meaning of the membership requirements, such as identifying the appropriate people to fill the roles of scientist, nonscientist, and nonaffiliated member, can be more difficult than anticipated. This chapter discusses IRB membership requirements and some of the practical challenges in meeting those requirements, and offers some ideas for potential members.

Introduction

An IRB is charged with safeguarding the rights and welfare of people who participate in human subjects research. In order to meet this charge, IRB members evaluate the safety and appropriateness of proposed research, including the procedures and methods to be employed. The regulations that govern human subjects research specify certain characteristics that are needed in the composition of an IRB to ensure that the review of research is thorough. The regulatory framework for IRB composition establishes a set of minimum standards but does not prescribe IRB member roster features in great detail. Many factors are involved in shaping an appropriate IRB roster, including the research portfolio of an institution, the setting in which research is conducted, the types of research conducted, and the communities and populations (especially vulnerable ones) that are likely to be the subjects of the research. This chapter explores some of the factors that shape IRB member selection, not only to ensure compliance with the minimum standards set by the regulations but also to help achieve effective human subjects protections.

The Common Rule [45 CFR 46.107] and Food and Drug Administration (FDA) regulations [21 CFR 56.107] describe the requirements for the composition of an IRB:

(a) Each IRB shall have at least five members, with varying backgrounds to promote complete and adequate review of research activities commonly conducted by the institution. The IRB shall be sufficiently qualified through the experience and expertise of its members (professional competence), and the diversity of its members, including race, gender, and cultural backgrounds and sensitivity to such issues as community attitudes, to promote respect for its advice and counsel in safeguarding the rights and welfare of human subjects. . . .

(b) Each IRB shall include at least one member whose primary concerns are in scientific areas and at least one member whose primary concerns are in nonscientific areas.

(c) Each IRB shall include at least one member who is not otherwise affiliated with the institution and who is not part of the immediate family of a person who is affiliated with the institution.

Member Expertise and Diversity

The regulations require IRB members to be qualified through expertise and diversity to ensure reviews of research that appropriately consider issues impacting the rights and welfare of subjects [21 CFR 56.107(a); 45 CFR 46.107(a)]. Conceptualizations of expertise and diversity are subjective, and an IRB should feel empowered to interpret this regulatory requirement in a way that optimizes the quality and efficiency of reviews. Ethical discussions are rarely black and white; instead, these discussions involve shades of gray, and people's experiences, education, culture, and beliefs influence how nuanced these ethical discussions are.

Expertise is not defined in the regulations and is not equated with scientific designation, meaning that expertise should be considered broadly to include a member's training, education, and life experience. Members have expertise when they have an understanding of professional and social norms and expectations that apply to research topics, settings, or populations. Expertise in the studies under review allows for knowledge of those norms and expectations to be applied to the ethical discussions. When reviewing a study, many of the determinations that need to be made are based on the appropriateness of proposed procedures. In order to evaluate appropriateness, a member needs to have some expertise in the research, discipline, procedures, and/or population.

Diversity tempers expertise by ensuring that subjective interpretations of professional and social norms are considered from different perspectives to achieve quality reviews. Diversity is also not defined in the regulations, and suitable diversity of membership will depend on institutional culture, research portfolios, and subject populations. There are a multitude of ways that an IRB can be diverse, including those stated in the regulations (race, gender, cultural background, and sensitivity to community attitudes), but might also include professions, sexual orientation, immigration status, or any other characteristic that is likely to improve the quality of reviews. An IRB that fails to have the necessary expertise and experience among its members not only fails to comply with the regulations but also fails to be an effective body. An IRB that researchers believe lacks the knowledge needed to evaluate research will not succeed in gaining researcher allies crucial to an effective human research protections program nor be able to cultivate a culture of compliance. Having among its membership knowledgeable and respected practitioners and scholars, as well as diverse representation from the communities in which the research is conducted, serves to bolster the reputation of an IRB and can create bridges between compliance and research aspects of studies. Ultimately, these can improve the experiences of subjects as well as strengthen public trust in the research enterprise.

Nonscientific, Nonaffiliated, and "Community" Members

In addition to expertise and diversity, the federal regulations require that there be "at least one member whose primary concerns are in nonscientific areas" as well as "at least one member who is not otherwise affiliated with the institution and who is not part of the immediate family of a person who is affiliated with the institution" [21 CFR 56.107; 45 CFR 46.107]. Unique to these two roles is the focus on what they are not, rather than what they are. As such, many IRBs struggle with who should appropriately fill these roles and how to define the expectations for these roles. Many IRBs have one member who checks both boxes, but this is not expected or required. Bauer (2001) recommends that IRBs have more than one member who fills these roles, because having a group of these members can increase the efficiency of the IRB.

In common parlance, nonaffiliated members are often referred to as "community" members; however, while the regulations refer to "sensitivity to such issues as community attitudes" [21 CFR 56.107; 45 CFR 46.107], the term "community member" is not to be found. Nevertheless, an IRB that draws upon the research participants' community for nonscientific and nonaffiliated members might benefit not only in terms of reputational integrity and public relations but also in terms of having expertise pertinent to the local context (community attitudes as well as values, mores, and life circumstances) for the research under review. Composing an IRB roster with this in mind can serve to strengthen an IRB's diversity and bring different viewpoints on the merits of any research proposal.

In an effort to understand what the nonscientist and nonaffiliated members contribute to the IRB, Klitzman (2012) interviewed 46 IRB chairs, directors, administrators, and members. He concludes that institutions vary widely with regard to their understanding of these roles, as well as their expectations for these members (Klitzman, 2012). Additionally, Klitzman highlights that these roles are often interpreted as "community members" with the responsibility to represent the viewpoints of communities where research occurs. Speers and Rose (2012) emphasize the term "community member" as the ideal role that IRBs should strive to fill. They offer several examples of organizations, including the Association for the Accreditation of Human Research Protections Programs (AAHRPP), that explicitly state the ethical importance of having community representation on the IRB to ensure that research is acceptable to the communities in which the research is to occur (Speers & Rose, 2012). AAHRPP standards include, in addition to the nonscientist and the nonaffiliate, "one or more members who represent the general perspective of participants" in the composition of an IRB (AAHRPP, 2019). AAHRPP's examples of who might have the perspective of the subjects include a former or current research subject or a research subject advocate.

🖉 8-7

Although the nonscientist and nonaffiliated members are chosen for what they are not, there are a number of characteristics they should have. Allison, Abbot, and Wichman (2008) surveyed IRB members at the NIH Intramural Research Program and included questions about the most important qualities of effective nonscientist (including affiliated and nonaffiliated) members. They reported that important qualities included assertiveness, self-confidence, willingness to ask questions, and ability to speak up (Allison et al., 2008). Arguably, these characteristics are similar to the types of characteristics that IRBs would look for in any members, so perhaps nonscientist and nonaffiliated members need not be singled out for special or unique abilities beyond those of any good IRB member. With regard to what nonscientist and nonaffiliated members bring to the review process, there was an emphasis on IRBs having these members review informed consent processes and documents exclusively, although this practice varied by IRB (Allision et al., 2008; Klitzman, 2012; Speers & Rose, 2012). Speers and Rose (2012) clearly state that they deem it unacceptable for any IRB member's duties to be limited, because the intent of having diversity on an IRB is to have different perspectives on the same issues, and limiting a reviewer's duties prevents that reviewer from offering his or her perspectives on other aspects of a study.

IRBs should take steps to ensure that nonscientist and nonaffiliated members feel empowered to review the entirety of any research proposal, because they have just as much to contribute to a discussion of the ethical merit of a study as other members. Additionally, Bauer (2001) highlighted unique contributions that these members bring to the review of a proposal, including the identification of coercive and opportunistic recruitment plans, misstatement of the risks and benefits, and aspects that could undermine privacy, among others. IRBs value the contributions that the nonscientist and nonaffiliated members make to the mission and responsibility of the IRB, and IRBs should ensure that these members are supported in performing their function, provided with training and tools for doing so, and encouraged to bring all that they have to offer to ensure the highest ethical standards for research are met.

The federal regulations do not define what exactly is meant by *nonscientist* and *nonaffiliated*, so IRBs should feel empowered to critically think about what these roles mean in their institutional culture and research portfolio context and then define these roles in their institutional <u>policies</u>. While it is important to ensure that IRBs meet the requirements in the regulations, IRBs also have a responsibility to consider what would assist them in ensuring an appropriate ethical review of the research they are responsible for reviewing.

✎ 2-3

Scientist Members

Scientist members are those whose training, background, and occupation are from a behavioral or biomedical research discipline (Secretary's Advisory Committee on Human Research Protections [SACHRP], 2011). Individuals with an MD or PhD will often be considered scientist members because their backgrounds often include research experience and/or training. However, anyone with behavioral or biomedical research training, background, or occupation would be considered a scientist member even if they do not have an MD or PhD.

When considering IRB membership, it is important to include scientist members with sufficient knowledge of the specific discipline(s) of the research under the IRB's purview, and an institution's research portfolio can be used as a way to identify needed expertise. Additionally, serving on the IRB may be an incentive to affiliated researchers because the training and education that IRB members receive may be valuable to their own research agendas. An important consideration with scientist members, particularly scientist members whose own research is reviewed by the IRB they serve on, is the potential for <u>conflicts of interest</u> on studies (e.g., when the scientist member is the principal investigator of a study). The FDA cautions that when members frequently have conflicts and must recuse themselves from deliberation and voting, it can impact the expertise of the IRB and the quality of the reviews (FDA, 1998).

✎ 12-7

In these cases, having multiple members with backgrounds in related research areas may be beneficial.

Other Special Members

In addition to the considerations for IRB membership discussed previously, there are some other types of members who might be appropriate for an IRB.

Vulnerable Populations

If an IRB regularly reviews research that involves <u>vulnerable subjects</u>, then IRB membership should include individuals who are knowledgeable about those subjects [21 CFR 56.107(a); 45 CFR 46.107(a)].

🖉 9-1

Representatives for pregnant women and fetuses, prisoners, and children: <u>Pregnant women and fetuses</u>, <u>prisoners</u>, and <u>children</u> are highlighted as vulnerable populations in the regulations [45 CFR 46 subparts B, C, and D]. Depending on the types of research the IRB reviews, appropriate representatives may consist of medical experts in the progression of disease in, or development of, pregnant women and fetuses or children, or it may consist of a social science perspective familiar with the lived experience of pregnant women and educational experiences of children. Prisoners have a unique situation in which their daily experiences vary quite dramatically from those of nonprisoners. DHHS regulations have additional criteria for IRB membership when reviewing research with prisoners: "a) A majority of the IRB shall have no association with the prison(s) involved, apart from their membership on the Board. b) At least one member of the Board shall be a prisoner, or a prisoner representative with appropriate background and experience to serve in that capacity, except that where a particular research project is reviewed by more than one Board only one Board need satisfy this requirement" [45 CFR 46.304(a-b)]. Some IRBs seek membership from among formerly incarcerated individuals, while others have included defense lawyers, social workers, or advocates with experience working with incarcerated populations.

🖉 9-4 🖉 9-5 🖉 9-6

Representatives for other vulnerable populations: Other vulnerable groups mentioned in the regulations include handicapped or mentally disabled persons, subjects vulnerable to <u>coercion or undue influence</u>, individuals with <u>impaired decision-making capacity</u>, or <u>economically or educationally disadvantaged</u> persons [21 CFR 56.107(a); 45 CFR 46.107(a)]. The specific characteristics for members who would meet the requirement to represent these populations will depend on the research portfolio that the IRB is responsible for reviewing. An IRB that regularly reviews research involving a given vulnerable population should consider having a member of that group among its permanent membership if possible. However, when an IRB only occasionally reviews research involving such populations, absent a regulatory requirement to have an actual IRB member (such as a prisoner representative, which is required by the regulations for certain projects), the IRB should seek appropriate outside consultation to ensure that the deliberation of that research is informed by the necessary experience and expertise that its membership may lack. Consultation is discussed later in greater detail.

🖉 9-8, 9-9
🖉 9-7
🖉 9-9

Lawyers

It may be important for an IRB to have an active or retired lawyer or someone with legal expertise as a member. Many states have laws governing research in addition to the federal regulations, so someone with legal expertise can assist the IRB with ensuring reasonable interpretation of laws. Additionally, some research portfolios include research on novel or sensitive topics such as sexual behavior or drug use, where the legal considerations needed for IRB review of risks may not be obvious. For example, a member with legal expertise may bring the IRB's attention to the nuances of state and federal laws that could impact research on cannabis or stem cells. Many institutions benefit from having an office of legal counsel, and while legal interpretation may be obtained through those offices, an IRB should recognize that internal counsel's primary responsibility is often to protect the institution, whereas the IRB's responsibility is to protect the people participating in research. For some IRBs it will be sufficient to seek outside consultation from a legal professional only when needed.

Students

⊘ 9-2

Many IRBs are located at universities, and research is often conducted in student populations. Having a student member on an IRB can benefit both the IRB as well as the student. IRBs benefit because students bring fresh and often younger perspectives to the review process, as well as the student subject perspective to research proposals that recruit from the student body. Additionally, medical IRBs can benefit from medical student members as they can help serve as a check on medical jargon or other technical issues that need to be simplified. The students benefit from service on the IRB because many times the students interested in serving on the IRB are future researchers, and they may learn firsthand how the IRB process and ethical conduct of research apply to their future studies. Some practical considerations for student members include the transient nature of student populations, the short duration of most courses of study, and the competing interests and demands upon a student's time.

Staff

Many IRB offices choose to have some or all of the staff serve as IRB members. Staff may be utilized to reduce the amount of time for reviews; to alleviate burden on IRB members with other competing institutional responsibilities (e.g., faculty, clinicians, researchers); and/or to reduce the need for volunteer members whose service to the IRB is an act of goodwill. Staff may often make

⊘ 5-3 ⊘ 5-5 exempt determinations and may also conduct expedited reviews depending on the model for that IRB.

While this is common practice for practical reasons, it is important to take steps to ensure that the reviews are being conducted in the spirit of the regulations that emphasize the need for different perspectives during review of research. Staff may fall victim to group-think, meaning that one perspective is being considered while reviewing and the benefits of diverse perspectives might be missing. The benefit of diversity on an IRB is to ensure that different perspectives are considered while reviewing and pondering ethical issues.

⊘ 8-4 When IRB staff are engaged as IRB members, the education and training provided to them is important. Many resources are available for this purpose, including the present volume and its previous editions and study guides; online courses designed for IRB professionals, and preparation for the Certified IRB Professional (CIP) exam.

Institutions that utilize IRB staff as board members would do well to spell out in their policies and standard operating procedures any limitations on what the staff members can review or approve. Clear guidelines can ensure that the IRB staff are protected from undue pressure from faculty and administration while also ensuring that the process does not give the appearance of a conflict of interest.

🖉 12-7

Alternates

An IRB roster may include voting members and alternate members. Alternate members can conduct reviews in the same way that voting members do but would only be allowed to vote on determinations at a convened meeting when a voting member was not present. Many IRBs utilize alternate members to ensure that appropriate expertise is available, while maintaining flexibility in member expectations or reviewer load. Alternate members can only represent a voting member with similar characteristics. For example, if a nonscientist is not available to attend a convened meeting, the alternate would also need to be a nonscientist. A scientist member would not be able to be an alternate for a nonscientist member.

Consultants

The regulations encourage the use of experts who are not IRB members (and who are not allowed to vote) when their expertise would assist the IRB in the review of complex issues in research **[21 CFR 56.107(f); 45 CFR 46.107(e)]**. When an IRB recognizes that it lacks the necessary expertise or experience to evaluate the safety or appropriateness of a given procedure, methodology, drug, device, community norms, or other aspect of the research, outside consultation should be sought. For example, if a study is to be undertaken in an international setting for which the IRB lacks experience, they might seek an individual who has lived or worked in that country to assist in determining that the study's aims, procedures, and consent processes are consistent with cultural norms and local laws (such consultation, however, should not be presumed to take the place of local ethical review from within the jurisdiction). Another example can be seen in the academic medical center model where the IRB relies on institutional arrangements whereby radiation safety committees, biosafety departments, or biomechanical engineering officers review aspects of the devices, agents, or procedures to be employed and convey their findings to the IRB for its use in evaluating the study and its components.

🖉 10-9

Committee Size and Composition

One of the most practical aspects of IRB composition is the number of members needed to adequately review the research portfolio while at the same time ensuring that quorum is manageable. An IRB needs at minimum five members **[21 CFR 56.107(a); 45 CFR 46.107(a)]**, but it also needs diverse membership to ensure adequate review of the types of research and populations used in research, which often results in more than five members. Quorum is the number of members who are needed to conduct a convened meeting and is a majority of voting members (IRB policy should specify quorum requirements). Additionally, quorum includes the characteristics of the members needed in order to conduct reviews, meaning that more than half of the members (or alternates thereof), including at least one nonscientist must be present, but

🖉 2-3

additional members are also needed in certain circumstances. For example, to review research with vulnerable populations, members with expertise in research with those populations are needed (or required in some cases, as in the case of research conducted in prisons, for which a prisoner representative must be present). An IRB's policy may go beyond regulatory requirements and also require other members to be present, such as nonaffiliated members, in order to conduct the meeting. Having an IRB that has a large roster of voting members may make obtaining quorum more onerous than convening a quorum of a leaner committee, whereas having a small roster may sacrifice necessary representation.

It may be sufficient for a small institution with a modest research portfolio, confined to a fairly small area of interest, or comprising fairly uniform methodologies and similar disciplines, to have a small board composed of the requisite five members. However, for a large research university with several graduate schools and multiple departments devoted to social, behavioral, and biomedical sciences, it may be necessary to have a large committee to represent all of the various research disciplines and to have the expertise to be familiar with the various methodologies used by those disciplines. Similarly, a teaching hospital or academic medical center's board may require several members to accomplish effective review of the research it sees, assuming it conducts research involving investigational drugs or devices and medical, surgical, and behavioral interventions. One approach that many IRBs use to address the size and diversity issue is to have a smaller roster of voting members and a larger roster of alternate members that can be utilized for meetings, to ensure quorum as well as to have adequate representation for the research under review at a meeting.

Education

🔖 8-4

An important aspect of cultivating and maintaining valuable and qualified members is member education. Members serving for the first time on an IRB, regardless of their designation or experience with research, will not be familiar with all of the details and nuance of regulations, laws, policy, and forms. Additionally, members who have been serving for many years can veer away from a solid review or may not be familiar with recent changes in the regulations or other issues impacting research, such as developments in technology.

The first important step in developing strong reviewers is to ensure that members receive adequate education and training when they begin reviewing. IRB member education can take many shapes; what is appropriate for a given board will depend on the staff and resources provided for the IRB, as

---

Things to Consider When Composing an IRB

- Ensure appropriate expertise for the types of research and populations that are part of the research portfolio.
- Ensure that enough members are available to review based on the size of the research portfolio and expectations regarding review times.
- Potentially have representatives on the IRB from the highest submitting departments.
- Include representation from the communities from which research subjects are drawn.
- Consider the role of IRB staff as members and the ways that they should contribute to IRB review.

well as the complexity of the research portfolio before the board and the IRB members' baseline understanding, training, experience, and level of education. New member orientations that may or may not include an online training component are common. IRBs can also consider having new members conduct concurrent reviews in partnership with an experienced IRB member. Continuing education is important to ensure that members maintain and build their knowledge. Continuing education for members can include presentations on important topics, attending webinars, or perhaps bringing interesting reviews for a group discussion. Contextual education is also important, and effective IRB professionals will recognize when a new study or new program of research being considered by the IRB warrants ensuring that the IRB application distributed to IRB members is adequate in terms of completeness and clarity. Providing some supplementary materials or training may be necessary to raise the IRB membership's level of understanding of a given study topic or experimental technique in order to satisfy the IRB's charge of having the necessary expertise and experience to determine whether or not the regulatory criteria for approval are met. Although there are many approaches to education, the important thing is to educate members in a way that is reasonable for the IRB and staff.

Member Compensation

Conducting reviews is a significant commitment, and many institutions recognize the work by compensating their IRB members for time spent on reviews and for meeting attendance. Compensation of IRB members differs among institutions in who receives compensation, what they are compensated for, how much compensation is received, and what type of compensation is offered. In the case of affiliated members, service on the IRB may be considered fulfillment of institutional responsibilities, and they may be compensated by course releases or reduction in service on other committees. Nonaffiliated members may be compensated for expenses incurred while serving the IRB (e.g., paying for parking), or they may be given a dollar amount per review, per meeting, or annually. Chairpersons or other members whose IRB responsibilities consume a large portion of their time may receive monetary compensation in addition to the other types of compensation discussed previously. Not all institutions are able to compensate members through monetary means, so creative approaches to recognizing the work of members may be needed. For example, continuing education that also meets professional certification requirements can help members in their roles both on the IRB and outside of the IRB. Additionally, IRBs should consider writing personalized letters of recognition that can be used for tenure and promotion or in other professional portfolios.

Evaluation

Evaluating IRB composition is important to ensure that reviews are being conducted in a timely manner, that expertise matches the research portfolio, and that the IRB is running like a well-oiled machine. That means not only finding new members to serve but also ensuring that current members are up to par and trimming the IRB if needed. Accreditation standards typically require some formal evaluation, either through self-evaluation or evaluation by a chair or director, in order to review effectiveness, efficiency, and satisfaction of stakeholders and to find areas for improvement (AAHRPP, 2019). Conducting a regular review of the IRB membership through member self-evaluations, staff feedback,

🖉 2-7

🖉 8-7

turnaround time calculations, and consultation with the Institutional Official and IRB chair(s) is an important way to ensure that the IRB is doing the best possible work for protecting subjects.

Conclusion

An IRB is only as good as the members who compose it. As with many deliberative bodies, any configuration or quorum of an IRB is merely the sum of its parts. For this reason, assembling the appropriate varieties of training, experience, and education is key. Careful curation of IRB membership is important to ensure effective and efficient reviews as well as to preserve community trust. In composing an IRB, it is important to consider characteristics of the institution, research portfolio, and potential IRB members. A strong IRB is an integral element in protecting the rights and welfare of the people who participate in research.

References

Allison, R. D., Abbott, L. J., & Wichman, A. (2008). Nonscientist IRB members at the NIH. *IRB: Ethics & Human Research, 30*(5), 8–13.

Association for the Accreditation of Human Research Protection Programs, Inc. (AAHRPP). (2019). *Evaluation instrument for accreditation.* www.aahrpp.org/apply/resources/annual-report-documents/evaluation-instrument-for-accreditation

Bauer, P. E. (2001). A few simple truths about your community IRB members. *IRB: Ethics & Human Research, 23*(1), 7–8.

Food and Drug Administration (FDA). (1998). *Institutional review boards frequently asked questions: Guidance for institutional review boards and clinical investigators.* www.fda.gov/regulatory-information/search-fda-guidance-documents/institutional-review-boards-frequently-asked-questions#IRBMember

Klitzman, R. (2012). Institutional review board community members: Who are they, what do they do, and whom do they represent? *Academic Medicine, 87*(7), 975–981.

Secretary's Advisory Committee on Human Research Protections (SACHRP). (2011). *Attachment B: Recommendation on IRB membership and definition of non-scientist under 45 CFR 46 and 21 CFR 56.* www.hhs.gov/ohrp/sachrp-committee/recommendations/2011-january-24-letter-attachment-b/index.html

Speers, M. A., & Rose, S. (2012). Labeling institutional review board members does not lead to better protections for research participants. *Academic Medicine, 87*(7), 842–844.

The IRB Chair

R. Peter Iafrate
Francis J. DiMario, Jr.

Abstract

Safe and ethical human subjects research requires researchers to engage subjects only after a thorough review and approval by an IRB, which stands as an integral component of the institution's human research protection program (HRPP). The person who directs the proceedings of an organized IRB meeting is referred to as the IRB chair, chairman, or chairperson. The IRB chair must be an individual with appropriate stature in the institution, who is knowledgeable of the human subjects protection regulations, and who has experience in human subjects research. The IRB chair is typically someone who has been an experienced member of an IRB, and the primary role is to assure fidelity to the process. The IRB chair will have varying responsibilities based on the extent to which the organization conducts human subjects research. The purpose of this chapter is to discuss the roles and responsibilities of the IRB chair within the overall HRPP of an organization.

Introduction

The IRB chair directs the proceedings and discussion of full board meetings to ensure that review and approval of full board or committee submissions are in accordance with the ethical principles of the *Belmont Report*; the appropriate regulatory requirements (i.e., **45 CFR 46.111** for federally funded research and **21 CFR 56.111** when the research is regulated by the Food and Drug Administration [FDA]); and abide by the HIPAA Privacy Rule (i.e., **45 CFR 160** and **45 CFR 164 subparts A and E**), state laws, and institutional policies. The chair's role includes, but is not limited to, making sure that ample time is allowed for discussion of each study being reviewed; that regulatory determinations are made as required; that there is a properly constituted vote for each study; and that members who have a <u>conflict of interest</u> leave the room during the final deliberation and vote. Additional proceedings that may be overseen by the chair during a convened full board meeting include the adjudication of researcher noncompliance; presentation of conflict of interest management plans; educational updates; and determining the need for auditing a protocol for cause.

🔗 1-1

🔗 12-7

2-1   The HRPP is a comprehensive system designed to ensure the protection of the rights and welfare of human research subjects. The HRPP incorporates institutional leadership, research administration, any and all of the components utilized in conducting human research, along with the researchers, study staff, and other relevant offices. The IRB chair may interface with researchers, institutional officials, and other components of the HRPP to enact appropriate action plans and policy discussions.

Roles of an IRB Chair

The role of the IRB chair may differ greatly depending on the research portfolio of the institution, the number of IRBs or IRB panels an institution has, and how robust the HRPP is at the institution.

The HRPP at an institution may be virtually nonexistent and consist only of an administrative assistant. However, the HRPP can be an expansive department with a director and 20 to 30 staff providing various IRB-related functions. Most institutions have some degree of computerization of their research efforts, and thus the support of information technology staff is key to any successful human research oversight program.

Hopefully, as the research portfolio increases, so does the financial support of the IRB from the institution. The research enterprise can vary from relatively few protocols at an institution with a single IRB that meets sporadically, to large universities having in excess of 15,000 active human subjects research protocols. An institution with a research portfolio this large may have more than seven IRBs or IRB panels, with at least one panel meeting every week. The scope of research at an institution can also vary widely. Institutional IRBs can oversee a wide range of research types that cover many medical, social-behavioral, and scientific disciplines, and thus may require not only more IRB members but also those with specialized content expertise from diverse backgrounds. Institutions may choose to stratify the reviews and boards by type and have, for example, an oncology board or a pediatric board, etc.

3-1

3-4

IRB chairs must manage their time wisely since most serve in the role on a part-time basis while maintaining a "day job." Although most IRB-related issues are not truly urgent, on occasion they are (e.g., emergent use of an investigational drug or serious researcher noncompliance that may require a protocol to be suspended). The IRB chair or an appropriate board member designee must be available to review and act accordingly in such circumstances. How much time needs to be devoted to serving as an IRB chair varies widely and may be in part dependent upon research types, protocol volumes, the number of IRB panels at an institution, and the turnaround time desired for completed reviews. The time commitment for this role is discussed further later.

Responsibilities of the IRB Chair

Some institutions limit the IRB chair to the role of directing the full IRB committee meeting, with other functions divided among different administrative positions. Although such a system can function effectively in protecting human research subjects, the lack of a strong institutional leadership role for the IRB chair is likely to reduce the overall effectiveness of the IRB in promoting a culture of respect for and compliance with human subjects protections. In all cases, the IRB chair must be knowledgeable about the regulations that govern human research and related topics. Some of these regulations are listed in

Table 3.2-1 Essential Regulatory Knowledge Base

Food and Drug Administration 21 Code of Federal Regulations (CFR)	Federally Funded Research

■ 21 CFR 50: Human Subject Protection
■ 21 CFR 54: Financial Disclosure
■ 21 CFR 56: Institutional Review Boards
■ 21 CFR 312: Investigational New Drug Application
■ 21 CFR 803: Medical Device Reporting
■ 21 CFR 812: Investigational Device Exemptions
	■ 45 CFR 46
	  ○ 45 CFR subpart A: Basic Policy ("Common Rule")
	  ○ 45 CFR 46 subpart B: Protection for Pregnant Women, Human Fetuses & Neonates
	  ○ 45 CFR 46 subpart C: Protection for Prisoners
	  ○ 45 CFR 46 subpart D: Protection for Children
	■ 21 CFR 164: Health Insurance Portability and Accountability Act (HIPAA)
	■ 34 CFR 99: Family Educational Rights and Privacy Act (FERPA)

International rules	Veterans Administration
■ ICH E6: Good Clinical Practice (GCP)	■ 38 CFR 16: VA regulations for human subjects research protections

Table 3.2-1. An IRB chair must work to become sufficiently knowledgeable in these domains; if not, they should not agree to serve as the IRB chair. In all cases, the IRB chair must remain objective in their deliberations.

An IRB chair may potentially be involved in the following activities:

1. Review and approve non–full board submissions in accordance with the ethical principles of the *Belmont Report*, the regulatory requirements of **45 CFR 46.111**, state laws, and institutional policies.
2. Participate in initial orientation of new members.
3. Assist in the continuing education of IRB members.

   🔗 8-4

   a) Assist in the training of IRB members about new policies and guidance.
   b) Periodically formally evaluate the IRB members on their committee activities.
   c) Provide guidance to IRB members during the review process at board meetings and outside of meetings when appropriate.
4. Discuss with the institutional official (IO) and/or HRPP director any needs of the committee for additional members or support or any issues with member performance.
5. Work closely with the HRPP staff to make sure the meeting agenda items are accurate and that the most appropriate reviewers are assigned to specific items.
6. Review correspondence as requested.
7. Provide consultation and guidance to the HRPP staff as needed.
8. Identify areas of the HRPP that require policy development and implementation, guidance, and/or updated procedures.

   🔗 2-3

9. Review and provide comments about proposed policies.
10. Seek outside consultation when needed.
11. Review initial allegations of serious and/or continuing noncompliance to determine whether to refer the incident for full board deliberation or to others within the institution.

    🔗 7-6

12. Review single-subject exceptions to determine whether it is acceptable for the researcher to deviate from the approved protocol for a single subject.

    🔗 7-5

13. Confer with researchers who wish to apply the FDA Expanded Access Emergency Use provisions, and review post-emergency use reports.

    🔗 11-4

14. Provide leadership to ensure that the rights and welfare of human subjects participating in research reviewed by the IRB are protected.

⊘ 3-3   15. Conduct <u>convened meetings</u>, and review and approve the minutes documenting IRB discussions and findings.

16. Administer board decisions and maintain the independence of the IRB.

17. Maintain a current knowledge of, and assure compliance with, relevant regulations, laws, and policies related to the protection of human subjects.

18. Serve as an interface between researchers, administrators, and the IRB.

⊘ 5-7   19. Become capable in directing the <u>full board</u> to make determinations in accordance with the regulations.

⊘ 11-5; 11-2   20. Understand the role of the IRB in relation to <u>Humanitarian</u> Use Device, <u>Investigational</u> New Drug, and <u>Investigational Device Exemption</u> requirements.
⊘ 11-3

⊘ 12-6   21. Adjudicate <u>conflict of interest</u> management plans.

Becoming or Choosing an IRB Chair

Meeting Skills

At a minimum, the IRB chair must have the leadership and time management skills to direct discussions at the full board meeting. This may emanate from prior experience running similar kinds of meetings. The ability to foster open and collaborative discussion among IRB members while maintaining a directed focus on the issues at hand is paramount. The cultivation of a team effort and a culture of respect among the board members will result in an efficient and rewarding experience. The chair must allow members time to present their issues, but guard against a filibuster from individual members. In other instances, the chair may even need to draw out opinions from board members who are less vocal or less confident within the group. The chair must stay engaged at all times, monitor the board's deliberations, and guide the board should the discussion veer off topic, stagnate, or go down a path that is not consistent with the appropriate regulations. Redirecting discussion toward identifying whether and/or how the researcher can meet criteria for approval and maintain research subject safety should be the primary goal.

Interpersonal Skills

To be effective, an IRB chair should be able to interact under difficult circumstances with people from many different backgrounds, areas of expertise, and levels of experience. In most settings, the IRB functions as a volunteer committee that will develop its own culture. As such, it is more productive for the IRB chair to serve as a role model for the membership to follow. In order for the IRB to make good decisions in an efficient time frame, the members need to discuss issues in an atmosphere of trust that encourages openness, debate, and new insights. It is not easy to continually encourage an atmosphere that promotes consensus on critical issues the IRB evaluates. However, an IRB chair whose interpersonal style leads to tension or disorganization will inhibit the IRB review process.

If the IRB works within an HRPP, the IRB chair must work closely with the other HRPP components. At times, conditions may involve time pressure and other stressful influences. Each component of the HRPP will have its own dynamics, but optimal IRB function requires that each member of the HRPP leadership work as a team to ensure the protection of human research subjects. Operating the IRB efficiently and in compliance with all applicable laws and regulations will be difficult if the IRB chair and HRPP staff do not work well together.

Another challenge to the IRB chair's interpersonal skills lies in their interactions with researchers. In many organizations, the IRB chair is expected to discuss IRB concerns with researchers and/or research coordinators. At times, these discussions can develop into moderately contentious situations between the IRB and the research community. This is often a difficult job under the best of circumstances, and an IRB chair with the wrong background or weak interpersonal skills will not be able to insist upon compliance with the correct regulatory requirements and also foster an environment that promotes ethical research conduct.

Leadership and Respect

It is important for the IRB chair to have a background and reputation that encourages respect from the IRB membership, the administration, and local researchers. To have a meaningful impact on the protection of human subjects, the IRB must promote a culture of respect and compliance with the IRB process and for issues related to research ethics. It is difficult to do this if researchers do not respect the IRB leadership, especially the IRB chair. For this reason, it is important that the IRB chair be a person with sufficient institutional standing and perceived integrity to command the respect of the research community. In most cases, the IRB chair should wear their "power" lightly. The IRB chair should be recognized as an authority on the protection of human research subjects and have strong background, knowledge, and expertise in both human subjects research methods and human subjects research regulations.

An IRB chair who is familiar with both methodological and regulatory aspects of human subjects research will be able to focus the IRB on the important regulatory requirements as best applied to and within the framework of ethical research conduct. The IRB chair must represent the views of the full membership of the IRB and be viewed as a respected member of the peer-review process. The chair must therefore be approachable by the research community for consultation and guidance on protocol design in accordance with ethical principles, local acceptability, and regulatory compliance prior to researcher submission for formal approval. This kind of interface will encourage the development of mutual respect between the chair and the research community. By extension, the chair must be willing to listen, act collegially, and deliberate consistently and in an unbiased manner.

An IRB chair who is a respected colleague of local researchers is likely to facilitate the ability of the IRB to make difficult decisions and will enhance the respect for the IRB within the research community.

Time Commitment and Compensation

The time commitment required to serve as an IRB chair will depend on factors such as the volume of IRB activity, the constitution of the HRPP and IRB support staff, the number of institutional IRB panels, and the ethical issues raised by the protocols. In addition to these factors, the chair's experience in the position and the institutional responsibilities expected of the IRB chair will help determine the time commitment needed. Moreover, the IRB chair may serve on other committees within the HRPP, such as clinical trial support, compliance oversight, and others involved with research administration.

Public Responsibility in Medicine and Research (PRIM&R) conducts periodic surveys of IRBs around the United States. In their 2017 survey of 200 different types of IRBs, they received 656 responses. These data showed that new protocols per year can range from 1 to over 1,000, and at least two-thirds of the IRB volume is work conducted outside of the full board. Full-time HRPP (IRB support) staff at institutions ranged from zero to more than 15, with 30% of institutions having one to two full-time staff. Although 56% of respondents indicated they had a single IRB, 7% had more than seven (Public Responsibility in Medicine and Research, 2017).

⬤ 5-5

These results clearly show a broad range of IRB activity, and thus it is difficult to make a general statement regarding an IRB chair's time commitment. The chair must adequately address pre-IRB meeting, IRB meeting, and post-IRB meeting needs. In addition, the chair must review nonsubstantive researcher responses to contingencies made by the board, evaluate researcher noncompliance reports and allegations, review <u>expedited</u> items, provide education, serve as an institutional representative among the HRPP leadership and be available for many ad hoc demands. In some cases, the chair and/or the board may designate one or more experienced board members or staff to assist in some of these activities.

⬤ 5-6

The administrative burden and resulting time commitment of the IRB chair may be reduced by adopting an HRPP staff-driven model for the IRB system, whereby, depending on their level of training and expertise, the IRB staff may be able to work with researchers and other research personnel to address submission deficiencies before the protocol is reviewed by the IRB chair and/or full committee. Also, <u>limited</u> IRB review for minimal risk protocols could be completed by full-time HRPP staff who are also official members of the full board. This can greatly decrease the workload of an IRB chair.

With a wide range of IRB configurations comes a wide range of compensation agreements for IRB chairs. The 2017 PRIM&R survey found that 20% of responding IRB chairs indicated they received no additional compensation for their IRB role (Public Responsibility in Medicine and Research, 2017). Those who were compensated received that compensation in the form of salary offsets, travel funding, teaching load reduction, or annual stipends. It is common for institutions to discuss professional commitments in terms of a unit called an FTE (full-time equivalent). IRB chairs in charge of IRBs that review approximately 200 new protocols per year likely spend 0.15 to 0.25 FTE on work directly related to their role as IRB chair. At institutions where the IRB chair receives salary support for IRB service, salary support at the 0.15 to 0.25 FTE level is not unusual. In some institutions, the IRB chair is a full-time, salaried position.

Status Within the Institution

An institution must assure that the IRB is able to function in an independent and credible manner. As such, at some academic institutions, professorial rank may be an important factor to consider when choosing or accepting the position of an IRB chair. Another factor to consider is whether a faculty member's appointment is tenured.

Similarly, within nonacademic institutions, the IRB chair should hold some level of authority or responsibility within that institution. A departmental director or a physician is a typical candidate.

A related but different issue is job security. When an IRB is functioning properly, it is not unusual for it to make decisions that are unpopular with powerful researchers or upper-level administrators. An IRB chair with a junior or intermediate academic or positional rank may feel concern that senior individuals unhappy with an IRB decision might act to compromise the chair's job security or chances for future promotion. A good relationship with the IO is key to avoid having the IRB chair feel threatened when making unpopular decisions.

Serving as an IRB chair may have a negative effect on academic or work productivity. As discussed previously, serving in this role will likely require a major time commitment, on the order of 0.1 to 0.25 FTE. For many faculty members, a commitment of this magnitude will come at the expense of teaching, research, or other activities that have traditionally been required for academic promotion. Performing well as the IRB chair should be viewed as an important academic accomplishment and a worthwhile contribution to the institution, on par with acting as a research collaborator or directing an innovative educational program. However, many institutional bylaws and promotion committees do not acknowledge this potential equivalence or give much weight to committee service, including chairing the IRB. Therefore, when a junior or mid-level faculty member is a candidate for IRB chair, it is important to consider the effect that the time commitment associated with this service will have on the chance of academic promotion in the future.

You're an IRB Chair, Now What?

Institutional Official Support

One major key to being a successful IRB chair is having an engaged and supportive IO. The IO is the individual who is legally authorized to act for the institution and, on behalf of the institution, obligates the institution to comply with the terms of the Federalwide Assurance (FWA), the legal agreement that institutions must have in order to receive federal research funds.

✒ 8-1

The IO is responsible for ensuring that the HRPP functions effectively and that the institution provides sufficient resources and support necessary to comply with all requirements applicable to research involving human subjects. If your institution does not have an FWA, someone within the institution should function in the IO capacity. The IO should be an individual of sufficient rank who has the authority to ensure that all obligations of the HRPP are carried out effectively and efficiently without coercion.

Before agreeing to become an IRB chair, you should meet with your IO to obtain a sense of their commitment to and support of the HRPP and you as the chair. Although the IRB chair's role is to ensure that human research is ethical and that regulatory requirements are applied to all submitted protocols, it is the IO's role to establish a culture of regulatory compliance and "have the back" of the IRB chair when significant conflicts arise. Establish a good working relationship with the IO, agree on what the IO wants to know and when, but choose your interactions wisely; you have to do your job yourself. However, when significant issues arise, providing your IO with a "heads up" will serve you, the IO, and the institution well. This will build confidence and trust between you and your IO.

Learn the Rules

Being an IRB chair is a significant responsibility. Not only are you protecting study subjects, you are also protecting the researchers, the IRB, and your institution. You must be willing to invest the time in learning the many rules and regulations that govern human subjects research. You must become a local expert in this field. Important regulations to review can be found in Table 3.2-1.

You will need to be knowledgeable about state laws and institutional policies dealing with human subjects research and related topics. You may also have to engage your institution's legal counsel and privacy officer for assistance. Context and local interpretation are important. Often the IRB is placed in the position of ensuring that other institutional policies are complied with (e.g., privacy rules, investigational drug rules, billing rules, conflict of interest, etc.).

Keeping abreast of the regulatory environment and engaging other IRB chairs, vice-chairs, and HRPP staff about their regulatory implementation and processes is important. Consistency is key but should never substitute for correctness. Benchmarking with other institutions and attending local, state, or national conferences will help mold your interpretations and may provide ideas on how to more efficiently and effectively maintain regulatory compliance.

Assess Your IRB Landscape

To become an effective IRB chair, you need a knowledgeable and dedicated support staff. You also need dedicated IRB members who have both knowledge of regulations and specific content expertise to span the types of research protocols that your IRB reviews. The following are areas you need to assess:

- ✪ 2-1
- ✪ 5-5
- ✪ 5-6

- _HRPP_: Understand the various roles, and have good working relationships with the support staff for the IRB, your IO, legal counsel, and a privacy officer with whom you can interact when necessary. Additionally, certain HRPP staff can be appointed as IRB members in order to provide <u>expedited</u> and <u>limited</u> IRB reviews.
- _Software support_: Does the IRB have a software program that is used to submit protocols and store all protocol-related information? If so, develop a good working knowledge of that system. If not, ensure the IRB has an effective paper-based system with rules to ensure all documents are properly stored.
- _IT consultation_: Determine the availability of IT expertise to assist in pre-review of proposed data storage and transfer requirements in individual protocols that the IRB reviews. This will be critical for the data security of web-based platforms and for ensuring HIPAA compliance.
- _Types of protocol submissions_: Know where the IRB workload comes from. Knowledge of the various departments or fields that submit protocols to your IRB should help you decide the content expertise needed within your board.

- ✪ 2-7

- _Metrics_: The more information you have to assess the IRB's workload and efficiency, the more you will be able to help to continually <u>improve the IRB process</u> at your institution. Software programs that provide workload volumes, turnaround times, the amount of work that goes to the full board vs. that completed outside of the full board, and other key information will allow the IRB and IRB chair to determine what process improvements will enhance the efficiency of the IRB. These data are also key to refuting unsubstantiated claims of IRB inefficiency and regulatory burden.
- _Need for vice-chairs_: A heavy workload, desired turnaround times, and limitations on the IRB chair's availability may indicate the need for one or more IRB vice-chairs. The vice-chair's primary value is with the work done outside of full board meetings.

Before, During, and After IRB Meetings

Full board meetings are what most researchers and research staff recognize as the IRB's main function. To effectively run a meeting, one should be prepared. As IRB chair, there is work to do before, during, and after an IRB meeting.

Before the meeting: Make sure you have reviewed the agenda of the meeting to identify the most appropriate reviewers or to obtain outside consultation to address a gap in content expertise within the board. Prepare potential learning points or educational material that might be pertinent. Discuss with the IRB staff any potential sensitive, unusual, or confrontational issues to anticipate, and invite the research team, legal counsel, or privacy officer (as appropriate) to help resolve the issue at the meeting. Alert other board members regarding these particular issues if they are assigned as reviewers. When possible, meet with researchers and/or their study staff long before the IRB meeting to address anticipated controverted issues or clarify what is not easily understood. This can be done by the IRB chair or designee. A prereview of protocols conducted by the IRB staff can resolve many of these issues prior to the protocol's being reviewed by the convened board.

During the meeting: Running an IRB meeting can sometimes feel like air traffic control. You need to manage the time, balancing giving the board members time to present their review and issues, while knowing when the discussion has stalled and a vote needs to be taken. You can establish with the board a chair's prerogative—a time when the chair will stop the discussion without hurting anyone's feelings. Part of the chair's role is to ensure that all regulatory issues are addressed. If the board is straying off topic, or if it appears a decision might be going down a path that does not adequately follow federal, state, or local rules, as the chair, you need to intervene. Such an event is often a teaching opportunity, when the chair can review a certain regulation or topic with the board. In some cases, the IRB staff may assist in that oversight at board meetings. If issues come up that might require a change in local policy, it is best to defer making a policy decision during the meeting and instead address it later when the issue can be thoroughly evaluated.

After the meeting: There are items following the board meeting that may need the attention of the IRB chair. Typically, the IRB staff ensure that proper minutes have been taken and recorded. However, there may be some communications that the chair may need to have with researchers after the meeting regarding protocols that the board had issues with, and the review of nonsubstantive contingency responses. The need for policy and procedure changes or the creation of new ones may have been postponed during the meeting for discussion with other chairs, vice-chairs, and HRPP staff.

Regulatory Noncompliance

Inevitably, an IRB chair will be made aware of an event of research <u>noncompliance</u>. This can come from a researcher's self-report, a study subject, a whistleblower, an IRB audit, or some other source. It is best to address the issue directly with the principal investigator (PI) of the study, recognizing that what you are told may not be the correct or entire story. Noncompliance may be minor and just need to be documented; other times the IRB chair may need to suspend the study. If it is not urgent, the chair may decide to have the issue reviewed by the full board in order to obtain ratification of a decision or for the board to determine what further course of action should be taken. OHRP, FDA, and other agencies and sponsors often have reporting requirements based on the severity of the noncompliance. Confidentiality must be maintained for all involved, especially for the study subject or whistleblower. When the noncompliance is determined to be significant, reports to the IO and perhaps the Risk Management Office may be appropriate.

🔗 7-6

Continuing Education

For IRB chairs who are expected to function as comprehensive IRB profession-als, continuing education will be a requirement of the job. Federal research regulations are constantly being revised, and the interpretation of existing reg-ulations is an ongoing process. Most IRBs review research that presents a wide range of complex ethical issues. IRBs are under increasing demand to function more efficiently in an environment of limited resources. All of these factors require that the chair of the IRB become a student of the disciplines of research ethics and research regulation.

To stay informed, most IRB chairs need to read journals and reference books that specifically deal with IRB issues. Another important source of in-formation is discussion with other members of the IRB community, especially other IRB chairs. Periodic attendance at national IRB-related meetings or other sponsored educational activities (at least once every 2 years is ideal) is bene-ficial. PRIM&R provides an excellent source for continuing education for IRB chairs and HRPP staff. PRIM&R's annual conferences provide an invaluable source of information and networking with other IRBs, IRB chairs, and govern-mental agencies. The Office for Human Research Protections (OHRP) and FDA also provide regional conferences on specific topics.

Other sources of continuing education include online monthly publica-tions such as the Human Research Report. Online discussion platforms, such as PRIM&R's IRB Forum (www.irbforum.org), are useful for exchanging ideas, asking questions, and understanding norms of IRB practice. Signing up for OHRP and FDA informational feeds to your email is also beneficial.

Finally, no matter how experienced an IRB chair becomes, it is helpful when addressing issues or interpreting the regulations to visit other institutions' IRB websites or to reach out to the IRBs and IRB chairs of similar institutions.

Conclusion

The IRB chair is responsible for ensuring the protection of human research sub-jects through the appropriate development and implementation of IRB policies and procedures. In addition, the IRB chair must engender respect for the IRB process by possessing the necessary knowledge and expertise about research practices and ethics, as well as federal, state, and local regulations. The leader-ship role of the IRB chair within an institution requires that the IRB chair has shared authority over IRB policy and procedure in collaboration with other in-stitutional officials and HRPP components. The IRB chair should be considered a professional position that requires a comprehensive set of knowledge, skills, and expertise as outlined in this chapter.

Reference

Public Responsibility in Medicine and Research. (2017). IRB workload and salary survey. www.primr.org/ProgramArchives_Detail.aspx?id=13147&type=Workload and Salary Surveys&actualtype=Human

CHAPTER 3-3

The IRB Meeting

Kimberly A. Lyford
Lorri E. Wettemann

Abstract

It takes considerable time, resources, and effort to assemble the full committee, and thus the IRB should use meetings to undertake reviews that by regulation require the attention of the convened membership. To achieve this goal requires forethought and planning, efforts by the IRB support staff and member reviewers to obtain complete materials, as well as guidance throughout the meeting. The meeting should provide a forum for discussion of ethical concepts and should enable the members to fulfill their service in a respectful academic environment.

Introduction

In this chapter, we will discuss management aspects of the IRB meeting, including arranging and running the meeting, following the agenda, IRB member responsibilities and roles, and voting considerations.

Arranging the Meeting

The length and frequency of meetings should be determined with an eye to balancing the efficiency of reviews, the responsiveness of the IRB, and the workload for the membership.

Length of IRB Meetings

The length of an IRB meeting should be sufficient to conduct the IRB business that requires the attention of the full committee. The meeting should be an efficient and effective use of time. It is important that the committee stay on track and adhere to the agenda as much as possible, while allowing enough time for adequate discussion. The IRB chair, with the assistance of the IRB staff, should identify discussions that have strayed off topic or appear to be stalled, and take action to re-focus the group or direct them toward a decision. An inefficient IRB meeting wastes committee members' time and creates a situation in which it is difficult to recruit and retain high-quality individuals for IRB service.

🔗 2-4
🔗 3-2

Should there be shorter meetings at more frequent intervals or longer meetings less frequently? Assuming IRB meeting time is used productively, the main argument in favor of long meetings (4 to 5 hours) is an increase in administrative efficiency. Of course, this efficiency must be balanced against the tendency for committee members to lose their ability to concentrate and participate in discussion for extended periods of time. IRB decision making often involves an understanding of complex and controversial ethical and regulatory issues, and discussion and deliberation are intellectually demanding, even for experienced IRB members. The efficiency and effectiveness of the IRB may be compromised by meetings that last too long. Many institutions schedule meetings for 4 hours per session to optimize efficiency and to accommodate members with busy schedules; however, if the committee is often unable to complete the review of all agenda items or runs over the scheduled period of time, consider reducing the overall agenda or increasing the frequency of the meetings.

Frequency of IRB Meetings

The appropriate frequency of full-committee meetings will be determined by the duration of the meeting, the efficiency of the review process, and the workload. One important piece of information to consider is that the number of studies and other items requiring review at a <u>convened meeting</u> are received by the IRB on a weekly or monthly basis. Even though more frequent, shorter meetings may allow for manageable agendas, make it easier for members to stay focused, and decrease the overall research review interval, it may be more difficult to schedule more frequent meetings. Many IRBs meet once per month, because it is often easier for IRB members to fit a monthly meeting into their schedules on an ongoing basis. Depending on the size of the committee, this may be a simpler logistical arrangement for the IRB administrators and staff as well.

5-7

Research Review Interval

The research review interval is the period of time from submission of a review item (initial application, modification, or new information) to the time the investigator is informed of the review outcome. This may also be referred to as "turnaround time" or "IRB responsiveness." This is an important <u>measure</u> to consider when determining if the IRB meeting schedule is effective, and it may have implications for the institution's research program. Excessive IRB turnaround times may compromise a researcher's ability to secure research contracts that benefit both the institution and research subjects, decrease researcher enthusiasm for doing research, and compromise respect for the IRB review system. Additionally, responses to <u>modifications</u> and important new information, such as safety updates, <u>unanticipated problems</u>, and <u>noncompliance</u>, should occur in a timely fashion and may require the review of the full committee.

2-7

7-1
7-3 *7-6*

Meeting Time Choice and Member Availability

As noted earlier, it is essential that members be able to concentrate and focus during the meeting for significant periods of time. Some members or committees may work well in late afternoon or early evening meetings, especially those with light agendas. However, many members are better able to conduct a thorough and efficient review at the beginning of the workday when they are most alert and able to focus and may be distracted during meetings held later in the day. Finding a convenient time for all members' schedules may be a difficult task. IRBs that are having trouble with attendance should consider whether the time of day of the meeting is the problem. The importance and expectation of regular attendance should be discussed during new member onboarding, since near-perfect attendance is important for establishing quorum and the authority to make determinations as a committee. Good attendance is also important for new members, because the bulk of education is experiential.

🖉 2-5

Alternate Reviewer System

Members who are unable to commit to attending every meeting may find a compatible colleague, who has the same general expertise, to share committee membership and with whom they can rotate regularly. In this scenario, the individuals alternate their attendance and do not typically attend the same meeting. This arrangement can work very well, provided both regularly attend the meetings to which they are scheduled and are committed to the work and the associated education. One member is listed as primary and the second as the alternate. This arrangement helps distribute the workload (reviews and meeting time) and creates a collaborative setting for the two members within their department or section. The individuals should schedule time to check in with each other for the purpose of achieving fluidity and consistency in reviews.

🖉 3-1

IRB Meeting Space

The appropriate setting for IRB meetings should optimize the work of the members and represent the importance of the activity. The location should be easily accessible with adequate parking. An appropriate choice may be to meet on the institution's campus, keeping in mind access for members who are not faculty or staff of the institution. The setting should be large enough for the entire committee and administrators to be comfortable and to accommodate guests. The meeting space should be well lighted, with power available (preferably, at their seats) to allow members to charge their laptops during long meetings. Ideally, the room should have the ability to initiate and receive conference calls and a way to project study materials for the entire committee to review simultaneously. Noise from adjacent spaces should be minimal. The temperature of the room should be controllable; this may be more important with larger groups and/or smaller rooms. A room with one large meeting table that seats all members and a couple of IRB administrators is the preferred arrangement. Having all members at the table is a symbol of equality and cooperation and provides equal access to the discussion space. This helps the chair identify the need for additional discussion, especially with members who have soft voices or those who command less attention. Additional seating should be available within the meeting space for other attendees and observers.

Deciding on Meeting Logistics

When determining the logistics of the meeting, it is essential to first work with the chair to determine what works best for their schedule and determine the feasibility of different days and times, and then consider how this will work with the rest of the committee. When the chair and the IRB administrator are considering changes to the schedule, they should consider polling the members to determine support and feasibility for any change in frequency and/or length of meetings. Once the optimal length of the full committee meeting has been decided, the number of reviews for the committee to undertake may be estimated, including initial applications, proposed modifications to approved

🖉 3-2

research, and annual continuing reviews. The time to accomplish full committee tasks such as review of minutes, subcommittee reports, and continuing

🖉 8-4 education must also be considered.

Guests at the IRB Meeting

As part of the work of the committee, the IRB may invite guests to attend convened meetings, such as investigators to discuss their proposals, consultants, new human research protections program administrators and staff, and others. The IRB may also receive requests from individuals who wish to engage in discussion with the committee, and others who wish to simply observe the meeting. IRB administrators may be asked to accommodate individuals who have an interest in the work of the committee as part of their own academic scholarship or employment. The committee should not be caught unaware by

🖉 2-4 guest attendees or observers at the meeting. The agenda should include the name, title, and reason for attendance of each guest, and the chair should introduce the guests at the beginning of the meeting. If it is not possible to plan in advance, last-minute guests can be managed by simply seeking permission of the chair and verbally informing the IRB members at the meeting.

Because the guest or observer will be privy to the deliberations, votes, and member comments, as well as intellectual property such as protocols or device schematics, the guest should sign a nondisclosure agreement prior to attendance. It is helpful if the IRB administrator takes a moment to walk through the agreement when it is presented to the guest, and that the agreement provide examples of prohibited sharing. If possible, this discussion should occur outside the IRB meeting, either just prior to the meeting, or in the days preceding the meeting. The IRB administrator and/or chair may wish to spend extra time with certain guests prior to the meeting to learn more about that individual's own interest in research ethics and the work of the IRB. These opportunities can be enlightening and may serve as a type of outreach to the research community, which is time well spent.

Following the Agenda

At the IRB meeting, an IRB administrator tracks attendance and notifies the

🖉 2-5 chairperson when quorum is reached. Quorum is defined in the regulations as a majority of the membership being present, including at least one member

🖉 3-1 whose primary concerns are in nonscientific areas [45 CFR 46.108(b)]. The chair will call the meeting to order and direct the committee's attention to the agenda.

The Agenda

🖉 2-4 The agenda is created prior to the meeting by the IRB staff, based on the prereviewed items ready for review, the expertise of the members attending the scheduled meeting, and the expected workload of each member. A consultant may submit a written assessment to provide guidance on issues that may not fall under the expertise of any attending IRB member, which the assigned reviewer may present to the committee. The agenda presents a suggested order of reviews, and contains notes and comments to guide reviewers regarding special considerations and determinations that need to be made. Other agenda items

🖉 2-6 may include the review of minutes from the last IRB meeting, subcommittee meeting schedules, and reports.

Determinations Related to the Research Population

Special populations require extra consideration of risk level and appropriate aims and safeguards, as well as plans for permission and assent. The regulations require the IRB to protect the rights and welfare of disabled persons regardless of the level of risk involved in the research [45 CFR 46.111(b)]. Whether or not an individual with impaired decision-making ability should be enrolled in a research study and who may provide permission for that individual are determinations best made by the convened committee. Some state laws specifically address the circumstances in which decisionally impaired individuals may be involved in research as well as who may legally sign for the individual. In 45 CFR 46.403, the IRB is charged with determining the risk level of research involving children. The regulations require the committee to approve risk-based plans for permission from one or both parents or a guardian, as well as documentation of the assent of the minor, as appropriate depending on the age of the child [45 CFR 46.408]. Research involving prisoners must be reviewed by a board that includes a prisoner advocate or representative as part of the membership [45 CFR 46.304]; best practices suggest that these reviews occur at a convened full committee meeting.

⌗ Section 9

⌗ 9-7

⌗ 9-6

⌗ 9-5

Determinations Related to Research Involving Drugs and Devices

The committee may find the investigational use of a drug product that is lawfully marketed in the United States to be exempt from the requirement to file an investigational new drug (IND) application, if certain criteria apply under 21 CFR 312.2(b). In a clinical investigation involving an investigational device, the committee may determine that the device as used in that investigation is a nonsignificant risk device [21 CFR 812.2(b)(1)(ii)]. Occasionally, an IRB will be asked to review a humanitarian use device (HUD) program. The IRB may determine that a consent form is required for participation in the program (Section 3052; 21st Century Cures Act, 2016).

⌗ 11-2
⌗ 11-3

⌗ 11-5

IRB Member Education

Education should be provided to each IRB member as a foundation for participation in reviews for the IRB meeting. Members can be provided with books, links to regulatory resources, and training in using the electronic platform for IRB review. New members can observe several meetings as part of the education process prior to undertaking a review assignment. Topics related to current events in human research and human subjects protections regulation can be presented by members (in turn) at the IRB meetings, to foster ongoing shared education. Guidance documents that cover the review expectations for initial applications, modifications to approved research, and annual continuing review can be provided and may be followed when preparing reviews and during the meeting (see "Resources and Guidance" later).

⌗ 8-4

Review Assignments

In preparation for the scheduled meeting, the IRB administrator should determine if any of the members have a conflict of interest (COI) with any of the studies on the agenda. The member with a COI will not take part in, or be

⌗ 12-7

2-5   present for, the deliberations or the vote, and may not be counted for <u>quorum</u>. If this will present a problem for quorum, especially if the review will occur at a time that other members may be missing, a plan should be developed to ensure quorum for the vote prior to the meeting. At the meeting, the order of review may be revised as needed to be responsive to needs.

Resources and Guidance

7-1
7-3   In order to effectively review research protocols, <u>modifications</u> of research, and <u>adverse events</u> in accordance with the federal regulations, IRB members need to be able to consult resources and guidance in preparation for and during the meeting. Member review sheets and checklists are effective tools. Resource doc-
5-4   uments with clear outlines of the <u>criteria for approval</u>, the required elements
6-2   of <u>consent</u>, the considerations for special populations, checklists for making determinations, published guidance from the Office of Human Research Protections (OHRP) and the Food and Drug Administration (FDA), as well as applicable state laws, should be centrally located and easily obtainable. Agenda comments may include reminders for access to these resources.

Other Agenda Items

The agenda often includes other items for the review and consideration of the
2-7   committee or notifications. These may include reports of <u>quality improvement</u>
5-5   <u>and assurance activities</u>, reports of <u>expedited</u> review actions, lists of minor
7-6   <u>noncompliance</u>, correspondence with federal agencies or others, proposed changes to institutional standard operating procedures, nominations of new members, and institutional information or changes.

IRB Member Responsibilities and Roles

Committees rely on each of their members to do their part to enable the meeting to be effective and efficient. Members need to plan their time to be able to meet these expectations.

IRB Member Preparation

IRB members are expected to conduct their assigned reviews prior to the meeting, preferably with enough time to make sure the information is complete and ask questions of the researchers, either directly or through the IRB office staff. Each member is responsible to review all documentation for the research to be reviewed at the meeting, to the extent necessary to make an informed opinion, and to be prepared to participate in discussions and to ask questions. Some members prefer to begin their review by reading the consent document, followed by the protocol, and finally the supporting documents. A reviewer template with the criteria for approval and the elements of consent may be useful as a checklist and framework for review notes. During the meeting, assigned reviewers are expected to summarize their review clearly for the committee and for documentation in the minutes, and may be called upon to answer any questions other committee members may ask regarding the proposed research activities. Some electronic platforms allow information
2-5   regarding the review to be entered in real time during the meeting by a <u>staff member</u>.

Primary and Secondary Member Review Structure

Many IRBs find that the primary and secondary reviewer system improves the quality and efficiency of IRB review. In this system, a limited number of reviewers, usually two, are assigned to each protocol to be reviewed at the full committee meeting, often based on each reviewer's area of expertise. Although each IRB member must review materials to be prepared for discussion of the agenda items, the assigned primary and secondary reviewers are responsible for having reviewed all the materials in detail, including, if necessary, asking questions of the researchers before the meeting; presenting a brief summary of the study; and answering questions raised by other IRB members at the meeting. The primary and secondary reviewers often focus on different parts of the review, addressing the regulatory <u>criteria for approval</u> based on their individual focus and point of view as described later. By corresponding prior to the meeting and pursuing answers to questions with researchers, these reviewer teams are able to resolve numerous issues together and to distill the concerns down to truly pertinent ethical questions.

🔗 5-4

The primary and secondary review structure is utilized largely for initial applications. Modifications and continuing reviews may often be accomplished with a single assigned primary reviewer; however, if a modification is extensive, a primary and secondary reviewer assignment may be prudent. The discussion that follows, regarding the roles of the primary and secondary reviewer, focuses on initial application reviews.

The Primary Reviewer

The primary reviewer, an IRB member with direct expertise pertaining to the research, is responsible for reviewing the experimental design of the study, the eligibility criteria, the aims, and the statistical plan, which are usually all part of the protocol document. Specific tasks of the primary reviewer include the following:

- Providing a determination regarding the level of risk presented to the research subjects and commenting on the appropriate minimization of risks and balance of possible benefits
- Providing insight into the potential value of the proposed research to the patient population and/or the community at large
- Presenting information provided regarding experimental drugs or devices being tested and the previous research that has been accomplished
- Making a recommendation about any determinations that need to be made regarding a drug or a device
- Ensuring the research is appropriately powered, with interim analyses and stopping rules allowing for the safety of participants
- Summarizing the issues that need to be addressed and providing recommendations for the vote and determinations

The Secondary Reviewer

The secondary reviewer, often a <u>nonscientist member</u>, or a nonaffiliated member who is not employed by the academic or medical establishment associated with the IRB, is responsible for reviewing the consent form; recruitment materials, including pamphlets and advertisements; and participant guidebooks, instructions, and support materials. Because nonscientists and

🔗 3-1

nonaffiliated members are usually the best representatives of potential participants in the research study, their reviews are extremely valuable to the committee in assessing the readability and understandability of these documents. Like the primary reviewer, the secondary reviewer presents their review to the committee, raising any ethical concerns and questions for the committee to discuss.

The Role of the Chair in Primary and Secondary Reviews

3-2 Once the reviewers have presented their summaries, the <u>IRB chair</u> may open the discussion to the full committee for questions and comments and allow the reviewers to respond. Ideally, a discussion ensues in which members feel comfortable disagreeing with their colleagues or expressing their confusion and/or concerns about important issues. Once the discussion has reached a conclusion with no new concerns, the chair asks the primary reviewer for a summary of the controverted issues (if any) and a recommendation for the vote.

Voting

Members Present for Reviews and Votes

Attention must be paid to committee member presence during the meeting. Quorum must be maintained during convened meetings [**45 CFR 46.108(b)**], and a member with applicable expertise and a nonscientist member must be present to participate in all reviews and votes [**45 CFR 46.107** and **45 CFR 46.108**]. Items to record include members absent from the discussion and vote, votes for and against approval, and recusals and abstentions from the vote. Re-

9-6; 9-5 viewers who represent <u>children</u> or <u>prisoners</u> must attend meetings where research involving those populations will be reviewed, and they must be present for votes on those research protocols.

Voting Options

45 CFR 46.109(a) addresses the determinations the IRB may make regarding a research proposal, specifying that "an IRB shall review and have authority to approve, require modifications in (to secure approval), or disapprove all research activities covered by this policy." The FDA regulations have analogous wording. **45 CFR 46.108(b)** requires a majority of IRB members (a quorum) to convene a committee meeting and requires that an action receive a majority of the votes, or more than half, of those present at the meeting. All votes are recorded and reported in the minutes. Whether approval has required any changes or not, the approval is valid for 1 year unless the committee designates a shorter period, due to the risks of the study.

Institutions develop their own set of voting options to best suit their needs; common voting options include the following:

- *Approved*: The research has been approved as submitted. The investigator is not required to change any aspect of the protocol or consent document. The approval date is the date of the convened meeting.
- *Minor revisions required to secure approval*: The full committee has decided that minor changes are needed, but does not need to review the materials again, unless the researcher does not provide "simple concurrence" with

the minor revisions requested. The simple requests are outlined in a letter to the researcher. Because the requests are no more than minor changes, review of the response can be completed via an <u>expedited</u> review by the chair or designated reviewer. If an investigator does not provide simple concurrence, the response must go back to a <u>convened meeting</u> for review. A final approval letter may be sent to the researcher once the response is approved. The IRB may decide that the approval date is the date of the meeting at which the revisions were required or that the approval date is the date when the reviewer decides simple concurrence has been provided, as long as the policy is outlined in the IRB standard operating procedures (Department of Health and Human Services [DHHS], 2010). Some IRBs edit study materials, making specific minor revisions requested by the committee, which are limited to edits that bring consent forms and advertising in line with local templates, and issuing an approval with the revised documents. This procedure bypasses notice of these minor administrative edits and the agreement of the principal investigator. In this case, the approval date is the date of the meeting.

● 5-5

● 5-7

- *Not approved*: The magnitude and/or number of concerns, questions, and problems is such that requesting only minor revisions is not appropriate. Some IRBs consider the study "tabled," and others use the term "deferred" if the committee finds that the materials provided are inadequate for their consideration and ability to approve the research. Other IRBs term the action "substantial revisions required" or "disapproved." The notification letter to the researcher should describe the reasons that the study could not be approved in specific enough detail to allow the researcher to work toward submitting the study for review again. All resubmissions must be reviewed by the full committee.

Administrative staff must ensure that all letters written to the researchers on behalf of the committee accurately describe the committee's concerns and requests, as well as make clear that the research may not begin until the committee has issued a letter of approval.

The Call to Vote

Votes are called by the IRB chair, calling first for those in favor of the recommendation and then for those opposed. The members have several options at the time that a vote is called.

- *Recuse*: If a member has a <u>conflict of interest</u> with any part of the study, the member may not participate in the initial review or any continuing review or action, except to provide information to the committee. The member must leave the room and not vote. This is considered a recusal. A member who is recused may not be included in the count for quorum.

● 12-7

- *Abstain*: If a member does not have a conflict of interest, but feels unable to vote for any reason, the member may abstain from the vote. A member who abstains is included in the count for quorum.
- *Absent*: If a committee member is not in the room when the vote is taken, the member is considered absent from the vote. A member who has left the meeting room may not be included in the count for quorum.

The committee depends on the administrative staff to look out for recusals and those who abstain or are absent from the vote, and to ensure that <u>quorum</u> exists for the vote.

● 2-5

Conclusion

Effective IRB meetings depend on carefully planned logistics, member preparation for the meeting, clear presentations of the research, discussion of ethical considerations, a properly managed vote, and clearly communicated determination conditions (if any). These elements not only facilitate efficiency and effectiveness in IRB operations, but help to ensure a respectful relationship with researchers. The maintenance of this positive connection with researchers, and an honoring of the IRB members' service to the ethical principles that define IRB work, are parallel goals of each meeting.

References

21st Century Cures Act. (2016). H.R. 34, 114th Congress. www.gpo.gov/fdsys/pkg/BILLS-114hr34enr/pdf/BILLS-114hr34enr.pdf

Department of Health and Human Services (DHHS). (2010). *Approval of research with conditions: OHRP guidance.* www.hhs.gov/ohrp/regulations-and-policy/guidance/guidance-on-irb-approval-of-research-with-conditions-2010/index.html

Social Science and Discipline-Specific IRBs

Victor M. Santana
Julie F. Simpson

Abstract

IRBs are often characterized by the type of research they review. Although IRBs may review all types of research conducted at an institution, two common distinctions are between biomedical IRBs, which primarily review biomedical research, and IRBs that review primarily social science research, which are often referred to as Social, Behavioral, and Educational Research (SBER) IRBs. Frequently, IRBs are further distinguished by a specific discipline, such as an IRB within an academic department (e.g., a psychology IRB) or a school/college, or for a specialty, such as an oncology IRB. In the past, a single-model IRB, which reviews both biomedical and social science research, was endorsed. In this chapter, we explain the benefits of the recent growth and adoption of topic-specific IRBs, specifically for SBER IRBs or discipline-specific (e.g., oncology) IRBs. Whether an institution has one or more IRBs that review all types of research or one or more topic-specific IRBs will depend on several considerations, which are discussed at the end of this chapter.

Definitions

Social science is the study of human society and of individual relationships in, and to, society. Academic disciplines that usually conduct social science research include sociology, psychology, anthropology, economics, and education. The terms *behavioral science* and *social science* are used interchangeably. In contrast to the social science focus on interpersonal relationships, biomedical sciences study human physiology and the treatment or understanding of disease. A dictionary definition of biomedical science is "the application of the principles of the natural sciences to medicine" (The Free Dictionary, n.d.). Health sciences and human services disciplines, such as nursing, occupational therapy, and social work, also conduct social science research.

Social Science IRBs

The nature of an institution often determines what type of IRB is appropriate to review the studies conducted by its researchers. For example, the second author's institution is a land-, sea-, and space-grant public university that does not have a medical school or any PhD programs in its College of Health and Human Services. Consequently, most of the research conducted by this institution's researchers is social/behavioral in nature. Therefore, the institution has an SBER IRB rather than a biomedical IRB.

⊘ 10-1
⊘ Section 9

According to federal regulations, SBER IRB members, like members of all IRBs, should have the expertise to review the types of studies that are proposed. Generally, this not only includes academic discipline expertise, such as psychology or sociology, but also expertise in both quantitative and <u>qualitative research</u> designs and methodologies, as well as familiarity with the <u>populations</u> commonly involved in SBER research, including children, individuals with cognitive disabilities, prisoners, students, and employees. As is generally true for groups of people with decision-making responsibilities, diversity in experiences and perspectives among IRB members will most likely enhance the quality of the decisions made.

⊘ 11-6

⊘ 9-6
⊘ 9-7 ⊘ 9-2

Education research often requires expertise in issues that specifically arise in this field (i.e., K–12 and higher education settings), as well as in the federal regulations with which the institution must comply. Such federal regulations include the Family Educational Rights and Privacy Act, the Protection of Pupil Rights Amendment, Title IX, and (often to a lesser extent) the <u>Health Insurance Portability and Accountability Act</u>. SBER IRBs should also have familiarity with their state's mandatory reporting laws, because these are frequently relevant to social science research, particularly research involving <u>minors</u>, the elderly, <u>incapacitated adults</u>, and <u>students</u> (e.g., hazing).

⊘ 12-5

⊘ 11-2, 11-3

Like biomedical IRBs, SBER IRBs should remain abreast of applicable technologies (both the topics and tools used in such studies), as well as emerging issues that researchers are interested in studying. Contemporary examples include recreational and medical marijuana use, immigration, artificial intelligence, social media, and data privacy. Furthermore, because sponsors are increasingly encouraging interdisciplinary or collaborative research and collaborations across disciplines are needed to address complex societal problems, SBER IRBs, particularly at larger institutions, are more frequently encountering research proposals that involve both biomedical and social science components. Examples are behavioral studies that include electroencephalograms, functional magnetic resonance imaging, or mobile health (i.e., <u>mHealth</u>) components, as well as behavioral interventions to ameliorate the effects of disease and/or treatment. Depending on the specific features of these studies, they may fall under the purview of the Food and Drug Administration (FDA) by investigating a regulated product, such as a <u>drug, medical device, or biologic</u>.

⊘ 3-1

Reviewing a study involving a product regulated by the FDA requires knowledge that many SBER IRBs do not have on hand or the capacity to acquire. Accordingly, SBER IRBs should have a plan for how to handle any research for which they do not have expertise (FDA related or otherwise) within the membership. Strategies include recruiting <u>IRB members</u> with the requisite expertise (if such components will be reviewed regularly), engaging appropriate consultants (e.g., a clinician), requesting a biomedical IRB from a neighboring institution to review the protocol and provide feedback, or requiring such studies be reviewed by a commercial IRB. The frequency of requests to review such studies, as well as other institutional factors (discussed at the end of the chapter), will determine how a traditional SBER IRB responds in the long term (e.g., evolve into a combined biomedical and social science IRB).

Discipline-Specific IRBs

Recently, an evolution of IRB models has occurred with the aim of helping to streamline the review process. Because biomedical research is increasingly a collaborative effort among different institutions and groups, a number of IRBs are now discipline–disease focused within individual institutions, or at a national level, or are part of a <u>centralized</u> ethical review model. Operationally, these IRBs provide a mechanism for ethical review of studies under a particular discipline–disease group or for all sites participating in more than one study in multisite research. Many of these initiatives have resulted from government policies, with the goal of improving efficiency and bringing focused expertise into the review process. Two recent examples include the NIH-sponsored large-scale national effort known as the *All of Us* Research Program and the National Cancer Institute (NCI) Central IRB (CIRB) that reviews and oversees the clinical trials emanating from the National Cancer Trial Network, which are inherently multicenter research studies.

⊘ Section 4

The *All of Us* Research Program proposes to collect data from a representative pool of the U.S. population to learn more about how individual differences in lifestyle, environment, and biological makeup influence health and disease through survey research and prospective clinical trials across many themes (allofus.nih.gov). The goal of this initiative is to study over 1 million participants from representative populations in the United States. Similarly, the four NCI CIRBs are constituted along various areas of research expertise. The Pediatric, Early Phase Emphasis, Late Phase Emphasis, and Cancer Prevention and Control CIRBs are managed through a central infrastructure that applies similar standards and operational support across all of the CIRBs. The effect of this centralization is measurable, and published data suggest that CIRB affiliation is associated with faster reviews (33.9 calendar days faster on average) and less research staff effort (6.1 hours fewer; Wagner, Murray, Goldberg, Adler, & Abrams, 2010). However, this finding is somewhat controversial because these protocol review timelines do not take into account any local administrative reviews that must occur before full activation of a protocol at an individual site (Katz & Smith, 2010).

These models propose to create uniformity and depth and breadth of expertise in the review process for clinical trials that may be unique in their risk and benefit characteristics (e.g., genomic testing for prognostic and treatment assignments, first human drug or biologic evaluations, vulnerable populations, and rare diseases). Another value of these models is the timeliness of the review process and reduction of redundancy of reviews, although comparative data on the quality of such reviews has not been prospectively evaluated.

A criticism of the discipline–disease-focused model is identifying and managing conflicts of interest in the review process, since some discipline-specific reviewers may be inherently vested in the research and often participate in the national groups sponsoring these studies. This criticism, however, is also applicable to smaller single-institution IRBs in which institutional expertise is found in a small group of researchers, and potential problems can be managed by adhering to well-established <u>conflict of interest</u> rules. Others have argued that this model can become so focused that it negates potential participation

⊘ 12-7

and insights by others who are not discipline experts. From both ethical and regulatory standpoints, this can be mitigated by assuring that these discipline–disease-focused IRBs have adequate member representation from other constituent groups. For example, both the *All of Us* and NCI CIRBs have voting members that represent nonscience disciplines, including subject advocates and ethicists. Similarly, for the centralized model, the review process must provide meaningful consideration of relevant local factors for the communities in which the research will be conducted. With the increasing complexity and innovation in biomedical research, no one IRB model can be uniformly appropriate for all needs. Thus, advancing our thinking of new prototypes for ethical review of human research is justified.

Considerations for Institutions

Advantages and Disadvantages of Different IRB Models

Each IRB model has advantages and disadvantages (**Table 3.4-1**), as outlined in the preceding discussion. How these different models are structured will differ according to institutional research volumes and portfolios, organizational factors, resources, and possibly accreditation status.

Volume and Types of Research

Institutions should create an IRB structure that best serves their volume and portfolio of human subjects research projects. Large institutions with medical schools or those with large doctoral degree-granting health sciences schools/colleges may require several biomedical IRBs, as well as at least one SBER IRB to serve its nonbiomedical researchers. Large institutions with medical schools that do not have a combined biomedical-SBER IRB or a separate SBER IRB may face the challenge of biomedical IRBs that do not understand and frequently do

Table 3.4-1 Advantages and Disadvantages of Topic-Specific IRBs

Advantages	Disadvantages
Specialization allows for quality and efficiency of reviews, with reviewers familiar with the types of studies under review	The lack of input from a wide range of expertise and perspectives may result in less comprehensive review
May improve IRB member satisfaction by not having to keep current with a wide range of issues and regulations not connected to expertise	The Common Rule does not recognize, or provide any guidance specific to, particular disciplines or specialties
Frequency and magnitude of risk often differ among disciplines/specialties, as does type of harm	Ethical standards are based on risk, not discipline/specialty, and all types of harms need to be addressed
Topic-specific IRBs may engage consultants for particular protocols in areas in which the IRB does not have expertise; IRBs may also engage commercial IRBs for studies in which they do not have the requisite expertise	Issues may overlap in a single project, particularly with the rise in interdisciplinary and collaborative research, requiring knowledge beyond the topic-specific IRB's area of specialty
Multiple topic-specific IRBs may provide a useful way to divide workload at institutions with high volumes of research	The specificity of topical IRBs may limit administrative flexibility in assigning workload among IRBs at high-volume institutions

not approve relatively simple social science (often <u>qualitative</u>) research studies. In the face of these challenges, institutions should ensure that they are effectively and efficiently serving the needs of all of their researchers and adequately protecting the rights and welfare of the research subjects involved in the institution's research activities via an appropriately structured IRB system.

🖉 10-1

Organizational Factors

Organizational factors, such as structure, leadership, precedent or history, values, and prevailing culture, will most likely play a role in the IRB structure adopted. Stasis or inertia may be very difficult to overcome. When change is needed (e.g., when changes occur in an institution's research portfolio that its existing IRB system cannot adequately support), it may require strong, informed leadership to realize the importance of making changes (e.g., creating separate, topic-specific IRBs to serve the new research interests of the institution). Recognizing what organizational factors are involved in institutional decision making for an institution's IRB system, their relative importance, and role is key to ensuring the system's effectiveness.

Institutional Resources

The availability of resources may play an important role in determining an institution's IRB structure. Key resources include expertise, funding, and staff. Regardless of the structure adopted, an institution must commit sufficient resources to support the desired system for it to be successful and to serve the needs of the institution's researchers and research subjects.

Conclusion

The type, scope, and complexity of current research in the social, behavioral, and biomedical sciences requires new approaches to facilitate ethical review while maintaining high standards. Institutions and sponsors of research are well served when they consider various models for effectively constituting IRBs to serve the needs of their research subjects and researchers. A number of factors and considerations, as outlined in this chapter, provide a basis for evaluating which models best fulfill regulatory mandates, seek to enhance subject protections, and accomplish overall research goals.

References

The Free Dictionary. (n.d.). "Biomedical science." WordNet 3.0, Farlex clipart collection. (2003-2008). www.thefreedictionary.com/biomedical+science

Katz, M. S., & Smith, M. L. (2010). Central institutional review board-facilitated review metrics omit critical components. *Journal of Clinical Oncology, 28*(6), e105.

Wagner, T. H., Murray, C., Goldberg, J., Adler, J. M., & Abrams, J. (2010). Costs and benefits of the National Cancer Institute Central Institutional Review Board. *Journal of Clinical Oncology, 28*(4), 662–666.

Single/Central IRBs

IRB Reliance Agreements

Barbara E. Bierer
David G. Forster

Abstract

When an institution relies on an external IRB that it does not operate, the institution and the IRB must document the institution's reliance on the IRB and the responsibilities that each entity will undertake, as required by the Common Rule [45 CFR 46.103(e)]. This chapter describes the different ways in which the reliance can be documented and focuses on the most common method used, the reliance agreement. In addition, this chapter explores some of the key considerations regarding reliance agreements, including the scope of the agreement and how responsibilities are divided between the IRB and the institution.

Introduction

Over time, human subjects research has become more collaborative, and clinical research is increasingly multi-institutional. Historically, the IRB of each institution engaged in research would conduct its own review and issue required changes to the protocol and/or the informed consent document, and those changes usually would need to be reviewed again by every institution's IRB until a concordant, common protocol and informed consent document were finalized. This process led to significant delays and resource expenditures, without evidence of enhanced human subjects protections (National Institutes of Health, 2006). In 2016, the National Institutes of Health (NIH) announced a policy that mandated single IRB (sIRB) review for most multisite, nonexempt human subjects research the agency funded, with a final effective date of January 25, 2018 (NIH, 2016). The NIH intended that the sIRB requirement would reduce administrative burden and shorten the time to approval without compromising human subjects protections and research oversight. In addition, the Office for Human Research Protections (OHRP) requires sIRB review as part of the 2018 Common Rule [45 CFR 46.114(b)], similar to the NIH policy, expanding this requirement for most multisite research funded or conducted by the federal government. The Common Rule requires institutions that rely on an IRB operated by another institution to document the arrangement, commonly referred to as a "reliance agreement." The purpose of these reliance agreements is to document the respective roles and responsibilities of each of the entities involved in the review and oversight of human subjects research.

The process for creating, reviewing, and executing reliance agreements varies based on the structure of the relying institution and its internal policies and procedures regarding agreements. Many institutions have delegated responsibility for developing and signing the agreements to a trained and knowledgeable person within the administrative office that supports IRB operations such as the IRB director, IRB administrator, or a designated reliance manager.

This chapter addresses the types of reliance agreements, various arrangements that might exist, and the content and documentation of these agreements. Although this chapter primarily focuses on IRB authorization agreements (IAAs), it also reviews other ways to document the reliance agreement, such as the less common individual investigator agreements used to cover the activities of individual researchers who are either affiliated with an institution that does not have a <u>Federalwide Assurance</u> (FWA) or unaffiliated with an institution (e.g., in community-based research).

⊘ 8-1

The shift to serving as an IRB for an external institution, on the one hand, and to relying on external IRBs, on the other, requires significant organizational changes. For example, IRBs will need to assume new responsibilities for ensuring compliance with state and local regulations, for decisions (and documentation of decisions) on behalf of external institutions and researchers with whom they are not familiar, and for communication with and oversight of those parties. Similarly, institutions that had embedded many of their institutional responsibilities for oversight of researchers and research in the "IRB office" have now been forced to restructure the institutional roles to disambiguate the IRB functions (regulatory review and approval of the research) from the other functions required to protect the rights and welfare of subjects, including researcher training and education, coordination of ancillary reviews (e.g., radiation safety, institutional biosafety), quality assurance and quality improvement, and auditing and monitoring. How these institutional and IRB functions can be executed is not codified in reliance agreements. This topic is further explored in the two following chapters, entitled "Responsibilities of the Reviewing IRB" and "Responsibilities of the Relying Institution."

When a Reliance Agreement Is Required

An IRB reliance agreement is required whenever (1) an institution is engaged in human subjects research that is conducted, supported, or otherwise subject to regulation by any federal department or agency that takes appropriate administrative action to make the policy applicable to such research, *and* (2) the IRB responsible for the review of the aforementioned research is not operated by the institution engaged in human subjects research. The requirement for reliance agreements arises from **45 CFR 46.103(e)** of the Common Rule, which states:

> For nonexempt research involving human subjects covered by this policy (or exempt research for which limited IRB review takes place pursuant to §46.104(d)(2)(iii), (d)(3)(i)(C), (d)(7), or (d)(8)) that takes place at an institution in which IRB oversight is conducted by an IRB that is not operated by the institution, the institution and the organization operating the IRB shall document the institution's reliance on the IRB for oversight of the research and the responsibilities that each entity will

undertake to ensure compliance with the requirements of this policy (e.g., in a written agreement between the institution and the IRB, by implementation of an institution-wide policy directive providing the allocation of responsibilities between the institution and an IRB that is not affiliated with the institution, or as set forth in a research protocol).

Reliance Agreement Format

The Common Rule states that the reliance agreement can be documented in several different formats, such as written agreement, an institution-wide policy directive, or within a protocol. However, IAAs are the most common means of documentation of a written agreement between the relying institution and the reviewing IRB. Some institutions incorporate additional contractual terms into the IAA.

RELIANCE AGREEMENTS FOR EXEMPT RESEARCH UNDER 2018 COMMON RULE

Note that exempt research that involves limited IRB review under **45 CFR 46.104(d)(2)(iii), (d)(3)(i) (C), (d)(7), or (d)(8)** of the revised Common Rule requires a reliance agreement whenever the reviewing IRB (aka the IRB of record) is not operated by the institution. This differs from the earlier Common Rule requirements, under which a reliance agreement was not necessary for any exempt research; the basis for the change emanates from the introduction of limited review procedures in the 2018 Common Rule.

Reliance Agreement Scope

Reliance agreements can be limited to a single research project or a certain body of studies (e.g., oncology studies) or can cover all research conducted by the signatories. The choice will depend on the type of research being conducted and the expected future relationship between the involved parties. For example, the Central Institutional Review Board for the National Cancer Institute (NCI CIRB) reviews NCI-funded, multisite, adult and pediatric oncology studies on behalf of collaborating institutions (NCI CIRB, n.d.). If the nature of the relationship between the parties is evolving or uncertain, the scope is often broad so that the reviewing IRB can review research for the relying institution without the need to modify the agreement.

Reliance Agreement Content

Because the regulations do not specify the content of reliance agreements, they can be quite short, such as the OHRP sample agreement.

This short sample agreement relies on the regulations to provide the roles and responsibilities of the relying institution and the reviewing IRB. However, many responsibilities that institutions would want elucidated in an agreement are not specified by the regulations; thus, many institutions prefer to document certain additional expectations of the parties and include standard contractual elements (such as protection of confidential and proprietary information, indemnification provisions, limitation of liabilities, insurance requirements, use of name, formal legal notice, fees and billing, term and termination, and survival requirements). Additionally, some agreements outline requirements that survive expiration or termination of the agreement, such as procedures for managing unanticipated problems, or serious or continuing noncompliance; access to records; expectations for corrective actions, audits, record keeping; and confidentiality.

🔗 7-3 🔗 7-6

If the reliance agreement applies only to federally supported research, the agreement does not need to reiterate regulatory requirements (e.g., requiring the IRB to perform continuing review at least once per year for research that requires continuing review), because these activities are required by the regulations, and repeating them in the reliance agreement does not strengthen their applicability. However, if the agreement will apply not only to federally funded research but also to research that is not federally supported, then it may be important to specify such expectations and responsibilities. For example, the agreement might need to specify the requirement for IRBs to maintain compliant board membership and IRB records, to conduct initial and continuing review, and to review changes to the research. The agreement should avoid statements such as "the IRB will follow all standard operating procedures (SOPs) of the institution" or that the institution "will follow all SOPs of the IRB," because the two entities will have separate sets of SOPs specific to their activities, responsibilities, records management, and workflow processes.

The reliance agreement should balance the need for specificity with the challenges of redrafting and executing modifications to the agreement when certain circumstances change. For instance, the agreement should not contain detailed administrative requirements that are likely to change as the type of research covered by the agreement changes or if regulations or guidance are updated. Details such as specific consent form language or the processing of Health Insurance Portability and Accountability Act (HIPAA) authorizations are best documented outside of the reliance agreement, such as in policy or SOPs.

Reliance agreements often contain additional contractual elements beyond those required by regulation, and those elements help to clarify the expectations of the relying institution or reviewing IRB, particularly where flexibility is allowable. Examples of these contractual elements include:

- Regulations and SOPs that will apply to the reliance process
- Scope of the agreement, especially any limitations to the research it covers
- Documentation of which IRB will be the reviewing IRB or how the reviewing IRB will be designated and documented
- Responsibility for notifications, including IRB decisions and determinations; process for review of unanticipated problems, complaints, serious and/or continuing noncompliance, and other events and potential reporting responsibilities

IRB AUTHORIZATION AGREEMENT

Sample text for an institution with an FWA to rely on the IRB/IEC of another institution (institutions may use this sample as a guide to develop their own agreement).

Institution or Organization Providing IRB Review:
Name (Institution/Organization A): _____
IRB registration number: _____
Federalwide Assurance (FWA) number, if any: _____

Institution Relying on the Designated IRB (Institution B):
Name: _____
FWA number: _____
The officials signing below agree that
_____ (name of Institution B) may rely on the designated IRB for review and continuing oversight of its human subjects research described here (*check one*):
(____) This agreement applies to all human subjects research covered by Institution B's FWA.
(____) This agreement is limited to the following specific protocol(s):
Name of research project: _____
Name of principal investigator: _____
Sponsor or funding agency: _____
Award number, if any: _____
(____) Other (describe): _____
The review performed by the designated IRB will meet the human subjects protection requirements of Institution B's OHRP-approved FWA. The IRB at Institution/Organization A will follow written procedures for reporting its findings and actions to appropriate officials at Institution B. Relevant minutes of IRB meetings will be made available to Institution B upon request. Institution B remains responsible for ensuring compliance with the IRB's determinations and with the terms of its OHRP-approved FWA. This document must be kept on file by both parties and provided to OHRP upon request.

Signature of signatory official (Institution/Organization A):

_____
Date: _____
Print full name: _____
Institutional title: _____
Signature of signatory official (Institution B):

_____
Date: _____
Print full name: _____
Institutional title: _____

Department of Health and Human Services (DHHS). (2017). *Individual investigator agreement.* www .hhs.gov/ohrp/register-irbs-and-obtain-fwas/forms/individual-investigator-agreement/index.html

- Privacy and confidentiality provisions
- <u>Conflict of interest</u> (COI) determinations, including their identification and assessment; creation and communication of management plan, if necessary; assessment of any limitations to the research as a consequence of the potential COI; and modifications to the informed consent language, if any

  ⚭ 12-6, 12-8
- Maintenance of liability insurance for conduct of human clinical research
- Rights, responsibilities, and abilities of the collaborating parties to request, require, conduct, and review audits and site visits as necessary
- Communication and consideration of institutional policies, local and state law, regulations and guidance

The roles and responsibilities of the reviewing IRB and relying institutions included in reliance agreements between institutions are further outlined in **Table 4.1-1**, modeled on the widely used SMART IRB Master Common Reciprocal IRB Agreement discussed later in this chapter. Although many responsibilities naturally fall to the relying institution or the reviewing IRB, there are many issues that can be conducted by either party.

Responsibilities of the Reviewing IRB

The responsibilities that fall solely to the IRB are often captured in the agreement. For example, the IRB must be registered with OHRP and the Food and Drug Administration (FDA), as appropriate to the research it reviews; maintain the registration for the period that it oversees the research; remain in good standing with OHRP, FDA, and other relevant agencies; and commit to inform the relying institution of any suspension or restriction of the IRB's authorization to review studies, including but not limited to a suspension or restriction of the IRB's registration. While not required by the regulations, a potential requirement is some demonstration of IRB quality (e.g., <u>accreditation</u>, such as by the Association for the Accreditation of Human Research Protection Programs, AAHRPP).

⚭ 8-7

The agreement should codify that the IRB will report to the relying institution any agency request to inspect or copy records regarding research conducted at the institution and to cooperate with the institution in the preparation and conduct of any regulatory inspection. However, the IRB should not commit to allowing the institution to control an agency inspection of the IRB. IRBs are directly regulated by FDA and OHRP and should control their own inspections. Conversely, the IRB should not control any agency inspections that take place at the relying institution.

The IRB should be required to provide relevant records to the relying institution as reasonably requested. These requests may involve, among others, sharing minutes of the meeting in which the study was reviewed, determination letters, and copies of communications to the principal or site researchers. The IRB must provide, as appropriate, any information the institution requests for external or internal audits or agency inspections.

When the reliance agreement ends, the IRB must retain a copy of its records for at least 3 years after the completion of the research [**45 CFR 46.115(b)**]. Copies can be provided to the relying institutions, but the agreement cannot require the IRB to provide "all copies" without allowing the IRB to maintain its own records for the time period as required by the regulations. It is prudent to clarify in advance if there will be costs for providing copies or returning the IRB records, if the institution decides that it needs copies of the records.

IRBs are required to take into consideration institutional policies, local and state law, regulations, and guidance, as communicated by the relying institution.

Table 4.1-1 Roles and Responsibilities of the Reviewing IRB and Relying Institutions under the SMART IRB Agreement[1]

	Reviewing IRB(s) The IRB of Record with authority for IRB review and oversight	**Relying Institution(s)** A Participating Institution that cedes IRB review to a Reviewing IRB
IRB Registration	Maintain current IRB registration with OHRP.	Not Applicable (NA)
IRB Membership	Maintain IRB membership that satisfies requirements of federal policy and other applicable regulations/policies.	NA
Policies and Procedures	Make policies and procedures available to the Relying Institution(s), when applicable and upon request.	NA
IRB Review and Oversight	Perform initial and continuing reviews, and reviews of amendments, unanticipated problems that may involve risks to subjects or others, and potential noncompliance, in accordance with the requirements of "Relying Institution's or Institutions' FWA(s)" and applicable regulations/policies.	Accept Reviewing IRB's decisions and requirements and require its research personnel to provide information that the Reviewing IRB requires for continuing review.
Local Considerations	Consider local requirements communicated by Relying Institution(s).	Communicate to the Reviewing IRB requirements of its FWA and any applicable state or local laws, regulations, institutional policies, standards, or other local factors, including local ancillary reviews that affect the conduct or approval of the Research at the Relying Institution.
Recordkeeping	▪ Maintain records of membership, review activities, determinations, other records, as required by regulation/policy. ▪ Make records accessible to Relying Institution(s), upon reasonable request, including portions of meeting minutes relevant to the research and the Relying Institution.	Require its research personnel to maintain all research records, including informed consent documents and HIPAA authorizations, in accordance with applicable federal, state, and local regulations.
HIPAA	▪ Default: Serve as Privacy Board, when a study falls under the HIPAA Privacy Rule. ▪ Flexibility: may make alternate arrangements (some/all Relying Institutions perform Privacy Board determinations). ▪ Ensure protected health information (PHI) will not be used/disclosed unless written authorization obtained from participants, waiver of alteration of authorization granted, or use of limited data set pursuant to a data use agreement. ▪ When authorization required, provide authorization language.	▪ With Reviewing IRB, establish whether separate or combined consent/HIPAA authorization will be used. ▪ Provide institution-specific language to the Reviewing IRB. ▪ Notify Reviewing IRB of specific local requirements and restrictions on use and disclosure of PHI that could prevent Reviewing IRB from approving a request for waiver of authorization for the institution.
Consent Forms	▪ Provide Relying Institutions/Site Investigators approved informed consent templates (when required). ▪ Permit customization of limited site-specific sections. ▪ Provide final, approved consent form(s) to Relying Institutions/Site Investigators (directly or via designee, e.g., Lead Study Team).	Provide Reviewing IRB with site-specific information requested/identified in the customizable sections of the Reviewing IRB's consent form.

	Reviewing IRB(s) The IRB of Record with authority for IRB review and oversight	**Relying Institution(s)** A Participating Institution that cedes IRB review to a Reviewing IRB
Conflicts of Interest (COI)	<ul><li>Consider Relying Institution's determinations and management plans.</li><li>Incorporate management plan into deliberations, as applicable.</li><li>May impose additional prohibitions or requirements more stringent or restrictive than proposed by a Relying Institution.</li><li>Will not modify plan/mandated disclosure to subjects without discussion with and acceptance by Relying Institution.</li></ul>	<ul><li>Maintain & share COI policies.</li><li>Perform COI analysis (unless alternate arrangement agreed upon).</li><li>Communicate COI determinations to Reviewing IRB.</li><li>Abide by Reviewing IRB COI determinations.</li></ul>
IRB Decisions, Changes, Lapses in Approval	Promptly notify Overall Principal Investigator (PI), Site Investigator(s), and Relying Institution(s) of determinations; review decisions; changes; lapses in approval and applicable corrective action plans.	May not initiate any research or change to the Research, except where necessary to eliminate apparent immediate hazards to subjects, without Reviewing IRB's prior approval.
Unanticipated Problems, Injuries, Complaints	Promptly notify Overall PI, Site Investigators, and Relying Institution(s) about findings of and actions related to:<ul><li>Unanticipated problems involving risks to subjects or others.</li><li>Subject injuries related to research participation.</li><li>Significant subject complaints.</li></ul>	Require Site Investigator(s) to promptly notify Reviewing IRB of unanticipated problems that may involve risks to subjects or others, or any subject injuries related to research participation, or any significant subject complaints at the Relying Institution.
Injury Coverage	NA	Ensure provisions of any applicable grant or contract that address financial coverage for research-related injuries in connection with Research funded in whole or in part by a non-federal entity are consistent with the approved Research protocol and consent form or that approved protocol and consent form, if more protective of human subjects, will control.
Complaints	NA	Ensure mechanism exists by which local Research participants or others may communicate complaints about the Research to a local contact.
Noncompliance, Suspension/ Termination of Approval, Restriction/Suspension of Authority	Promptly notify Overall PI, Site Investigators and Relying Institution(s) about findings of and actions related to:<ul><li>Apparent serious and/or continuing noncompliance</li><li>Serious and/or continuing noncompliance, including any steps it deems necessary for remediation at the Relying Institution</li><li>Suspension or termination of IRB approval.</li></ul>	Promptly notify Reviewing IRB of potential noncompliance with applicable regulations or with the IRB's requirements/ determinations, and of any suspension/ restriction of its research personnel's authority to conduct the Research.

(continues)

Table 4.1-1 Roles and Responsibilities of the Reviewing IRB and Relying Institutions under the SMART IRB Agreement[1] (Continued)

	Reviewing IRB(s) The IRB of Record with authority for IRB review and oversight	**Relying Institution(s)** A Participating Institution that cedes IRB review to a Reviewing IRB
Audits, Investigations, Corrective Actions	May choose to: ■ Conduct audits of the research; ■ Request Relying Institution conduct audit/investigation and report its findings; OR ■ Work with Relying Institution to conduct an audit/investigation. If conducting audit or investigation, promptly notify and report findings of fact to Relying Institution and inform of any corrective actions.	■ Cooperate with and require its research personnel to cooperate with any audit or investigation by the Reviewing IRB/Institution. ■ If asked to do so, conduct own audit/investigation or work cooperatively with the Reviewing IRB/Institution to conduct audit/investigation and report back findings of fact to Reviewing IRB/Institution within a reasonable timeframe. ■ Comply with and require its research personnel to comply with all corrective actions required by the Reviewing IRB/Institution; may adopt more stringent additional corrective actions.
Reporting	■ Notify Relying Institution if report is required to a regulatory agency, sponsor, funding agency, and/or other oversight authority. ■ Typically, draft report and provide involved Relying Institution(s) opportunity to review before sending to external recipients. ■ Not obligated to adopt comments of a Relying Institution.	■ Promptly provide any comments on draft report. ■ If requested, promptly prepare draft report and provide Reviewing IRB/Institution with opportunity to review and comment. ■ If making own additional report, provide copy to Reviewing IRB/Institution.
Communications with Regulatory Agencies	Promptly notify Relying Institution(s) of any communications received from the FDA, OHRP, and/or other regulatory agencies regarding: ■ Unanticipated problems ■ Suspension or termination of IRB approval ■ Serious and/or continuing noncompliance ■ Other regulatory compliance concerns regarding the research.	■ Promptly notify Reviewing IRB/Institution of communications received by or between Relying Institution and FDA, OHRP, and/or other regulatory agencies, regarding unanticipated problems, noncompliance, or other compliance concerns regarding the research. ■ Require Overall PI/Site Investigator(s) to do the same.
Congruence of Federal Grant Applications/Contract Proposals	Review congruence of any federal grant application or contract proposal with the Research submitted for review, when required by federal regulations or oversight agencies (unless other arrangements are made).	NA

[1] Reproduced with permission from Cobb, N., Witte, E., Cervone, M., Kirby, A., MacFadden, D., Nadler, L., & Bierer, B. (2019). The SMART IRB platform: A national resource for IRB review for multisite studies. *Journal of Clinical and Translational Science*, 3(4), 129–139. doi:10.1017/cts.2019.394

🔗 Section 6
🔗 12-2

Therefore, IRBs must have the capability to maintain distinct consent form versions for each institution or study team (e.g., in the case of small clinical practices). Institutional requirements that often affect <u>consent form</u> language include <u>payments to subjects</u>, compensation for research-related injury, and appropriate local contacts for subject questions or complaints. In addition, many institutions also wish to require additional specific language in the consent form, such as particular wording regarding risks and benefits, alternate treatments, COIs, or HIPAA compliance. The reviewing IRB will need to determine whether the specific language requested is appropriate, understandable, and consonant with the rest of the informed consent. There may be site-specific religious and cultural norms (e.g., Catholic institutions that have a position on the use of birth control) that require unique language on an institutional basis. Any specific institutional template language should be documented outside of the reliance agreement. As noted previously, if such requirements are detailed specifically in the agreement, it becomes difficult to change.

The IRB must have processes in place to consider and document <u>COI</u> determinations, including institutional management plans and required consent language. To the extent that COIs may affect the consent form, the agreement should allow for the IRB to assess COIs (or determine) and approve disclosure to subjects, when appropriate. Furthermore, if the reviewing IRB determines that the review by the relying institution is insufficient (or has not been performed), the agreement should allow the IRB to impose additional conflict management requirements, which should be communicated to the relying institution. The relying institution remains responsible for monitoring compliance with the management plan or withdrawing from the ceded IRB review for that specific protocol if it cannot comply with the IRB's requirements.

12-6, 12-8

The scope of information that the reviewing IRB will communicate to the relying institution, federal agencies, and others should be addressed. For example, the reliance agreement might specify that the IRB notify the relying institution (and vice versa) promptly of any <u>unanticipated problems</u> involving risks to subjects or others, any serious or continuing <u>noncompliance</u>, and any suspension or termination of IRB approval. These requirements are in the regulations, so need not be included in the reliance agreement itself; however, institutions commonly document timelines for reporting (e.g., "promptly," "within 5 business days," etc.) in the agreement.

7-3
7-6

Some institutions wish to be notified of all reported adverse events or subject injuries and request inclusion of such language in a reliance agreement. Requiring IRBs to review all reported adverse events or subject injuries is burdensome and ineffective because the majority of adverse events are anticipated, do not result in IRB action, and are not required to be reported to the IRB by regulation or guidance. IRBs should work with relying institutions to specify which adverse events and injuries (e.g., those that constitute unanticipated problems) the IRB will report and the timeline for those reports.

Responsibilities of the Relying Institution

Many of the relying institution responsibilities reflect and mirror the IRB responsibilities. The reliance agreement should detail the responsibilities of the relying institution so that performance expectations are clear. The relying institution must maintain an <u>FWA</u> if federally funded research is involved and identify the institutional official who is responsible for, and has authority to ensure, research compliance. The institution should also maintain a <u>human research protection program</u> and ensure that researchers are appropriately qualified and <u>trained</u> in human research protections.

8-1

2-1

8-5

The reliance agreement should specify key notifications that the relying institution should make to the reviewing IRB and potential time frames for the communication, including the following:

- If the institution's FWA is modified (or lost) or the institutional official (IO) is changed

- Any agency request to inspect or copy records regarding research conducted at the institution under the oversight of the reviewing IRB
- When the institution takes action to suspend or restrict a research project, a researcher, or other research staff or becomes aware of such suspensions or restrictions
- The discovery of potential serious or continuing noncompliance or an unanticipated problem that involves risks to subjects or others

The relying institution should maintain policies regarding the disclosure and management of COIs related to research and provide management plans and consent language to the IRB as requested. As noted previously, the agreement should require a relying institution to provide the IRB with information regarding "local context," including any specific language needed for the identified site-specific sections of the consent forms that will be approved by the IRB. The institution should also provide the IRB with information necessary for review of local information, including applicable local and state laws (e.g., who can serve as the legally authorized representative, age of majority, etc.), local standards, relevant institutional policies, qualifications of the researcher and research staff, and local community considerations (Department of Health and Human Services [DHHS], 2013). The communication of local context is usually accomplished through an IRB submission form or other checklist or survey (e.g., smartirb.org/sites/default/files/Relying-Site-Survey-POCs.pdf).

The reliance agreement should make clear that it is the relying institution's responsibility to coordinate local review by ancillary committees relevant to the ceded research (e.g., institutional biosafety committee, radiation safety, and pharmacy) and require the institution to report any resulting changes in research or findings to the reviewing IRB that could affect the IRB's review of the study.

The reliance agreement should specify which records the reviewing IRB will maintain and for how long, and whether, how, and when documents will be shared with the relying institution. In addition, the reliance agreement should specify the expectation that the relying institution will cooperate with the IRB in the preparation and conduct of any inspection, <u>audit</u>, or site visit. Some institutions will maintain some level of duplicate files, ranging from a simple listing of outsourced protocols to maintaining a complete shadow file of all documents approved by the IRB and provided to the researcher. Several factors may influence this decision, including the institution's approach to risk management, its knowledge of and comfort with the reviewing IRB, its knowledge of and comfort with the researcher and the research program, and the convenience of access to the IRB's records.

🖉 8-6

Finally, because a researcher could bypass institutional review entirely, submitting directly to an external IRB, the institution will need policies and a process in place to ensure that the research has received appropriate institutional consideration and the institution is comfortable participating in the research. This expectation is often codified in a policy that stipulates a researcher's responsibility to complete not only the IRB submission form but also to engage an institutional sign-off process. Typically, these policies and processes are not described in the reliance agreement, because they are specific to the relying institution and do not involve the relying IRB.

Responsibilities of Either the IRB or the Relying Institution

Many responsibilities can be assigned to either the reviewing IRB or the relying institution. One is the process to receive and respond to subject inquiries and complaints. Regardless of which party is responsible, the agreement should provide for prompt communication of the receipt of any subject inquiry or complaint and a process for the IRB and institution to cooperate in investigation and resolution.

🔗 7-6

An agreement may allow for either the IRB or institution to be responsible for the reporting of unanticipated problems, serious or continuing noncompliance, or IRB suspensions or terminations to OHRP, FDA, and other Common Rule agencies. Regardless of which party is responsible for reporting, the parties should cooperate in sharing information and collaborating in developing the report prior to its submission. Cooperation may require confidentiality agreements to be in place. Nothing in the agreement should prevent the other party from making its own report.

🔗 7-3 🔗 7-6

The reliance agreement should specify which entity assumes responsibility related to the HIPAA Privacy Rule. Many of the HIPAA requirements that apply to research can be the responsibility of either party, and the decision regarding which party conducts them depends, to a certain extent, on whether a separate HIPAA authorization form will be used. If the HIPAA authorization will be a separate document from the informed consent form for the research, the responsibility for review of the HIPAA authorization form may be assigned to the IRB or the relying institution, with some exceptions (e.g., the U.S. Department of Veterans Affairs [VA] regulatory requirements do not currently allow the IRB to assume oversight of HIPAA authorization language). If two separate forms are used, it is important to ensure that the two documents are consistent in terms of what protected health information will be shared and who has permission to access that information, and the reliance agreement should specify which party will determine the concordance of the information. If the HIPAA authorization language is embedded in the informed consent form, then the IRB would have responsibility for reviewing that language as part of its review and approval of the final consent form.

🔗 11-6

The responsibility for the review of waivers and alterations of authorization under the HIPAA Privacy Rule can be assigned to an IRB or a privacy board. The waivers and alterations could be conducted by the reviewing IRB, the relying institution's IRB acting as a privacy board, a privacy board at the relying institution, or a privacy board at an external institution.

While routine (i.e., not-for-cause) audits are usually performed by the institution, responsibility for the conduct of for-cause audits can be assigned to the IRB or relying institution (or designee). Some institutions prefer to conduct audits using their own resources, such as using a compliance or legal office, whereas other institutions prefer the reviewing IRB or another external entity to perform such audits to avoid institutional conflicts. The agreement may be flexible regarding responsibilities for audits and when such audits might be required. More specific information about how the audits are conducted and any applicable reimbursement for their costs, however, are best outlined in supplementary SOPs or addenda to the agreement.

🔗 7-4

The reliance agreement should address the need for the reviewing IRB to consider local context information from the relying institution. Examples of local context information relevant to the ceded review include specific requirements of state or local law, regulations, or policies; social or cultural issues, particularly relevant to discrete and insular communities; and whether the researchers have the appropriate training and qualifications as well as the appropriate resources to conduct the research (e.g., staffing, medical equipment, and emergency equipment). Gathering information for analysis of local research context can be assigned in the agreement to either party or can be collected jointly.

SMART IRB: A National Platform for IRB Reliance

Given the increasing frequency of sIRB review of multisite trials, U.S. institutions were faced with a proliferation of one-off, individually negotiated reliance agreements to conduct collaborative research. The terms and responsibilities outlined in each of these agreements differed, requiring legal review, negotiation, and approval. Furthermore, researchers and research teams were often conducting multiple trials under the purview of different IRBs, each with different expectations, presenting a challenge to compliance. To address this problem, the NIH National Center for Advancing Translational Sciences (NCATS) funded a program to develop a national IRB reliance agreement, with the vision to harmonize and systematize these reliance relationships and, ultimately, to reconcile and unify processes and procedures to conduct multisite research efficiently, without compromise to human subjects protections. That program evolved into a national system termed the Streamlined, Multisite, Accelerated Resources for Trials (SMART) IRB platform (www.SMARTIRB.org), the core of which was a master reliance agreement (Cobb et al., 2019).

The agreement specifies the eligibility requirements for participation in the SMART IRB Agreement, and the signatory institutions agree to be bound by the terms and conditions of the Agreement. The SMART IRB Agreement functions as a "treaty" agreement among all signatories, such that any two or more entities that have signed onto the agreement can engage in reliance without executing an additional agreement between or among the parties: all are signatories to one master agreement. This reduces administrative burden, saves repetitive institutional approvals, and may shorten the time to initiating research.

The SMART IRB Agreement serves as an example of an agreement in which terms and conditions have been accepted by a large number and differing types of institutions engaged in human subjects research. How the SMART IRB Agreement outlines specific roles and responsibilities is outlined in Table 4.1-1. There are elements of flexibility embedded in the SMART IRB Agreement that must be agreed upon between the reviewing IRB and relying institution(s). For instance, either the IRB or relying institution can serve as the privacy board for the study, the HIPAA authorization can be either a combined consent or two separate documents, and either the IRB or institution can be responsible for required reporting to any external entity (e.g., federal agencies, sponsors, etc.). When the SMART IRB Agreement is used as a reliance agreement, institutions must document the specific study or studies it covers and how the flexible terms will be implemented. In conjunction with the master agreement, SMART IRB developed a comprehensive suite of SOPs specific to setting up reliance agreements.

Individual (or Independent) Investigator Agreements

A less common form of a reliance agreement is required when an individual researcher (i.e., investigator) wishes to participate in research, but that researcher is associated with an institution that does not have an FWA, or is not associated with an institution at all (e.g., community-based research). Any institution that agrees to extend its FWA to an individual researcher should execute an individual investigator agreement (IIA) that clearly outlines the responsibilities of and expectations for the individual researcher, including training, qualifications, expectations for research conduct, and reporting requirements. The IIA allows an unaffiliated researcher to participate in federally funded research with an institution that has the infrastructure required to engage in research. The use of IIAs is particularly useful when the research involves researchers in community settings (e.g., private dental clinics, community mental health clinics, dialysis units), or individuals, including contractors associated with corporations, consulting firms, nonprofit foundations, and other external organizations, who are conducting research on behalf of the institution. Typically, the IIA is signed by the individual engaged in human subjects research and the responsible institutional official of the institution extending its FWA to cover that individual(s). Any agreement should clearly outline the responsibilities of and expectations for the individual researcher, as the institution will be accountable for his or her performance and conduct. A standard template for an IIA is available on the OHRP website, or institutions can develop their own agreement (DHHS, 2017). If the institution then relies on an external IRB for review of the research, the IIA is either maintained by the reviewing IRB (providing a copy to the relying party) or appended to the research protocol.

Conclusion

The use of external IRBs must be documented in a written agreement that outlines the roles and responsibilities of each entity. The elements of the reliance agreement must reflect the regulatory requirements for documentation and may include other contractual arrangements between the institutions.

As the number of these reliance agreement increases, greater complexity is introduced, in that each IRB may have somewhat different processes and procedures with which researchers and their teams must comply. Communication channels, educational resources, and other tools (e.g., checklists, templates, etc.) may be particularly helpful. A national platform for IRB reliance, SMART IRB, is striving to simplify and harmonize processes and procedures. Harmonizing expectations, roles, and responsibilities, canonized in the reliance agreement, will help decrease administrative burden while maintaining human subjects protections.

References

Central Institutional Review Board for the National Cancer Institute (NCI CIRB). (n.d.). *Welcome to the CIRB.* www.ncicirb.org

Cobb, N., Witte, E., Cervone, M., Kirby, A., MacFadden, D., Nadler, L., & Bierer, B. (2019). The SMART IRB platform: A national resource for IRB review for multisite studies. *Journal of Clinical and Translational Science, 3*(4), 129–139. doi:10.1017/cts.2019.394

Department of Health and Human Services (DHHS). (2013). *Secretary's Advisory Committee on Human Research Protections. Attachment A: Consideration of local context with respect to increasing use of single IRB review.* www.hhs.gov/ohrp/sachrp-committee/recommendations/2013-january -10-letter-attachment-a/index.html

Department of Health and Human Services (DHHS). (2017). *Individual investigator agreement.* www.hhs.gov/ohrp/register-irbs-and-obtain-fwas/forms/individual-investigator-agreement /index.html

National Institutes of Health (NIH). (2006). *National conference on alternative IRB models: Optimizing human subject protection.* https://osp.od.nih.gov/wp-content/uploads/2013/08 /irbconf06rpt.pdf

National Institutes of Health (NIH). (2016). *Final NIH policy on the use of a single institutional review board for multi-site research.* Notice Number: NOT-OD-16-094. grants.nih.gov/grants /guide/notice-files/not-od-16-094.html. Amended by Notice Number: NOT-OD-17-076, June 16, 2017. https://grants.nih.gov/grants/guide/notice-files/NOT-OD-17-076.html

Responsibilities of the Reviewing IRB

Ann Johnson
Megan Kasimatis Singleton

Abstract

This chapter focuses on the role of the reviewing IRB when a single IRB model is used. Use of a single IRB (sIRB) is required for cooperative research subject to the Common Rule, with some exceptions. Additionally, some funding agencies or industry partners may require use of an sIRB for multisite research. Given these requirements, many IRBs may consider serving as a reviewing IRB. This chapter outlines models for serving as a reviewing IRB, the general responsibilities of reviewing IRBs and how they may be implemented, and the factors each IRB should consider when contemplating serving in the role of a reviewing IRB for multisite research.

Single IRB Models

The specific context within which an IRB may take on the role of reviewing IRB for multisite research, also referred to as a single IRB (sIRB), varies greatly. Some IRBs serve as the reviewing IRB for all multisite research conducted under a consortium or for a specific research network (e.g., StrokeNet or NeuroNext). Other IRBs assume the role of the reviewing IRB for research targeting specific disease groups (e.g., Central IRB for the National Cancer Institute) or as part of a funded initiative (e.g., Trial Innovation Network). In contrast, some IRBs may choose to serve as the reviewing IRB only for a single study and define specific circumstances in which the IRB is willing to assume this role (e.g., when their institution is the prime awardee for a multisite initiative or when the project is limited to a few sites). For some IRBs, serving as a reviewing IRB is part of routine business practice, as is often the case for commercial or independent IRBs.

Deciding When to Serve as a Reviewing IRB

The decision to serve as a reviewing IRB requires careful assessment. When IRBs agree to serve as the reviewing IRB, they should be confident they have the capacity and expertise to serve in this role and the resources needed to effectively execute the responsibilities of the reviewing IRB. Acting as a reviewing IRB often can lead to additional costs and workload for the IRB office, as well as the institutional offices that support the IRB, and increase the complexity of the IRB review process. Some institutions will determine they do not have capacity to ever serve as a reviewing IRB, whereas others may be willing to consider requests on a case-by-case basis. This section details some of the considerations IRBs must make when determining whether to assume the role of a reviewing IRB.

IRB and Institutional Workload Capacity and Training

An IRB and its institution should assess how much additional workload will be generated when taking on the responsibilities of a reviewing IRB. Increased workload can come in many forms but generally presents itself as the additional requirements for the following:

- Staff time needed for responding to requests for reliance, negotiating and implementing reliance agreements, and collecting and disseminating any additional reliance documentation necessary for each study
- Staff and voting member time needed for reviewing and processing the information submitted for sites participating in the multisite study both at initial review and throughout the life of the study
- Support time contributed to the IRB by other institutional offices, which may include legal counsel, compliance and auditing personnel, conflicts of interest review committees and fiscal personnel

New training needs also must be factored into the additional workload. IRB staff and voting members often require training in order to perform the new responsibilities, whereas researchers and study personnel interacting with the reviewing IRB also may require training and education on use of the sIRB model and process.

Defining the Scope of the Reviewing IRB

An IRB may decide it wishes to define the types of studies for which it is willing to serve as the reviewing IRB. This may be helpful in ensuring that the IRB's resource and review capacity fits the types of research for which it will accept the reviewing IRB role.

When an IRB assesses the set of studies it will agree to review, it should consider the following:

- Is there a limit to the number of research sites the IRB can effectively review and oversee?
- Is the IRB willing to review research of any risk level or research discipline?
- Is the IRB equipped to review multisite research involving vulnerable populations (e.g., children, prisoners, individuals with impaired decision-making capacity)?

9-6 9-5 9-7

- Does the IRB have a special expertise or area of focus for which it could serve as the reviewing IRB (e.g., pediatric research, planned emergency research, research involving specific disease conditions)?
- Is the IRB willing to act as a reviewing IRB for nontraditional or inexperienced research sites, such as private clinics, nonacademic facilities, businesses, secondary schools, or community organizations? Research at these types of sites may involve extra, unfamiliar tasks for the site, such as securing a <u>Federalwide Assurance (FWA)</u>, training site personnel on human research protections, and disclosing financial conflicts of interest. Because of the sites' unfamiliarity of these tasks, the reviewing IRB may need to take on the extra responsibility of guiding sites through this work. Additionally, because such sites may be unlikely to have internal research oversight mechanisms, such as conflict of interest review processes and compliance monitoring capabilities, the reviewing IRB (or the reviewing IRB's home institution) may need to assist with or perform these tasks.

  🖉 8-1

- If the IRB is part of a research institution, is the IRB willing to act as a reviewing IRB for studies when its home research institution is not a participating site? An IRB has an institutional interest in representing its own institution as a reviewing IRB when the institution participates in a multisite study. However, this interest may not extend to wholly unaffiliated research sites, where concerns over use of institutional resources, institutional liability, and institutional reputation may give reason for the IRB to decline the reviewing IRB role when its institution is not a participating site in the research.
- Is the IRB willing to act as a reviewing IRB for sites <u>outside of its home country</u>? Given the diversity of research laws and regulations worldwide, the IRB must assess its ability to effectively review a site according to these laws and be responsive to local researchers who may need to interact with the IRB staff for help with questions or concerns.

  🖉 10-9

Sufficiency of Systems for Communication, IRB Submission, and IRB Review

An IRB also should assess the process it uses for communication, IRB submission, and IRB review to ensure it can handle the increased workload and complexity of a reviewing IRB's responsibilities for multisite research. Suitable systems can be paper-based or electronic but must be sufficient to receive information from relying institutions and communicate IRB determinations back to those relying site researchers, either directly to them or through a lead study team or coordinating center. IRB applications may need to be modified to collect more specific information about the participating sites, and the IRB review processes may need to be modified to document site-specific regulatory determinations. At a minimum, reviewing IRBs will need to ensure their communications provide sufficient information about regulatory determinations (e.g., category of approval for pediatric research, whether waivers of consent were granted, nonsignificant risk determinations) for the relying institution and its researchers to understand what has been approved for their site. The reviewing IRB also must have the capacity to create and track site-specific versions of the informed consent form, tailored to include locally required language (e.g., compensation for injury, contact information, and costs), and other site-specific materials (e.g., recruitment materials).

Accreditation or Quality Assessment

When contemplating serving as a reviewing IRB, it is important for institutions to consider that many relying institutions will expect a reviewing IRB to demonstrate a high-quality review and administrative performance. A reviewing IRB should determine whether independent accreditation or <u>assessment of IRB quality</u> is necessary as a method to demonstrate the reviewing IRB's ability to perform the sIRB functions. This can provide assurance to the relying institutions, as well as the reviewing IRB, that responsibilities will be properly executed and that human subjects protections regulations be appropriately applied. Relying institutions or research consortia may propose an acceptable <u>accreditation</u> or <u>quality assessment</u> of the reviewing IRB as a condition of the reliance agreement, and the reviewing IRB should be prepared with documentation of their assessment.

🖉 2-7

🖉 8-7 🖉 2-7

Developing a Process to Review Specific Requests to Serve as the Reviewing IRB

If an institution determines it has the capacity to serve as the reviewing IRB and is willing to consider requests to serve in this role, it must develop a process for receiving and reviewing requests to serve in this capacity. Commercial or independent IRBs have processes in place to request their services. Noncommercial IRBs also should develop a process for receiving and reviewing requests for their services as a reviewing IRB for multisite research. Because the plan for such services often must be included in an application for federal funding or contracts with industry partners, the process for requesting services typically occurs prior to any formal submission of a protocol to the IRB for review.

An important component of the review of requests to serve as the reviewing IRB is an assessment of whether each planned relying institution is engaged in human subjects research. For example, institutions that will only serve as a physical location where research may be conducted or may be simply referring potential subjects to the study team for information about study participation may not be engaged and would thus not need to rely on the reviewing IRB.

The reviewing IRB should designate authorized individuals to review the requests and assess whether the IRB has the capacity to provide the reviewing IRB services requested. The decision to serve as the reviewing IRB should be made at the institutional level and requires <u>formal documentation</u>. Individual researchers, with some exceptions (e.g., private practices), cannot decide on behalf of an institution that an IRB will serve in the role of a reviewing IRB.

🖉 4-1

IRB Review Fees

An IRB may consider charging review fees when acting as a reviewing IRB. Commercial IRBs support their entire operation with such review fees. However, an institution-based IRB may receive funding support from multiple sources, such as through facilities and administrative funding from grants. Because of the additional work a noncommercial IRB may assume when reviewing on behalf other institutions, an institution might consider implementing review fees to cover these costs.

The National Institutes of Health (NIH), as described in "Scenarios to Illustrate the Use of Direct and Indirect Costs for Single IRB Review under the NIH Policy on the Use of a Single IRB for Multi-site Research," allows for the financial costs of sIRB review to be covered by a grant using direct and/or indirect costs, and outlines acceptable scenarios for cost allocation (NIH, 2016). Additional discussion on fees and costing models is provided in the SMART IRB (2018b) "Points to Consider: Fees and Costing Models under the NIH sIRB Policy." An assessment of the specific fees required to serve as a reviewing IRB should be established up front as part of the agreement to serve as a reviewing IRB.

Understanding and Establishing the Responsibilities of the Reviewing IRB

An IRB that decides to serve as a reviewing IRB must understand and be able to execute its responsibilities. These responsibilities include both core IRB review responsibilities that it would perform for local researchers, but which are expanded to cover multiple sites, and new responsibilities unique to the role of the reviewing IRB. This section outlines the responsibilities of the reviewing IRB that align with the core responsibilities of any IRB, the expanded role an IRB must assume as a reviewing IRB, and optional responsibilities an IRB may choose to assume in its capacity as a reviewing IRB.

Establishing the Role and Responsibility of the Reviewing IRB

A critical first step is for the reviewing IRB to establish a specific plan for how it will work with relying institutions and study teams. These responsibilities are typically delineated in the <u>reliance agreement</u>. It is important for the roles and responsibilities of both the reviewing IRB and relying institution to be clear to guide how the reviewing IRB interacts with and processes relying institution information through its review functions. As part of establishing roles and responsibilities, the reviewing IRB should consider what role, if any, the overall principal investigator (PI) or coordinating center PI may have in facilitating the sIRB review process. Having roles and responsibilities clearly documented will help the reviewing IRB to carry out its responsibilities and ensure relying institutions and site study teams know what to expect when working with the reviewing IRB.

🖉 4-1

Core IRB Review Responsibilities

Any IRB, independent of whether it acts as the reviewing IRB for a multisite research study or the specific model utilized for sIRB review, must assume certain responsibilities. For federally supported and/or Food and Drug Administration (FDA)-regulated research, these responsibilities generally include the following:

- Maintaining current IRB registration with the Office for Human Research Protections (OHRP) in compliance with the applicable regulations
- Maintaining <u>IRB membership</u> that satisfies the requirements of applicable regulatory requirements, with assurance that there is sufficient expertise or access to expertise to review the research for which the IRB will serve as the reviewing IRB, which includes any expertise needed to assess the proposed research according to the social and cultural attitudes and norms of the potential subject population(s)

🖉 3-1

- Performing initial and continuing review of all research for which the IRB is a reviewing IRB in accordance with applicable regulatory requirements, which includes review of <u>amendments</u> and <u>continuing review</u> applications, where required

🖉 7-1 🖉 7-2

- Reviewing <u>unanticipated problems</u> posing risks to subjects or others

🖉 7-3

🔗 Section 2

🔗 2-3

- Communicating its determinations to researchers
- Maintaining <u>records</u> of its membership, its review activities and determinations, and other records as required by applicable federal regulations
- Maintaining <u>policies and procedures</u> as required per applicable regulations and institutional policies
- Making determinations as to whether research should be suspended or terminated, when applicable
- Ascertaining the acceptability of proposed research in terms of applicable institution-specific policies and resources, as well as local and federal laws

Core IRB Review Responsibilities Affected by Serving as a Reviewing IRB

While many of the core review responsibilities are the same for an IRB serving as a reviewing IRB for multisite research as when it reviews single-site research, there are two specific areas where the responsibility of the reviewing IRB expands because of its responsibility for relying institutions: the responsibility (1) to communicate with relying institutions and researchers and (2) to consider, as part of site onboarding and through the life of the study, unique local site context information that may impact the IRB's decision making related to those sites.

Communication and documentation

Communication with researchers, including to provide IRB determinations and decisions and obtain information relevant to its review, is an essential function of any IRB. When the responsibility to communicate with researchers extends to multiple sites and research teams, the reviewing IRB must establish clear communication channels. As part of this responsibility, it is critical that reviewing IRBs ensure that research teams at each relying institution are aware of and have access to the reviewing IRB's policies and procedures and understand expectations for working with the reviewing IRB.

This communication effort often requires partnership with lead/coordinating teams. Generally, reviewing IRBs adopt one of two common approaches to communicating with researchers: (1) direct communication between the reviewing IRB and relying site researchers and study teams or (2) interaction through a centralized study contact, such as a lead researcher, a coordinating center, or a contract research organization. Many researchers are accustomed to having a direct line of communication with their local IRBs, and it may be viewed as a burden or an unnecessary step to have all communication funneled through a central contact. However, for large trials with many researchers, a central study contact may provide the benefit of more consistent IRB-related communication across a study. While the communication methods can be influenced by the size and type of study being reviewed, it is up to each reviewing IRB to determine its preferred or required communication style and ensure appropriate resources are allocated to its maintenance.

It may be helpful for reviewing IRBs to create a formal communication plan that can be disseminated to relying institutions. This communication plan should document key communication responsibilities and the responsible party for each required action. For example, the plan might outline which party will provide determinations of the IRB to relying site study teams and which party will communicate site-specific local context information to the reviewing IRB, such as detailed in the SMART IRB "Template Communication Plan" (SMART IRB, n.d.). Whatever mechanism the reviewing IRB selects for providing information, it must ensure that each relying site has access to its approval determinations and that any requirements of its approvals are clearly communicated to relying site researchers. Where site-specific determinations are required, the reviewing IRB must ensure its documentation (e.g., meeting minutes and correspondence) reflects these necessary determinations.

The added communication responsibilities extend not only to relying site researchers but also to the institutions themselves, because each reviewing IRB must develop a plan to promptly inform relying institutions of any determinations of suspension, termination, and findings of an <u>unanticipated problem</u> posing risks to subjects or others or serious/ continuing <u>noncompliance</u>. The reviewing IRB must also be prepared to provide IRB meeting minutes or other required documents to the relying institutions upon request (e.g., when the relying institution is conducting an internal audit of research at their site). Establishing the communication pathways up front and ensuring relying institutions are aware of how these communications will occur is the role of a reviewing IRB.

🖉 7-3
🖉 7-6

Review of local context information

Federal regulations specify that an IRB must have the ability to "ascertain the acceptability of proposed research" in terms of institution-specific policies, resources, and local laws; in addition, the IRB must be "sufficiently qualified" to assess research according to the social and cultural attitudes and norms of the potential subject population, usually referred to as *local context* [**45 CFR 46.107(a)** and **21 CFR 56.107(a)**]. The <u>reliance agreement</u> outlines the division of responsibilities between the reviewing IRB and the relying institution and typically makes clear that it is the responsibility of the relying institution to identify and communicate local context issues to the reviewing IRB. However, it is the responsibility of the reviewing IRBs to establish a process for collecting and reviewing this information throughout the life of the study; local context considerations may be triggered by a study modification or an event that may have been reported for one site.

🖉 4-1

Reviewing IRBs vary in their approach to collecting and verifying local context information with relying sites. Various tools are available to assist with the collection of local context information including questionnaires and online surveys. Some information about a site is static and nonstudy specific and has been referred to as an institutional profile. Examples of institutional profile information include those developed by the IRB Reliance Exchange (2020) and SMART IRB (2018a). Some electronic systems have been developed to capture static information about a site and make it available electronically to the reviewing IRB. Each study also may trigger unique local considerations that must be collected from the relying institutions on a study-specific basis. For example, site variations in what is considered standard or usual care could affect the reviewing IRB's assessment of risks of a study intervention for that site. Likewise, differences in state law regarding the circumstances when minors may consent for themselves, or the age of majority, may impact the type of consent process and documentation that the reviewing IRB must review and approve. Even if the information provided is incomplete or irrelevant to the conduct of this study at the site, the reviewing IRB may need to seek clarification from the relying institution or study team.

The following examples illustrate the variation in types of local context information and how differences in the types of local context considerations may alter whether this information must be collected on a study-specific basis or could be provided more generally:

a. Any unique characteristics of a community in which a relying institution is located may be relevant local context information that a reviewing IRB would need to consider. For example, does the community predominantly comprise a religious group with specific norms? Does it comprise individuals from different cultural backgrounds with differing expectations for privacy? These community characteristics usually do not change rapidly and remain relatively static. The reviewing IRB would be able to rely on information provided about the characteristics of the community surrounding a relying institution for multiple studies conducted at the site without the need to collect it frequently. This could be collected through an overall information sheet about the relying institution or obtained from databases containing a site's institutional profile.

b. What is considered usual care or part of standard practice at an institution, in contrast, can vary across institutions in specific ways and may change rapidly. For protocols that presume, for example, that a specific intervention represents "usual care" or standard practice at each site, it would be important to verify the accuracy of this information on a study-specific basis. Because this type of information would generally not be found in an overall profile for a specific relying institution, the reviewing IRB must develop a method to collect this information separately on a study-specific basis.

⌗ Section 6

⌗ 11-6

⌗ 2-1

As part of its process to collect local relying institution information, each reviewing IRB must establish a pathway to collect site-specific consent language, when the study involves <u>informed consent</u>. There may be components of the site-specific consent language that are dictated by the policy of the relying institution, such as research-related injury language and <u>Health Insurance Portability and Accountability Act (HIPAA)</u> authorization language. However, there also may be site-specific consent language that is not prescribed by policy that nonetheless needs to be included, such as site-specific costs to subjects or procedures for obtaining compensation and reimbursement. Representatives of the human research protection program (<u>HRPP</u>) or legal counsel at the relying institution may have a role in verifying the accuracy of the site-specific consent language provided to the reviewing IRB, most likely in situations delineated in institutional policy. The relying site study personnel may also have a role in providing site-specific language. Additional information about the role of the relying institution in communicating local context considerations to the reviewing IRB is further delineated in Chapter 4-3, "Responsibilities of the Relying Institution."

Approval of Participating Sites

Once the reviewing IRB has established a process for collecting site-specific local context information, it must define the way in which individual relying institutions will be reviewed and approved. While the reviewing IRB's assessment of local context information provided by relying institutions often may be handled via an expedited review, it is important for each reviewing IRB to establish the criteria for when a site addition may be processed via an expedited review or requires review by a convened IRB. This is especially important where study procedures may vary across institutions and the regulatory determinations required per site may differ. The addition of a participating site may be eligible for <u>expedited review</u> if there are no specific local context considerations that would impact the <u>criteria for approval</u> and the only site-specific consent language changes are minor variations to previously approved consent language. In contrast, <u>convened IRB review</u> of a relying site may be needed if the local context information provided by the relying institution may impact the criteria for approval. For example, if a relying institution indicates that the overall study recruitment plan would not allow for equitable subject selection at the site given the characteristics of the local community, convened IRB review would be warranted. In this example, if the study were greater than minimal risk, since the criterion for equitable subject selection is called into question, the convened IRB must establish if the criteria for approval are met for the site.

    ⊘ 5-5
    ⊘ 5-4

    ⊘ 5-7

    An IRB should assess its capacity to design a process that effectively documents, considers, and acts upon the local context issues that are relevant to site and specific studies it reviews. The IRB may need to expand the diversity and representation capacity of its <u>voting membership</u> in order to broaden its qualifications for reviewing research in different communities or seek advice from a consultant where additional review expertise is needed. For example, a reviewing IRB willing to serve in this capacity for a location <u>outside of its home country</u> may need a consultant to help understand local cultural norms around consent and appropriate subject recruitment.

    ⊘ 3-1

    ⊘ 10-9

    As part of its approval of participating sites, a reviewing IRB also must determine the pathway it wishes to use for consent form creation. Two common models include: (1) the reviewing IRB creates a site-specific consent form using information supplied by the relying institution or (2) the relying institution must create its own site-specific consent form and supply it to the reviewing IRB. Each model has advantages and disadvantages. By controlling the development of site-specific consent forms, reviewing IRBs may retain more version control; however, they must also assume additional workload burden associated with consent form creation. The reviewing IRB may elect to utilize an approach that best aligns with the resources it has available. A reviewing IRB may also consider if and how to limit language changes in specific sections of the informed consent document to reduce the variance in documents across sites, potentially allowing for a more streamlined review of these documents. This has been accomplished by some reviewing IRBs by disallowing institution-specific changes to sections of language that are not expected to differ across sites, such as study procedures, risks, and benefits, as well as statements about voluntary participation and the right to withdraw.

Executing the Core Functions of the Reviewing IRB

Although many of its core responsibilities remain the same when serving as a reviewing IRB, reviewing IRBs may develop specific strategies for executing them to accommodate multisite research. Key considerations for executing core functions as a reviewing IRB follow.

Initial Protocol Review

For many reviewing IRBs, the initial protocol review is the one component of the IRB review process that is most similar to the review of single-site research, because in this case the primary responsibility of the reviewing IRB is to assess the approvability of the research using applicable human subjects protection requirements. Many reviewing IRBs choose to limit the initial review to only include a review of the protocol, a master template consent, and any materials that will be used study-wide, such as standardized recruitment materials, rather than review of site-specific information. In this model, often called a parent-child model, the protocol, consent, and associated study documents typically are not released to relying institutions to use for their local context review until the study itself has been initially approved by the reviewing IRB. Other reviewing IRBs may choose to gather site-specific information up front and conduct an initial review of the protocol and any identified relying institutions at the same time. A potential drawback of this approach may be that relying institutions expect to see the protocol in its final approved form before completing a final local context review, meaning a local context review may be required both before and after the reviewing IRB has approved the study.

Amendments or Modifications

*7-1

Under an sIRB model, reviewing IRBs also must consider how to process changes to approved research (e.g., amendments or modifications). Reviewing IRBs should establish who has the authority to submit changes that will affect the study as a whole and which types of site-specific changes will be permitted. For example, if a core component of a research study is to evaluate a specific recruitment methodology, site-specific variations to the recruitment plan may not be able to be submitted at the site level and may need to be considered more broadly as part of a study-wide change. It is often helpful to establish processes for study-wide amendments versus site-specific changes with the lead study team/coordinating center team, who can help to reinforce expectations with relying institution study teams. Additionally, as part of amendment review, reviewing IRBs need to consider whether changes to the study prompt new local context considerations.

Reviewing IRBs should be explicit regarding whether they will assume responsibility for review of study team changes and the circumstances when study team changes must be submitted to the reviewing IRB versus the relying institution for review. Generally, reviewing IRBs should be responsible for reviewing changes in PI at relying institutions and changes in study team

*12-6

members that result in identification of a new or updated conflict of interest. A detailed plan for who will be responsible for the review of other study team changes should be established with relying institutions and communicated to study teams at all relying institutions.

Continuing Review

*7-2

Reviewing IRBs also must develop procedures for processing continuing review submissions for multisite research, when continuing review is required. While generally there is only one continuing review application that provides an assessment of the study in its entirety, site-specific information about progress and updates should be provided so the reviewing IRB may assess whether the criteria for approval continue to be met for each site, or if any concerns with specific sites may need to be addressed. Generally, site-specific information would include details that could feed into an overall study report (e.g., a summary of site-specific <u>deviations</u>, subject <u>complaints</u>, and enrollment information). Because it is important that a study (including the lead site and all relying institutions) has only one approval period, the reviewing IRB will need to establish a process for what occurs if a site does not supply its information for a <u>continuing review</u> in a timely way (e.g., whether that site be suspended and all others approved). Additionally, reviewing IRBs must develop strategies for considering whether cumulative progress data across study sites suggest any changes may be needed for the study to continue. Since in its role as a reviewing IRB, the sIRB may have access to more data for the study as a whole than was previously available when serving as the IRB for a single site, reviewing IRBs should consider how to best evaluate this study-wide data. Notably, even when continuing review is not determined to be required, a reviewing IRB may still seek progress reports or site-specific updates if this is determined to be appropriate to enable ongoing oversight for the study.

🔗 7-5 🔗 7-6

🔗 7-2

Reportable Events

Reviewing IRBs are responsible for reviewing events that could qualify as <u>unanticipated problems</u> posing risks to subjects or others occurring at all sites. In addition, reviewing IRBs often assume the added role of making regulatory determinations as to whether an incident of noncompliance rises to the level of serious and/or continuing <u>noncompliance</u> and therefore may require that a wider range of events be reported to the IRB for review. The reviewing IRB must establish processes to consider how an event reported at one site may impact the overall study and whether changes to the study are required for continued approval. Additionally, where concerns are raised about individual site noncompliance, the reviewing IRB may need to determine whether site suspension or termination may be warranted. Where appropriate, the reviewing IRB may wish to request the relying institution to perform an internal audit or conduct an independent audit of the study itself in order to appropriately assess any reported noncompliance. It is important that when concerns are identified, the reviewing IRB informs the relying institution, because the relying institution may have access to information that would be critical to the reviewing IRB's assessment (e.g., information about prior similar noncompliance of a researcher).

🔗 7-3

🔗 7-6

Because reportable events often require the development of a corrective action plan to address the event, the reviewing IRB should have mechanisms to solicit input from affected institutions related to any proposed site-specific corrective action plan prior to its review. Local HRPPs are important partners in the review of such events and can help provide context about local operations or expectations to inform the IRB's decision making, and they may be best positioned to inform the development of appropriate corrective action plans.

Common Additional Responsibilities a Reviewing IRB May Assume

A reviewing IRB may elect to assume additional responsibilities. Typically, the specific scope of work a reviewing IRB has agreed to undertake is defined in the <u>reliance agreement</u>.

🔗 4-1

Serving as the HIPAA privacy board: In this role, a reviewing IRB would be responsible for making determinations on behalf of relying institutions that are covered entities in compliance with the HIPAA Privacy Rule related to the use and disclosure of protected health information (PHI) in research. This would include (a) determining when written authorization will be obtained from each subject for the use of PHI and (b) granting waivers or alterations of authorization for use and disclosure of PHI when appropriate and applicable.

⌗ 11-6

Audits and investigations of the activities of relying institutions: While not a required role, in order to feel comfortable assuming additional oversight for relying institutions, some reviewing IRBs may choose to take a more active role in routine and/or for-cause audits of relying site study teams. Audits may include physical or remote review of research records and related study information, meeting with representatives from the relying institution and study team, and working with a relying institution to develop corrective action plans.

⌗ 7-4

Drafting and submitting letters to federal oversight entities: While not required by regulation, many reviewing IRBs will assume a lead role in drafting and submitting any reports required to a federal oversight agency (e.g., OHRP, FDA), sponsor, funding agency, and/or other oversight authority. This would include reports of any findings of serious or continuing noncompliance, unanticipated problems involving risks to human subjects or others, and any suspensions or terminations of IRB approval. Many reviewing IRBs will assume the responsibility for submitting these reports on behalf of the relying institution because of their role in assessing and making determinations about the event; this responsibility may be outlined in the reliance agreement. Reviewing IRBs that assume this role should work closely with the relying institution to draft and finalize these reports to ensure the accuracy of the information presented and organizational acceptance of any corrective action plans proposed for the researchers or relying institution.

⌗ 4-1

Review of studies to ensure concordance with any applicable grants or contracts: While the IRB is not responsible for ensuring concordance between studies and federal grants supporting research, many institutions have determined that the IRB is best positioned as part of its review process to perform this assessment. Reviewing IRBs may take on the added responsibility of ensuring congruence of federal grant applications and contracts with the application submitted to the IRB for review. When this role is assumed, the reviewing IRB should formally establish that it will perform this function in any arrangement with the relying institution and develop a mechanism to document that this assessment was performed.

Conclusion

In order to effectively assume the responsibility of a reviewing IRB, IRBs considering serving in this capacity should carefully evaluate the resources, expertise, and education needed to fulfill this role. Reviewing IRBs must develop robust processes for working with relying institutions and study teams and performing their core and expanded review responsibilities. Strong partnerships with relying institution HRPPs and lead/coordinating center study teams are essential to ensure reviewing IRBs can perform this important function and uphold the highest standards for human subjects protections.

References

IRB Reliance Exchange. (2020). *Institutional profile quick guide*. www.irbexchange.org/p/wp-content/uploads/2018/10/IREx_InstitutionalProfile_QuickGuide_20180320.pdf

National Institutes of Health (NIH). (2016). *Scenarios to illustrate the use of direct and indirect costs for single IRB review under the NIH policy on the use of a single IRB for multi-site research grants.* nih.gov/grants/guide/notice-files/NOT-OD-16-109.html

SMART IRB. (n.d.). *Template communication plan for SMART IRB*. Smartirb.org/sites/default/files/Communications_Plan_Form.pdf

SMART IRB. (2018a). *Institutional profile.* smartirb.org/sites/default/files/Institutional-Profile-20180726.pdf

SMART IRB. (2018b). *Points to consider: Fees and costing models under the NIH's IRB policy*. Smartirb.org/sites/default/files/Fees-and-Costing-Models.pdf

Responsibilities of the Relying Institution

Nichelle Cobb
Martha F. Jones

Abstract

This chapter explores the ways that an institution can establish and maintain appropriate human subjects protections in collaboration with external IRBs. Reliance on an external IRB may be required by a funding entity or because of federal regulations, such as the Common Rule requirement for use of a single IRB review for cooperative research. In other cases, an institution may voluntarily use an external IRB to review all or some of its human subjects research portfolio, such as when it lacks resources to maintain an internal IRB, when it does not have the expertise to review certain research, or as a strategy to manage institutional conflicts of interest relevant to a research study. Regardless of whether it uses an external or internal IRB to oversee its research, an institution remains responsible for having a comprehensive program to protect the human subjects who participate in that research. When relying on an external IRB, the institution must understand and delineate the roles and responsibilities of the external IRB versus those that it retains.

Selecting a Reviewing IRB

An institution must first decide whether it is willing to rely on a review conducted by an external IRB and, if so, under what circumstances. Some institutions choose to use an external IRB for all IRB reviews. Other institutions only allow reliance for certain types of research or decide to use an external IRB on a case-by-case basis. Institutions should develop policies and procedures that identify when an external IRB review may be used, any allowed or preferred IRBs, the acceptable terms and review process for reliance agreements, who can determine when research can be ceded, and who has authority to sign reliance agreements.

🔗 4-1

Determining When to Rely on an External IRB

In developing policies and procedures about when an external IRB may be used, an institution should consider the following:

- Whether, if an internal IRB exists, it has the expertise and capacity to review some or all research conducted at the institution, including serving as the reviewing IRB for multisite research where use of a single IRB may be required or desired.
- Situations when an external IRB must be used in order to participate in the research, such as when an industry sponsor expects all sites to use the same commercial (independent) IRB or because funding entities or federal regulations require the use of a single IRB for multisite research.
- ✐ 8-7 Expected qualifications for an external IRB, including whether the IRB must be <u>accredited</u>.
- If any tribal, state, or local laws or other requirements prohibit use of an external IRB.
- Whether research risk level, type of research, location of the research, or personnel involved should be taken into account as part of the decision whether to use an external IRB.
- ✐ 12-8 The potential use of an external IRB when the institution has a <u>conflict of interest</u> relevant to the research, as part of a management plan to mitigate the conflict.

Assessing External IRBs

Institutions should ensure that any IRB overseeing research regulated by the Food and Drug Administration (FDA) or conducted or supported by the Department of Health and Human Services (DHHS) is registered with the Office for Human Research Protections (OHRP) and, if the IRB is associated with an institution (as opposed to being an independent IRB), that its institution has a current
✐ 8-1 <u>Federalwide Assurance (FWA)</u>. In addition to these considerations, many factors may influence the selection of an external IRB. These include the following:

- *The expertise and experience of the reviewing IRB with the type of research proposed*: Certain studies may be more suited to particular IRBs.
- *The originator of the research*: Some institutions use independent IRBs to oversee industry-generated and -sponsored research but retain oversight of investigator-initiated studies.
- *Where the primary award is held*: The institution that holds an award often, but not always, provides IRB review.
- *An assessment of the processes the IRB has in place to ensure compliance with regulatory and ethical requirements necessary to effectively protect human subjects*:
✐ 8-7 This may include determining whether <u>accreditation</u> has been earned. Accreditation, such as by the Association for the Accreditation of Human Research Protection Programs (AAHRPP), can indicate a certain level of resources, infrastructure, and commitment to support human subjects protections and compliance with applicable regulations.
- *The number of sites involved and complexity of the study*: Some IRBs may not have the capacity to review research that includes a large number of participating sites or sites located outside their local area.
- *Estimated costs*: The research budget may influence whether the fees an IRB charges can be accommodated.

Defining Responsibilities

When institutions use an external IRB, they must document that arrangement. In the case of nonexempt multisite research subject to the Common Rule regulations, <u>reliance arrangements</u> must be documented by a written agreement that outlines the responsibilities of the relying institution and the <u>external IRB</u> with regard to how they will meet regulatory requirements. The reliance agreement, or reliance terms included in other agreements such as a subaward or subcontract, should clearly define the responsibilities of the external reviewing IRB and those that remain with the institution. Relying institutions retain significant responsibilities when IRB review is ceded, including "ensuring compliance with the IRB's determinations and with the Terms of its OHRP-approved FWA" (DHHS, 2017) and "for safeguarding the rights and welfare of human subjects and for complying with [the Common Rule]" [**45 CFR 46.114(a)**]. Although FDA regulations do not explicitly require documentation of reliance arrangements, the agency's guidance recommends putting in place an "agreement signed by the parties" (FDA, 2006).

🖉 4-1

🖉 4-2

Identifying and Tracking Research Reviewed by an External IRB

Relying institutions need to implement systems to collect information and track their research portfolio in order to meet their oversight responsibilities when using an external IRB. Often IRB or research application systems or processes may be shortened and adapted to an "administrative" or "registration" application that collects key institutional information about a study that will be reviewed by an external IRB. This information may include the demographics of the research such as study title, principal investigator (PI), research team members and their human subjects protection education or training status, funding details, and conflict of interest information. The administrative application also may include key documents (e.g., the study abstract, protocol, and template consent documents) to allow the relying institution to identify local context issues that should be communicated to the reviewing IRB or that trigger local ancillary reviews (e.g., pharmacy, biosafety, radiation safety). These administrative applications should be used to fulfill the responsibilities of the relying institution rather than for the institution to conduct a shadow IRB review or duplicate information that is the reviewing IRB's responsibility.

An institution should consider what information its researchers should provide to local personnel and offices, not just at the time a study is initially ceded but throughout the life of a study. For example, the institution may require researchers to communicate some reportable events (e.g., <u>noncompliance</u> that is potentially serious or continuing or <u>unanticipated problems</u>) to local offices that monitor study compliance or oversee clinical trials. Additionally, if a reviewing IRB determines a study does not need to undergo <u>continuing review</u>, the relying institution may wish to require that their study teams provide periodic updates (e.g., an annual check-in) and report when the study is closed at their site to an appropriate local office, in order to ensure compliance with applicable regulations and have an accurate picture of their current research portfolio.

🖉 7-6

🖉 7-3

🖉 7-2

Responsibility for a Human Research Protection Program

The use of an external IRB underscores the need for institutions to decouple institutional from IRB review requirements and create an integrated program that provides protections regardless of the location of the reviewing IRB. Many institutions now have positions with human research protection program (HRPP) titles, such as HRPP director or HRPP manager, that may directly oversee IRB operations but often include responsibility for quality assurance functions (e.g., post-approval monitoring) and other non-IRB functions related to human subjects research (e.g., education and training). This need for distributed responsibilities between the IRB and other institutional components is exemplified by AAHRPP's standards for accreditation, which assign responsibilities to the institution (AAHRPP uses "organization"), the IRB or ethics committee, and researchers and research staff. AAHRPP standards, in parallel with DHHS requirements, assign responsibility to the institution that is engaged in research for the protection of the rights and welfare of research subjects.

🔗 2-1
🔗 2-7
🔗 7-4
🔗 8-5

Because institutions often leverage IRBs as gatekeepers for many compliance functions beyond what is required by the regulations for IRB oversight, the use of external IRBs requires institutions to rethink the roles and actions that are at times presumed to be under the IRB's purview. When institutions rely on an external IRB, they are responsible for ensuring compliance with the IRB's determinations and with their own FWAs, as well as for safeguarding the rights and welfare of human subjects (AAHRPP, 2019). Without local IRB review to assist with oversight of human subjects research, institutions need to use other processes, such as researcher education and monitoring functions, to meet compliance obligations. Aspects of research compliance oversight that usually remain the responsibility of relying institutions, and thus require mechanisms and processes to meet these obligations, are described in more detail later, and include the following:

- Credentialing, education, and training of researchers and their support staff
- Receiving notification of injuries to human subjects or subject complaints
- Conducting monitoring, quality assessment, and quality improvement programs and implementing corrective action plans as necessary
- Conducting ancillary reviews (see **Table 4.3-1** for examples of ancillary reviews)
- Ensuring compliance with the terms of the reliance agreement
- Providing coordination and liaison functions between the researcher and the external IRB

Credentialing, Education, and Training

Verification of the qualifications and credentials of researchers often remains the responsibility of the relying institution, because it is the entity most likely to be knowledgeable about the qualifications of their staff. The responsibility may reside with a human resources office, a research administration office, or a combination of multiple institutional areas. As part of assessing personnel education (e.g., for human subjects protection) and training (e.g., to perform their research role), the relying institution also should monitor and communicate any restrictions on their research personnel's authority or ability to conduct the research to the reviewing IRB throughout the life of the study. Because some reviewing IRBs do not require submission of personnel changes, or limit personnel updates to certain study team members (e.g., site PI), relying

🔗 8-5

Table 4.3-1 Common Institutional Ancillary Reviews

Review Area*	Review Focus	Who Conducts the Review
Feasibility and scientific or scholarly merit	Feasibility review often assesses whether the research team has or has access to: ■ Sufficient time and personnel to devote to the research ■ A subject population available to meet enrollment goals in the time frame of the study ■ Adequate financial support for the study ■ Access to facilities, space, and equipment that are appropriate for the research ■ The ability and credentials to complete study procedures Scientific and scholarly review often focuses on the rationale or basis for the research, appropriateness of study design, analysis plan, and whether study objectives can be met (e.g., a sufficient population exists and can be recruited, study is adequately powered).	Reviews might be performed by the researchers' departments or units to which they belong or specialized committees designated to conduct such reviews, including scientific review committees.
Pharmacy	Availability of drugs for a research study or the control and dispensing of investigational drugs	Investigational drug service or other pharmacy review
Fiscal, such as billing compliance, contracts, budget	Review may include: ■ Assessing whether study procedures may be billed to Medicare, Medicaid, and other third-party payers ■ Ensuring clinical trial agreements or other funding agreements are consistent with consent form language (e.g., compensation for injury) ■ Evaluating whether the proposed research budget is adequate	Often dispersed across several functions, such as sponsored programs, departments, and billing compliance offices
Use of biospecimens	Review might assess whether existing biospecimens can be used in research or whether biospecimens collected for research purposes can be shared with external researchers	May include sign-off from a pathology department or biospecimen bank as well as an assessment of the need for a material transfer agreement.
Data security, which may include electronic health record access	Assessment of transmission and storage of, or access to, identifiable data to ensure adequate data security controls are in place	May be conducted by a formal data security review process or controlled by institutional policies
Conflicts of interest	Assessment of potential financial conflicts of interest relevant to research as well as the creation of management plans, when appropriate	May be conducted by a formal conflict of interest committee or office
Researcher-held investigational new drug (IND) or investigational device exemption (IDE)	Often includes confirming training in place for researchers who hold INDs or IDEs and monitoring compliance with FDA requirements for IND- or IDE-holders	IND/IDE support programs or pharmacy or device committees
ClinicalTrials.gov	Assessment regarding whether a study must be registered at ClinicalTrials.gov per FDA requirements and ongoing updates after initial registration	May be a function of a quality assurance program or a function specifically focused on compliance with FDA ClinicalTrials.gov requirements
Radiation safety	Review of research that involves ionizing radiation as a research procedure that is not part of subjects' routine care or that uses radiology resources	Might be performed by a radiology department specialized committee designated to conduct such reviews
Biological safety	Review of research that involves the use of recombinant DNA, gene therapy, or biohazardous agents	Usually performed by an institutional biological safety committee

*Other types of ancillary reviews might include processes or committees that assess embryonic stem cell research, clinical research review committees, nursing resource reviews, and engineering reviews.

institutions may be responsible for tracking personnel changes. Relying institutions may delegate primary responsibility for monitoring personnel changes to their study teams but should ensure they are aware of this expectation and have mechanisms to perform such oversight.

Subject Injuries and Complaints

When subject injuries happen, whether they are expected or unexpected, institutions must ensure that appropriate response and care occur and that costs are handled in compliance with information provided during the consent process. The institution also retains responsibility to answer questions related to injuries 7-6 or <u>complaints</u> and work with relevant external IRBs and other components of the institution to resolve any concerns or complaints of subjects.

Quality Assurance and Quality Improvement

7-4 Quality assurance and quality improvement can include a variety of <u>activities</u>, such as routine research monitoring (e.g., for compliance with institutional requirements), conducting for-cause audits of researcher records at the request of an IRB to ensure compliance with the IRB's determinations, and creation and monitoring of corrective action plans to address problems that arise in research. An external IRB typically will not (or cannot) commit resources or personnel to conduct on-site monitoring of a relying institution research site. Consequently, the responsibility for monitoring compliance with the requirements of the external IRB generally remains with the relying institution. Moreover, monitoring for compliance with local policies and procedures resides with the institution rather than the external IRB. Consequently, institutions need to ensure that they have or have access to appropriate personnel to perform compliance monitoring for human subjects research.

Reliance arrangements often require relying institutions to be able to conduct for-cause audits of their researchers. While many institutions have internal programs that can conduct random and for-cause audits, not all have such resources, and thus some may need to engage outside individuals to meet this requirement. Expectations regarding who will monitor compliance and how it will be monitored for research reviewed by an external IRB should be clearly assigned and documented.

7-3
7-6 Problems that arise in research, such as <u>unanticipated problems</u>, serious noncompliance, or continuing <u>noncompliance</u>, often lead to the need for a corrective action plan. External IRBs vary in whether they create corrective action plans, collaborate with relying institutions regarding developing such plans, or delegate responsibility to relying institutions to create these plans. Regardless of which party creates them, the relying institution generally is responsible for ensuring the implementation of and compliance with any corrective action plans imposed by an IRB and thus needs processes and mechanisms to meet this responsibility. Additionally, relying institutions are likely to be the parties responsible for responding to federal oversight inquiries and requirements for correction.

Ancillary Reviews

When only internal IRBs are used for review, it is common for IRB applications to flag ancillary requirements that must be completed before IRB review continues or can be finalized or before a study can begin. For institutions relying on an external IRB, the IRB review process can no longer be used as the means to ensure researchers comply with institutional requirements. Institutions thus must have mechanisms in place to identify and communicate ancillary (i.e., non-IRB) requirements to their researchers as well monitoring to ensure they have been met. Table 4.3-1 outlines common ancillary reviews and responsibilities for each.

Ensuring Compliance with the Terms of the Reliance Agreement

Because <u>reliance agreements</u> vary in the specific responsibilities assumed by a relying institution, relying institutions should have processes in place for ensuring they comply with the terms of their reliance agreements and conduct periodic assessments of their adherence to any reliance agreements. Common variations in reliance arrangements include expectations for types of information reviewing IRBs require to identify local context issues, what events to report to the IRB and timelines for reporting them, who reports certain determinations to federal agencies (e.g., serious or continuing noncompliance and unanticipated problems), and timelines for reporting.

🖉 4-1

Communicating Local Context Issues to Reviewing IRBs

Relying institutions usually are responsible for providing local context information to a reviewing IRB that may affect that IRB's review of a study. Local context may encompass any applicable state or local laws, regulations, institutional policies, standards, or other local factors, including local ancillary reviews, relevant to the ceded research that would affect the conduct or approval of the study at the relying institution. This responsibility includes providing any language required in consent documents by the institutions, such as compensation for injury language. Reviewing IRBs vary in the type of local context information they request from relying institutions and how they collect it, but some common items requested by IRBs include the following:

- FWA number and components listed under the FWA
- Whether the institution is a covered entity under the HIPAA Privacy Rule (and, if so, whether the institution permits HIPAA language to be incorporated into consent documents)
- Age of majority in the institution's state and when minors can consent for themselves and the institution's policy on the use of short forms
- Any site-specific ancillary reviews that could have an impact on IRB review for the site
- Any local requirements or state laws that can have an impact on study protocol implementation (e.g., age of majority, how data will be accessed or stored, who can make the initial contact of research subjects) or the content of associated documents (e.g., compensation for injury language in consent forms)
- Drug/device storage and control policies
- Information about any financial conflicts of interest (COIs) that may affect IRB review of research

In regard to <u>COIs</u>, the relying institution needs to be able to communicate any COI determinations, prohibitions, and management plans relevant to the ceded research to the reviewing IRB throughout the life of the study. This means that the relying institution must have a process for identifying new COIs (e.g., due to personnel changes) or changes in COIs. If a relying institution does not

🖉 12-6, 12-8

have a COI process, then it must work with the reviewing IRB to determine an acceptable arrangement.

Event Reporting

Expectations regarding event reporting should be outlined in a reliance agreement, standard operating procedures governing a reliance arrangement, or within the <u>IRB's policies</u> that are available to the relying institution and researchers. Relying institutions should ensure their research teams are aware of reporting policies for the various external IRBs they use and should monitor for compliance with the external IRB's reporting requirements. Additionally, relying institutions should ensure they are aware of whether they or the external IRB are responsible for reporting the IRB's determinations of serious noncompliance, continuing noncompliance, unanticipated problems, suspensions of research, or terminations of research to federal agencies and any timelines for reporting them. Although IRBs are often responsible for making reports to federal agencies when these are required, many reliance agreements require IRBs to allow relying institutions a period to comment on draft reports before they are submitted to federal agencies.

🔗 2-3

Coordination Between Researchers and External IRBs

Many institutions have created reliance teams or liaison positions, which might reside within an IRB or other office within the HRPP, to assist research teams who work with external IRBs. These positions might provide education for researchers regarding the reliance process and the requirements of the external IRB, institutional requirements that must be met prior to study activation, and researcher responsibilities in the case of multisite research.

HIPAA Privacy Rule and External IRBs

When using an external IRB, institutions that are covered entities should consider whether they will request an external IRB to perform reviews required under the <u>Health Insurance Portability and Accountability Act</u> of 1996 (HIPAA) Privacy Rule, specifically consideration of partial and complete waivers of authorization as well as alterations of authorization. Not all IRBs agree to take on these privacy board functions to address HIPAA Privacy Rule requirements. When a reviewing IRB will not act as a privacy board, the relying institution must determine, in the case of research that may require waivers or alterations of authorization, the entity that will be responsible for this function, such as a local IRB, local privacy board, or the privacy board at another institution.

🔗 11-6

Institutions also must determine whether they will include authorization language within consent documents or require stand-alone authorizations be signed by subjects and discuss their preference with an external IRB. Some external IRBs are willing to review consent documents that include authorization language while others are not. Any arrangements related to HIPAA privacy board functions should be outlined in any reliance arrangement. Finally, when institutions are covered entities they remain responsible for compliance with the HIPAA Privacy Rule, such as ensuring a data use agreement is executed for the disclosure of limited data sets or a business associate agreement is in place when required, monitoring for appropriate use and disclosure of protected health information (PHI), and training personnel regarding HIPAA Privacy Rule requirements.

Conclusion

The components of an effective HRPP fit together to protect the rights and welfare of human subjects and ensure compliance with the determinations of the various IRBs overseeing research conducted at an institution. Reliance on an external IRB does not obviate the responsibility of the institution to oversee the conduct of the research, the actions of the researchers, or the protection of human subjects.

References

Association for the Accreditation of Human Research Protection Programs (AAHRPP). (2019). *Procedures & standards*. www.aahrpp.org/apply/resources/procedures-and-standards

Department of Health and Human Services, Office for Human Research Protections (DHHS). (2017). *Institutional Review Board (IRB) authorization agreement*. www.hhs.gov/ohrp/register-irbs-and-obtain-fwas/forms/irb-authorization-agreement/index.html

Food and Drug Administration (FDA). (2006). *Using a centralized IRB review process in multicenter clinical trials: Guidance for industry*. www.fda.gov/regulatory-information/search-fda-guidance-documents/using-centralized-irb-review-process-multicenter-clinical-trials

PART 5

Review of Research

Activities That Are Not Human Subjects Research

Lori Roesch
Belinda Smith

Abstract

One of the most challenging assessments a human research protection program (HRPP) or IRB professional may be asked to make is to determine whether or not a project should be classified as human subjects research (HSR). Having definitions, tools, and an organized process will aid the requestors and help ameliorate some of the challenges. The purpose of this chapter is to explain relevant concepts, identify regulations and guidance that provide the framework for the development of local resources for making HSR determinations, and identify types of activities that are not HSR.

Introduction

Activities that meet the federal definitions of research involving human subjects are subject to IRB oversight. The IRB has no regulatory authority to oversee activities that are legitimately classified as something other than HSR. The Department of Health and Human Services (DHHS) Office for Human Research Protections (OHRP) and the Food and Drug Administration (FDA) recommend that organizations have policies in place that identify the individual or entity authorized to determine whether or not activities are HSR (DHHS, 2016a). Most often, it is the organization's <u>HRPP</u> that is charged with making these determinations. The individual(s) determining whether an activity constitutes research involving human subjects should have the authority to represent the organization and have no direct involvement in the activity being examined. It is considered best practice for the HRPP to develop standard operating procedures and tools that describe how the organization decides when it is acceptable to classify a project as not research, or not human subjects research, and to provide written determinations to requestors. It is important for the HRPP to have these resources readily available for members of the organization.

🔗 3-1

When deciding whether an activity is research involving human subjects, one must consider the regulations, laws, codes, and guidance that the organization follows. Many organizations oversee or conduct activities that are covered by two or more sets of laws, regulations, codes, and guidance. In these cases, the organization must apply all relevant definitions of *research* and *human subject* or develop a plan that guides the HRPP in determining which definitions apply in specific research instances. It is best practice for the HRPP to define a process for making a "not HSR" determination for activities not covered by laws, regulations, codes, or guidance. Such activities may be subject to other requirements such as privacy regulations, professional standards, and ethical obligations.

🔗 11-6
🔗 1-1

Framework for Making a Determination

In order to determine whether an activity would require IRB oversight or qualify for an exemption determination, one must systematically and sequentially assess whether a project meets the definition of both (1) research *and* (2) human subjects. The order of these considerations is important, and the outcome could be different if not done sequentially.

Decision 1: Is the Activity Research?

🔗 11-6

The Common Rule at **45 CFR 46.102(l)** and the Health Insurance Portability and Accountability Act (HIPAA) (DHHS, 2013) define *research* as "a systematic investigation, including research development, testing, and evaluation, designed to develop or contribute to generalizable knowledge." When evaluating a specific project, it is useful to think of this definition as involving two key elements: (1) whether the project involves a *systematic investigation* and (2) whether the design, meaning the goal, purpose, or intent, of the investigation is to develop or contribute to *generalizable knowledge*.

The first of these elements—the use of a systematic investigation—may be a characteristic of both research and nonresearch projects. Public health practice, quality assessment (QA) and quality improvement (QI) programs, resource utilization reviews, and outcome analyses are examples of nonresearch activities that frequently use statistical analyses and other scientific methods to collect and analyze data in a manner that is identical to that of research studies. All medical activities involve a systematic approach to data collection and analysis, but the use of a systematic investigation does not mean that an activity should be classified as research.

The second element of the definition of research is that the primary reason for conducting the activity is to develop or contribute to generalizable knowledge. Just as with the first element of the definition of research (a systematic investigation), this second element is not unique to research activities. For example, the main purpose of most education programs is to bring new knowledge to as many people as possible. Similarly, an integral part of many quality assessment and improvement

FDA DEFINITIONS

The FDA uses the term *clinical investigation* to define scope of activities considered to be research. Clinical investigation means "any experiment that involves a test article and one or more human subjects and that either is subject to requirements for prior submission to the FDA, or the results of which are intended to be later submitted to, or held for inspection by, the Food and Drug Administration as part of an application for a research or marketing permit." **[21 CFR 56.102(c)]**

Human subject means an individual who is or becomes a participant in research, either as a recipient of the test article or as a control. A subject may be either a healthy individual or a patient. **21 CFR 56.102(e)**

projects is the dissemination of results to people who may be in a position to benefit from or act on this kind of information.

The regulations require an activity to have both features, a systematic investigation for which the primary goal is to develop or contribute to generalizable knowledge, to be classified as research. Having only one of these properties means that the activity is not research and should not be handled as such from the IRB standpoint. Since these two key features, systematic investigation and generalizable knowledge, are not defined in regulations, it is considered best practice to include working definitions germane to one's organization in standard operating procedures to ensure the proper categorization of the activity.

Decision 2: Is the Research Activity Human Subjects Research?

After a project has been determined to meet the definition of research, the next decision is whether the project involves human subjects. The Common Rule states:

1. *Human subject* means a living individual about whom an investigator (whether professional or student) conducting research:
   (i) Obtains information or biospecimens through intervention or interaction with the individual, and uses, studies, or analyzes the information or biospecimens; or
   (ii) Obtains, uses, studies, analyzes, or generates identifiable private information or identifiable biospecimens. **[45 CFR 46.102(e)(1)]**
   It further defines these terms as follows:
2. *Intervention* includes both physical procedures by which information or biospecimens are gathered (*e.g.,* venipuncture) and manipulations of the subject or the subject's environment that are performed for research purposes.
3. *Interaction* includes communication or interpersonal contact between investigator and subject.
4. *Private information* includes information about behavior that occurs in a context in which an individual can reasonably expect that no observation or recording is taking place, and information that has been provided for specific purposes by an individual and that the individual can reasonably expect will not be made public (*e.g.,* a medical record).
5. *Identifiable private information* is private information for which the identity of the subject is or may readily be ascertained by the investigator or associated with the information.
6. An *identifiable biospecimen* is a biospecimen for which the identity of the subject is or may readily be ascertained by the investigator or associated with the biospecimen. **[45 CFR 46.102(e)(2)-(6)]**

Office for Human Research Protections (2017) Federal Policy for the Protection of Human Subjects. https://www.federalregister .gov/documents/2017/01/19/2017-01058/federal-policy-for-the-protection-of-human-subjects#p-1290

An activity will require IRB review if it is determined to be both research and involve human subjects. To aid the determination, OHRP provides a decision chart entitled, "Is an Activity Research Involving Human Subjects Covered by 45 CFR Part 46?" (DHHS, 2020).

Except for some special types of projects (e.g., FDA Expanded Access, humanitarian use devices), activities that do not meet the federal definitions of *research* and *human subject* do not require (as a matter of regulation) IRB review or oversight.

🔗 11-4
🔗 11-5

Activities That Are Not Research or Human Subjects Research

Select activities have been "deemed not to be research" under the Common Rule. When all conditions are met, these four activities are deemed not to be research [**45 CFR 46.102(l)(1-4)**]:

1. "Scholarly and journalistic activities (e.g., oral history, journalism, biography, literary criticism, legal research, and historical scholarship), including the collection and use of information, that focus directly on the specific individuals about whom the information is collected" [**45 CFR 46.102(l)(1)**] and not on generalizing the information or findings to other individuals.

   OHRP draft guidance explains how scholarly and journalistic activities must be conducted solely for the primary intent of the activity in question to not be considered human subjects research. For example, an oral history project being done solely for collecting oral history interviews for archiving in a repository to be made available to the public for future use and historic preservation would not be considered research. However, a project that is designed to contribute to generalizable knowledge that happens to involve the use of oral histories and is being conducted for both purposes (i.e., contributing to generalizable knowledge and collecting oral history interviews), whether the interviews will be deposited into an archive, may still meet the definition of research and require IRB review (DHHS, 2018a).

2. "Public health surveillance activities, including the collection and testing of information or biospecimens, conducted, supported, requested, ordered, required, or authorized by a public health authority." [**45 CFR 46.102(l)(2)**] The intent is to prevent the regulation from impeding a public health authority's ability to accomplish its mandated mission to protect and maintain the health and welfare of the population.

   According to OHRP guidance, the applicability of the public health surveillance activities exclusion depends on the purpose of the project, the context in which it is conducted, and the role of the public health authority (DHHS, 2018b).

   Such activities are limited to those necessary to allow a public health authority to identify, monitor, assess, or investigate potential public health signals, onsets of disease outbreaks, or conditions of public health importance (including trends, signals, risk factors, patterns in diseases, or increases in injuries from using consumer products). Such activities include those associated with providing timely situational awareness and priority setting during the course of an event or crisis that threatens public health (including natural or man-made disasters). See OHRP Public Health Surveillance guidance for additional information on this exclusion (DHHS, 2018b).

3. "Collection and analysis of information, biospecimens, or records by or for a criminal justice agency for activities authorized by law or court order solely for criminal justice or criminal investigative purposes." [**45 CFR 46.102(l)(3)**]

4. "Authorized operational activities (as determined by each agency) in support of intelligence, homeland security, defense, or other national security missions." [**45 CFR 46.102(l)(4)**]

Quality Improvement or Research?

In 2006, the Hastings Center published a report recognizing QI as "any systematic, data-guided activity that is designed to bring about the immediate improvement of care in a local setting" and further noting that, while QI uses a wide variety of methods, they all involve deliberate actions to improve care, guided by data reflecting the effects (Hastings Center, 2006). QI is focused not on defining the standard of care or best practice but rather on identifying problems associated with the standard of care, implementing and monitoring corrective action, and studying its effectiveness. In contrast, research is focused on seeking knowledge that may inform or define the standard of care or best practice.

It is sometimes challenging for the researcher and the reviewer to determine whether a QI project also meets the definition of research involving human subjects. OHRP has issued relevant guidance in the form of FAQs, which provide the following interpretations (DHHS, 2019):

- DHHS regulations do not apply to QI activities whose purposes are limited to: "(a) implementing a practice to improve the quality of patient care, and (b) collecting patient or provider data regarding the implementation of the practice for clinical, practical, or administrative purposes."
- DHHS regulations do not apply to QI activities if their purposes are limited to: "(a) delivering healthcare, and (b) measuring and reporting provider performance data for clinical, practical, or administrative uses."
- "Intent to publish is an insufficient criterion for determining whether a quality improvement activity involves research." However, in certain cases, a quality improvement project may constitute human subjects research. For example, if a project involves introducing an untested clinical intervention for purposes which include not only improving the quality of care but also collecting information about patient outcomes for the purpose of establishing scientific evidence to determine how well the intervention achieves its intended results, that quality improvement project may also constitute nonexempt human subjects research under the DHHS regulations.

These interpretations may be extrapolated to QI activities conducted in non-healthcare settings such as education, academia, or community.

If a project is originally initiated as a local QI project but the findings are of interest and the project investigator chooses to expand the findings into a human subjects research study, IRB review is required at that time. The project investigator turned researcher should clearly indicate to the IRB that the data were originally collected as part of a QI project. The IRB should be prepared to handle this type of review and take the next steps as required of all human subjects research projects (e.g., consideration of whether the activity is exempt or requires expedited or convened IRB review; whether consent is required or waiver of consent is appropriate, etc.).

When Is Informed Consent or Authorization a Consideration?

HIPAA allows projects conducted within a covered entity with the intent of obtaining information related to treatment, payment, or healthcare operations to be conducted without additional patient authorization. Patients should be made aware of these uses of their data via the privacy notice required by HIPAA. A QI project

🔗 11-6

may be appropriately initiated without patient authorization or consent; however, consideration must be given to whether or not healthcare workers should be aware of and possibly required to consent to the project. These are decisions that must be well thought out by the initiators of the QI teams at the institution.

On the other hand, human subjects research is not covered under the HIPAA "treatment, payment, or health care operations" [**45 CFR 164.501**] exemptions, and therefore, if research is being conducted, the requirements for waiving informed consent and/or waiving the requirements for documentation of informed consent must be met.

✏ 6-4 ✏ 6-5

Other Activities That Are Often Deemed Not Research or Human Subjects Research

IRB review is required when an activity meets both the federal definition of *research* and *human subjects*. Some activities only partially meet the applicable definitions, and these are commonly designated as not human subjects research ("not HSR"). However, such activities may be subject to privacy regulations or other organizational policies.

Quality Assessment

Quality assessment involves activities that are designed to determine whether aspects of practice are being performed in line with established standards.

Quality Assurance

Quality assurance is defined as "a program for the systematic monitoring and evaluation of the various aspects of a project, service, or facility to ensure that standards of quality are being met" (Merriam-Webster, 2019). It generally requires participation of or information on all or most individuals receiving a particular treatment or undergoing a particular practice or process. In some states, this term is used in health care, specifically for reviewing, analyzing, or evaluating patient- and/or provider-specific data that may indicate the need for changes in systems or procedures that would improve the quality of care. The review is often triggered by predetermined "thresholds/criteria." Generally, the analysis is conducted by an entity authorized to act on the findings to make improvements. The knowledge generated is typically for immediate local application.

Case Reports and Case Series

A physician requests access to his or her patient's medical record to prepare a "case report" for publication in a medical journal. The first step is to determine whether the project contains both of the elements from the regulatory definition of research (a systematic investigation and the intent to contribute to generalizable knowledge). In our opinion, it is not reasonable to suggest that the organization of information for a case report constitutes a systematic investigation to the extent that would be expected of a research project. Because the first element of the regulatory definition of research is not present, this project is not research and, therefore, is beyond the regulatory authority of the IRB. In our opinion, this kind of case report project is most appropriately classified as an educational or descriptive activity. Care should be taken, however, to distinguish a case report from an "n-of-1" research study in which there is systematic manipulation of an intervention to produce generalizable results.

When discussing the classification of case series projects, many people ask whether the inclusion of more than one patient, client, or individual requires that the project be classified as research. In our opinion, the number of individuals is not a defining factor. Descriptive activities of anecdotal experiences often involve discussion of the course of a group of patients. It is the use of statistical methods, such as subgroup comparisons, and tests for prognostic factors that are the distinguishing features of a systematic investigation. In the absence of the basic elements of a systematic investigation of a scientific question, the case report project should be classified as an educational or descriptive activity rather than research, regardless of the number of individuals that form the basis for the discussion. However, some organizations have established a threshold of a report of four or more individuals to require IRB review. Any organizational limits should be described in the tools provided to project investigators.

Some journal editors, such as the International Committee of Medical Journal Editors (ICMJE), may expect "IRB approval" for case report and case series projects when they are published. It is our opinion that a written determination stating that the project does not meet the definition of research involving human subjects will meet journal editor requirements. In the event a case report or case series cannot be published or presented without the potential for identifying the patients (including publication of patients with a rare disease), HIPAA privacy rules apply, and permission from the patient(s) must be obtained before use of the data (ICMJE, 2019).

Medical Practice and Innovative Therapy

A commonly cited definition of *medical practice* describes an activity that is designed solely to enhance the well-being of an individual patient. A type of medical practice that is often confused with research is a class of activities that has been called "innovative therapy." Innovative therapy describes an activity that is designed solely to benefit an individual patient(s), but for which the ability of the activity to result in the desired outcome is, to some degree, unproven. Levine has suggested that a better term for this class of activity is "non-validated practice" (Levine, 2008). As long as the intent remains focused on patient well-being and does not evolve into systematic assessment with results, conclusions, and dissemination, the activity is not research. In addition, FDA information sheets indicate that "off-label" use of a marketed product when the intent is the "practice of medicine" does not require the submission of an investigational new drug application (IND), investigational device exemption (IDE), or review by an IRB (FDA, 1998).

🔗 11-2
🔗 11-3

Public Health Practice

Public health practice is similar to medical practice for the benefit of others, in that the activity involves people who do not directly benefit from the intervention. The most common situation in which there is confusion about the distinction between a public health practice and research is with public health practices that require the review of identifiable private information about health status. Examples of public health practices that often do not involve research include surveillance (e.g., monitoring of diseases) and program evaluation (e.g., immunization coverage or use of clinical preventive services such as mammography).

Resource Utilization Review

Medical record review is often conducted to evaluate the use of resources in a specific healthcare activity. Terms such as *cost control* are used to describe this class of activity, but the terms *utilization review* or *resource utilization review* are more general and often more accurately reflect the fundamental goal of projects in this category. Although a research project may involve review of resource utilization, a resource utilization review usually refers to a nonresearch activity.

Education

The transferring of information from one group of people to another is a common activity in all aspects of society. As we explained earlier in this chapter, the regulatory definition of research focuses on the desire to develop or contribute to "generalizable knowledge." The reason to mention education in the context of a discussion about the definition of research is that it is important to recognize that the goal of most educational activities is to spread or "generalize" knowledge. The fact that an activity is undertaken for the specific purpose of teaching somebody something does not mean that the activity involves research.

Classroom Assignments

Class projects designed for educational purposes that teach research methods or demonstrate course concepts do not meet the definition of research. The activities take place within the term of the course and are not intended to create new knowledge or contribute to generalizable knowledge. Instructors have an obligation to ensure students involved in course projects meet professional and ethical standards.

Program Evaluation

Program evaluation is a systematic method for collecting, analyzing, and using information to answer questions about projects, policies, and programs, particularly about their effectiveness and efficiency. Findings are expected to direct improvements to the program or project, rather than contribute to generalizable knowledge, and so do not meet the definition of research.

Use of Decedent Data

Federal research regulations requiring IRB oversight only apply to living individuals. Data obtained from individuals who are deceased prior to the conduct of the research are in existence prior to collection. However, organizations may exclude fetal tissue from this not-HSR determination process and require IRB review to ensure such research meets the highest ethical standards, state laws, and funding agency requirements. For instance, the NIH Policy for Human Fetal Tissue Research requires informed consent from donors for any NIH-funded research using human fetal tissue (NIH, 2018a, 2019).

Research with Publicly Available Data Sets

Publicly available data sets provide open access to information for research purposes without conditions of use and may be deemed not HSR, since the information in such data sets is typically not identifiable or, by definition, private.

Coded Private Information or Specimens Use in Research

🔗 10-10   Private information or <u>biological specimens</u> are not considered individually identifiable when they cannot be linked to specific individuals by the researcher(s). According to guidance:

"OHRP does not consider research involving **only** coded private information or specimens to involve human subjects as defined under 45 CFR 46.102(f) if the following conditions are both met:

1. the private information or specimens were not collected specifically for the currently proposed research project through an interaction or intervention with living individuals; and
2. the investigator(s) cannot readily ascertain the identity of the individual(s) to whom the coded private information or specimens pertain because, for example:
   a. the investigators and the holder of the key enter into an agreement prohibiting the release of the key to the investigators under any circumstances, until the individuals are deceased (note that the HHS regulations do not require the IRB to review and approve this agreement);
   b. there are IRB-approved written policies and operating procedures for a repository or data management center that prohibit the release of the key to the investigators under any circumstances, until the individuals are deceased; or
   c. there are other legal requirements prohibiting the release of the key to the investigators, until the individuals are deceased." (DHHS, 2008a)

Often, the specimens or information is obtained from a public or commercial source or from an "honest broker" or "bank custodian," who acts as a neutral intermediary, providing a firewall between the subject and the researcher. If the individual providing the data or specimen is involved in the conduct, analysis, or reporting of the research, the activity would be considered human subjects research. This is also the case when anyone involved in the research can readily identify subjects through treatment relationships, has prior knowledge of scheduled procedures involving procurement of desired specimens, or access to the code or information that may be used to re-identify subjects. Providers frequently require data use agreements to outline the restrictions and terms of use. The NIH decision chart (**Figure 5.1-1**) may aid in determining whether research involving private information or biological specimens constitutes research with human subjects (DHHS, 2020). Last, some funding agencies have policies, such as the NIH Genomic Data Sharing (GDS) Policy, that require IRB review for select activities that technically do not meet the DHHS federal definitions of human subjects research (NIH, 2014).

Criteria for deidentification of protected health information (PHI) differ, as some codes are considered identifiable under the Privacy Rule and not under the Common Rule. (For more information, see Chapter 11-6, "HIPAA and Research.)

Relevant Questions to Ask When Making a Human Subjects Research Determination

In order for the reviewer to make a written determination regarding whether an activity is or is not human subjects research, we suggest that information be requested from the project investigator relevant to the following general considerations:

- Is the activity designed (and/or implemented) for organizational purposes in support of the organization's mission? The intent should be clear in the purpose/

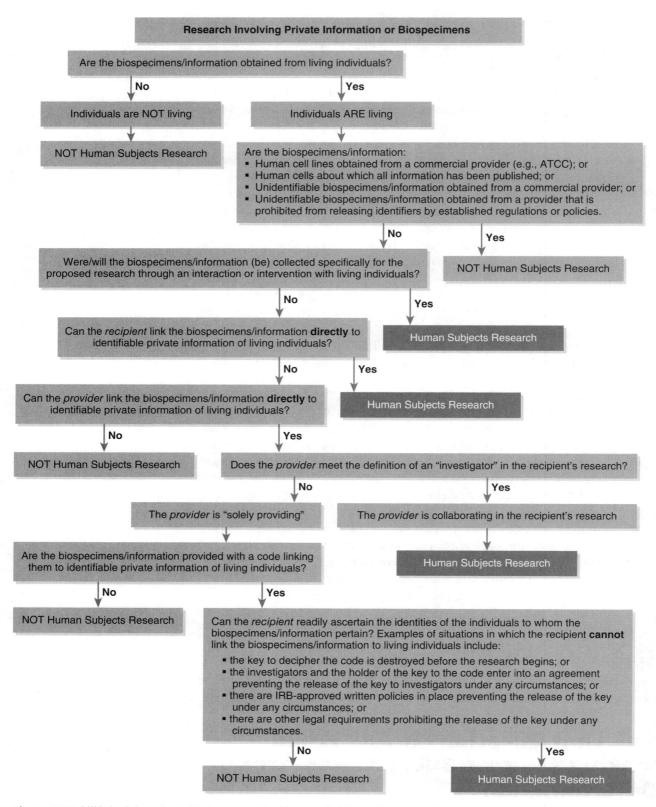

Figure 5.1-1 NIH decision chart 01: Is an Activity Human Subjects Research Covered by 45 CFR Part 46?

National Institutes of Health (NIH). (2005). Decision Chart for Research Involving Private Information or Biological Specimens. https://grants.nih.gov/grants/policy/hs/PrivateInfoOrBioSpecimensDecisionChart.pdf

aim statement for the specific project. In general, QI projects are aimed at improving local systems of care (nongeneralizable), and results are intended to be rapidly implemented. If the intent is to promote "betterment" of a process of care, clinical outcome, etc., then the project may be considered QI.

- Are the activity's findings designed to be used by and within the organization?
- Is the activity designed for the purpose of contributing to generalizable knowledge that expands the knowledge base of a scientific discipline or other scholarly field of study?
- Has the activity been funded by a federal/external agency as "human subjects research," thus requiring IRB oversight? Governmental agencies, such as NIH, have the final say as to whether an activity is considered research (NIH, 2018b). If there is question, seek a determination from the funding agency.
- Does the activity meet the FDA definition of a *clinical investigation requiring IRB review*? (see Sidebar, FDA Definitions). Design characteristics indicative of clinical investigations include use of double-blind or randomized intervention, placebo controls, an element that may be considered outside of standard of care, or involving individuals who would not normally receive the intervention under study.
- Will the project impose risks or burdens beyond the standard of practice in order to make the results generalizable?

Once the determination is made, it is important to communicate the determination to the project investigator. It is also important to inform the requestor that if the purpose or design of the activity changes or is modified significantly, IRB review may be required at that time. The changes should be brought forward for a new determination.

Doesn't Publication Make It Research?

Historically, when considering whether a project met the definition of research, HRPPs/IRBs often based the determination on the assumption that publication of results in a scientific journal met the threshold of contributing to generalizable knowledge. OHRP's FAQ on this topic clearly states that the intent to publish is an insufficient criterion for determining whether a quality improvement activity involves research (DHHS, 2019). Planning to publish an account of an activity does not necessarily mean that the project fits the definition of research; people seek to publish descriptions of nonresearch activities for a variety of reasons if they believe others may be interested in learning about those activities. Conversely, a project may involve research even if there is no intent to publish the results.

It is appropriate to inform project investigators that nonresearch activities can be published, but it is necessary to remind them that the term *research* cannot be contained within the publication. If the term *research* is used to describe the project, IRB review is required, and journal editors may inquire about the status of IRB review. A best practice would be to include the phrase "a quality improvement initiative" in the title of the presentation or publication.

Would You Conduct This Project as Planned If You Knew You Would Never Receive Any Form of Academic Recognition for It?

To classify projects accurately as either research or nonresearch, a critical factor may be the extent to which the project is being conducted to benefit people other than those who will participate directly in the activity. Questions about the publication or presentation of results in an academic forum are the most useful way to evaluate research intent, but the focus of the question should be different from what it was historically.

The important question is not whether the project investigator might want to publish or present results in the future, but rather if the project would be done as planned if academic recognition is definitely not a possibility. Members of the HRPP community have recommended that the following question be used to determine whether a project that involves a systematic investigation, and that is likely to develop generalizable knowledge, should be classified as research from the regulatory standpoint:

> Would this project be conducted as proposed if the project investigator knew that they would never receive any form of academic recognition for the project, including publication of results in a medical journal or presentation of the project at an academic meeting?

> If prohibition from receiving any form of academic recognition for the project would affect the conduct of the project in any way, then research is likely a motive for the activity to a degree that the project should be classified as research from the regulatory standpoint.

Conclusion

The evaluation of whether a project meets the criteria for it to be deemed human subjects research is an often challenging yet crucial role of the HRPP. It is important to understand that nonresearch activities may use scientific methods and produce results that are suitable for publication in a medical journal; however, these elements in and of themselves are not sufficient to be considered research. A fundamental goal of research is to learn something that will benefit future individuals (not the subjects enrolled in the research study) and expand the knowledge base of the scientific or scholarly community. Applying research regulations to nonresearch activities can be like trying to put a square peg in a round hole, and it may unnecessarily divert limited HRPP resources and attention from the primary objective of ensuring the protection of human subjects. Having a set of well-defined processes and tools for making these determinations is invaluable for the project investigators and the organization.

References

Department of Health and Human Services (DHHS). (2008a). *Coded private information or specimens use in research: Guidance*. www.hhs.gov/ohrp/regulations-and-policy/guidance/research-involving-coded-private-information/index.html

Department of Health and Human Services (DHHS). (2013). *Office for Civil Rights: Summary of the Health Insurance Portability and Accountability Act*. www.hhs.gov/hipaa/for-professionals/privacy/laws-regulations/index.html

Department of Health and Human Services Protections (DHHS). (2016a). *Institutional review board (IRB) written procedures: Guidance for institutions and IRBs draft guidance*. www.hhs.gov/ohrp/regulations-and-policy/requests-for-comments/guidance-for-institutions-and-irbs/index.html

Department of Health and Human Services (DHHS). (2018a). *Scholarly and journalistic activities deemed not to be research: Draft guidance*. www.hhs.gov/ohrp/regulations-and-policy/requests-for-comments/draft-guidance-scholarly-and-journalistic-activities-deemed-not-to-be-research/index.html

Department of Health and Human Services (DHHS). (2018b). *Activities deemed not to be research: Public health surveillance draft guidance.* www.hhs.gov/ohrp/regulations-and-policy/requests-for-comments/draft-guidance-activities-deemed-not-be-research-public-health-surveillance/index.html

Department of Health and Human Services (DHHS). (2019). *Quality improvement activities FAQs.* www.hhs.gov/ohrp/regulations-and-policy/guidance/faq/quality-improvement-activities/index.html

Department of Health and Human Services (DHHS). (2020). *Chart 01: Is an activity human subjects research covered by 45 CFR Part 46?* www.hhs.gov/ohrp/regulations-and-policy/decision-charts-2018/index.html#c1

Food and Drug Administration (FDA). (1998). *"Off-label" and investigational use of marketed drugs, biologics, and medical devices.* www.fda.gov/regulatory-information/search-fda-guidance-documents/label-and-investigational-use-marketed-drugs-biologics-and-medical-devices

Hasting Center. (2006). *The ethics of using QI methods to improve health care quality and safety.* www.thehastingscenter.org/wp-content/uploads/The-Ethics-of-Using-QI-Methods.pdf

International Committee of Medical Journal Editors (ICMJE). (2019). *Protection of research participants.* www.icmje.org/recommendations/browse/roles-and-responsibilities/protection-of-research-participants.html

Levine, R. J. (2008). The nature, scope, and justification of clinical research. In E. Emanuel, C. Grady, R. A. Crouch, R. Lie, F. G. Miller, & D. Wendler (Eds.), *The Oxford textbook of clinical research ethics.* Oxford University Press.

Merriam-Webster Dictionary. (2019). *Quality assurance.* www.merriam-webster.com/dictionary/quality%20assurance

National Institutes of Health (NIH). (2005). *Decision chart for research involving private information or biological specimens.* grants.nih.gov/grants/policy/hs/PrivateInfoOrBioSpecimensDecisionChart.pdf

National Institutes of Health (NIH). (2014). *Genomic data sharing policy.* osp.od.nih.gov/scientific-sharing/genomic-data-sharing/

National Institutes of Health (NIH). (2018a). *Policy on human fetal tissue research.* grants.nih.gov/grants/policy/nihgps/html5/section_4/4.1.14_human_fetal_tissue_research.htm

National Institutes of Health (NIH). (2018b). *Grants policy statement.* grants.nih.gov/grants/policy/nihgps/html5/section_4/4.1.15_human_subjects_protections.htm

National Institutes of Health (NIH). (2019). *Changes to NIH requirements regarding proposed human fetal tissue research.* grants.nih.gov/grants/guide/notice-files/NOT-OD-19-128.html

Human Subjects Research Not Subject to the Common Rule: Flexibility and Alternate Paths

Linda (Petree) Mayo

Sharon Zack

Abstract

In the preamble to the 2018 Common Rule, the Department of Health and Human Services (DHHS) included the plan to eliminate the option to extend an institution's Federalwide Assurance (FWA) to non-federally funded human research. Although this change to the FWA application process has not occurred at the time of this writing, the Office for Human Research Protections (OHRP) nevertheless has never required or encouraged institutions to choose this option. Choosing not to strictly apply federal regulations to all human subjects research (HSR) provides institutions with opportunities to apply flexible and specific equivalent protections intended to reduce administrative burden and streamline review processes. The purpose of this chapter is to learn how to integrate flexibility into IRB policies in a way that reflects fundamental ethical principles such as respect for persons and beneficence and how to clearly delineate research that can be reviewed under flexible policies.

Background

With the implementation of the 2018 Common Rule in January of 2019, DHHS planned to implement a proposed nonregulatory change to the assurance mechanism, eliminating the option for institutions to voluntarily extend the FWA to non-federally funded research. The preamble to the 2018 Common Rule notes that, "As a result, the final rule continues to allow institutions the same wide degree of flexibility that they currently have with regard to making

✐ 8-1

other similar determinations regarding ethical oversight of research not regulated by the Common Rule" (Federal Register, 2017, Preamble, p. 7156). Prior to that time, U.S. institutions had the option to voluntarily pledge to conduct all nonexempt human subjects research, regardless of funding source, in compliance with the Common Rule or the Common Rule and subparts B, C, and D of 45 CFR 46—often referred to as "checking the box" on the assurance form. In 2013, OHRP reported that two-thirds of U.S. institutions elected to apply the Common Rule to all of their research (Blatt, Makle, & Stith-Coleman, 2013).

With the elimination of this option—or, until this change is implemented, when institutions "uncheck the box"—research at an institution that is neither conducted nor supported by a Common Rule agency is no longer subject to OHRP oversight. This enables institutions to use flexible approaches for the management and oversight of non-federally funded research, with the goal of reducing administrative burden while maintaining equivalent protections of human research subjects. Some institutions that were early adopters of flexible policies (or "flex policies") include the University of Michigan (University of Michigan, 2019) and the University of Southern California (U.S.C., 2019). The efforts of the U.S.C.-based Flexibility Coalition are reflected in many of the 2018 Common Rule changes specific to exemptions and continuing review.

Institutions and Flex Policies

2-1

Before implementing flex policies within a human research protection program (HRPP), it is important to consider whether it is prudent in the context of an institution's overall research portfolio. For example, if the vast majority of studies are federally funded, the HRPP may be more efficient and less subject to errors if it reviews all human research under a single set of policies. Another consideration is frequency of collaborative research that requires engagement in IRB reliance agreements. If the institution enters into reliance agreements for a significant number of studies, flex policies may be discouraged, as some agreements may mandate or expect review under Common Rule regulations. Alternatively, institutions providing federally mandated single IRB services may want to ensure that their reliance agreements, if used, clearly identify whether nonregulated studies will be reviewed under flex policies. Other considerations include contractual obligations or restrictions that preclude eligibility for use of flex policies.

Section 4
4-1

4-2

Identifying Eligible Studies

5-1

It is important to clearly distinguish studies that are eligible to be reviewed using flex policies from those that are not. The institution's policies and procedures should clearly identify who is authorized to determine whether studies are subject to the requirements of 45 CFR 46 and lay out clear processes and criteria for using flex policies. Many institutions use a checklist to determine and document eligibility for flex policies. A sample checklist is shown in **Figure 5.2-1**.

Developing Flexible Policies

2-3

There are various ways to implement flexibility into IRB policies and procedures. For instance, an institution might begin with language from federal regulations and then indicate where policies and procedures for non-federally funded research may differ from federal regulations. Flex policies should meet

Available Flexibility Initiatives-Checklist

Section I: MANDATORY

"Unchecked Box"	*Notes*
Uncheck all boxes on Federalwide Assurance (FWA) **or** check box for Subpart A but uncheck Subparts B, C, D (allows for different flexibilities)	
Flex Policy	
For studies that are no greater than minimal risk	
For studies with no federal funding	
Provide equivalent protections to subjects commensurate with risk level	
Exclusions to Flexibility	
Exclude greater than minimal risk studies	
Exclude no-cost extension studies	
Exclude projects in which a student is paid or supported from a federal training grant or otherwise paid or supported from the faculty advisors' federal funds	
Exclude federally-sponsored studies, including federal training grants	
Exclude studies with FDA-regulated components	
Exclude studies with contractual obligations or restrictions that preclude eligibility in this policy	
Exclude studies with clinical interventions Exclude studies using prisoners as subjects Exclude studies seeking or obtaining Certificates of Confidentiality	
Standard Operating Procedures (SOPs)	
Flex policy can be integrated in IRB Policies and Procedures (e.g., revise applicable sections) or be a stand-alone policy Implement campus-specific policy, if necessary (Socio-Behavioral Research vs. Biomedical)	

Figure 5.2-1 Sample checklist to determine and document eligibility for flex policies.
Used with permission from University of Southern California OPRS.

local needs and restrictions, such as consideration of whether to apply them to both social, behavioral, and educational research (SBER) and biomedical research, or whether to implement one overarching flex policy versus integrating flexibility throughout all relevant policies and procedures. An institution might choose to develop one policy for all research not covered by the FWA. This policy would include eligibility criteria, as noted previously, and would delineate review standards that deviate from federal regulations (such as additional exempt or expedited review categories, less frequent or no continuing review, less stringent application of subpart regulations, alternative consent waiver options, etc.). Alternatively, a specific flex policy, such as one on conducting research with <u>vulnerable populations</u>, can specify that non-federally funded minimal risk research will not be reviewed under subpart regulations. Regardless of how flexibility is implemented, it is imperative to have a robust staff preview process to ensure appropriate triage of federally funded and Food and Drug Administration (FDA)-regulated research.

⬥ Section 9

It is important to ground flex policies on the same foundational ethical principles on which the Common Rule is based and to consider using (or continuing to use) the criteria at 45 CFR 46.111 as a basis for approval of all human research. Flexibility can include a less rigorous application of subpart B, C, and D regulations, such as eliminating application of subpart B for most, if not all, minimal risk research involving pregnant women; accepting only one parent signature for child participation where two are normally required under regulation; and waiving child assent.

🖉 9-4
🖉 9-6

🖉 5-5   Institutions may consider using expedited review procedures for minimal risk studies that would not otherwise be eligible for expedited review under the provisions at 45 CFR 46.110(b)(1)(i). Examples include research that nominally exceeds the standards for expedited review, such as minimally invasive tissue collection, performance of intense exercise (e.g., VO2 max), blood draws via indwelling catheter, or radiation exposure of ≤1 mSv per year.

🖉 5-3   Similarly, flex policies may be used to exempt categories of research not explicitly addressed in the regulations at 45 CFR 46.104. Examples include minimal risk surveys involving children as subjects or research involving the collection of nonsensitive data via video or audio recording or use of noninvasive eye-tracking technology.

When considering and developing processes that expand the use of expedited review procedures or exemption, thought should be given to the composition of the institution's overall research portfolio and the reviewers' (whether IRB members or HRPP staff) understanding of risks of common procedures. Steps should be taken to ensure that IRB reviewers feel comfortable with less rigorous requirements and that there is consensus that adequate protections are being applied. It is also important to consider the researchers' expertise in addition to any compliance-related issues when implementing less rigorous policies.

Developing Flexible IRB Processes

There are also opportunities to incorporate flexibility in the IRB submission and review process. Policies should allow for the least restrictive level of review and allow qualified staff (e.g., those who are CIP-certified) to serve as designated reviewers. Flexibility empowers IRB staff by giving them responsibilities that are typically assigned to IRB members. Institutions can make choices in how they process and review amendments, renewal submissions, and in reporting procedures for studies approved under flex policies. Some may decide that only amendments involving a potential increase in risk of harm to subjects need to be reviewed by the IRB, while all other amendments can be reviewed by the HRPP or other qualified staff. It is important to note that staff do not need to be IRB members in order to be designated reviewers under flex policies. Regarding initial applications for IRB review, IRBs can be more permissive with respect to the amount of detail they typically require in a minimal risk protocol so that review of modifications to the research are not necessary (e.g., the range of subjects to be enrolled instead of an exact number; general recruitment strategies instead of specific scripts).

🖉 7-1

🖉 5-3   Recently, one innovative HRPP piloted an exemption self-determination tool for exempt categories 1, 2, and 3. In this model, the researcher is permitted to issue a system-generated exemption determination letter based on responses to key questions within qualifying exemption categories. This IRB does not review self-determined exempt studies; however, the institution did implement a post-determination validation process by IRB staff to ensure that the exemption criteria are being applied in accordance with regulatory requirements and that the potential risk to human subjects remains minimal (University of Michigan, 2019).

Institutions may consider similar self-determination models for other types of human subjects research that are not subject to federal regulations.

Consistent with the effort to reduce administrative burden on the researcher and IRB, institutions might consider eliminating or reducing common nonregulatory requirements related to IRB review such as "approval stamping" informed consent documents and recruitment materials and formally approving meeting minutes. Institutions might also consider relaxing engagement requirements for unfunded collaborative research, including limiting the use of IRB reliance agreements; instead, alternative forms of communication can be used to document collaborations. Last, IRB policies might allow a brief (30-day) grace period after expiration of the previous approval, for processing of the application for continuing approval, before study activities must stop.

Postapproval Monitoring

When continuing review is not required under 45 CFR 46.109(f), many institutions may still choose to maintain oversight of minimal risk human research by creating a brief status report to check in on the study and/or extend the research approval period beyond the current term. This can be done simply through email communication. This same procedure can be implemented under flex policies for studies that might otherwise require continuing review under 45 CFR 46. In addition, IRBs that do require formal continuing review of non-federally funded research can consider flexibility in determining the length of IRB approval. Policies can also employ more flexible criteria for determining when a study can be closed to ongoing monitoring and review. If closure requirements are met, studies can be administratively closed by IRB staff.

Research studies that are outside the scope of the FWA are not subject to the same requirements as studies under federal oversight for reporting of serious or continuing noncompliance, suspensions or terminations, adverse events, or reporting of unanticipated problems involving risk to subjects or others. Institutions with flex policies do not need to report those matters to the federal agencies, but instead should follow established internal institutional reporting requirements.

Finally, it is important to keep records and metrics specific to research approved under flex policies to document quality assurance and to assess whether implementation of such policies resulted in improvements to the program.

⊘ 7-4

⊘ 7-2

⊘ 7-7

Informed Consent

There are many opportunities for flexibility with regard to the informed consent process. Researchers may use simple information sheets that may or may not include federally required elements, depending on the nature of the study. The requirement for signature can be waived for most, if not all, minimal risk research. The IRB can also eliminate the use of federally mandated requirements when granting waivers or modifications of some or all of the elements of informed consent. Requirements surrounding the use of legally authorized representatives to enroll subjects may also be flexible in certain jurisdictions.

⊘ Section 6

⊘ 6-4

Special Populations

When conducting research with pregnant women, institutions may decide not to apply subpart B, if the IRB considers it appropriate. Institutions can also

⊘ 9-4

apply flexible policies with regard to specific criteria under subpart B, such as for minimal risk research in which pregnant women are only incidentally included and there is no prospect of direct benefit. Other flex approaches include only requiring permission from the mother for research with fetuses and neonates. It is also important to note that the FDA regulations do not include subpart B, so flexibility can even be considered when reviewing FDA-regulated research.

● 9-5   Some institutions choose not to allow research with <u>prisoners</u> to be reviewed under flex policies. The inclusion of prisoners should not be a barrier to the use of flex policies. Institutions may choose to voluntarily apply the substantive portions of subpart C, while exercising flexibility in the scope. For example, policies may narrow the definition of *prisoner* and may not consider persons in transitional custody (e.g., halfway houses, electronic monitoring, and house arrest) or subjects who become incarcerated incidentally after enrollment to be prisoners (West Virginia University, 2019). Still others may choose not to apply subpart C regulations to research involving only secondary analysis of existing prisoner data. In addition, institutions are not required to certify approval under subpart C to OHRP for nonregulated research.

● 9-6   Research studies involving <u>children</u> are subject to the regulations and tiered review standards at **45 CFR 46 subpart D**. But for those following flexible policies, the Association for the Accreditation of Human Research Protections Programs (AAHRPP) will accept some research involving children as subjects to qualify for additional exempt determinations (e.g., survey and interview procedures; AAHRPP, n.d., Tip Sheet 27). Requirements for assent and parental permission may be altered or waived for reasons other than those outlined in **45 CFR 46.408(c)** and may not necessarily require an alternative mechanism for protecting some children (such as older adolescents and minors attending college) or require documentation of child assent (the latter of which most IRBs require, but federal regulations do not).

Conclusion

● 1-1   OHRP encourages flexibility in the preamble to the revised Common Rule (Federal Register, 2017). When considering flexibility in HRPP procedures, institutions should always keep in mind the ethical principles delineated in the *Belmont Report* (National Commission, 1979). It is important to create robust prereview and quality assurance processes to ensure research is reviewed under appropriate applicable regulations and policies. Organizations should be thoughtful in their approach to incorporating flex policies and do so where it reduces the greatest amount of administrative burden without compromising the protection of human subjects.

References

Association for the Accreditation of Human Research Protections Programs, Inc. (AAHRPP). (n.d.). *Tip sheet 27: Guidance on equivalent protections.* https://admin.aahrpp.org/Website%20 Documents/Tip_Sheet_27_Guidance_on_Equivalent_Protections.pdf

Blatt, H., Makle, J., & Stith-Coleman, I. (2013). *When the assurance comes a "knocking": Everything you need to know about OHRP's FWA and IRB registration process.* www.hhs.gov/ohrp/sites /default/files/ohrp/education/training/OHRP%20Webinars/assurances_webinar_handout2 .pdf

Federal Register. (2017). Vol. 82, No. 12. 45 CFR 46 and Preamble. www.govinfo.gov/content /pkg/FR-2017-01-19/pdf/2017-01058.pdf

National Commission for the Protection of Human Subjects of Biomedical and Behavioral Research. (1979). *The Belmont Report: Ethical principles and guidelines for the protection of human subjects in biomedical and behavioral research*. www.hhs.gov/ohrp/regulations-and-policy/belmont -report/index.html

University of Michigan, Research Ethics and Compliance. (2019). *HRPP flexibility initiatives: The Michigan initiative*. https://research-compliance.umich.edu/human-subjects/hrpp-flexibility -initiatives

University of Southern California (USC), Office for the Protection of Research Subjects. (2019). *Flexibility coalition: About*. https://oprs.usc.edu/hspp/flexibility-coalition/ West Virginia University, Office of Human Research Protection. (2019). *Flex model procedures*. https://oric .research.wvu.edu/files/d/cc838a1c-a1af-490a-ab2f-fe900ec05317/wvu-flexibility-model -procedures-v10-05-30-19.pdf

CHAPTER 5-3

Exempt Research

Teresa Doksum
Courtney Jarboe

Abstract

The Common Rule recognizes that many types of research—including many social, behavioral, and educational studies—pose little, if any, risk to subjects. To minimize regulatory burden on these types of studies, the regulations allow for exemption from the requirements of 45 CFR 46 if studies meet certain criteria. This chapter explains how IRBs determine whether or not a study is eligible for exemption, who can make this determination, and the eight categories of exemptions. It also describes issues for IRBs to consider in making these determinations and what other protections may still be needed to protect the welfare and rights of research subjects.

What Is Exempt Human Subjects Research?

The Common Rule allows some types of social, behavioral, and educational research (SBER) studies, as well as some studies involving biospecimens, to be "exempt" from the regulatory requirements [45 CFR 46.104(d)]. The purpose of exemptions is to minimize unnecessary oversight of research studies that are of benefit to the public but that pose minimal risk to subjects. The Common Rule includes eight exemption categories, some of which require "limited IRB review" to ensure protections are in place for exempt studies that have informational risks.

🖉 5-6

DEFINITION: INFORMATIONAL RISKS

The risk of harm to subjects from the loss of confidentiality of their personal information.

The regulations allow IRBs to develop their own policies regarding whether, and how, they apply the exemptions. IRBs should have clear policies and procedures to ensure consistent application of the exemptions within their institution. For example, some institutions may not allow the use of exempt categories

🖉 2-3

7 and 8 related to the storage, maintenance, and secondary use of identifiable private information or identifiable biospecimens using broad consent. In addition, in the context of collaborative research, one institution's IRB may exempt a study while another institution's IRB may not, because it has a policy of not granting exemptions. This scenario is most likely for federally funded research conducted in <u>other countries</u>, most of which do not use exemptions. IRBs should have a policy for how to handle studies that are eligible for exemption according to U.S., but not local, policies.

10-9

Considerations in Making Exempt Research Determinations

Who Makes Exempt Research Determinations?

The Common Rule does not specify who can make exempt research determinations, and IRBs vary considerably in their exemption policies and practices. For example, some institutions allow researchers to determine whether a study is eligible for exemption and others do not; some offer additional exemptions for non-federally funded research. The Department of Health and Human Services (DHHS) Office for Human Research Protections (OHRP) recommends that (1) "because of the potential for conflict of interest, investigators not be given the authority to make an independent determination that human subjects research is exempt" and (2) IRBs specify in their policies who within their institution can make the determination (DHHS, 2019a). The forms used by many IRBs include an option for researchers to request exemption under the various categories; however, a trained administrative staff person (with authority to make the determination) then reviews and confirms that the study meets the criteria. The final authority to determine if a study is eligible for exemption rests with the Common Rule agency conducting or funding the research (Federal Register, 2017, Preamble p. 7183).

What Information Do IRBs Need to Make Exempt Research Determinations?

Given the complexity of the exemption options and criteria, IRBs should ensure that their policies, processes, and forms elicit sufficient details about the study to make an accurate exemption determination. For example, IRBs should consider all planned research activities across all stages of the research study, since the overall study would not be eligible for exemption if any single research activity did not fall into one of the exemption categories [45 CFR 46.104(a)]. IRBs should also request to see data collection instruments to assess risks (e.g., informational risks, risk of psychological harm). Since many research studies

---

DEFINITION: PSYCHOLOGICAL HARMS

Note: Although the definition of psychological harms given here is from archived guidance, it may be useful for IRBs to consider.

"Participation in research may result in undesired changes in thought processes and emotion (e.g., episodes of depression, confusion, or hallucination resulting from drugs, feelings of stress, guilt, and loss of self-esteem). These changes may be either transitory, recurrent, or permanent. Most psychological risks are minimal or transitory, but IRBs should be aware that some research has the potential for causing serious psychological harm." (DHHS, 2001)

evolve over time, IRBs should prospectively assess any proposed changes to the original study design that might affect eligibility for exemption and issue an updated determination (DHHS, 2019a).

IRBs should also have enough information about the study to identify which other laws, regulations, and policies apply to the research (e.g., other countries, federal, state, tribal, local) that could affect eligibility for exemption.

Are Studies Involving Vulnerable Populations Eligible for Exemption?

The involvement of a <u>vulnerable population</u> does not automatically disqualify studies from an exemption. The Common Rule allows for the involvement of most vulnerable populations covered by <u>subparts B</u>, <u>C</u>, and <u>D</u> (**Table 5.3-1**), assuming the study activities meet the requirements of an exemption. IRBs should consider the nature or characteristics of the vulnerability to determine

🔗 9-1

🔗 9-4 🔗 9-5 🔗 9-6

Table 5.3-1 Application of Exemption Categories to Subpart Populations

Exemption Category	Subpart B Fetuses, Pregnant Women, and Human In Vitro Fertilization 45 CFR 46.104(b)(1)	Subpart C Prisoners 45 CFR 46.104(b)(2)	Subpart D Children 45 CFR 46.104(b)(3)
1 Normal Educational Practices and Settings	Each of the exemptions may be applied	None of the exemptions may be applied "except for research aimed at involving a broader subject population that only incidentally includes prisoners"	May be applied
2i Educational Tests, Surveys, Interviews, or Observations: Anonymous			May only be applied to "educational tests and observation of public behavior when the investigator(s) do not participate in the activities being observed"
2ii Educational Tests, Surveys, Interviews, or Observations: not sensitive			
2iii Educational Tests, Surveys, Interviews, or Observations: not anonymous but has limited IRB review			May not be applied
3 Benign Behavioral Interventions with Adults			May not be applied
4 Secondary Research for which Consent Is Not Required			May be applied
5 Public Benefit or Service Programs			May be applied
6 Taste and Food Quality Evaluation and Consumer Acceptance Studies			May be applied
7 Storage or Maintenance for Secondary Research for Which Broad Consent Is Required			May be applied
8 Secondary Research for Which Broad Consent Is Required			May be applied

🔗 9-7

whether the involvement of the population would qualify or disqualify the study from an exemption. For example, a study involving a benign behavioral intervention with adults who <u>lack capacity</u> to consent would not qualify for exemption under category 3 because the adult would be unable to provide prospective agreement.

2018 COMMON RULE: EXEMPTIONS FOR PRISONERS

One major change in the 2018 Common Rule is to allow exemptions for studies that might involve prisoners only incidentally, rather than as the main study population. For example, an exempt longitudinal study involving annual surveys with subjects from a nonincarcerated population may maintain exempt status even if some of those subjects become incarcerated at the time of an annual survey.

How Should IRBs Handle Ethical, Privacy, or Legal Issues for Exempt Research?

Some studies that are eligible for exemption may still need an IRB member, professional staff, or similar expert to assess the need for consent or to address privacy or legal issues. IRB experts are often the best trained to identify these issues, so some IRBs characterize their review as ethical/privacy/legal review rather than review for compliance with human subjects regulations. For example, studies that involve linking in-person surveys with administrative data

🔗 Section 6

may still need written <u>consent</u> according to the privacy laws governing the administrative data. In these cases, the IRB may deem the research exempt but choose to maintain oversight via their policy; alternatively, they may choose not to exempt the research.

🔗 8-5

IRBs may require human subjects <u>training for researchers</u>, even if they only conduct exempt research. In addition, other agencies, such as the National Institutes of Health (NIH), may also require training (NIH, n.d.). When making exempt determinations, IRBs should also check that the research team is up-to-date on any required trainings.

Food and Drug Administration Regulations Do Not Exempt Research from IRB Review

🔗 11-1

Food and Drug Administration (FDA) <u>regulations</u> for the protection of human subjects do not have categories of research that qualify for exempt status like those listed in the Common Rule. The FDA does not exempt any research under its jurisdiction from IRB review, except research in emergency circumstances and taste and food quality studies (the same as exemption category 6 under the DHHS regulations). Because the FDA primarily regulates clinical trials involving investigational drugs, biologics, and medical devices, there is no need for expanded exemptions. The FDA announced in 2018 an intent to harmonize its regulations wherever possible with the 2018 Common Rule (FDA, 2018). IRBs should stay apprised of future announcements or guidance from the FDA about any changes that may affect FDA-regulated research.

Categories of Exempt Research

The Common Rule includes eight categories of exempt research in **45 CFR 46.104(d)**. To help IRBs determine whether a study meets the criteria for an exemption, each of the following sections describes the purpose of the exemption, defines key terms, and provides examples of studies that do or do not qualify for the exemption. OHRP also provides a series of decision charts, one for each exemption category, to assist institutions with exemption determinations (DHHS, 2020).

Exemption 1: Normal Educational Practices and Settings

> Research, conducted in established or commonly accepted educational settings, that specifically involves normal educational practices that are not likely to adversely impact students' opportunity to learn required educational content or the assessment of educators who provide instruction. This includes most research on regular and special education instructional strategies, and research on the effectiveness of or the comparison among instructional techniques, curricula, or classroom management methods **45 CFR 46.104(d)(1)**.

The purpose of Exemption 1 is to minimize the regulatory burden for research on "normal educational practices" in school settings (e.g., elementary, secondary, postsecondary). "Normal educational practices" refers to instructional techniques already in use or classroom management (DHHS, 2019b). The exemption recognizes that most studies of this type can improve education for the public good with little risk to subjects. Examples of research that would fall under this category would be a study to evaluate the use of accepted or revised standardized tests or evaluation of a continuing education program. However, a randomized controlled trial with the control group receiving the "normal educational practice" and the experimental group receiving a new or innovative practice would not fall under this exemption.

CHANGES TO EXEMPTION 1 IN THE 2018 COMMON RULE

The exemption includes a minor update from the pre-2018 Common Rule: the addition of two restrictions that studies must meet in order to be eligible for this exemption, namely, that they are not likely to adversely impact (1) students' opportunity to learn required educational content or (2) the assessment of educators who provide instruction. The purpose of these restrictions is to exclude research studies that "might draw enough time and attention away from the delivery of the regular educational curriculum that they could have a detrimental effect on student achievement" (Federal Register, 2017, Preamble p. 7186). These types of studies would require review by the IRB to ensure the research had procedures in place to mitigate this risk.

Exemption 2: Educational Tests, Surveys, Interviews, or Observations

> Research that only includes interactions involving educational tests (cognitive, diagnostic, aptitude, achievement), survey procedures, interview procedures, or observation of public behavior (including visual or auditory recording) if at least one of the following criteria is met:
>
> (i) The information obtained is recorded by the investigator in such a manner that the identity of the human subjects cannot readily be ascertained, directly or through identifiers linked to the subjects;
>
> (ii) Any disclosure of the human subjects' responses outside the research would not reasonably place the subjects at risk of criminal or civil liability or be damaging to the subjects' financial standing, employability, educational advancement, or reputation; or
>
> (iii) The information obtained is recorded by the investigator in such a manner that the identity of the human subjects can readily be

ascertained, directly or through identifiers linked to the subjects, and an IRB conducts a limited IRB review to make the determination required by §46.111(a)(7) 45 CFR 46.104(d)(2).

CHANGES TO EXEMPTION 2 IN THE 2018 COMMON RULE

The updates to this exemption category include the requirement for limited IRB review for **45 CFR 46.104(d)(2)iii** and the addition of "educational advancement" to the list of disclosure-related risks, such as those associated with educational test results. The exemptions under **45 CFR 46.104(d)(2)i** and **ii** can be applied to some research with children, according to the restrictions listed in Table 5.3-1.

Exemption 2 applies to commonly used SBER data collection methods that do not pose informational risks, either because subjects' answers cannot be linked to their identities or they do not elicit sensitive information that could put subjects at risk of liability or harm if disclosed outside the research team. This exemption does not apply to research that includes noninformational risks such as psychological risks or those associated with vulnerable populations (e.g., interviews with veterans about symptoms of posttraumatic stress disorder). IRBs vary in their use of this exemption for focus groups, with some not using this exemption for focus groups due to the privacy risks inherent in group discussions. This exemption includes research that collects identifiable information, but only if the research undergoes limited IRB review according to **45 CFR 46.111(a)(7)**. The intent behind this provision is to allow exemption of most survey research, regardless of the sensitivity level of the data or whether the research team has identifiers linkable to subjects' data, since the main risk of this research is informational and can be mitigated through robust data security procedures reviewed by the IRB.

🔖 5-6
🔖 10-4

Exemption 3: Benign Behavioral Interventions Including Adults

(i) Research involving benign behavioral interventions in conjunction with the collection of information from an adult subject through verbal or written responses (including data entry) or audiovisual recording if the subject prospectively agrees to the intervention and information collection and at least one of the following criteria is met:

(A) The information obtained is recorded by the investigator in such a manner that the identity of the human subjects cannot readily be ascertained, directly or through identifiers linked to the subjects;

(B) Any disclosure of the human subjects' responses outside the research would not reasonably place the subjects at risk of criminal or civil liability or be damaging to the subjects' financial standing, employability, educational advancement, or reputation; or

(C) The information obtained is recorded by the investigator in such a manner that the identity of the human subjects can readily be ascertained, directly or through identifiers linked to the subjects, and an IRB conducts a limited IRB review to make the determination required by §46.111(a)(7).

(ii) For the purpose of this provision, benign behavioral interventions are brief in duration, harmless, painless, not physically invasive, not likely to have a significant adverse lasting impact on the subjects, and the investigator has no reason to think the subjects will find the interventions offensive or embarrassing. Provided all such criteria are met, examples of such benign behavioral interventions would include having the subjects play an online game, having them solve puzzles under various noise conditions, or having them decide how to allocate a nominal amount of received cash between themselves and someone else.

(iii) If the research involves deceiving the subjects regarding the nature or purposes of the research, this exemption is not applicable unless the subject authorizes the deception through a prospective agreement to participate in research in circumstances in which the subject is informed that he or she will be unaware of or misled regarding the nature or purposes of the research **45 CFR 46.104(d)(3)**.

Exemption 3 says that research that only includes adults and involves the collection of information from benign behavioral interventions—interventions that are "brief in duration, harmless, painless, not physically invasive, not likely to have a significant adverse lasting impact on the subjects, and the investigator has no reason to think the subjects will find the interventions offensive or embarrassing" [45 CFR 46.104(d)(3)(ii)]—may be exempt if certain conditions are met. First, subjects must prospectively agree to participate in the intervention and agree to the collection of information. This means that to qualify for the exemption, research must only include adults who have the decision-making capacity to consent to research. If the research involves deception, the subject must also prospectively agree to being deceived.

Second, the data must be collected by oral response, written response, and/or audiovisual methods. As a result, certain data collection methods are not allowed under this exemption category, including the collection of data from wearable devices such as smartwatches or Fitbits. The collection of blood, blood pressure, pulse rate, serum cortisol data, and bodily fluids via introduction of a tool or sensor into the body (e.g., buccal swab) would also not meet the requirements for this exemption, as these activities are considered either a medical intervention or physically invasive (DHHS, 2017a). In addition, for this exemption to apply, one of the following criteria must be met: (1) the information collected is recorded in a deidentified manner; (2) disclosure of the subjects' responses outside of the research would not place the subject at risk; or (3) the information collected is recorded in an identifiable manner, and the IRB conducts a limited IRB review according to **45 CFR 46.111(a)(7)**.   🔗 5-6

The purpose of this exemption, which was new in the 2018 Common Rule, is to reduce regulatory burden and oversight for low-risk social and behavioral research activities, such as laboratory-based studies that measure or control a single variable or factor (e.g., studies of cognition, attitudes, learning; Riley & Akbar, 2017). For example, a study that evaluates the effect of music on test takers would likely be exempt under this category. If there is uncertainty about whether a research study meets the conditions of this exemption, including whether an intervention is benign, the IRB should consult a subject matter expert such as a psychologist or behavioral scientist, or an IRB administrator, for further guidance.

SACHRP INTERPRETATION OF "BENIGN BEHAVIORAL INTERVENTIONS"

The Secretary's Advisory Committee on Human Research Protections (SACHRP) has provided the following further specification of "benign behavioral interventions," but this has not been adopted as official guidance:

"Research procedures that are employed in the study of psychological states and processes, cognition, ideas and attitudes, or behavior, and do not include physical (bodily) tasks or physical manipulations (e.g., range of motion activities, physical exercise) unless these are minor activities that are incident to the behavioral intervention and do not increase risk." (DHHS, 2017a)

Exemption 4: Secondary Research for Which Consent Is Not Required

Secondary research uses of identifiable private information or identifiable biospecimens, if at least one of the following criteria is met:

(i) The identifiable private information or identifiable biospecimens are publicly available;

(ii) Information, which may include information about biospecimens, is recorded by the investigator in such a manner that the identity of the human subjects cannot readily be ascertained directly or through identifiers linked to the subjects, the investigator does not contact the subjects, and the investigator will not re-identify subjects;

(iii) The research involves only information collection and analysis involving the investigator's use of identifiable health information when that use is regulated under 45 CFR parts 160 and 164, subparts A and E, for the purposes of "health care operations" or "research" as those terms are defined at 45 CFR 164.501 or for "public health activities and purposes" as described under 45 CFR 164.512(b); or

(iv) The research is conducted by, or on behalf of, a Federal department or agency using government-generated or government-collected information obtained for nonresearch activities, if the research generates identifiable private information that is or will be maintained on information technology that is subject to and in compliance with section 208(b) of the E-Government Act of 2002, 44 U.S.C. 3501 note, if all of the identifiable private information collected, used, or generated as part of the activity will be maintained in systems of records subject to the Privacy Act of 1974, 5 U.S.C. 552a, and, if applicable, the information used in the research was collected subject to the Paperwork Reduction Act of 1995, 44 U.S.C. 3501 *et seq* **45 CFR 46.104(d)(4)**.

Exemption 4 covers the reuse for research purposes of identifiable information or identifiable biospecimens that were originally collected for some other research study or for nonresearch purposes, or that will be collected at a future date, if certain conditions are met (DHHS, 2017b). The research use of data or specimens that were collected for other purposes is known as "secondary research use." Secondary use research activities must meet one of the following conditions in order to be exempt:

⊘ 12-3

- The identifiable private information or identifiable biospecimens are publicly available.
- The information is recorded in a way that the identity of the subjects cannot be readily ascertained, and the researcher will not attempt to contact or reidentify the subjects.
- The research involves only the collection or analysis of protected health information (PHI) from a covered entity, meaning that the PHI is already subject to the Health Insurance Portability and Accountability Act of 1996 Privacy Rule (HIPAA).
- Research is conducted by, or on behalf of, a federal department or agency using government-generated or government-collected information obtained for nonresearch purposes.

Even when a study meets the criteria for this exemption, it is important to be aware of other federal, state, or local regulations that require informed consent or additional protections for subjects. Although they might be considered exempt under the Common Rule, FDA regulations require IRB review for activities that involve the use of data regarding subjects or control subjects, or data regarding the use of a device on human specimens (identified or unidentifiable) submitted to or held for inspection by FDA (DHHS, 2017b). In addition, states may have special protections for the use or collection of sensitive information that may require consent (DHHS, 2017b).

The <u>HIPAA</u> condition of this exemption (condition 3) also requires careful evaluation. Information obtained from biospecimens, but not the collection of biospecimens, can qualify for the HIPAA exemption. If a researcher plans to collaborate with other institutions or organizations, IRBs should consider whether the researcher will disclose PHI and if those institutions are covered entities. Disclosures from a covered entity to a noncovered entity result in the loss of HIPAA protections (DHHS, 2017b). It may be permissible to allow exemption if the researcher under a covered entity plans to share PHI with a second covered entity, as long as HIPAA authorization or a waiver or alteration of authorization to allow the disclosure is approved by the privacy board (often the IRB serves in this role; DHHS, 2017b).

🖉 11-6

CHANGES TO EXEMPTION 4 IN THE 2018 COMMON RULE

Prior to the 2018 Common Rule, only secondary research use of information that already existed at the time of IRB submission could be considered exempt. This limitation often resulted in the IRB requiring expedited review for low-risk research activities, just because the data didn't exist at the time of IRB submission. The 2018 Common Rule eliminates the limitation to existing data under this category.

Exemption 5: Public Benefit or Service Programs

Research and demonstration projects that are conducted or supported by a Federal department or agency, or otherwise subject to the approval of department or agency heads (or the approval of the heads of bureaus or other subordinate agencies that have been delegated authority to conduct the research and demonstration projects), and that are designed to study, evaluate, improve, or otherwise examine public benefit or service programs, including procedures for obtaining benefits or services under those programs, possible changes in or alternatives to those programs or procedures, or possible changes in methods or levels of payment for benefits or services under those programs. Such projects include, but are not limited to, internal studies by Federal employees, and studies under contracts or consulting arrangements, cooperative agreements, or grants. Exempt projects also include waivers of otherwise mandatory requirements using authorities such as sections 1115 and 1115A of the Social Security Act, as amended.

(i) Each Federal department or agency conducting or supporting the research and demonstration projects must establish, on a publicly accessible Federal Web site or in such other manner as the department or agency head may determine, a list of the research and demonstration projects that the Federal department or agency conducts or supports under this provision. The research or demonstration project must be published on this list prior to commencing the research involving human subjects **45 CFR 46.104(d)(5)**.

CHANGES TO EXEMPTION 5 IN THE 2018 COMMON RULE

The 2018 Common Rule added several clarifying statements to make it easier to expand the use of this exemption for: (1) "public benefit or service programs that a Common Rule department or agency does not itself administer or conduct through its own employees or agents, but rather supports through a grant or contact program. Therefore, the exemption applies to research and demonstration projects supported through, for example, federal grants or cooperative agreements" (Federal Register, 2017, Preamble p. 7195); (2) research designed to improve the benefit or service program; and (3) projects with waivers of otherwise mandatory requirements.

Exemption 5 applies to federally conducted or supported research on public benefit or service programs such as Medicaid, unemployment, and Social Security. The rationale for this exemption is that federal research on public programs is of benefit to the public, and federal privacy laws such as the Privacy Act mitigate any informational risks via requirements to protect research subjects' information. However, IRBs should still assess and address other potential risks such as those associated with vulnerable populations. In order to promote transparency with the public about federal research that will not be subject to IRB oversight, the Common Rule includes a requirement that federal agencies must publicly post projects eligible for Exemption 5 prior to the start of the research.

Exemption 6: Taste and Food Quality Evaluation and Consumer Acceptance Studies

Taste and food quality evaluation and consumer acceptance studies:

(i) If wholesome foods without additives are consumed, or

(ii) If a food is consumed that contains a food ingredient at or below the level and for a use found to be safe, or agricultural chemical or environmental contaminant at or below the level found to be safe, by the Food and Drug Administration or approved by the Environmental Protection Agency or the Food Safety and Inspection Service of the U.S. Department of Agriculture **45 CFR 46.104(d)(6)**.

There are two types of research activities that are allowed under Exemption 6. Taste tests of wholesome foods (with no additives) and research that requires humans to consume plants or animals raised for food products may qualify for exemption. For example, research that involves taste testing of two varieties of apples to determine an individual's preference would qualify for exemption if the apples do not contain any additives or chemicals. Other research that evaluates the effects of environmental contaminants may also be exempt if the researcher can provide evidence that the contaminant levels are within the guidelines set forth by the Environmental Protection Agency (EPA) or the Food Safety and Inspection Service of the U.S. Department of Agriculture (USDA). In addition, research that involves taste testing grass-fed beef and beef with a phosphate additive to retain moisture and protect flavor could be exempt as long as the additive is below the guidelines set forth by the FDA. However, if additives are included with the intent to submit an FDA marketing application, this exemption cannot be applied. Institutions should also consider whether taste testing of alcohol products such as wine (that otherwise would qualify for Exemption 6) would be determined exempt or require further IRB review and oversight. Some institutions require IRB review of wine or alcohol testing to ensure compliance with legal drinking age laws and that there are adequate procedures for monitoring consumption and the safety of participants.

Exemption 7: Storage or Maintenance for Secondary Research for Which Broad Consent Is Required

> Storage or maintenance for secondary research for which broad consent is required: Storage or maintenance of identifiable private information or identifiable biospecimens for potential secondary research use if an IRB conducts a limited IRB review and makes the determinations required by §46.111(a)(8) **45 CFR 46.104(d)(7)**.

Exemptions 7 and 8, which were new to the 2018 Common Rule, provide a regulatory framework for exempting from regular IRB review the storage, maintenance, and future use of identifiable private information or identifiable biospecimens, if broad consent is obtained at the time of specimen or data collection. Prior to the revisions to the Common Rule in 2018, there were two primary ways for researchers to conduct secondary research using already collected identifiable private information or identifiable biospecimens without having to get IRB approval and obtain traditional informed consent for the secondary use: (1) request a waiver of consent from the IRB; or (2) strip the information or biospecimens of identifiers before using them for research, so that the research would no longer count as human subjects research. These two exemption categories (7 and 8) introduce broad consent for future research as an alternative to traditional informed, study-specific consent.

🔗 6-9

🔗 6-4

Exemption 7 says that the storage or maintenance of identifiable private information or identifiable biospecimens for future secondary research use is eligible for exemption if two conditions are met: (1) broad consent for that storage, maintenance, or secondary research use is obtained from the subject, as outlined in **45 CFR 46.116(d)**; and (2) the IRB conducts a limited IRB review to determine whether broad consent was appropriately obtained and documented and to assess the adequacy of the protections for subject privacy and the confidentiality of data, according to **45 CFR 46.111(a)(8)**.

🔗 5-6

When subjects provide broad consent for storage and maintenance of their identifiable private information or identifiable biospecimens for secondary use—for instance, in a data repository or biobank—researchers do not need to obtain their study-specific informed consent for each future research use, and those future research uses would be exempt under category 8 described next (DHHS, 2017c).

🔗 12-3 🔗 10-10

Exemption 8: Secondary Research for Which Broad Consent Is Required

> Secondary research for which broad consent is required: Research involving the use of identifiable private information or identifiable biospecimens for secondary research use, if the following criteria are met:
>
> (i) Broad consent for the storage, maintenance, and secondary research use of the identifiable private information or identifiable biospecimens was obtained in accordance with §46.116(a)(1) through (4), (a)(6), and (d);
>
> (ii) Documentation of informed consent or waiver of documentation of consent was obtained in accordance with §46.117;

(iii) An IRB conducts a limited IRB review and makes the determination required by §46.111(a)(7) and makes the determination that the research to be conducted is within the scope of the broad consent referenced in paragraph (d)(8)(i) of this section; and (iv) The investigator does not include returning individual research results to subjects as part of the study plan. This provision does not prevent an investigator from abiding by any legal requirements to return individual research results **45 CFR 46.104(d)(8)**.

Exemption category 8 allows IRBs to exempt secondary research proposing the use of the subject's identifiable biospecimens and identified private information, if it was collected using <u>broad consent</u> for storage and maintenance for possible secondary use, in accordance with Exemption 7.

🔗 6-9

Before the study can be determined exempt, the IRB must conduct a <u>limited IRB review</u> to determine that there are adequate provisions to protect the privacy of subjects and the confidentiality of data and that the proposed study's use of identifiable biospecimens and data is within the scope of the broad consent for which the biospecimens and data were originally obtained. The IRB has discretion to determine how it will decide whether the proposed research activities fall within the parameters of the research described in the broad consent document. Also, to qualify for this exemption, the investigator cannot plan to return individual research results to the subjects. SACHRP has suggested that in the event there are clinically meaningful results that are not related, but found in the course of study participation, researchers can disclose the information to subjects (DHHS, 2017c).

🔗 5-6

Conclusion

Exemptions provide opportunities for IRBs to focus on their mission of protecting the rights and welfare of human subjects in low-risk studies, such as via limited IRB review. Exempt determinations have always been one of the more challenging responsibilities of IRBs and, as a result, likely one of the main sources of variation among IRBs that researchers find confusing and frustrating. To facilitate consistent application of exemption determinations and to foster communication with researchers, IRBs should make transparent any policies, procedures, or tools the IRB will use to make the exempt determinations. Documentation as to how the study meets exemption criteria should also be completed in the event of inquiry regarding the determination. For collaborative research, IRBs should carefully document their rationale for determining that a study is eligible for an exempt category and communicate their findings to each other. In addition, if the IRB is unsure as to whether an activity meets exemption criteria, it should seek consultation from subject matter experts or regulatory guidance as it becomes available.

References

Department of Health and Human Services (DHHS). (2001) *Institutional Review Board Guidebook. Chapter III Basic IRB Review.* biotech.law.lsu.edu/research/fed/ohrp/gb/irb_chapter3.htm

Department of Health and Human Services (DHHS). (2017a). *Secretary's Advisory Committee on Human Research Protections. Attachment B — Recommendations on benign behavioral intervention: A guidance and educational tool for benign behavioral interventions.* www.hhs.gov/ohrp/sachrp-committee/recommendations/attachment-b-august-2-2017.html

Department of Health and Human Services (DHHS). (2017b). *Secretary's Advisory Committee on Human Research Protections. Attachment B — Recommendations on the interpretation and application of §_.104(d)(4), the "HIPAA exemption."* www.hhs.gov/ohrp/sachrp-committee/recommendations/attachment-b-december-12-2017/index.html

Department of Health and Human Services (DHHS). (2017c). *Secretary's Advisory Committee on Human Research Protections. Attachment C — Recommendations for broad consent guidance.* www.hhs.gov/ohrp/sachrp-committee/recommendations/attachment-c-august-2-2017/index.html

Department of Health and Human Services (DHHS). (2019a). *Exempt research determination FAQs.* www.hhs.gov/ohrp/regulations-and-policy/guidance/faq/exempt-research-determination/index.html

Department of Health and Human Services (DHHS). (2019b). *Revised Common Rule Q&As: Exemptions.* www.hhs.gov/ohrp/education-and-outreach/revised-common-rule/revised-common-rule-q-and-a/index.html#exemptions

Department of Health and Human Services (DHHS). (2020). *Human Subject Regulations Decision Charts: 2018 Requirements.* www.hhs.gov/ohrp/regulations-and-policy/decision-charts-2018/index.html

Federal Register. (2017). Vol. 82, No. 12. 45 CFR 46 and Preamble. www.govinfo.gov/content/pkg/FR-2017-01-19/pdf/2017-01058.pdf

Food and Drug Administration (FDA). (2018). *Impact of certain provisions of the Revised Common Rule on FDA-regulated clinical investigations.* www.fda.gov/regulatory-information/search-fda-guidance-documents/impact-certain-provisions-revised-common-rule-fda-regulated-clinical-investigations

National Institutes of Health (NIH). (n.d.). *Frequently asked questions human subjects: Human subjects education.* grants.nih.gov/policy/hs/faqs.htm#5782

Riley, W. T., & Akbar, F. (2017). Revision to the Common Rule: Implications for behavioral and social sciences research. *Observer, 30*(5). www.psychologicalscience.org/observer/revisions-to-the-common-rule-implications-for-behavioral-and-social-sciences-research

Criteria for Approval

Monika S. Markowitz

Jeremy J. Corsmo

Abstract

The Common Rule criteria for approval are an ethically grounded guide to the IRB's final determination of whether or not a study or its modification warrant approval. This chapter provides a discussion of each of the criteria, comparison to the criteria in Food and Drug Administration (FDA) regulations, and comparison to the pre-2018 Common Rule. Using the criteria as more than a simple checklist or check-off for documentation purposes is recommended in order to optimize the IRB's comprehensive review. The criteria also serve to educate investigators about information that the IRB requires in order to justify approval of the research.

Introduction

The criteria for IRB approval, in the Common Rule at **45 CFR 46.111** and the FDA regulations at **21 CFR 56.111**, have become a well-known mantra for human research protection programs (HRPPs). In recent years, HRPPs have become increasingly interested in and oriented toward consistency and quality improvement. As such, IRBs are also becoming more rigorous in directly applying the criteria for approval in their review of studies as a means for documenting their reflection on ethical considerations during the review of the research. Initial review, continuing review, and review of modifications are all subject to the criteria for approval. Each of the approval criteria reflects one or more of the *Belmont* principles, which serve as the ethical foundation of the federal regulations for the protection of human subjects (National Commission, 1979). When the IRB is positioned to approve FDA-regulated research, the FDA criteria for approval at **21 CFR 56.111** apply. **Table 5.4-1** lists the criteria for IRB approval in the two versions of Common Rule regulations (pre-2018 and 2018) as well as the criteria in the FDA regulations. Differences between the pre-2018 Common Rule and the 2018 Common Rule are highlighted in the middle column, and differences between the 2018 Common Rule and FDA regulations are highlighted in the right column.

🔗 7-2 🔗 7-1

🔗 1-1

Table 5.4-1 Criteria for Approval: Common Rule and FDA Regulations

Common Rule Pre-2018 Requirements 45 CFR 46.111	Revised Common Rule (2018 Requirements) 45 CFR 46.111	FDA 21 CFR 56.111
(a) In order to approve research covered by this policy the IRB shall determine that all of the following requirements are satisfied:		
(1) Risks to subjects are minimized: (i) By using procedures which are consistent with sound research design and which do not unnecessarily expose subjects to risk, and (ii) whenever appropriate, by using procedures already being performed on the subjects for diagnostic or treatment purposes.	(1) Risks to subjects are minimized: (i) By using procedures that are consistent with sound research design and that do not unnecessarily expose subjects to risk, and (ii) Whenever appropriate, by using procedures already being performed on the subjects for diagnostic or treatment purposes. NO CHANGE	(1) Risks to subjects are minimized: (i) By using procedures which are consistent with sound research design and which do not unnecessarily expose subjects to risk, and (ii) whenever appropriate, by using procedures already being performed on the subjects for diagnostic or treatment purposes. SAME as Revised COMMON RULE
(2) Risks to subjects are reasonable in relation to anticipated benefits, if any, to subjects, and the importance of the knowledge that may reasonably be expected to result. In evaluating risks and benefits, the IRB should consider only those risks and benefits that may result from the research (as distinguished from risks and benefits of therapies subjects would receive even if not participating in the research). The IRB should not consider possible long-range effects of applying knowledge gained in the research (for example, the possible effects of the research on public policy) as among those research risks that fall within the purview of its responsibility.	(2) Risks to subjects are reasonable in relation to anticipated benefits, if any, to subjects, and the importance of the knowledge that may reasonably be expected to result. In evaluating risks and benefits, the IRB should consider only those risks and benefits that may result from the research (as distinguished from risks and benefits of therapies subjects would receive even if not participating in the research). The IRB should not consider possible long-range effects of applying knowledge gained in the research (e.g., the possible effects of the research on public policy) as among those research risks that fall within the purview of its responsibility. NO CHANGE	(2) Risks to subjects are reasonable in relation to anticipated benefits, if any, to subjects, and the importance of the knowledge that may be expected to result. In evaluating risks and benefits, the IRB should consider only those risks and benefits that may result from the research (as distinguished from risks and benefits of therapies that subjects would receive even if not participating in the research). The IRB should not consider possible long-range effects of applying knowledge gained in the research (for example, the possible effects of the research on public policy) as among those research risks that fall within the purview of its responsibility. SAME as Revised COMMON RULE
(3) Selection of subjects is equitable. In making this assessment the IRB should take into account the purposes of the research and the setting in which the research will be conducted and should be particularly cognizant of the special problems of research involving vulnerable populations, such as children, prisoners, pregnant women, mentally disabled persons, or economically or educationally disadvantaged persons.	(3) Selection of subjects is equitable. In making this assessment the IRB should take into account the purposes of the research and the setting in which the research will be conducted. The IRB should be particularly cognizant of the **special problems of research that involves a category of subjects who are vulnerable to coercion or undue influence,** such as children, prisoners, **individuals with impaired decision-making capacity,** or economically or educationally disadvantaged persons.	(3) Selection of subjects is equitable. In making this assessment the IRB should take into account the purposes of the research and the setting in which the research will be conducted and should be particularly cognizant of the **special problems of research involving vulnerable populations,** such as children, prisoners, **pregnant women, handicapped, or mentally disabled persons,** or economically or educationally disadvantaged persons.

Common Rule Pre-2018 Requirements 45 CFR 46.111	Revised Common Rule (2018 Requirements) 45 CFR 46.111	FDA 21 CFR 56.111
(4) Informed consent will be sought from each prospective subject or the subject's legally authorized representative, in accordance with, and to the extent required by §46.116.	(4) Informed consent will be sought from each prospective subject or the subject's legally authorized representative, in accordance with, and to the extent required by, §46.116. <u>NO CHANGE</u>	(4) Informed consent will be sought from each prospective subject or the subject's legally authorized representative, **in accordance with and to the extent required by part 50.**
(5) Informed consent will be appropriately documented, in accordance with, and to the extent required by §46.117.	(5) Informed consent will be appropriately documented **or appropriately waived** in accordance with §46.117.	(5) Informed consent will be appropriately documented, in accordance with **and to the extent required by §50.27.**
(6) When appropriate, the research plan makes adequate provision for monitoring the data collected to ensure the safety of subjects.	(6) When appropriate, the research plan makes adequate provision for monitoring the data collected to ensure the safety of subjects. <u>NO CHANGE</u>	(6) **Where** appropriate, the research plan makes adequate provision for monitoring the data collected to ensure the safety of subjects.
(7) When appropriate, there are adequate provisions to protect the privacy of subjects and to maintain the confidentiality of data.	(7) When appropriate, there are adequate provisions to protect the privacy of subjects and to maintain the confidentiality of data. (i) **The Secretary of HHS will, after consultation with the Office of Management and Budget's privacy office and other Federal departments and agencies that have adopted this policy, issue guidance to assist IRBs in assessing what provisions are adequate to protect the privacy of subjects and to maintain the confidentiality of data.** (ii) [Reserved]	(7) **Where** appropriate, there are adequate provisions to protect the privacy of subjects and to maintain the confidentiality of data.
No #8	(8) **For purposes of conducting the limited IRB review required by §46.104(d)(7)), the IRB need not make the determinations at paragraphs (a)(1) through (7) of this section, and shall make the following determinations:** (i) **Broad consent for storage, maintenance, and secondary research use of identifiable private information or identifiable biospecimens is obtained in accordance with the requirements of §46.116(a) (1)-(4), (a)(6), and (d);** (ii) **Broad consent is appropriately documented or waiver of documentation is appropriate, in accordance with §46.117; and**	No #8

(continues)

Table 5.4-1 Criteria for Approval: Common Rule and FDA Regulations (*continued*)

Common Rule Pre-2018 Requirements 45 CFR 46.111	Revised Common Rule (2018 Requirements) 45 CFR 46.111	FDA 21 CFR 56.111
	(iii) **If there is a change made for research purposes in the way the identifiable private information or identifiable biospecimens are stored or maintained, there are adequate provisions to protect the privacy of subjects and to maintain the confidentiality of data.**	
(b) When some or all of the subjects are likely to be vulnerable to coercion or undue influence, such as children, prisoners, pregnant women, mentally disabled persons, or economically or educationally disadvantaged persons, additional safeguards have been included in the study to protect the rights and welfare of these subjects.	(b) When some or all of the subjects are likely to be vulnerable to coercion or undue influence, such as children, prisoners, **individuals with impaired decision-making capacity,** or economically or educationally disadvantaged persons, additional safeguards have been included in the study to protect the rights and welfare of these subjects.	(b) When some or all of the subjects, such as children, prisoners, **pregnant women, handicapped, or mentally disabled persons,** or economically or educationally disadvantaged persons, are likely to be vulnerable to coercion or undue influence additional safeguards have been included in the study to protect the rights and welfare of these subjects.
		(c) **In order to approve research in which some or all of the subjects are children, an IRB must determine that all research is in compliance with part 50, subpart D of this chapter**.

The Common Rule and FDA criteria were virtually identical until the promulgation of the revised Common Rule in 2018, which applies to research that is regulated or funded by any of the 16 Common Rule agencies. Institutions are not obligated to apply these criteria for review of research that does not fall under the Common Rule or FDA regulations, unless state law provisions apply. However, motivated by accreditation standards, a desire for standardization, or simply because the Common Rule regulations are anchored in ethical principles, many HRPPs use the Common Rule criteria for IRB approval for the review of all human subjects research, regardless of funding source. If a very large clinical trial is funded by a Common Rule federal agency as well as nonfederal sponsors, the Common Rule regulations and criteria for approval apply to the study. We begin with a brief explanation of each criterion at 45 CFR 46.111 and then discuss how the criteria are incorporated into IRB review.

Common Rule Criteria for Approval at 45 CFR 46.111

The first two criteria for approval deal with the IRB's assessment of risk within a study protocol and are based in the *Belmont* principle of beneficence (National Commission, 1979). The criteria are intended to work together to reflect a comprehensive evaluation of risk by the IRB. If the risk of the research is found to be unjustifiably high or not appropriately addressed in the research plan or in responses from the researcher, the IRB should not approve the study as submitted.

1: Risks to Subjects Are Minimized

45 CFR 46.111(a)(1) Risks to Subjects are minimized:
(i) By using procedures that are consistent with sound research design and that do not unnecessarily expose subjects to risk, and
(ii) Whenever appropriate, by using procedures already being performed on the subjects for diagnostic or treatment purposes.

Federal Policy for the Protection of Human Subjects: Preamble to the Revised Common Rule (2017). Federal Register Vol. 82, No. 12: 7149 - 7259. https://www.govinfo.gov/content/pkg/FR-2017-01-19/pdf/2017-01058.pdf

The first approval criterion has two sections. Both must be addressed in order for the IRB to determine that criterion 1 has been satisfied.

The first section establishes that:

Risks to subjects are minimized by using procedures that are consistent with sound research design and that do not unnecessarily expose subjects to risk . . . .

Ascertaining that a research protocol is consistent with sound research design is part of the review by the IRB. Although many protocols are subjected to formal scientific review before submission to the IRB, as part of an agency funding evaluation or by a scientific review committee within the HRPP's organization, the IRB itself must be confident that sound research design has been fully considered and is appropriate to address the aims of the research. "Sound" research design means that the proposed execution of a study aligns with research questions, methods, and analysis that are known or accepted within the discipline or are otherwise justifiable.

Assessment of research design by the IRB is a controversial aspect of the IRB's responsibility and can be a source of discord in the research community. Researchers consider themselves well versed in their fields and may take offense at their research design being questioned by the IRB or a single IRB reviewer in the case of <u>expedited review</u>. The IRB, as a disinterested body of experienced and multidisciplinary individuals, provides an objective lens through which to evaluate a study's scientific methodology. In its review to address this criterion, the IRB considers whether there is another way to do the research that fulfills its aims and also reduces risks to subjects but does not introduce unintended consequences of exposure to risk. If specific questions about risks, and ways to minimize them, are not addressed to the IRB's satisfaction, the IRB would not be carrying out its responsibility if it approves the study.

5-5

Some study designs obligate the IRB to consider a number of aspects, including results from preclinical studies, use of intervention and control arms (including use of <u>placebo</u>), blinding and randomization procedures, and the number of proposed subjects. For the latter, a biostatistician may be needed to ascertain the "n" that is required to power a study in order to achieve statistical significance, especially for a high-risk study. Utilizing more subjects than is statistically warranted unnecessarily exposes more individuals to risks posed by the study. On the other hand, not utilizing enough subjects to adequately answer the research question may invalidate the study's results, thereby exposing prospective subjects to unnecessary risk.

10-11

The second section of criterion 1 establishes the requirement that:

> Risks to subjects are minimized whenever appropriate, by using procedures already being performed on the subjects for diagnostic or treatment purposes.

The procedures used to collect information are part of the study design. The researcher decides what data is needed and how to collect it in order to answer the research question. Data collection procedures should not indiscriminately repeat similar procedures to which a subject has been or will be exposed. For clinically oriented research, the collection of data can be planned to coincide with procedures or clinical activities already being done as part of the "standard of care" for a patient. Although the term "standard of care" has legal implications that are beyond the scope of this chapter, the term is typically meant to convey the expected or customary care practices that are used to diagnose or treat an illness or disease. For example, if blood draws are clinically indicated at regular intervals, collection of a blood sample for research purposes can be coordinated with a scheduled blood draw in order to minimize the discomfort and risk from an additional needle stick. For research that involves investigation of tumor cells, the specimen collection should be coordinated with the time of surgical biopsy, when feasible, to avoid an additional risky procedure for research purposes. IRB reviewers should also be attuned to proposed research activities within a social, behavioral, or educational study that are unnecessarily repetitive, lengthy, or intrusive.

2: Risks to Subjects Are Reasonable in Relation to Anticipated Benefits

> **45 CFR 46.111(a)(2)** Risks to subjects are reasonable in relation to anticipated benefits, if any, to subjects, and the importance of the knowledge that may reasonably be expected to result. In evaluating risks and benefits, the IRB should consider only those risks and benefits that may result from the research (as distinguished from risks and benefits of therapies subjects would receive even if not participating in the research). The IRB should not consider possible long-range effects of applying knowledge gained in the research (e.g., the possible effects of the research on public policy) as among those research risks that fall within the purview of its responsibility.

Department of Health and Human Services. 21CFR56.111. Accessed at https://www.accessdata.fda.gov/scripts/cdrh/cfdocs/cfcfr/cfrsearch.cfm?fr=56.111

The second criterion for IRB approval of research is often evaluated together with criterion 1. However, there are important considerations unique to this approval criterion. The inclusion of approval criterion 2 in the federal regulations can be traced directly to *Belmont*'s fundamental ethical principle of beneficence, which practically translates to maximizing benefits and minimizing risks (National Commission, 1979). When determining whether approval criterion 2 has been satisfied, IRBs can look to both the text of the regulation and the supporting *Belmont* principle of beneficence. Criterion 2 is broken down into two sections that together contribute to the IRB's determination that this approval criterion has been satisfied.

The regulation begins by establishing the requirement:

🔗 1-1

> Risks to subjects are reasonable in relation to anticipated benefits, if any, to subjects, and the importance of the knowledge that may reasonably be expected to result.

When determining whether the risks associated with participation in research are reasonable, IRBs should first consider risk in relation to any potential direct benefits the individual subjects may receive from their participation in the research. IRBs are not to consider hypothetical or other possible long-term abstract benefits that the subject may experience in the future.

Second, IRBs should consider risk in relation to the importance of the knowledge that may result from the research. A question is whether IRBs should take a position that exposing subjects to even minimal risk is acceptable if the research is not reasonably expected to generate new knowledge. Consider the example of student-based research, which frequently involves studies with well-settled research conclusions. Student-based research often poses concern about exposing subjects to risks or burdens with no possibility of benefit to the subjects themselves. IRBs generally appreciate the importance of students' experiential learning about the human research process. As a result, IRBs are often amenable to making a reasonable risk/benefit determination of student research that poses some risk and no benefit, especially if there is adequate assurance of subjects' autonomy in deciding whether to participate in the study.

The second section of criterion 2 directs that

> In evaluating risks and benefits the IRB should consider only those risks and benefits that may result from the research (as distinguished from risks and benefits of therapies subjects would receive even if not participating in the research).

This approach to separating research into therapeutic and nontherapeutic components in order to independently evaluate the risks and benefits of participating in the research is often a challenging aspect of reviewing research. Using a component analysis methodology, risks and benefits of identified research-only components of the study are evaluated with the goal of establishing whether there is a favorable risk/benefit ratio of participating in the research, specifically. Although instruction on how to fully leverage component analysis methodology in conducting IRB review is beyond the scope of this chapter, the Secretary's Advisory Committee on Human Research Protections (SACHRP) has considered this topic extensively (FDA, 2012).

In evaluating the research risks in relation to benefits, the IRB should consider all risks that may reasonably result from participation in the research. This includes both physical risks (e.g., clinical side effects, complications, allergic reactions, etc.) and nonphysical risks (e.g., psychological/emotional risks, socioeconomic risks, privacy/confidentiality risks, etc.). Such consideration applies to all arms of a study: the treatment or experimental arm, the nonexperimental arm, and placebo arm, as appropriate.

3: Selection of Subjects Is Equitable

> **45 CFR 46.111(a)(3)** Selection of subjects is equitable. In making this assessment the IRB should take into account the purposes of the research and the setting in which the research will be conducted. The IRB should be particularly cognizant of the special problems of research that involves a category of subjects who are vulnerable to coercion

or undue influence, such as children, prisoners, individuals with impaired decision-making capacity, or economically or educationally disadvantaged persons.

Federal Policy for the Protection of Human Subjects: Preamble to the Revised Common Rule (2017). Federal Register Vol. 82, No. 12: 7149 - 7259. https://www.govinfo.gov/content/pkg/FR-2017-01-19/pdf/2017-01058.pdf

⊘ 1-1

Of all the criteria for approval, criterion 3 addresses the *Belmont* principle of justice most directly. In its explanation of the principle, the <u>Belmont Report</u> describes a need to scrutinize the selection of research subjects to ensure that certain groups are not "being systematically selected simply because of their easy availability, their compromised position, or their manipulability, but rather for reasons directly related to the problem being studied" (National Commission, 1979). According to *Belmont*, the principle of justice also incorporates the need to ensure that the research "not provide advantages only to those who can afford them and that such research should not unduly involve persons from groups unlikely to be among the beneficiaries of subsequent applications of the research" (National Commission, 1979).

"Equitable" subject selection addresses more than equality. Whereas "equality" means that all individuals are considered and treated the same, "equitability" takes into account that individuals are different and should be treated fairly given those differences but not necessarily the same. Equitability in subject selection entails thoughtful consideration of which population categories are in fact necessary and appropriate to answer the research questions. In addition, equitable subject selection means that the risks and benefits of research participation are fairly distributed. For example, subjecting a population in a low-income country to the risks of a clinical trial involving an expensive drug, without the possibility of eventually benefitting from such participation, is generally viewed as unjust. Some types of population groups, such as those described in the criterion text, as well as others, may be vulnerable to undue influence or coercion in the research context, preventing them from fully exercising their autonomy.

⊘ 9-1

The terms "undue influence" and "coercion" are often incorrectly used interchangeably in referring to inappropriate pressure experienced by some subject groups. Undue influence involves offers for research participation that are "too good to refuse," influencing a subject to act against his or her better judgment. Coercion involves a perceived threat that something bad will happen if one does not agree to participate. <u>Vulnerability</u> to undue influence or coercion is often a function of unequal status or a power differential between the researcher and the subject, due to factors such as the subject's health condition, cognitive ability, age, sex, race, language, education, socioeconomic circumstances, or association with a historically marginalized group. Payment for study participation frequently raises concerns of undue influence. For example, inordinately high <u>payment</u> for participation in a study with significant risk may impact the extent

⊘ 12-2

REMOVAL OF PREGNANT WOMEN AS A CATEGORY OF "VULNERABLE POPULATIONS"

The 2018 Common Rule removed pregnant women as a category of subjects vulnerable to coercion or undue influence. Subpart B of the DHHS human research regulations at 45 CFR 46 remains in place, detailing a set of regulatory requirements to be considered when pregnant women will be targeted for enrollment in research. It is often applied regardless of funding source. Criterion 3 in the FDA regulations refers to pregnant women not as vulnerable, but rather as a population which poses a "special problem" in research.

to which consent by economically disadvantaged persons is voluntary. The lure of payment may cloud their decision making about whether participating in such a study is right for them. The IRB is in a position to assess whether the amount of payment, given the type of study and the proposed recruitment population, poses undue influence over participation. Proposed recruitment of patients, students, employees, or members of the military may involve perceived or actual coercion to participate because prospective subjects may feel they were pushed to participate or fear that refusal could negatively impact their health care, grades, employment, or role in the military. IRB assessment of the proposed subject categories and the recruitment scenarios is necessary to minimize the effect of possible undue influence or coercion in subject selection.

The term "cognitive impairment" in criterion 3 broadly describes a permanent, temporary, or fluctuating condition that affects the ability to think and make a decision about something that affects oneself. The IRB is charged to consider the research context—the purpose and setting of the research—in order to take into account the extent to which the <u>decision-making ability</u> of subjects as a group may be impaired or compromised not only during a moment in time but also over the course of a study. Examples abound in which cognitive abilities within population groups can vary. Consider research seeking to enroll persons who have recently received a life-changing diagnosis or who are in severe pain. Neither of these groups may be able to fully comprehend the details of a proposed study at the time of presentation. However, with the passage of some time, or even the administration of pain relief, individuals in both groups may be much more able to cognitively focus on the offer of study participation.

                        🖉 9-7, 9-8

In another example, consider the possible variation in cognitive ability for a study looking at the performance of daily living activities among elderly individuals over 80 years of age. Among this group of prospective subjects, there is likely a wide range of decisional capacity. Similarly, consider a study about drug addiction that will target users of illicit substances, who may or may not have functional capacity to decide about study participation. The IRB is reminded to be cognizant of special life challenges of certain categories of subjects. At the same time, the IRB must be aware that narrow views of decisional ability may not only violate an individual's autonomy, but may also impact the equitability of subject selection by unjustly excluding certain groups from participation in research. This reminder pertains particularly to keeping an open mind about the range of decisional abilities among those who are deemed educationally or <u>economically disadvantaged</u>. Prospective subjects in both of these groups should not be considered decisionally impaired solely due to their life circumstances. It is incumbent upon researchers and the IRB to ensure that there are few, if any, barriers to equitable study participation and that the research is explained in language that is lay accessible.

                        🖉 9-9

IRBs should be particularly aware of research that proposes the recruitment of <u>vulnerable groups</u> simply because they are an available or even captive audience and not because their group is a focus of the research questions. Casting a large recruitment net in such circumstances may seem to provide a good chance of study enrollment but is not conducive to voluntary informed consent or ethically sensitive equitability considerations.

                        🖉 9-1

Likewise, the IRB needs to be aware of plans to enroll subjects of limited proficiency in the language of the research <u>setting</u>. Although equal opportunity to participate in studies of potential therapeutic benefit appeals strongly to the principle of justice, language differences may in fact prevent some persons from being enrolled because they are not able to fully understand what the study requires, or they may be unable to communicate research-related adverse

                        🖉 6-8

events. In such a situation, the IRB is in the position of considering whether regard for beneficence—preventing harm for individuals and possibly all subjects enrolled in a study—has greater weight than the principle of justice, unless safeguards against language obstacles are written into the research protocol. Examples of safeguards include the use of clinical navigators, who are specifically charged with guiding a subject through a study, or the presence of similar language skills among the research team.

⊘ 9-5 ⊘ 9-6

The text in criterion 3 specifically mentions the subject categories of <u>prisoners</u> and <u>children</u>, whose restricted or developing autonomy may make them vulnerable to undue influence or coercion in subject selection. Concerning prisoners and children, respectively, subpart C in 45 CFR 46 and subpart D in both DHHS and FDA regulations address regulatory considerations. It is worth noting that neither persons with impaired <u>decision-making capacity</u> nor economically or educationally <u>disadvantaged</u> persons are otherwise covered by specific regulatory subparts.

⊘ 9-7
⊘ 9-9

4 and 5: Informed Consent Will Be Sought and Documented

> **45 CFR 46.111 (a)(4)** Informed consent will be sought from each prospective subject or the subject's legally authorized representative, in accordance with, and to the extent required by, §46.116.
>
> **45 CFR 46.111 (a)(5)** Informed consent will be appropriately documented or appropriately waived in accordance with §46.117.

Federal Policy for the Protection of Human Subjects: Preamble to the Revised Common Rule (2017). Federal Register Vol. 82, No. 12: 7149 - 7259. https://www.govinfo.gov/content/pkg/FR-2017-01-19/pdf/2017-01058.pdf

⊘ Section 6

⊘ 1-1

Approval criteria 4 and 5 both address informed consent. The concept of <u>informed consent</u> is a cornerstone of the ethical conduct of human subjects research. Like the other approval criteria, these two are grounded in the principles of the *Belmont Report*, specifically, the principle of respect for persons (National Commission, 1979). Unlike the previous approval criteria, the regulatory text does not provide much information. It states that informed consent will be sought and directs the IRB to the relevant sections of the regulations pertaining to the required and additional elements of informed consent [**45 CFR 46.116**] and the requirements for documentation or waiver of informed consent [**45 CFR 46.117**]. Refer to section 6 in this volume for an extensive discussion about informed consent considerations.

⊘ 6-2

In reviewing the process for how researchers will seek informed consent from each prospective subject (or the subject's legally authorized representative), IRBs must ensure the presence of the required regulatory <u>elements</u> and additional elements, as appropriate, in consent documents. IRBs should evaluate the consent process and associated documents as they relate to the setting in which consent will be obtained. In a mobile/digital world, the setting is frequently not the traditional one-on-one private location wherein the researcher and potential subjects review the consent forms together. Due to evolving and dynamic consent procedures, IRBs should be familiar with, and open to, reviewing a variety of modalities for obtaining initial and ongoing informed consent and addressing the elements in **45 CFR 46.116**.

The IRB's review of the informed consent process often tends to be, somewhat mistakenly, overly focused on the wording of the informed consent form(s).

Interestingly, however, the text in criteria 4 and 5 does not mention an informed consent "form." Rather the text states that "informed consent" is sought in criterion 4 and documented in criterion 5. By not specifically referencing an informed consent form, the criteria instead establish the IRB's consideration of informed consent as a process. Such consideration starts with review of how prospective subjects are informed about a study and how they are recruited and enrolled. It also includes consideration of the required regulatory elements, how or whether a legally authorized representative will be utilized for some or all subjects, whether a <u>short form</u> consent process is indicated for the study, and how or whether consent documentation occurs. The IRB is in a position to determine whether some or all of the required elements of informed consent in **45 CFR 46.116** can be <u>waived</u>, and whether <u>documentation of consent</u> can be waived according to **45 CFR 46.117**.

🔗 6-8

🔗 6-4 🔗 6-5

IRBs should keep in mind that waiving some or all elements of informed consent, or waiving documentation, can occur whether or not a physical informed consent form is actually utilized. The IRB's recognition of informed consent as a process also entails consideration of whether subjects continue to understand and agree to their ongoing participation in a research study, especially for a long-standing or longitudinal study. In order for the IRB to review ongoing consent to participate, the research plan or protocol should provide information on the manner and frequency in which subjects are reminded that they are research subjects, that their participation is voluntary, and that they can withdraw from the study at any time.

Aside from a misdirected focus on the informed consent form instead of the process, IRBs can also lose sight of the fact that the informed consent criteria are only 2 of the 8 approval criteria. If, for example, the IRB does not determine that research risks are minimized, risks and benefits are reasonably balanced, privacy and confidentiality issues are addressed, and vulnerable populations appropriately protected, inviting subjects to participate would be unethical and informed consent, therefore, invalid. The *Belmont* principles, as exemplified in the criteria for approval, work together in their enactment of ethical research.

6: Data Monitoring for Subject Safety

> **45 CFR 46.111(a)(6)** When appropriate, the research plan makes adequate provision for monitoring the data collected to ensure the safety of subjects.

Federal Policy for the Protection of Human Subjects: Preamble to the Revised Common Rule (2017). Federal Register Vol. 82, No. 12: 7149 - 7259. https://www.govinfo.gov/content/pkg/FR-2017-01-19/pdf/2017-01058.pdf

The sixth approval criterion, which is tied to the *Belmont* principle of beneficence, requires IRBs to make decisions about oversight of ongoing research in terms of how and/or whether collected data is monitored. The regulation begins with the clause "when appropriate," which allows IRBs to determine that certain types of research may not need to include provisions for monitoring the data collected in order to ensure the safety of subjects. Consequently, it is important for IRBs to understand which types of research will need definitive provisions for monitoring data to ensure subject safety. Several federally based references are available to help guide IRBs in establishing their local requirements. These include the National Institutes of Health (NIH) Policy for Data and Safety Monitoring (NIH, 2000), Further Guidance on a Data and Safety

Monitoring for Phase I and Phase II Trials (NIH, 1998), and the Agency for Healthcare Research and Quality (AHRQ) Data and Safety Monitoring Policy (AHRQ, 2011).

In general, two features of a study determine whether it is appropriate to monitor the data collected to ensure the safety of subjects: (1) level of risk and (2) whether the proposed research involves research interventions. A common IRB practice is to require that all research determined to be "greater than minimal risk" include adequate provisions for monitoring the data to ensure subject safety. It is also common for IRBs to require that all research involving research interventions, even if minimal risk, make adequate provisions for monitoring the data to ensure subject safety.

Once an IRB has established the types of research that appropriately require provisions for safety monitoring, the IRB is faced with determining what constitutes "adequate provision." IRBs should keep in mind that there are multiple approaches to providing data and safety monitoring, including mechanisms like a single independent monitor, separate systems for review of safety data, regular discussion of the data by the research team, internal vs. external monitoring, and simple review of the data by the principal investigator. The <u>monitoring plan</u> should be explained by the researcher in sufficient detail in the protocol. Results of monitoring are then reported to the reviewing IRB consistent with IRB safety reporting requirements. With regard to what constitutes "adequate provision," the federally based references mentioned previously have fairly robust guidance establishing when formal data and safety monitoring boards or committees (DSMBs or DSMCs) would represent "adequate provision." For greater than minimal risk studies, an independent, formally chartered DSMB or DSMC is generally considered to be the most comprehensive approach to monitoring the data for subject safety. An IRB may also require a data and safety monitoring plan, at its discretion, for minimal risk studies that involve multiple consent groups, new or untested researchers, or for unusual study designs. A monitoring plan for a minimal risk study will likely not utilize a formal DSMB or DSMC. A requirement for a data and safety monitoring plan can be lifted after review of the first data and safety monitoring report, at continuing review, or whenever the IRB is comfortable doing so. **Figure 5.4-1** illustrates a continuum of appropriate data monitoring as risk to subjects increases.

The continuum begins with a baseline level of safety monitoring resulting from the researcher's obligation to comply with the reviewing IRB's internal safety reporting policies regarding potential <u>unanticipated problems</u>

🔗 7-4

🔗 7-3

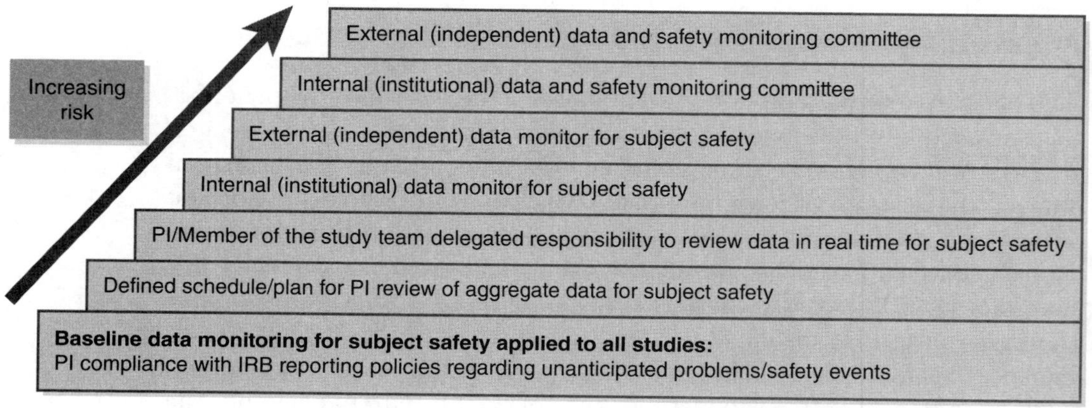

Figure 5.4-1 Continuum of appropriate data monitoring, as risk to subjects increases.

and other safety events. In multisite studies, locally mandated data and safety monitoring may be very limited in terms of actual safety oversight that can be provided, since study-wide safety data is not generally available to researchers at individual sites. It is therefore important for IRBs to carefully assess the provisions for data and safety monitoring in multisite research to ensure that there is adequate and appropriate oversight at the central or sponsor level.

7: Adequate Provisions to Protect Privacy and Confidentiality

45 CFR 46.111(a)(7) When appropriate, there are adequate provisions to protect the privacy of subjects and to maintain the confidentiality of data.

(i) The Secretary of HHS will, after consultation with the Office of Management and Budget's privacy office and other Federal departments and agencies that have adopted this policy, issue guidance to assist IRBs in assessing what provisions are adequate to protect the privacy of subjects and to maintain the confidentiality of data.

Federal Policy for the Protection of Human Subjects: Preamble to the Revised Common Rule (2017). Federal Register Vol. 82, No. 12: 7149 - 7259. https://www.govinfo.gov/content/pkg/FR-2017-01-19/pdf/2017-01058.pdf

Criterion 7 addresses the increasingly fluid concepts of privacy, confidentiality, and data security that pose ongoing challenges as technologies of data generation, analysis, storage, and sharing evolve. Genetic analysis of biospecimens poses additional challenges, as reidentifying specific individuals from previously deidentified specimens becomes increasingly possible. Storing physical paper research data in a locked file cabinet in a locked office with limited access, which was once a standard form of data security, is now almost quaint. While some research, such as low-risk surveys or educational interventions, may still lend themselves to traditional data security measures, most research data is collected and stored in sophisticated electronic formats. Breaches to data security can pose significant risks to the protection of privacy and maintenance of confidentiality; limiting the possibility of such breaches minimizes the risk of privacy violations. An increasing emphasis on cooperative research, data sharing, and development of large databases, such as those used for genome-wide association studies, requires meaningful review of data security plans.

⚭ 12-4
⚭ 10-10

Protecting privacy of information and maintaining the confidentiality of data are tied to the *Belmont* principles of respect for persons and beneficence. Privacy, which broadly refers to protection of a subject's control over others' access to the subject's person and identity, is distinguished from confidentiality, which refers to how and by whom information about a subject is accessed or used. In the case of privacy concerns, the IRB is interested in knowing how the researcher intends to protect a subject's control or expectation over how or whether their identity or identifiable information might be revealed. In the case of confidentiality, the IRB should ascertain that the researcher has made appropriate provisions for how subjects' data will be stored and shared with, or used by, others. A research protocol should provide information about both how privacy is protected and how confidentiality of data is maintained. Criterion 7 converges on several of the other criteria for approval, such as minimizing risks and risk/benefit consideration

⚭ 1-1

(criteria 1 and 2) and addressing how privacy and confidentiality are addressed in the consent and consent documentation processes (criteria 4 and 5).

🔗 11-1

Criterion 7 represents the first significant divergence between the Common Rule and FDA regulations (see Table 5.4-1). Although both sets of regulations address protecting privacy and maintaining confidentiality, the Common Rule indicates that the Secretary of DHHS will, after appropriate consultation, issue guidance to assist IRBs in assessing "what provisions are adequate to protect the privacy of subjects and to maintain the confidentiality of data" [45 CFR 46.111(a)(7)]. Points that DHHS suggests will be addressed in its guidance are found in the preamble to the 2018 Common Rule (Federal Register, 2017, p. 7207). The guidance will purportedly advise the IRB how to think about privacy and confidentiality in a context of changing technological capabilities, including potential identification of a specific individual from data or samples that were previously considered to be deidentified. Although the guidance is not available at the time of this volume's publication, it is possible, given recent efforts to harmonize the Common Rule and FDA regulations, that subsequent guidance will be jointly issued by the Office for Human Research Protections (OHRP) and FDA.

8: Criteria for Limited IRB Review of Exempt Category 7

> **45 CFR 46. 111(a)(8)** For purposes of conducting the limited IRB review required by §46.104(d)(7)), the IRB need not make the determinations at paragraphs (a)(1) through (7) of this section, and shall make the following determinations:
>
> (i) Broad consent for storage, maintenance, and secondary research use of identifiable private information or identifiable biospecimens is obtained in accordance with the requirements of §46.116(a)(1)-(4), (a)(6), and (d);
>
> (ii) Broad consent is appropriately documented or waiver of documentation is appropriate, in accordance with §46.117; and
>
> (iii) If there is a change made for research purposes in the way the identifiable private information or identifiable biospecimens are stored or maintained, there are adequate provisions to protect the privacy of subjects and to maintain the confidentiality of data.

Federal Policy for the Protection of Human Subjects: Preamble to the Revised Common Rule (2017). Federal Register Vol. 82, No. 12: 7149 - 7259. https://www.govinfo.gov/content/pkg/FR-2017-01-19/pdf/2017-01058.pdf

🔗 5-6 🔗 5-3

The final criterion for IRB approval is unique to the Common Rule at the time of publication of this volume. Criterion 8 establishes the determinations the IRB must make to conduct "limited IRB review," specifically as it pertains to exempt category 7. As a reminder, exempt category 7 deals with storage or maintenance of identifiable private information or identifiable biospecimens for secondary research using the broad consent mechanism. This type of research scenario requires "limited IRB review," which involves only the consideration of approval criterion 8, and does not require consideration of approval criteria 1 through 7 discussed earlier. Limited IRB review may be done using an expedited review mechanism. (Reference to limited IRB review also appears in exempt categories 2, 3, and 8; however, these exemptions are subject to approval criterion 7, not criterion 8).

🔗 6-9

🔗 5-5

In general, the elements that make up approval criterion 8 are fairly straightforward. Specifically, subsections (i) and (ii) require the IRB to confirm that broad consent was obtained or will be obtained in a manner consistent with the sections of the regulations that established the required components of broad consent. The elements also require that research subjects' broad consent is documented in a manner that is consistent with the regulations.

Subsection (iii) refers to IRB consideration of whether "adequate provisions to protect the privacy of subjects and to maintain the confidentiality of data" remain if there are proposed modifications to the manner of storage or maintenance of identifiable private information and/or identifiable samples. Such modifications include changes to storage systems or formats, location, accessibility, or changes to responsible personnel. Unlike criterion 7 dealing with privacy and confidentiality, criterion 8 does not mention issuance of guidance to describe what are "adequate provisions." It is possible that the awaited guidance may also be applied to this approval criterion.

Additional Safeguards for Vulnerable Populations

> **45 CFR 46.111(b)** When some or all of the subjects are likely to be vulnerable to coercion or undue influence, such as children, prisoners, individuals with impaired decision-making capacity, or economically or educationally disadvantaged persons, additional safeguards have been included in the study to protect the rights and welfare of these subjects.

Federal Policy for the Protection of Human Subjects: Preamble to the Revised Common Rule (2017). Federal Register Vol. 82, No. 12: 7149 - 7259. https://www.govinfo.gov/content/pkg/FR-2017-01-19/pdf/2017-01058.pdf

The IRB approval criteria close with a discussion of additional safeguards to protect the rights and welfare of potentially vulnerable subjects. This provision charges IRBs to think beyond subparts B, C, and D, to consider *any* populations that may be vulnerable to coercion or undue influence. The text of **45 CFR 46.111(b)** gives the same list of types of subjects who may be vulnerable to coercion or undue influence as does criterion 3. The regulation directs IRBs to ensure that there are additional safeguards included within the research plan and procedures to protect the rights and welfare of these subjects in consideration of their vulnerabilities to coercion or undue influence. Whereas criterion 3 is about vulnerability in subject selection, given the purposes of the research and the setting in which it will be conducted, **45 CFR 46.111(b)** reminds IRBs to be diligent about protecting the rights and welfare of vulnerable subjects throughout the conduct of the research.

IRBs are charged with identifying potentially vulnerable populations as well as identifying what might be appropriate additional safeguards to protect their rights and welfare. These additional protections can take many forms and extend beyond those considered in criterion 3 regarding subject selection. With regard to coercion, IRBs should generally focus on minimizing or mitigating the conditions that can create potential for coercion. For instance, in the case of subjects who are also patients, the IRB should consider whether having the consent process carried out by the patient's physician may be perceived as coercive, to the extent that the patient-subject may fear they will receive inferior medical care if they refuse to participate. The IRB should also be thoughtful about whether the patient-subject is at liberty to withdraw from the study at any time without fear of reprisal. Requiring someone other than the subject's physician to conduct the initial and ongoing consent conversations and being

Section 9

attentive to mechanisms described in the research plan to ensure ongoing voluntariness are ways to address concerns about possible coercion.

IRBs also focus on reducing the potential for undue influence. For example, IRBs should look at <u>payments</u> used as an initial recruitment incentive, being attentive to whether the amounts being offered are likely to skew potential subjects' perception of risks. In addition, IRBs should consider the proposed payment schedule for studies that require continued interventions or study visits over time. As a general rule, incremental payments provide a better safeguard for the subject's right to voluntarily continue participation than does a lump-sum payment at the end, which may make the subject feel pressured to stay in the study against their better judgment in order to receive payment. IRBs have latitude to be creative with solutions that meet the unique circumstances of the research in order to safeguard subjects who may be vulnerable to coercion or undue influence.

⊘ 12-2

Incorporating the "111 Criteria for Approval" into the IRB Review Process

The 111 criteria for IRB approval of research have, at their core, a grounding in the basic ethical principles from the *Belmont Report*. However, practically incorporating the consideration of these criteria into an IRB's review of research is not always easy. A main reason is that although approval of the research according to the criteria at 45 CFR 46.111 represents the required regulatory finding that an IRB must make in order to achieve compliance with the federal regulations, the regulations do not require that the IRB actually document their findings that the research has met *each* specific criteria in order to grant the approval. Discussions with IRB administrators will likely yield many different opinions on whether an IRB should document their consideration of each of the 111 criteria. However, regardless of whether the IRB decides to generate specific documentation of its assessment of each of the 111 criteria, having IRB members structure their review of research according to the 111 criteria has several benefits. Beyond ensuring that the IRB is reliably meeting regulatory requirements, using the 111 criteria to structure and focus its review minimizes possible distractions the IRB may experience in its review and oversight of the research. Additionally, when IRBs are faced with deciding whether to defer or even disapprove a protocol, it is important for the IRB to document the rationale for the disapproval or deferral within the context of the 111 criteria.

IRBs may use a variety of checklists to ensure that all regulatory requirements are met, including the elements of informed consent and the subpart requirements. Using a checklist approach to address the criteria for approval is no different. The 111 criteria can be made available to the <u>convened IRB</u> and individual reviewers in a variety of formats, such as a large wall poster or copies of laminated pages of the criteria in the IRB meeting area; projection on a screen during <u>IRB meetings</u>; or included on a required review sheet within an electronic system. The objective is for the IRB reviewers to turn their attention to the criteria that must be met for a research plan or modification to be approved. Directing the IRB to the criteria for approval at the conclusion of its protocol review ensures that the IRB's regulatory responsibility is being met and allows documentation of IRB action. Invoking the criteria as the final decision-making mechanism also facilitates consistency in review, by ensuring that each research plan is reviewed according to a uniform procedure that utilizes the same criteria for approval. Consistency in IRB adherence to approval criteria is important

⊘ 5-7

⊘ 3-3

across similar types of research, such as clinical trials, as well as across different types of research, such as biomedical and social science studies.

Despite the common IRB practice of utilizing checklists, use of a checklist based solely on the regulatory text in the criteria for approval will not in itself ensure adequate IRB review. After all, the text of each criterion is relatively brief, but each invokes a number of ethical concepts and requires the application of informed judgment. Use of checklists for IRB review should be supplemented by adequate <u>education of IRB members</u> so that they are equipped to understand the meaning of the criteria and can interpret and apply the criteria. The failure of IRB members to understand the intention of each criterion can result in incomplete consideration of the approval criteria, especially in a high-risk study, in which possible risks take many forms, as further described later.

🖉 8-4

Of all the approval criteria, criteria 1 and 2 are the most nuanced in their directive to assure that risk is minimized and that it is reasonable. Minimizing risk by ensuring procedures of sound research design, as well as no unnecessary exposure to risk, may require ancillary reviews concurrent with IRB review. These include review by the institutional biosafety committee if therapeutically oriented research involves recombinant DNA, or the radiation safety committee if the research involves exposure to radiation for either therapeutic or nontherapeutic purposes. Another important concurrent review is for <u>conflict of interest</u> and its management. The risk of harm to research subjects or the threat to a study's integrity due to unmanaged bias by a conflicted researcher can be serious. The IRB should give substantial consideration as to whether a conflict of interest management plan is adequate to protect subjects as well as the objectivity of the research.

🖉 12-6

Another consideration for making determinations incorporated in criteria 1 and 2, but not explicitly stated, involves ensuring the appropriate qualifications of the research team to safely conduct the research. Although human subjects protection education for researchers is not specifically required in the Common Rule, the term of assurance number 3 in the <u>Federalwide Assurance</u> (FWA) filed through the OHRP requires compliance with the relevant regulations for both domestic and non-U.S. institutions (DHHS, 2017). Because knowledge about the ethical principles and regulations facilitates compliance, most institutions require all researchers engaged in the research to complete <u>human subjects protection training,</u> typically a purchased online training course or an internally developed training program. Completion of institutionally required training is generally verified by the IRB administrative office. However, ensuring that the principal investigator and other engaged researchers have the scientific knowledge and/or experience to safely conduct the research is an IRB responsibility. The type and amount of knowledge and/or experience deemed necessary depend on the risk assessment of the research. Whereas the researchers for a first-in-human clinical trial researching an investigational drug or device should be highly experienced and the principal investigator an expert clinician, the researchers for a study involving human blood collection for basic science research do not warrant the same level of experience or expertise with human subjects research.

🖉 8-1

🖉 8-5

The IRB may learn of institutional circumstances that present ethical issues for multiple studies, but because of their broad applicability to the research environment, appear to be beyond the scope of the criteria for approval. IRBs should keep in mind that when subjects' rights and welfare are at risk of being negatively affected by institutional circumstances, those circumstances may be relevant to the criteria for approval and may be within the IRB's purview. Some examples include IRB awareness of insufficient resources, such as staffing or emergency equipment for addressing adverse events at a research location or knowledge that one or more greater than minimal risk studies are being run by overcommitted researchers whose attentiveness may be compromised. Both of these circumstances may affect the risk assessment for multiple studies. As another example, the IRB may become aware of institutional obstacles to payment of research subjects that can affect subjects' voluntary participation. These types of institutional circumstances, which implicate one or more *Belmont* principles, and hence one or more criteria for approval, may require the IRB's referral to other HRPP entities for resolution.

Conclusion

Adherence to the criteria for approval is required by the Common Rule. At the same time, the criteria for approval are instrumental to the comprehensive ethical review of a research plan by the IRB. Although the regulatory text detailing each of the criteria is relatively brief, the discussion in this chapter demonstrates that many of the criteria are complex. It is critical for ethical review and approval of research to educate the IRB to utilize the criteria for approval, understand the criteria's relation to the *Belmont* principles, and appreciate the multiple considerations contained within the criteria. Balancing full consideration of the criteria for approval with an institution's desire for efficiency and consistency in review can be a challenge for every IRB.

References

Agency for Healthcare Research and Quality (AHRQ). (2011). *AHRQ data and safety monitoring policy.* (NOT-HS-11-015). grants.nih.gov/grants/guide/notice-files/NOT-HS-11-015.html

Department of Health and Human Services (DHHS). (2017). *DHHS Office for Human Research Protections: Terms of assurance: Federalwide Assurance (FWA) for the protection of human subjects.* www.hhs.gov/ohrp/register-irbs-and-obtain-fwas/fwas/fwa-protection-of-human-subjecct/index.html

Federal Register. (2017). Vol. 82, No. 12. 45 CFR 46 and Preamble. www.govinfo.gov/content/pkg/FR-2017-01-19/pdf/2017-01058.pdf

Food and Drug Administration (FDA). (2012). *Presentation to the Secretary's Advisory Committee on Human Research Protections: Component analysis.* www.fda.gov/media/84798/download

National Commission for the Protection of Human Subjects of Biomedical and Behavioral Research. (1979). *The Belmont Report: Ethical principles and guidelines for the protection of human subjects of research.* www.hhs.gov/ohrp/regulations-and-policy/belmont-report/read-the-belmont-report/index.html

National Institutes of Health (NIH). (1998). *NIH policy for data and safety monitoring.* (NOT-98-084). grants.nih.gov/grants/guide/notice-files/not98-084.html

National Institutes of Health (NIH). (2000). *Further guidance on data and safety monitoring in Phase I and Phase II Trials.* (NOT-OD-00-038). grants.nih.gov/grants/guide/WeeklyIndex-subjecct/index.html

Expedited Review of Research

David Borasky

Nancy Olson

Abstract

The Common Rule and the Food and Drug Administration (FDA) regulations for the protection of human subjects include a pathway for reviewing research that does not warrant review by the full IRB at a convened meeting. This pathway, known as expedited review, is described in the Common Rule at **45 CFR 46** and the FDA regulations at **21 CFR 56**. Under expedited review, certain types of research may be reviewed by the IRB chairperson or by one or more experienced reviewers designated by the chairperson. This chapter reviews the regulations governing expedited review procedures and describes how this type of review should be implemented.

What Is Expedited Review?

Expedited review is a type of review whereby a subset of the IRB—the IRB chairperson or one or more experienced IRB members designated by the chairperson—review proposed research in lieu of review by the convened IRB. This pathway allows certain proposed minimal risk research, as well as minor changes to approved research, to be reviewed without waiting for a meeting of the convened IRB. Under expedited review, the designated reviewer(s) apply all applicable regulations (Common Rule and/or FDA), including the criteria for approval and the requirements for informed consent, and have the authority to either approve the submission or require modifications as a condition of securing IRB approval. Expedited reviewers may not disapprove research; if the reviewer(s) cannot approve the research it must be referred to a meeting of the convened IRB for further review.

    The 2018 revisions to the Common Rule included changes to the expedited review regulations that have not been adopted by the FDA at the time of this publication. The most significant change is that, under the revised regulations (the 2018 Requirements), there is an assumption that all activities and examples on the list of expedited categories are no greater than minimal risk,

🔗 5-7

🔗 5-4
🔗 6-2

and therefore the burden on the reviewer is to determine if or when a proposed activity on the list is greater than minimal risk. This differs from the pre-2018 requirements according to which the reviewer was expected to separately verify that that proposed research was both on the list and that it involves no more than minimal risk. The revised regulations were also modified to further encourage the utilization of expedited review. **45 CFR 46.115(a)(8)** now requires documentation of the rationale for an expedited reviewer's determination under **45 CFR 46.110(b)(1)(i)** that the research under review falls within one of the categories on the expedited review list but is more than minimal risk.

⊘ 5-6
⊘ 5-3

In addition, under the 2018 Common Rule, expedited review procedures may be used to conduct the limited IRB review that is required for certain exempt categories of research **[45 CFR 46.110(b)(1)(iii)]** (Department of Health and Human Services, 2018).

What Is Eligible for Expedited Review?

The Common Rule and FDA regulations allow the use of expedited review for two general types of submissions to the IRB: (1) research that is no more than minimal risk and all procedures and methods are included on the list of categories maintained by the Department of Health and Human Services (DHHS) and (2) minor changes to previously approved research during the period for which approval is authorized.

Research That Is No More Than Minimal Risk and on the List of Categories Maintained by DHHS

The first permitted type of expedited review is the review of research identified on the expedited review list. The current expedited review list was last revised in 1998 and includes seven categories of activities that may be initially approved via expedited review and two categories for the expedited continuing review of research that was initially approved by the convened IRB (DHHS, 1998). For the expedited review of research under one or more of the seven categories on the list, there is a presumption that all of the proposed research activities are no greater than minimal risk. Under the pre-2018 Common Rule, the IRB member(s) conducting expedited review had to find that the proposed activities involve no more than minimal risk. Under the 2018 Common Rule, the IRB member(s) conducting expedited review may proceed with the review unless the reviewer determines that the study involves more than minimal risk. This subtle shift in approach—from having to find that an activity on the list was indeed minimal risk, to the presumption that it is—foreshadows a revision to the expedited review categories, giving all of the categories the presumption of minimal risk. However, the list was not revised with the 2018 Common Rule revision and has not been revised at the time of publication. Until there is a new list, OHRP has reconciled this issue by stating that the instructions in the current list, which require a determination that an activity on the list is minimal risk, remain in effect until the list is revised (DHHS, 2019).

Given the presumption that activities on the list are no greater than minimal risk, it is necessary to review the definition of minimal risk. Under both the Common Rule and FDA regulations, minimal risk means "that the probability and magnitude of harm or discomfort anticipated in the research are not greater in and of themselves than those ordinarily encountered in daily life or during the performance of routine physical or psychological examinations or tests" [45 CFR 46.102(j); 21 CFR 50.3(k)]. When applying this definition, reviewers are cautioned to avoid a relativistic approach. The threshold for minimal risk should not fluctuate based on an individual's condition in a way that allows procedures to be viewed as minimal risk for a research subject, when the same procedures would not be considered minimal risk if they were performed on a healthy person in daily life. At the same time, applying this definition also means that there will be procedures that are minimal risk for some populations and not others. For example, a cardiac stress test may be minimal risk in a population of physically active young adults but greater than minimal risk for adults with known cardiac disease. IRB member(s) conducting expedited review must be satisfied that the research activities being approved are all no greater than minimal risk.

The last two categories on the current list allow for expedited review for the continuing review of research previously approved by the convened IRB in certain circumstances. One of the categories allows expedited review based on the current state of the research with respect to implementation: for example, research where the remaining research activities are limited to data analysis. The second category of expedited continuing review is for research that was initially reviewed by the convened IRB, and the IRB determined that the research was minimal risk.

✏ 7-2

Minor Changes to Previously Approved Research

The second permitted type of expedited review is the review and approval of minor changes to previously approved research, during the period for which approval is authorized. The regulations do not define a "minor change." Reasonable interpretations of a minor change include the addition of procedures that are described in one of the expedited categories, modifications that add no more than minimal risk to subjects, and modifications that do not substantively alter the research design.

Expedited Review Categories (DHHS, 1998)

Category 1

Clinical studies of drugs and medical devices only when condition (a) or (b) is met.

(a) Research on drugs for which an investigational new drug application (21 CFR Part 312) is not required. (Note: Research on marketed drugs that significantly increases the risks or decreases the acceptability of the risks associated with the use of the product is not eligible for expedited review.)

(b) Research on medical devices for which (i) an investigational device exemption application (21 CFR Part 812) is not required; or (ii) the medical device is cleared/approved for marketing and the medical device is being used in accordance with its cleared/approved labeling.

Given the nature of most clinical investigations of FDA-regulated drugs and devices, there will be few submissions that qualify for category 1 expedited review.

Category 2

Collection of blood samples by finger stick, heel stick, ear stick, or venipuncture as follows:

(a) from healthy, nonpregnant adults who weigh at least 110 pounds. For these subjects, the amounts drawn may not exceed 550 ml in an 8 week period and collection may not occur more frequently than 2 times per week; or

(b) from other adults and children, considering the age, weight, and health of the subjects, the collection procedure, the amount of blood to be collected, and the frequency with which it will be collected. For these subjects, the amount drawn may not exceed the lesser of 50 ml or 3 ml per kg in an 8 week period and collection may not occur more frequently than 2 times per week.

When applying category 2, reviewers should pay careful attention to the proposed volumes and frequency of sample collection to ensure that they remain within the limits of the category. When the proposed subject population falls under category 2(b), special expertise may be needed to confirm that the collection of samples is minimal risk, given the specifics of the subject population and the circumstances in which the samples are obtained.

Category 3

Prospective collection of biological specimens for research purposes by noninvasive means.

Examples: (a) hair and nail clippings in a nondisfiguring manner; (b) deciduous teeth at time of exfoliation or if routine patient care indicates a need for extraction; (c) permanent teeth if routine patient care indicates a need for extraction; (d) excreta and external secretions (including sweat); (e) uncannulated saliva collected either in an unstimulated fashion or stimulated by chewing gumbase or wax or by applying a dilute citric solution to the tongue; (f) placenta removed at delivery; (g) amniotic fluid obtained at the time of rupture of the membrane prior to or during labor; (h) supra- and subgingival dental plaque and calculus, provided the collection procedure is not more invasive than routine prophylactic scaling of the teeth and the process is accomplished in accordance with accepted prophylactic techniques; (i) mucosal and skin cells collected by buccal scraping or swab, skin swab, or mouth washings; (j) sputum collected after saline mist nebulization.

The numerous examples provided in this category should be generally well understood. Reviewers may consider the proposed use of the specimens and whether the use may be greater than minimal risk, taking into account mechanisms put in place by the research team to mitigate risks related to the use of the specimens.

Category 4

Collection of data through noninvasive procedures (not involving general anesthesia or sedation) routinely employed in clinical practice, excluding procedures involving x-rays or microwaves. Where medical devices are employed, they must be cleared/approved for marketing. (Studies intended to evaluate the safety and effectiveness of the medical device are not generally eligible for expedited review, including studies of cleared medical devices for new indications.)

Examples: (a) physical sensors that are applied either to the surface of the body or at a distance and do not involve input of significant amounts of energy into the subject or an invasion of the subjects' privacy; (b) weighing or testing sensory acuity; (c) magnetic resonance imaging; (d) electrocardiography, electroencephalography, thermography, detection of naturally occurring radioactivity, electroretinography, ultrasound, diagnostic infrared imaging, doppler blood flow, and echocardiography; (e) moderate exercise, muscular strength testing, body composition assessment, and flexibility testing where appropriate given the age, weight, and health of the individual.

Examples provided should be generally well understood. Reviewers should be mindful of the excluded procedures (e.g., sedation, x-ray).

Category 5

Research involving materials (data, documents, records, or specimens) that have been collected, or will be collected solely for nonresearch purposes (such as medical treatment or diagnosis). (NOTE: Some research in this category may be exempt from the HHS regulations for the protection of human subjects. 45 CFR 46.101(b)(4). This listing refers only to research that is not exempt.)

This category applies to research using retrospectively or prospectively collected materials that were obtained for nonresearch purposes. When the materials will be maintained in an identifiable manner, the reviewer should ascertain that there are adequate provisions to protect the privacy of subjects and to maintain the confidentiality of data, to the extent that the risk to subjects is not greater than minimal risk. It is also noted that the revised DHHS regulations have expanded the categories of <u>exemption</u> so that some activities   🖉 5-3 that could previously be expedited under category 5 may now qualify for one or more exempt category.

Category 6

Collection of data from voice, video, digital, or image recordings made for research purposes.

IRB reviewers should be satisfied that the proposed use of the information does not expose subjects to risks that are greater than minimal. When the materials will be maintained in an identifiable manner, the reviewer should ascertain that there are adequate provisions to protect the privacy of subjects and to maintain the confidentiality of data to the extent that the risk to subjects is not greater than minimal risk.

Category 7

Research on individual or group characteristics or behavior (including, but not limited to, research on perception, cognition, motivation, identity, language, communication, cultural beliefs or practices, and social behavior) or research employing survey, interview, oral history, focus group, program evaluation, human factors evaluation, or quality assurance methodologies. (NOTE: Some research in this category may be exempt from the HHS regulations for the protection of human subjects. 45 CFR 46.101(b)(2) and (b)(3). This listing refers only to research that is not exempt.)

IRB reviewers should determine that the collection and use of the data remain minimal risk. When information will be collected in a group setting, such as a focus group survey, the reviewer should consider whether subjects are being asked to disclose information that could reasonably place the subjects at risk of criminal or civil liability or be damaging to the subjects' financial standing, employability, or reputation.

Category 8

Continuing review of research previously approved by the convened IRB as follows:

where (i) the research is permanently closed to the enrollment of new subjects; (ii) all subjects have completed all research-related interventions; and (iii) the research remains active only for long-term follow-up of subjects; or where no subjects have been enrolled and no additional risks have been identified; or where the remaining research activities are limited to data analysis.

Forms used by the IRB to collect information for continuing review should be designed to collect the information in a manner that facilitates the application of category 8. This includes obtaining precise information about the status of the research with respect to initiation, enrollment, and the nature of ongoing research activities. In addition, the IRB must ascertain whether additional risks have been identified since the last review.

Category 9

Continuing review of research, not conducted under an investigational new drug application or investigational device exemption where categories two (2) through eight (8) do not apply but the IRB has determined and documented at a convened meeting that the research involves no greater than minimal risk and no additional risks have been identified.

This category is typically employed with protocols that are clearly minimal risk but did not fit an existing expedited category at the time of initial review. For example, a study assessing perceptions of individuals whose hands are exposed to cold stimulation may be minimal risk, but there is no category for the exposure to cold stimulation.

Conclusion

The regulations were written with an understanding that not all research activities require the attention of a convened IRB. One pathway for the review of certain minimal risk research is the expedited review procedure. IRBs should be encouraged to utilize expedited review whenever applicable. However, careful attention should be given to ensure that reviews are completed by one or more experienced IRB members. Expedited categories must be applied appropriately, and the IRB must adopt a method for keeping all members advised of research proposals that have been approved under the expedited review procedure, as required by DHHS regulations at **45 CFR 46.110(b)(2)(c)** and FDA regulations at **21 CFR 56.110(c)**.

References

Department of Health and Human Services (DHHS). (1998). *Expedited review categories: Categories of research that may be reviewed by the institutional review board (IRB) through an expedited review procedure.* www.hhs.gov/ohrp/regulations-and-policy/guidance/categories-of-research-expedited-review-procedure-1998/index.html

Department of Health and Human Services (DHHS). (2018). *Revised Common Rule Q&As.* www.hhs.gov/ohrp/education-and-outreach/revised-common-rule/revised-common-rule-q-and-a/index.html

Department of Health and Human Services (DHHS). (2019). *2018 Requirements FAQs.* www.hhs.gov/ohrp/regulations-and-policy/guidance/faq/2018-requirements-faqs/index.html

Limited IRB Review

Helene Lake Bullock

Ada Sue Selwitz

Abstract

The purpose of this chapter is to discuss limited IRB review, which is required for four exemption categories of research as outlined in the Common Rule. In limited review, the reviewer(s) is not required to apply all of the standard approval criteria listed in **45 CFR 46.111** of the regulations. Limited IRB review is applicable for studies that meet four exemption categories, which retain research subjects' identifiable private information or use identifiable biospecimens. The criteria for limited IRB review include determining that privacy protections and confidentiality are adequate. In addition, for two of the exemption categories, the limited IRB review must determine that broad consent requirements are met.

Basic Requirements for Conducting Limited IRB Review

The Common Rule requires limited IRB review for select <u>exemption</u> categories. Best practice suggests that limited IRB review be conducted by the IRB chair or an IRB member(s) familiar with privacy protections and confidentiality considerations (Department of Health and Human Services [DHHS], 2018). The reviewer (or reviewers) must apply the criteria of approval that are specifically listed in the regulations for each exemption category. The reviewer(s) is not required to apply all of the standard <u>IRB approval criteria</u> listed in **45 CFR 46.111**.

🔗 5-3

🔗 5-4

Exemptions That Require Limited IRB Review and the Applicable Determinations

There are four exemption categories subject to the limited IRB review requirement:

- [45 CFR 46.104(d)(2)] Research that only includes interactions involving educational tests (cognitive, diagnostic, aptitude, achievement), survey procedures, interview procedures, or observations of public behavior (including visual or auditory recording) if …(iii) The information obtained is recorded by the investigator in such a manner that the identity of the human subjects can readily be ascertained, directly or through identifiers linked to the subjects, and an IRB conducts a limited IRB review to make the determination required by §46.111(a)(7). The determination required by §46.111(a)(7) is that, when appropriate, there are adequate provisions to protect the privacy of subjects and to maintain the confidentiality of data. (Note: This research cannot be subject to subpart D.)

- **[45 CFR 46.104(d)(3)(i)]** Research involving benign behavioral interventions in conjunction with the collection of information from an adult subject through verbal or written responses (including data entry) or audiovisual recording if the subject prospectively agrees to the intervention and information collection and … (C) The information obtained is recorded by the investigator in such a manner that the identity of the human subjects can readily be ascertained, directly or through identifiers linked to the subject, and an IRB conducts a limited IRB review to make the determination required by §46.111(a)(7), as outlined previously. (Note: This research cannot be subject to subpart D.)

- **[45 CFR 46.104(d)(7)]** Storage or maintenance for secondary research for which broad consent is required: Storage or maintenance of identifiable private information or identifiable biospecimens for potential secondary research use if an IRB conducts a limited IRB review and makes the three determinations required by §46.111(a)(8). The three determinations listed in **45 CFR 46.111(a)(8)** are as follows:

    (i) Broad consent for the storage, maintenance, and secondary research use of the identifiable private information or identifiable biospecimens was obtained in accordance with §46.116(a)(1) through (4), (a)(6), and (d);

    (ii) Broad consent is appropriately documented or waiver of documentation of consent is appropriate consistent in accordance with §46.117;

    (iii) If there is a change made for research purposes in the way the identifiable private information or identifiable biospecimen are stored or maintained, there are adequate provisions to protect the privacy of the subjects and to maintain the confidentiality of the data.

- **[45 CFR 46.104(d)(8)]** Secondary research for which broad consent is required: Research involving the use of identifiable private information or identifiable biospecimens for secondary research use, if the following criteria are met:

    (i) Broad consent for the storage, maintenance, and secondary research use of the identifiable private information or identifiable biospecimens was obtained in accordance with §46.116(a)(1) through (4), (a)(6), and (d);

    (ii) Documentation of informed consent or waiver of documentation of consent was obtained in accordance with §46.117;

    (iii) An IRB conducts a limited IRB review and makes the determination required by §46.111(a)(7) and makes the determination that the research to be conducted is within the scope of the broad consent referenced in paragraph (d)(8)(i) of this section; and

    (iv) The investigator does not include returning individual research results to subjects as part of the study plan. This provision does not prevent an investigator from abiding by any legal requirements to return individual research results.

The Limited IRB Review Process

The following are elements of a limited IRB review process:

- The expedited review mechanism may be used, which means that the IRB chair or an experienced IRB member performs the limited IRB review. A convened IRB can fill this function as well (DHHS, 2018).
- The limited IRB reviewer only applies the specific criteria required for each exempt category and determines if the applicable criteria are met. These criteria include **45 CFR 46.111(a)(7)**, which references protection of privacy of subjects and confidentiality of data, and/or **45 CFR 46.111(a)(8)** which focuses on obtaining, documenting, or waiving documentation of broad consent, or whether the research is consistent with broad consent.   6-9
- The IRB reviewer needs the appropriate expertise to make the required determinations. For example, depending upon the study, IRBs may include an IT expert as a reviewer to ensure maintenance of confidentiality by use of appropriate security controls.
- The IRB reviewer who conducts limited IRB review may require modification(s) to the proposed research prior to approval or determine that the study meets the applicable criteria and is eligible for exemption.
- There is no yearly or continuation review required for studies approved via limited IRB review (DHHS, 2018).
- If the study is not eligible for the exempt category proposed, the study may be reviewed using expedited or convened IRB procedures. Limited IRB review is not a regulatory requirement for nonexempt studies.

  5-3

Administration of Limited IRB Review

Effective administration of a limited IRB review system requires the same components as those required for nonexempt review. The IRB and the IRB staff develop and maintain written limited IRB policies, including standard operating procedures. The electronic system and/or paper reviewer forms must address limited IRB review issues. The capture of information from an electronic system or paper forms must be adequate to enable limited IRB review. Guidance or training of IRB members and researchers should include which exempt research categories require limited IRB review and points to consider in addressing the requirements. A system to support researcher compliance with the requirements as outlined by the limited IRB review may be needed as part of the overall human subjects research protection program.

Limited IRB Review and Privacy

Privacy pertains to a person's desire to control the access of others to themselves or to information about themselves. For example, a person may not want to be seen entering a place that might stigmatize them, such as a pregnancy counseling center that is clearly identified as such by signs on the front of the building. Limited IRB review should evaluate the research proposal for strategies to protect privacy, including how the researcher will identify, contact, and recruit subjects; how information will be accessed and managed; and plans for deidentification and possible reidentification of identifiable subject information or biospecimens.

🔗 6-9   For the categories of exempt research that require <u>broad consent</u>, limited review of privacy also includes consideration of the collection of identifiable information or biospecimens, including appropriate documentation of informed

🔗 6-5   consent or <u>waiver of informed consent</u>, secondary research use of the information/biospecimens, and that the research is conducted within the scope of the broad consent.

Limited IRB Review and Confidentiality

Confidentiality pertains to data and the researcher's agreement with the subject about how the subject's identifiable private information or identifiable biospecimens will be managed. Limited IRB review should evaluate the research proposal for strategies to maintain confidentiality of identifiable data, including controls on storage, handling, and sharing of data. The long-range plan for protecting the confidentiality of research data, including a schedule for retention or destruction of identifiers associated with the data, should also be evaluated.

For the broad consent categories, limited review of confidentiality also includes consideration of storage and maintenance of identifiable information/biospecimens collected; potential risk of harm should the information be lost, stolen, or compromised; security measures to protect the confidentiality and integrity of the information/biospecimens; secondary research use of the information/specimens; and confidentiality of the data should any change be made for research purposes regarding storage or maintenance of the information/biospecimens.

Information to Collect for a Limited IRB Review

To ensure that the limited IRB review process is thorough, sufficient information must be gathered from the researcher to enable the review. This can be achieved by using a form, or in the case of an electronic system, a page containing questions that the researcher answers to provide information regarding the data or biospecimens collected from research subjects. Factors that will assist a limited IRB review include (but are not limited to) the following:

- Information on the identifiable information/biospecimen(s) to be collected, and a list of the source(s) of the information, such as a list of any data that will accompany the specimen or be extracted from the medical record
- Plan to protect the identifiable information/biospecimens
- Information on management and physical storage of specimens and data, such as where the identifiable information/biospecimens will be stored and how access is secured
- Information on the mechanism for how biospecimens will be shared (internally/externally), including procedures for coding, deidentification, encryption, and/or data-use agreements
- Description of who will have access to the identifiable information/biospecimens, such as internal researchers, external collaborators, commercial industry, IRB, sponsors, Food and Drug Administration, data safety monitoring boards, and any others given authority by law

- Description of the retention plan for maintaining the data and/or biospecimens and, if applicable, the plan for destroying the data at the earliest opportunity consistent with the conduct of the research
- Explanation for why the research could not practically be conducted without access to and/or use of the proposed identifiable information/biospecimens
- Reasonable efforts to limit identifiable information/biospecimens to the minimum necessary to accomplish the intended purpose of the use, disclosure, or request; an explanation for why the identifiable private information obtained for this study is the minimum information needed to meet the research objectives
- Description of what the potential risk of harm is to research subjects, should the information/biospecimens be lost, stolen, compromised, or otherwise used in a way contrary to the expectations of the research under the exemption; risks associated with a breach of confidentiality include impacts on privacy, insurability, and/or stigmatization
- Description of tracking subject choices where options are provided within the broad consent
- Subject study withdrawal procedure as it relates to data retention and data sharing
- Whether secondary research could involve genetic or genomic research or creation of cell lines
- Copy of the broad consent document or a justification for waiving documentation of broad consent
- Description of the process for obtaining broad consent
- Plan for how to manage data breach or the information getting into the wrong hands

Conclusion

The Common Rule requires limited IRB review for select exempt categories, which collect identifiable private information or identifiable biospecimens. During the limited IRB review, the IRB must make the determinations specifically outlined in the regulations, such as ensuring that protection of subject privacy and maintenance of confidentiality of the data are adequate. Collection of relevant information to be able to conduct limited IRB review is crucial, as is knowledge of the exempt categories that qualify for the review.

Reference

Department of Health and Human Services (DHHS). (2018). *Revised Common Rule Q&As*. www.hhs.gov/ohrp/education-and-outreach/revised-common-rule/revised-common-rule-q-and-a/index.html

Full Committee Review

Martha F. Jones
Amy Waltz

Abstract

Federal regulations require nonexempt research be reviewed by a convened IRB, or full committee, unless the research is eligible for expedited review. This chapter discusses key aspects of full committee review. Discussion of preview activities includes understanding what research requires full board review, choosing a committee structure, and providing materials. The authors also address the IRB's conduct of the review, including organizing the meeting to facilitate the IRB's discussion and review..

Identifying Research Requiring Full Board Review

The Common Rule provides the basis of human research protections for most institutions. The Common Rule requires IRB review for nonexempt human subjects research by the full board or by expedited review. The <u>expedited</u> review procedures are available for minimal risk research falling into one or more published categories. According to the Common Rule and the expedited categories (Department of Health and Human Services [DHHS], 1998), research that is not eligible for expedited review must be initially reviewed by the full board. Research may require full board review because it does not meet one of the regulatory definitions of minimal risk and thus is determined to be greater than minimal risk; it does not fall into a category for expedited review; the expedited reviewer does not believe that the <u>criteria for approval</u> are met; or because local policies require full board review.

🔗 5-5

🔗 5-4

Full Board Review Based on a Determination of Greater Than Minimal Risk

Greater than minimal risk research is not eligible for expedited review and must be reviewed by the full committee. The regulations do not define "greater than minimal risk" but instead provide two definitions of minimal risk, one

EXEMPT VERSUS NONEXEMPT RESEARCH

Exempt research, research fitting the categories described in **45 CFR 46.104**, is exempt from the regulations and does not require IRB review, full committee or otherwise. As such, this chapter will not address exempt research. All references to "research" should be read to mean nonexempt human subjects research, as defined by the federal regulations.

for nonprisoner populations and a slightly different definition for the prisoner population. Thus, greater than minimal risk is interpreted to be research that *does not* meet the regulatory definition of minimal risk for the applicable population under study:

> "*Minimal risk* means that the probability and magnitude of harm or discomfort anticipated in the research are not greater in and of themselves than those ordinarily encountered in daily life or during the performance of routine physical or psychological examinations or tests. [45 CFR 46.102(j)]

> *Minimal risk for prisoners* means the probability and magnitude of physical or psychological harm that is normally encountered in the daily lives, or in the routine medical, dental, or psychological examination of healthy persons. [45 CFR 46.303(d)]"

Although the general (nonprisoner) definition does not reference "healthy persons," it is generally interpreted that the healthy person should be used as the standard in this definition.

Depending on the chosen model of IRB review, an initial determination of risk may be made at various steps in the review process. A trained IRB staff person could initially triage research studies to expedited review or full board review. When this process is used, the final determination of risk is made by either the expedited reviewer or the full board. For example, if the triage person routes a study to expedited review, the designated expedited reviewer could still determine that the study is greater than minimal risk and route the research to a full board review.

Some institutions allow the researcher to note in the IRB application whether they believe the study is minimal risk or greater than minimal risk, and/or the applicable expedited category, if minimal risk. The IRB or IRB reviewer must make the final determination of risk level (or expedited category), but the researcher's choice can be used as an initial triage mechanism for operational efficiency. Other possible review paths include having all research initially screened by a designated expedited reviewer to determine which studies meet criteria for expedited review, and which should be reviewed by the full board or via a subcommittee to make this determination. The full board should document its final determination of minimal risk or greater than minimal risk in the meeting <u>minutes</u>.

🔗 2-6

Full Board Review Based on Falling Outside the Regulatory Expedited Categories

The Common Rule includes language that implies a presumption of minimal risk if the research appears on the expedited review list [45 CFR 45.110(i); 45 CFR 46.115(a)(8)]. The list of expedited categories published by the Office for Human Research Protections (OHRP) requires that the research present no more than minimal risk *and* that all activities involved in the research be covered by one or more of the categories on the list (DHHS, 1998). For research

🔗 5-5

to be approved through <u>expedited review</u>, the designated reviewer would need to make two distinct determinations: (1) that all activities met the definition of minimal risk and (2) that all activities fall into one or more of the expedited categories. Thus, research in which all activities could be deemed minimal risk, but (for example) one procedure was not consistent with the expedited categories, could not be approved through an expedited review process and would require full board review. A common example is research involving any type of x-ray, such as a dual energy x-ray absorptiometry (DEXA) scan. Today, these scans are typically considered minimal risk and are a part of everyday medical practice. However, because they are specifically not included in the list of expedited categories, research in which these scans are conducted would need to go to the full board for initial review. As such, the full board may be required to review research that could be minimal risk but that includes procedures not found in the current expedited categories.

The 2018 Common Rule enacted a requirement for regular review of the categories of research that could be approved through expedited review, removing the requirement for a separate determination that research in these categories are minimal risk. Under this provision, research reviewed under expedited categories codified subsequent to the 1998 list will not need a separate minimal risk determination. However, the 2018 Common Rule allows that research that appears to fall under one or more expedited categories could still be determined by the designated expedited reviewer to be greater than minimal risk, thus routing the research to a full board review. When this occurs, the reviewer's rationale must be documented [45 CFR 46.115(a) (8)] and should be provided to the full committee for consideration during its review.

Research That the Expedited Reviewer Feels Does Not Meet the Criteria for Approval

The regulations do not allow expedited reviewers to disapprove research [45 CFR 46.110(b)(2)]. If the expedited reviewer cannot find that the research meets the regulatory criteria for approval at **45 CFR 46.111** or the additional **subparts B, C,** or **D,** the research must be referred to the full board for review. In such cases, the reviewer's comments, and any response from the researcher, should be provided to the full board for its review.

✎ 5-4

Research Where Local Policies Require Full Board Review

Although the federal regulations are sometimes described as the "floor," or minimal requirements, for review and oversight of human subjects research, they do not preclude individual IRBs or institutions from developing additional requirements for the protection of human subjects. An institution and its IRB may choose to review all research through the full board mechanism and not utilize an expedited review process at all. When making this choice, consideration should be made as to whether this unduly slows the review process without adding additional protection for human subjects.

More often, it may be appropriate for certain types of research to be sent to the full board even if they otherwise would qualify for expedited review. For example, if expedited reviewers do not have appropriate expertise to review vulnerable populations such as children or individuals with impaired decision-making capacity, even minimal risk studies of these populations may be more appropriately reviewed by the full board if it has relevant expertise. Another example

✎ 9-6
✎ 9-7

🔗 10-4   is a study that would normally fall into an expedited category, such as <u>survey research</u>, where the survey is asking very sensitive questions, the risk of which would be better assessed by the full board. Though not required by the regula-

🔗 9-5   tions, <u>prisoner</u> research is often sent to the full board even if it would otherwise qualify for expedited review, especially for initial review purposes.

When review procedures require or allow for full board review that could otherwise be reviewed through expedited mechanisms, local policies should clearly define what research should be reviewed by the full board, the review process, and any required determinations.

Overall, institutions should ensure that the designated reviewers and/or full board members who are responsible for determining whether research is reviewed through an expedited or full board process are trained in the appli-

🔗 2-7   cable definitions, regulations, and policies. A process of <u>quality assurance</u> is useful to ensure not only compliance with all requirements, but consistency across reviewers, full boards, and a variety of research studies.

Conducting IRB Review

Research not otherwise eligible for review via expedited procedures is presented to the full board for consideration. The primary responsibility of the

🔗 5-4   board is to review the research to determine whether the regulatory <u>criteria for approval</u> have been met, as well as any requirements under subparts B, C, and/

🔗 3-3   or D as applicable. While the structure of the committee <u>meeting</u> will vary from institution to institution, the requirements of the discussion should achieve the regulatory required determinations.

How the determinations are made can occur in a variety of ways. The IRB must make determinations about each of the criteria for approval described in the regulations. If all the criteria for approval and any applicable subpart requirements are not met, the research cannot be approved, regardless of other "outside" considerations. For example, research that seems very appropriate from a scientific design standpoint cannot be approved if risks have not been minimized even if a determination has been made that the risk/benefit ratio is

🔗 Section 9   appropriate. Likewise, targeting a <u>vulnerable population</u> to simply make the research easier to conduct or less costly would not meet the criteria for approval, regardless of the scientific importance of the research.

The process for determining that all required criteria and subparts have been met may vary across full boards. Generally, one or more members of the board present the research to the board, including a summary of the research, whether the research appears to meet the criteria for approval, any questions or concerns about the research, and conclude with a recommended action for the board. In this model, the presenter(s) have thoroughly reviewed the entire application and documented that each criterion and applicable subpart(s) have been met. Alternatively, the presenter(s) and/or full board can walk through each criterion during the meeting. The committee members then share their opinions about the questions and concerns raised and raise any new questions or concerns prompted by the discussion. Finally, a chair or member calls for a vote.

Directing the full board's discussion is an extremely important, but dif-

🔗 3-2   ficult, job. This task often falls to the <u>chair</u>, but staff may also serve in this facilitator role. The facilitator must be able to encourage discussion, redirect the discussion on important points, or call the discussion to a close, as necessary.

Focus on the Criteria for Approval

The full board discussion should primarily focus on the <u>criteria for approval</u> and determining whether the research at issue meets those criteria. Reviewers should use the criteria for approval as the basis for their presentation to the rest of the board, identifying any concerns. While full board members may also share suggestions on research design or discuss institutional issues or local approval requirements, these topics should be secondary to the criteria for approval.

🔗 5-4

In order to ensure the criteria for approval are the primary drivers of the discussion, the criteria should be highlighted and easily accessible for reference to the full board members. Consider providing a reviewer checklist designed around the criteria, listing the criteria for approval near the full board reviewer materials, or even hanging the criteria in the meeting room or printing table copies for reviewers to reference.

Identify and Resolve Controverted Issues

One of the goals of the IRB discussion is to identify and resolve controverted issues. Controverted issues are "those that cause controversy and dispute among the IRB membership during a convened meeting [and] . . . usually are the result of opposition to some aspect of the proposed research" (DHHS, 2017, section III.E). Any number of issues may give rise to a controverted issue. The IRB discussion should address these issues in a comprehensive manner, and the facilitator should ensure that all viewpoints are raised and discussed until the board is able to resolve the issue. If the IRB feels that it lacks the information necessary to come to resolution, the questions or concerns should be posed to the researcher.

It is important to note that resolution does not require unanimous agreement. While some controverted issues may be resolved during the discussion itself, some may be controversial enough that IRB members simply will not be able to agree on the same viewpoint or decision. The facilitator should be able to recognize when further debate on an issue is no longer valuable and either redirect the discussion to another topic or call for a vote. The final resolution of a controverted issue may simply be a majority vote for IRB action. Many would argue that a well-functioning IRB will have periodic votes that reflect dissenting opinions.

If an IRB identifies a similar controverted issue in multiple research studies, institutions may consider offering additional resources to the IRB on that topic: a review of the approach taken by similar institutions to the topic, requesting an external opinion from a bioethicist or institutional counsel, or working with research community members to draft guidance.

Be Specific in Which Criteria for Approval Are Not Met and Requirements for Modifications

When the full board determines that all criteria for approval are not met, reviewers should identify the specific criterion (or criteria) or subpart requirement that is not met and why. Reviewers should be careful to point out specific changes that need to be made, and the facilitator may need to ask questions to clarify the reviewers' requests to ensure that modifications can be clearly communicated to the research team.

TIPS FOR DIRECTING THE FULL BOARD DISCUSSION

- Create a culture in which members' viewpoints are valued.
- Discourage interruptions when members are talking.
- Discourage negative reactions such as "you just don't understand research."
- Specifically request feedback from members who are less extroverted and provide time for their viewpoint.
- If a particular member is being left out or overwhelmed, ask him/her to provide written comments.
- Ask members to specifically identify which criterion (or criteria) is driving their requests for modifications.
- Ask members to share their rationale or thought process, not just their conclusion, so that other members can react to the salient points and staff can clearly describe the discussion in the meeting minutes.
- Remind members that unanimity is not the goal.

If the discussion begins to be repetitive, with the same arguments raised repeatedly, end the discussion by calling for a motion or vote.

Taking Full Board Action

The full board's discussion should culminate in a vote on the action to be taken. While institutions may identify a number of specific actions based on institutional needs, full board actions generally fall into one of three categories: approval (possibly with pending changes), request for modifications in order to secure approval, and disapproval.

- *Approval*: Approval indicates that the research meets all criteria for approval as written, as well as any applicable subpart requirements, and may proceed as of the date of approval.
- *Approval pending changes:* When the full board determines that all criteria for approval and applicable subpart requirements will be met after very specific, directive changes are made, the full board can approve the research pending these changes being made and resubmitted. If the researcher agrees to the required changes, the research does not need to be reviewed again by the full board, as long as a designated reviewer verifies that the requirements of the board have been met. If the researcher does not make the required changes, the research would need to return to the full board for further review. Requests by the full board for "clarifications" or more information would not qualify as specific, directive changes and could not be approved pending changes if these requests impact the determinations of whether criteria for approval or subparts have been met. See **Table 5.7-1** for additional examples.

Table 5.7-1 **Recommendations for Researcher Communication**

Instead of:	... consider:
Redesign the protocol to provide additional safeguards for subjects.	The risk of low platelet counts is not adequately minimized by the current protocol. Revise the protocol to require that platelet counts be conducted and reviewed on all subjects prior to subjects' receipt of dose 3.
	The protocol does not include adequate protection procedures for subjects who may be depressed. Revise the protocol to include a plan for when subjects are identified as depressed or possibly depressed.
The study team needs more appropriate expertise.	The current study team does not include all expertise required to adequately identify and minimize the risks posed by the study drug. Identify a cardiologist to be added to the study team whose role will include review of all cardiac-related adverse events.
The informed consent document needs to be rewritten in lay language.	The informed consent is not written in language understandable by most subjects in the target population. Revise the section "What will happen to you in this study" to describe the study procedures in 8th-grade-level language.
The data safety monitoring plan is insufficient.	The plan for monitoring data does not provide sufficient review to ensure ongoing safety of subjects. Revise the data safety monitoring plan, page 3, to require that the data safety monitoring committee meet quarterly instead of annually.

- *Request for modifications in order to secure approval (sometimes called "tabling," or "deferring"):* If the full board determines that modifications to the research are needed before the criteria for approval or subpart requirements can be met, the research cannot be approved. The full board should identify the required changes in a specific and meaningful way that is actionable for the research team. The full board's communication must include the justification or basis for the modifications (DHHS, 2017, section III.D).
- *Disapproval:* Disapproval indicates that the criteria for approval are not met. The full board must communicate the reason for the disapproval and allow an appeal process.

Conclusion

Conducting full board review is a primary responsibility of an IRB, but approaches to doing so vary widely across organizations. Institutions and IRBs must create custom procedures for conducting full board review that comply with federal regulatory requirements and are appropriate for their organization's size and structure. Key activities include determining whether full board review is required, implementing successful strategies for leading meeting discussions, documenting issues and their resolutions, and making final determinations. By applying the concepts and practical approaches presented in this chapter, institutions can facilitate a robust and compliant approach to full board review.

References

Department of Health and Human Services (DHHS). (1998). *OHRP expedited review categories.* www.hhs.gov/ohrp/regulations-and-policy/guidance/categories-of-research-expedited-review-procedure-1998/index.html

Department of Health and Human Services (DHHS). (2017). *Minutes of institutional review board (IRB) meetings: Guidance for institutions and IRBs.* www.hhs.gov/ohrp/minutes-institutional-review-board-irb-meetings-guidae-institutions-and-irbs.html-0

PART 6

Informed Consent

The Functions of Informed Consent

Nir Eyal
Monica Magalhaes

Abstract

Informed consent is one of the core elements of research regulation and human subjects protection. This chapter discusses four core ethical functions of informed consent: protecting subjects' *welfare*, respecting their *autonomy*, providing *transparency*, and fostering *trust* in the research enterprise. Among researchers, there is a conventional idea of what a consent process looks like—providing a detailed document aiming at full disclosure of relevant information, full comprehension of that information by subjects, and written documentation of consent by a signature. Understanding the core functions of informed consent can guide IRBs away from this one-size-fits-all set of requirements and help them determine what would be an appropriate consent process for each specific study, when there might be reason to require more than would be conventionally expected, and when studies would remain ethically justified with less.

The "Conventional" Picture of Informed Consent

Informed consent, a core element of research regulation and human subjects protection, is shorthand for informed, voluntary, and capacitated consent. This introductory chapter invites readers to consider the philosophical foundations of informed consent through the lens of the set of functions that an informed consent process should serve in order for research to be ethical. In our view, this functional approach provides a useful structure to help IRB members think through their decisions about which qualities the consent process of a particular study must display in order to be ethical and which are less important.

The <u>Belmont Report</u> (National Commission, 1979) identifies three ethical principles as particularly relevant to human subjects research: respect for persons (respect for the autonomy of individuals and protection of those with

🖉 1-1

diminished autonomy), beneficence (maximizing benefits and minimizing harms), and justice (regard for the fair distribution of benefits and harms created by human subjects research). As *Belmont* itself states, however, these broad principles can be and have been interpreted in different and sometimes contradictory ways: beneficence can be read as a duty to do harm only if it will lead to a proportionate benefit or as a duty to do no harm at all. Justice, or the idea of fairness in distribution of benefits and harms, is philosophically contentious: a fair distribution can be understood to mean an equal distribution, or a distribution according to need, or according to individual contribution, or to individual desert, or to some other criterion. Later theory is likewise emphatic that the resulting principles require further specification (Beauchamp & Childress, 2009). We hope that consideration of the functions of informed consent in research can help specify any underlying principles.

Belmont also sets out three requirements for human subjects research that guide IRBs: informed consent, assessment of risks and benefits, and fair subject selection. Later theory and documents on ethical human subjects research point out additional or somewhat altered requirements. This chapter focuses on informed consent, but it should be immediately clear that no consent process alone, however demanding, is *sufficient* for justifying studies of human subjects. If the consensus in the field is right, there are things that we cannot justifiably do to people, even with their full consent. The central question about informed consent to study participation, and the one that this chapter expounds, accordingly focuses on studies that the IRB finds to have a reasonable risk/benefit ratio and to be justified at the bar of all other ethical requirements besides that of informed consent. In these circumstances, the question facing the IRB becomes: What kind of informed consent process, if any, should we require researchers to put in place, given the proposed study's particular characteristics?

To start our discussion of this question, let us differentiate three notions of informed consent:

- *Informed consent as a* **decision**: The acts by which a potential subject, having sufficient understanding of what participation entails, of the risks and benefits of participation, and of alternatives to participation, voluntarily opts to participate in a study.
- *Informed consent as a* **form**: A written or electronic document containing information about the study, which is a common means by which researchers convey information to the subject and record the subjects' decision to participate in research (for example, when subjects sign the form).
- *Informed consent as a* **process**: The acts by which researchers impart this information to a potential subject, potentially ensure his or her comprehension, and, if necessary, produce a written or electronic record of his or her informed consent. The informed consent *process* is the focus of this chapter.

Belmont's account of informed consent contains three elements: information (disclosure, especially of the risks involved in the study); comprehension (manner of disclosure in relation to subject's capacity of comprehension, measures to test comprehension when warranted by the level of risk, provisions for cases where subject has limited capacity for comprehension); and voluntariness (agreement to participate free from coercion, pressure, or undue influence).

In practice, these elements have crystallized into a certain picture of a proper informed consent process. In what we shall call the "conventional" picture of the informed consent process, a detailed consent form discloses all relevant information (or at least aims to do so, based on scientific understanding as it exists at the time of the study); potential subjects read and fully comprehend that information; and they sign the consent form to express their consent decision.

This chapter proposes a somewhat different picture: Informed consent processes exist to serve specific ethical functions. The necessity and relative importance of the informed consent process, as well as its ideal form in human subjects research, vary according to what would best serve the functions of consent in the relevant study. The circumstances of a particular study may also shape the relative relevance and importance of each of these functions.

This chapter starts by listing the major ethical functions of informed consent to research and then uses them to poke holes in the conventional picture of the requirement of informed consent to research.

Major Ethical Functions of Informed Consent to Research

Here are what we see as the main functions of the informed consent process (adapted from Dickert et al. [2017] which presents a more complex framework):

1. *Protecting subjects'* **welfare** *(including their health)*: Because the proper goal of research is to produce generalizable knowledge rather than to benefit individual subjects, even perfectly permissible studies can pose net risks to subjects (that is, risks to subjects that exceed expected benefits to them). Studies do so, legitimately, in order to generate substantial social benefits. Still, net risks to subjects can be excessive, and the first line of defense against excessive risks to subjects is the IRB's requirement of a reasonable risk/benefit ratio. Informed consent protects subjects' welfare by offering a double check on this first line of defense, because it is rare for a competent, free, and informed person to knowingly take on enormous net personal risks for trivial social causes. In addition to this protection against "objectively" excessive risks to subjects' health and welfare, the requirement of informed consent can serve more "subjective" determinants of welfare. Each potential subject has privileged insight into what is good for them and how the risks of a particular study would affect them specifically. By requiring disclosure of relevant risks and benefits and allowing potential subjects to decline to take part in research that carries risks that they are not willing to take, informed consent requirements shield subjects against medical or other welfare risks that are excessive by their own standards and given their own potentially idiosyncratic values and preferences.

2. *Respecting subjects'* **autonomy**: Even in the absence of (net) risks to health and welfare, autonomy transgressions can wrong research subjects (Beauchamp & Childress, 2009; Dworkin, 1988; Faden et al., 1986). We generally consider it impermissible to force a person to undergo an invasive exam or procedure against their will in either a research or a clinical setting, even when this procedure is expected to benefit the person "objectively" or by their own value system (and even if it would somehow protect the subject's personal autonomy in the long run). In a research context, because the primary goal is not to benefit subjects, the prohibition against enrollment without authorization is even stronger, as forced participation in research may amount to using subjects as a means to serve an end that they typically will not share: producing knowledge to benefit others, potentially at great risk to themselves (Emanuel et al., 2000; Walen, 2020). Protecting subjects' autonomy through informed consent helps ensure that research is in agreement with subjects' autonomous will.

3. **Transparency**: Informed consent processes also provide potential subjects with information on what the study involves and aims to achieve, what

participation entails, the risks and benefits of participating, and other relevant aspects of the study. Transparency is essential to subjects' ability to evaluate the acceptability of welfare risks and to make autonomous decisions about study participation, the importance of which is discussed earlier. Transparency also furthers accountability and the integrity of the research enterprise, which matter both in their own right and for maintaining public trust in scientific research (see function 4 next).

4. *Protecting public* **trust** *in scientific research*: A consistent record of living up to functions 1 to 3 honors the trust that past research subjects and funders have placed in researchers and in research institutions and fosters further societal trust in research and in medicine. If studies were to consistently place subjects at high risk without their consent, mislead them into giving such consent, or even enroll them with formal "consent" but under circumstances that may be seen as pressure to consent, this would presumably reinforce suspicion of researchers' motivations and, given the relationship between trust and perception of risk (Siegrist, 2019), increase reluctance to participate in research or fully rely on the medical system that uses that research. A climate of mistrust in research may also erode support for public funding of studies.

In any given study, these functions will usually overlap. For example, transparency about the nature, goals, and risks/benefits of a study is also required for subjects to make autonomous decisions, protect their welfare interests, and judge whether the research is consistent with their values. The functions may also clash, as when transparency requires highly detailed informed consent documents that undermine subjects' comprehension and autonomous decision making.

The rest of this chapter argues that considering informed consent in light of its appropriate functions should sometimes lead IRBs to depart from certain conventional expectations from informed consent to study participation. The following examples of such circumstances are not meant to be exhaustive, or even compelling. They merely illustrate how the functions can help structure IRB members' nuanced reasoning when making decisions about consent in particular studies.

Ethical Human Subjects Research Does Not Always Require Written Documentation of Consent

In the conventional view, informed consent processes require subjects to sign a form to record their consent. Rather than demand signatures as a one-size-fits-all policy, IRBs have discretion to require less or require more.

Requiring a signature can certainly serve the functions of informed consent, by signaling the importance of the decision at hand to the subject, and hence the personal commitment entailed by choosing to participate in research. This may have the effect of focusing the subject's attention more intensely, amplifying his or her scrutiny of both what we called "objective" and "subjective" welfare risks, and making the decision about participation more autonomous. Trust in the enterprise of scientific research may also be reinforced when the public expects a clear-cut mark of consent such as a signature for recruitment into risky studies.

🔗 6-5 Still, IRBs might require less than is conventionally expected and <u>waive the signature</u> altogether if participants are illiterate (their oral consent can be recorded) or where written consent increases the main risk to subjects, for example, when a survey recruits persons living with HIV in a setting with extreme HIV stigma in which requiring a signature might, despite best efforts, expose subjects' HIV status. It is also legitimate to waive the signature requirement in order to reduce the burden on researchers and subjects when risk to autonomy or welfare, and therefore arguably also to trust, is minimal. Two surveys of U.S. respondents have found a preference for verbal consent over traditional written consent in pragmatic trials (Dickert et al., 2018a, 2018b). IRBs can waive the signature on a consent form in certain circumstances, including when a study presents only minimal risks to subjects and involves no procedure that would require written consent outside a research setting [45 CFR 46.117(c)(1)(ii)]. Many pragmatic trials are cases in point. Although regulations in most cases require some written information to be given to subjects (even if not that it be signed), there is a margin of discretion for IRBs to decide to supplement this with other means of disclosure (see next section).

    Conversely, in a higher-risk interventional study or one where therapeutic misconception may be of particular concern, the IRB might want to require more than a signature. In many ongoing early-phase studies that test potential strategies for curing HIV, subjects living with HIV who are doing well on antiretroviral medications take large risks by participating, such as experimental drug toxicity, interruptions of their antiretroviral regimens, and more (Deeks et al., 2016; Eyal, 2017; Eyal & Kuritzkes, 2013). Not only are these trials risky to participants, there are reasons to be particularly concerned about the therapeutic misconception and other inappropriate motivations for participation when the alluring words "HIV cure" are mentioned. High rates of declared willingness to participate in cure-related trials (Dubé et al., 2017; Henderson et al., 2018) may indicate that many potential subjects overestimate their chances of cure and/or underestimate study risks (Eyal, 2018). Given both risks to subjects' health and risk of therapeutic misconception that might cloud autonomous decisions, an IRB might want to exceed the conventional documentation requirement. The IRB might, for instance, require that subjects, in addition to signing a consent form, also write out a statement like "I am aware that I am unlikely to be cured and could suffer adverse effects."

    In sum, if there is no clear gain, or there is a clear loss, in terms of the key functions of informed consent from requiring written documentation of consent, it is permissible to waive it. If there would be gains from requiring written documentation in excess of the conventional signature, this is also something that IRBs may consider.

Ethical Human Subjects Research Does Not Always Require Consent Forms

The conventional informed consent requirements include a signed consent form that conveys information on certain key topics. Rather than adhere to this conventional requirement as a one-size-fits-all policy, IRBs have discretion to require more or require less. Regulations demand that key information about the study be presented in a manner that facilitates comprehension and decision making [45 CFR 46.116(5)(i)]. The form in which this information is presented, in our view, should be determined by what best serves the functions of consent. An IRB can, for example, waive the requirement for a signed form but still require that subjects be provided with written information about the study [45 CFR 46.117(c)(2)].

In terms of the functions of informed consent, the consent form (with or without requirement of a signature) is one possible means to ensure disclosure of information. To that extent, the form is an instrument of transparency, trust, autonomy, and the protection of welfare. But disclosure and transparency that allow subjects to make judgments about their welfare and thus autonomous decisions could also be achieved by other means of conveying the relevant information, such as a conversation, a video, or a website. In practice, there is usually no great cost to providing written information, which can then be supplemented by other means. In most circumstances, therefore, there may be no compelling reason for the IRB to require less than is conventional. In principle, though, if for whatever reason producing or distributing this information would be burdensome and threaten the viability of the study, the same protection of the functions of consent could be achieved through alternate means.

Still, it is possible that the traditional written presentation of the consent form may express the importance of the decision (as argued previously regarding signatures), thus promoting subjects' autonomous decision making. This may seem particularly important to IRBs for studies that are more than minimal risk, where, as discussed earlier, IRBs may decide to require more than is conventional. The printed form, which subjects can keep and refer to and which cannot be altered by researchers, may contribute to accountability and trust. Different desiderata may therefore be at play, and IRB members must exercise nuance and judgment.

Ethical Human Subjects Research Does Not Always Require Full Disclosure

As understood conventionally, informed consent processes aim for full disclosure. But what constitutes "full" disclosure? Current regulations afford the IRB discretion over when to require detailed disclosure and when to allow disclosure to be more general. The Common Rule requires specific information to be disclosed [45 CFR 46.116(b)] but does not require a given level of detail. In other words, the IRB has discretion over how much subjects need to be told in order for their consent to count as informed.

It might seem as though more detailed disclosure necessarily means greater transparency and therefore better protection of welfare, autonomous decision making, and trust. However complex, technical language that is not easily comprehensible to most subjects is not an effective means of disclosing information and may do more harm than good to genuine transparency, autonomy, and welfare. The longer and more complex the disclosure, the greater the potential for essential information about the research and its value-laden aspects to get diluted in less relevant information. Unnecessarily complex forms may also be perceived as mere legal cover, undermining trust. The Common Rule recognizes that the functions of consent are not always better served by more (and more detailed) disclosure and require a summary of "key" information about the study written in simple language.

🔗 6-3

🔗 10-3

Maximal disclosure is simply impossible in research that requires deception, where subjects' advance knowledge of the exact nature of the research would make the study impossible. Behavioral studies involving deception are commonly permitted, but deceiving subjects in interventional studies that would put them at high medical risk is rarely allowed (the scientific or social value of such a study would have to be extreme to justify the risks to subject welfare and autonomy and the potential serious damage to trust). Either way, the Department of Health and Human Services recommends that researchers carrying out studies involving deception, which cannot practically be carried out after an informed consent process, provide "pertinent information" to subjects after the fact [45 CFR 46.116(f)(3)]. This preserves a measure of transparency even in the absence of truthful disclosure at the most relevant time for autonomous decision making about study participation; namely, prior to the decision on whether to participate.

Even when no deception is required by the aims of the study, detailed disclosure is sometimes simply unnecessary. In a recent survey study investigating HIV patients' interest in participating in risky HIV cure studies (by a research group in which we participate), a simple two-sided information sheet covering basic questions ("Why is this study being done?" "What will happen if I take part in this research study?") in general terms was all the disclosure required by the IRB. This was arguably an appropriate level of disclosure to require. Clearly, however, a similar sheet would not be sufficient disclosure in a risky HIV cure intervention study.

The absence of health risks does not mean, however, that disclosure is unnecessary. The functions of consent can help identify the occasions when disclosure remains important. Reanalysis of biospecimens carries no medical risk to subjects and under the Common Rule can be subject to broad consent requirements. In the famous Havasupai court case, however, the failure to disclose the potential future uses of biospecimens undermined subjects' autonomy to decide whether to participate based on their own values. The repercussions of this lack of disclosure led to a widely publicized lawsuit, which probably undermined trust in research among American Indians. More generally, failures or perceived failures to respect the welfare and autonomy of subjects from identifiable and often underserved populations may be one contributing factor to the lower rates of research participation of many racial and ethnic minorities and its far-reaching repercussions for their care.

🖉 6-9
🖉 1-2

Ethical Human Subjects Research Does Not Always Require Full Comprehension by Subjects

Subjects who comprehend more are better able to decide autonomously and protect their own welfare. Better understood research is more transparent and more likely to foster trust. That said, IRBs can, in some situations, permissibly require less than full comprehension. However, the case for requiring less than full comprehension does not stem from the ethical functions of consent but from the practical difficulties of achieving full comprehension and the resulting effects that requiring it may have on the fairness and feasibility of subject recruitment and therefore on the fairness, viability, and validity of research.

When subjects are more likely to directly benefit than to be harmed from participating in a trial, it has been argued (Sreenivasan, 2003) that therapeutic misconception, which can clearly undermine comprehension, does not invalidate consent: that it is permissible to enroll them in the study even if they mistakenly believe that the balance of risks is even more favorable than it actually is. Otherwise, because the therapeutic misconception is so widespread and, often, recalcitrant, perfectly justified and benign medical studies might become impossible. While generally it does not betray subjects' trust to enroll them in a beneficial study that they consider more beneficial than it actually is, it is up to the IRB to exercise judgment on whether allowing beneficial studies when the subject is known to have therapeutic misconception is liable, in particular circumstances, to undermine societal trust in research.

In other cases, full comprehension is so important that it may justify compromises of other aspects of informed consent, such as full disclosure. As already mentioned, IRBs should prefer short consent forms that potential subjects are likely to comprehend, over long, detailed forms that maximize disclosure at the expense of comprehension. Full comprehension is even more important when risks are more than minimal. In the extreme case of risky research on potentially curative interventions for HIV, where there is high concern about therapeutic misconception and other inappropriate motivations for participation, it may make sense to avoid the word "cure" altogether, so as not to create false expectations, even when that word accurately discloses the goal of the research enterprise (Eyal & Kuritzkes, 2013; Peay & Henderson, 2015; Rennie et al., 2015). In such cases, revealing an intermediate goal of the study (say, to determine whether a form of immunotherapy achieves certain endpoints) rather than its ultimate goal (to develop a curative intervention) may be construed as less than full disclosure. However, in our view, given the presence of high welfare and autonomy risks, in such cases it may be justified to sacrifice full disclosure in the interest of avoiding therapeutic misconception, thus keeping consent as autonomous as possible.

When a study is high risk, participation itself is burdensome and demanding, or when the risk of therapeutic misconception is suspected to be high, robust demands of comprehension (which may incorporate elements like testing subjects' understanding of the risks and benefits) should often be used to screen potential subjects.

Ethical Human Subjects Research Does Not Always Require Consent

⊘ 6-4

Finally, in U.S. law, when reviewing a proposed study, IRBs have the choice to waive informed consent altogether. The conditions set by the Common Rule on when IRBs have discretion to waive consent are consistent with the account we have presented: waiving informed consent is allowed when the study would not be practical without the waiver, risk to subjects are minimal, and, crucially, the waiver does not "adversely affect the rights and welfare of the subjects." As mentioned previously, the regulations also require that when informed consent is waived "pertinent information" be provided after the fact whenever appropriate [45 CFR 46.116(f)(3)]. Consistent with the current chapter's functional approach, the Common Rule allows IRBs to waive informed consent precisely when the study does not require the informed consent process to safeguard welfare and autonomy. The requirement for retrospective provision of information safeguards transparency. Together, the safeguarding of these functions by means other than informed consent protects trust in the research enterprise. In our view, it is for this reason that a study meeting these conditions constitutes ethical research even without informed consent. Philosophical accounts of the conditions for informed consent waivers can be found in Gelinas et al. (2016) and Eyal (2019).

Conclusion

The fundamental ethical functions of informed consent processes in research on human subjects—welfare, autonomy, transparency, and trust—are often, but not always, well served by informed consent processes as conventionally construed. These ethical functions can guide IRBs' decisions on when to follow conventional expectations and when to depart from them. They can also help IRBs articulate their reasons for following or deviating from convention.

References

Beauchamp, T., & Childress, J. (2009). *Principles of biomedical ethics* (6th ed.). Oxford University Press.

Deeks, S. G., Lewin, S. R., Ross, A. L., Ananworanich, J., Benkirane, M., Cannon, P., Chomont, N., Douek, D., Lifson, J. D., Lo, Y. R., Kuritzkes, D., Margolis, D., Mellors, J., Persaud, D., Tucker, J. D., Barre-Sinoussi, F., International AIDS Society Towards a Cure Working Group, Alter, G., Auerbach, J., Autran, B., …, Zack, J. (2016). International AIDS Society global scientific strategy: Towards an HIV cure 2016. *Nature Medicine, 22,* 839–850.

Dickert, N. W., Eyal, N., Goldkind, S. F., Grady, C., Joffe, S., Lo, B., Miller, F. G., Pentz, R. D., Silbergleit, R., Weinfurt, K. P., Wendler, D., & Kim, S. (2017). Reframing consent for clinical research: A function-based approach. *American Journal of Bioethics, 17*(12), 3–11.

Dickert, N. W., Wendler, D., Devireddy, C. M., Goldkind, S. F., Ko, Y. A., Speight, C. D., & Kim, S. (2018a). Consent for pragmatic trials in acute myocardial infarction. *Journal of the American College of Cardiology, 71*(9), 1051–1053.

Dickert, N. W., Wendler, D., Devireddy, C. M., Goldkind, S. F., Ko, Y. A., Speight, C. D., & Kim, S. Y. (2018b). Understanding preferences regarding consent for pragmatic trials in acute care. *Clinical Trials, 15*(6), 567–578.

Dubé, K., Evans, D., Sylla, L., Taylor, J., Weiner, B. J., Skinner, A., Thirumurthy, H., Tucker, J. D., Rennie, S., & Greene, S. B. (2017). Willingness to participate and take risks in HIV cure research: Survey results from 400 people living with HIV in the US. *Journal of Virus Eradication, 3*(1), 40–50 [e21].

Dworkin, G. (1988). *The theory and practice of autonomy.* Cambridge University Press.

Emanuel, E. J., Wendler, D., & Grady, C. (2000). What makes clinical research ethical? *JAMA, 283,* 2701–2711.

Eyal, N. (2017). The benefit/risk ratio challenge in clinical research, and the case of HIV cure: An introduction. *Journal of Medical Ethics, 43*(2), 65–66.

Eyal, N. (2018). What can the lived experience of participating in risky HIV cure-related studies establish? *Journal of Medical Ethics, 44*(4), 277–278.

Eyal, N. (2019). Informed consent. *Stanford Encyclopedia of Philosophy.* https://plato.stanford.edu/archives/spr2019/entries/informed-consent/

Eyal, N., & Kuritzkes, D. R. (2013). Challenges in clinical trial design for HIV-1 cure research. *Lancet, 382*(9903), 1464–1465.

Faden, R., Beauchamp, T., & King, N. (1986). *A history and theory of informed consent.* Oxford University Press.

Gelinas, L., Wertheimer, A., & Miller, F. (2016). When and why is research without consent permissible? *Hastings Center Report, 46*(2), 35–43.

Henderson, G. E., Peay, H. L., Kroon, E., Cadigan, R. J., Meagher, K., Jupimai, T., Gilbertson, A., Fisher, J., Ormsby, N. Q., Chomchey, N., Phanuphak, N., Ananworanich, J., & Rennie, S. (2018). Ethics of treatment interruption trials in HIV cure research: Addressing the conundrum of risk/benefit assessment. *Journal of Medical Ethics, 44*(4), 270–276.

National Commission for the Protection of Human Subjects of Biomedical and Behavioral Research. (1979). *The Belmont Report: Ethical principles and guidelines for the protection of human subjects of research.* www.hhs.gov/ohrp/regulations-and-policy/belmont-report/read-the-belmont-report/index.html

Peay, H. L., & Henderson, G. E. (2015). What motivates participation in HIV cure trials? A call for real-time assessment to improve informed consent. *Journal of Virus Eradication, 1*(1), 51–53.

Rennie, S., Siedner, M., Tucker, J. D., & Moodley, K. (2015). The ethics of talking about "HIV cure." *BMC Medical Ethics*, *16*, 18.

Siegrist, M. (2019). Trust and risk perception: A critical review of the literature. *Risk Analysis*. doi:10.1111/risa.13325

Sreenivasan, G. (2003). Does informed consent to research require comprehension? *Lancet*, *362*, 2016–2018.

Walen, A. (2020) Using, risking, and consent: Why risking harm to bystanders is morally different from risking harm to research subjects. *Bioethics*, *34*(9): 1–7. https://doi.org/10.1111/bioe.12743.

CHAPTER 6-2

The Elements of Informed Consent

Heather H. Pierce

Abstract

Informed consent is a cornerstone of human subject protections, and reviewing the information that will be provided to prospective research subjects represents a significant component of the IRB's responsibility. The elements of informed consent, as defined through regulation, provide the basis for the required information that a research subject or that individual's legally authorized representative will receive. An IRB must review a proposed consent document or process to ensure that each element is included or considered and that as a whole the document contains the information a reasonable person would need to make an informed choice about whether or not to participate in the research. This chapter outlines the elements of informed consent required by the regulations and explores the IRB's responsibilities for ensuring proposed informed consent processes meet these requirements.

The IRB's Role in the Informed Consent Process

Before deciding to become a research subject, an individual is given information that describes the nature of the research and what it would mean to be a part of the study. What someone needs to know and how each piece of information will be weighted in their decision making depends in part on the type of research and the demands it places on the subject. Is it a one-time survey, a dietary intervention, or a clinical trial of a new drug? Is the person a healthy volunteer or a very ill patient? As a general principle, no person should be a research subject without being *informed* about the research and providing voluntary *consent* to participate.

Ideally, this process comprises two distinct activities for each research study: (1) the identification of a particular set of information as likely to be important to anyone trying to make the decision about participation and (2) an engagement between an individual and a research team member that both facilitates and verifies understanding of what it means to enroll in the research. The IRB has important responsibilities related to the first activity, which provides a critical foundation for the protection of human rights and welfare in research. Because the IRB is not involved in the conversations with each research subject to ensure voluntary informed consent (the second activity), its role in developing the consent process that will be used is crucial.

The IRB's review of a proposed informed consent process should not be approached as an exercise in regulatory compliance alone. Although the lengthy consent requirements lend themselves well to checklists and templates, the IRB can, and should, have significant influence on how information is formatted and presented to a prospective subject, including the words used to describe risks of participation and how clearly the drafted materials communicate to prospective subjects what they will be asked to do during the study.

Federal Regulations Governing Informed Consent

The Common Rule's requirements on informed consent found at 45 CFR 46.116 specify the types of information that must be provided to a research subject, as well as how to present that information. This chapter focuses on the fundamental required elements of informed consent, according to the Common Rule. Circumstances in which the IRB chooses to waive or alter these elements are discussed in Chapter 6-4, and the special case of the use of "broad consent" is discussed in Chapter 6-9. The fundamental required elements of consent are divided in the regulations into general requirements, basic elements, and additional elements.

General Requirements

The Common Rule sets forth some general requirements that should guide researchers in how they craft informed consent documents and processes and guide IRBs in their review of those documents and processes [45 CFR 46.116(a)]. These general requirements, which are separate from the specific elements described later, speak to *how* information should be presented to subjects, rather than providing substantive guidance on *what* must be included in the consent process. Collectively, these general provisions require the following [45 CFR 46.116(a)]:

(1) that a researcher obtain "legally effective informed consent of the subject or the subject's legally authorized representative" (LAR) prior to involving a person in research;

(2) that consent be obtained "only under circumstances that provide …sufficient opportunity to discuss and consider whether or not to participate and that minimize the possibility of coercion or undue influence";

(3) that the information be provided "in language understandable to the subject or the legally authorized representative";

(4) that the information provided is what a "reasonable person would want to have in order to make an informed decision about whether to participate";

🔗 6-3

(5) (i) that the key information for making a decision is presented in a "concise and focused" way at the beginning of the process;

(5) (ii) that the informed consent process as a whole presents information in a way that "facilitates . . . understanding of the reasons why

one might or might not want to participate" in the research; and

(6) that participants are not asked via "exculpatory language . . . to waive or appear to waive" any legal rights.

IRB review of a proposed consent process to determine if it complies with these general requirements is less straightforward than evaluating the relevance or sufficiency of the specific required elements outlined later, since the general requirements concern primarily how the information is provided to potential subjects. Requiring that informed consent be written to facilitate understanding demands thinking about the consent process from the perspective of potential subjects (Rosenfeld, 2019). It requires presenting the information in a way that will help a potential subject understand the reasons why they might or might not want to participate in this particular research study—that is, what might be said in favor of, and against, participating. The general requirements therefore urge researchers and IRBs to think of the informed consent process as a decision aid, rather than a mere list of facts about the study left to the subject to interpret. Approaching informed consent in this way demands thinking carefully about the prospective subjects being asked to make decisions and what they might want to know about this particular study.

Thinking about how to present information does not lend itself well to checklist-type mechanisms for ensuring compliance; however, IRBs can facilitate informed consent processes that meet these general requirements by providing guidance, sample consent materials, and even templates that encourage and guide researchers to take the subject's perspective and to organize and present information in a way that fosters subject understanding and decision making. At the same time, depending on the nature of the research, the IRB may need to ask additional questions about when and how discussions about the research will take place with prospective subjects.

Some of the provisions under the general requirements require special IRB attention. For instance, the IRB needs to assess whether the circumstances in which consent is obtained minimize the possibility of undue influence and coercion. Making this determination will require the IRB to not only understand how the research procedures, risks, and benefits are described in the consent process; it will require understanding *who* will be requesting consent; the relationship of that individual to the potential subject; where, when, and how consent will be obtained; and assessment of how those factors might affect the voluntariness of the decision. Is the subject being recruited to a phase III drug trial in their doctor's office by their personal physician? Might they therefore feel pressured to agree to enroll, out of fear that their physician might be upset with them if they do not? Is there the potential, given the setting, that the subject will not adequately understand the purpose of the research and that they might be randomized to a placebo? The Office for Human Research Protections frequently asked questions on informed consent include several points about how the IRB can assess the potential for undue influence and coercion (DHHS, 2019).

The IRB also needs to evaluate whether the consent process happens in a "language understandable to the subject." To make this assessment, the IRB

WHAT IS LEGALLY EFFECTIVE INFORMED CONSENT?

The Department of Health and Human Services (DHHS) defines legally effective informed consent as consent that meets the Common Rule regulatory requirements and is consistent with applicable laws of the jurisdiction in which the research is conducted (DHHS, 2019). Faden and Beauchamp (1986) have offered the following definition: "legally effective informed consent means consent from a legally competent person." Competence may be as simple as the ability to evidence a preference or as difficult as the ability to "(1) show an accurate understanding, (2) weigh its risks and benefits, and (3) make a prudent decision in light of such knowledge" (Faden & Beauchamp, 1986).

6-4

INTERPRETING THE "REASONABLE PERSON" STANDARD

Dresser has suggested that interpretation and application of the reasonable person standard calls for researchers and IRBs to learn more about what potential subjects want to know about the research they are invited to join, and to consult with people who have served as study subjects about their personal experiences (Dresser, 2019). Rosenfeld has interpreted the reasonable person standard as providing a counterbalance to the focus on facilitating subject understanding of the reasons why they might or might not want to participate, and the idea that some information will be "key" to such decisions. These latter considerations seem to point in the direction of significant "tailoring" of informed consent to subjects' needs and preferences. But of course informed consent forms must be standardized for any one study. The notion of a reasonable person, then, provides a "minimal standard for participant understanding against which a single consent form can be written" (Rosenfeld, 2019).

should ensure not just that the document or process is conducted, for instance, in Spanish for Spanish speakers. The IRB also has a responsibility to ensure that the language in which study procedures, risks, and benefits are described is at the appropriate comprehension level for the potential subjects. The IRB should thus pay attention to factors such as the subject populations' numeracy, science literacy, and reading level. Researchers may not always be best positioned to explain their research in simple, nontechnical terms, so guidance and tools from the IRB on how to do so is crucial.

The general requirements also stipulate that what is provided to a potential subject during the informed consent process is information that a "reasonable person" would want to know in order to make an informed decision about participating in the research. Although the "reasonable person" standard has been a fixture of tort law for years, it was a new addition to the 2018 Common Rule, and little guidance has been provided regarding how IRBs should determine what a reasonable person would want to know (Odwazny & Berkman, 2017). Absent such guidance, the "reasonable person" is a standard that individuals IRBs will have to negotiate and refine over time (see sidebar, Interpreting the Reasonable Person Standard).

Finally, the general requirements forbid the inclusion in informed consent of "exculpatory language" through which a subject is asked to waive any of their legal rights or to release the study sponsor or other parties from liability. This requirement can confuse IRBs, because the informed consent *can* include, per basic element 8 discussed later, statements such as: that there are no plans to compensate subjects for any commercial products that result from research on their biospecimens, or that subjects or their insurance may be responsible for costs of treatment if they are injured during participation in the study. Informed consent is meant to let potential subjects know what they can expect from participating in the research as planned, so that they can decide if participating makes sense for them. But in consenting to participate in research as described, subjects do not, and, indeed, cannot, give up their rights under our legal system, including, for instance, the right to hold other parties liable for injury.

The Basic Elements of Informed Consent

Unless the IRB has approved a <u>waiver or alteration</u> of the informed consent requirements, the informed consent process must include each of the basic elements described. Although these elements do not need to be presented in this order, each element must be addressed.

The basic elements of informed consent, outlined at **45 CFR 46.116(b)**, are:

(1) A statement that the study involves research, an explanation of the purposes of the research and the expected duration of the subject's participation, a description of the procedures to be followed, and identification of any procedures that are experimental;

(2) A description of any reasonably foreseeable risks or discomforts to the subject;

(3) A description of any benefits to the subject or to others that may reasonably be expected from the research;

(4) A disclosure of appropriate alternative procedures or courses of treatment, if any, that might be advantageous to the subject;

(5) A statement describing the extent, if any, to which confidentiality of records identifying the subject will be maintained;

(6) For research involving more than minimal risk, an explanation as to whether any compensation and an explanation as to whether any medical treatments are available if injury occurs and, if so, what they consist of, or where further information may be obtained;

(7) An explanation of whom to contact for answers to pertinent questions about the research and research subjects' rights, and whom to contact in the event of a research-related injury to the subject;

(8) A statement that participation is voluntary, refusal to participate will involve no penalty or loss of benefits to which the subject is otherwise entitled, and the subject may discontinue participation at any time without penalty or loss of benefits to which the subject is otherwise entitled; and

(9) One of the following statements about any research that involves the collection of identifiable private information or identifiable biospecimens:

(i) A statement that identifiers might be removed from the identifiable private information or identifiable biospecimens and that, after such removal, the information or biospecimens could be used for future research studies or distributed to another investigator for future research studies without additional informed consent from the subject or the legally authorized representative, if this might be a possibility; or

(ii) A statement that the subject's information or biospecimens collected as part of the research, even if identifiers are removed, will not be used or distributed for future research studies.

Although many of these items are straightforward, it is again important to remember that the basic elements should, in any single consent process, be addressed in a way that facilitates understanding of the reasons why a reasonable person might or might not want to participate in the research. Keeping that in mind will determine the order in which the basic elements are presented, the language used to discuss them, and, in some cases, the level of detail provided. For example, required element 2 addresses the reasonably foreseeable risks or discomforts to the subject. Note that this element does not say that a complete list of *all* possible risks of the study must be described. The IRB should help researchers determine *which* risks are important to disclose and how, using the guiding ideas of what the reasonable person would want to know and what might be most useful information to a person's decision about whether or not to participate.

Additional Elements of Informed Consent

In some cases, additional elements must also be included in the consent process. When any of these elements apply to the proposed research or circumstances of the individual's participation, this information needs to be incorporated into the informed consent process. In reviewing an informed consent process for compliance with the Common Rule, the IRB should not consider these additional elements as optional but rather as required elements if they apply to the particular study. This means that if an IRB finds that a particular additional element is applicable to the research study, it cannot be omitted from the informed consent process without an IRB undertaking the process set forth in the regulations for waiving or altering consent, just as it would have to do before omitting any of the basic elements.

The additional elements of informed consent, as outlined in **45 CFR 46.116(c)** are as follows:

(1) A statement that the particular treatment or procedure may involve risks to the subject (or to the embryo or fetus, if the subject is or may become pregnant) that are currently unforeseeable;

(2) Anticipated circumstances under which the subject's participation may be terminated by the investigator without regard to the subject's or the legally authorized representative's consent;

(3) Any additional costs to the subject that may result from participation in the research;

(4) The consequences of a subject's decision to withdraw from the research and procedures for orderly termination of participation by the subject;

(5) A statement that significant new findings developed during the course of the research that may relate to the subject's willingness to continue participation will be provided to the subject;

(6) The approximate number of subjects involved in the study;

(7) A statement that the subject's biospecimens (even if identifiers are removed) may be used for commercial profit and whether the subject will or will not share in this commercial profit;

(8) A statement regarding whether clinically relevant research results, including individual research results, will be disclosed to subjects, and if so, under what conditions; and

(9) For research involving biospecimens, whether the research will (if known) or might include whole genome sequencing (i.e., sequencing of a human germline or somatic specimen with the intent to generate the genome or exome sequence of that specimen)

⊘ 12-1 The Common Rule does not require the <u>return of research results</u> to subjects. If a proposed research study has the potential to reveal clinically relevant findings, then additional consent element 8 becomes relevant, and the informed consent must include a statement about whether such findings will be returned or not. According to the regulations, an informed consent process could say that researchers may come across clinically relevant information in the course of the research but that if they do, the information will not be returned to subjects. Including such a statement in the consent allows a potential subject to decide whether that arrangement is acceptable to them; if it is not, then they can decide not to enroll in the research (see sidebar, Return of Research Results).

Together, the general requirements, basic elements, and additional elements represent the totality of regulatory requirements for the informed consent process. However, there are few limits on what is allowed to be included in a consent document, which

RETURN OF RESEARCH RESULTS

Some have argued that by not requiring researchers to plan to return clinically relevant results, the Common Rule lags behind an emerging consensus that at least some research results should be returned to subjects as a matter of gratitude, respect, beneficence, and/or reciprocity (National Academies of Science, Engineering, and Medicine, 2018; Multi-Regional Clinical Trials Center, 2017). Indeed, some IRBs may not be comfortable with this approach and will need to decide whether they want to have an institutional policy requiring the return of results, and in what conditions.

can be used to <u>serve many purposes</u>. The IRB may require still other items be included, such as disclosures of conflicts of interest held by the <u>investigator</u> or the <u>institution</u>. The organization overseeing the research may have its own template language to add, and clinical trial sponsors may add yet more information.

🔗 6-1
🔗 12-6
🔗 12-8

Application of the Elements of Informed Consent to IRB Review

The elements of consent listed in the Common Rule are designed to ensure that prospective research subjects have the information they need to decide whether to participate in (or remain in) a research study. In most cases, the IRB will be reviewing a written document that the researchers or sponsors propose to provide to prospective research subjects. As has been noted, an IRB should consider not only the content of that document, but also how the informed consent process as a whole will present the information to a prospective subject. Especially in the context of research that presents significant risks to subjects or involves novel study designs, the IRB should consider whether the proposed informed consent process is likely to lead to a clear understanding of the research, the risks, and the obligations for the subjects.

It has been long recognized that asking someone to read a complicated document is not a reliable way to convey important information. Multiple studies have demonstrated that informed consent documents are often lengthy, difficult for participants to understand, and not consistently clear in the explanation of critical information (Nathe & Krakow, 2019). The changes in the 2018 Common Rule attempted to address this problem in a couple of ways, namely, by discussing the organization, presentation, and prioritization of the information, and by requiring the process begin with "a concise and focused presentation of the key information" that would help someone decide whether or not to participate in the research. Although this summary could well provide a welcome antidote to the concern that a vital piece of information could be buried a dozen pages into a dense and highly technical form, the <u>key information</u> section itself, along with the addition of four new elements to add to the process, may only serve to make the document even longer.

🔗 6-3

Scholarship in <u>adult learning techniques</u> and advances in <u>electronic consent</u> tools may provide researchers with <u>more effective ways</u> to ensure that consent is truly informed. This can put an IRB in a challenging situation. Although the regulations do not require that the information be provided in a single form, the structure of the rules and relative ease of developing and reviewing a document may serve to discourage researchers from proposing novel methods of providing information to participants. When the proposed informed consent process seeks to inform individuals about the research through means other than a document, whether through videos, oral presentation, interactive tools, or other approaches, the IRB may be concerned about being able to document that each of the elements will be adequately addressed. In addition, the Common Rule mandates that an "IRB-approved consent form" for each clinical trial be posted on a publicly available website [45 CFR 46.116(h)], a requirement that has caused some IRBs to assume that for clinical trials, all consent information must be on a form. Despite these challenges, the IRB should exercise restraint before summarily rejecting informed consent processes that propose an approach other than a form or document.

🔗 6-7 🔗 6-6
🔗 6-10

Informed Consent and Identifiability

The basic elements of informed consent include a requirement to help research subjects understand the potential future uses of their identifiable private information or biospecimens. An IRB should pay close attention to how this information is presented in the informed consent process and whether the promises made to subjects match the intended uses of that information or those biospecimens described in the protocol, especially in cases where the research involves the collection of identifiable biospecimens.

It is important to note that the definition of "identifiable" is neither purely objective nor static. Information or biospecimens are deemed identifiable if the identities of the research subjects that are their source are associated with them, or if those subjects' identities "may readily be ascertained by the investigator" [45 CFR 46.102(e)(5) and (6)]. Whether an investigator can readily ascertain the identity of an individual from the data or biospecimens being studied is highly context dependent. Furthermore, the Common Rule requires that the agencies that have implemented the regulations regularly "reexamine the meaning of identifiable private information . . . and identifiable biospecimen" [45 CFR 46.102(e)(7)(i)]. As technologies and reidentification techniques evolve, it is likely that some biospecimens considered not identifiable at the time of initial IRB review will be deemed identifiable in later years. Clarifying a researcher's intentions for storage and use of this material and ensuring alignment between consent process and study protocol can address future concerns.

🖎 10-10

Harmonization of Informed Consent Elements Across Agencies

The 2018 Common Rule has not, as of the publication of this volume, been harmonized with the regulations on informed consent for clinical investigations regulated by the U.S. Food and Drug Administration (FDA) at **21 CFR Part 50 subpart B**. Therefore, the basic elements of informed consent regarding whole genome sequencing and the three final additional elements related to biospecimens and the return of clinically relevant research subjects noted earlier, do not have analogous requirements in FDA regulations. The 21st Century Cures Act of 2016 directed the Secretary of DHHS to harmonize differences between the Common Rule and FDA regulations, which include the elements of informed consent (21st Century Cures Act, 2016). Prior to a formal rulemaking process which would be required to modify FDA regulations, in 2018 FDA released a guidance document expressing the agency's intention to harmonize the informed consent requirements with the Common Rule and clarifying that the basic and additional elements of informed consent in the revised Common Rule "are not inconsistent with FDA's current policies and guidances" (FDA, 2018). If an IRB is reviewing proposed research that falls under the purview of both the Common Rule and FDA, it should ensure that the informed consent process meets the more extensive requirements of the Common Rule.

Conclusion

Although the requirements set forth in the Common Rule provide the elements an informed consent process must include, the development of an informed consent process can be subject focused, employing resources and the knowledge of the research team to identify the most pertinent information about the study to provide the most effective way to communicate that information and the most accurate way to assess if the information was understood. When the IRB and the research team are partners in struggling through these difficult questions, the elements of informed consent can act as building blocks, both to protect human subjects and to engage those individuals as participants in the process of advancing discovery.

References

21st Century Cures Act. (2016). Pub. L. No. 114–255, 130 Stat. 1033.

Department of Health and Human Services (DHHS). (2019). *The Office for Human Research Protections: Informed consent FAQs.* www.hhs.gov/ohrp/regulations-and-policy/guidance/faq/informed-consent/index.html

Dresser, R. (2019). The reasonable person standard for research disclosure: A reasonable addition to the Common Rule. *Journal of Law, Medicine, & Ethics, 47*(2), 194–202.

Faden, R. R., & Beauchamp, T. L. (1986). *A history and theory of informed consent.* Oxford University Press.

Food and Drug Administration (FDA). (2018). *Impact of certain provisions of the revised Common Rule on FDA-regulated clinical investigations.* www.fda.gov/media/117042/download

Multi-Regional Clinical Trials Center of Brigham and Women's Hospital and Harvard (MRCT). (2017). *Return of individual results to participants: Principles.* https://mrctcenter.org/wp-content/uploads/2017/12/2017-11-20-Return-of-Individual-Results-Principles-Nov-2017.pdf

Nathe, J. M., & Krakow, E. F. (2019). The challenges of informed consent in high-stakes, randomized oncology trials: A systematic review. *MDM Policy & Practice, 4*(1), 2381468319840322.

National Academies of Science, Engineering, and Medicine (NASEM). (2018). *Returning individual research results to participants: Guidance for a new research paradigm.* The National Academies Press.

Odwazny, L. M., & Berkman, B. E. (2017). The "reasonable person" standard for research informed consent. *American Journal of Bioethics, 17*(7), 49.

Rosenfeld, S. J. (2019). Informed consent and the revised Common Rule: The benefits and challenges of the updated Common Rule. *Harvard Medical School Bioethics Journal.* https://bioethics journal.hms.harvard.edu/summer-2019/informed-consent-and-revised-common-rule

Key Information

Jonathan M. Green
Stephen Rosenfeld

Abstract

The Common Rule requires that informed consent documents begin with a key information section, providing the prospective subject with a "concise and focused presentation" of the information that is most important in deciding whether or not they should participate in the research. In this chapter, we provide a description of this requirement and our understanding of the rationale and ethical basis. We discuss how to determine what might be considered key information and the challenges faced by researchers and IRBs in meeting this regulatory requirement.

Regulatory Text

45 CFR 46.116(a)(5): Except for broad consent obtained in accordance with paragraph (d) of this section:

(i) Informed consent must begin with a concise and focused presentation of the key information that is most likely to assist a prospective subject or legally authorized representative in understanding the reasons why one might or might not want to participate in the research. This part of the informed consent must be organized and presented in a way that facilitates comprehension.

(ii) Informed consent as a whole must present information in sufficient detail relating to the research, and must be organized and presented in a way that does not merely provide lists of isolated facts, but rather facilitates the prospective subject's or legally authorized representative's understanding of the reasons why one might or might not want to participate.

Purpose

There is general agreement among researchers and IRBs that informed consent documents frequently do not adequately assist prospective subjects in making a decision as to whether or not to join a research study (Beardsley et al., 2007; Grady, 2015; Paasche-Orlow et al., 2003). Ideally, the informed consent

267

document should be a decision-making aid that allows the potential subject to evaluate the study and determine if enrollment is consistent with their goals and values. Instead, potential subjects are often presented with documents that are unreasonably long (in some cases up to 40 or 50 pages), excessively legalistic, and presented in a manner that is difficult, if not impossible, to understand.

While the key information provision of the Common Rule does not address all the problems of informed consent documents, it does attempt to ensure that there is at least one portion of the document that is readily understandable to the prospective subject and is explicitly written to facilitate their decision making. The preamble to the 2018 Common Rule makes this rationale explicit:

> In considering changes to the general requirements set forth in §46.116(a), we considered arguments put forth by some that consent forms have evolved to protect institutions rather than to provide potential research subjects with the most important pieces of information that a person would need in order to make an informed decision about whether to enroll in a research study. Instead of presenting the information in a way that is most helpful to prospective subjects—such as explaining why someone might want to choose not to enroll—these individuals argued the forms may function more as sales documents or as a means to protect against institutional liability. We also considered a growing body of literature that suggests informed consent forms have grown too lengthy and complex, adversely affecting their ability to effectively convey the information needed for prospective participants to make an informed decision about participating in research. (Federal Register, 2017, Preamble p. 7211)

Ethical Principles and Challenges

Respect for persons is one of the three overarching ethical principles described in the *Belmont Report* (National Commission, 1979) and includes the principles of autonomy and protection of those incapable of exercising self-determination (i.e., "vulnerable populations"):

> An autonomous person is an individual capable of deliberation about personal goals and of acting under the direction of such deliberation. To respect autonomy is to give weight to autonomous persons' considered opinions and choices while refraining from obstructing their actions unless they are clearly detrimental to others. To show lack of respect for an autonomous agent is to repudiate that person's considered judgments, to deny an individual the freedom to act on those considered judgments, or to withhold information necessary to make a considered judgment, when there are no compelling reasons to do so.
>
> However, not every human being is capable of self-determination. The capacity for self-determination matures during an individual's life, and some individuals lose this capacity wholly or in part because of illness, mental disability, or circumstances that severely restrict liberty. Respect for the immature and the incapacitated may require protecting them as they mature or while they are incapacitated (National Commission, 1979)

Belmont divides research subjects into two classes—those who can exercise autonomy and those who cannot. Members of the latter class are defined as not being "capable of self-determination." Note that this is not simply an internal characteristic, reflecting the intellectual or emotional capability of the individual, but may also reflect their position in society. *Belmont* makes this point explicit in its discussion of prisoners, who are not fully capable of self-determination because of their limited ability to act freely, not because of limits in their decision-making power.

While philosophically compelling, there are practical problems with implementing a simple dualistic approach to who can exercise autonomy, problems that *Belmont* recognizes. As noted previously, the report explicitly discusses the problem of prisoners, who have the intellectual capacity to make decisions for themselves but whose imprisonment may materially change the context and consequences of their decisions. To avoid such situations, the report proposes that the decision to participate be made under circumstances free of *coercion* and *undue influence*. *Belmont* describes these factors as "unjustifiable pressures" and notes: "A continuum of such influencing factors exists, however, and it is impossible to state precisely where justifiable persuasion ends and undue influence begins" (National Commission, 1979).

With the notable but perhaps rare exception of individuals who are motivated to participate in research purely for altruistic reasons, research subjects *always* come to a study with other motivations. These motives may include hope for treatment of intractable or incurable disease, lack of therapeutic alternatives, the opportunity for marginalized members of society to receive high-quality medical care, and economic gain. Any of these motives has the potential to move a consent *conversation,* along the continuum described earlier, from "justifiable persuasion" to "undue influence." The content of the informed consent document has traditionally been restricted to the particulars of the research study, at least partly to avoid these concerns, but the context of a decision (including the beliefs and biases that individuals on both sides of the conversation bring) gives facts meaning. An informed consent document that simply discloses such facts about the study and does not address "the reasons why one might or might not want to participate in the research" risks using the subject's signature to memorialize a preexisting bias, rather than using the document as an opportunity for informing and enhancing voluntariness.

Using the informed consent document to simply disclose facts about the study also means that responsibility for the integrity of the *consent process* is delegated to the researcher or member of the study team who is responsible for explaining the study to the potential subject. *Belmont* recognizes this consequence but limits its discussion to the consequences for *comprehension*:

> Because the subject's ability to understand is a function of intelligence, rationality, maturity and language, it is necessary to adapt the presentation of the information to the subject's capacities. Investigators are responsible for ascertaining that the subject has comprehended the information. While there is always an obligation to ascertain that the information about risk to subjects is complete and adequately comprehended, when the risks are more serious, that obligation increases. On occasion, it may be suitable to give some oral or written tests of comprehension (National Commission, 1979)

Thus, of the three elements of informed consent identified in *Belmont* (information, comprehension, and voluntariness), the first is addressed by the content of the informed consent document (written by the sponsor or investigator and reviewed by the IRB); the second is left to the researcher (although the IRB is tasked with confirming that the language is "understandable"); and the third is partly addressed by eschewing coercion and undue influence. To some extent, the IRB has a role in removing such language from the consent document, but the main responsibility falls to the researcher in the context of the consent discussion itself.

The Problematic Role of the Researcher

Prior to the 2018 revisions to the Common Rule, the responsibilities of the researcher vis-à-vis informed consent were described in **45 CFR 46.116**:

> Except as provided elsewhere in this policy, no investigator may involve a human being as a subject in research covered by this policy unless the investigator has obtained the legally effective informed consent of the subject or the subject's legally authorized representative. An investigator shall seek such consent only under circumstances that provide the prospective subject or the representative sufficient opportunity to consider whether or not to participate and that minimize the possibility of coercion or undue influence. The information that is given to the subject or the representative shall be in language understandable to the subject or the representative. No informed consent, whether oral or written, may include any exculpatory language through which the subject or the representative is made to waive or appear to waive any of the subject's legal rights, or releases or appears to release the investigator, the sponsor, the institution or its agents from liability for negligence.

The researcher's specific obligations were limited to the following:

- Providing sufficient opportunity for meaningful consideration
- Seeking consent in *circumstances* that minimize the possibility of coercion or undue influence
- Using language in the consent that is *understandable* to the subject or representative

Although the regulations called for minimization of coercion or undue influence in the circumstances of the consent process, for practical reasons review boards have applied this criterion *to the form*. Such an approach is limited (as discussed earlier), and the only form-specific criterion in the regulations is that the language used be "understandable." Understandability is a characteristic of the language used, and in practice, structuring informed consent this way leaves it up to the potential subject to actually make the effort to understand. The researcher has no responsibility under the regulations to ensure that the consent form has actually been understood.

This limitation of the consent process has long been recognized, and several approaches have been proposed and used to mitigate it, particularly in higher risk studies. These include tests of comprehension, as originally suggested in the *Belmont Report*, as well as "teach-back" (Flory et al., 2004; Schenker et al., 2011); however, the use of both of these approaches has been limited by the anticipated burden they would place on the research enterprise.

⊘ 6-7

Even this limited delegation of responsibility to the researcher is not without problems. Researchers virtually always come to the consent process with a bias toward participation—a bias whose impact may be enhanced by educational and power differences and, in some circumstances, by the doctor–patient relationship. The practice of limiting the contents of the informed consent document to objective information about the study and relying on the "consent process" to appropriately address subject perspectives means that the critical elements of comprehension and voluntariness are entrusted to those individuals whose known conflicts the IRB was created to oversee.

The key information provisions of the 2018 Common Rule attempt to address these challenges in two ways. First, they add new required content to the consent form: the key information section. Second, they change the requirement that language simply be "understandable," to requiring that information be presented in a way that "facilitates comprehension." The new content itself does not follow the model of the pre-2018 Rule, which simply provided a list of topics, or elements, that had to be disclosed. Instead, the updated Rule requires that researchers or other authors of consent forms make the effort to see the research from the subjects' perspective and provide "the key information that is most likely to assist a prospective subject . . . in understanding the reasons why one might or might not want to participate in the research." [45 CFR 46.116(1)(i)].

What Constitutes Key Information?

The regulatory text does not specify what information is key, but the discussion in the preamble identifies some categories of information that are likely to be considered key for most studies (Federal Register, 2017, Preamble p. 7214):

Key Information Categories

1. The fact that consent is being sought for research and that participation is voluntary
2. The purposes of the research, the expected duration of the prospective subject's participation, and the procedures to be followed in the research
3. The reasonably foreseeable risks or discomforts to the prospective subject
4. The benefits to the prospective subject or to others that may reasonably be expected from the research
5. Appropriate alternative procedures or courses of treatment, if any, that might be advantageous to the prospective subject

Importantly, this relatively specific list is included in the preamble, *not* in the regulatory text, and the preamble further explains that placement decision as follows:

> We recognize the advantages of allowing institutions to design informed consents, consistent with §46.116(a)(5)(i), that are tailored to particular research studies to assist prospective subjects in understanding the most fundamental aspects of the informed consent. For this reason, the final rule does not strictly specify the types of information that should or should not be included to satisfy §46.116(a)(5)(i), or the length of such concise and focused presentations. This flexibility is responsive to public comments recommending against a rigid approach to enable institutions and individuals to tailor informed consents to the circumstances of particular studies. (Federal Register, 2017, Preamble p. 7213)

The Secretary's Advisory Committee on Human Research Protections (SACHRP) released recommendations on this provision in October 2018 (Department of Health and Human Services, 2018). In its deliberations, SACHRP considered at length what might constitute key information and how this could be determined for any given study. The committee examined several approaches and concluded that there was no general tool or algorithm that could identify the key information for any specific trial. Nonetheless, important themes emerged from this discussion, including that key information should be viewed from the perspective of the potential subject and, perhaps most importantly, that the new informed consent requirements be viewed as an opportunity to improve upon current practices. SACHRP urged the regulatory agencies to allow for flexibility and creativity as the community works to find the best method to meet this new requirement.

SACHRP also addressed the question of whether the elements of consent discussed in the preamble are in themselves necessary and sufficient to meet the key information requirement. It determined that although, in some circumstances, the points from the preamble may be adequate, in many circumstances additional information may be necessary or some points may be unnecessary (DHHS, 2018). For example, elements of study design such as randomization or use of a placebo are likely to be key for many studies. In clinical investigations studying the safety and efficacy of a new treatment for which an accepted therapy exists, it may be important to draw attention to how the investigational treatment differs from standard of care. For some studies, it may be advisable to provide information on discomforts and inconveniences, such as the time commitment required or the need to abstain from specific activities. In minimal risk studies, a statement of risk may not be needed. The committee concluded that researchers and institutions should refrain from taking a template approach to compliance that assumes that if the elements from the preamble are addressed they have met the regulatory requirement; they should instead make a good faith effort to determine what is most important to the population enrolling in this study (DHHS, 2018).

Some statement of risks of harm and potential benefits is likely to be considered key information for many studies, but duplicating the exhaustive list of risks that would typically appear later in the form is unlikely to be helpful to potential subjects. In assessing which risks and benefits might be considered key, SACHRP advised that risks or potential benefits that are likely to be used *alone* by a subject as a criterion to decide whether or not to enroll, or that differ from those of standard clinical care, are more likely to be important. SACHRP also advised providing a more meaningful description of potential benefits than the typical vague statement of "you may or may not benefit" that is common in many consent documents (DHHS, 2018).

Given the complexity of determining what information might be considered key for any given study, SACHRP developed a list of questions that could be used by researchers to identify for their study what information might be most important (DHHS, 2018):

- What are the main reasons a subject will want to join this study?
- What are the main reasons a subject will not want to join this study?
- What is the research question the study is trying to answer? Why is it relevant to the subject?
- What aspects of research participation or this particular study are likely to be unfamiliar to a prospective subject, diverge from a subject's expectations, or require special attention?
- What information about the subject is being collected as part of this research?
- What are the types of activities that subjects will do in the research?
- What impact will participating in this research have on the subject outside of the research? For example, will it reduce options for standard treatments?
- How will the subjects' experience in this study differ from treatment outside of the study?
- In what ways is this research novel?

This list was not meant to be exhaustive, and researchers and IRB members should consider additional questions to prompt them in developing and assessing the key information.

Presentation of the Key Information

The regulations do not specify the format in which the key information must be presented to the prospective subject. Although informed consent documents are typically in a narrative format, there is no reason that alternative presentations could not be used. For example, a tabular format might be used to describe the pros and cons of participation or to contrast an investigational treatment with standard clinical care. Graphic presentations can be an effective means to communicate complex concepts, and investigators should be encouraged to incorporate these when appropriate. Electronic consent provides new opportunities for presenting information in meaningful and accessible formats that can facilitate understanding and are useful not just for the key information section but the entire consent document.

Although one of the most common complaints about current informed consent documents is that they are too lengthy, this new requirement is likely to increase, not decrease, the length of the document. The regulations do not require researchers to repeat information in the body of the consent if it is included in the key information, but it may be advisable to do so if it would facilitate subject understanding. For example, repeating risk information that was considered "key" along with the complete list of risks in the body of the consent gives the subject one place in which all the risks were listed. Conversely, for relatively simple protocols, the key information section itself may meet all the requirements for full consent.

Remaining Challenges

Informed consent documents are used in a wide range of human subjects research, ranging from low-risk studies of healthy individuals in which the only intervention may be the collection of information via a survey instrument, to extremely complicated interventional studies investigating new therapeutic drugs or devices. Similarly, the individuals enrolled in studies vary just as widely. This array of possibilities suggests that it will be impossible to develop a general and complete specification *a priori* of what information should be considered key for all persons enrolling in any given trial.

The importance and utility of the key information section are likely to be greater in some circumstances than others. For example, clinical trials in which individuals must choose between receiving therapy for their condition as part of a research protocol or pursuing treatment in a nonresearch setting require potential subjects to make one of the most complicated and vexing decisions faced by a person suffering from a serious disease. In this case, the patient must be able to assess the benefits and burdens of the research as compared to routine clinical care, place them in the context of their particular circumstances, and make a decision whether or not to enroll that is most consistent with their needs, goals, and values.

Consider an individual with a newly diagnosed malignancy, who is considering enrollment in a trial of an investigational agent that has shown promise in inducing long-term remission. Standard treatment exists, but many patients relapse within 5 years. Although the investigational treatment appears quite promising, the side effects can be life-threatening, whereas the standard therapy is generally well tolerated. Participation in the research requires several invasive biopsy procedures that are not typically done as part of standard care, as well as a much greater frequency of follow-up visits and imaging studies.

It is likely that consent documents written under the pre-2018 Common Rule would focus virtually exclusively on describing the experimental regimen, outlining the various procedures, and detailing the risks. The description of alternatives would almost be certainly limited to a few lines at the most. Satisfying the 2018 Common Rule key information requirement would necessitate clearly contrasting all aspects of the experimental protocol with standard of care, including not only the risks and potential efficacy of the investigational drug with the standard of care regimen, but also drawing attention to how other aspects of the patient's, experience would differ. In the absence of this, patients are being asked to make decisions based on incomplete data, which risks both selecting an option that may not be aligned with their goals, as well as generating unrealistic expectations.

Contrast this scenario with the decision of a healthy volunteer to join a study in which the only intervention is a survey and a single MRI session. The potential impact of a "wrong" decision (if a wrong decision even exists) is minimal. Thus, "getting the key information section right" is much more important in the former situation than the latter.

As noted previously, the individuals who consider enrollment in a study are as varied as the types of studies themselves, and no single informed consent document can capture what is most important to all possible subjects. The unique characteristics of each person are likely to determine, at least in part, what is key for them, which may in turn be irrelevant or unimportant for others. For example, the rare risk of high-pitch hearing loss or peripheral neuropathy is likely to be key to a concert violinist, but may not be as important to others. In recognition that the consent form cannot anticipate all such circumstances, **45 CFR 46.116(a)(4)** directs that the consent form, including the key information section, provide "the information that a reasonable person would want to have in order to make an informed decision about whether to participate." Like "key information," the "reasonable person" standard is not further defined in the regulations but provides a standard against which to write studywide consent forms. Ideally, the *process* of informed consent, during which the researcher engages directly with the potential subject, provides an opportunity to solicit and discuss what is most important to a given individual. However, no regulatory mandate can ensure that this occurs, and IRBs rarely exercise their option to observe the consent process. Again, like the key information requirement itself, the reasonable person standard provides flexibility at the cost of uncertainty. It is likely the research community will need time and data to better understand how to implement both of these provisions of the updated rule.

From a practical perspective, the requirements also have implications for how consent forms are written. Both the key information and reasonable person standards require the IRB to consider the research from the perspective of potential subjects. This perspective may or may not be provided by the requirements for IRB membership, which have generally been interpreted to require that <u>IRB members</u> be selected based on their ability to review *the research*. The IRB membership requirements *do* include provisions for understanding the contexts of research with populations "vulnerable to coercion or undue influence" **[45 CFR 46.107(a)]**, and a more nuanced understanding that such <u>vulnerability</u> may extend beyond the categories explicitly identified (children,

🔗 3-1

🔗 Section 9

prisoners, individuals with impaired decision-making capacity, and economically or educationally disadvantaged persons) may be helpful.

The requirement for considering the subject perspective is not necessarily only a matter of judgment, but it also could be informed by data. But research into the informed consent process to date has not provided data that is generalizable enough to be useful in this context, and there are no existing funding resources that would enable such a research program. The requirement at **45 CFR 46.116(h)** that one version of the consent form for clinical trials be made publicly available on a federal website will help facilitate such future research.

Conclusion

The informed consent provisions in the Common Rule should be a stimulus to the research oversight community to rethink how we obtain informed consent from potential research subjects. While regulation alone cannot solve the many problems with the current approach to informed consent, these changes can serve as an impetus to researchers and IRBs to take a step back and examine their practices and, ideally, develop new ways to accomplish what informed consent should be—a process that allows individuals to make a decision whether to enroll in research that is most consistent with their personal goals and values.

References

Beardsley, E., Jefford, M., & Mileshkin, L. (2007). Longer consent forms for clinical trials compromise patient understanding: So why are they lengthening? *Journal of Clinical Oncology, 25*(9), e13–e14.

Department of Health and Human Services. (2018). Secretary's Advisory Committee on Human Research Protections. Attachment C: New "key information" informed consent requirements. www.hhs.gov/ohrp/sachrp-committee/recommendations/attachment-c-november-13-2018/index.html

Federal Register. (2017). Vol. 82, No. 12. 45 CFR 46 and Preamble. www.govinfo.gov/content/pkg/FR-2017-01-19/pdf/2017-01058.pdf

Flory, J., & Emanuel, E. (2004). Interventions to improve research participants' understanding in informed consent for research: A systematic review. *JAMA, 292*(13), 1593–1601.

Grady, C. (2015). Enduring and emerging challenges of informed consent. *New England Journal of Medicine, 372*(9), 855–862.

National Commission for the Protection of Human Subjects of Biomedical and Behavioral Research. (1979). *The Belmont Report: Ethical principles and guidelines for the protection of human subjects in biomedical and behavioral research.* www.hhs.gov/ohrp/regulations-and-policy/belmont-report/index.html

Paasche-Orlow, M. K., Taylor, H. A., & Brancati, F. L. (2003). Readability standards for informed-consent forms as compared with actual readability. *New England Journal of Medicine, 348*(8), 721–726.

Schenker, Y., Fernandez, A., Sudore, R., & Schillinger, D. (2011). Interventions to improve patient comprehension in informed consent for medical and surgical procedures: A systematic review. *Medical Decision Making, 31*(1), 151–173.

Waiving Informed Consent

Karen Christianson

Elizabeth Kipp Campbell

Abstract

This chapter discusses waivers and alterations of informed consent under the Common Rule and the Food and Drug Administration (FDA) regulations relating to protection of human subjects. Also addressed are waivers of parental permission and waivers of pediatric assent under subpart D. This chapter does not attempt to address the rules or policies of various other federal agencies (such as the Department of Defense) or state or local law. Readers should be aware that there are other pathways under which consent may not be required.

Introduction and Scope of Chapter

Informed consent is central to the _Belmont Report_ principle of respect for persons and is fundamental to the protection of human subjects. As stated in _Belmont_, "Respect for persons requires that subjects, to the degree that they are capable, be given the opportunity to choose what shall or shall not happen to them. This opportunity is provided when adequate standards for informed consent are satisfied" (National Commission, 1979).

1-1

Given the presumptive requirement to obtain informed consent, the circumstances under which an IRB may waive informed consent in its entirety are limited. However, U.S. regulating bodies recognize that there are circumstances when valuable research would be precluded if informed consent were required and provide provisions for IRBs to waive the requirement for informed consent when certain criteria are satisfied. Likewise, U.S. regulations provide for alterations of consent, in which one or more of the elements of consent are omitted or altered, when those same criteria are satisfied. This chapter discusses waivers and alterations of informed consent under the Common Rule and FDA regulations. Also addressed are waivers of parental permission and waivers of pediatric assent under subpart D.

9-6

This chapter does not attempt to address the rules or policies of various federal agencies (such as the Department of Defense) or state law. Readers

5-3

11-4, 11-7

6-5

should be aware that the Common Rule and FDA requirements for informed consent (and thus for waivers or alterations of the requirement) do not apply to exempt research. Readers should also understand that there are other regulatory pathways under which consent may not be required but that do not fall under the definition of "waiver," such as the FDA exceptions for emergency use and planned emergency research, outlined in **21 CFR 50.23** and **21 CFR 50.24**; waivers of the requirement issued by the Department of Health and Human Services (DHHS) Secretary or other federal departments or agencies; and under enforcement discretion decisions such as those issued by the FDA for certain in vitro diagnostic (IVD) research. Also not addressed in this chapter are the criteria that allow the IRB to waive documentation of the consent process.

Screening, Recruiting, or Determining Eligibility

Although not a true waiver of consent, under the Common Rule, an IRB may approve a study in which a researcher will obtain information or biospecimens for the purpose of screening, recruiting, or determining the eligibility of prospective subjects without the informed consent of the prospective subject, if one of the following two criteria are met:

> 1) The researcher will obtain information through oral or written communication with the prospective subject or legally authorized representative, or
> 2) The researcher will obtain identifiable private information or identifiable biospecimens by accessing records or stored identifiable biospecimens [**45 CFR 46.116(g)**]

Likewise, the FDA does not consider preliminary review of records to evaluate trial eligibility to be part of a "clinical investigation," and thus a waiver of informed consent for these preliminary activities would not be required under FDA regulations. Information recorded prior to seeking informed consent should be limited to the information necessary to establish eligibility (e.g., presence or absence of medical conditions, date of onset, lab results) and the patient's contact information (FDA, 2014). At the time this chapter was written, the FDA had not promulgated any guidance regarding the use of biospecimens for screening.

11-6

Organizations should be aware that, in addition to the Common Rule and FDA considerations outlined previously, the Health Insurance Portability and Accountability Act (HIPAA) may also apply to screening or recruitment activities when the records or biospecimens are held by a covered entity and include protected health information (PHI; or in the case of biospecimens, are labeled or provided with PHI). Action on the part of an IRB or a privacy board, such as a partial waiver of the requirement for HIPAA authorization, may be necessary before PHI can be accessed for screening, even when a waiver of consent is not necessary under the Common Rule or FDA GCP for the same activity.

Waivers and Alterations of Consent

The Common Rule includes two categories under which informed consent may be waived or altered: the "General" category at **45 CFR46.116(f)** and the "Public Benefit and Service Programs" category at **45 CFR 46.116(e)**.

In order for an IRB to waive or alter consent under the "General" provision, the IRB must determine and document that all of the following criteria are satisfied:

1) The research involves no more than minimal risk to the subjects;
2) The research could not practicably be carried out without the requested waiver or alteration;
3) If the research involves using identifiable private information or identifiable biospecimens, the research could not practicably be carried out without using such information or biospecimens in an identifiable format;
4) The waiver or alteration will not adversely affect the rights and welfare of the subjects; and
5) Whenever appropriate, the subjects or legally authorized representatives will be provided with additional pertinent information after participation. **[45 CFR 46.116(f)]**

A more in-depth discussion of the "General Waiver" criteria is included later in this chapter.

Under the "Public Benefit and Service Programs" provision, in order for the IRB to waive or alter consent, it must determine and document the following:

1) The research or demonstration project is to be conducted by or subject to the approval of state or local government officials and is designed to study, evaluate, or otherwise examine:
   a) Public benefit or service programs;
   b) Procedures for obtaining benefits or services under those programs;
   c) Possible changes in or alternatives to those programs or procedures; or
   d) Possible changes in methods or levels of payment for benefits or services under those programs; and
2) The research could not practicably be carried out without the waiver or alteration. **[45 CFR 46.116(e)]**

Importantly, under both the General and Public Benefit provisions, an IRB *cannot*:

1. Waive consent for the storage, maintenance, or secondary research use of identifiable private information or identifiable biospecimens if an individual was asked to provide broad consent in accordance with **45 CFR 46.116(d)** and refused to provide broad consent **[45 CFR 46.116(e)(1); 45 CFR 46.116(f)(1)]**.
2. Approve an alteration of consent that includes the omission or alteration of any of the general requirements for informed consent described at **45 CFR 46.116(a)** (e.g., the requirement that subjects or their legally authorized representatives are provided with information that a reasonable person would want to have in order to make an informed decision about whether or not to participate **[45 CFR 46.116(a)(4)]** or the requirement that informed consent begin with a concise and focused presentation of <u>key information</u> **[45 CFR 46.116(a)(5)(i)]**; or, if broad consent is used, omit or alter any of the elements required under **45 CFR 46.116(d)**.

✐ 6-3

<u>Broad consent</u> refers to the regulatory option available under the 2018 Common Rule to seek consent for the storage, maintenance, and secondary research use of identifiable information or identifiable biospecimens in adherence with alternative requirements outlined in **45 CFR 46.116**.

✐ 6-9

As of 2019, the FDA had published a proposed rule to permit waivers or alterations of informed consent for certain minimal risk clinical investigations (FDA, 2018). The proposed rule uses almost the same criteria as the "General" provision of the Common Rule, but *excludes* the criterion regarding the use of identifiable private information or identifiable biospecimens (criterion 3 in the "General" list). Until the FDA rule is finalized, guidance remains in effect, which states that the FDA does not object to IRB approval of waivers or alterations of informed consent when the IRB finds and documents that (FDA, 2017):

1. The clinical investigation involves no more than minimal risk (as defined in 21 CFR 50.3(k) or 56.102(i)) to the subjects;
2. The waiver or alteration will not adversely affect the rights and welfare of the subjects;
3. The clinical investigation could not practicably be carried out without the waiver or alteration; and
4. Whenever appropriate, the subjects will be provided with additional pertinent information after participation.

Importantly, just as the Common Rule includes limitations on alterations of consent, under the FDA's proposed rule, an IRB cannot approve an alteration that involves the omission or alteration of the consent element for clinicaltrials.gov at 21 CFR 50.25(c) when the research is an "applicable clinical trial" under the Public Health Service Act.

IRB Evaluation of the "General" Waiver Criteria

To aid with interpretation of the criteria for waivers and alterations of consent, IRBs and researchers are encouraged to consult Charts 12 and 13 of the Office for Human Research Protections (OHRP) decision charts (DHHS, 2020), as well as several other resources. The Secretary's Advisory Committee on Human Research Protections (SACHRP) produced recommendations in 2008 that remain relevant (DHHS, 2008), and the preamble to FDA's proposed rule provides insight (FDA, 2018), as does the preamble to the 2018 Common Rule (Federal Register, 2017). The following provides a discussion of each criterion, relevant background, and factors an IRB may consider.

Criterion 1: The Research Involves No More Than Minimal Risk to the Subjects

Minimal risk is defined in the Common Rule and FDA GCP regulations as meaning "that the probability and magnitude of harm or discomfort anticipated in the research are not greater in and of themselves than those ordinarily encountered in daily life or during the performance of routine physical or psychological examinations or tests" [45 CFR 46.102(j); 21 CFR 50.3].

The evaluation of whether an activity is minimal risk is much more complex than it appears on the surface. Much debate has taken place regarding proper interpretation and application of this criterion, particularly regarding the meaning of "ordinarily encountered in daily life" and of "routine physical or psychological examinations or tests." Adding to this debate is the constant evolution in what is "ordinary" and "routine," and how to best identify the ordinary and routine when studies or registries or repositories for future research may be open for many years, even decades. For example, the risk that individual subjects may be able to be reidentified from supposedly deidentified data has increased over time as the volume, types, and availability of data that is collected about individuals for a variety of purposes has increased, and the scientific methodology to cull, combine, and use this <u>data</u> has advanced. The question this evolution raises is whether the risk of identification should be considered a risk "ordinarily encountered in daily life." Likewise, as social and cultural norms evolve over time, perceptions of whether certain data is "sensitive" or "private" may also change. Research that meets the "minimal risk" criterion today may not in the future, and vice versa.

⊘ 12-4

To understand the intended application of the criterion, one can look to the discussion included in preambles at the time of the rule making and other historical sources. While no longer considered active guidance, the *Institutional Review Board Guidebook*, last updated by OHRP in 1993, is one source for understanding the intended application of the criterion (DHHS, 1993). Chapter III.A of the Guidebook discusses IRB risk/benefit analysis and provides insight into the concept of minimal risk and the assessment of risk. The Guidebook provides the following example of minimal risk: "For example, the risk of drawing a small amount of blood from a healthy individual for research purposes is no greater than the risk of doing so as part of routine physical examination" (DHHS, 1993). Note the use of the words "healthy" and "small amount."

IRBs should keep in mind that the risks of drawing blood and other "routine" procedures may not be minimal risk for certain subjects or under certain circumstances. For example, the risk of blood draws may not be minimal risk for subjects with conditions or on medications that impact clotting or for those with underlying or treatment-induced anemias. The Guidebook also includes discussion of the assessment of risk and emphasizes that IRBs must differentiate risks that may result from the research from risks to which subjects would be exposed even if not participating in the research and recognizes that this may require "very thin line drawing" (DHHS, 1993). For example, a subject with a given condition may be expected to have imaging procedures as part of their routine care. As a research subject, the schedule or type of imaging (e.g., magnetic resonance imaging [MRI] with or without contrast) may be dictated by the research protocol, whereas in routine care, those matters would be decided by the treating clinician. As such, even though the individual would be undergoing imaging whether or not they participated in research, the risks associated with the imaging in the research may be different from those that the person would encounter if not participating in the research and must be considered as risks of the research by the IRB. On the other hand, if the protocol-dictated imaging is based on clinical guidelines that the provider routinely adheres to, the risk analysis may change. This analysis may be further complicated by variability in "standard of care" among providers or sites. The IRB Guidebook also draws attention to the fact that risks may be introduced or increased by the design of the research (e.g., random assignment, double-blinding) and by the methods used to gather and analyze data, not just by the interventions or procedures that subjects undergo.

SACHRP outlined a set of recommendations related to waivers of informed consent and interpretation of minimal risk in a letter to the Secretary in January 2008, with a set of case studies illustrating their recommendations appended (DHHS, 2008). Although it is important to recognize that these recommendations were never formalized into OHRP guidance, there is also no interpretive guidance that contradicts these recommendations, so it is reasonable for IRBs to take the recommendations into consideration. Among other recommendations, SACHRP advises that "In its estimate of research-related risk, the IRB should carefully consider the characteristics of the subjects to be enrolled in the research including an evaluation of subject susceptibility, vulnerability, resilience and experience in relation to the anticipated harms and discomforts of research involvement" (DHHS, 2008).

Furthermore, building upon the healthy person discussion in the IRB Guidebook, SACHRP notes that, "While the harms and discomforts ordinarily encountered differ widely among individuals and individual populations, an ethically meaningful notion of 'harms and discomforts ordinarily encountered' should reflect background risks that are familiar and part of the routine experience of life for 'the average person' in the 'general population.' It should not be based on those ordinarily encountered in the daily lives of the proposed subjects of the research or any specific population" (DHHS, 2008). In other words, the standard for whether risks or discomforts are routine risks or risks of everyday life should not be based upon the routine experiences of a sick or otherwise vulnerable subject population. Being offered the opportunity to give informed consent is a presumed right, and IRBs and researchers should not be more tolerant of waiving this right for those who are sick or otherwise vulnerable simply because their lives routinely involve exposure to more risk than the average person.

Consistent with the Guidebook and SACHRP, FDA has also referenced the "healthy person" standard in regard to determinations of minimal risk, beginning with a response to comments in the preamble to the 1981 final rule, Part 50: Protection of Human Subjects; Informed Consent, in which FDA amended its definition of minimal risk to match that used in the Common Rule. The FDA noted that this definition "takes into account the fact that the risks in the daily life of a patient are not the same as those of a healthy individual, and uses the risks in daily life as the standards for minimal risk" (FDA, 1991). In the same preamble, in response to comments suggesting the FDA allow exceptions from the requirements for informed consent, FDA noted their position and their agreement with the National Commission "that even in no-risk or low-risk studies, respect for the rights and dignity of human subjects would require informed consent before participation in any clinical investigation" (FDA, 1991). Reflective of this position, and tied to its statutory authority under the Food, Drug, and Cosmetics Act, FDA has historically only permitted exceptions from requirement for informed consent under tightly defined circumstances and had no provisions for general waivers or alterations. This changed with the passage of the 21st Century Cures Act in December 2016, and subsequent issuance of FDA guidance in 2017. FDA does not expand upon its interpretation of "minimal risk" in its 2017 guidance or in the preamble to FDA's current proposed rule allowing waivers (FDA, 2018), but the proposed rule does include a solicitation for additional stakeholder input on the types of clinical investigations for which sponsors would anticipate requesting a waiver or alteration of informed consent. It is possible that additional insight will be provided when the final rule is published.

🔖 11-1

Criterion 2: The Research Could Not Practicably Be Carried Out Without the Requested Waiver or Alteration

This is a key criterion for IRBs to assess when determining whether to allow a waiver of consent. Despite a lack of definition of what "practicably" means, historically many IRBs have considered it in terms of its most literal meaning of "not possible" to conduct the research without the waiver. For example, for retrospective studies with large sample sizes and large geographic distribution, it may be the case that the research could not be conducted without a waiver of consent. Conversely, for prospective studies in which there is interaction with subjects, it becomes more difficult to make a reasonable argument that it is not practicable to obtain consent and thus conduct the study. That said, there may be some circumstances in which obtaining consent might threaten the validity of the study data or raise ethical concerns, thereby rendering the conduct of the study with traditional consent impracticable. A waiver of consent in such circumstances may be deemed appropriate.

Notably, DHHS has declined to define "practicably," despite many requests by the community that it do so, offering instead in the preamble to the 2018 Common Rule their conclusion that the requirements for waivers and alterations "appropriately honor respect for persons and balances this with other ethical principles" (Federal Register, 2017, Preamble p. 7226). The FDA and SACHRP both emphasize that the practicability criterion states that it would be impracticable to *conduct the research* without the waiver, not that it would be impracticable to obtain consent. SACHRP also advises that practicability "should not be determined solely by considerations of convenience, cost, or speed" (DHHS, 2008).

Criterion 3: If the Research Involves Using Identifiable Private Information or Identifiable Biospecimens, the Research Could Not Practicably Be Carried Out Without Using Such Information or Biospecimens in an Identifiable Format

Whereas the assessment of "practicably" in this criterion rests on similar considerations as for criterion 2, OHRP also provides the following insight in its FAQs regarding the 2018 Common Rule:

> The purpose of this additional criterion is that if the research could be done using non-identifiable information, then that is what should be done. In these cases, researchers shouldn't be using identifiable information because it increases the risk of breaches of privacy or confidentiality. (DHHS, 2018)

WAIVER CRITERION 3: ADDITIONAL CONSIDERATIONS

This criterion was added with the 2018 Common Rule and is not applicable to ongoing studies that have not been transitioned to comply with the 2018 Requirements, nor, as noted earlier, is it included in the FDA's proposed rule. However, FDA specifically solicited comment regarding inclusion of this criterion so it is possible it could be incorporated into FDA's final rule. Additionally, as of 2019, the Department of Justice (DOJ) had not signed onto the revised Common Rule; thus, this criterion would not apply to research subject to DOJ regulations.

Criterion 4: The Waiver or Alteration Will Not Adversely Affect the Rights and Welfare of the Subjects

This criterion reflects the idea that the primary ethical imperative in human subjects research is to ensure that the rights of potential research subjects are respected and their well-being protected, regardless of how valuable the research in question may be. Therefore, it is important for IRBs to consider under what conditions not seeking traditional consent for a research study would, itself, undermine subjects' rights or negatively affect their welfare. In thinking about this criterion, it may be helpful for IRBs to consider whether the potential subject population would believe that their rights were violated if they knew about the waiver. It is also important to assess whether these subjects might have any legal rights that must be considered under other federal, state, or local laws and regulations, especially if those other legal rights might supersede the ability to grant a waiver or alteration.

In considering potential adverse effects, it should be noted that the potential for a breach of confidentiality is the principal risk in many of the types of research for which waivers are requested (e.g., research involving the use of medical records or residual clinical specimens). In such cases, information about subjects that might identify them is being utilized in the research; if not carefully safeguarded, this information could be made public without subjects' permission or knowledge. Thus, it is the researcher's obligation to explain to the IRB how they will protect the subject's privacy and the confidentiality of their information. Ultimately, it is up to the researcher to provide a reasonable explanation for why a waiver of consent would *not* negatively impact the subjects, despite such risks, and to describe what measures will be taken to ensure that subjects' rights and welfare are protected.

Criterion 5: Whenever Appropriate, the Subjects or Legally Authorized Representatives Will Be Provided with Additional Pertinent Information After Participation

The final criterion for waivers or alterations of consent has been a source of difficulty for many researchers and IRBs, particularly as it relates to full waivers. Challenging questions include: Under what circumstances would it be appropriate to provide subjects with information about research that they were never informed of, much less agreed to participate in? What information is "pertinent"? Although the criterion must always be considered, leeway is provided for IRBs to determine whether postparticipation disclosure of information is appropriate given the specific research and circumstances.

🔗 10-3

Perhaps the most commonly cited example to illustrate when postparticipation disclosure of additional information may be appropriate is for research involving <u>deception</u>, in which the true purposes of the research or the specific research procedures involved are not disclosed during the initial consent process, because the information may alter behavior and bias results. Participation in such research is commonly followed by a debriefing session in which the subject(s) are informed of the true purpose or nature of the research or research procedures, and they may be offered the opportunity to withdraw consent for the use of their data. In other words, they are provided with "additional pertinent information after participation."

🔗 12-1

Another example is when consent is waived for the research use of specimens originally collected for other purposes, such as clinical care. When such research is likely to generate findings that may be relevant to the health or well-being of subjects, researchers and IRBs should consider whether <u>disclosing this information</u> would be warranted. In such circumstances, researchers and IRBs should carefully consider the plan for disclosure to ensure that it is appropriate.

Waiver of Parental/Guardian Permission

🔗 9-6

In accordance with *Belmont* and the federal agencies that have adopted subpart D, <u>children</u> who are subjects of research require additional protections. One of those additional protections is parental permission. Similar to waivers of consent for competent adults, there are some circumstances under which parental permission may be waived. In addition to the provisions previously noted for waivers of consent that also apply to parental permission, the DHHS regulations contain a provision that states that if the IRB determines that parental or guardian permission is not a reasonable requirement to protect the subjects of a particular study, the IRB may waive this permission requirement [subpart D – Additional Protections for Children Involved as Subjects in Research, **45 CFR 46.408(c)**]. However, the IRB must also ensure that there is an appropriate mechanism for protecting the children, as a substitute for parental permission. Additionally, the waiver must not be inconsistent with federal, state, or local laws. This is a particularly salient point, as many states and municipalities have laws addressing required permissions.

In evaluating the choice of the most appropriate mechanism to substitute for parental permission, the IRB should examine the nature and purpose of the study procedures, the risks and benefits to the child subjects, as well as their age, maturity, status, and condition. This allows the IRB to find a mechanism that makes sense for the characteristics of study and of the particular children who will participate in the study. An appropriate alternate mechanism for a research study that includes adolescents seeking treatment for a sexually transmitted disease will likely differ from the appropriate mechanism for a research study that includes physically abused preschoolers.

An often-cited example of a study that would meet the criteria for waiving parental permission is a study of neglected or abused children, where it is apparent that seeking parental permission is inappropriate. Waivers of parental permission are also sometimes sought for studies in which the child subject is participating in research on a topic for which parental permission would not be required in the nonresearch arena, primarily related to adolescents seeking medical care. For example, in some states a study of adolescents seeking birth control would not require parental permission.

Of note, provisions for waivers of consent for public benefit and service programs, as well as the provision for when parental permission is not a reasonable requirement, do not apply to FDA-regulated research. Additionally, the FDA's proposed rule and current guidance are silent regarding waivers of parental permission for minimal risk research. However, should the FDA's proposed rule be finalized as currently written, it appears that such waivers would be permissible. Subpart D **21 CFR 50.55 (e)** states, "In addition to the determinations required under other applicable sections of this subpart D, the IRB must determine, in accordance with and to the extent that consent is required under part 50, that the permission of each child's parents or guardian is granted." Because FDA's proposed rule would insert the provision for waivers or alterations into part 50 at **21 CFR 50.22**, it would follow that parental permission would not be required if the IRB determined that the criteria for a waiver are satisfied.

Waiver of Child Assent

Just as parental permission is a protection for children as vulnerable research subjects, a second protection for child subjects in research is conducting an assent. However, the IRB may waive the requirement for assent in any of the following conditions [**45 CFR 46.408(a)**]:

🔗 9-6

1. The IRB determines that the capability of some or all of the children is so limited that they cannot reasonably be consulted
2. The intervention or procedure holds out the prospect of direct benefit that is important to the health or well-being of the children and is available only in the context of the research

3. The standard consent waiver criteria of subpart A, described earlier in this chapter are met [consistent with **45 CFR 46.116** or subpart D **21 CFR 50.55(d)**]

With regard to the first condition, in making this determination the IRB should consider the ages, maturity, and psychological states of the children involved in the research. Additionally, the IRB may make this decision across the board for all children in the research, for a subset of children, or for each child individually.

The second condition speaks directly to approval category **45 CFR 46.405** and **21 CFR 50.52**, "research involving greater than minimal risk but presenting the prospect of direct benefit to the individual subjects." As noted previously, this condition includes the additional caveats that the IRB must not only make a determination that there is a direct benefit (or the prospect of such) to the child, but must also determine that this benefit is important to the child's well-being. Furthermore, the IRB must determine that this benefit may *only* be obtained by participating in the research study, a significantly higher standard than the simple standard for direct benefit.

As with waivers of parental permission, waivers of child assent must not be inconsistent with federal, state, or local laws. For example, many states have statutes regarding a minor's "right to object" or other similar laws.

Importance of IRB Documentation

The Common Rule and the proposed FDA rule require that IRBs "find and document" that the criteria permitting a waiver or alteration are satisfied (e.g., in IRB minutes and/or reviewer checklists). Because the criteria for waivers require interpretation and judgment, documentation of the rationale behind such determinations can be helpful in the event of an audit, inspection, or accreditation review and when explaining decisions to investigators and collaborating organizations. Such documentation also assists with consistency in decision making across IRB reviewers.

References

Department of Health and Human Services (DHHS). (1993). *Institutional review board guidebook.* www.hhs.gov/ohrp/education-and-outreach/archived-materials/index.html

Department of Health and Human Services (DHHS) (2008). Secretary's Advisory Commission on Human Research Protections. *SACHRP letter to HHS Secretary: Recommendations related to waiver of informed consent and interpretation of "minimal risk."* www.hhs.gov/ohrp/sachrp-committee/recommendations/sachrp-recommendations/index.html

Department of Health and Human Services (DHHS). (2018). *Revised Common Rule Q&As.* www.hhs.gov/ohrp/education-and-outreach/revised-common-rule/revised-common-rule-q-and-a/index.html

Department of Health and Human Services (DHHS). (2020). *Human Subject Regulations Decision Charts: 2018 Requirements.* www.hhs.gov/ohrp/regulations-and-policy/decision-charts-2018/index.html

Federal Register. (2017). Vol. 82, No. 12. 45 CFR 46 and Preamble. www.govinfo.gov/content/pkg/FR-2017-01-19/pdf/2017-01058.pdf

Food and Drug Administration (FDA). (1991). *FDA policy for the protection of human subjects.* www.fda.gov/science-research/clinical-trials-and-human-subject-protection/fda-policy-protection-human-subjects

Food and Drug Administration (FDA). (2014). *Informed consent information sheet: Guidance for IRBs, clinical investigators, and sponsors (draft).* www.fda.gov/regulatory-information/search-fda-guidance-documents/informed-consent

Food and Drug Administration (FDA). (2017). *IRB waiver or alteration of informed consent for clinical investigations involving no more than minimal risk to human subjects: Guidance for sponsors investigators, and institutional review boards.* www.fda.gov/media/106587/download

Food and Drug Administration (FDA). (2018). *Institutional review board waiver or alteration of informed consent for minimal risk clinical investigation (proposed rule).* Federal Register Docket No. FDA-2018-N-2727. www.federalregister.gov/documents/2018/11/15/2018-24822/institutional -review-board-waiver-or-alteration-of-informed-consent-for-minimal-risk-clinical

National Commission for the Protection of Human Subjects of Biomedical and Behavioral Research. (1979). *The Belmont Report: Ethical principles and guidelines for the protection of human subjects in biomedical and behavioral research.* www.hhs.gov/ohrp/regulations-and-policy /belmont-report/index.html

Waiving Documentation of Consent

Jonathan E. Miller
Brenda L. Ruotolo

Abstract

The Federal Policy for the Protection of Human Subjects (Common Rule) and the Food and Drug Administration (FDA) human subjects regulations require that informed consent be documented by way of a written consent form signed by the subject or the subject's legally authorized representative, with a written copy provided to the person signing the form, unless the IRB determines that certain conditions are met for a waiver of these requirements. This chapter describes the federal regulatory options under which an IRB may waive documentation of consent [45 CFR 46.117(a); 21 CFR 50.27].

Regulatory Pathways for Waiver of the Requirement to Obtain Documentation of Consent

When the Common Rule or FDA regulations, or both, apply to the research, the informed consent process must be documented with a written informed consent form that is signed by the subject or the subject's legally authorized representative, with a signed copy provided to the subject, unless the IRB determines that these documentation requirements can be waived under applicable regulatory provisions.

Under the Common Rule, these documentation requirements apply to all nonexempt research, as well as to the exemption related to broad consent, found at 45 CFR 46.104(d)(8). The Common Rule includes three provisions under which the IRB may waive the documentation requirements.

⌗ 5-3

An IRB may waive the requirement for the investigator to obtain a signed informed consent form for some or all subjects if it finds any of the following:

> (i) That the only record linking the subject and the research would be the informed consent form and the principal risk would be potential harm resulting from a breach of confidentiality. Each subject (or legally authorized representative) will be asked whether the subject wants documentation linking the subject with the research, and the subject's wishes will govern;
>
> (ii) That the research presents no more than minimal risk of harm to subjects and involves no procedures for which written consent is normally required outside of the research context; or
>
> (iii) If the subjects or legally authorized representatives are members of a distinct cultural group or community in which signing forms is not the norm, that the research presents no more than minimal risk of harm to subjects and provided there is an appropriate alternative mechanism for documenting that informed consent was obtained. **[45 CFR 46.117(c)]**

The FDA regulations only provide one option for waiver of documentation of consent. This waiver provision is equivalent to the second Common Rule provision.

> (1) The IRB may, for some or all subjects, waive the requirement that the subject, or the subject's legally authorized representative, sign a written consent form if it finds that the research presents no more than minimal risk of harm to subjects and involves no procedures for which written consent is normally required outside the research context. **[21 CFR 56.109(c)(1)]**

The informed consent process is an integral part of the protection of human subjects in research, and as such, documentation of that process is an important component. However, there are circumstances in which documentation of the consent process in the form of a signature on a consent document does not provide an appreciable contribution to the subjects' protection. This is the basis for the option of waiving documentation when the study procedures are no greater than minimal risk and are equivalent to procedures performed outside of the research environment without written consent. In addition, documentation of the consent process may actually increase the risk of harm to subjects in circumstances where confidentiality could be placed at risk by virtue of the subject having a signed form. The provisions for waiver of documentation of consent give IRBs the option to waive these requirements for the benefit of the subjects and perhaps for the convenience of both subjects and researchers, when appropriate (See Appendix 3 for a comparison of waiver options).

When the documentation requirements are waived under any of these provisions, the IRB may require the researcher to provide subjects or legally authorized representatives with a written statement regarding the research **[45 CFR 46.117(c)(2); 21 CFR 56.109(d)]**. This written statement might be a paper or electronic copy of the informed consent form without signature lines and signatures, or an information sheet. Information displayed on

CHANGES FROM PRE-2018 REQUIREMENTS TO REVISED COMMON RULE

Of note, the third option for waiving documentation of consent is new with the 2018 Common Rule and addresses the need for IRBs to be respectful of and consider cultural norms. For IRBs that continue to manage studies approved under the pre-2018 Requirements, only the first and second provisions may be considered because only those were included in the pre-2018 Requirements. There are minor revisions to the first provision between the pre-2018 and 2018 Requirements, but the general requirements are concordant. There were no changes to the second provision with the 2018 revision.

a screen or sent as an email are examples of electronic options that would meet this requirement, as long as the information is in a format and on a device where the subject can refer back to it at a later time or has an option for printing. For waivers under **45 CFR 46.117(c)(1)(i)**, for subjects who request to have documentation that connects them with the study, a consent form or information sheet with signatures would provide such documentation. When electronic media is being utilized, such as in an online survey or a mobile app, this requirement can also be met electronically through use of a digital signature.

When the IRB waives documentation of consent under any of these provisions, either at a <u>convened IRB meeting</u> or via the <u>expedited</u> or <u>limited IRB review</u> procedure, the IRB should document the determination and the specific criteria under which the waiver was granted. For convened IRB meeting determinations, this could be documented in the <u>meeting minutes</u>. For expedited or limited IRB reviews, the reviewer's determination may be documented in a number of ways such as via a reviewer's checklist or within the IRB's electronic management system. An example reviewer's checklist is provided as an appendix to this chapter. Documentation should make clear that the convened IRB or designated IRB member conducting the review has made the determination, as opposed to the decision having been made by (nonmember) IRB office staff.

Similarly, when documentation of consent has been waived by the IRB under **45 CFR 46.117(c)(1)(iii)**, the researcher should have procedures in place for documenting that informed consent was obtained. While not required, such documentation is best practice when documentation of consent has been waived under other regulatory provisions.

⊘ 5-7 ⊘ 5-5 ⊘ 5-6

⊘ 2-6

Examples for Each of the Waiver Options That Illustrate How They Can Be Applied

Example 1: A study in which the only document linking the subject to the research is the consent form, and the principal risk of harm is breach of confidentiality [45 CFR 46.117(c)(1)(i)]

The association between alcohol use and stress is well established, and this combination may in turn increase the risk for intimate partner violence. A researcher will conduct a study to gain a more in-depth understanding of these interrelated factors as a first step toward development of individual- and couple-level interventions aimed at reducing the risk for intimate partner violence. Study procedures include an online screener to determine eligibility, and in-person interviews with women who are interested in participating in the study after seeing flyers that ask if they "have ever felt afraid when their partner is drinking."

Potential subjects will read an information sheet online prior to completing the online screener. Checking a box that they are over age 18 years and wish to complete the screener will provide access to the screening tool. Eligible individuals will be provided with information to schedule an interview. When each subject arrives for the interview, the researcher will review the information sheet with her and will discuss any questions or concerns before obtaining verbal consent. A copy of the information sheet, which will not contain her name, signature, or other identifying information, will be offered to the subject. Each subject will also be asked if she wants documentation linking her to the study, which could be realized through signatures on the information sheet, with a copy provided to the subject. The subject's wishes will govern. The research is federally funded and was reviewed and approved by the IRB after January 21, 2019.

In this example, the study was initially reviewed at a convened meeting of the IRB because it involved a population at high risk of being victims of violence. The IRB determined that the existence of a consent form that described the purpose of the research and included the subject's signature could place the subject at risk of physical harm if her partner found the signed consent form or there was a breach of confidentiality and her partner learned of her participation in the study. The risk of emotional or reputational harm that could occur if family members, friends, or community or professional acquaintances learned of her participation was also a factor in the determination. Accordingly, the requirement for the subject's signature on a consent form was waived in accordance with the provision permitted under **45 CFR 46.117(c)(1)(i)**.

The researcher proposed, and the IRB approved, a process whereby the researcher would ask each subject if she wanted documentation linking her with the research. If so, the consent process would be documented by the subject signing a copy of the information sheet. For those who do not wish to have documentation linking them with the research, the researcher will provide detailed notes about the consent process in the research records.

The determinations of the IRB were documented in the minutes of the IRB meeting, which are maintained in a secure electronic system.

Example 2A: A minimal risk study where written documentation of consent is not required outside of the research context [45 CFR 46.117(c)(1)(ii)]

A research study seeks to assess patterns of exercise and eating habits and whether there is a correlation to body mass index, from a broad range of college students. Recruitment methods include flyers posted in student spaces, an ad in an online student newspaper, and a broadcast email, all of which direct interested students to attend one of several open sessions to complete study procedures. Modest compensation is offered. Study procedures are limited to face-to-face interviews with the students and noninvasive physical measurements, specifically height and weight. The researcher will review study information with students and obtain verbal consent, after which the interview and measurements will take place. Students will be provided with a copy of an information sheet about the research. The research is federally funded and was reviewed and approved by the IRB after January 21, 2019.

In this example, the study was reviewed through an expedited review process because it presented no more than minimal risk of harm to subjects, and all procedures were within the parameters of the <u>expedited review</u> categories. The IRB member-reviewer determined that the study met the criteria for waiver of documentation of informed consent under **45 CFR 46.117(1)(c)(ii)** because it was minimal risk, and neither interview procedures nor having height and weight recorded are procedures for which written informed consent is required outside of the research context.

The study approved by the IRB member-reviewer included a description of the manner in which the researcher would document the consent process: on a form that had been prepared for this purpose and which included the subject's name, date, and time of consent, and assignment of a unique study identifier. The data collection form on which the subject's interview responses and physical measurements would be documented contained the unique study identifier and not the subject's name.

🔗 5-5

The IRB member-reviewer used a checklist to confirm that waiver criteria were met and documented all determinations that were made in the institution's secure electronic system for IRB reviews, in accordance with established procedures.

Example 2B: A minimal risk study where written documentation of consent is not required outside of the research context [21 CFR 56.109(c)(1)]

A mobile medical application (MMA) that is subject to FDA oversight will be used to allow subjects who have a specific medical condition to track their symptoms, experiences of living with the condition, and strategies for managing symptoms. The researcher plans to use the data to develop self-help strategies that can be provided through the MMA to facilitate better self-management of symptoms, engage subjects in the process of developing such strategies, and connect subjects to patient advocacy resources.

Recruitment will be through flyers on relevant websites, brochures in clinic waiting areas, and through patient advocacy groups. Interested individuals will be directed to an online site, through which information about the study is available. In addition to being provided with required consent elements, visitors to the site will be asked if they are at least 18 years old and, if they respond affirmatively, will be asked to confirm through checking a box that they have read the information and wish to participate. Subsequently, they will be provided with a link to the MMA that can be downloaded to their device.

In this example, the MMA met the criteria for expedited review because it presented no more than minimal risk of harm to subjects, and the medical device that is involved does not require an investigational device exemption application to the FDA. The MMA records the subject's responses to the questions regarding age of majority, review of the information about the study, and willingness to participate. However, the subject is not asked to sign a consent document. The IRB member-reviewer determined that the study met the criteria for waiver of documentation of informed consent under FDA requirements [21 CFR 56.109(c)(1)] because it was minimal risk, and self-reporting of symptoms is not a procedure for which written documentation of informed consent is required outside of the research context.

The IRB member-reviewer documented all determinations that were made in the institution's secure electronic system for IRB reviews, in accordance with established procedures.

If this study were to be conducted within a covered entity, or in the covered component of a hybrid entity, each as defined by the Health Insurance Portability and Accountability Act (HIPAA), it would be necessary to assess whether the self-report constitutes protected health information (PHI). An alteration to the requirement for HIPAA authorization, if HIPAA was determined to be applicable, could manifest in the form of a waiver of documentation, if permitted in accordance with the covered entity's policies.

⌀ 11-6

Example 3: A study where subjects are members of a distinct cultural group or community in which signing forms is not the norm; the research presents no more than minimal risk of harm to subjects, and there is an appropriate alternative mechanism for documenting that informed consent was obtained [45 CFR 46.117(c)(1)(iii)]

A researcher will conduct interviews with adolescent Rohingya girls living in Cox's Bazar, a large refugee settlement in Bangladesh, to understand their sexual and reproductive health-related needs and priorities as a first step toward exploring the feasibility of implementing a targeted intervention in UNICEF-supported safe spaces within the settlement. The researcher will use a written script that will be conveyed in the local language to obtain verbal consent. For subjects under 18 years of age, verbal permission from a parent or caregiver will be obtained, before obtaining verbal assent from the adolescent. The research is federally funded and was reviewed and approved by the IRB after January 21, 2019.

🔗 5-5

In this example, the risk of harm to subjects was considered to be no more than minimal, and the study was reviewed by an <u>expedited review</u> process. The IRB member-reviewer determined that it was not reasonable in this instance to require a signature on a consent form and waived the requirement for such documentation in accordance with the cultural exception permitted under **45 CFR 46.117(c)(1)(iii)**. Key factors in the determination were that the local language (Rohingya) is not a written language, literacy among the population is very low, and verbal consent is standard practice in the community. In addition, the IRB member-reviewer considered that there could be unintended harm by having a subject sign or thumbprint a document that they cannot read, particularly in an area where there is limited trust in government authorities.

The researcher was required to document the verbal consent process in dated and signed research notes but was not required to provide subjects or parents/caregivers with a written statement regarding the research. Because Rohingya is not a written language, a written statement would have to be in another language, and the document would not be a resource or reference for the subjects.

🔗 9-6

<u>Subpart D</u> of 45 CFR 46, Additional Protections for Children Involved as Subjects in Research, requires documentation of permission by parents or guardians, and documentation of assent by children, in accordance with and to the extent permitted by **45 CFR 46.117** [**45 CFR 46.408(d)**; **45 CFR 46.408(e)**]. The IRB reviewer determined that waiver of documentation of consent was acceptable for both the adolescent girls and their parents or guardians.

The determinations of the IRB member-reviewer were documented in accordance with the IRB's standard operating procedures, in a reviewer notes section within a secure electronic system.

This research was reviewed under the Common Rule, which included the addition of the provision for waiving the requirement to obtain documentation of consent for cultural reasons.

EXAMPLE 3 AND PRE-2018 REQUIREMENTS

If the research in Example 3 had been reviewed and approved by the IRB under the pre-2018 Common Rule Requirements, the request for waiver of documentation of consent would have had to be considered under the more general provision for minimal risk research for which written documentation of consent is not required outside of the research context **[45 CFR 46.117(c)(1)(ii)]**. Although this provision could have been utilized, and remains in the 2018 Common Rule, the cultural provision is more appropriate.

Verbal and Implied Consent

The most common outcome of waiving the requirement to obtain documentation of informed consent when there is verbal interaction between the researcher and the subject is that verbal consent is obtained. This could occur when both the researcher and subject are in the same location or when each is in different locations and communicating by telephone or through other electronic media. Note that if verbal consent is documented via electronic means such as audio- or video-recording, a waiver of documentation would still be necessary, because the regulations require a written informed consent form approved by the IRB and signed by the subject or the subject's legally authorized representative. In cases where there is no verbal interaction between the researcher and the subject (e.g., through an online process), consent may be implied by an action that the subject takes after reading information about the study (see sidebar: "Implied Consent") or provided through an electronic process that does not qualify as a legal signature.

Other Considerations

In addition to the regulatory provisions noted and illustrated in these examples, IRBs must also consider other applicable federal or international regulations, state and local laws, and institutional policies when determining whether a waiver of documentation of consent is an option. IRBs should have a <u>policy</u> in place that establishes guidelines for documentation of informed consent in the review of research that is not subject to federal regulations and for which there are no other statutory requirements for such documentation.

If research is conducted in a covered entity or in the covered component of a hybrid entity, each as defined by HIPAA, and PHI will be used, an IRB that has made a determination to waive documentation of consent must also consider whether documentation of <u>HIPAA</u> authorization is required. Depending on institutional policy and interpretation of HIPAA regulations, the covered entity's privacy board may approve an alteration of the authorization requirement to waive the documentation requirement for HIPAA authorization.

> **IMPLIED CONSENT**
>
> Application of waiver provisions **45 CFR 46.117(c)(1) (ii)** or **21 CFR 56.109(c)(1)**, when the study is minimal risk and written documentation of consent is not required outside of the research context, could also take the form of a process that is sometimes referred to as "implied consent." For example, a researcher conducting a nonexempt survey may distribute the survey by mail or email to prospective subjects. If the survey materials clearly state that by responding to the questions and mailing the survey back the recipients have agreed to participate in the research, consent is implied by the subject's return of the completed survey. In situations like this, the IRB must have approved and appropriately documented a waiver of documentation of informed consent under **45 CFR 46.117(c)(1)(ii)** or **21 CFR 56.109(c)(1)**.

● 2-3

● 11-6

Conclusion

Federal regulations for the protection of human subjects respect the principle of autonomy while also providing options for flexibility, through waiver of the requirement for a signature on a consent form and providing subjects with a written copy, in certain limited circumstances. IRBs should be aware of these provisions and their respective criteria to avoid creating unnecessary obstacles to research.

Reference

Department of Health and Human Services (DHHS). (2019). *Informed consent FAQs: Can consent or parental permission ever be "passive" or "implied"?* www.hhs.gov/ohrp/regulations-and-policy /guidance/faq/informed-consent

Appendix 1

Waiver of Documentation Decision Tree

Reproduced from www.hhs.gov/ohrp/regulations-and-policy/decision-charts-2018/index.html#c14

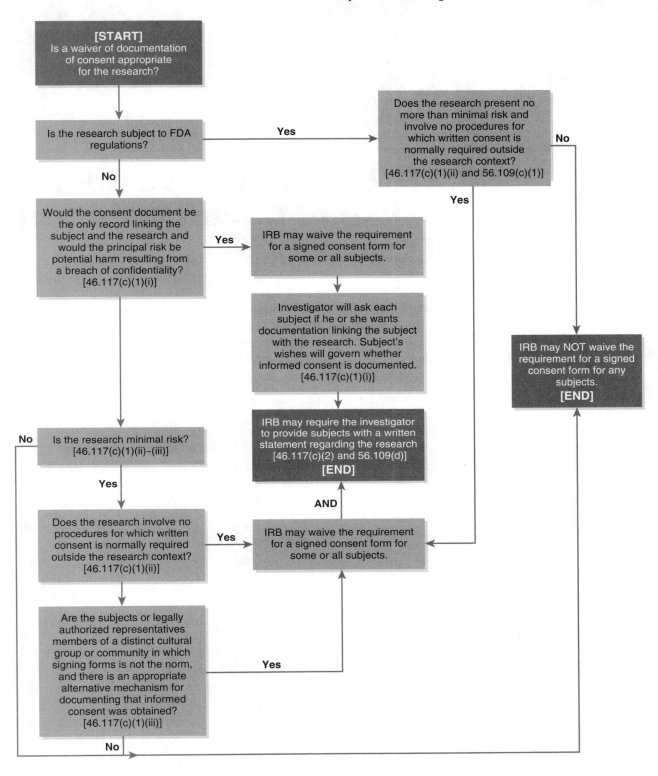

Appendix 2

IRB Reviewer Checklist: Waiver of Documentation of Consent

Waiver of the requirement to obtain signatures on a written informed consent form and, as applicable, to provide a written copy to the person signing the informed consent form must meet one of the following criteria. All regulatory references are to the 2018 Common Rule (45 CFR 46, Subpart A), unless otherwise indicated.

- ☐ The waiver meets the requirements of 45 CFR 46.117(c)(1)(i). All of the following must be true:
  - ☐ The only record linking the subject and the research would be the informed consent form,
  - ☐ The principal risk would be potential harm resulting from a breach of confidentiality, and
  - ☐ The study is not subject to the FDA regulations.

  Each subject (or legally authorized representative) will be asked whether the subject wants documentation linking the subject with the research, and the subject's wishes will govern. Indicate how researchers will document this link if the subject wishes (e.g., signature on the consent form or information sheet).

  _____

  _____

- ☐ The waiver meets the requirements of 45 CFR 46.117(c)(1)(ii) and/or 21 CFR 56.109(c)(1). All of the following must be true:
  - ☐ The research presents no more than minimal risk of harm to subjects, and
  - ☐ The research involves no procedures for which written consent is normally required outside of the research context.

- ☐ The waiver meets the requirements of 45 CFR 46.117(c)(1)(iii). All of the following must be true:
  - ☐ The subjects or legally authorized representatives are members of a distinct cultural group or community in which signing forms is not the norm,
  - ☐ The research presents no more than minimal risk of harm to subjects,

❐   There is an appropriate alternative mechanism for documenting that informed consent was obtained, and

❐   The study is not subject to the FDA regulations.

Describe how the researcher will document for each subject that informed consent was obtained.

_____

_____

If documentation of consent is waived via one of the provisions noted here, does the IRB require that the researcher provide subjects or legally authorized representatives with a written statement regarding the research?

Yes   No   Not applicable (documentation not waived)

Appendix 3

At-a-Glance Comparison of Waiver Options

Waiver Option	Regulatory Applicability	Conditions	Required Documentation	Other Requirements
The informed consent form would be the only record linking the subject, and the principal risk would be potential harm resulting from a breach of confidentiality.	Allowed under Common Rule [45 CFR 46.117(c)(1)(i)]	None	Each subject (or legally authorized representative) will be asked whether the subject wants documentation linking the subject with the research, and the subject's wishes will govern.	The IRB may require the investigator to provide subjects or legally authorized representatives with a written statement regarding the research [45 CFR 46.117(c)(2)].
The research involves no procedures for which written consent is normally required outside of the research context.	Allowed under Common Rule [45 CFR 46.117(c)(1)(ii)] and/or FDA regulations [21 CFR 56.109(c)(1)]	Minimal risk research only	None	
The subjects or legally authorized representatives are members of a distinct cultural group or community in which signing forms is not the norm.	Allowed under Common Rule [45 CFR 46.117(c)(1)(iii)]	Minimal risk research only	There must be an appropriate alternative mechanism for documenting that informed consent was obtained.	

Electronic Informed Consent

Kindra Cooper

Joshua Fedewa

Abstract

Electronic informed consent (eConsent) involves the use of an electronic system to communicate study information and obtain and document informed consent. eConsent may be as simple as converting a paper consent document into a digital format (PDF) and obtaining an electronic signature or as complex as a multimedia presentation involving subject interaction. The literature describes how research subjects often fail to understand the goals of research or concepts like randomization and voluntary participation. eConsent has been widely studied in the interest of improving consent processes. As with any new approach, studies have shown that eConsent has distinct advantages, such as the ability to appeal to multiple learning styles, but comes with challenges as well. While the regulatory requirements related to the content of eConsent (i.e., the elements of informed consent) are the same as for traditional consent, eConsent processes are subject to additional regulatory requirements. IRBs should understand the requirements that apply to eConsent and ensure that studies utilizing eConsent satisfy these requirements. In this chapter, we define eConsent, summarize the literature on its advantages and challenges, establish the regulatory requirements, explain the responsibilities of an IRB reviewing eConsent, and discuss operational considerations regarding implementation.

Introduction: What Is eConsent?

As defined by the Department of Health and Human Services (DHHS) and the Food and Drug Administration (FDA), eConsent is "the use of electronic systems and processes that may employ multiple electronic media, including text, graphics, audio, video, podcasts, passive and interactive Web sites, biological recognition devices, and card readers, to convey information related to the study and to obtain and document informed consent" (FDA, 2016). eConsent varies in complexity and operation, but it is important to understand that merely creating an electronic version of a consent document (such as a PDF) is not eConsent. The regulatory definition of eConsent applies only where the consent is provided to subjects electronically and/or the process for obtaining and documenting consent is completed electronically (FDA, 2016).

A looser definition of eConsent is encountered within the literature (Friedlander et al., 2011; Lentz et al., 2016; Ramos, 2017; Rothwell et al., 2014). Some authors define eConsent as simply incorporating multimedia components into the consent in order to create "an interactive experience for participants aligned with their preferences, needs, and learning styles" (Vanaken & Masand, 2019).

Anecdotally, a lack of understanding among some sponsors and researchers regarding the regulation of eConsent may place IRBs experienced with eConsent in the role of educator on this complex topic. The literature, however, suggests that some IRBs remain reluctant to review eConsent and that confusion regarding the requirements for eConsent persists among some IRB professionals (Kane & Gallo, 2017). Meanwhile, eConsent tools are proliferating in the marketplace, and there is some evidence to suggest that at least a segment of research subjects prefers eConsent for reasons including the perceived approachability of a digital format (Frelich et al., 2015).

In light of these trends and the various definitions of eConsent encountered in the literature, it is important that IRB professionals understand what qualifies as eConsent from a regulatory perspective, when additional regulations apply, and what steps sponsors, researchers, and IRBs can take to ensure that eConsent is implemented appropriately.

Advantages and Challenges of eConsent

Despite hopes that eConsent can provide an opportunity to overcome the limitations of the paper form, including length and accessibility (Kane & Gallo, 2017), the literature on eConsent is mixed as to its advantages.

Advantages of eConsent

DHHS and FDA suggest that electronic communication may promote subject understanding during consent (FDA, 2016). Similarly, Anderson and colleagues conducted focus group interviews in which subjects expressed that eConsent could "show, not just tell" study information, facilitating greater comprehension (Anderson et al., 2017). Vanaken and Masand suggest that eConsent appeals to multiple learning styles, which may further encourage understanding and retention (Vanaken & Masand, 2019). The Clinical Trials Transformation Initiative asserts that eConsent allows for a "Tiered Consent Model," in which content is presented to participants in segments (Lentz et al., 2016). Elsewhere in the literature, subjects confirm that segmented delivery of content promotes enhanced understanding of consent materials (Madathil et al., 2013).

Ramos (2017) demonstrates that subjects may perceive an electronic format as "less intimidating and more to the point" than paper forms. Subjects in the focus groups conducted by Anderson and colleagues reported that use of eConsent could allow subjects to slow down and help to mitigate the pressure they felt to sign quickly (Anderson et al., 2017). Both familiarity and reduced time pressure may promote comfort, leading to increased comprehension. Subjects in Anderson's focus groups also stated that feeling rushed to provide consent leaves subjects feeling used (Anderson et al., 2017). Thus, if eConsent allows greater time for contemplation, it may also benefit subjects by supporting autonomous decision making.

Advantages of eConsent accrue to study teams as well. In a pilot study of eConsent used by legally authorized representatives (LARs) in an acute stroke investigation, eConsent significantly reduced the time between initial contact and randomization (Haussen et al., 2017). eConsent tools that allow subjects to obtain additional information for themselves—by accessing hyperlinks or optional content (Anderson et al., 2017)—may also lead to more or better questions from subjects, improving subject engagement and understanding. Participant survey responses in the study conducted by Vanaken and Masand (2019) provide support for this hypothesis. Subjects in that study expressed a perception that eConsent tools may enhance their ability to flag consent information they find confusing in order to raise these issues with study staff at a later time, perhaps because unlike paper forms, digital consent tools are searchable. As such, if eConsent promotes subject understanding and encourages subjects to ask more or better questions during the consent process, use of eConsent may also lead to improved study compliance on the part of subjects.

The speed of eConsent appears to benefit both subjects and study teams. DHHS and FDA indicate that eConsent may allow for "rapid notification to . . . subjects of any amendments pertaining to the informed consent that may affect their willingness to continue to participate" (FDA, 2016). Use of electronic technology to obtain and document consent may also allow for real-time consent monitoring (Parrish, 2017), rapid data transfer, and streamlined data management, suggesting a potential time savings to study teams (Frelich et al., 2015). eConsent may also promote time savings by permitting easy retrieval of subject-specific responses to opt-ins for future and optional research (Madathil et al., 2013). Rapid retrieval of information from eConsent platforms may also foster more efficient regulatory compliance (Vanaken & Masand, 2019). Finally, the flexibility of eConsent, which permits consent to be obtained and documented both at the study site and remotely, may increase access to and participation in clinical trials (Moore et al., 2017).

Challenges of eConsent

While some literature suggests that eConsent improves subject understanding of consent, other studies contradict these findings, casting doubt on whether eConsent results in improved subject comprehension and illustrating the ways in which eConsent may create challenges within research.

A pair of studies have shown little difference in subject comprehension when eConsent is compared with traditional processes and paper forms (Ramos, 2017; Rothwell et al., 2014). Some subjects may prefer paper documents, just as others feel more comfortable with digital versions. In addition, use of eConsent without a paper alternative may unfairly limit the ability of some subjects to participate in research. DHHS and FDA indicate that eConsent may not be appropriate for older subjects or for subjects who lack familiarity with technology or have physical limitations (such as poor motor skills, poor eyesight, etc.) (FDA, 2016). Lack of familiarity with technology was cited as a barrier to participation by subjects in Anderson's focus groups as well (Anderson et al., 2017).

eConsent may also create barriers to subject comprehension. Whether subjects will be as inattentive to eConsent as they are to the terms of use and privacy policies that accompany their use of mobile applications, for example, remains an open question (Doerr et al., 2016; see also Moore et al., 2017). Researchers may mitigate this risk by implementing interactive components, multimedia elements, or assessments and quizzes within eConsent tools (Doerr et al., 2016; FDA, 2016; Moore et al., 2017).

Subjects themselves also express the concern that remote consent may diminish the quality of subjects/site interaction (Vanaken & Masand, 2019). Reduced interaction or poor-quality interaction may impair the establishment of trust between researchers and subjects (Anderson et al., 2017).

The literature also raises privacy and security concerns regarding eConsent (Haussen et al., 2017; Moore et al., 2017; Vanaken & Masand, 2019). DHHS and FDA suggest that the electronic storage of subject data increases risks that subject information could fall prey to hacking or other forms of remote exploitation (FDA, 2016). Privacy and security challenges associated with eConsent also have ramifications for study teams. As DHHS and FDA permit eConsent to be conducted remotely, security complications arise around verifying that the individual providing consent is either the person who will participate in the research or that person's representative (FDA, 2016). In addition, researchers relying on third-party applications to support their eConsent process should anticipate questions from the IRB, institution, and study subjects regarding the platform and privacy policies of the third-party vendor (Moore et al., 2017). To adequately answer these questions, researchers must develop an understanding of these services and tools. Researchers may also need to provide documentation to the IRB confirming that third-party platforms and privacy policies are compliant with applicable regulations.

Exclusion of technologically naïve subjects from studies using eConsent (Anderson et al., 2017; FDA, 2016) may also have implications for researchers, who are responsible for ensuring equitable subject selection [45 CFR 46.111; 21 CFR 56.111]. In addition, there are significant costs associated with the development of multimedia eConsent tools. In cases where researchers will need to obtain images, video, and other content for multimedia presentations in more than one language, costs multiply. Should researchers elect not to incur the cost of developing eConsent in multiple languages, the population excluded from research employing these tools could grow exponentially.

Finally, study teams maintain concerns that these technologies may increase time spent in training to use, access, and manage eConsent systems (Vanaken & Masand, 2019). Questions regarding the consequences should an eConsent platform fail contribute to skepticism among some researchers that eConsent will require more time than it promises to save (Vanaken & Masand, 2019).

ADVANTAGES AND CHALLENGES OF ECONSENT

Potential advantages of eConsent:

- Increased subject comprehension
- Enhanced subject autonomy
- Reduced time between recruitment and randomization
- Increased subject engagement
- Increased subject compliance
- Speed of electronic communication
- Time savings in data management and regulatory compliance
- Flexibility to obtain and document consent remotely

Potential challenges of eConsent:

- Impaired subject comprehension

- Exclusion of some subjects from research participation
- Inattentiveness to digital content
- Risks to confidentiality and privacy
- Verifying the identity of subjects consenting remotely
- Reduced subject/researcher interaction with remote eConsent
- Impaired trust between subjects and researchers
- Equitable subject selection
- Time associated with learning and maintaining an eConsent platform
- eConsent system failure

Regulation of eConsent

As with traditional consent, when eConsent is used for participation in Common Rule or FDA-regulated research, the requirements established for consent in the Common Rule and/or 21 CFR parts 50 and 56 apply. Thus, consent obtained electronically must be informed, voluntary, and provided with comprehension in order to be valid. Additionally, the content of eConsent and the processes used to obtain and document eConsent must be reviewed and approved by the IRB (**45 CFR 46.109**; **21 CFR 56.111**; FDA, 2016).

Part 11

Unlike paper consent, eConsent may also be regulated by **21 CFR 11**, also known as "part 11." Part 11 establishes the standards by which FDA considers electronic records and signatures equivalent to paper records and handwritten signatures **[21 CFR 11.1(a)]**. The requirements of part 11 apply to electronic records "created, modified, maintained, archived, retrieved, or transmitted" under FDA regulations **[21 CFR 11(b)]**. Part 11 also applies to the electronic systems that produce electronic records and is intended to do so broadly, that is, to systems that are custom built or commercially available, mobile or not (FDA, 2017). Research regulated exclusively under the Common Rule is not subject to part 11, but part 11 does apply to research regulated by both the Common Rule and the FDA. An IRB may also adopt the requirements of part 11 as a single standard of review for all studies under its oversight.

PART 11 DEFINITIONS

- *Electronic system*: Systems, including hardware and software, that produce electronic records. (FDA, 2016)
- *Electronic record*: [A]ny combination of text, graphics, data, audio, pictorial, or other information representation in digital form that is created, modified, maintained, archived, retrieved, or distributed by a computer system. **[21 CFR 11.3(b)(6)]**
- *Electronic signature*: [A] computer data compilation of any symbol or series of symbols executed, adopted, or authorized by an individual to be the legally binding equivalent of the individual's handwritten signature. **[21 CFR 11.3(b)(7)]**
- *Biometrics*: [A] method of verifying an individual's identity based on measurement of the individual's physical feature(s) or repeatable action(s) where those features and/or actions are both unique to that individual and measurable. **[21 CFR 11.3(b)(3)]**

Food and Drug Administration. (2017). Use of Electronic Records and Electronic Signatures in Clinical Investigations Under 21 CFR Part 11 – Questions and Answers. Guidance for Industry. www.fda.gov/media/105557/download.

In the context of human subjects research, an eConsent tool or platform is an electronic system, a digital consent form is an electronic record, and the act by which a participant "signs" the eConsent constitutes an electronic signature. Biometrics, such as fingerprints, are one means of creating an electronic signature.

Part 11 requires electronic systems to ensure the veracity and confidentiality of electronic records submitted to FDA **[21 CFR 11.10]**. Under part 11, systems must be validated to ensure accuracy, reliability, consistent intended performance, and the ability to detect invalid or altered reports **[21 CFR 11.10(a)]**. Access to these systems must be limited to authorized individuals **[21 CFR 11.10(d)]**. Systems subject to part 11 are required to use secure, computer-generated, time-stamped audit trails to record the date and time that records within the system are created, modified, or deleted, as well as the identity of the individual initiating these actions **[21 CFR 11.10(e)]**. Part 11 also requires that systems be capable of producing accurate and complete copies of all records created by and housed within the system and do so for the retention period required by FDA for each record **[21 CFR 11.10(b); 21 CFR 11.10(c)]**.

Records subject to part 11 must clearly indicate the name of the signer, the date and time when the signature was created, and the meaning attached to the signature—in other words, what the signer is agreeing or attesting to by signing the record. Part 11 also requires that electronic records and signatures be linked to ensure that signatures cannot be removed, copied, or transferred from the record, as a guard against tampering **[21 CFR 11.70]**.

Part 11 requirements regarding electronic signatures are designed to ensure that signatures may not be altered, copied, or forged (FDA, 2017). Therefore, eSignatures must be unique to one individual and may not be used by or reassigned to anyone else **[21 CFR 11.100(a)]**. Part 11–compliant signatures may be created using biometrics or two distinct identification components **[21 CFR 200]**. Examples of biometrics and identification components are included in the section of this chapter on "IRB Responsibilities in Review of eConsent." Finally, eSignatures regulated by part 11 may only be collected and recorded by an electronic system after the identity of the individual creating the signature has been verified **[21 CFR 11.100(b)]**.

HIPAA

🔗 11-6

eConsent is subject to regulation under the <u>Health Insurance Portability and Accountability Act</u> (HIPAA; DHHS, 2013): "If the entity holding the subject's personal information is a covered entity under the Health Insurance Portability and Accountability Act of 1996 (HIPAA) (Public Law No. 104-191) . . . or acting as a business associate of a HIPAA-covered entity, the requirements in the HIPAA Privacy, Security, and Breach Notification Rules apply (see 45 CFR parts 160 and 164)" (FDA, 2016). Where HIPAA applies, electronic signatures must also meet the requirements of the Electronic Signatures in Global and National Commerce Act (E-Sign Act, 2000), and electronic systems housing subject information must comply with the HIPAA privacy, security, and breach notification rules **[45 CFR parts 160 and 164]**. Notably, compliance with the HIPAA security rule typically requires that information stored within regulated systems be encrypted (FDA, 2016). Where these conditions are met, HIPAA authorizations for research may be obtained electronically (FDA, 2016).

IRB Responsibilities in Review of eConsent

IRB regulatory responsibilities in review of eConsent fall into five categories: (1) evaluating eConsent under part 11, (2) ensuring the appropriateness of the eConsent process, (3) assessing the adequacy of eConsent content, (4) verifying that modifications to eConsent continue to adhere to the criteria for IRB approval, and (5) record retention of eConsent materials.

Part 11

When eConsent is proposed for a study subject exclusively to the Common Rule, the review process outlined in this section of the chapter does not apply. In these cases, the IRB should verify with the sponsor that the proposed eSignature will be legally valid in the jurisdiction where the study will be conducted (FDA, 2016) and move on to assess the process, content, and other requirements for eConsent. When eConsent is proposed for a study subject to FDA regulations, alone or in combination with the Common Rule, or where an IRB has adopted part 11 as a single standard of review, the IRB must evaluate whether eConsent systems and signatures are part 11 compliant.

According to DHHS and FDA guidance, IRBs, researchers, and sponsors "[M]ay rely on a statement from the vendor of the electronic system used for obtaining the electronic signature that describes how the signature is created and that the system meets the relevant requirements contained in 21 CFR part 11" (FDA, 2016). The ability to rely on a vendor statement relieves the IRB of the obligation of becoming an expert in the intricate, technological requirements of the statute, such as assessing whether an electronic system is appropriately validated or the sufficiency of an audit trail. Reliance on a vendor statement does not entirely relieve the IRB of its responsibility to evaluate part 11 compliance, however. The DHHS guidance permitting sponsors or IRBs to rely on a vendor statement also suggests that IRBs independently assess elements of part 11 compliance (FDA, 2016). Thus, one way to describe the obligations of the IRB relative to part 11 compliance is "trust but verify." The most straightforward means of adopting this direction would to be implement a two-part review.

First, the IRB should obtain a vendor statement attesting to part 11 compliance. Guidance is silent regarding the form and content of vendor statements, and IRBs take a variety of approaches to these documents. One approach requires that statements be issued by a third-party auditor hired by the vendor to assess the part 11 compliance of the eConsent system (Parrish, 2017). Another approach requires an attestation provided from the vendor. The IRB might also obtain the sponsor's attestation that the sponsor has been appropriately assured as to part 11 compliance. Whatever the approach, it is unlikely that reliance on a bare assurance of compliance would be adequate in the eyes of regulators (Parrish, 2017). Best practice likely requires that attestations speak to the elements of part 11 directly. A list of these elements is included in the "IRB Checklist for Part 11 Compliance," later in this chapter.

Second, the IRB should independently evaluate elements of part 11 compliance identified by guidance: signature creation and the functionality of the system regarding hard copy documents. Confirmation that signatures are created using biometrics or two distinct identification components **[21 CFR 11.200(a)]** can be accomplished by asking the sponsor to describe the method of signature creation. eSignatures created using biometrics may utilize fingerprints, hand geometry (finger length and palm site), iris and retinal patterns, voiceprints, or another measurement of an individual's physical feature(s) or repeatable action(s) as long as those features or actions are unique to the individual, measurable, and unlikely to change over time [21 CFR 200(3)(b); FDA, 2016]. eSignatures not created using biometrics may be established using a combination of government-issued identification documents, computer-readable identification cards, unique username and password combinations (FDA, 2016), and handwritten signatures created with an eSignature device or written into the digital consent using a stylus. These examples appear in guidance, and as only identification codes and passwords appear in the text of the statute, IRBs should expect these lists to evolve with technology. *Critically, eSignatures that do not meet these requirements may only be used in FDA-regulated studies that qualify for a waiver of documentation of consent* [21 CFR 50.27; FDA, 2016; see also 21 CFR 11.2].

The IRB should also confirm that an eConsent system can produce a full and complete hard copy of the consent document and that the hard copy document includes all information conveyed to subjects via hyperlink or multimedia components in the eConsent (FDA, 2016). Including confirmation of this functionality among the IRB requirements of the vendor statement or sponsor attestation is the least complicated means of addressing this suggestion.

IRB CHECKLIST FOR PART 11 COMPLIANCE

Obtain a vendor statement regarding part 11 compliance. A vendor statement addressing the statutory elements of part 11 would include attestation to the following:

- eSignatures are part 11 compliant.
- eConsent systems can produce an accurate and complete copy of the current version of the consent on demand, including all information conveyed by hyperlink or multimedia elements.
- System can produce versions of all consents reviewed and approved by the IRB throughout the conduct of the trial and maintain these document for the duration required by FDA.
- Systems employ secure, computer-generated, time-stamped audit trails to record the times and dates at which IRB-approved content is uploaded to the system, study staff modify content or elements of the system, and subjects provide their signature—and to document the identity of each individual performing these tasks.
- System access is restricted to authorized users.
- Where HIPAA applies, data will be transmitted and stored by the system in an encrypted format and be compliant with the E-Sign Act and the HIPAA Security Rule.

Independently assess signature creation and hard copy functionality:

- eSignatures are created using biometrics or at least two identification components.
- Hard copy functionality is included in the IRB's requirements for vendor statements.

Remember:

- Part 11 applies to FDA-regulated research or where an IRB has adopted part 11 as a single standard of review.

eSignatures that are not part 11 compliant may only be used in FDA-regulated studies that qualify for a waiver of documentation of consent.

eConsent Processes

Whether researchers use eConsent or traditional consent, the IRB must ensure that consent is obtained under circumstances providing the subject (or their representative) with enough time to contemplate participation and minimizing the potential for coercion or undue influence [**45 CFR 46.116**; **21 CFR 50.20**]. Informed consent must also be appropriately documented unless the study qualifies for a <u>waiver</u> of documentation of consent [**45 CFR 46.117**; **21 CFR 50.27**]. These obligations have implications for IRB review of eConsent.

🔗 6-5

According to guidance, the IRB should verify that prior to initiating an eConsent process, subjects are informed as to the nature of information that will be provided and an estimate of how much time the consent process is likely to require (FDA, 2016). This information allows subjects to decide where and when to view the eConsent, particularly if eConsent is being obtained remotely, and whether they wish to access the consent in private. Understanding how long the process will take allows subjects to devote enough time to develop an understanding of the research and come to an informed decision regarding participation.

The IRB should understand which type of device will obtain and document eConsent (e.g., tablet, laptop, mobile phone) and how subjects will access the eConsent (e.g., mobile app, invitation via email, webpage). Regarding the functionality of eConsent, the IRB should confirm the tool is easy to navigate, provides users with the ability to move back and forth within the content, and permits users to stop and start the process as desired. Omission of these features may result in diminished subject comprehension, inability to revisit key study information, or pressure on subjects to provide consent without adequate time for reflection. One means of assessing functionality is to require that the IRB be provided with a working link to the eConsent tool. An IRB may also review screenshots depicting how the tool operates.

When eConsent is obtained at a study site, guidance clarifies that study staff may help subjects to navigate eConsent tools as appropriate (FDA, 2016). Understanding whether eConsent will be obtained on-site or remotely, therefore, may also inform the IRB's assessment of eConsent functionality.

Compliance with part 11 mandates that a subject may not sign an eConsent until their identity has been verified. At the research site, study staff may verify a subject's identity prior to obtaining the subject's electronic signature (FDA, 2016). For example, staff could ask to see a subject's government-issued ID before permitting the subject to sign. With remote eConsent, the system used to obtain the subject's signature must include functionality to verify a subject's identity (FDA, 2016). One approach would be to employ an eConsent tool requiring subjects to upload a photograph of their government-issued ID before the tool may accept a signature. The IRB should understand how a subject's identity will be verified prior to providing their signature.

For research regulated solely under the Common Rule, the Office for Human Research Protections (OHRP) acknowledges that verifying that the person providing consent is either the research subject or the subject's legally authorized representative may not always be feasible or required (FDA, 2016). As such, "OHRP encourages investigators to apply a risk-based approach to the consideration of subject identity," adding, "social and behavioral minimal risk research will not typically warrant such verification" (FDA, 2016). When Common Rule research meets specific requirements, informed consent [**45 CFR 46.116(f)**] or <u>documentation</u> of consent [**45 CFR 46.117**] may be <u>waived</u> for minimal risk research. Thus, when

🔗 6-5
🔗 6-4

eConsent is proposed for research governed exclusively by the Common Rule, the IRB might consider whether either waiver would apply before confirming with the sponsor that the proposed eSignature will be legally valid in the jurisdiction where the research takes place (or, where an IRB elects per its own policy to hold all eConsent to the requirements of part 11, before obtaining a vendor statement regarding part 11 compliance).

⚓ 9-6

If the study includes <u>children</u>, the IRB should assess whether eConsent content is age appropriate and whether the functionality of the eConsent would affect the child's ability to provide assent (e.g., whether the tool is difficult to use). Unless the assent of the minor is not required for the study **[21 CFR 50.55(c)]** or the study qualifies for a waiver of assent **[21 CFR 50.55(d)]**, the IRB should determine that the tool includes functionality to obtain (and document, unless waived) both the minor's assent and the parent or guardian's consent (FDA, 2016).

Researchers may not delegate the responsibility for obtaining informed consent to an electronic system (FDA, 2016). Thus, with remote eConsent, IRBs should consider whether the process includes follow-up with researchers **[21 CFR 50;** FDA, 2016**]**. More specifically, the IRB should ensure that remote eConsent plans allow subjects to ask questions of researchers prior to providing consent and throughout the study. Follow-up with study personnel may be accomplished in-person or through a combination of messaging, telephone calls, and video conferencing. When live chat or video conferencing is used, guidance suggests that "investigators and study personnel should remind subjects to conduct the eConsent discussion in a private location to help ensure privacy and confidentiality" (FDA, 2016). When eConsent is used at the study site, study staff may review the eConsent and answer subject questions as they would with a paper form.

A copy of the eConsent document, including all information accessed by hyperlink, etc., must be provided to subjects **[45 CFR 46.117(a)**; **21 CFR 50.27(a)]**. The copy should include the subject's signature and the date of signature. Copies of the eConsent may be distributed in hard copy or as an attachment via email (FDA, 2016). If participants receive their copy electronically, guidance dictates that the consent should include language advising subjects of the risks associated with storing or viewing the document on a personal electronic device, particularly if that device is "shared with other users or is lost, hacked or subject to a search warrant or subpoena" (FDA, 2016). As such, the IRB should verify how subjects will receive the consent, require that the copy be signed, and, if subjects will receive the document electronically, ensure that appropriate language has been added to the consent.

IRB CHECKLIST FOR REVIEW OF ECONSENT PROCESSES

Confirm:

- Subjects are informed of the nature of the information contained in the consent and the time required to complete the consent prior to the start of the process.
- What type of device subjects will use to provide consent and how subjects will access the eConsent.
- The eConsent tool allows subjects to move back and forth through consent content, as well as to stop and restart the process.
- Subject's identity will be verified before the subject's signature is obtained.
- The eConsent tool is age appropriate and includes functionality to obtain and document parental consent and a minor's assent (as applicable).

- Whether subjects will provide consent at the study site or remotely.
- Whether remote eConsent processes allow for follow-up with investigators.
- Subjects will receive a copy of the consent in hard copy or electronically.

Remember:

- When consent is obtained at the study site, staff may assist subjects in navigating an eConsent tool (as appropriate).
- Investigators may not delegate responsibility for obtaining consent to an electronic system.
- If subjects will receive a copy of the consent document electronically, language regarding risks of electronic transmission should be added to the consent form.

eConsent Content

In assessing eConsent content, the IRB must ensure that subjects are provided with sufficient information to come to an informed decision regarding participation, presented in language they are able to understand, free from exculpatory language or language that waives or appears to waive their legal rights in the event of investigator, sponsor, or institutional negligence [**45 CFR 46.116**; **21 CFR 50.20**; see also **21 CFR 56.111**].

As with traditional consent materials, IRBs should review the content of eConsent against the required <u>elements</u> of informed consent [**45 CFR 46.116**; **21 CFR 50.25**]. IRB review should extend to all consent documents (electronic and paper) and informational or recruitment materials, including any videos, internet-based presentations, graphics, audio, or other digital media elements included in these materials. Where eConsent incorporates assessments or other checks on subject comprehension, the questions or elements used to verify subject comprehension should also be provided for IRB review. eConsent content submitted for IRB review must be approved in its final version and must be identical to the content provided to subjects in hard copy versions of the consent (FDA, 2016). Given the length and complexity of consent documents, the IRB should consider requiring an attestation from the sponsor that electronic content is a full and accurate version of the hard copy consent.

 6-2

If an eConsent includes content accessed via hyperlink or hover text or is conveyed using graphics or other multimedia elements, the IRB should establish that these elements function and that the content conveyed via these elements is acceptable. A working link or login to the eConsent tool facilitates IRB review of these elements. Guidance also provides that the IRB should understand what content will be viewed by participants within the eConsent and what content, if any, will be provided outside of the eConsent (i.e., recruitment materials, study information; FDA, 2016). Understanding what content will be included within the eConsent allows the IRB to determine whether the requirements for informed consent have been satisfied.

IRB CHECKLIST FOR REVIEW OF ECONSENT CONTENT

Confirm:
- eConsent content includes all required elements of informed consent established at **45 CFR 46.116** and **21 CFR 50.25**.
- eConsent content is identical to hard copy consent content.
- What content will be viewed by subjects as part of the consent and what materials will be viewed separately (recruitment items, etc.).

- Information provided to subjects regardless of format or location—text, video, web-based, graphics, audio, digital media, hyperlink, hover text, multimedia presentations, etc.—is accurate and acceptable under the regulations.
- Hyperlinks, hover text, and multimedia elements operate as intended.

Remember:

- Materials viewed by participants, including recruitment items and study materials, must be reviewed and approved by the IRB prior to use.
- Content approved by the IRB must be in final form.
- The IRB may require attestation from the sponsor that eConsent and hard copy content are identical.

Modifications to eConsent

7-1

The IRB must review and approve <u>modifications</u> to eConsent prior to use of the revised processes or materials by investigators [**45 CFR 46.108**; **21 CFR 56.108**]. In reviewing modifications to eConsent, the IRB is responsible for ensuring that content and processes remain compliant with the requirements for informed consent [**45 CFR 46.116**; **21 CFR 50.20**; see also **21 CFR 56.111**]

Review of revisions to eConsent, as with traditional consent, is typically limited to the aspects being modified. As such, the IRB would not be required to reassess the adequacy of electronic signatures under part 11 unless the sponsor was proposing to change the method by which signatures are created. Similarly, an animated component of a multimedia eConsent would only need to be re-reviewed if changes were being made to the animated content specifically. There is no requirement that modifications to eConsent take electronic form (FDA, 2016). For example, a study using eConsent at enrollment may later opt to provide subjects with an IRB-approved hard copy consent if updates to consent content become necessary.

Modifications to eConsent should be reviewed according to the regulations and guidance summarized in the IRB checklists for review of eConsent processes and eConsent content, discussed earlier in the chapter.

IRB CHECKLIST FOR REVIEW OF MODIFICATIONS TO ECONSENT

Confirm:

- Revised eConsent content and processes continue to meet the criteria for IRB approval.

Remember:

- Revised eConsent processes or content must be approved by the IRB prior to implementation.
- IRB review of revisions to eConsent is typically limited to the content or elements being revised.
- Modifications to eConsent are not required to be electronic.

IRB Record Keeping

IRB record-keeping obligations apply to eConsent just as they do to paper documents. To meet the requirements established in **45 CFR 46.115** and **21 CFR 56.115**, IRBs must maintain copies of all approved consent documents, paper and electronic, and retain them for a minimum of 3 years after a trial has concluded. Maintaining copies of content that exists online poses a challenge to the IRB as websites by their nature evolve over time. To satisfy its regulatory obligations, the IRB must "maintain the version of the [w]eb site . . . that contains the study-related information that the IRB reviews and approves, either electronically or as a hard copy (see 45 CFR 46.115 and 21 CFR 56.115)" (FDA, 2016).

IRB CHECKLIST FOR ECONSENT RECORD KEEPING

Confirm that:

- Copies of IRB-approved eConsent materials are retained for at least 3 years after the study concludes.

Remember:

- The IRB should retain the version of web-based consent materials reviewed and approved by the IRB.

Operational Considerations in IRB Review of eConsent

Not all IRBs currently permit the use of eConsent in studies under their oversight (Kane & Gallow, 2017). Whether this will change as eConsent becomes more commonplace remains unknown. Regardless, adoption of eConsent has implications for the operation of an IRB.

Small IRBs should assess the appetite for eConsent within their institutional communities given the additional resources that review of eConsent may require. They should also consider the adequacy of their institution's technology infrastructure if these tools are intended for deployment on site. IRBs of all sizes should consider the impact of adopting eConsent on human resources. IRB members and staff will require education regarding the regulatory requirements for IRB approval of eConsent. An institution may also need to revise its human research protection program plan and IRB <u>policies and procedures</u> prior to adopting eConsent review. An IRB new to eConsent may also need to hire area-specific expertise from legal, compliance, and technology sectors in order to assess the adequacy of eConsent proposals.

Given the additional challenges associated with remote consent, IRBs might assess their comfort with the practice and establish when it would be acceptable in studies under their oversight. For example, an IRB could choose to limit approval of remote eConsent to minimal risk research.

OHRP and FDA recommend that researchers seek IRB feedback regarding eConsent processes and materials prior to finalization (FDA, 2016). IRB pre-review of eConsent conserves resources for sponsors and researchers. Prere-view of eConsent, however, may require the IRB to review both draft and final content, doubling its efforts. For <u>single IRBs</u> reviewing eConsent plans and materials on behalf of sites with unique requirements, time required for review will be driven not only by the potential for a two-part review process, but also by the number of sites and the extent of customization required by those sites.

2-3

Section 4

Conclusion

Demand for eConsent is growing, and the literature cautiously suggests that eConsent may offer benefits to researchers and subjects (FDA, 2016; see also

Anderson et al., 2017; Friedlander et al., 2011; Ramos, 2017; Rothwell et al., 2014; Vanaken & Masand, 2019). The literature also suggests, however, that researchers perceive IRBs as being "anti-innovation" (Anderson et al., 2017) and inexperienced with alternative and multimedia consent tools specifically (Kane & Gallo, 2017). Researchers in Anderson's focus groups expressed doubt that IRBs would approve nontraditional consent processes (Anderson et al., 2017), and a survey of IRB chairs suggested that some IRBs are unfamiliar with these tools and perhaps reluctant to embrace them (Kane & Gallo, 2017). Key findings by Kane and Gallo (2017) include:

- 98% of chair respondents had never reviewed a multimedia consent process.
- 65% of chair respondents work for IRBs that do not allow eConsent.
- Pervasive ambiguity exists regarding whether their IRB would approve a nontraditional consent, as well as uncertainty regarding the regulatory requirements for eConsent.

These studies have limitations. The Anderson study was small, and the IRB chairs surveyed by Kane and Gallo self-selected into that study. It is also possible that IRB chairs in the Kane and Gallo study were unfamiliar with eConsent in part because researchers are not widely using eConsent and are therefore not submitting eConsent proposals for IRB review. Nevertheless, as demand for use of electronic technology grows within the research space and the functionality of these technologies expands, it seems inevitable that IRBs will be required to develop greater comfort and literacy regarding eConsent.

References

Anderson, E. E., Newman, S. B., & Matthews, A. K. (2017). Improving informed consent: Stakeholder views. *AJOB Empirical Bioethics, 8*(3), 178–188.

Department of Health and Human Services (DHHS). (2013). *Office for Civil Rights: Summary of the Health Insurance Portability and Accountability Act.* www.hhs.gov/hipaa/for-professionals/privacy/laws-regulations/index.html

Doerr, M., Suver, C., & Wilbanks, J. (2016). Developing a transparent, participant-navigated electronic informed consent for mobile-mediated research. *SSRN Electronic Journal.* Dx.doi.org/10.2139/ssrn.2769129

Electronic Signatures in Global and National Commerce Act (E-Sign Act). (2000). Public Law No. 106-229. www.govinfo.gov/content/pkg/PLAW-106publ229/pdf/PLAW-106publ229.pdf

Food and Drug Administration (FDA). (2016). *Use of electronic informed consent: Guidance for institutional review boards, investigators, and sponsors.* www.fda.gov/media/116850/download

Food and Drug Administration (FDA). (2017). *Use of electronic records and electronic signatures in clinical investigations under 21 CFR Part 11 – questions and answers.* Guidance for Industry. www.fda.gov/media/105557/download.

Frelich, M. J., Bosler, M. E., & Gould, J. C. (2015). Research electronic data capture (REDCap) electronic informed consent form (eICF) is compliant and feasible in a clinical research setting. *International Journal of Clinical Trials, 2*(3), 51.

Friedlander, J. A., Loeben, G. S., Finnegan, P. K., Puma, A. E., Zhang, X., de Zoeten, E. F., Piccoli, D. A., & Mamula, P. (2011). A novel method to enhance informed consent: A prospective and randomised trial of form-based versus electronic assisted informed consent in paediatric endoscopy. *Journal of Medical Ethics, 37,* 194–200.

Haussen, D. C., Doppelheuer, S., Schindler, K., Grossberg, J. A., Bouslama, M., Schultz, M., Perez, H., Hall, A., Frankel, M., & Nogueira, R. G. (2017). Utilization of a smartphone platform for electronic informed consent in acute stroke trials. *Stroke, 48,* 3156–3160

Kane, E., & Gallo, J. (2017). Perspectives of IRB chairs on the informed consent process. *AJOB Empirical Bioethics, 8*(2), 137–143.

Lentz, J., Kennett, M., Perlmutter, J., & Forrest, A. (2016). Paving the way to a more effective informed consent process: Recommendations from the Clinical Trials Transformation Initiative. *Contemporary Clinical Trials, 49*, 65–69.

Madathil, K. C., Koikkara, R., Obeid, J., Greenstein, J. S., Sanderson, I. C., Fryar, K., Moskowitz, J., & Gramopadhye, A. K. (2013). An investigation of the efficacy of electronic consenting interfaces of research permissions management system in a hospital setting. *International Journal of Medical Informatics, 82*(9), 854–863.

Moore, S., Tassé, A.-M., Thorogood, A., Winship, I., Zawati, M., & Doerr, M. (2017). Consent processes for mobile app mediated research: Systematic review. *JMIR MHealth and UHealth, 5*(8), e126.

Parrish, M. (2017). Adopting eConsent in research: Security, privacy, and other considerations. [Quorum IRB whitepaper]. Out of print.

Ramos, S. R. (2017). User-centered design, experience, and usability of an electronic consent user interface to facilitate informed decision-making in an HIV clinic. *Computers, Informatics, Nursing, 35*(11), 556–564.

Rothwell, E., Wong, B., Rose, N. C., Anderson, R., Fedor, B., Stark, L. A., & Botkin, J. R. (2014). A randomized controlled trial of an electronic informed consent process. *Journal of Empirical Research on Human Research Ethics, 9*(5), 1–7.

Vanaken, H., & Masand, S. N. (2019). Awareness and collaboration across stakeholder groups important for eConsent achieving value-driven adoption. *Therapeutic Innovation and Regulatory Science, 53*(6), 724–735.

Assessing Informed Consent Communication

Elizabeth A. Bankert

Abstract

This chapter discusses the importance of assessing and improving communication between the research team and the potential research subject during the informed consent process and culminates in a description of an education program developed as a resource for research team members to help them improve consent communications. The education program includes a discussion of ethical and regulatory information, describes the importance of understanding health literacy, and advocates for the use of the "teach back" technique during the consent process.

Introduction

Ensuring individuals are provided the opportunity to make an informed decision about whether or not to enroll in a research study is a cornerstone of conducting ethical research. The question of how we ensure that consent is valid and that a signature on the consent document represents a truly informed research subject has been a topic of discussion in the research community for decades.

The *Belmont Report* defines the three key components of the consent process as information, comprehension (information provided in a way that is understandable), and voluntariness (National Commission, 1979). Obtaining valid consent addresses the ethical concept of respect for persons as described in *Belmont*, in that it allows individuals to make autonomous decisions related to whether the potential risks and benefits of study participation are acceptable to them personally. Although informed consent must be obtained before participation in the study begins, the process should be thought of as ongoing throughout a study, with subjects being made aware that they are always free to leave the study.

🔗 1-1

Researchers may rely heavily on the consent form to provide information to prospective subjects. However, dependency on a document without additional means of evaluating the level of comprehension may not be the most effective way to obtain valid consent. The research community has long acknowledged that consent forms have increased in length, detail, and complexity, which may actually reduce, rather than increase, comprehension.

It remains incumbent on research staff to engage prospective research subjects in discussions about their potential role in the study and then provide enough time for reflection before subjects decide whether to enter the study. Initial and subsequent interactions serve as opportunities to build a trust-based rapport with the prospective subject. Researchers are responsible for educating potential subjects, helping them consider their options, and ensuring that they understand the purpose of the research, the risks and potential benefits of participation, and what is expected of them.

In 2009, the Food and Drug Administration (FDA) published "Guidance for Industry: Investigator Responsibilities—Protecting the Rights, Safety, and Welfare of Study Subjects" (FDA, 2009). Within the document, the FDA states that when delegating tasks, researchers "should ensure that there is adequate training for all staff participating in the conduct of the study," and that staff "are competent to perform or have been trained to perform the tasks they are delegated" (FDA, 2009). Furthermore, the guidance indicates that during inspections, the FDA identified instances in which *obtaining informed consent* was being conducted by individuals lacking adequate training and supervision. Research team members need to be knowledgeable in all aspects of conducting a research study, including obtaining informed consent. It follows there should be a plan to <u>educate</u> researchers on this vital role.

🔗 8-5

The 2018 Common Rule notes that the "prospective subject or their representative must be provided with the information that a reasonable person would want to have in order to make an informed decision about whether to participate, and an opportunity to discuss that information" [45 CFR 46.116 (a)(2)]. It is worth noting that this is the first time "an opportunity to discuss" the information provided appears in the Common Rule. In the past, IRBs and researchers tended to focus on ensuring that there was a comprehensive consent document. Requiring that there be "an opportunity to discuss" will hopefully provide motivation to the research community to remember that consent is a process and to reconsider the means by which consent is obtained. Using the "teach back" method described in the next section is one way to provide the "opportunity to discuss" that is mentioned in the regulations.

Although there is an abundance of ethical guidance and regulatory requirements regarding informed consent, factors such as time constraints, pressure from sponsors to meet enrollment goals, and increasingly complex consent documents all contribute to ongoing concerns related to obtaining valid informed consent in the research setting. The next section provides a brief description of the importance of health literacy and the teach back technique, as described in the healthcare setting.

Healthcare Setting: Health Literacy and Teach Back

The Institute of Medicine defines health literacy as "the degree to which individuals have the capacity to obtain, process, and understand basic health information and services needed to make appropriate health decisions" (Department of Health and Human Services [DHHS], 2015). Research shows that patients remember and understand less than half of what clinicians explain to them and that well-educated people may become functionally health illiterate when diagnosed with a serious disease (Schillinger et al., 2003).

The video "Health literacy and patient safety: Help patients understand" (www.youtube.com/watch?v=ubPkdpGHWAQ) provides a vivid depiction of concerns in the clinical setting. In one scene, a healthcare provider asks a young mother what dose of medicine she would give her 4-year-old child if the child's fever persists. The mother answers "1.5 tablespoons." We then see a close-up of the prescription indicating the correct dose as "1.5 teaspoons." Another scene depicts a woman who says, "When they gave me medicine, I didn't take it right. I admit that. I didn't have the nerve to ask and I didn't want anyone to know I can't read." Another woman takes several daily medications; however, because she does not understand the timing, she takes "16 pills every morning," so she knows she "gets them all." These examples show that understanding the level of comprehension of every patient is an important aspect of providing good health care.

"Teach back" is a communication method used by healthcare providers to determine whether a patient or caretaker understands what is being explained to them. Teach back involves the healthcare provider asking a patient to explain in their own words what they need to know or do, based on what they have heard. By encouraging dialogue in a conversational manner, the clinician can learn how well they have explained a concept. If a patient is not able to explain or recall using their own words, the clinician repeats important information (perhaps in an alternative manner). In this way it becomes the responsibility of the healthcare provider to communicate via a dialogue, rather than assuming a patient understands following a monologue that simply provides information.

The teach back method has been shown to improve communication and patient comprehension. "Asking that patients recall and restate what they have been told" is one of the 11 top patient safety practices based on the strength of scientific evidence (Shojania et al., 2001). While the use of closed-ended questions such as "Do you understand?" or "Do you have any questions?" will most likely be answered with a yes or no, the teach back method creates an opportunity for dialogue, which, in turn, provides a better opportunity to ensure there has been successful communication of the necessary information.

Utilizing teach back in clinical practice is depicted in the video "Physician Experience about Learning Teach-back," in which the physician indicates that he considered himself a good teacher (vimeo.com/50438603). He takes time with his patients to describe their health conditions; however, when he asks the patients to describe those conditions back to him in their own words, he is able to appreciate that his patients are not, in fact, understanding important aspects of their care. The physician goes on to explain that we are all lifelong learners and that by using teach back and asking his patients questions, he now can be more confident that patients are understanding important concepts. Finally, the physician notes that he considers the use of teach back a "component of caring."

Education Program for Researchers

Recognizing that there was a dearth of education programs aimed specifically at educating researchers about obtaining valid consent, a team composed of research and IRB staff at Dartmouth created the VoICE (Valid Informed Consent Education) education program. The program translates techniques used in the healthcare setting that are proven to enhance patient comprehension, to the research setting, including the teach back technique. The program is an in-person interactive workshop with research team members.

Each research study is unique, and the settings for obtaining consent can vary. The workshop provides an opportunity to discuss the specifics of a particular study and gives researchers tools that can be used for future research studies. For example, a study enrolling patients with diminished capacity raises different issues and requires a different approach than a study enrolling capacitated oncology patients. Since one size does not fit all, the program addresses these variations as well as acknowledges the intrinsic difficulty in obtaining valid consent.

The program begins by describing the ethical and regulatory basis for obtaining valid consent. It then discusses the "who, what, where, when, and how" of obtaining valid consent. "Who," "when," and "where" are often study specific and should be discussed within the research team prior to approaching prospective subjects. The "what" translates to what is the essential information a potential research subject should understand prior to enrollment in this study. And the "how" encompasses how we ensure that the potential research subject comprehends the research study prior to decision making. Thinking about the "how" leads us to consider health literacy and the goals of the teach back method.

The education program utilizes the videos described earlier and transfers the methods employed in the teach back technique to the research setting. Applied in the research setting, teach back involves the researcher explaining a key element of the research and using an open-ended phrase to encourage dialogue, such as: "If you call your sister tonight, tell me how you would explain the purpose of this research study to her." Or, "To ensure I am doing my job correctly in explaining this research study to you, please tell me what you understand about the risks."

As in the healthcare setting, it is important to understand that this technique is not a test of the prospective subject, but rather a test of how well the researcher explained a concept. Often, the research team member presents information (e.g., in a consent form) without making an effort to understand the comprehension level of the prospective subject. Using teach back turns the tables by placing the responsibility of providing a clear explanation of the key elements of the research on the research staff, rather than assuming that a one-way delivery of information and a signed consent form is sufficient. In teach back, the prospective research subject is asked to confirm their understanding of the key elements of the research study by describing them in their own words.

During our pilot program, it was determined that mastering the teach back technique and the use of open-ended phrases takes practice. As such, part of the VoICE education program includes time to consider what the most important elements of a particular research study may be and time to actually rehearse the teach back method with colleagues. We also ascertained that it was important to begin the consent discussion with language such as the following:

> "We are about to discuss a research study. There are reasons to participate in this research study, but the study may not be right for everyone. It is not the kind of situation where we can just tell you what you should do. It is important that you make the final decision about taking part in this study, and that means I need to adequately explain what the study is all about. We know this is new information for you, and people often need to ask questions and hear things explained more than once before they feel like they understand what they want to know."

This type of language sets the stage for a dialogue rather than a monologue.

During the pilot program, some research staff voiced concern that the teach back method may lengthen the consent process. In reality, however, the research staff agreed that although the teach back method changed the process, it did not necessarily lengthen it, because the team understood the level of comprehension of the prospective subject and could determine how much further discussion may or may not be needed.

We also encourage the use of creating a master consent form. The master consent form can be used to embed teach back questions at key points throughout the consent document, thereby reminding the research staff to pause and assess the level of comprehension of the research subject on those issues. Creating a master consent form requires the research team to take time to review all aspects of the study, and it presents an opportunity to consider how a potential subject may react to the information. For example, whether the study requires multiple visits beyond that of the standard of care, the distance to the medical center, and whether or not they are able to drive, might be important considerations for a particular patient. Selecting the most important items a potential research subject should understand and then embedding teach back questions throughout a master consent form can remind researchers of the importance of a thorough discussion of particular issues prior to requesting enrollment into a research study.

The Future

The Common Rule requires that informed consent begin with a "concise and focused presentation of key information" that will help prospective subjects understand the reasons they may or may not want to participate in the study [45 CFR 46.116(a)(5)(I)]. The regulations do not specify which information is <u>key</u> but rather make it clear that what information is key will depend on the specific nature of the study and the characteristics of the potential subject. As IRBs consider how best to operationalize the key information requirement, they might do well to look to the teach back method and the training program outlined previously. If key information is the *most important information* for a prospective subject to understand to make a research participation decision, then that information should be the focus of the consent discussion and the use of teach back. The consent document might then contain other (important) information, including other <u>required elements</u>. If the teach back method is utilized with each piece of key information, the level of comprehension of research subjects may be increased in a meaningful way, thereby allowing each subject to make a well-informed decision relevant to their needs and interests.

⬤ 6-3

⬤ 6-2

Conclusion

Because of the undeniable necessity for, and potential complications stemming from, the informed consent process, IRBs may want to consider providing an education program that can assist research team members in understanding health literacy and techniques for obtaining valid consent. It is the responsibility of the research team to ensure that the prospective subject understands the study. <u>Improving</u> the consent process may require further innovative options to confirm that prospective subjects grasp key elements of the research. The conversation is ongoing in the research community, and this chapter serves as a reminder that "informed consent is often exceedingly difficult to obtain in any complete sense. . . . Nevertheless, it remains a goal toward which one must strive" (Beecher, 1966).

⬤ 6-10

References

Beecher, H. K. (1966). Ethics and clinical research. *New England Journal of Medicine, 274*, 1354–1360.

Department of Health and Human Services, Office of Disease Prevention and Health Promotion (DHHS). (2015). *Health literacy online: A guide to simplifying the user experience.* health.gov /healthliteracyonline/

Food and Drug Administration (FDA). (2009). Guidance for industry: Investigator responsibilities— protecting the rights, safety, and welfare of study subjects. www.fda.gov/regulatory-information /search-fda-guidance-documents/investigator-responsibilities-protecting-rights-safety-and-welfare -study-subjects

National Commission for the Protection of Human Subjects of Biomedical and Behavioral Research. (1979). *The Belmont Report: Ethical principles and guidelines for the protection of human subjects in biomedical and behavioral research.* www.hhs.gov/ohrp/regulations-and-policy /belmont-report/index.html

Schillinger, D., Piette, J., Grumbach, K., Wang, F., Wilson, C., Daher, C., Leong-Grotz, K., Castro, C., & Bindman, A. B. (2003). Closing the loop: Physician communication with diabetic patients who have low health literacy. *Archives of Internal Medicine, 163*(1), 83–90.

Shojania, K. G., Duncan, B. W., McDonald, K. M., Wachter, R. M., & Markowitz, A. J. (2001). Making health care safer: A critical analysis of patient safety practices. *Evidence Report/Technology Assessment (Summary), 43*, i-x, 1–668.

Short Form Consent

Anastasia Doherty

Fariba Houman

Abstract

When the research subject cannot read the consent form, both the Common Rule and the Food and Drug Administration (FDA) regulations have provisions for the use of a short form consent (SFC) in the presence of a witness. This chapter describes the SFC and reviews when it is appropriate to use, who can serve as a witness, and how signatures are documented. The chapter also discusses special situations and points for IRBs to consider when evaluating the appropriateness of the SFC.

Introduction

The principle of justice, as stated in the _Belmont Report_, requires that individuals who are unable to understand the primary language used in a research study be afforded the same opportunities to participate in research as those able to understand the primary language, when they may receive some benefit. Inclusion of all segments of the population also reduces bias in research and makes the findings more generalizable (National Commission, 1979). Unless the study qualifies for <u>waiver</u> of consent, the Common Rule and the FDA regulations require that researchers obtain legally effective informed consent of all subjects or their legally authorized representatives (LARs). For this reason, the Common Rule and the FDA regulations have provisions for an oral presentation and the use of an SFC in a language that is understandable to prospective subjects [45 CFR 46.117(b)(2); 21 CFR 50.27(b)(2)], providing sufficient detail that allows them to make an informed decision about whether or not to participate in research (Department of Health and Human Services [DHHS], 1995; FDA, 1998).

    The SFC is not, despite its name, a simpler or abbreviated way to obtain consent. The SFC requires a "short" form in addition to the full consent form (referred to as a "summary" in this context), the presence of a witness, and the witness's signatures on both forms.

🔗 1-1

🔗 6-4

323

SHORT FORM CONSENT [45 CFR 46.117(B)(2)]

A short form written informed consent form stating that the elements of informed consent required by §46.116 have been presented orally to the subject or the subject's legally authorized representative, and that the key information required by §46.116(a)(5)(i) was presented first to the subject, before other information, if any, was provided. The IRB shall approve a written summary of what is to be said to the subject or the legally authorized representative. When this method is used, there shall be a witness to the oral presentation. Only the short form itself is to be signed by the subject or the subject's legally authorized representative. However, the witness shall sign both the short form and a copy of the summary, and the person actually obtaining consent shall sign a copy of the summary. A copy of the summary shall be given to the subject or the subject's legally authorized representative, in addition to a copy of the short form.

Using Translated Full Consent Form Versus the Short Form

Full consent form: If the research study is specifically seeking to enroll populations who speak other languages, or if the researcher knows in advance that certain populations speaking other languages are likely to be eligible to participate, the full consent form should be translated (unless there are justifiable reasons not to include individuals who speak other languages, such as survey instruments only being validated in the primary consent language; DHHS, 1995; FDA, 1998). An interpreter fluent in both languages should participate in the consent process for the duration of the study. For clinical studies, the use of a medical interpreter is highly recommended. At times, someone from the study team who speaks both languages may serve as the interpreter. When the full consent form is translated, the researcher should document the use of the interpreter. This can be done by having the interpreter sign and date the consent form to signal their presence during the consent process or as a note to file documenting the date, time, and interpreter's information.

Short form: When the prospective subject/legally authorized representative (LAR) cannot read the consent form, the regulations say that IRBs may allow the use of a short form. Institutions have their own policies as to whether and when a short form can be used. IRBs generally allow the use of the SFC when enrolling individuals who do not speak the primary language of the research study for studies deemed by the IRB to carry minimal risk. IRBs may also allow use of the SFC in greater than minimal risk studies that offer the prospect of benefit that is not otherwise available outside of research, and where there is no time to translate the full consent form prior to enrollment. Some IRBs allow use of the SFC for obtaining consent from subjects with a

COST OF TRANSLATION

Federal sponsors allow inclusion of the costs of translation and interpreter fees. Institutions should also consider adding a budget line to include these costs in the clinical trial agreements that they negotiate with corporate sponsors. Here is sample language:

"XXX Institution's Institutional Review Board will ordinarily require the preparation of a translated consent form into the appropriate language, for recruitment of any non-English speakers included in the Study. If such translation is necessary, XXX shall present Sponsor with an invoice for translation services, which Sponsor shall pay to XXX within thirty (30) days of receipt. The parties acknowledge that said translation costs are not included in the Budget."

low literacy level or low vision. In these cases, the short form in the subject's primary language is used to document their consent in a manner consistent with applicable state law. IRBs often approve and post a variety of short forms in common languages spoken in the location of the research and have them available for use by researchers, but the IRB would need to review and approve a new translated short form prior to use.

What Is a Short Form?

When signed by the subject/LAR, the "short form" is an attestation that the consent process was carried out orally and the subject/LAR has voluntarily given consent to participate in research. As such, the short form includes the basic required elements of informed consent [45 CFR 46.116; 21 CFR 50.25] and mentions that the interpreter has covered other additional pertinent information (such as presence of a clinical trial registry, compensation [if any] for research-related injury, additional costs, optional studies such as future use of data and specimens), if applicable. If there are check boxes or optional sections in the full consent form, the person obtaining consent asks the subject/LAR those questions with the assistance of the interpreter and marks the choices on the subject's behalf.

What Is the Summary Form?

The federal regulations require that IRBs approve a written summary of what is to be presented orally to subjects during the SFC. The "summary" is typically the same as the IRB-approved "long" or "full" consent form. The Common Rule at 45 CFR 46(a)(5)(ii) requires that key information about the research study be presented first to the subject in an organized way that will facilitate comprehension and making an informed decision about participating in research [21 CFR 50]. FDA regulations have not yet been revised to harmonize with the 2018 Common Rule. Because the presentation of key information only serves to streamline the presentation and to improve understanding, a short form template that is revised to state that key information will be presented first is also suitable for use with FDA-regulated studies (FDA, 2018).

🔖 6-3

Requirement for a Witness

Both the Common Rule and the FDA regulations require a witness to the oral presentation in the SFC process. The role of the witness is to be present during the entire consent process and note that the subject/LAR was given an opportunity to ask questions. The witness is typically an experienced interpreter who is fluent in both the primary language of the consent and the language spoken by the subject/LAR. FDA guidance recommends that an impartial third party, not otherwise connected with the study, serve as the witness (FDA, 2014). Some IRB policies allow a family member to serve as witness. While not considered a best practice, the IRB may allow a bilingual family member to serve as witness if, for example, the subject refuses the presence of an impartial witness. The family member, however, is not suitable to fulfill the role of an interpreter, as interpreting research descriptions and concepts requires experience and familiarity with medical and technical terminology. In contrast, if the person obtaining consent is fluent in the language of the subject/LAR, they can fulfill the role of interpreter, but another impartial witness must be present during the consent process.

IRBs are encouraged to review their local laws (e.g., state law) regarding the definition of a witness and define what it means to serve as a witness in their institutional SFC policy and guidance. This is particularly important as some interpreters may refuse to serve as witness, because acting as a witness has different meanings in other settings.

For example, the FDA guidance defines the purpose of the witness as attesting "to the voluntariness of the subject's consent and the adequacy of the consent process by ensuring that the information was accurately conveyed and that the subject's questions were answered" (FDA, 2014). The International Medical Interpreters Code of Ethics specifies, "Interpreters will refrain from accepting assignments beyond their professional skills, language fluency, or level of training" (International Medical Interpreters Association, 2006). Interpreters who are asked to serve as witnesses might feel that they are being asked to attest to the accuracy and completeness of the information that was presented, when their role is only to translate orally the information that the person obtaining consent was presenting.

IRBs are encouraged to provide periodic trainings for the interpreter service staff to help them understand the role of the interpreter when they serve as a witness in the SFC process and what a signature means in this context. **Figure 6.8-1**, which illustrates the witness role in the short form consent process, can be adapted as a poster for use in the interpreters' lounges or offices and research consent areas. The poster defines the witness role as (1) being present during the consent process, (2) confirming the oral presentation was given in a language that was understandable to subject/LAR, and (3) confirming the subject/LAR had the opportunity to ask questions.

Documentation: Who Signs What Form?

When the subject/LAR signs and dates the short form in the language they understand, they attest that the information in the full consent was given orally and that they are giving voluntary consent to participate in research. The subject/LAR does not sign the full (summary) consent form or any applicable Health Insurance Portability and Accountability Act (HIPAA) authorization that is not in the language they understand. IRBs are advised to grant an alteration of the HIPAA authorization if HIPAA is applicable. If a child is present and does not speak/read the language of the primary assent form, the child may sign the short form if the IRB has required documentation of assent. The full consent form is signed by the person obtaining consent. The interpreter signs both the short and the full consent form (summary form) as the witness. IRBs are advised to ensure that the witness signature line is preceded by the definition of witness. This can be added to the IRB's consent form templates.

Another way to remember the signature requirements is that each person signs and dates the form in the language they understand. The person obtaining consent signs and dates the full consent form (summary form), the subject/LAR signs and dates the short form in their native language, and the witness signs and dates *both* the short form *and* the full consent (summary) form on the

11-6

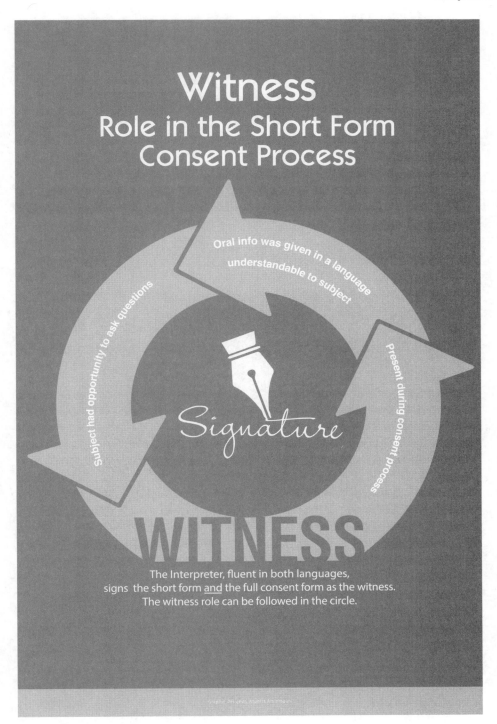

Figure 6.8-1 Witness role in the short form consent process.

Courtesy of Anahita Amini.

witness line (**Figure 6.8-2**). The subject/LAR receives *two* copies: a copy of the short form and a copy of the full (summary) consent form.

Special Consideration 1: Whose Short Form Is Used?

In the context of <u>single IRB</u> review, unless the IRB of record requires the use of their short forms, the local short forms can be used, as these may better

🔗 Section 4

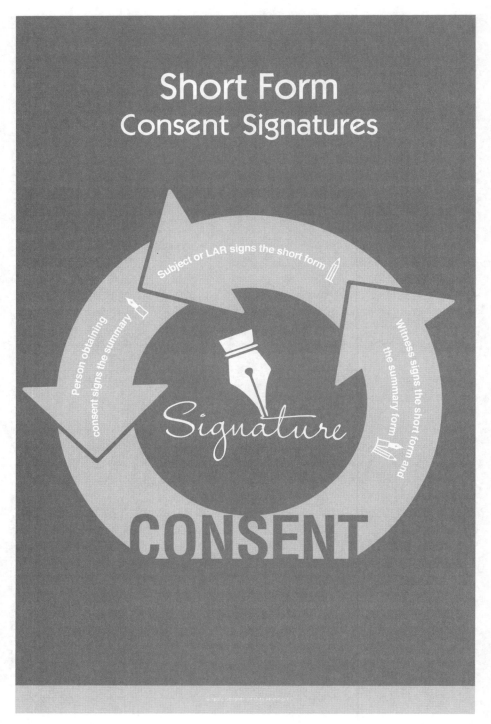

Figure 6.8-2 Short form consent signatures.
Courtesy of Anahita Amini.

represent the diversity of the local languages. A point to consider when relying on another IRB is that the main study consent form will likely have that IRB of record's contact information, and the short form will have the local IRB's contact information, resulting in two different IRB contacts. Because the IRB is contacted about subjects' rights in research, this should not be a concern, and the subject can be referred to the IRB of record, if warranted. IRBs should enlist the help from interpreter services when fielding calls from subjects.

Special Consideration 2: When the Interpreter Is Remote

With an increasing number of non-English speakers participating in research in the United States, institutions often contract a third-party remote business to provide interpreter services. This is because in-person interpreters are not always available due to competing priorities, and institutions may not have the resources to hire trained and native speakers to serve as interpreters for the few subjects who speak uncommon languages. When the interpreter is available only through phone or video, the documentation of the witness signature becomes a challenge.

The <u>waiver</u> of consent documentation requirements in the Common Rule require that IRBs make certain determinations and document in writing why a subject signature may not be necessary for a given consent process. In the case of the remote interpreter, the waivers of documentation criteria do not apply to the interpreter/witness signature. There is currently no provision in the federal regulations to waive the witness signature when using the SFC.

✎ 6-5

The remote interpreter may be unwilling to accept special requests to sign the witness signature line on research consent forms. Sometimes the web- or teleconference with the interpreter may be interrupted, and another interpreter is reached upon reconnecting. For these reasons, the IRB has to adopt a specific procedure for documenting the signature of the witness in accordance with what state law considers the intent to sign. The procedure would involve defining what it means to act as witness and asking the remote interpreter if the person obtaining consent can sign on their behalf. IRBs will need to work with legal counsel, their interpreter services, and the company providing language services to come up with a solution that meets regulatory requirements. The IRB may also want seek guidance from FDA and the Office for Human Research Protections (OHRP). Because the process is complicated and may not be used very often, IRBs are advised to implement a checklist and training modules for research staff involved in obtaining consent.

Conclusion

Researchers and the IRB should carefully consider the ethical/legal ramifications of enrolling subjects when the subject/LAR does not speak or read in the language of the consent form. The SFC process follows the same guidelines as the full consent process. In addition, a witness must be present during the entire consent process to attest that the presentation was in a language the subject/LAR understood and that they had the opportunity to ask questions. IRBs need to define the term *witness* and communicate it to the interpreter services, and they must train researchers in the proper use of the SFC. When the SFC process is utilized, IRBs should also consider other issues such as translation of other forms and ability to communicate with families on emergent issues during the course of the study.

Acknowledgments

The authors would like to acknowledge Susan Kornetsky and Stephen Rosenfeld for discussion and comments on the concepts presented.

References

Department of Health and Human Services (DHHS). (1995). *Informed consent of subjects who do not speak English*. www.hhs.gov/ohrp/regulations-and-policy/guidance/obtaining-and-documenting -infomed-consent-non-english-speakers/index.html

Food and Drug Administration (FDA). (1998). *A guide to informed consent*. www.fda.gov/regulatory -information/search-fda-guidance-documents/guide-informed-consent#nonenglish

Food and Drug Administration (FDA). (2014). *Informed consent*. www.fda.gov/regulatory-information /search-fda-guidance-documents/informed-consent#shortform

Food and Drug Administration (FDA). (2018). *Impact of certain provisions of the revised Common Rule on FDA-regulated clinical investigations*. www.fda.gov/regulatory-information/search-fda-guidance -documents/impact-certain-provisions-revised-common-rule-fda-regulated-clinical-investigations

International Medical Interpreters Association. (2006). *Code of ethics*. www.imiaweb.org/code/

National Commission for the Protection of Human Subjects of Biomedical and Behavioral Research (1979). The Belmont Report: Ethical Principles and Guidelines for the Protection of Human Subjects in Biomedical and Behavioral Research. www.hhs.gov/ohrp/regulations -and-policy/belmont-report/index.html

Broad Consent

Julie Kaneshiro
Michele Russell-Einhorn

Abstract

The 2018 Common Rule allows for the use of broad consent as a tool to facilitate the storage and maintenance of identifiable data and identifiable biospecimens and secondary research with identifiable data and identifiable biospecimens. Broad consent does not apply to the collection of identifiable data or identifiable biospecimens through a research interaction or intervention. There are specific restrictions relating to a subject's declination of broad consent, as well as restrictions on using broad consent when a researcher intends to report research results. This chapter discusses some of the key features of broad consent that institutions and researchers might want to consider before choosing to exercise this new option offered by the 2018 Common Rule.

The Concept of Broad Consent Before and After January 20, 2019

To understand the concept of broad consent as it is used in the Common Rule, it is helpful to look at the history of the term and, specifically, what is new in the 2018 Common Rule. The term *broad consent* was used before it was included in the revised Common Rule, but it has a specific regulatory meaning in the 2018 Common Rule. Under the pre-2018 Requirements, individuals were sometimes asked to consent to having their identifiable private information or identifiable biospecimens stored and used for a wide range of future research. Sometimes such consent was referred to in practice as "broad consent," even though the pre-2018 rule does not include this term. This type of consent for a wide range of future research has been used to establish research repositories, which were sometimes created under a formal research study, to facilitate future research. However, in order for such "broad consent" obtained under the pre-2018 rule to cover a specific research study that uses identifiable material from such a repository, the consent needed to satisfy the standard elements of informed consent for the specific study. Satisfying the standard elements of informed consent for a specific study can be difficult when consent to establish a research repository is often

🔗 10-10, 12-3

🔗 6-2

general and broad, specifically because the particular studies to be conducted with the materials from the repository are unknown at the time consent is sought.

🔗 12-3

The 2018 Common Rule further facilitates <u>secondary research</u> by including a specific regulatory standard for broad consent, which provides new options for conducting secondary research with identifiable private information

🔗 10-10

or identifiable <u>biospecimens</u>. Secondary research refers to research that uses information or biospecimens that were originally collected for a different purpose, such as for a different research study or clinical care. Broad consent does not apply to research that *collects* information or biospecimens through an intervention or interaction with an individual. Broad consent is one of a few regulatory options for conducting secondary research. For example, conducting secondary research with nonidentifiable private information or nonidentifiable biospecimens continues to fall outside of the purview of the Common Rule. In

🔗 6-4

addition, it is permissible for an IRB to <u>waive</u> informed consent for secondary research that uses identifiable private information or identifiable biospecimens, provided the IRB determines that all of the waiver criteria are satisfied.

If researchers choose to seek broad consent under the 2018 Common Rule instead of a waiver of consent from an IRB, broad consent has the potential to give individuals more control over researchers' use of their identifiable private information and identifiable biospecimens, while also facilitating the conduct of secondary research. However, the permissibility of a broad consent to cover a wide variety of as yet unknown research studies could make some individuals less likely to agree to provide broad consent. In addition, the need to track those who refuse to provide broad consent may make the option less appealing to a researcher than other available options. This chapter discusses some of the key features of broad consent that institutions and researchers might want to consider before choosing to exercise this new option offered by the 2018 Common Rule.

Broad Consent Elements

Broad consent under the 2018 Common Rule is a separate consent provision at **45 CFR 46.116(d)**, and its requirements are distinct from the requirements for standard informed consent at **45 CFR 46.11(6)(b)** and **(c)**. There are, how-

🔗 6-2

ever, some <u>elements</u> of standard informed consent (including some basic and additional elements of consent) that are incorporated into the required broad consent elements. In addition, the broad consent provision includes required elements that are unique to broad consent and are intended to respond to certain issues that are likely to be present in future research.

As clarified by the Office for Human Research Protections (OHRP),

Under the revised Common Rule, broad consent is also required to comply with most of the general elements of informed consent outlined 45 CFR 46.116(a). These include: obtaining informed consent before involving a human subject in a research activity; only seeking informed consent under circumstances that provide the prospective subject sufficient opportunity to discuss and consider whether or not to participate; providing information to potential subjects in a way that is understandable to the subject; providing prospective subjects with all of the information that a reasonable person would want to have in order to make an informed decision about participation; and not including certain types of exculpatory language in informed consent. (OHRP, 2018a)

Importantly, all of the elements that are described for broad consent must be included. None of the broad consent elements can be altered or omitted.

BROAD CONSENT ELEMENTS

1. The information required in paragraphs (b)(2), (b)(3), (b)(5), and (b)(8) and, when appropriate, (c)(7) and (9) of this section.
   This element of broad consent includes disclosing certain information also included under the basic elements of consent: reasonably foreseeable risks; reasonably expected benefits to subjects or others; confidentiality safeguards; and that participation is voluntary and may be discontinued without penalty. In addition, this element of broad consent includes disclosing certain information included under the additional elements of consent, when appropriate: a statement about commercial profit and whether subjects will or will not share in it; as well as whether research might include whole genome sequencing.
2. A general description of the types of research that may be conducted with the identifiable private information or identifiable biospecimens. This description must include sufficient information such that a reasonable person would expect that the broad consent would permit the types of research conducted.
3. A description of the identifiable private information or identifiable biospecimens that might be used in research, whether sharing of identifiable private information or identifiable biospecimens might occur, and the types of institutions or researchers that might conduct research with the identifiable private information or identifiable biospecimens.
4. A description of the period of time that the identifiable private information or identifiable biospecimens may be stored and maintained (which period of time could be indefinite), and a description of the period of time that the identifiable private information or identifiable biospecimens may be used for research purposes (which period of time could be indefinite).
5. Unless the subject or legally authorized representative will be provided details about specific research studies, a statement that they will not be informed of the details of any specific research studies that might be conducted using the subject's identifiable private information or identifiable biospecimens, including the purposes of the research, and that they might have chosen not to consent to some of those specific research studies.
6. Unless it is known that clinically relevant research results, including individual research results, will be disclosed to the subject in all circumstances, a statement that such results may not be disclosed to the subject.
7. An explanation of whom to contact for answers to questions about the subject's rights and about storage and use of the subject's identifiable private information or identifiable biospecimens, and whom to contact in the event of a research-related harm **[45 CFR 46.116(d)]**.

Secretary's Advisory Committee on Human Research Protections. (2017). Recommendation to the HHS Secretary, Appendix C, Recommendations for Broad Consent Guidance. https://www.hhs.gov/ohrp/sachrp-committee/recommendations/attachment-c-august-2-2017/index.html.

Differences Between Broad Consent and Specific Consent

Although the broad consent elements include some of the same underlined elements of consent required for standard informed consent, the circumstances when broad consent may be used as an alternative to standard informed consent are limited. Broad consent may only be used under the 2018 Common Rule for the storage, maintenance, and secondary research use of identifiable private information

● 6-2

or identifiable biospecimens (collected for either research studies other than the proposed research or for nonresearch purposes). Broad consent does not apply to research that collects information or biospecimens through a research intervention or interaction with living individuals. Consent for the original or primary study that involves a research intervention or interaction must satisfy the standard consent requirements [**45 CFR 46.116(c)** and **(d)**].

Applying Broad Consent to Information or Specimens Originally Collected for Nonresearch Purposes Versus Applying Broad Consent in a Research Context

Broad consent for secondary research can be sought for information or biospecimens (1) originally collected for a nonresearch purpose, such as clinical care or education, or (2) originally collected as part of a different research study.

An institution or organization might choose to seek broad consent for the secondary use of information or biospecimens collected for a nonresearch purpose, if it anticipates that such information or biospecimens will be used for secondary research studies. For example, a hospital might seek broad consent from all patients who have a blood test for clinical purposes to also allow the specimen to be stored in a repository that could be used for secondary research studies.

Similarly, a researcher might choose to seek broad consent for the secondary use of information or biospecimens originally collected for a different study. For example, if a researcher is carrying out a research study that the researcher anticipates will collect or generate identifiable private information or identifiable biospecimens that might be used in future research, the researcher could seek broad consent for the secondary use of these materials at the same time that consent is sought for the original or primary research study (OHRP, 2018b). Broad consent can be combined with the standard consent for the primary study (as long as it is clear that the broad consent does not cover the collection of information or biospecimens through a research interaction or intervention, such as collection through a research survey or research biopsy). Alternatively, broad consent can be sought through a separate form, assuming documentation of consent has not been <u>waived</u>. Regardless of whether broad consent is combined with the consent for the primary study, research subjects generally should be given the choice to provide broad consent or decline to provide broad consent and still be permitted to consent to participate in the primary study.

🔗 6-5

Applying Broad Consent to Non-FDA Regulated, Non-Federally Funded Research

Although the regulatory requirements related to broad consent only apply to research that is covered by the 2018 Common Rule, broad consent that meets the regulatory standards could be voluntarily utilized for research not governed by the Common Rule. This might be done to facilitate secondary research covered by the Common Rule. For example, a non-federally funded researcher who is conducting a clinical trial might seek broad consent for the secondary use of identifiable private information or identifiable biospecimens that will be collected as part of the trial, if the researcher envisions that these identifiable research materials will be useful for researchers covered by the Common Rule, such as those supported by a grant from a Common Rule department or agency to conduct secondary research. In addition, seeking broad consent might promote individuals' ability to control researchers' use of their identifiable private information or biospecimens, regardless of whether the research would be covered by the Common Rule.

It should be noted that at the time this chapter was written, the Food and Drug Administration (FDA) had not modified its regulations to incorporate the 2018 Common Rule's broad consent provisions. Therefore, it is unknown at this time whether broad consent will be an option for FDA-regulated research.

Exemptions Relating to Broad Consent

There are two <u>exemptions</u> that apply specifically to situations in which broad consent was obtained, thus permitting storage, maintenance, and secondary research use of identifiable private information or identifiable biospecimens without expedited or full board IRB review (**Table 6.9-1**). These relate to the storage or maintenance of identifiable private information or identifiable biospecimens for secondary research (Exemption 7) and the secondary research use of such identifiable material (Exemption 8). They are not available for the *collection* of identifiable private information or identifiable biospecimens through a research intervention or interaction.

🖉 5-3

Exemption 7 states:

(7) Storage or maintenance for secondary research for which broad consent is required: Storage or maintenance of identifiable private information or identifiable biospecimens for potential secondary research use if an IRB conducts a limited IRB review and makes the determinations required by [**46.111(a)(8)** and **45 CFR 46.104(d)(7)**].

Exemption 8 states:

(8) Secondary research for which broad consent is required: Research involving the use of identifiable private information or identifiable biospecimens for secondary research use, if the following criteria are met:

(i) Broad consent for the storage, maintenance and secondary research use of the identifiable private information or identifiable biospecimens was obtained in accordance with 46.116(a)(1) through (4), (a)(6), and (d);

(ii) Documentation of informed consent or waiver of documentation of consent was obtained in accordance with 46.117;

(iii) An IRB conducts a limited IRB review and makes the determination required by 46.111(a)(7) and makes the determination that the research to be conducted is within the scope of the broad consent referenced in paragraph (d)(8)(i) of this section; and

(iv) The investigator does not include returning individual research results to subjects as part of the study plan. This provision does not prevent an investigator from abiding by any legal requirements to return individual research results [**45 CFR 46.104(d)(8)**].

Table 6.9-1 Comparison of Exemptions 7 and 8

Exemption 7: Storage and Maintenance	Exemption 8: Secondary Research Use
Broad consent was obtained in accordance with the regulations.	Broad consent was obtained in accordance with the regulations.
Broad consent is appropriately documented or documentation of broad consent is waived in accordance with the regulations.	Broad consent is appropriately documented or waived in accordance with the regulations.
If changes to the storage or maintenance were made for research purposes, there are adequate provisions to protect the privacy of subjects and to maintain the confidentiality of data.	There are adequate provisions to protect the privacy of subjects and to maintain the confidentiality of data.
	The research to be conducted is within the scope of the broad consent.
	The researcher does not plan to return individual research results to subjects.

Note that the restriction relating to research results only applies to individual research results, not aggregate research results, and references a "plan" to return results, as opposed to the actual return of results.

While 7 and 8 are exemptions, the IRB must make a determination, *through a limited IRB review process, that the requirements for each of these exemptions have been confirmed* and that privacy and confidentiality protections are appropriate before approving of research actions under these exemptions.

✎ 5-6

Refusal to Give Broad Consent

Broad consent introduces the concept of "refusal to consent," with associated future consequences. An IRB may not waive or alter consent where an individual has "refused to consent" to a request for broad consent [45 CFR 46.116(f)].

This restriction, however, applies to storage, maintenance, and secondary research use of *identifiable* private information or *identifiable* biospecimens. Thus, the data or specimens could be stored and used for future research, notwithstanding the refusal to give broad consent, as long as it is *deidentified*; or if the information does not meet the definition of "private" information. This is because secondary research on nonidentifiable private information or information that is not private is not human subjects research and falls outside of the purview of the Common Rule.

The word "refusal" is defined as an activity that demonstrates an indication to not accept something. Refusal to consent may be viewed as an explicit action of not providing permission as opposed to the passive activity of simply never returning the consent form or throwing it in the trash. It is recommended that IRBs and institutions adopt guidance regarding what will count as a refusal and how nonresponse will be interpreted at their institution (Secretary's Advisory Committee on Human Research Protections, 2017).

The scope of the refusal to consent should be limited to the broad consent offered to the prospective subject, specifically, restricted to both the specific researcher and the purposes set out in that specific broad consent.

Waiver of Consent

There are certain situations in which an IRB may <u>waive</u> or alter the requirement to obtain informed consent. This is described in **45 CFR 46.116 (f)**, which includes specific requirements relating to situations in which an individual was asked to provide broad consent for the storage, maintenance, and secondary research use of identifiable private information or identifiable biospecimens consistent with the requirements in **45 CFR 46.116(d)**.

📎 6-4

If a subject provided broad consent, then there is no reason for an IRB to waive consent for the storage, maintenance, or secondary research use of the data or biospecimens, as this was already agreed to with the broad consent and may fall within the exempt categories of 7 and 8, provided all of the conditions of the exemptions are satisfied.

If, however, an individual refused to provide broad consent (and note that the word used in the regulation is *refused,* indicating an affirmative decision not to participate), then that individual's identifiable private information or identifiable biospecimens cannot be used in research pursuant to a waiver of consent. This, too, is consistent with the concept of broad consent in that the request is for permission to use data or biospecimens for secondary research, and a refusal is an indication that consent was specifically rejected for that purpose.

Similarly, an IRB may not alter the requirements of informed consent if a broad consent procedure has been used and an individual has refused to consent to the broad consent [**45 CFR 46.116 (f)(2)**].

Tracking Requirements for Broad Consent

If an individual refuses to provide broad consent, such refusals must be honored, which requires that a tracking system for refusals be established. Because the regulations prohibit the use of a waiver of consent where an individual has refused to provide broad consent for the storage, maintenance, or secondary research use of identifiable private information or identifiable biospecimens, the scope of the broad consent must be clear, and an entity that uses broad consent must have a system to track refusals of consent to a proffered broad consent. The absence of any system to track these refusals would mean that an IRB could inappropriately grant a waiver of consent for the storage, maintenance, or secondary research use of identifiable private information or identifiable biospecimens for a subject who previously refused to consent.

Chart reviews are a good example. If an individual declined broad consent for the storage, maintenance, and secondary research use of their data and biospecimens from their participation in a research study relating to an investigational agent for breast cancer, no other researchers can access their data relating to their participation in that breast cancer research study. The only way that this can be managed is by having a system that can track consent refusals such that subjects are protected from unrelated research requests.

Combining a Broad Consent and a Standard Consent

Section 116 of the 2018 Common Rule, "General Requirements for Informed Consent," includes an initial section titled "General" [**45 CFR 46.116(a)**], followed by a section "Basic elements of informed consent" [45 CFR 46.116(b)], and then a section "Additional elements of informed consent" [45 CFR 46. 116(c)]. Following these sections are the requirements for broad consent, specifically: "Elements of broad consent for the storage, maintenance, and secondary research use of identifiable private information or identifiable biospecimens" [45 CFR 46.116(d)].

This sets up a configuration that permits two different types of research informed consent. Consent that falls under Section 116(b) will be referred to as "specific consent"; broad consent refers to the type of consent described in Section 116(d). Can a specific consent be combined with a broad consent? Yes, as long as the integrity of the individual differences and requirements of the two is maintained.

Generally, a specific consent is for a specific research purpose that involves an interaction or intervention with human subjects. The specific consent is for the collection of data or biospecimens. A broad consent is only for the purpose of storing or maintaining identifiable private information or identifiable biospecimens or for secondary research use. It cannot be used as a vehicle to collect or obtain the data or biospecimens.

Thus, as noted in the regulation, broad consent cannot be used to actually obtain the data or the biospecimens through a research intervention or interaction. Specific research consent should be obtained for the collection of information or biospecimens through a research intervention or interaction, and information or biospecimens initially collected for nonresearch purposes (e.g., for clinical care or during the course of surgery) should follow any relevant nonresearch requirements. Broad consent is the tool that permits a *next research use* of the data or biospecimens after the first interaction/intervention.

Thus, a broad consent could indeed be combined with a specific consent. Where data is collected for clinical care, a broad consent easily will fit in with a clinical consent because the data or biospecimens were collected for the purpose of clinical care. But, if at the time an individual is being treated clinically they are asked questions regarding their preferences for certain drugs, that has nothing to do with their clinical care, and that information would be stored and later used for secondary research, that activity would not be consistent with the requirements of broad consent.

Participation in an activity for which specific consent is sought should not be conditioned upon agreement to the broad consent, because that would essentially transform the broad consent into a tool for the procurement of the private identifiable information or identifiable biospecimens.

Conclusion

The broad consent permitted by the regulations can serve as a useful tool for the creation of a repository that could facilitate numerous research projects involving the secondary research use of identifiable private information or identifiable biospecimens without the need to obtain expedited or full board IRB review. That said, use of the broad consent requires access to systems that can track refusals to consent. Therefore, institutions and researchers should consider the requirements and implications associated with broad consent when deciding whether to use this new option offered by the 2018 Common Rule.

References

Office for Human Research Protections. (2018a). *Q and A: Does broad consent have to comply with all the usual elements of consent?* www.hhs.gov/ohrp/education-and-outreach/revised-common -rule/revised-common-rule-q-and-a/index.html#informed-consent

Office for Human Research Protections. (2018b). *Q and A: Can an investigator ask subjects for broad consent for future research at the time of obtaining standard consent for a present study?* www .hhs.gov/ohrp/education-and-outreach/revised-common-rule/revised-common-rule-q-and-a /index.html#informed-consent

Secretary's Advisory Committee on Human Research Protections. (2017). *Recommendation to the HHS Secretary: Appendix C, recommendations for broad consent guidance.* www.hhs.gov/ohrp /sachrp-committee/recommendations/attachment-c-august-2-2017/index.html

Improving Informed Consent

Christine Grady

Abstract

Informed consent is a process meant to give research subjects an opportunity to make informed and voluntary decisions about enrolling or continuing in research. The process consists of disclosure of study information, subject understanding and deliberation, and subjects' voluntary decisions, usually authorized by a signature on a written consent form. Unfortunately, the practice of informed consent often falls short of its intended goals. Disclosure of information is variable in amount, clarity, and complexity; subjects often have limited understanding of significant information; and choices are not always voluntary. IRBs have a major role in improving the research informed consent process by working with researchers to assure that information disclosed is appropriate, clear, and understandable; that research teams pay attention to how well subjects understand; and that subjects are in a position to make choices. This chapter explores some of the ways IRBs can help to improve research informed consent.

Introduction

Informed consent is the process of providing potential subjects with sufficient information about a research study to allow them to make an informed decision about participating, facilitating understanding of that information, providing an opportunity for potential subjects to ask questions and to consider whether or not to participate, and then asking them to communicate a choice about participation (Food and Drug Administration [FDA], 2014). This process thus involves disclosure of information, understanding, voluntary choice, and authorization. The _Belmont Report_ clearly articulated the desired goal of informed consent: "Respect for persons requires that subjects, to the degree that they are capable, be given the opportunity to choose what shall or shall not happen to them. This opportunity is provided [through] informed consent" (National Commission, 1979).

🔗 1-1

Unfortunately, empirical evidence and experience show that in practice, informed consent often does not achieve its goal of facilitating the informed and voluntary choice of research subjects. There is documented wide variation in how information is disclosed (Beardsley et al., 2007; Paasche-Orlow et al., 2003); in how much subjects understand (Mandava et al., 2011; Tam et al., 2015); and in how decisions are made and influenced (Mammotte & Wassenaar, 2017). The process of informed consent is variable and complex, and the quality and outcome can be difficult to define and measure. Although researchers, IRBs, and others have tried various ways to improve the process of informed consent, there is still need for improvement. IRBs should focus on the goals of informed consent when reviewing information in written consent forms and other documents shared with subjects, as well as the proposed process for obtaining consent, in order to determine whether they are appropriate and likely to facilitate subject understanding and choice. One study of IRB chairs learned that the IRB focus is largely on the written documentation of informed consent than on subject comprehension (Kane & Gallo, 2017). Although it is easier for the IRB to determine whether all of the risks of a research study are listed on the consent document, for example, it is more important to consider whether the overall risk disclosure is clear and understandable and how researchers will know whether subjects understand the risks and factor them into participation decisions. IRBs have an important role in assuring that the quality of informed consent is high, and they should work with researchers and research teams to both monitor and take steps to improve the process of informed consent.

This chapter will briefly review what is known about disclosure, understanding, and voluntariness in research informed consent and explore ideas for IRBs to contribute to improving informed consent in research (**Table 6.10-1**).

Table 6.10-1 IRB Considerations for Improving Informed Consent

Informed Consent	Description	Considerations for the IRB
Disclosure of study information	Study information, both written and oral, should include purpose, research procedures, risks, benefits, alternatives, and other pertinent information. Disclosure should take into account subjects' language, education, familiarity with research, and cultural values.	Are the amount, detail, and complexity of information to be disclosed appropriate for the study and the subject population, taking into account age, education, language, and culture of the subjects? Are the regulatory elements satisfied? How will the information be disclosed to subjects? By whom? And where?
Understanding	Understanding of the purpose, risks, benefits, alternatives, and requirements of the research and appreciating how they apply.	How will the research team assess understanding? What should the subjects understand?
Voluntary decision making	Freedom from coercion and undue influence. Freedom to choose not to enroll.	Are there influences that might be controlling or unduly affecting subjects' decisions about research participation? Can subjects safely say no?
Authorization	Usually given by a signature on a written consent document.	Will subjects be asked to sign the written consent form? Does the IRB waive documentation of consent under certain circumstances? (See Chapter 6-5.)

Disclosure of Study Information

Research teams disclose and discuss study information with prospective research subjects and provide written documents, including informed consent forms, advertisements and recruitment materials, and other written or visual materials, to convey information about the study. The IRB reviews, often suggests modifications, and ultimately approves the informed consent process and documents before they are used.

Early in developing a research study, researchers decide how much and what information to include in the consent form, guided by the required elements listed in the federal regulations **[45 CFR 46.116; 21 CFR 50.25]**. Even *Belmont* noted, however, that a simple listing of items does not help us judge how much and what sort of information should be provided to subjects. IRBs view the regulatory elements as a minimum standard and may suggest additional information to facilitate subjects' enrollment decisions. The IRB also should review where, by whom, when, and how information will be presented to subjects and take into account the circumstances of the subject population and the research setting (these details will vary, for example, if the research is planned in an emergency room, a busy clinic, a classroom, or via the internet). *Belmont* noted that ". . . the manner and context in which information is conveyed is as important as the information itself" (National Commission, 1979).

6-2

In addition to assessing the content of consent forms, IRBs should consider the length, complexity, readability, and clarity of these forms to determine whether they are readable and understandable to the target subject population. Importantly, more than one-third of U.S. adults, about 77 million people across all racial and ethnic groups, have basic or below basic health literacy, and more than half of U.S. adults have basic or below basic quantitative literacy and thus difficulty understanding numerical presentations of risk and benefit data (FDA, 2014). Specific subjects or groups of subjects might be at higher risk of low health literacy or numeracy (Anderson et al., 2017).

Empirical studies have shown that consent forms are long and have increased in length over time (Albala et al., 2010; Beardsley et al., 2007; Tarnowksi et al., 1990). Furthermore, consent forms are often complex, written at a high reading level, and contain legalistic language, making them less likely to be read or understood. Even after IRB review, studies show that consent forms and consent templates often are written at about the 11th grade level or higher (Grossman et al., 1994; Paasche-Orlow et al., 2003; Sharp, 2004), and they are sometimes missing required elements or information considered relevant to a particular study (Abeysena et al., 2012; Horng et al., 2002; Silverman et al., 2001). Although fewer studies have documented how information is shared orally with potential research subjects, it is likely to be quite variable (Koyfman et al., 2016).

What Can the IRB Do?

IRBs could help improve disclosure of information in informed consent by paying attention to consent form content, length, readability, and format. Ironically, however, IRBs sometimes contribute to making consent forms longer and more complex. IRBs often develop and encourage or require the use of boilerplate language or templates. The IRB should assure that boilerplate or template language is straightforward, clear, understandable, and appropriate to the context. IRBs evaluate whether the required underlined elements of informed consent are included in the consent form and whether there is other important information

6-2

that subjects should know in order to decide about participation. The Common Rule requires that consent forms begin with a concise and focused presentation of "key information" to help subjects understand the reasons they may or may not want to participate [45 CFR 46.116(a)(5)(i)]. The hope is that concise and understandable key information will give subjects the information they need to make a decision, although evaluation of both how key information is implemented and how it might help subjects is needed. IRBs might be involved in experimenting with different ways to present key information and/or studying subjects' perspectives.

6-3

Many advise using plain language guidelines for effective consent forms. The federal plain language guidelines direct writers to know their audience and organize the content of information from that perspective; to use short paragraphs, sentences, and words; simple language; active voice; a personal tone; concrete ideas or images; headings; and white space (Federal Plain Language Guidelines, 2011). Words familiar to the subject population should be used to define or replace scientific or medical terms, and acronyms and abbreviations should be avoided. Charts, pictures, flowcharts, and graphics can facilitate understanding, whereas small fonts, single-spaced text, and large chunks of text without headings can hamper it. Electronic documents are more likely to be read if they are short and engaging (Department of Health and Human Services [DHHS], 2016).

IRBs can assess consent form readability using several commercially available tools, such as Flesch-Kincaid (National Cancer Institute [NCI], 2017; Paasche-Orlow et al., 2013). In addition to written materials, IRBs can review electronic or video presentations of information to assess their appropriateness and clarity for subjects. IRBs could evaluate their own practices by periodically reviewing a sample of approved documents to see how often they approved a consent form with a missing element, overly technical language, absence of relevant risks, exculpatory language, or other deficiencies. IRBs can learn from studies about effective disclosure, which emphasize that more is not always better, that timing matters, and that technology can be helpful (Schenker & Meisel, 2011).

Understanding of Study Information

After information is disclosed to subjects and questions and concerns are addressed, subjects should have the information they need to deliberate about the study, understand important elements, and make a decision. Understanding is more than just knowledge or recitation of facts; it requires that subjects absorb the information disclosed in the consent process and think about how it applies to their own interests and preferences. Accordingly, understanding is said to require both knowledge and appreciation, where knowledge is about relevant information, and appreciation is about how it applies. For example, a subject who knows "this is a randomized placebo-controlled trial" has knowledge, but if they believe that their doctor will ensure that they get the medication they need in the trial, the subject lacks appreciation. Subjects often operate under a therapeutic misconception, defined by Appelbaum and colleagues as when a research subject misunderstands the purpose of research as individualized treatment for their own benefit (Appelbaum & Lidz 2008). Commentators have explored the extent to which different types of misunderstandings might invalidate informed consent (Horng & Grady, 2003).

There is little agreement about how much a subject should understand about a study in order to give consent (Wendler & Grady, 2008). Most agree that the threshold for understanding rises as risks increase. *Belmont*, for example, notes "While there is always an obligation to ascertain that the information about risk to subjects is complete and adequately comprehended, when the risks are more serious, that obligation increases. On occasion, it may be suitable to give some oral or written tests of comprehension" (National Commission, 1979). Generally, it is unrealistic to expect subjects to know everything written in the consent form or to remember all study details after reading the consent information and discussing it with the research team. Research decisions may be like decisions in other areas of life. As Levine notes, we may seek lots of information to make an informed decision about buying a car, for example, but once the decision is made, we forget much of what we might have learned (Levine, 1986). Nonetheless, there are certain elements of study information that seem more critical for subjects to understand when they are deciding whether to enroll; at a minimum, they should know that they are enrolling in research, that there are some risks, that it is their choice, and that they can withdraw without penalty.

A large body of evidence, however, shows that even after subjects give consent to research, they have variable and often limited understanding of study information (Mandava et al., 2012; Tam et al., 2015). Depending on the study, as few as 27% of subjects (and up to 100%) appear to understand the purpose or nature of research (Joffe et al., 2001; Krosin et al., 2006; Pace et al., 2005a), and a similar range understand research risks (Joffe et al., 2001; Leach et al., 1999; Tam et al., 2015; Weinfurt et al., 2012). Many fewer subjects seem to understand research procedures such as randomization (Harrison et al., 1995; Pace et al., 2005b; Tam et al., 2015). A 2015 meta-analysis of studies measuring subject understanding of components of informed consent in clinical trials found that none of the required elements of informed consent was understood by more than 75% of subjects, including that participation was voluntary, and only about half understood the concepts of randomization or placebo (Tam et al., 2015).

These data cause concern about the quality of informed consent and raise unsettling questions about how much subjects should understand about a study, how we should measure understanding, what should happen if certain information is not understood, and how we can improve understanding of significant study information.

Various strategies have been tested in multiple studies to try to improve understanding in research informed consent. In a systematic review of informed consent studies conducted before 2004, Flory and Emanuel showed that studies of multimedia strategies (e.g., audiotapes, videotapes, interactive computers) demonstrated no consistent or significant improvement in understanding and that fewer than half (6 of 15) of the reviewed studies with enhanced consent forms (modified style, format, length, or complexity) found significant improvement in understanding (Flory & Emanuel, 2004). From their review, the most promising strategies for increasing understanding involved more person-to-person contact (through extended discussions [in 3 of 5 studies] or test/feedback strategies [in 5 of 5]), although data were limited (Flory & Emanuel, 2004). A subsequent systematic review and meta-analysis concluded that enhanced consent forms and extended discussions were the most effective in improving subject understanding (Nishimura et al., 2013). The enhanced consent form studies in their analysis included studies that tested simplified forms; forms with low reading levels; some that added pictures, graphics, or color; and some that created booklets and supplementary materials. Although some multimedia strategies were effective, they did not consistently or significantly

6-7

improve understanding, and there were too few test/feedback strategies to really know. Nishimura and colleagues also recognized that because science is increasingly complex and contemporary research involves genomics, biobanking, and other sophisticated technologies, there is a pressing need to find effective strategies to increase subject understanding.

As a result of their meta-analysis, Nishimura et al. recommend direct comparisons in randomized studies of shorter versus longer consent forms. In the largest randomized trial (n = 4,229) to date of a standard versus a simpler and shorter written consent form, there was no difference in understanding between subjects randomized to the standard form and those randomized to the concise form (Grady et al., 2017). Recent studies of electronic consent, although still quite limited, have shown that although the consent process takes longer, understanding is sometimes better, and some subjects are more satisfied with the process (Harle et al., 2019; Rothwell et al., 2014; Rowbotham et al., 2013).

🔗 6-6

What Can the IRB Do?

IRBs should be aware that data about understanding after research informed consent shows that subjects have variable understanding at best, and limited understanding of some key research concepts. Furthermore, IRBs should know about factors that can affect subject understanding, including age, education, cognitive capacity, literacy, pain, and familiarity with research. When reviewing consent forms and proposed processes and evaluating the likelihood that subjects will understand the information, IRBs should consider characteristics of the subject population, the study complexity, the circumstances in which the study will be conducted, and how study information will be disclosed. IRBs can recommend shortening, clarifying, or emphasizing information provided and can also recommend or require independent capacity assessments, independent consent monitoring, and/or formal and informal methods of assessing understanding as appropriate (**Table 6.10-2**). An informal

Table 6.10-2 Selected Strategies That the IRB Can Use or Stipulate in Order to Enhance Informed Consent

Subject advocates or advisory boards	Subject advocates can review consent language and advise regarding appropriate disclosure strategies and incentives.
Readability assessments	The use of Flesch-Kincaid reading level, for example, or other tools to assure reading level is appropriate to subject population.
Independent capacity assessment	Assessment of a subject's capacity to provide their own consent, usually done by a psychiatrist, neurologist, or ethics consultant using a standard tool such as the MacArthur Competence Assessment Tool for Clinical Research.
Consent monitoring	A person independent of the research team monitors the consent process to assure that adequate and understandable information is provided, that the subject has an opportunity to ask questions and is satisfied that they are answered, that the subject knows they can choose not to participate, request more time, or obtain more information.
Assessments of understanding	Informal or formal measures of subject understanding of study information.
Confidential procedures for consent or refusal	Strategies to allow subjects to say no without others (family, doctors, tribe members) knowing why.

open-ended understanding <u>assessment</u> might include questions such as "What do you expect to happen in this study?" "What is the best and the worst thing that could happen?" "Could you say no?" "What would happen if you said no?" Formal assessments of understanding might include written quizzes or tests with a passing threshold. Consent monitors could assure that adequate information is provided, that prospective subjects are given the opportunity to ask questions and these are answered appropriately, and that consenting subjects have sufficient understanding of the study information to make a decision. IRBs could evaluate whether repetition of information by researchers and research coordinators, the opportunity to talk with other providers or subjects, sending information to prospective subjects in advance, and other strategies influence retention or understanding.

🖉 6-7

Voluntary Decision About Research Participation

Informed consent requires disclosure, understanding, and a voluntary decision. Although ethically very important, it is difficult to determine when a decision is sufficiently voluntary, and it is challenging to measure the voluntariness of a decision. What does it mean to make a voluntary decision? According to the federal regulations, researchers must not only provide understandable information to subjects but also ensure that prospective subjects have ". . . sufficient opportunity to discuss and consider whether or not to participate and . . . minimize the possibility of coercion or undue influence." [45 CFR 46.116 (a)(2)]. Faden and Beauchamp (1986) describe an autonomous voluntary decision as independent or free from controlling influences, especially control by others. Not all influences are controlling, however, "The presence of influences does not mean that a decision is not voluntary. A decision is involuntary only if it is subject to a particular type of influence that is external, intentional, illegitimate, and causally linked to the choice of the research subject" (Appelbaum et al., 2009).

Multiple factors could influence a subject's decision about participation in research, and some of these could be controlling. Subjects might be in positions where it is hard to make a voluntary choice. <u>Prisoners</u>, members of the military, <u>students</u>, and employees (among others) may not feel they are able to say no to an invitation to participate in research, especially if they perceive that their superior wants them to participate, or there might be consequences to refusing. Saying no may also be difficult for subjects who are invited to participate by a doctor or other health professional with whom they have a relationship and/or from whom they are receiving care. Subjects sometimes feel pressure from family members or friends that influence their choice. Women in some situations and cultures may not have the authority to make their own decisions, including about research participation (Osamor & Grady, 2016). Some commentators have expressed concerns that trust in healthcare providers or deference to their recommendations, having limited or restricted alternative options, money or other enrollment incentives, and perhaps even serious illness could hamper one's ability to make a voluntary choice (Appelbaum et al., 2009). Evidence to date shows that people can and do still make informed and voluntary decisions in the face of <u>serious illness</u>, restricted options, and <u>payment</u>.

🖉 9-5
🖉 9-2

🖉 9-8 🖉 12-2

In an attempt to assess the voluntariness of research enrollment decisions, studies measure how often subjects decline to join a study after receiving study information. Some studies have asked whether subjects felt any pressure to enroll and if so, from whom or from what they felt pressure. In studies to date, the percentage of subjects who report feeling pressure from another person is generally low (Pace et al., 2005b). Although data are limited, the fraction of subjects who report feeling pressure from something else, such as illness or their financial situation, is often higher (e.g., 58% from child's disease; Pace et al., 2005b).

A third measure used in some empirical studies is the extent to which subjects know that they can refuse to enroll or can change their mind and withdraw without penalty. The percentage varies from 90% of Swedish women in a gynecological trial who said they knew they could refuse (Lynoe et al., 2004); to 71% of Thai participants in an HIV study (Pace et al., 2005a); and 90% of U.S. cancer patients (Joffe et al., 2001), who knew they could withdraw. In an interesting study of the informed consent of women offered HIV testing in South Africa, most said that they knew they could quit at any time, but almost all said the hospital would not let them quit; the authors concluded that the women's consent was informed but not voluntary (Abdool Karim et al., 1998). A situation like this should be further explored.

What Can the IRB Do?

In evaluating a proposed subject population, IRBs should consider whether subjects are in a dependent position or would be likely to defer to their superiors, doctors, researchers, or families. If so, IRBs can put additional protections in place. IRBs can stipulate who can obtain consent from subjects (e.g., only those who are trained) and who cannot (e.g., supervisors or those in dual relationships). IRBs can also work with researchers to ensure that subjects know they have the right to decline participation or withdraw from a study, and also that they are given the opportunity to say no, confidentially if needed. Throughout the course of a study, subjects can be reminded of their rights and that participation in research is voluntary. It might be useful to evaluate various elements of the subject's voluntary choice either immediately after informed consent, or at any time during or after participation in the research. Did the subject feel any pressure to enroll and from whom or what? Did the subject know they could say no? Did the subject themself agree to take part in the research? Who made or helped with the enrollment decision? Because subjects may in some cases delegate the authority to make decisions, the IRB should also ask if the subject freely delegated the decision to take part in research to a third party.

Conclusion

Informed consent for research is ethically important as a process that gives subjects the information and the opportunity to decide whether or not they want to participate and remain in in a research study. Data suggests that informed consent could be improved. Consent forms are often long and complex; understanding of study information is variable and subjects often have difficulty understanding certain features of research; and many participants do not know (or feel) that they can decline or withdraw. Data show that spending more time talking to subjects may enhance their understanding of study information. Shorter, less complex, and more engaging methods of providing study information may also help understanding. The quality of informed consent could be assessed by examining the content and methods of information disclosure, the extent to which research subjects understand, and whether they made a voluntary decision. IRBs tend to preferentially focus on information to be disclosed and pay less attention to how it will be presented or how the research team will know that the subjects' decision is both informed and voluntary. More research would help to improve our understanding of research informed consent, how it varies (and should vary) in diverse clinical settings, and effective ways to enhance subjects' understanding, decision making, and research experience.

References

Abeysena, C., Jayamanna, K., & Dep, S. (2012). Completeness of consent forms in research proposals submitted to an ethics review committee. *Indian Journal of Medical Ethics, 9*(2), 100–103.

Abdool Karim, Q., Abdool Karim, S. S., Coovadia, H. M., & Susser, M. (1998). Informed consent for HIV testing in a South African hospital: Is it truly informed and truly voluntary? *American Journal of Public Health, 88*, 637–640.

Albala, I., Doyle, M., & Appelbaum, P. S. (2010). The evolution of consent forms for research: A quarter century of changes. *IRB: Ethics & Human Research, 32*(3), 7–11.

Anderson, E., Newman, S., & Matthews, A. (2017). Improving informed consent: Stakeholder views. *AJOB Empir Bioeth, 8*(3), 178–188.

Appelbaum, P. S., & Lidz, C. W. (2008). Twenty-five years of therapeutic misconception. *Hastings Center Report, 38*, 5–6.

Appelbaum, P. S., Lidz, C. W., & Klitzman, R. (2009). Voluntariness of consent to research. A conceptual model. *Hastings Center Report, 39*(1): 30–39.

Beardsley, E., Jefford, M., & Mileshkin, L. (2007). Longer consent forms for clinical trials compromise patient understanding: So why are they lengthening? *Journal of Clinical Oncology, 25*(9), e13–e14.

Department of Health and Human Services (DHHS). (2016). *Use of electronic informed consent: Questions and answers.* www.hhs.gov/ohrp/regulations-and-policy/guidance/use-electronic -informed-consent-questions-and-answers/index.html

Faden, R., & Beauchamp, T. (1986). *A history and theory of informed consent.* Oxford University Press.

Federal Plain Language Guidelines. (2011). https://plainlanguage.gov/guidelines/

Flory, J., & Emanuel, E. J. (2004). Interventions to improve research participants' understanding in informed consent for research: A systematic review. *JAMA, 292*, 1593–1601.

Food and Drug Administration (FDA). (2014). Informed consent guidance for IRBs, clinical investigators, and sponsors. www.fda.gov/regulatory-information/search-fda-guidance-documents /informed-consent

Grady, C., Touloumi, G., Walker, A. S., Smolskis, M., Sharma, S., Babiker, A., Panatazis, N., Tavel, J., Florence, E., Sanchez, A., Hudson, F., Papadopoulous, A., Emanuel, E., Clewett, M., Munroe, D., Denning, E., & INSIGHT START Informed consent study group. (2017). A randomized trial comparing concise and standard consent forms in the START trial. *PLoS ONE, 12*(4), e0172607.

Grossman, S. A., Piantadosi, S., & Covahey, C. (1994). Are informed consent forms that describe clinical oncology research protocols readable by most patients and their families? *Journal of Clinical Oncology, 12*(10), 2211–2215.

Harle, C. A., Golembiewski, E. H., Rahmanian, K. P., Brumback, B., Krieger, J. L., Goodman, K. W., Mainous, A. G., & Moseley, R. E. (2019). Does an interactive trust-enhanced electronic consent improve patient experiences when asked to share their health records for research? A randomized trial. *Journal of the American Medical Informatics Association, 26*(7), 620–629.

Harrison, K., Vlahov, D., Jones, K., Charron, K., & Clements, M. L. (1995). Medical eligibility, comprehension of the consent process, and retention of injection drug users recruited for an HIV vaccine trial. *Journal of Acquired Immune Deficiency Syndromes and Human Retrovirology: Official Publication of the International Retrovirology Association, 10*(3), 386–390.

Horng, S., Emanuel, E. J., Wilfond, B., Rackoff, J., Martz, K., & Grady, C. (2002). Descriptions of benefits and risks in consent forms for phase 1 oncology trials. *New England Journal of Medicine, 347*(26), 2134–2140.

Horng, S., & Grady, C. (2003). Misunderstanding in clinical research: Distinguishing therapeutic misconception, therapeutic misestimation, and therapeutic optimism. *IRB, 25*(1), 11–16.

Joffe, S., Cook, E. F., Cleary, P. D., Clark, J. W., & Weeks, J. C. (2001). Quality of informed consent: A new measure of understanding among research subjects. *Journal of the National Cancer Institute, 93*(2), 139–147.

Kane, E., & Gallo, J. (2017). Perspectives of IRB chairs on the informed consent process. *AJOB Empir Bioeth, 8*(2), 137–143.

Koyfman, S. A., Reddy, C. A., Hizlan, S., Leek, A. C., Kodish, A. E., & Phase I Informed Consent (POIC) Research Team. (2016). Informed consent conversations and documents: A quantitative comparison. *Cancer, 122*(3), 464–469.

Krosin, M. T., Klitzman, R., Levin, B., et al. (2006). Problems in comprehension of informed consent in rural and peri-urban Mali, West Africa. *Clinical Trials, 3*(306), e13.

Leach, A., Hilton, S., Greenwood, B. M., Manneh, E., Dibba, B., Wilkins, A., & Mulholland, E. K. (1999). An evaluation of the informed consent procedure used during a trial of a *Haemophilus influenzae* type B conjugate vaccine undertaken in The Gambia, West Africa. *Social Science & Medicine* (1982), *48*(2), 139–148.

Levine, R. J. (1986). *Ethics and regulation of clinical research* (2nd ed.). Urban and Schwarzenberg.

Lynoe, N., Nasstrom, B., & Sandlund, M. (2004). Study of the quality of information given to patients participating in a clinical trial regarding chronic hemodialysis. *Scandinavian Journal of Urology and Nephrology, 38*, 517, e20.

Mamotte, N., & Wassenaar, D. (2017). Voluntariness of consent to HIV clinical research: A conceptual and empirical pilot study. *Journal of Health Psychology, 22*(11), 1387–1404.

Mandava, A., Pace, C., Campbell, B., Emanuel, E., & Grady, C. (2012). The quality of informed consent: Mapping the landscape. A review of empirical data from developing and developed countries. *Journal of Medical Ethics, 38*, 356–365.

National Cancer Institute (NCI). (2017). *Using online and manual readability tools to assess the reading level of informed consent documents.* ctep.cancer.gov/protocolDevelopment/docs/NCI _Informed_Consent_Template_Readability_Assessments.pdf

National Commission for the Protection of Human Subjects of Biomedical and Behavioral Research. (1979). *The Belmont Report: Ethical principles and guidelines for the protection of human subjects of research.* www.hhs.gov/ohrp/regulations-and-policy/belmont-report/index.html

Nishimura, A., Carey, J., Erwin, P. J., Tilburt, J. C., Murad, M. H., & McCormick, J. B. (2013). Improving understanding in the research informed consent process: A systematic review of 54 interventions tested in randomized control trials. *BMC Medical Ethics, 14*, 28.

Osamor, P. E., & Grady, C. (2016). Women's autonomy in health care decision-making in developing countries: A synthesis of the literature. *International Journal of Women's Health, 8*, 191–202.

Paasche-Orlow, M. K., Brancati, F. L., Taylor, H. A., Jain, S., Pandit, A., & Wolf, M. S. (2013). Readability of consent form templates: A second look. *IRB, 35*(4), 12–19.

Paasche-Orlow, M. K., Taylor, H. A., & Brancati, F. L. (2003). Readability standards for informed consent forms as compared with actual readability. *New England Journal of Medicine, 348*(8), 721–726.

Pace, C., Emanuel, E. J., Chuenyam, T., et al. (2005a). The quality of informed consent in a clinical research study in Thailand. *IRB: Ethics and Human Research, 27*(1), 9–17.

Pace, C., Talisuna, A., Wendler, D., et al. (2005b). Quality of parental consent in a Ugandan malaria study. *American Journal of Public Health, 95*, 1184, e9.

Rothwell, E., Wong, B., Rose, N. C., Anderson, R., Fedor, B., Stark, L. A., & Botkin, J. R. (2014). A randomized controlled trial of an electronic informed consent process. *Journal of Empirical Research on Human Research Ethics, 9*(5), 1–7.

Rowbotham, M. C., Astin, J., Greene, K., & Cummings, S. R. (2013). Interactive informed consent: Randomized comparison with paper consents. *PLoS One, 8*(3), e58603.

Schenker, Y., & Meisel, A. (2011). Informed consent in clinical care: Practical considerations in the effort to achieve ethical goals. *Journal of the American Medical Association, 305*(11), 1130–1131.

Sharp, S. M. (2004). Consent documents for oncology trials: Does anybody read these things? *American Journal of Clin Oncology, 27*(6), 570–575.

Silverman, H., Hull, S. C., & Sugarman, J. (2001). Variability among institutional review boards' decisions within the context of a multicenter trial. *Critical Care Medicine, 29*(2):235–241.

Tam, N. T., Huy, N. T., le Thoa, T. B., Long, N. P., Trang, N. T., Hirayama, K., & Karbwang, J. (2015). Participants' understanding of informed consent in clinical trials over three decades: Systematic review and meta-analysis. *Bulletin of the World Health Organization, 93*(3), 186–198.

Tarnowski, K. J., Allen, D. M., Mayhall, C., & Kelly, P. A. (1990). Readability of pediatric biomedical research informed consent forms. *Pediatrics, 85*(1), 58–62.

Weinfurt, K., Seils, D. M., Sulmasy, D. P., Astrow, A. B., Hurwitz, H. I., Cohen, R. B., & Meropol, N. J. (2012). Research participants' high expectations of benefit in early-phase oncology trials: Are we asking the right question? *Journal of Clinical Oncology, 30*(35), 4396–4400.

Wendler, D., & Grady, C. (2008). What should research participants understand to understand they are participants in research? *Bioethics, 22*, 203–208.

IRB Review of Approved Protocols

Modifications to Approved Research

Emily Eldh
Chris S. Witwer

Abstract

The IRB must review and approve changes to previously approved research in order to ensure that the regulatory criteria for IRB approval continue to be met and that the risk/benefit ratio remains appropriate in light of the proposed changes. This chapter discusses the regulatory background, submission process, and IRB review of modifications to previously approved research, as well as IRB review outcomes and documentation.

Introduction

The IRB must review and approve changes to previously approved research in order to ensure that the <u>regulatory criteria</u> for IRB approval continue to be met and that the risk/benefit ratio remains appropriate in light of the proposed changes. These changes may be referred to interchangeably as modifications, amendments, revisions, addenda, updates, and additions.

🔗 5-4

The researcher is responsible for proposing any changes for IRB review and approval prior to implementation, except when the changes are necessary to avoid immediate hazards to subjects. The IRB staff are responsible for managing the IRB review process and communicating the IRB's decision to the researcher.

Regulatory Overview

Under the Common Rule, the IRB must establish and follow written procedures for "ensuring prompt reporting to the IRB of proposed changes in a research activity, and for ensuring that investigators will conduct the research activity in accordance with the terms of the IRB approval until any proposed changes have been reviewed and approved by the IRB, except when necessary to eliminate apparent immediate hazards to the subject" [45 CFR 46.108(a)(3)(iii)].

Similarly, the Food and Drug Administration (FDA) requires IRBs to follow written procedures "for ensuring prompt reporting to the IRB of changes in research activity, and for ensuring that changes in approved research, during the period for which IRB approval has already been given, may not be initiated without IRB review and approval except where necessary to eliminate apparent immediate hazards to the human subjects." [21 CFR 56.108(a)(3, 4)].

🖉 2-3   To comply with these regulations, the IRB staff must prepare and maintain <u>written procedures</u> to address these obligations. Procedures should describe processes for the submission, review, and approval of proposed revisions.

It is important that researchers be made aware of the obligation to prospectively submit proposed revisions for IRB review and of the requirement to secure IRB approval prior to implementing those proposed revisions. One way to make researchers aware is to include the obligation in initial IRB approval documents, although IRB staff may adopt additional methods such as education programs or other outreach.

🖉 Section 4   Effective January 2020, cooperative research reviewed under **45 CFR 46** must rely upon review by a <u>single IRB</u>, including proposed modifications of the research.

Submission of Study Revisions

Study changes are submitted to the IRB staff by the researcher or a member of the study team with the authority to submit modifications on behalf of the researcher. The revision request must be submitted in accordance with the reviewing IRB office's infrastructure. Some IRB offices utilize paper forms, whereas others require electronic modification requests or the editing of existing materials housed within the IRB office's electronic system. Although the tools used to submit changes will vary by IRB office, all proposed changes should include a clear description of and justification for the proposed revisions, as well as a description of any variation in the level of risk to human subjects.

To assist IRB reviewers with their evaluation of the proposed changes, the IRB staff will typically require tracked-change versions of any revised documents and/or a summary description of the changes. Additional information may also be important to include in a modification request, such as who initiated the revision (e.g., sponsor), subject status, or enrollment status of the study.

All IRB-approved study materials should be updated when the proposed revision affects their content. These may include the study plan, informed consent and assent form(s), advertisements, surveys, subject materials, and any other documents previously approved by the IRB. The researcher also should have considered whether any changes in the research could affect the subjects' willingness to continue participating in the research, and if so, the researcher should have proposed to the IRB what information will be communicated to subjects.

Assessment of Proposed Modifications

The IRB office must triage proposed modifications to determine what type of review is required (**Figure 7.1-1**). Generally, changes can be divided into two

Please identify the type(s) of changes PROPOSED by checking all that APPLY:		
Type of Amendment	**Examples**	**Proposed**
Increased risk to subjects	New risk identified; changes made as result of updated Investigator Brochure, serious adverse event, or IND/IDE report	☐
Dose escalation amendment	Open/close a preexisting dose level; change in cohort	☐
Status change	Re-opening to enrollment; moving from Phase I to Phase II	☐
Therapy changes	Study modifications that result in a change in preparation, administration, route, or dose; a change in premedications; and/or a change in the dose modification plan	☐
Eligibility changes	Change to the inclusion or exclusion criteria in the study	☐
Recruitment of subjects	Change in the way subjects are recruited; new or revised advertisement	☐
Scientific changes	Adding a new arm; changing objectives; changing statistical analysis; adding correlative studies; increase or decrease in overall accrual goal	☐
Data, data collection, and data collection materials	Revised study diaries, questionnaires, or surveys given to subjects; addition or removal of data points or visits in the case report forms	☐
Editorial, administrative changes	Change in contact information; change in site subjects; typographical errors corrected; clarifications made to previously approved research	☐

Figure 7.1-1 An example modification application that may help the IRB office triage submissions for the correct IRB review.

Courtesy of Dana-Farber Cancer Institute, Used with permission.

types: minor revisions (involving no more than minimal risk) and major, or substantive, revisions (more than a minor change to the study and/or involving increased risks to subjects).

Minor Revisions

Minor revisions are changes made to study procedures that are no more than minimal risk or other changes that do not increase risks to subjects. Minimal risk means that the probability and magnitude of harm or discomfort anticipated in the research are not greater in and of themselves than those ordinarily encountered in daily life or during the performance of routine physical or psychological examinations or tests.

An IRB's policies and procedures may specify the types of revisions that can be reviewed as a minor change, such as the following:

- Updated telephone numbers
- Changes in study staff
- Typographical revisions to the recruitment materials
- Minor reduction in the number of research subjects
- Addition of minimal risk questions in a survey

Major Revisions

Unless the entire study qualifies for an <u>expedited</u> review process, revisions that involve increased risk to subjects or that significantly affect the design of

⏺ 5-5

the study are considered major revisions and must be reviewed by the convened IRB.

An IRB's policies and procedures will typically require that the following examples be considered a major change:

- New risk identified that may affect a subject's willingness to participate in the research
- Adding a new disease group, a new drug, and/or a research intervention
- Major change to the inclusion or exclusion criteria in the study
- Changing the consent form to include newly identified side effects or adverse events related to the study drug/intervention
- Adding a conflict of interest management plan

IRB Review Process

🖉 2-3

The IRB office's policies and procedures will help determine the level of review that is needed. One IRB office may allow certain changes without prospective IRB review (e.g., administrative updates), whereas another IRB office may require that all changes be prospectively reviewed by the IRB, no matter how minor.

🖉 5-3
🖉 5-1

IRB offices may also differ in their revision review requirements relating to studies previously determined to be exempt from the Common Rule or not human subjects research (NHSR).

🖉 5-5 🖉 5-7

When changes to previously approved research require IRB review, the revision request will be reviewed via either the expedited or convened review process, as specified in the regulations.

The IRB office should receive the following from researchers when changes to approved research are being proposed: the information needed to understand what the proposed changes are, the rationale or justification for those proposed changes, whether and how the proposed changes affect the risks to study subjects, and a description of any safeguards that will be implemented to minimize any additional risks. Some revisions are so substantive they may require an additional study arm or a separate study. Adding a separate study would require a new protocol and generally cannot be handled as a modification of previously approved research.

🖉 Section 6

If the revision includes a change in the consent form, a revised consent form should be submitted as part of the revision request. The IRB reviewer(s) must determine whether the change affects previously enrolled study subjects and whether it might affect their willingness to continue in the study. The IRB reviewer(s) should determine whether it is necessary to repeat the consent process or notify the subjects of the changes and under what circumstances (e.g., at next study visit, immediately, etc.).

Research Originally Approved Under an Expedited Review Procedure

When the entire study is eligible for expedited review, any proposed changes that maintain the expedited category of the study can continue to be reviewed via the expedited review procedure. Changes to a nonexempt study that push it out of an expedited review category will require convened board review, unless the proposed revisions would exempt the research from the human protection regulations.

Research Originally Approved by the Convened IRB

Federal regulations allow an IRB reviewer to use the expedited review procedure to review "[m]inor changes in previously approved research during the period for which approval is authorized." [**45 CFR 46.110(b)(1)(ii)**]. An expedited review process may be used to review such minor modifications, even when the study was initially reviewed by the convened IRB. Any change that is more than a minor change to research that was previously reviewed by the convened IRB must also be reviewed by the convened IRB.

IRB Review Outcomes

The IRB may approve the revision as submitted or may request modifications to the proposed revision prior to approving the change. Possible IRB review outcomes include the following:

- Approval
- Conditional approval or approval with conditions (or modifications)
- Deferral (open-ended questions are unresolved)
- Disapproval (note that only the full board may disapprove research)
- Tabling (when information is missing or there is an administrative error delaying review)

The IRB must consider whether subjects must be notified of changes in the research (**Figure 7.1-2**). The IRB will then determine what new information shall be communicated to subjects, the timing of that communication, and how it should be communicated. Communicating changes to subjects can be accomplished through various methods, including the following:

- Verbal notification via telephone or in person (with documentation in the study file)
- Notification letter
- Revised informed consent document
- Consent addendum

IRB determinations and considerations regarding notifying or seeking re-consent from subjects

---

Is it necessary to notify or seek re-consent from subjects?
- If no
  - Indicate so in IRB determination letter
- If yes, new subjects only
  - Consider methods: revised consent or verbal notification
- If yes, all currently enrolled subjects actively participating in research interventions
  - Consider methods: revised consent, verbal notification, or notification letter
- If yes, all currently enrolled subjects in follow-up
  - Consider methods: consent, verbal notification, or notification letter
- If yes, all subjects off study
  - Consider methods: verbal notification or notification letter

---

Figure 7.1-2 IRB determinations and considerations regarding notifying or seeking re-consent from subjects

Courtesy of Dana-Farber Cancer Institute, Used with permission.

IRB Documentation

An IRB shall notify investigators and the institution in writing of its decision to approve or disapprove the proposed research activity, or of modifications required to secure IRB approval of the research activity. If the IRB decides to disapprove a research activity, it shall include in its written notification a statement of the reasons for its decision and give the investigator an opportunity to respond in person or in writing. [45 CFR 46.109(d)]

The original revision request and all accompanying documents must be maintained in the study file within the IRB office. When new or revised informed consent or assent form(s) are approved as part of the revision, the revised forms will typically include the new IRB approval date or version number.

For IRB offices employing electronic IRB systems, researchers should be encouraged to retrieve the most recently approved version of study documents, such as informed consent forms, directly from the IRB's electronic systems rather than relying on paper copies or versions stored locally on individual computers. Doing so helps ensure that the most current versions of these documents are consistently used throughout the study, minimizing the risk of noncompliance.

All IRB members must be informed of research approved through the expedited review process, including minor revisions to previously approved research. The IRB office may accomplish this by providing a report of all expedited reviews to the committee members at the next possible convened IRB meeting.

Additional Considerations for Ongoing Research

Typically, subject enrollment may continue as previously approved by the IRB while proposed changes to the research are under IRB review. If, however, the proposed changes affect the future enrollment of subjects or new risks have been identified, the researcher and/or the IRB staff may place a study's enrollment on hold while awaiting IRB review of the proposed change(s).

It is important to note that when a researcher wishes to enroll a subject who does not meet all the IRB-approved inclusion criteria, the researcher must not waive the inclusion criterion without prior IRB approval. Revising any aspect of the study, even for a single subject, requires prospective IRB approval. If modifications are implemented without IRB approval, this must be reported to ⊘ 7-5 ⊘ 7-6   the IRB as a <u>deviation</u> from the approved research or as <u>noncompliance</u>, per the reviewing IRB's policies and procedures.

Once a revision request is approved, documented, and the outcome communicated to the researcher, the researcher is obligated to follow the revised IRB-approved research plan moving forward. Any further revisions also require submission and IRB approval prior to implementation.

Conclusion

IRBs and researchers must understand that federal regulations require IRB approval of any changes to previously approved research prior to implementation of the proposed revisions. IRB offices have differing procedures for processing proposed study modifications, but all IRB offices share the obligation to ensure that changes are not initiated without IRB approval, except when necessary to eliminate apparent immediate hazards to human subjects.

Continuing Review

Linda Coleman
Meghan Scott

Abstract

IRB review and approval of a new study is intended to ensure that the ethical principles and applicable standards that govern human subjects research are considered and applied. During the initial review process, the IRB should determine the level and frequency of continuing review, which should be relayed to the researcher via the final approval letter. For research that is Food and Drug Administration (FDA) regulated and/or federally funded, there are specific regulations that discuss the requirements for continuing review. For research that is not FDA regulated or federally funded, the institution may choose to adhere to the regulations or develop internal institutional policies and procedures. This chapter provides an overview of continuing review requirements as defined by federal regulations and applicable international guidelines for studies reviewed and approved by an IRB. The chapter also considers options for implementing the requirements in light of different regulatory standards and organizational practices.

What Is Continuing Review?

Continuing review is a mechanism by which the researcher provides a report to the IRB regarding a study's progress. Because it is not often possible to predict the complex evolution of a study at the time a study is initially reviewed by the IRB, continuing review allows the IRB the opportunity to determine whether the study continues to meet approval requirements and to monitor study progress to ensure that safeguards are in place to protect the rights and welfare of study subjects. It also provides the IRB with the opportunity to reapply the ethical principles outlined in the _Belmont Report_ (National Commission, 1979) and applicable human research standards.

🖉 1-1

Federal Regulations and International Guidelines

The U.S. Federal Policy for the Protection of Human Subjects, or "Common Rule" (administered by the Office for Human Research Protections [OHRP]), and the FDA human subjects protection regulations define the IRB's obligations and considerations for both the initial review of a study and ongoing approval during the life of that study, including determinations regarding informed consent, risks, potential benefits, equitable subject selection, and safeguards for human research subjects. Additionally, the 2016 International Council for Harmonisation (ICH) Good Clinical Practice (GCP) guidelines reiterate an IRB's initial review and ongoing review obligations (ICH, 2016a).

🔗 8-2

The Common Rule

According to the Common Rule, the IRB is required to conduct continuing review for a study under its purview at least annually until the study is closed with the IRB, unless an exception applies where continuing review is not required [**45 CFR 46.109(f)(1)**]:

> Unless an IRB determines otherwise, continuing review of research is not required in the following circumstances:
> 1. Research eligible for expedited review in accordance with §46.110;
> 2. Research reviewed by the IRB in accordance with the limited IRB review described in §46.104(d)(2)(iii), (d)(3)(i)(C), or (d)(7) or (8);
> 3. Research that has progressed to the point that it involves only one or both of the following, which are part of the IRB-approved study:
>   • Data analysis, including analysis of identifiable private information or identifiable biospecimens, or
>   • Accessing follow-up clinical data from procedures that subjects would undergo as part of clinical care.

🔗 5-5 🔗 5-6

Even when annual continuing review is not required because one of these exceptions applies (e.g., studies eligible for expedited or limited IRB review), the IRB still retains the authority to require continuing review. This decision must be documented with sufficient rationale.

The pre-2018 Common Rule requires continuing review of research by an IRB no less than annually, but no exceptions apply [pre-2018 Requirements, **45 CFR 46.109(e)**]. Therefore, if an institution has studies sponsored by federal agencies that have not signed on to the 2018 Common Rule, or Common Rule agency–sponsored studies that have not been transitioned to the 2018 Requirements, the pre-2018 Common Rule continuitng review requirements apply. The IRB will need to consider options for tracking studies and implementing the various requirements because of the different regulatory standards.

OHRP guidance outlines review criteria for the IRB to consider when conducting continuing review (DHHS, 2010). It states the following:

> HHS regulations set forth the criteria for IRB approval of research (45 CFR 46.111, 46.204-207, 46.305, and 46.404-409). . . .

> When conducting continuing review, the IRB should start with the working presumption that the research, as previously approved, [continues to satisfy the criteria for IRB approval of research]. The IRB

should focus on whether there is any new information provided by the investigator, or otherwise available to the IRB, that would alter the IRB's prior determinations, particularly with respect to the IRB's prior evaluation of the potential benefits or risks to the subjects. The IRB also should assess whether there is any new information that would necessitate revision of the protocol and/or the informed consent document. IRBs have the authority to disapprove or require modifications in (to secure re-approval of) a research activity that does not [continue to] meet the above criteria (45 CFR 46.109(a)). If research does not satisfy all of the above criteria, the IRB must require changes that would result in research satisfying these criteria, defer taking action, or disapprove the research. When conducting continuing review and evaluating whether research continues to satisfy the criteria for IRB approval of research, IRBs should pay particular attention to the following four aspects of the research: Risk assessment and monitoring; Adequacy of the process for obtaining informed consent; Investigator and institutional issues; and Research progress.

Food and Drug Administration

The FDA requires the IRB to conduct continuing review at least annually until the study is closed with the IRB [21 CFR 56.109 (f)]:

> If a study is reviewed and approved by the IRB and is subject to FDA requirements, the IRB is required to "conduct continuing review . . . at intervals appropriate to the degree of risk, but not less than once per year . . ."

The FDA also provides guidance (FDA, 2012):

> When conducting continuing review, the IRB should start with the assumption that the research, as previously approved, satisfied all of the criteria under 21 CFR 56.111. The IRB should focus on any new information provided by the investigator or sponsor, or otherwise available to the IRB, that may alter the IRB's prior determinations, particularly with respect to the IRB's prior evaluation of the potential benefits or risks to the subjects. The IRB also should assess whether there is any new information that would necessitate revision of the protocol and/or the informed consent document. If the IRB determines that a research activity no longer meets the criteria for approval under 21 CFR 56.111, the IRB is not permitted to reapprove it, but may either disapprove it or require modifications in order to secure re-approval (21 CFR 56.109(a)).
>
> . . . when conducting continuing review and evaluating whether research continues to satisfy the criteria for IRB approval of research, IRBs should pay particular attention to the following areas: 1) Risk Assessment; 2) Adequacy of Informed Consent; 3) Local Issues, and 4) Trial Progress.

While the Common Rule provides an exception from continuing review requirements for certain types of studies, no such exception exists (as of this writing) for FDA-regulated studies. The FDA, however, "intends to undertake notice and comment rulemaking to harmonize, to the extent applicable, FDA's regulations with the revised Common Rule" (FDA, 2018a).

International Council for Harmonisation

🔗 8-2   The <u>International Council for Harmonisation</u> of Technical Requirements of Pharmaceuticals for Human Use (ICH), ICH Harmonised Guideline, Integrated Addendum to ICH (R1) Guideline for Good Clinical Practice E6 (R2)

> . . . is an international ethical and scientific quality standard for designing, conducting, recording and reporting trials that involve the participation of human subjects. Compliance with this standard provides public assurance that the rights, safety, and well-being of trial subjects are protected, consistent with the principles that have their origin in the Declaration of Helsinki, and that the clinical trial data are credible. (ICH, 2016a)

The ICH GCP guideline (E6, R2) requires review and approval by an IRB for a study to commence (section 3.1.2; ICH, 2016b) and requires continuing review at least once per year (section 3.1.4; ICH 2016b). "The IRB/IEC should conduct continuing review of each ongoing trial at intervals appropriate to the degree of risk to human subjects, but at least once per year" (ICH, 2016b). Section 4.10.1 also reiterates this expectation: "The investigator shall submit written summaries of the trial status to the IRB/IEC annually, or more frequently, if requested by the IRB" (ICH, 2016b). ICH GCP E6 R2 was adopted by the United States on March 1, 2018 (FDA, 2018b). Agencies in other countries have also adopted this ICH guideline and are listed on the ICH.org website.

Determining the Level of IRB Review: Full Board or Expedited

Initial Full-Board Review

🔗 5-7   Studies that are initially reviewed by a <u>convened meeting</u> of the IRB will continue to be reviewed at a convened meeting at the time of continuing review. For studies subject to FDA regulations or the pre-2018 Common Rule, at the
🔗 5-5   time of continuing review, <u>expedited</u> review is allowed if those studies were initially reviewed at a convened IRB meeting under expedited categories 8 and 9 (DHHS, 1998; FDA, 1998), as follows:

- Category 8: Continuing review of research previously approved by the convened IRB as follows:
  (a) Research is permanently closed to the enrollment of new subjects; all subjects have completed all research-related interventions; and research remains active only for long-term follow-up of subjects; or
  (b) no subjects have been enrolled and no additional risks have been identified; or
  (c) the remaining research activities are limited to data analysis.
- Category 9: Continuing review of research not conducted under an investigational new drug application or investigational device exemption where categories 2 through 8 of the expedited review categories do not apply; however, the IRB has determined and documented at a convened meeting that the research involves no greater than minimal risk and no additional risks have been identified.

The expedited review categories are established by the FDA **[21 CFR 56.110]** and the Secretary of DHHS (pre-2018 Requirements, **45 CFR 46.110**). For studies subject to the 2018 Common Rule, research that is eligble for expedited review does not require annual continuing review.

Initial Expedited Review

For studies subject to FDA regulations or the pre-2018 Common Rule, research activities that initially qualified as minimal risk and underwent initial <u>expedited</u> review and approval may continue to be reviewed under expedited review procedures at continuing review, unless the study no longer qualifies for expedited review because of changes to the research (e.g., changes to the research that cause the study to be more than minimal risk, etc.). For studies subject to the 2018 Common Rule, research activities that initially qualified as minimal risk and underwent initial expedited review and approval do not require continuing review of any sort, unless the study no longer qualifies for expedited review because of changes to the research.

⌖ 5-5

Issues the IRB Evaluates at Continuing Review

For studies that require continuing review, it is useful for the IRB to ask specific questions to facilitate the continuing review process. Some of the topics or questions an IRB may consider are described in the list that follows. As noted in OHRP guidance, "the amount of time the IRB spends on the continuing review of a particular study will vary depending on the nature and complexity of the research, the amount and type of new information presented to the IRB and whether the investigator is seeking approval of substantive changes to the research protocol or informed consent document" (DHHS, 2010).

Accrual

- Has accrual progressed as planned? If not, will this impact the ability of the researcher to complete the study?
- If the study objectives cannot be met and the study involves more than minimal risk interventions, is it reasonable to continue accrual?
- If the study is a multisite trial, has the researcher provided you with trial-wide accrual data in addition to local accrual data?

Unanticipated toxicity

- How many serious and unexpected toxicities have occurred since the trial's initiation?
- If the toxicities (in type or number) are linked to the study intervention, are new toxicity risks described in the consent form?
- Will the information about unanticipated toxicity(s) impact the risk/benefit ratio and continued study approval?

Subject complaints

- Were there concerns about approach or contact for the study?
- Have subjects withdrawn because of disappointing interactions with the study team?

- Is there a need to modify procedures or reeducate staff because of these concerns?
- Do study team members know whom to contact with questions about the rights of research subjects?

New information or findings relating to risk/benefit assessment

- Are safety and risk factors for subjects adequately described in the consent form based on findings to date? If not, is the informed consent process or document still acceptable, or does it require revision?
- Has any new institutional policy, regulation, or other standard been instituted since the last IRB review? If so, does this influence the future conduct of the study?

Interval of renewal

- Should continuing review be done annually or more frequently? The risk to subjects determines the renewal frequency.

Continuing Review Administration Considerations

Timing of IRB Review

The IRB must have a system in place for tracking time frames of protocol approvals and ensuring that renewal notices are sent out to researchers in a timely manner to ensure that continuing review occurs no less than annually (or the time frame established by the IRB).

Deadlines for Renewal

Reminder notices should be sent to researchers 2 or 3 months before the IRB-designated continuing review date. In addition, the continuing review notices and the receipt of continuing review information should be tracked. Specifying what information to submit is also important. For example, asking specific questions to facilitate continuing review is an efficient way for the researchers and IRB to evaluate data from the study and to make determinations about the study's continued approvability by the IRB. Researchers should also be advised regarding the consequences of failing to comply with continuing review requirements, such as study suspension, possible loss of funding and/or publication, or reporting of noncompliance to sponsors or funding agencies.

Policies and Procedures for When Continuing Review Is Not Required by Regulation

Even when annual continuing review is not required, organizations may wish to develop ongoing administrative check-in processes in lieu of continuing review to satisfy local requirements and to remind researchers of their ongoing responsibilities for conducting research. Administrative check-in processes can serve as important reminders for researchers and study staff regarding their ongoing obligations, such as the following:

- Submitting modifications to ongoing research to the IRB prior to implementation

- Submitting reportable events, such as potential <u>noncompliance</u> or <u>unanticipated problems</u> involving risks to subjects or others
- Informing the IRB of the current study status and alerting the IRB when the research is complete
- Ensuring local training requirements are met

🔗 7-6
🔗 7-3

An administrative check-in process may be implemented in a number of ways. Organizations may consider the following when deciding whether and how to implement a check-in process:

- How frequently will check-ins occur (e.g., annually, every 3 years, every 5 years)?
- If utilizing an electronic IRB system, can automated notifications be sent to reduce the administrative burden on IRB staff?
- Will a response be required from the researcher or study team? If yes, what are the consequences if a researcher does not respond?
- Who will review responses from the researcher (i.e., IRB staff, IRB chair)?
- Were any institutional requirements checked at the time of continuing review? If so, can these be tied to an administrative check-in process (e.g., confirming current training for researchers, checking posting of IRB-approved consent to clinicaltrials.gov)?

While organizations may differ in their approaches to monitoring studies when continuing review is not required by regulations, efforts should be taken to reduce the administrative burden to researchers and IRB staff (as envisioned by the regulators) for these minimal risk activities.

Conclusion

Consistent with ethical principles, ongoing monitoring of a study is an important aspect of the IRB's role in protecting the rights and welfare of research subjects. By establishing policies and practices that focus on evaluating study progress, the IRB will be able to comply with applicable regulations, guidance, and organizational requirements.

Acknowledgment

Karen M. Hansen contributed to this chapter.

References

Department of Health and Human Services (DHHS). (1998). *OHRP expedited review categories.* www.hhs.gov/ohrp/regulations-and-policy/guidance/categories-of-research-expedited-review -procedure-1998/index.html

Department of Health and Human Services (DHHS). (2010). *Guidance on continuing review-IRB continuing review of research.* www.hhs.gov/ohrp/regulations-and-policy/guidance/guidance-on -continuing-review-2010/index.html#section-b1

Department of Health and Human Services (DHHS). (2016). *Federal policy for the protection of human subjects ('Common Rule').* www.hhs.gov/ohrp/regulations-and-policy/regulations /common-rule/index.html

Food and Drug Administration (FDA). (1998). *Categories of research that may be reviewed by the institutional review board (IRB) through an expedited review procedure.* www.fda.gov/science -research/clinical-trials-and-human-subject-protection/categories-research-may-be-reviewed -institutional-review-board-irb-through-expedited-review

Food and Drug Administration (FDA). (2012). *IRB continuing review after clinical investigation approval. guidance for IRBs, clinical investigators, and sponsors.* www.fda.gov/science-research/guidance-documents-including-information-sheets-and-notices/information-sheet-guidance-institutional-review-boards-irbs-clinical-investigators-and-sponsors

Food and Drug Administration (FDA). (2018a). *Impact of certain provisions of the revised common rule on FDA-regulated clinical investigations guidance for sponsors, investigators, and institutional review boards.* www.fda.gov/regulatory-information/search-fda-guidance-documents/impact-certain-provisions-revised-common-rule-fda-regulated-clinical-investigations

Food and Drug Administration (FDA). (2018b). *E6(R2) Good Clinical Practice: Integrated addendum to ICH E6(R1) guidance for industry.* www.fda.gov/regulatory-information/search-fda-guidance-documents/e6r2-good-clinical-practice-integrated-addendum-ich-e6r1

International Council for Harmonisation of Technical Requirements for Pharmaceuticals for Human Use (ICH). (2016a). *Guideline for Good Clinical Practice E6 (R2).* www.ich.org/page/efficacy-guidelines

International Council for Harmonisation of Technical Requirements for Pharmaceuticals for Human Use (ICH). (2016b). *ICH harmonised guideline. Integrated addendum to ICH E6(R1): Guideline for Good Clinical Practice E6(R2).* database.ich.org/sites/default/files/E6_R2_Addendum.pdf

National Commission for the Protection of Human Subjects of Biomedical and Behavioral Research. (1979). *The Belmont Report: Ethical principles and guidelines for the protection of human subjects of research.* www.hhs.gov/ohrp/regulations-and-policy/belmont-report/read-the-belmont-report/index.html

Unanticipated Problems Involving Risks to Subjects or Others

Lisa Denney

Kathy McClelland

Nancy Olson

Ernest D. Prentice

Abstract

This chapter describes the regulatory requirements for reporting unanticipated problems involving risks to subjects or others ("unanticipated problems") in nonexempt human subjects research to the IRB and offers suggestions to support the IRB review process.

Introduction

There are always risks to participating in research, and as a research study progresses, it is likely that subjects will experience problems. The challenge is to determine whether or not a problem is caused by or related to the study. The purpose of continuing to review and monitor ongoing studies is to ensure that the risk/benefit relationship continues to be acceptable and that the rights and welfare of the subjects continue to be protected. In order to do this, it is of paramount importance that, as a study progresses, the IRB is notified of unanticipated problems. The IRB will review the event and, if necessary, make recommendations to protect human subjects.

🔗 7-2 🔗 7-4

The Department of Health and Human Services (DHHS) Office for Human Research Protections (OHRP) and the Food and Drug Administration (FDA) require prompt reporting of any unanticipated problems to the IRB. To supplement the regulatory requirements, both OHRP and FDA have released guidance to help facilitate efficient and effective IRB review of unanticipated problems, "so that human subjects can be better protected from avoidable harm" and "to help differentiate between those adverse events that are unanticipated problems that must be reported to an IRB and those that are not" (DHHS, 2007; FDA, 2009).

Terminology and Definitions

Adverse Event

Though the OHRP and FDA documents do not define adverse event (AE), and the phrase does not appear in the applicable regulations, it is widely used and broadly accepted to mean "any untoward or unfavorable medical occurrence in a human subject, including any abnormal sign (for example, abnormal physical exam or laboratory finding), symptom, or disease, temporally associated with the subject's participation in the research, whether or not considered related to the subject's participation in the research" (DHHS, 2007). Simply put, an adverse event (or adverse effect or adverse experience) is some harm that occurs to a subject in a research study, whether or not that harm is directly related to the research.

Unanticipated Problems Involving Risks to Subjects or Others

In contrast, an "unanticipated problem involving risks to subject or others" (unanticipated problem, or UP) is an unexpected event that occurs in the context of research that might cause harm (that is, represents a risk of harm). An unanticipated problem may not actually result in any harm; actual harm to a subject is not a prerequisite in order for reporting to be required.

An unanticipated problem has the following characteristics (DHHS, 2007):

- It is "**unexpected** in terms of nature, severity, or frequency given (i) the research procedures described in the protocol-related documents … and (ii) the characteristics of the subject population being studied"
- It is "**related or possibly related to participation in the research** (… possibly related means there is a reasonable possibility that the incident, experience, or outcome may have been caused by the procedures involved in the research)" *and*
- It "suggests that the research places subjects or others at a **greater risk of harm** (including physical, psychological, economic, or social harm) than was previously known or recognized" [emphasis added].

AE Versus UP and Federal Reporting Requirements

The critical difference between an AE and a UP is that an AE is an actual harm that occurs but may or may not be related to the research, and a UP is a potential harm (a risk) that is related (or possibly related) to the research. Adverse events and unanticipated problems may overlap (**Figure 7.3-1**). Some, but not all UPs are also AEs, and some but not all AEs are also UPs.

The Common Rule at 45 CFR 46.108(a)(4)(i) and the corresponding FDA regulations at 21 CFR 56.108(b)(1) require the IRB to establish and follow

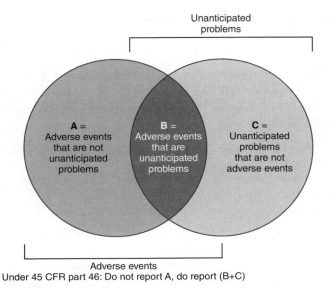

Figure 7.3-1 The relationship between adverse events and unanticipated problems.

Department of Health and Human Services (DHHS). (2007). *Unanticipated problems involving risks and adverse events guidance.*
www.hhs.gov/ohrp/regulations-and-policy/guidance/reviewing-unanticipated-problems/index.html.

written procedures for ensuring prompt reporting to the IRB, appropriate institutional officials, and the department or agency head, "of any unanticipated problem involving risks to subjects or others." Only unanticipated problems need to be reported by investigators to the IRB, or by the IRB to the department or agency.

However, a literal reading of the phrase "any unanticipated problem involving risks" would result in the reporting of all events, even minor, unexpected problems to the IRB. In 2007 and 2009, respectively, OHRP and FDA issued guidance on the reporting requirements, clarifying that only events that are unexpected, related or possibly related, *and* suggest greater risk of harm than previously known are unanticipated problems that require reporting to the IRB. Both guidance documents make it clear that only a subset of adverse events meet the reporting requirements of an unanticipated problem.

Prompt Reporting

The Common Rule [45 CFR 46.108(a)(4)(i)] and the corresponding FDA regulations [21 CFR 56.108(b)(1)] require "prompt reporting." The purpose of prompt reporting is to ensure that appropriate steps are taken in a timely manner to protect other subjects from avoidable harm.

The regulations do not define "prompt," and the appropriate time frame for satisfying the requirement for prompt reporting will vary depending on the specific nature of the unanticipated problem, the nature of the research associated with the problem, institutional requirements, and the entity to which reports are to be submitted.

OHRP recommends the following guidelines in order to satisfy the requirement for prompt reporting (DHHS, 2007):

1. Unanticipated problems that are serious adverse events should be reported to the IRB within 1 week of the investigator becoming aware of the event.

2. Any other unanticipated problems should be reported to the IRB within 2 weeks of the investigator becoming aware of the problem.
3. All unanticipated problems should be reported to appropriate institutional officials (as required by an institution's written reporting procedures), the supporting agency head (or designee), and OHRP within one month of the IRB's receipt of the report of the problem from the investigator.

OHRP allows, in certain cases, for reporting requirements to be "met by submitting a preliminary report to the IRB, appropriate institutional officials, supporting DHHS agency head (or designee), and OHRP, with a follow-up report submitted at a later date when more information is available" (DHHS, 2007). Determining appropriate timing for reporting is a judgment call for the institution, and preventing avoidable harms to other subjects should be a priority.

🔗 11-2 FDA investigational device exemption (IDE) regulations require a researcher to submit a report of any unanticipated adverse device effect to the sponsor and the reviewing IRB "as soon as possible, but in no event later than 10 working days after the researcher first learns of the event" [21 CFR 812.150(a)(1)]. The

🔗 11-3 investigational new drug (IND) regulations, on the other hand, are silent as to suggested timing of reporting requirements to the IRB.

🔗 Section 6 Prompt reporting of an unanticipated problem could prevent other subjects from experiencing a similar event and make the researcher more aware of the need for surveillance for a particular problem. If changes to the consent form result, it may help current subjects appropriately reevaluate their participation and new subjects make a more informed decision regarding entering a study.

IRB Review of Unanticipated Problems

🔗 2-3 Every IRB must have and follow written policies and procedures concerning the reporting and review of unanticipated problems. Although institutions develop local policies and dictate what should be reported, the policies and practices should closely follow regulatory requirements and guidance. Association for the

🔗 8-7 Accreditation of Human Research Protection Programs (AAHRPP) accredited institutions should also ensure that policies meet AAHRPP standards, using AAHRPP tip sheets as guidance. The flow chart in **Figure 7.3-2** may be used to determine whether an adverse event represents an unanticipated problem that must be reported under the Common Rule.

The researcher should provide information to the IRB in accordance with the IRB's written policies and procedures, which may include a detailed description of the event, including date and location of the event; time when the researcher became aware of the event; and any proposed changes to the protocol, consent form(s), and any other relevant documents, or the rationale for no changes being made.

The IRB will review the information and consider the potential impact on the research and whether the unanticipated problem being reported warrants changes to protect study participants. For example, may the research continue as is, or is a substantive protocol amendment required before the study may continue? May participants currently enrolled continue in the study as planned, or should they be provided with additional information and should additional consent be obtained? In this way, the IRB is assured that the risks are minimized, the benefits are maximized, and the risk/benefit relationship of the research continues to be acceptable.

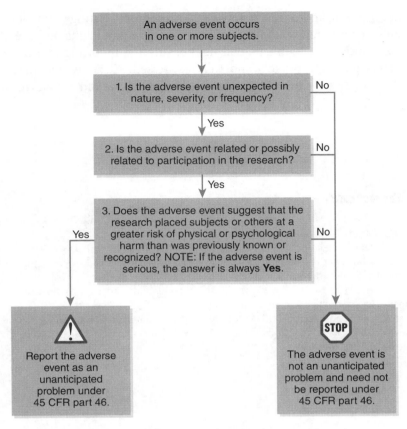

Figure 7.3-2 Determination of reporting requirements for adverse events.

Department of Health and Human Services (DHHS). (2007). *Unanticipated problems involving risks and adverse events guidance.* www.hhs.gov/ohrp/regulations-and -policy/guidance/reviewing-unanticipated-problems/index.html

Reporting by the Institution to Federal Agencies

Reporting requirements for unanticipated problems extend beyond the IRB and institutional officials. The Common Rule [45 CFR 46.108(4)(1)] and FDA regulations [21 CFR 56.108(b)(1)] require the institution to have and follow written procedures for prompt reporting of unanticipated problems to the appropriate "department or agency head." In the case of research that is subject to DHHS regulations, unanticipated problems must be reported to OHRP, which acts on behalf of the Secretary of DHHS. For research that is subject to FDA regulations, reporting is generally accomplished through established reporting channels from the researcher, to the sponsor, to FDA, in accordance with the requirements of all applicable FDA regulations. If, however, the researcher holds the investigational new drug application or investigational device exemption, they should report the unanticipated problem directly to FDA and to the researcher's IRB.

Conclusion

As a study progresses, the IRB must be assured that risks continue to be minimized, benefits continue to be maximized, and the risk/benefit relationship of the research continues to be acceptable. Review of unanticipated problems allows the IRB to assess the impact on continuation of the research, whether the informed consent form(s) requires revision, and whether additional consent should be sought from subjects already enrolled in the research. When institutions create and/or revise policy and procedures relating to unanticipated problems, a thorough reading of the regulatory requirements and the OHRP and FDA guidance documents will help ensure the reporting and review requirements are appropriately and fully addressed. Clear written procedures provide a process for the IRB and researchers to follow and maximize subject safety.

References

Code of Federal Regulations. (1999). Title 21, Chapter 1—Food and Drug Administration, DHHS; Part 312—Investigational New Drug Application.

Code of Federal Regulations. (2018). Title 21, Chapter 1—Food and Drug Administration, DHHS; Subchapter H—Medical Devices; Part 812—Investigational Device Exemptions.

Department of Health and Human Services (DHHS). (2007). *Unanticipated problems involving risks and adverse events guidance.* www.hhs.gov/ohrp/regulations-and-policy/guidance/reviewing -unanticipated-problems/index.html

Food and Drug Administration (FDA). (2009). *Guidance for clinical investigators, sponsors, and IRBs – adverse event reporting to IRBs – improving human subjects protection.* www.fda.gov /media/72267/download

Appendix

Sample Policy for IRB Review

1. Upon receipt of an unanticipated problem report, the IRB staff previews the submission and, if needed, contacts the investigator for corrections or additional information.
2. The IRB Chair or designated reviewer receives and reviews the report and makes an initial determination as to whether the event represents an unanticipated problem. If needed, the chair or designee may request additional information from the investigator, sponsor, or others (including study committees, such as data monitoring committees, data safety monitoring boards, or steering committees).
3. If the reviewer determines that the problem does not meet the definition of an anticipated problem, they will determine whether any additional actions are necessary to ensure the protection of subjects. As warranted, the reviewer may refer the matter to the convened IRB for review. The results of the review will be recorded in review notes and communicated to the investigator.
4. If the reviewer determines that the event may be an unanticipated problem, the report will be referred for review by the convened IRB. The convened IRB will determine whether the event is an unanticipated problem and whether any additional actions, such as those outlined below, are necessary to ensure the protection of subjects. If needed, the IRB may request additional information from the investigator, sponsor, or others (including study committees, such as data monitoring committees, data safety monitoring boards, or steering committees). The results of the review will be recorded in the IRB minutes and communicated to the investigator.
5. Based upon the circumstances, the IRB may take any of the following actions, or others, to ensure the protection of subjects:
   a. Require modifications to the protocol or plan or procedures for implantation of the research as described in the application and other materials submitted to the IRB.
   b. Revise the continuing review timetable.
   c. Modify the consent process.
   d. Modify the consent, permission, and/or assent document(s), as applicable.
   e. Require additional information be provided to currently enrolled subjects (e.g., whenever the information may relate to the subject's rights, welfare, or willingness to continue participation).

   f. Provide additional information to subjects who have completed the study.

   g. Require additional training of the investigator and/or study staff.

   h. Require that currently enrolled subjects provide additional consent to continue participation.

   i. Monitor the research.

   j. Monitor the consent process.

   k. Report or refer to appropriate parties (e.g., the Institutional Official, Office of Integrity and Compliance, Risk Management, Office of Information Security).

   l. Suspend IRB approval.

   m. Terminate IRB approval.

When the IRB determines that an event is an unanticipated problem, the IRB staff will follow the regulatory and institutional requirements for reporting to regulatory agencies, sponsors, and organizational officials. When appropriate, a preliminary report may be submitted while more information is obtained to inform the determination or actions.

Post-Approval Oversight

Leslie M. Howes

Eunice Y. Newbert

Abstract

An important aspect of any human research protection program (HRPP) is its ability to ensure ongoing institutional compliance with human subjects protection requirements. The purpose of this chapter is to discuss how an institution may leverage a quality assurance (QA)/quality improvement (QI) program's auditing function as one way to provide post-approval oversight of the researcher. This chapter will also review the regulatory basis for post-approval oversight, define and differentiate quality assurance and quality improvement, discuss the various types of oversight and QA/QI program models, describe how an institution may design a QA/QI program considering size and resources, and provide an overview of how to approach an investigator audit.

Regulatory Basis for Post-Approval Oversight

The Common Rule states that an IRB must conduct continuing review at "intervals appropriate to the degree of risk" and that an IRB has "authority to observe or have a third party observe the consent process and the research" [45 CFR 46.109(e); 45 CFR 46.109(g); 21 CFR 56.109(f)]. Regulations also require that an IRB ensure that the "research plan makes adequate provision for monitoring the data collected to ensure the safety of subjects" [45 CFR 46.111(a)(6); 21 CFR 56.111(a)(6)]. These citations highlight an institution's responsibility for ensuring compliance. As discussed further in this chapter, an institution may establish an auditing program as an approach to post-approval oversight.

This expectation is reinforced through the <u>accreditation</u> process. Incorporated in 2001, the Association for the Accreditation of Human Research Protection Programs (AAHRPP) established standards and elements required to achieve accreditation status. Included in AAHRPP's evaluation instrument is the obligation to "conduct audits or surveys . . . to assess compliance with organizational policies and procedures and applicable laws, regulations, codes, and guidance" (AAHRPP, 2018).

🔗 8-7

✎ 8-2 Perhaps the most clear support for post-approval oversight comes from the International Council for Harmonisation (ICH) Good Clinical Practice (GCP) guidance, an international ethical and scientific quality standard for designing, conducting, recording, and reporting trials that involve human subjects (ICH, n.d.). The Food and Drug Administration (FDA) guidance expects that GCP is followed "when generating clinical trial data that are intended to be submitted to regulatory authorities" and suggests broader application to "other clinical investigations" (FDA, 2018). A sponsor may also require study adherence to GCP. Such guidance is clear that the "investigator/institution should permit monitoring and auditing by the sponsor, and inspection by the appropriate regulatory authority(ies)" (ICH, n.d.).

Despite the support for evaluating researcher compliance, an institution has great latitude in executing this process. For example, one institution may find it appropriate to depend on researcher self-assessments, while another institution may choose to establish an internal QA/QI program, which includes an auditing function as part of its scope of service. A variety of factors may shape how an institution configures its audit program, including financial and human resources, structure and size, research portfolio, and known compliance vulnerabilities.

Types of Post-Approval Oversight

Different types of oversight are used in research, such as "audit," "monitoring," "inspection," and "data and safety monitoring." These terms are often used interchangeably because the basic purpose and activities involved are similar (**Table 7.4-1**). The main difference is the "independence, objectivity and frequency" of the oversight (Ruppert, 2004). Recognizing the differences is important in order to understand why audits are used as a quality assurance measure.

Audits give an institution the flexibility to customize a QA function to best fit its research culture and available resources. For example, in designing an audit program, an institution can define its own parameters, including what type of studies to audit, how many studies to audit, and how often to conduct audits. An institution may also amend these parameters based on aggregate audit data, as needed. It is important for an institution to periodically review audit findings not only to ensure program effectiveness but also to evaluate what an institution can do to improve performance moving forward—i.e., quality improvement.

Quality Assurance and Quality Improvement Defined

ICH defines quality assurance as "all those planned and systematic actions that are established to ensure that the trial is performed and the data are generated, documented (recorded), and reported in compliance with GCP and the applicable regulatory requirements" and identifies audits as an "independent" QA activity (ICH, n.d.). Quality improvement is generally defined as a systematic, formal approach to the analysis of performance and efforts designed to improve performance. As such, a robust auditing program will include both QA and QI features. QA/QI program activities generally fall into two categories: evaluating performance (QA) and improving performance (QI). Although QA/QI programs can take a variety of forms, often the cornerstone of a QA/QI program is its (investigator) auditing function, because it is an effective means to evaluate compliance and an opportunity to identify ways to improve performance (**Figure 7.4-1**).

Table 7.4-1 Comparing Types of Oversight

Oversight Type	Activities	Reason & Intent	May Result in	Who Provides Oversight	Required?
Audit	Assess Compliance, data collection and study conduct through on-site review of following (not limited to): ■ Approved protocol ■ Regulatory requirements ■ Sponsor SOPs ■ Institutional Policies ■ Good Clinical Practices ■ Subject records ■ Regulatory documents ■ Study conduct: research staff interviews and document review ■ Compare CRFs (de-identified data) with source documents (identifiable)	■ Quality Assurance ■ Can be conducted at any time during study "Compliance Snapshot" ■ Conducted by someone in-dependent of the study; cannot be study monitor ■ Evaluate study processes ■ Ultimate goal is to ensure study is conducted in compliance with applicable regulatory requirements and Good Clinical Practices pertaining to human subjects, protections.	■ Changes to study processes, design, and monitoring (SOPs, protocol) ■ Changes to policies and procedures (IRB/HRPP)	■ Sponsor ■ Institution: internal QA/QI program, IRB, HRPP	No regulation specifically requires a sponsor or institution conduct audits during a study.
Monitoring		■ Quality Control ■ Ongoing, planned, and frequent oversight ■ Conducted by someone familiar with the study, usually a sponsor-monitor ■ Evaluate site progress ■ Ultimate goal to ensure the reliability and validity of data used for analysis	■ Data corrections (queries) ■ Staff training and education	■ Sponsor	FDA requires sponsors of FDA-regulated research conduct ongoing monitoring
Inspection		■ Assess data integrity and reliability ■ Ensure overall compliance ■ Determine whether to accept supporting data	■ Accept or not accept data to support research for publication, marketing application	■ Regulatory authorities	No regulations specifically require inspections, though regulatory agencies have the authority to conduct inspections as they deem necessary.
Data and Safety Monitoring	Evaluation focuses on results: data, adverse events, and study progress	■ Ongoing, planned oversight of results ■ Protect subject/patient safety ■ IRB responsible for ensuring adequate plan	■ Study termination ■ Change in study design, stopping rules	■ Group of experts, independent of sponsor or lead investigator ■ One member is a statistician	Regulations require IRBs to ensure that the research plan includes an adequate ongoing monitoring of data

Modified from Ruppert, M. P. (2004). Defining the Meaning of 'Auditing' and 'Monitoring' & Clarifying the Appropriate Use of the Terms. AHIA/HICCA focus group. ahia.org/assets/Uploads/pdfUpload/WhitePapers/DefiningAuditingAndMonitoring.pdf

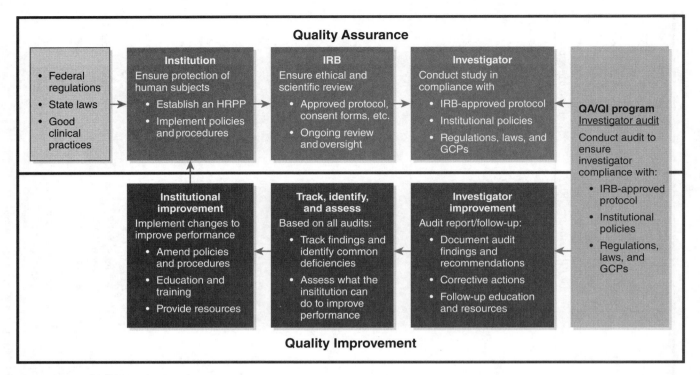

Figure 7.4-1 QA/QI continuous improvement.

Developing a QA/QI program

🔗 2-1   The planning of a QA/QI program should involve all stakeholders of the HRPP, including institutional officials, the IRB, and researchers. Establishing a QA/QI program as a collaboration will help to facilitate the perception that the program is intended to serve as an educational resource and not another punitive obstacle. It may also serve to leverage a common interest across various compliance units that intersect with IRB-related business.

Some key points to consider when developing a QA/QI program are as follows:

- *Institutional endorsement*: Before developing a program, it is important to understand what the institutional officials will support in terms of scope of authority and resources. The scope of who will be audited and what will be audited will be defined by institutional support. Consider what would happen if an audit is questioned or challenged: will the institutional officials back up your program?
- *Scope of authority*: Although this chapter focuses on auditing the researcher, it does not mean a QA/QI program is limited to investigator audits. Work with institutional officials to determine who within the HRPP will be audited.
- *Independence*: A distinguishing factor of an audit is that it is conducted by someone who is independent from the process being evaluated. If the QA/QI program is tasked with auditing the IRB, consider whether the QA/QI program could effectively carry out this mission if structured as a function of the IRB.
- *Resources*: The number of audits and scope of each audit (depth and length of each audit) are dependent on available resources.
- *Access to records*: The records available determine what a program is able to audit. Will the program have access to IRB records to help prepare for an audit? Will an auditor have access to study records, source documents, and medical records on site?

- *Study selection*: Define the scope of the audit. Resources and institutional endorsement will affect which studies are selected for audit. Selection criteria can include study type (e.g., greater than minimal risk, studies active for at least 1 year).
- *Approach*: Set a nonpunitive tone by structuring the audit process as an educational opportunity. Audits should not only identify what to correct, but help researchers implement corrective changes through education and providing resources. The QA/QI program should become a resource available during and after an audit.
- *Audit summary reports*: How will audit findings be summarized and reported to institutional officials? How often should summary reports be prepared (e.g., quarterly or annually)? Who will receive summary reports? Entities that receive and review the report should be able to implement decisive follow-up actions in a timely manner (see previous description of "Institutional Endorsement").

QA/QI Program Models

When considering where an audit program best fits within an HRPP, it is important to ensure that the program maintains the flexibility to provide independent and objective assessments. Once again, resources, scope of authority, and institutional endorsement will be factors in determining a program model (**Table 7.4-2**).

Table 7.4-2 QA/QI Program Models

Model	Description
Function of an IRB	QA/QI initiatives and services considered the responsibility of the IRB office (in addition to IRB administrative duties). Pro: good option if resources are limited (e.g., available staffing and/or space) or the number of studies do not justify an independent program or dedicated full-time employee. Con: would not be able to audit the IRB without perception of bias; the researcher may perceive that not-for-cause audits are related to the IRB review process (initial or continuing).
Independent program (separate from IRB)	QA/QI initiatives and services provided by dedicated staff and independent of IRB responsibilities. Pro: facilitates broader evaluation of HRPP/IRB without any bias or conflict. An audit program that is independent from both the researcher and IRB role can identify deficiencies resulting from the researcher-IRB relationship by improving the review process and facilitating communication. Pro: when a QA/QI program is able to audit all entities of an HRPP, it emphasizes that the onus of compliance is not solely on the researcher. Con: this structure may be cost prohibitive for smaller institutions where HRPP staff cover multiple roles/responsibilities.
External group	QA/QI services by contract with an outside consultant or contract research organization (CRO). Pro: may be good option for smaller institutions with minimal studies that do not justify dedicating resources to an audit program. Con: an external auditor may have additional obstacles of not being familiar with the institutional research culture and policies and procedures and may not easily access research and medical records and navigate electronic systems.
Collaborative	QA/QI services are shared among participating programs as part of a collaborative group. Pro: may be good option for a smaller institution with limited resources or to introduce objectivity. Con: same as External Group model above; also this model does not guarantee equal benefit/balance of resources.

Anatomy of an Investigator Audit

Although QA/QI programs can take a variety of forms, a key feature is its investigator/researcher auditing function. Take time to thoughtfully plan and organize the audit process to ensure it will adequately capture the information needed to make sound determinations of compliance. Note that what is considered "adequate" will depend on the institutional endorsement and scope of authority. The threshold of what is considered noncompliant can vary greatly, so work closely with institutional officials to understand what the institutional threshold will be. Having an organized audit plan will help on-site efficiency, avoid redundancy, and foster consistency among auditors and between audits. Ensuring consistency in audit practices is important to the reliability of key findings and trends, which may be used in making larger, institutional changes (e.g., policy changes, available resources, educational materials).

An investigator audit may be broken down into four distinct stages: preparation, on-site engagement, report and resolution, and follow-up. A summary of the key tasks associated with each stage is described next.

Preparation

Depending on the nature of the audit, it may first be necessary to identify a study to review. This is often an essential starting point for a not-for-cause audit. In contrast, for-cause audits are often prompted by an IRB or Institutional Official request and typically involve situations where additional information is needed in order to facilitate IRB review—e.g., researcher noncompliance or subject complaint. Although not-for-cause audits may be the result of researcher request, most are likely in response to institutional triggers. Such triggers are useful in encouraging auditing for voluntary or developing QA/QI programs that have not yet established their reputation. See **Table 7.4-3** for some examples of audit triggers and requestors, which differ depending on the type of audit.

Once a study is identified, some level of notification is necessary. The nature of the audit may help determine how much advance notice and instruction are appropriate. For example, an institution may provide shorter notice with for-cause audits—e.g., 24 hours—but allow greater advance notice with the

🔗 7-6

Table 7.4-3 Audit Triggers and Requestors

Audit Type	Triggers	Requestors
For-cause	Potential compliance concern Potential subject safety concern	IRB Institutional official
Not-for-cause	External audit preparation Prior compliance concerns—e.g., follow-up of prior for-cause audits Institutional compliance concerns, e.g., sponsor-investigator studies; studies transitioned or subject to the Common Rule 2018 Requirements Evaluation of new or revised policy	Principal investigator/ study staff IRB QA/QI program (per program scope/ authority)

not-for-cause variety—e.g., 2 to 4 weeks. At a minimum, this notification should explain how the QA/QI program has identified the study for an audit and what is expected, if anything, of the research team during the audit process. A note about records access: Access to facilities and study records is paramount to the success of an audit. As such, a QA/QI program is wise to outline the expectations about access in its initial notification of subsequent information prior to on-site engagement.

Prior to going on site, an auditor should be familiar with the study under review. This could be done by reviewing the IRB study file and, if applicable, IRB meeting minutes. Such a practice, however, requires that the HRPP structure permits the QA/QI program access to its records, whether those exist in hard copy or electronic format. This may be easier for smaller programs that share physical space and/or human resources. While not discussed in detail in this chapter, a QA/QI program may leverage this preparation into an IRB file audit. This practice could be an initial step for a program striving to expand its scope beyond researcher compliance.

> ## REAL-TIME COMPLIANCE
>
> When considering notification of audit, another relevant factor is a more philosophical question: is it valuable to the institution to evaluate *real-time* compliance? Or, is advance notice—and, therefore, the researcher's capacity to prepare—simply a means to an end when it comes to achieving compliance? Research illustrates that researcher self-assessment prior to on-site engagement can lead to greater compliance, i.e., fewer observations/findings (Wolf & O'Rourke, 2002).

On-Site Engagement

On-site engagement refers to the activities an auditor may perform *on site;* however, many audits can effectively occur remotely. Although not discussed in this chapter, available guidance from the Food and Drug Administration (FDA) discusses remote monitoring (FDA, 2013). Instead, the discussion that follows considers the customary practice whereby an auditor physically reviews documents at the study site(s).

Depending on the nature and/or scope of the audit, the auditor may carry out the following:

- Observe study conduct, including recruitment activities, consent process, and/or implementation of research procedures. When carrying out such activities, an auditor should seek prospective subject agreement prior to any observation.
- Review subject files. A QA/QI program should consider whether to review all available subject files or a sample. When a sample is found to be appropriate, consideration should be given to how files will be identified. To support auditor objectivity, selecting files at random is ideal, and applications exist to help facilitate this practice. For example, an online random sequence generator (such as at random.org) might be used to create a list of subject file numbers in random order. From there, an auditor could take the first 10% to review.
- Review regulatory documentation. Regulatory documentation is oftentimes maintained in a "regulatory binder." The regulatory binder refers to an organizational system that compiles all those documents—"essential documents" according to GCP—that demonstrate and support study compliance and protocol adherence. Such materials may be maintained as hard copy, electronically, or a combination.

On-site engagement most often concludes with an exit interview or simply a summary of preliminary findings. An exit interview can solicit valuable information that provides helpful context to the observations made on

REPORT DISTRIBUTION

At a minimum, the audit report is for the researcher and becomes part of the QA/QI program's records. In addition, an organization must determine when to include additional stakeholders, such as the institutional official and IRB, assuming they are not routinely copied. For example, a QA/QI program may adhere to a policy whereby the IRB is only copied on its for-cause audit reports, unless a not-for-cause report indicates potential serious/continuing noncompliance and/or unanticipated problems involving risk to subjects or others. A QA/QI program should carefully craft its distribution expectations, because it may have implications for what a researcher must share with a federal agency and/or sponsor.

site. For example, it may allow the auditor to better evaluate oversight of the study by the principal investigator (PI), confirm a particular practice in relation to what was observed during the audit, or facilitate understanding of the root cause of observed noncompliance. This exchange between the study team and the auditor also allows for the exchange of additional information and/or clarification, as necessary. When time allows, an auditor may take the opportunity to provide focused education to the researcher and study staff.

Report and Resolution

The auditor should distribute a report within a reasonable time frame, such as 2 weeks. As described in the *Quality Assurance and Quality Improvement Handbook for Human Research* (Howes et al., 2019), the following elements should be included in an audit report:

1. Cover page
   a. Protocol
   b. Investigator name
   c. Date of review
   d. Date of report
   e. QA/QI reviewer(s)
2. Introduction
   a. Purpose of site review
   b. Individuals present at meeting
   c. Material reviewed at the time of site review (e.g., regulatory documentation, all consent forms, and subject files for XX of YY subjects)
3. Observations
   a. Provide specific examples and sufficient detail so the site can identify individual errors
   b. Consider providing regulatory references and corrective actions
4. Conclusion
   a. Summarize the site review and provide contact for questions
   b. Consider identifying priorities for the site
   c. Consider "grading" the report
   d. If response from the site is required, identify timeline for response

Follow-up

Post-audit activities will vary across QA/QI programs. Some options may include the following:

- No further action for researcher and/or QA/QI program.
- Confirmation that corrective actions have been implemented. Such confirmation may be performed by the QA/QI program or through researcher attestation, depending on the scope of the audit and/or nature of corrective actions. For example, an organization may prefer that the QA/QI program return on site to confirm reconciliation for an audit in which the IRB determined there was serious <u>noncompliance</u>. Alternatively, researcher attestation may be sufficient for a not-for-cause audit where the primary finding was incomplete training documentation.

🖉 7-6

- <u>Education</u>. Depending on the observations made on site, QA/QI programs may return to offer focused training. Topics may complement those in need of further explanation, as highlighted in the audit report, but also cover areas of interest to the researcher and/or study staff.

🔖 8-5

Developing a Standard Operating Procedure for Investigator Audits

As mentioned previously, consistency among auditors and between audits is important to ensure overall reliability of key findings. Developing a standard operating procedure (SOP) for conducting investigator audits can facilitate overall consistency by providing written step-by-step instructions. Written SOPs can also foster transparency and trust with the research community by setting expectations.

The following are some considerations to include in an SOP for an investigator audit (for descriptions of corresponding templates, see **Table 7.4-4**):

- *Selection and notification*: Method of study and subject selection and process of notification. Templates may include notification memo and information sheet for researchers of what to expect during audit process.
- *Scope of audit*: List areas to be audited (e.g., consent process, recruitment, regulatory documents), documents required for audit (both for audit prep and on-site review), and who needs to be available during on-site audit. Templates may include audit checklist and researcher interview script.
- *Define noncompliance*: Identify what would be considered noncompliance or area of concern. Note that this should be consistent with institutional and IRB policies of noncompliance and reportable events.
- *Audit reports and researcher follow-up*: Outline process for required corrective actions and recommendation (best practices) and timeline for sending completed report and researcher follow-up (if required). Templates may include report template.

Table 7.4-4 Common Tools and Templates

Investigator QA Audit Common Tools and Templates	
Tool	**Purpose**
Audit notification memo Information sheet for what to expect during an audit	Makes audit preparation more efficient by automating the notification process Prepares researchers for what to expect and describes how to prepare to help minimize the number of questions a researcher may have before an audit
Audit checklist	Helps auditor prepare for an audit by providing a comprehensive list of things that need to be completed during the audit Defines the scope of an audit by including only the topics and items to be evaluated and the parameters of each Minimizes potential inconsistencies between auditors, which is important for identifying trends in overall performance
Interview script	Minimizes potential inconsistencies between auditors (i.e., can provide prompts to encourage consistency in how each auditor approaches each interview)
Audit report outline	Ensures consistency in reports Makes report writing a more efficient and organized process

- *Audit summary report (from all audits)*: Outline method to track findings. Provide a list of who should receive summary reports (e.g., institutional officials, IRB) and the frequency with which summary reports will be provided (e.g., quarterly, annually, after every 25 audits completed).

References

Association for the Accreditation of Human Research Protection Programs (AAHRPP). (2018). *AAHRPP evaluation instrument.* www.aahrpp.org

Food and Drug Administration (FDA). (2013). *Guidance for industry oversight of clinical investigations: A risk-based approach to monitoring.* www.fda.gov/media/116754/download

Food and Drug Administration (FDA). (2018). *E6(R2) Good Clinical Practice: Integrated addendum to ICH E6(R1) guidance for industry.* www.fda.gov/downloads/Drugs/Guidances/UCM464506.pdf

Howes, L. M., White, S. A., & Bierer, B. E. (2019). *Quality assurance and quality improvement handbook for human research.* Johns Hopkins University Press.

International Council for Harmonisation of Technical Requirements for Pharmaceuticals for Human Use (ICH). (n.d.). *Good Clinical Practice guidelines.* ichgcp.net

Ruppert, M. P. (2004). *Defining the meaning of "auditing" and "monitoring" and clarifying the appropriate use of the terms.* AHIA/HCCA focus group. ahia.org/assets/Uploads/pdfUpload/WhitePapers/DefiningAuditingAndMonitoring.pdf

Wolf, D., & O'Rourke, P. (2002). Ensuring investigator compliance and improving study site performance: Implementing a quality assurance and quality improvement program in academic health center. *Clinical Researcher, 2*(5).Report Distribution

Protocol Deviations and Eligibility Exceptions

Joy Jurnack

Kelley A. O'Donoghue

Abstract

The identification and management of protocol deviations can be challenging for IRBs, researchers, and sponsors. Lack of consistency and specificity in federal regulations regarding the definition of deviations and absence of specific guidance on review and reporting requirements contribute to a variety of approaches to the management of these occurrences in research. IRBs must develop specific definitions to cover a wide range of deviation events and ensure that researchers are educated on requirements to identify, report, and obtain prospective approval of deviations when appropriate.

Conduct of Research Under an Approved Protocol

Human subjects research must be conducted under a protocol approved by an IRB and, as applicable, a study sponsor. Both the Common Rule and the Food and Drug Administration (FDA) regulations require that the researcher carry out the research in compliance with the IRB-approved protocol. The FDA requires that a sponsor monitor the research for instances where the approved protocol is not followed. The researcher may also be responsible for adhering to the International Council for Harmonisation guidance on Good Clinical Practice (ICH-GCP), which endorses similar requirements regarding IRB approval and monitoring of study conduct. However, both the federal regulations and the ICH-GCP acknowledge that the protocol may change over time as the research is carried out and (in somewhat varied ways) identify how changes should be handled by the researcher, the IRB, and the sponsor. These changes are often referred to collectively as "deviations" from the approved protocol, whether intentional or unintentional, and include a wide variety of changes and exceptions. A comprehensive review of the similarities and differences in specific requirements and language used to address deviations is provided in

🔗 8-2

the Secretary's Advisory Committee on Human Research Protections (SACHRP) recommendations to the DHHS Secretary (Department of Health and Human Services, 2012). The relevant text from the regulations and ICH-GCP are noted here:

> The Common Rule regulations require that the IRB "establish and follow written procedures for…ensuring that investigators will conduct the research activity in accordance with the terms of the IRB approval until any proposed changes have been reviewed and approved by the IRB, except when necessary to eliminate apparent immediate hazards to the subjects." [45 CFR 46.108(a)(3)(ii)]

> The FDA regulations require that the IRB "follow written procedures for ensuring that changes in approved research… may not be initiated without IRB review and approval except where necessary to eliminate apparent immediate hazards to human subjects." [21 CFR 56.108(a)(2)]

> The ICH-GCP states "The investigator should not implement any deviation from, or changes of the protocol without agreement by the sponsor and prior review and documented approval/favourable opinion from the IRB/IEC of an amendment, except where necessary to eliminate an immediate hazard(s) to trial subjects, or when the change(s) involves only logistical or administrative aspects of the trial (e.g., change in monitor(s), change of telephone number(s))" (ICH, 2016).

Defining Protocol Deviations

There is no single definition of "deviation" across the federal regulations and their associated guidance documents. This is reflected in the varied definitions and approaches that IRBs and sponsors have developed to identify and address these events. Often the terms "protocol violation" or "noncompliance" are used in place of or in addition to "protocol deviation" or "deviation." Some IRBs go further in categorizing deviations into "minor" or "major" and/or "serious" or "non-serious." These categorizations often are used to differentiate levels of risk or impact on the scientific validity of research. Regardless of the terminology used, IRBs should create a definition such that researchers clearly understand what the term encompasses, as well as when, how, and to whom they must report events included in the definition. In developing a definition, the IRB should also consider whether the research they oversee is conducted under the Common Rule, FDA regulations, and/or ICH-GCP to ensure compliance with the specific requirements of each.

The FDA's *Compliance Program Guidance Manual* provides an example of how a deviation could be defined, which may be used as a guide for IRBs developing their own definition:

> A protocol deviation/violation is generally an unplanned excursion from the protocol that is not implemented or intended as a systematic change. A protocol deviation could be a limited prospective exception to the protocol (e.g. agreement between sponsor and investigator to enroll a single subject who does not meet all inclusion/exclusion criteria). Like protocol amendments, deviations initiated by the clinical investigator must be reviewed and approved by the IRB and the sponsor prior to implementation, unless the change is necessary to eliminate apparent immediate hazards to the human subjects (21 CFR 312.66), or to

protect the life or physical wellbeing of the subject (21 CFR 812.35(a)(2)), and generally communicated to FDA. "Protocol deviation" is also used to refer to any other, unplanned, instance(s) of protocol non-compliance. For example, situations in which the investigator failed to perform tests or examinations as required by the protocol or failures on the part of study subjects to complete scheduled visits as required by the protocol, would be considered protocol deviations . . . (FDA, 2008)

An important idea in this definition is that a deviation is not usually considered to be a "systematic" change to the approved protocol. Rather it is a one-time change, perhaps to accommodate a single event or situation with a single subject. The systematic changes that commonly occur in research are often called "amendments" or "modifications" and denote a prospective change that is approved prospectively by the IRB and documented through a written protocol change that becomes a part of the overall approved protocol. However, IRBs may choose to include amendments or modifications as a subset of deviations or may define them as separate events from deviations.

🖉 7-1

The definition should also recognize that deviations may occur intentionally or unintentionally and can include deviations by the research team or the research subjects. Examples of common intentional deviations include when a researcher wants to enroll a subject that does not meet all eligibility criteria (e.g., they are outside of an age range, laboratory values are not within required limits, or insufficient time has elapsed since prior therapies), or a research subject needs to have their study visit outside of the visit window because they are traveling. Unintentional deviations can be quite varied and often can include those that relate to the subject not following the protocol. These might include not showing up for a scheduled study visit, not taking study drug appropriately, or not returning drug or study diaries as required. The research team may also be responsible for unintentional deviations, for example, by failing to do a required screening procedure, not noticing that an eligibility requirement has not been met, not conducting all required procedures at a study visit, or failing to maintain an accurate delegation log. These unintentional deviations may be recognized by the research team after they have occurred, or they may be identified through internal monitoring programs or externally by the sponsor or the FDA.

Procedures for Reporting and Review of Deviations

The IRB should develop written procedures for researchers to report deviations and to describe how the IRB will review the reports. The institution should also have procedures that require corrective and preventive action plans (CAPAs) be developed to address unintentional deviations. These procedures should identify who is responsible for developing the CAPAs and who confirms that they have been fully implemented.

🖉 2-3

Because deviations may include a wide range of events, it may be useful for the IRB to develop a table or matrix with examples of different types of deviations, which includes how quickly they should be reported, how they should be reported, and how they will be reviewed. This should be readily accessible to the researcher as a reference document, such as on a website to support compliance with the requirement. The IRB should also clearly state that reporting requirements to sponsors may differ and that the researcher is responsible for compliance with both the sponsor reporting requirements as well as the IRB requirements. In addition, if researchers are using multiple IRBs to oversee their research, they are responsible for understanding and tracking how each IRB defines a deviation and knowing the requirements for reporting, which will likely vary across IRBs.

Categorizing unintentional deviations into minor/major or serious/non-serious as discussed earlier may help researchers understand when to report to the IRB. For example, a study subject completing their study visit 1 day outside of the study window may be defined as a "minor" deviation, especially if it did not impact the safety of the subject or the integrity of the research. This type of deviation may not require immediate reporting to the IRB and may be included in a listing or summary of minor deviations at the time of continuing review. However, a major deviation might be a failure to obtain subject consent prior to research activities occurring. This deviation would be reportable on a more immediate basis (e.g., within 3 working days) through some type of "reportable event" form, which is then quickly reviewed within the IRB system.

⏴ 7-2

Intentional deviations should be reported to and approved by the IRB before they occur, unless it is a deviation to eliminate an immediate hazard. As previously discussed, a researcher requesting an eligibility exception or a change in treatment for a single subject are common examples of intentional deviations.

⏴ 5-5
⏴ 5-7

Approval of this type of deviation may occur through usual expedited or full board review processes, or IRBs may have a specialized review process to be able to quickly respond to these exception or deviation requests. For example, a single expedited reviewer may be tasked with reviewing all exception requests that are submitted on a specialized exception form, or requests requiring full board review may be prioritized on meeting schedules. IRBs should recognize that the regulations do not identify a review path for intentional deviations outside of the expedited or full board review requirements. IRBs who wish to review these quickly will need to develop efficient methods of conducting the regulatory expedited or full board reviews for these deviations.

⏴ 7-6 ⏴ 7-3

Deviations may also be considered noncompliance or unanticipated problems involving risks to subjects or others (UPIRTSO) under an IRB's definitions of those terms. For example, the deviation of failure to obtain written consent prior to a subject participating in research activities could meet the definition of serious noncompliance and be reportable as such to federal regulatory agencies. A deviation of a subject taking double the dose of an investigational product by accident may be considered UPIRTSO and also require regulatory reporting. IRBs should include processes and procedures to decide whether a deviation meets these other definitions.

Although not specifically an IRB responsibility, the IRB should encourage and support an institutional approach to requiring researchers to develop written procedures for identifying and tracking deviations, especially in research that is not sponsored and would thus need to develop their own procedures and tracking mechanisms.

Additional Considerations for Eligibility Exceptions

The Common Rule and the FDA regulations do not mention or define eligibility exceptions. When an IRB approves a protocol, the review of the eligibility criteria confirms that it meets the requirements for appropriate selection of subjects. The IRB considers whether the research is designed to include those individuals who will potentially benefit from participation and exclude those who may be at increased risk. Therefore, the idea of an eligibility exception may be particularly challenging to assess. According to the regulations, any modification to an IRB-approved protocol must be reviewed and approved by the IRB before it is implemented, "except when necessary to eliminate apparent immediate hazards to the subject" [45 CFR 46.108(a)(3)(iii)]. In this case, an eligibility exception does not eliminate harm because the patient/subject is not yet enrolled.

Typically, the information submitted to the IRB includes justification for the eligibility exception, and it should demonstrate that an appropriate risk/benefit ratio is maintained and that the scientific integrity of the study is not diminished. If there is a study sponsor, they would also need to approve any eligibility exceptions, and the IRB should consider whether these may occur in parallel or if the IRB would only consider those exceptions first approved by the sponsor.

Eligibility exceptions may also provide the researcher (and sponsor, as applicable) with insight into future protocol <u>amendments</u> needed to revise the eligibility criteria. When requested exceptions to the same eligibility requirements become frequent, the IRB should consider whether it will require such amendments prior to granting additional exceptions.

🖉 7-1

Conclusion

Researchers and IRB professionals should understand the concept of protocol deviations and have robust written <u>policies and procedures</u> defining these terms and the associated reporting requirements. These policies and procedures should be consistent with the regulatory requirements and guidance under which the research is conducted, and researchers must understand their responsibilities in obtaining prior approval for planned deviations and for monitoring, reporting, and correcting unintentional deviations.

🖉 2-3

Acknowledgment

The authors wish to thank Martha Jones for her contribution to this chapter.

References

Department of Health and Human Services (DHHS). (2012). *SACHRP letter to the HHS Secretary: Attachment C: Recommendation on protocol deviations*. www.hhs.gov/ohrp/sachrp-committee/recommendations/2012-march-30-letter-attachment-c/index.html

Food and Drug Administration (FDA). (2008). *Program 7348.811 Chapter 48-Bioresearch: Monitoring clinical investigators and sponsor-investigators*. www.fda.gov/media/75927/download

International Council for Harmonisation of Technical Requirements for Pharmaceuticals for Human Use (ICH). (2016). *Integrated Addendum to ICH E6(R1): Guideline for Good Clinical Practice E6(R2)*. Database.ich.org/sites/default/files/E6_R2_Addendum.pdf

Noncompliance and Complaints

Susie R. Hoffman

Lynn E. Smith

Abstract

Complaints about a study or allegations of noncompliance may range in seriousness from a subject's not receiving their study compensation to nonadherence to an IRB-approved protocol. The IRB may learn about complaints, or allegations from a subject, an internal audit, or a call from a whistleblower. Regardless of the source and severity of the issue, according to **45 CFR 46.108(a)(4)**, the IRB must have policies and procedures in place to investigate, report, and resolve the issue. This process may involve communications with internal compliance offices within the institution engaged in the human subjects research or require reports to external federal agencies. If the reviewing IRB is external to the institution engaged in human subjects research, communication between the IRB and the human research protection program (HRPP) of the institution will also be required.

Federal Regulations

The IRB must have <u>policies and procedures</u> in place to investigate, report, and resolve "unanticipated problems involving risks to subjects or others or any serious or continuing noncompliance with this policy or the requirements or determinations of the IRB"; and "[a]ny suspension or termination of IRB approval" [45 CFR 46.108(a)(4)]. In addition, "[a]n IRB shall have authority to suspend or terminate approval of research that is not being conducted in accordance with the IRB's requirements or that has been associated with unexpected harm to subjects. Any suspension or termination of approval shall include a statement of the reasons for the IRB's action and shall be reported promptly to the investigator, appropriate institutional officials, and the agency or department head" [45 CFR 46.113]. The Food and Drug Administration has similar language at **21 CFR 56.108** and **21 CFR 56.113**.

✐ 2-3

Institutional Policy

To provide consistency and compliance with the regulations, it is essential for HRPPs and the reviewing IRB to develop and follow policies regarding suspected noncompliance and complaints. Individuals with knowledge of federal regulations and institutional requirements should be involved in the creation of the policy. It is important that the policy interface with other institutional policies such as the scientific misconduct policy, the <u>conflict of interest</u> policy, and the <u>unanticipated problems</u> involving risks to subjects or others policy. Institutional policy should include definitions of key concepts to enable compliance, as suggested in the box.

🔗 12-6
🔗 7-3

NONCOMPLIANCE POLICY EXAMPLE

As part of its commitment to protecting the rights and welfare of human subjects in research, the institution reviews all reports of complaints or suspected noncompliance and takes any necessary action to ensure the ethical conduct of research. All investigators and other study personnel involved in human subjects research are required to comply with all laws and regulations governing their research activities, as well as with requirements and determinations of the HRPP.

Definitions

- *Noncompliance*: Failure to adhere to federal, state, or local regulations governing human subjects research, organizational policies related to human subjects research, or the requirements or determinations of the IRB. Noncompliance may be minor or sporadic, or it may be serious or continuing.
- *Serious noncompliance*: Noncompliance that, in the judgment of the convened IRB, creates an increase in risks to subjects; adversely affects the rights, welfare, or safety of subjects; or adversely affects the scientific integrity of the study. Willful violation of regulations and/or policies may also constitute serious noncompliance.
- *Continuing noncompliance*: A pattern of noncompliance that, in the judgment of the convened IRB, suggests a likelihood that instances of noncompliance will continue unless the IRB or organization intervenes.
- *Allegation of noncompliance*: An unproved assertion of noncompliance.
- *Finding of noncompliance*: An allegation of noncompliance that is proven true or a report of noncompliance that is clearly true. (For example, a finding on an audit of an unsigned consent document or an admission of an investigator of that the protocol/research plan was willfully not followed represent reports of noncompliance that would require no further action to determine their truth and therefore represent findings of noncompliance.) Once a finding of noncompliance is proven, it must be categorized as minor, serious, sporadic, or continuing.

Establishing Procedures

Following acceptance of the HRPP noncompliance policy by the institutional official (IO) and other key positions within the HRPP, individual offices will need to establish procedures for implementing the policy including a range of options depending on the relative seriousness of the report.

All reports are important to review; however, each instance need not be subjected to the same level of scrutiny. It is appropriate to investigate and respond to the complaint or report of suspected noncompliance relative to its level of seriousness. Some reports will clearly be more serious than others. For example, forming a subcommittee and conducting an extensive audit would not be appropriate for the isolated use of an outdated consent form.

More detailed suggestions or preferences may be included in institutional guidance documents. These guidance documents should include specifics of how different offices within the HRPP will work together if overlapping responsibilities are identified (e.g., when a report of noncompliance is determined to be scientific misconduct). Details may include information such as which office will take the lead in an investigation and which offices will submit reports to outside agencies.

✎ 2-1

If the study is overseen by an IRB outside of the institution engaged in human subjects research, it is also critical to include in the procedure or guidance document a plan for communication with the reviewing IRB regarding a complaint or a report of suspected noncompliance.

Distribution of the Policy and Procedures

After the policy and procedures are written it is imperative that they are distributed to the research community, including study team members, IRB staff and members, and institutional compliance offices. This may be accomplished in several ways, including publication on websites, in researchers' guides, or referred to in IRB approval letters. The policy and procedures may be combined into one document or separated with all policies in one document and procedures in a separate document.

Reporting Mechanisms

Institutions also need to establish a mechanism for the research community to report to the institution's IRB or HRPP a complaint or suspected noncompliance. Various mechanisms have been used by institutions, including providing phone numbers, email addresses, or hard copy addresses. These can be used to report in either an identifiable or anonymous fashion. To enhance efficiency, institutions may develop template reporting forms that can be used to submit a complaint or report of suspected noncompliance, and template letters that the institution's HRPP can use to prepare notification of such reports to sponsors, federal agencies, and/or the Association for the Accreditation of Human Research Protection Programs (AAHRPP). The reporting form may include the following:

✎ 8-7

- Study title
- Principal investigator name
- Date of the suspected noncompliance
- Date the study team became aware of the issue
- A thorough description of the issue
- Opinion of the study team regarding increased risk to subjects or if the rights and welfare of the subjects have been affected
- Corrective action plan, which may include planned modifications to the study, re-consent, and/or additional education
- Information to determine if a data breach may have occurred (if the IRB also serves as the Health Insurance Portability and Accountability Act (HIPAA) Privacy Board)
- Optional section for the name and contact information for the individual submitting the report

Receiving Allegations of Noncompliance

Sometimes, it is clear that an allegation of noncompliance has merit, and immediate action should be taken to protect human subjects, such as suspending research or enrollment. However, in some instances the allegation clearly does not reach this level of seriousness and can be handled via a different review process.

Establishing an Investigative Committee

There may be times when an allegation of noncompliance is brought forward, and it is not immediately clear whether the allegation has a basis in fact. When this occurs, it may be best to establish an investigative committee to gather facts through review of documentation and interviews with key personnel. The committee's charge is to determine whether the allegation has a basis in fact, and if so, whether the noncompliance is determined to be serious or continuing noncompliance. Smaller institutions may want to identify a key individual or individuals who will carry out the investigation in lieu of a committee (using essentially the same process). The IO, or designee, should appoint members to the investigative committee based on the expertise and background needed to evaluate the allegation; appoint a chair of the investigative committee; and charge the investigative committee with the question to be answered. The affected investigator should be notified that an investigation is being conducted, what the allegation is that is being evaluated, and the time frame for completion.

The investigative committee should carry out these procedures within 60 days, because allegations resulting in serious or continuing noncompliance may require prompt reporting to federal agencies, sponsors, or others. The investigative committee should first determine whether a suspension of the research is necessary to protect human subjects. After this determination, the committee should review the information to decide, based on a preponderance of the evidence and by majority vote, whether the allegation has a basis in fact.

Investigative Process

The committee should determine what information it will need to review and what individuals it will need to interview. The committee should begin to gather information and interview individuals as quickly as possible. If the investigative committee believes that a transcription of the interviews will be required to make a proper decision, the investigative committee should record all interviews. The committee should repeat information gathering and interviews as reasonable until a decision can be made. The investigative committee should provide a written report of the investigative committee's decision to the IO or designee.

Investigative Committee Findings

If the investigation finds that the allegation has no basis in fact, the investigation will be considered complete, and this determination should be communicated as appropriate. If the investigation finds a basis in fact, the committee should submit its finding in the written report to the IO, and the IRB should work with the investigators and study teams involved in the finding of noncompliance, as described next.

Reviewing Findings of Noncompliance

Findings of Noncompliance That Are Neither Serious nor Continuing

If there is a finding of noncompliance that is neither serious nor continuing, the IRB should work with the individual or group responsible for the noncompliance to develop and implement a suitable corrective action plan. If the individual or group responsible for the noncompliance is unwilling to work with the IRB to develop and implement a suitable corrective action plan, the IRB should consider the noncompliance to be continuing noncompliance and follow the procedures for serious or continuing noncompliance (described next).

Findings of Noncompliance That Are Determined to Be Serious or Continuing

Noncompliance that is determined to be serious or continuing should be reported to a <u>convened IRB</u> to determine what corrective actions, if any, need to be taken (see box for examples of possible actions), and to whom the serious or continuing noncompliance should be reported.

✎ 5-7

ACTIONS THAT MAY BE TAKEN BY THE CONVENED IRB

The convened IRB must determine whether any additional actions need to be taken when reviewing serious or continuing noncompliance, such as the following:

- Modifying the protocol
- Modifying the information disclosed during the consent process
- Providing additional information to current subjects when the information may relate to subjects' willingness to continue in the research
- Providing additional information to past subjects
- Obtaining re-consent of current subjects
- Increasing the frequency of continuing review
- Observing research activities or the consent process
- Requiring additional training of the investigator or study team
- Notifying investigators at other sites
- Terminating IRB approval
- Suspending IRB approval
- Transferring subjects to another investigator
- Arranging for clinical care outside the research
- Allowing continuation of some research activities under the supervision of an independent monitor or a different principal investigator
- Requiring follow-up of subjects for safety reasons
- Requiring adverse events or outcomes to be reported to the IRB and the sponsor
- Obtaining additional information
- Considering whether changes without prior IRB review and approval were consistent with ensuring subjects' continued welfare

---

When Action Is Taken to Suspend or Terminate Ongoing Research

When the IRB determines that an immediate suspension or termination of the research is necessary, the IRB should notify the investigator that all research activities must stop, including recruitment, advertisement, screening, enrollment, and consent procedures. The IRB should advise the investigator whether or not interventions, interactions, and collection or analysis of private identifiable information may be continued, if necessary, for the subjects' safety or welfare.

Reporting of Serious or Continuing Noncompliance

Serious or continuing noncompliance requires prompt reporting internally to the IO and appropriate department chair or dean and externally to sponsors (if applicable) and/or the Office for Human Research Protections (OHRP) and to the FDA when the research involves drugs, devices, or biologics. When reporting to federal agencies, it is best to report not only the issue of noncompliance but also the action plan that will be carried out to correct it.

Subject Complaints

Subject complaints that result in a finding of serious or continuing noncompliance should be processed according to review by a convened IRB, as described previously. Review of subject complaints might also result in a determination of an unanticipated problem that involves risk to subject or others.

7-3

Process to Handle Subject Complaints

When the IRB receives a question, concern, or complaint, the individual receiving it should document the nature of the question, concern, or complaint and the contact information of the person contacting the IRB. If possible, the IRB staff should respond to any questions or concerns and, when appropriate, should tell the person that they will follow up with them once they have been able to find additional information or an answer to their question, concern, or complaint. Following up with the subject is key to ensuring a culture of trust between the research institution and the research subject community. If the question, concern, or complaint cannot be easily resolved or answered, the investigative process described previously should be followed to determine if it suggests an issue of noncompliance.

IRB Review of Summary of Events at Time of Continuing Review

7-2

At the time of continuing review, the IRB should receive a summary of events, including the resulting resolution, of any noncompliance, complaints, and/or unanticipated problems involving risks to subjects or others or other adverse events.

Conclusion

Having a written policy and procedure in place to follow when a complaint or report of suspected noncompliance is received supports timely and appropriate review of each such report and helps ensure a consistent institutional approach to all allegations of noncompliance. Each report should be treated in a prompt, professional, confidential, and fair manner. Doing so promotes an environment in which individuals feel comfortable voicing their concerns, and researchers do not feel singled out when issues arise.

Closing a Study

John Baumann
Bethany Johnson

Abstract

Study closure is not addressed in the regulations and is only briefly mentioned in federal guidance. Despite the lack of regulatory requirements, institutions should be aware of the human subjects research being conducted by their personnel and under the oversight of their IRB. Therefore, policies and procedures should include a requirement for study closure, including explanations of when and how studies are closed with the IRB.

Regulations and Applicable Guidance

The two primary regulations under which IRBs operate are the Common Rule and FDA regulations: 45 CFR 46 and 21 CFR 56, respectively. However, in neither regulation is there a single reference to the obligation to or processes for "closing a study." The only reference to be found is in an information sheet for IRBs published by the FDA, which states "completion of the study is a change in activity and should be reported to the IRB," and this statement is guidance only, not a regulation (FDA, 1998).

Yet, in spite of the apparent lack of a regulatory mandate, virtually every human research protection program (HRPP) has instituted a requirement and process for closing out IRB approvals. From a strictly regulatory perspective, this may seem to be something of a paradox. The widespread inclusion of a "requirement" not found in the regulations is somewhat unusual in this era of reduction of administrative burden, in which many institutions have moved away from inclusion of virtually all nonregulatory requirements in their IRB policies and procedures. In fact, it is not uncommon for institutions to require extensive justification for introducing a nonregulatory requirement. However, from a practical, administrative, and quality assurance perspective, requiring study closure is a necessity. This chapter explores the why, when, and how of this "necessity."

🔗 2-1

Why Close Studies?

As indicated earlier, virtually every HRPP/IRB, whether it is large or small, and whether it focuses on clinical, translational, biomedical, or social/behavioral/ educational research, has a close-out process. An accurate picture of an institution's active research portfolio serves institutional and HRPP officials and should enhance human subject protections.

Knowledge

At the simplest level, institutions want to know what activities, including research, are being carried out in their names. No institutional official wants to get a call from the local newspaper, radio, or television station or an angry parent asking about a research project about which the official cannot provide relatively up-to-date information. An inability to respond to these inquiries is more than embarrassing; it may have significant and reputational impact.

Administrative Efficiency and Integrity

Being able to report how many and which studies are active enables HRPP leadership to align resources to workload and audit programs to select active studies for review. This information allows the institution to accurately report to both internal and external stakeholders the nature and amount of research its personnel are conducting.

Enhance Subject Protections

Most importantly, requiring closure of certain types of research can enhance human subject protections. Typically, when closure is required, study teams
⊘ 7-3   report information, such as final enrollment numbers, summaries of <u>adverse</u>
⊘ 7-6   <u>events</u>, a report of any <u>noncompliance</u> that occurred during the conduct of the study that did not otherwise require reporting to the IRB, and a brief statement regarding the outcomes of the study. Collecting this type of information allows the IRB to conduct a final review of accumulated information to ensure that regulatory requirements were met until completion of the study and that no additional risks arose that were not previously reported to the IRB. If any noncompliance or unexpected risks are discovered during review of study closure, the IRB can determine what actions, if any, are necessary to ensure subject protections and compliance with federal and institutional reporting requirements. This study-specific information, moreover, can and should be integrated with other close-out report information to form a collective portrait for planning
⊘ 2-7   HRPP <u>quality improvement</u> initiatives.

When to Close?

In addition to determining whether study closure is required, institutions must consider when study closure is appropriate. Study closure should not be permitted until the activities conducted by the study team no longer meet the definition of human subjects research. However, once use of identifiable information or biospecimens is completed, continued IRB oversight of the research is not required by the regulations, nor does IRB oversight serve to protect subjects. Additionally, a study may be closed because it was never and will not be initiated or because it was discontinued prior to its completion.

Institutions should provide specific guidance to researchers describing when study closure is appropriate. Commonly, researchers are instructed to report study closure when all access to and use of identifiable data are complete. Researchers are permitted to continue analysis of deidentified data, draft a manuscript or presentation, and pursue publication after closure of the study with the IRB.

It is important to note two cautions:

- Closing a study does not mean that the identifiable data has to be destroyed. In fact, many research agreements and institutional policies require such data to be securely maintained for a minimum or specified number of years. In such cases, the researcher certifies to the IRB at the time of closure that the identifiable data will be archived and not accessed. Any future access to the identifiable data would require either a new IRB submission or re-opening the closed study, depending on institutional policies.
- Just as research agreements often require the reporting of human subject complaints or problems for up to several years after the termination of the agreement, so should researchers report to the HRPP any human subject issues that come to their attention after closure of the study with the IRB.

How to Close?

The first major decision point in developing and implementing close-out processes involves determining to what studies closure applies: All research, including exemptions? All nonexempt research? Only greater than minimal risk research? While some institutions require a close-out process for all research, including exemptions, the most common approach is to require it for only nonexempt research, with exempt research given a presumed end date of a certain number of years after granting of exemption. Further questions must address whether the same process will be required for minimal and greater than minimal risk research and how (if at all) the elimination of the requirement for continuing review of minimal risk research impacts the implementation of the process.

✐ 5-3

Close-out reports for greater than minimal risk studies generally may request the following information:

- Total number of subjects who were enrolled, failed screening, or withdrew since the beginning of the study
- Reasons for subject withdrawal
- Information pertaining to any reportable events (either requiring prompt report or not requiring prompt report) since last IRB review
- Information pertaining to the data safety monitoring plan and available data safety monitoring reports, if applicable
- General information about study results, including trends and observations; whether subjects received benefits from participation; and whether there was any indication of a change in the risk to benefit assessment
- Significant findings from external sources, including literature reviews or external audits

For minimal risk research, some but generally not all of this information may be required. Institutions most often require submission of information regarding number of subjects participating, any unreported reportable events, and general information about study results; the remaining information may or may not have to be reported. Such reports are reviewed by the HRPP staff and accepted; no IRB review and approval are required (unless the closure report includes information related to unreported noncompliance, adverse events, or other reportable events that do require IRB review).

Conclusion

⊘ 8-4, 8-5
⊘ 2-7

Although study closure is not required by the regulations, close-out reports can be incorporated into an HRPP's overall <u>program of education</u> and <u>quality improvement</u>. Rather than just accepting and filing the reports, proactive HRPPs pull this information together and treat it as data for building educational outreach and quality improvement efforts. The process of requiring study closure can provide important information to help ensure the integrity and human subject protections that are the responsibility of the HRPP.

Reference

Food and Drug Administration (FDA). (1998). *Institutional review boards frequently asked questions: Guidance for institutional review boards and clinical investigators.* www.fda.gov/regulatory -information/search-fda-guidance-documents/institutional-review-boards-frequently-asked -questions

PART 8

Administration, Education, and Regulatory Issues

OHRP Federalwide Assurance

Irene Stith-Coleman

Abstract

This chapter describes the Federalwide Assurance (FWA) compliance process. By signing an FWA, an institution pledges to conduct its nonexempt Department of Health and Human Services (DHHS)-conducted or -supported human subjects research in compliance with the DHHS regulations at 45 CFR part 46. The Office for Human Research Protections (OHRP) approves FWAs for federalwide use, and other federal departments and agencies that have adopted the Federal Policy for the Protection of Human Subjects (Common Rule) accept an OHRP-approved FWA to cover the nonexempt research that they conduct or support. Since February 2005, the FWA has been the only type of assurance of compliance that OHRP accepts and approves. The revised Common Rule, which became effective June 19, 2018, modified the assurance requirements. The modified assurance requirements do not apply to research subject to the pre-2018 Requirements.

Assurance of Compliance

The FWA was introduced in 2000 to streamline and simplify the assurance process, and its use led to a significant decrease in administrative burdens for both submitting institutions and OHRP. The DHHS regulations require any institution engaged in nonexempt human subjects research conducted or supported by DHHS to provide OHRP written assurance of compliance with the 45 CFR 46 regulations. The only exception applies to international institutions. If OHRP determines that a procedural standard affords protections equivalent to the protections provided by 45 CFR 46, the institution may instead comply with such protections. The FWA also applies to research supported by any other federal department or agency that has adopted the Common Rule and relies on the FWA. The requirement for an FWA applies to both U.S. and international institutions. The institution must commit to follow the terms of the FWA, which can be found on OHRP's website (DHHS, 2016a). The institution also must certify to the federal department or agency conducting or supporting the research that such research has been reviewed and approved by an IRB. Details on scenarios that generally would result in an institution being considered engaged in nonexempt human subjects research and therefore be required to obtain an FWA, or scenarios that would result in an institution being considered not engaged in such a study and therefore not required to obtain an FWA, can be found on OHRP's website (DHHS, 2016b). As of this writing, of the 13,346 total active FWAs in OHRP's database, 9,634 (72%) are with U.S. institutions and 3,712 (28%) are with international institutions.

History of Assurances

From the mid-1970s to 2005, the Office for Protection from Research Risks (OPRR, the predecessor office to OHRP), and later OHRP, approved several different types of assurances including General Assurances, Single Project Assurances, Cooperative Project Assurances, and Multiple Project Assurances (MPAs). Of these, MPAs, first approved in the 1980s, were approved for federalwide use. OHRP began accepting and approving FWAs for federalwide use in 2000. Since February 2005, subsequent to a transition period of several years, the FWA has been the only type of assurance OHRP has accepted and approved.

In June 2011, OHRP implemented some significant changes to the FWA process, including the following: (1) increasing the standard FWA approval period from 3 years to 5 years; (2) permitting FWA institutions' signatory officials to electronically sign the FWA, eliminating the prior need for institutions to submit hard copy signature pages by postal mail or facsimile (for new FWA submissions, updates, and renewals); and (3) requiring institutions to electronically submit all FWAs using OHRP's electronic submission system, unless an institution lacks the ability to do so.

The assurance requirements were further revised when DHHS and 15 other federal departments and agencies published a revision to the Common Rule (the 2018 Requirements), in January 2017. The 2018 Requirements were amended January 22, 2018 and June 19, 2018, with an effective date of July 19, 2018 and a general compliance date of January 21, 2019. These changes include the following: (1) removal of the pre-2018 requirement that an institution provide a statement of ethical principles by which an institution will abide as part of the assurance process; (2) removal of the pre-2018 requirement that an up-to-date list of the IRB members and their qualifications be included in an institution's assurance (instead, the 2018 Requirements require an IRB or the institution to prepare and maintain a current list of IRB members); and (3) removal of the pre-2018 requirement that an institution designate one or more IRBs on its FWA. The 2018 Requirements assurance changes do not apply to studies that remain subject to the pre-2018 Requirements.

FWA Process

An institution's FWA is not project specific. Instead, an FWA covers all nonexempt human subjects research conducted at the FWA-submitting institution that is DHHS-conducted or DHHS-supported or supported by any other federal department or agency that has adopted the Common Rule and relies on the FWA (DHHS, 2017). The FWA is approved for a 5-year period and must be renewed, even if no changes have occurred, in order to maintain an active FWA.

An FWA institution must update its FWA within 90 days after changes occur to the legal name of the institution, the human protections administrator (HPA), or the signatory official (SO). All FWA renewals or updates that are submitted electronically and approved by OHRP begin new 5-year effective periods.

Legal Name of FWA Institution

When first applying for a new FWA, the institution must provide the institution's legal name and city, state or province, and country where the institution is located. OHRP uses this information to identify the specific institution to which the FWA applies. The FWA-submitting institution can also list one or more components over which the institution has legal authority that operate under a different name that would be covered by its FWA.

Human Protections Administrator

Identifying information (name, institutional title, address, telephone and fax numbers, and email address) of the institution's HPA must be included on an FWA application. That individual will serve as the primary contact person for the institution's system for protecting human subjects. The HPA should have comprehensive knowledge of all aspects of the institution's human subjects protections system, be familiar with the institution's commitments under the FWA, and play a key role in ensuring that the institution fulfills its responsibilities under the FWA.

Signatory Official

The signature, date, and identifying information (name, institutional title, address, telephone and fax numbers, and email address) of an official legally authorized to represent the institution, identified on the FWA as the signatory official (SO), must be provided. The SO must ensure that human subjects research covered by the FWA is conducted in accordance with the terms of assurance. The SO must electronically sign and date the FWA using the electronic submission system available through the OHRP website, unless the institution lacks the ability to submit its FWA electronically. Generally, the SO is someone at the level of president, chief executive officer, or vice president of a company, or at the level of president, provost, chancellor, vice president, or dean of an academic institution, unless another official has been specifically delegated with this authority.

Checking the Box

The practice that allows U.S. institutions to voluntarily elect on their FWAs to conduct all of their nonexempt human subjects research, regardless of funding source, in compliance with the Common Rule or the Common Rule and subparts B, C, and D of 45 CFR 46, is referred to as "checking the box." Checking the box gives the federal government the authority to enforce compliance with the Common Rule or with the Common Rule and subparts B, C, and D of 45 CFR 46, over all of the FWA institution's research with human subjects (DHHS, 2020). The preamble of the 2018 Common Rule states that a nonregulatory change will be made to the assurance mechanism to eliminate the option that enables institutions with an active FWA to "check the box."

(Federal Register, 2017, Preamble p. 7181). Institutions could, if they desire, continue for purposes of their own internal rules to voluntarily extend the regulations to all research conducted by the institution, but this voluntary extension would no longer be part of the assurance process, and such research would not be subject to OHRP. As of this writing, of the 9,634 active U.S. FWAs in OHRP's database, 60%, or 5,719, check the box to voluntarily apply the Common Rule or the Common Rule and subparts B, C, and D of **45 CFR 46** to all of its research, regardless of funding source. Twenty-eight percent apply the Common Rule, and 32% apply the Common Rule and subparts B, C, and D.

Conclusion

The FWA is an agreement between an institution and the federal government that it will conduct its human subjects research in accordance with the regulatory requirements for protection of human research subjects. It serves to assure the government, as the funder and steward of public research dollars, and the public, as potential research subjects or beneficiaries of research, that the research is being conducted in accordance with long-standing regulatory and ethical frameworks that have evolved over time. Since first introduced in 2000, the FWA process has been modified two times, in 2011 and 2018, to further simplify and streamline the assurance process while maintaining protections for those who are the subjects of research.

References

Department of Health and Human Services (DHHS). (2016a). *Forms*. www.hhs.gov/ohrp/register-irbs-and-obtain-fwas/forms/index.html

Department of Health and Human Services (DHHS). (2016b). *Regulations, policy, & posting*. www.hhs.gov/ohrp/regulations-and-policy/index.html

Department of Health and Human Services (DHHS). (2017). *Assurance process FAQs*. www.hhs.gov/ohrp/regulations-and-policy/guidance/faq/assurance-process/index.html

Department of Health and Human Services (DHHS). (2020). *FWA Form to 2020*. www.hhs.gov/ohrp/register-irbs-and-obtain-fwas/forms/fwa-form-2017/index.html

Federal Register. (2017). Vol. 82, No. 12. 45 CFR 46 and Preamble. www.govinfo.gov/content/pkg/FR-2017-01-19/pdf/2017-01058.pdf

International Council for Harmonisation

Lindsay McNair

J. Jina Shah

Abstract

The International Council for Harmonisation of Technical Requirements for Pharmaceuticals for Human Use (ICH) was created in 1990 as a joint regulatory industry initiative to harmonize regulatory requirements for the development of medicinal products between the United States, the European Union, and Japan. Although the United States has not adopted ICH guidelines as federal regulation, IRBs should be aware of what ICH requires regarding the responsibilities and procedures of IRBs, because biopharmaceutical sponsors who plan to submit study data in other countries must ensure that the study has been conducted in compliance with these guidelines. This chapter will review the history and structure of ICH guidelines and will outline key differences between ICH and Food and Drug Administration (FDA)/Department of Health and Human Services (DHHS) regulations with regard to IRB review and informed consent.

History of ICH, Members, and Objectives

The International Council for Harmonisation of Technical Requirements for Pharmaceuticals for Human Use, formerly the International Conference on Harmonisation, was created in 1990 as a joint regulatory industry initiative to harmonize regulatory requirements for the development of medicinal products between the United States, the European Union, and Japan (ICH, n.d.c). The reorganization, reforms, and renaming of ICH in 2015 resulted in the establishment of the ICH Association, which is a nonprofit legal entity under Swiss law (Roache, 2017). Objectives of the ICH include improving the efficiency of new drug development and registration processes, promoting public health, preventing duplication of clinical trials in humans, and minimizing the use of animal testing without compromising safety and effectiveness.

The ICH Assembly serves as the ICH governing body, with the intent of focusing global pharmaceutical regulatory harmonization work in one venue. With the reorganization came new members and observers to the Assembly, including both regulatory agencies and industry. As of November 2019, ICH has 16 members and 32 observers. Because of these changes, ICH is now a more global initiative to harmonize pharmaceutical regulatory requirements, and with this expanded scope has come expanded challenges.

An Overview of ICH Guidelines and the Process of Harmonization

There are four categories of ICH guidelines that are developed by "expert working groups." The guidelines in each are named by the first letter of the category (see Sidebar, Four Categories of ICH Guidelines) and are numbered sequentially. Revisions to guidelines have the letter R for revision and a number added to the name.

These guidelines have been written, and continue to be revised as needed, through a process of harmonization. The ICH harmonization process typically begins with selection of a topic on which a new or revised guideline is needed, followed by the drafting of a technical document. Next, input is provided by an expert working group (Step 1), which can include patient advocacy groups; endorsement (Step 2) by the Assembly; and regulatory consultation and discussion (Step 3), including public meetings convened by regulatory agencies. After adoption of the guideline (Step 4), the final step (Step 5) is implementation (ICH, n.d.b).

ICH Guidelines Related to Ethics: A Work in Progress

🔗 1-1

The efficacy guidelines with the most direct reference to ethics, E6 (Good Clinical Practices, or GCP) and E8 (General Considerations for Clinical Trials), have been identified as needing significant revision. Other efficacy guidelines also link to E6 and E8 and have explicit references to the Declaration of Helsinki and/or discussion of other ethical considerations (**Table 8.2-1**).

The increasing role of patient advocacy organizations in the process of developing ICH guidelines is a recent development that also promises to shape the guidelines with the voices of study participants and patients who may ultimately benefit from the clinical research. If the ICH guidelines are considered a road map to the conduct of scientifically sound studies, with an aim to help patients *through* research, then the Declaration of Helsinki, with its emphasis on ensuring protection of individual rights and well-being, serves as a counterbalance, protecting subjects *from* research that may hurt the individual or fail to advance medical science.

Regardless of the state of the efficacy guidelines at any particular time in the process of revision, what is certain is that they will relate to each other and likely still point to the Declaration of Helsinki as the ethical foundation.

FOUR CATEGORIES OF ICH GUIDELINES

Quality (Q): Stability, quality, manufacturing, and analytic procedures related to products.

Safety (S): Preclinical safety, pharmacology, genotoxicity, and reproductive toxicity studies.

Efficacy (E): Design, conduct, and safety of clinical trials. This is the category that has the most direct reference to ethical guidance, particularly E6 that covers Good Clinical Practice, and E8, General Considerations for Clinical Trials.

Multidisciplinary (M): Topics that do not fit into any of the others, such as the Medical Dictionary for Regulatory Activities (MedDRA) and Electronic Standards for the Transfer of Regulatory Information.

Table 8.2-1 ICH Efficacy Guidelines with Reference to Ethics

Efficacy Guideline	Main Topic	Ethical Reference	Other Ethical Considerations
E6	Good Clinical Practices (GCP)	Declaration of Helsinki (DoH)	Responsibilities, functioning, operations, procedures of IRBs Communication and informed consent as sponsor and researcher responsibilities Vulnerable populations
E8	General Considerations for Clinical Trials	E6 and DoH regarding protection of clinical trial subjects	Special considerations of vulnerable populations
E11	Pediatric populations	(R1) Institutional Ethics Committee (IEC)/IRB as in E6, recruitment should be free of inducements, population should represent demographics and disease being studied, assent should be obtained. Minimize risk and distress.	(R1 addendum) Minimal risk If a pediatric subject does not have direct benefit, lever of risks and burdens should be low and comparable to available treatment. There should be reasonable expectation of benefit to pediatric population. Clinical trial results should be publicly available to reduce unnecessary trials and inform clinical practice.
E7	Geriatric populations	Clinical testing programs should be carried out according to agreed ethical and scientific principles.	Clinical trial data should be available for populations that use the drug. Age-related differences should be studied.
E17	Multiregional clinical trials	E6 GCP	All sites should meet ethical standards. Safety information should be provided to ethics committees. Specific guidance is provided on use of active comparators.
E2A	Clinical safety data management: definitions and standards for expedited reporting	E6 GCP	Investigator Brochure should be updated to keep IEC/IRB informed of new safety information.
E3	Clinical study reports	DoH	Ethics, IEC/IRB, patient information and consent all to be in accordance with DoH.
E18	Biobanking	DoH	

Data from International Council for Harmonisation: Efficacy Guidelines. www.ich.org/page/efficacy-guidelines

What It Means for an IRB to Be ICH-Compliant

After the guidelines were finalized, several countries adopted them as law. In the United States, however, the FDA adopted the ICH only as guidance (Federal Register, 1997, pp. 25691–25709). Therefore, the ICH guidelines do not have the force of law in the United States and are not even regulations. In the Federal Register notice, FDA stated that the ICH guideline "does not create or confer any rights for or on any person and does not operate to bind FDA or the public. An alternative approach may be used if such approach satisfies the requirements of the applicable statutes, regulations, or both" (Federal Register, 1997). Therefore, compliance is voluntary, but as with any published FDA guideline, compliance is considered part of good clinical practice.

For drug manufacturers/sponsors, the advantage of complying with the ICH guidelines is that the FDA and equivalent government agencies in other countries will consider studies conducted in accordance with the ICH guidelines to meet the regulatory requirements of the drug approval processes for all of these countries. Therefore, biopharmaceutical sponsors who are conducting multinational studies or who plan to use the data from a United States–conducted study in international regulatory submission, will want to use IRBs that meet the ICH requirements. One of the requirements of the ICH guidelines is that "the sponsor obtain from the investigator/institution . . .[a] statement obtained from the IRB/IEC that it is organized and operates according to GCP and the applicable laws and regulations" (ICH E6, 5.11). There are some requirements of ICH that are not included in FDA or DHHS regulations, which an IRB would also have to follow, to be able to state that they are ICH-compliant. A sponsor could be adversely affected if a regulatory agency refuses to accept data in an application because the IRB that oversaw the research was not fully in compliance with the ICH IRB requirements.

While ICH E6R2 guidelines generally agree with the FDA regulations for IRBs and informed consent, there are a few areas in which the ICH guidelines have requirements that go beyond either FDA or DHHS (Common Rule) requirements. It is important to know what these differences are, because full compliance with ICH requires some changes in IRB operations. If the <u>written procedures</u> include (as they should) how the IRB complies with the various requirements of the ICH guidelines, they must be followed by the IRB. The FDA only inspects IRBs to the standards of the FDA regulations, not ICH, but FDA can cite an IRB for not following its own written procedures. **Table 8.2-2** outlines the differences between the responsibilities of the IRB as defined in ICH E6R2, and the FDA regulations that would already be applying to FDA-regulated research, and what IRBs may need to consider to be ICH-compliant.

⊘ 2-3

A few of the ICH guideline requirements for elements that must be included in the <u>informed consent</u> document go beyond the FDA requirements. Most of these additional elements are commonly seen in consent forms for biopharmaceutical research that is FDA-regulated, and IRBs that review this type of research will be used to seeing them and may even expect them as part of the complete disclosure of study information (for example, the chance of randomization into each study arm). However, to be fully ICH-compliant, the IRB would need to treat these as actual required <u>elements of consent</u>. **Table 8.2-3** outlines the elements of informed consent that are required by ICH E6R2, in addition to those required by FDA regulations.

⊘ Section 6

⊘ 6-2

IRB Responsibilities

There are several differences between the FDA and ICH regarding the responsibilities and duties of the IRB, as outlined in Section 3 of ICH E6R2.

Documents the IRB Must Review

The ICH provides a list of documents that the IRB should review. IRBs routinely review most of the materials listed. Compliance with ICH requires reviewing all the listed materials.

The IRB/IEC should obtain the following documents: trial protocol(s)/amendment(s), written informed consent form(s) and consent form updates that the investigator proposes for use in the trial, subject recruitment procedures (e.g., advertisements), written information to be

Table 8.2-2 Differences Between ICH Guidelines and U.S. Regulations Relevant to IRB Review

Topic	ICH E6R2	FDA Regulations	Notes
Definition of vulnerable subjects	Vulnerable subjects: "Individuals whose willingness to volunteer in a clinical trial may be unduly influenced by the expectation, whether justified or not, of benefits associated with participation, or of a retaliatory response from senior members of a hierarchy in case of refusal to participate. Examples are members of a group with a hierarchical structure, such as medical, pharmacy, dental, and nursing students, subordinate hospital and laboratory personnel, employees of the pharmaceutical industry, members of the armed forces, and persons kept in detention. Other vulnerable subjects include patients with incurable diseases, persons in nursing homes, unemployed or impoverished persons, patients in emergency situations, ethnic minority groups, homeless persons, nomads, refugees, minors, and those incapable of giving consent." (1.61)	"... vulnerable populations such as children, prisoners, pregnant women, handicapped, or mentally disabled persons, or economically or educationally disadvantaged persons." **[21 CFR 56.111(b)]**	IRBs must decide what types of special protections are required for these and other vulnerable populations and whether to extend protections to those not specifically named in the regulations or the ICH guidelines.
Signature by person conducting the consent discussion	"Prior to a subject's participation in the trial, the written informed consent form should be signed and personally dated by the subject or by the subject's legally acceptable representative, and by the person who conducted the informed consent discussion." (4.8.8)	The FDA regulations only require the signature of the subject and the date the subject signed the consent form. **[21 CFR 50.27(a)]**	Many IRBs already require the signature of the person obtaining consent on consent forms, especially for greater than minimal risk research. If not, it is easy to include a signature line labeled "person conducting informed consent discussion." This line should not be labeled "Investigator's Signature," as the investigator is not always the person who obtains consent.
Subject receipt of a signed and dated copy of the consent form	Requires that "the subject or the legally acceptable representative should receive a copy of the signed and dated written informed consent form." (4.8.11)	The FDA regulations state that the person signing the form will receive a copy of the form, but do not specify that it be a copy of the signed form. **[21 CFR 50.27(a)]**	IRB should include notice in the consent form that the subject will receive a signed and dated copy of the consent form. Persons obtaining consent must then ensure that this procedure is followed.

(continues)

Table 8.2-2 Differences Between ICH Guidelines and U.S. Regulations Relevant to IRB Review (Continued)

Topic	ICH E6R2	FDA Regulations	Notes
Assent of children and decisionally impaired adults	"When a clinical trial (therapeutic or non-therapeutic) includes subjects who can only be enrolled in the trial with the consent of the subject's legally acceptable representative (e.g., minors, or patients with severe dementia), the subject should be informed about the trial to the extent compatible with the subject's understanding and, if capable, the subject should assent, sign and personally date the written informed consent." (4.8.12)	FDA regulations require assent of children, when the children are judged capable of doing so. FDA regulations do not specifically require that incapacitated adults assent to research participation. **[21 CFR 50.55 subpart D]**	Most IRBs have considered obtaining the assent of decisionally impaired adults to be an additional protection, which they have required for this vulnerable population. To meet the ICH requirement, the IRB would have to institute a policy for formally considering assent whenever a protocol allows decisionally impaired adult subjects to be enrolled.
Impartial witness for illiterate subjects	"If a subject is unable to read or if a legally acceptable representative is unable to read, an impartial witness should be present during the entire informed consent discussion. After the written informed consent form and any other written information to be provided to subjects is read and explained to the subject or the subject's legally acceptable representative, and after the subject or the subject's legally acceptable representative has orally consented to the subject's participation in the trial, and, if capable of doing so, has signed and personally dated the informed consent form, the witness should sign and personally date the consent form. By signing the consent form, the witness attests that the information in the consent form and any other written information was accurately explained to, and apparently understood by, the subject or the subject's legally acceptable representative, and that informed consent was freely given by the subject or the subject's legally acceptable representative." (4.8.9)	The FDA addresses the documentation of informed consent for illiterate subjects by allowing the use of a short form consent document and a written summary for oral presentation. **[21 CFR 50.27(b)(2)]**	The ICH guideline goes beyond the FDA regulations in requiring that the witness be impartial and specifying to what the witness should attest. Most IRBs define impartial as not being connected with the study team. This allows relatives, nonstudy employees, and similar persons to fill this role. Whatever the definition, it should be included in the IRB written procedures and investigators must know who qualifies as impartial, and the IRB will have to determine a way for the signature to be documented.

Topic	ICH E6R2	FDA Regulations	Notes
Inclusion of decisionally impaired persons in nontherapeutic clinical trials	"Except as described in 4.8.14, a nontherapeutic trial (i.e., a trial in which there is no anticipated direct clinical benefit to the subject) should be conducted in subjects who personally give consent and who sign and date the written informed consent form." [4.8.13] "Nontherapeutic trials may be conducted in subjects with consent of a legally acceptable representative provided the following conditions are fulfilled: (a) The objectives of the trial cannot be met by means of a trial in subjects who can give informed consent personally. (b) The foreseeable risks to the subjects are low. (c) The negative impact on the subject's well-being is minimized and low. (d) The trial is not prohibited by law. (e) The approval/favorable opinion of the IRB/IEC is expressly sought on the inclusion of such subjects, and the written approval/favorable opinion covers this aspect. Such trials, unless an exception is justified, should be conducted in patients having a disease or condition for which the investigational product is intended. Subjects in these trials should be particularly closely monitored and should be withdrawn if they appear to be unduly distressed." (4.8.14)	FDA regulations and guidance do not specifically address this issue.	IRBs should ensure that subjects without capacity are not included in nontherapeutic trials, except in the conditions described.

Table 8.2-3 Elements of Informed Consent Required by ICH

Elements of Consent	ICH E6R2	FDA or DHHS requirements	Comments
Alternative treatments	Requires an explanation of "[t]he alternative procedure(s) or course(s) of treatment that may be available to the subject, and their important potential benefits and risks." (4.8.10(i))	Not required by FDA or DHHS regulations.	This is an area where many IRBs decide to limit their compliance with ICH. Many IRBs and researchers already struggle with the length of informed consent documents. Especially in therapeutic areas in which there may be a wide variety of alternatives, compliance with this requirement can add substantially to the consent document, and may make the document less informative for potential participants.
Confidentiality of medical records	Requires "[t]hat the monitor(s), the auditor(s), the IRB/IEC, and the regulatory authority(ies) will be granted direct access to the subject's original medical records for verification of clinical trial procedures and/or data, without violating the confidentiality of the subject, to the extent permitted by the applicable laws and regulations and that, by signing a written informed consent form, the subject or the subject's legally acceptable representative is authorizing such access." (4.8.10(n)) "The sponsor should verify that each subject has consented, in writing, to direct access to his/her original medical records for trial-related monitoring, audit, IRB/IEC review, and regulatory inspection." (5.15.2)	In seeking informed consent, the following information shall be provided to each subject: ... [5] A statement describing the extent, if any, to which confidentiality of records identifying the subject will be maintained and that notes the possibility that the Food and Drug Administration may inspect the records. **[21 CFR 50.25(a)(5)]**	Most consent forms approved by IRBs now permit access to *research records* by sponsors. Access of foreign regulatory agencies to research records is not troubling; however, access for both these entities to subjects' medical records is problematic for both IRBs and subjects. For the sake of compliance, it is an easy matter to change the wording in a consent form from "research records" to "research and medical records," but philosophically—and logistically—it may be of concern.

Elements of Consent	ICH E6R2	FDA or DHHS requirements	Comments
Probability of assignment to each study arm in a study.	The informed consent form should include: "[t]he trial treatment(s) and the probability for random assignment to each treatment" (4.8.10(c))	The informed consent form must include: "A statement that the study involves research, an explanation of the purposes of the research and the expected duration of the subject's participation, a description of the procedures to be followed, and identification of any procedures which are experimental." [21 CFR 50.25(a)(1)]	This difference can be addressed by including a description of each arm of the study in the consent form and including a statement about the likelihood of receiving each of the study arms.
Compensation for study-related injury	Requires an explanation of "[t]he compensation and/or treatment available to the subject in the event of trial-related injury" (4.8.10(j))	FDA only requires this information for research involving more than minimal risk. [21 CFR 50.25(a)(6)]	Most FDA-regulated clinical trials are greater than minimal risk and therefore already require a compensation for injury clause.
Description of subject's responsibilities	Requires an explanation of "[t]he subject's responsibilities" (4.8.10(e))		One of the unintended consequences of this requirement is to make the consent form look more like a contract between two parties, and this may confuse subjects about their right to withdraw.
Statement of no benefit	Requires an explanation of "[t]he reasonably expected benefits. When there is no intended clinical benefit to the subject, the subject should be made aware of this." (4.8.10(h))		Many IRBs also customarily include this information, so compliance with this requirement should not pose any problems.
Prorated payment in the consent form	Requires an explanation of "[t]he anticipated prorated payment, if any, to the subject for participating in the trial" (4.8.10(k))	Prorated payment is addressed in the FDA Information Sheet entitled "Payment to Research Subjects" (FDA, 2018)	While not a regulatory requirement, it is common practice to include information about prorated payments in consent forms.

provided to subjects, Investigator's Brochure (IB), available safety information, information about payments and compensation available to subjects, the investigator's current curriculum vitae and/or other documentation evidencing qualifications, and any other documents that the IRB/IEC may require to fulfill its responsibilities. (ICH E6R2, 3.1.2)

The FDA regulations do not specifically list in one place what documents an IRB should review. FDA requires the IRB to review the consent form [21 CFR 56.109(b)], and 21 CFR 56.115(a) requires the IRB to keep "copies of all research proposals reviewed, scientific evaluations, if any, that accompany the proposals, approved sample consent documents." (Of note, the ICH requirement that IRBs review "written information to be provided to subjects" is the basis for IRB review of documents such as participant drug diary forms and any other materials which will be participant-facing).

Availability of Written Procedures

ICH E6R2 3.4 states "The IRB/IEC may be asked by investigators, sponsors, or regulatory authorities to provide its written procedures and membership lists."

The FDA regulations do not contain a similar disclosure provision. Many IRBs consider their membership roster to be private and are concerned that disclosure of names may encourage attempts at inappropriate influence of board members. Some IRBs have addressed this concern by disclosing the roster with the names redacted and members described by credentials and role. Some IRBs also consider their written procedures as proprietary information; however, many groups advocate increased public sharing of the procedures used by IRBs, and many IRBs actually put their procedures and policies online.

IRB Appeals Process

Although the FDA regulations do not require an appeals process, the ICH requires it by stating that "the IRB/IEC [will have] procedures for appeal of its decisions/opinions" (ICH E6R2 3.3.9). A written appeals process for IRB decisions is a good practice, but it must be written in a way that does not contradict the FDA regulation which states that no other body may approve a study that the IRB has disapproved [21 CFR 56.112].

Conclusion

In the United States, compliance with the ICH E6R2 guidelines is voluntary for IRBs, because it is not federal regulation. For research institutions that conduct clinical trials of biopharma products, however, pharmaceutical sponsors often insist that the ICH requirements be met so that the data is accepted by regulatory bodies in countries where ICH compliance is mandatory. For IRBs to do this, they must assess their level of compliance and decide whether to make the changes necessary to their institutional policies. If they do not, they should be clear with sponsors that they are not ICH-compliant.

Acknowledgements

The authors wish to thank A. J. Allen for his contribution to the chapter outlines, and David Forster and Gary Chadwick, contributors of the second edition chapter.

References

Federal Register. (1997). International conference on harmonisation; good clinical practice: consolidated guideline; availability. www.federalregister.gov/documents/1997/05/09/97-12138/international-conference-on-harmonisation-good-clinical-practice-consolidated-guideline-availability

Food and Drug Administration (FDA). (2018). *Payment and reimbursement to research subjects: Guidance for institutional review boards and clinical investigators.* www.fda.gov/regulatory-information/search-fda-guidance-documents/payment-and-reimbursement-research-subjects

International Council for Harmonisation (ICH). (n.d.a). *Efficacy guidelines.* www.ich.org/page/efficacy-guidelines

International Council for Harmonisation (ICH). (n.d.b). *Formal ICH procedure.* www.ich.org/page/formal-ich-procedure

International Council for Harmonisation (ICH). (n.d.c). *Welcome to the ICH official website.* www.ich.org

Roache, A. (2017). *Overview of the International Council for Harmonisation (ICH) and reforms.* www.fda.gov/media/104916/download

Certificates of Confidentiality

John Heldens
Catherine Sutherland

Abstract

Certificates of Confidentiality (referred to as Certificates hereafter) are established by federal law as a means to protect the privacy of research subjects. As currently codified by the 21st Century Cures Act, Certificates prohibit researchers from disclosing identifiable, sensitive research information except under specific conditions (U.S. Congress, 2016). In 2017, the National Institutes of Health (NIH) streamlined the process for issuing Certificates for NIH-funded research (NIH, 2019a). For NIH-funded research, the protections required by Certificates are now documented as a term and condition of the funding award (NIH, 2019b). Researchers may still apply for Certificates for research that is not funded by NIH.

Legal Protections of Certificates of Confidentiality

The 21st Century Cures Act amended Title 42, U.S. Code, Section 241(d) Protection of privacy of individuals who are research subjects. Under the 2016 federal law, "identifiable, sensitive information…shall be immune from the legal process, and shall not, without the consent of the individual to whom the information pertains, be admissible as evidence or used for any purpose in any action, suit, or other judicial, legislative, or administrative proceeding [and] shall be subject to the protections afforded by this section for perpetuity." (**42 U.S.C. 241**; U.S. Congress, 2016).

🔗 1-2

Identifiable, Sensitive Information

The Common Rule uses the term "identifiable private information" as part of the definition of a human subject [**45 CFR 46.102(e)(5)**]. The Health

⏵ 11-6   Insurance Portability and Accountability Act (<u>HIPAA</u>) Privacy Rule uses the term "protected health information" (PHI) to define the data that are subject to the requirements of HIPAA (**45 CFR 160.103**; Department of Health and Human Services [DHHS], 2013a, 2013b). The 21st Century Cures Act uses the term "identifiable, sensitive information" to define the data to be protected under Certificates.

As detailed here, *identifiable, sensitive information* encompasses a broader set of data than either *identifiable private information* or *PHI*. Notably, the NIH policy on Certificates explicitly categorizes individual genomic data as identifiable, sensitive information, even if those data are not directly connected with identifiers such as PHI. IRB professionals are well advised to be familiar with the exact wording of the federal law and NIH policy.

From **Title 42 U.S.C. 241(d)(4)**:

> For purposes of this subsection, the term "identifiable, sensitive information" means information that is about an individual and that is gathered or used during the course of research described in paragraph (1)(A) and—
>
> (A) Through which an individual is identified; or
> (B) For which there is at least a very small risk, as determined by current scientific practices or statistical methods, that some combination of the information, a request for the information, and other available data sources could be used to deduce the identity of an individual.

From NIH policy, "What Is a Certificate of Confidentiality?" (NIH, 2019a):

> NIH considers research in which identifiable, sensitive information is collected or used to include:
>
> - Human subjects research as defined in 45 CFR 46, including exempt research except for exempt research when the information obtained is recorded in such a manner that human subjects cannot be identified or the identity of the human subjects cannot readily be ascertained, directly or through identifiers linked to the subjects;
> - Research involving the collection or use of biospecimens that are identifiable to an individual or for which there is at least a very small risk that some combination of the biospecimen, a request for the biospecimen, and other available data sources could be used to deduce the identity of an individual;
> - Research that involves the generation of individual level, human genomic data from biospecimens, or the use of such data, regardless of whether the data is recorded in such a manner that human subjects can be identified or the identity of the human subjects can readily be ascertained as defined in the Federal Policy for the Protection of Human Subjects (45 CFR 46); or
> - Any other research that involves information about an individual for which there is at least a very small risk, as determined by current scientific practices or statistical methods, that some combination of the information, a request for the information, and other available data sources could be used to deduce the identity of an individual, as defined in subsection 301(d) of the Public Health Service Act.

Take note that the NIH interpretation of *identifiable, sensitive information* explicitly includes research data that may be <u>exempt</u> or <u>may not be human subjects research</u> as defined by **45 CFR 46**. NIH policy on Certificates explains that "institutions and their investigators are responsible for determining whether research they conduct is subject to this Policy and therefore issued a Certificate" (NIH, 2019a).

⬤ 5-3 ⬤ 5-1

Responsibilities of Researchers and Institutions

The additional privacy protections afforded by Certificates are possible in large part due to specific responsibilities placed on institutions and their researchers. Certificates offer no protection if institutions or their researchers fail to abide by these responsibilities.

Under **42 U.S.C. 241**, any investigator conducting research covered by a Certificate:

- [S]hall not disclose or provide to any other person not connected with the research the name of such an individual or any information, document, or biospecimen that contains identifiable, sensitive information about such an individual and that was created or compiled for purposes of the research [42 U.S.C. 241(d)(1)(B)].
- [S]hall not, in any Federal, State, or local civil, criminal, administrative, legislative, or other proceeding, disclose or provide the name of such individual or any such information, document, or biospecimen that contains identifiable, sensitive information about the individual and that was created or compiled for purposes of the research [42 U.S.C. 241(d)(1)(D)].

Exceptions are permitted in the following circumstances. From **42 U.S.C. 241(d)(1)(C)**, institutions and researchers are permitted to make disclosures:

(i) required by Federal, State, or local laws, excluding instances described in [42 U.S.C. 241(d)(1)(D)];

(ii) necessary for the medical treatment of the individual to whom the information, document, or biospecimen pertains and made with the consent of such individual;

(iii) made with the consent of the individual to whom the information, document, or biospecimen pertains; or

(iv) made for the purposes of other scientific research that is in compliance with applicable Federal regulations governing the protection of human subjects in research.

There are some simple strategies for complying with these responsibilities. For example, if a researcher or IRB becomes aware of a subpoena, legislative action, or legal request for research data, they should contact general counsel at their institution and obtain legal advice and assistance. General counsel can review the request and determine the best approach for responding. Contacting general counsel in these situations is a simple "takeaway" message to convey when providing training on Certificates at your institution.

Regardless of whether there is a Certificate, researchers should not disclose identifiable information about their research subjects if the disclosure is not covered by the approved consent form, or without additional consent from the subject, or without additional IRB approval if the disclosure is for secondary research. When providing training on Certificates, another simple strategy is to emphasize the importance of maintaining responsible practices to protect all identifiable research data, even for research that is not covered by a Certificate.

The protections and responsibilities of a Certificate apply to the research data in perpetuity. For NIH-funded research, the Certificate applies to data collected under the funded activity. If a researcher collects data after their NIH funding ends, the new data collected is not covered by the Certificate unless a new Certificate is applied for and issued.

Researchers are responsible for informing any other institutions or researchers receiving identifiable, sensitive information about the Certificate protections and responsibilities, because the Certificate would continue to apply. Secondary research conducted with Certificate-protected information is subject to the same rules as the initial research.

Consent Forms

In general, NIH expects consent forms to include a discussion of Certificates for covered research. IRBs should have template consent wording regarding Certificates available for researchers to use what applicable. NIH has sample consent language posted (NIH, 2019c). Please note NIH may update this language.

From NIH policy, "Example Informed Consent Language" (NIH, 2019c):

> *This language is not required.*
>
> This research is covered by a Certificate of Confidentiality from the National Institutes of Health. This means that the researchers cannot release or use information, documents, or samples that may identify you in any action or suit unless you say it is okay. They also cannot provide them as evidence unless you have agreed. This protection includes federal, state, or local civil, criminal, administrative, legislative, or other proceedings. An example would be a court subpoena.
>
> There are some important things that you need to know. The Certificate DOES NOT stop reporting that federal, state or local laws require. Some examples are laws that require reporting of child or elder abuse, some communicable diseases, and threats to harm yourself or others. The Certificate CANNOT BE USED to stop a sponsoring United States federal or state government agency from checking records or evaluating programs. The Certificate DOES NOT stop disclosures required by the federal Food and Drug Administration (FDA). The Certificate also DOES NOT prevent your information from being used for other research if allowed by federal regulations.
>
> Researchers may release information about you when you say it is okay. For example, you may give them permission to release information to insurers, medical providers, or any other persons not connected with the research. The Certificate of Confidentiality does not stop you from willingly releasing information about your involvement in this research. It also does not prevent you from having access to your own information.

IRBs need to be able to identify NIH-funded research to make sure the approved consent forms include an acceptable description of Certificates.

As noted previously, research involving *identifiable, sensitive information* may be <u>exempt</u> and may even include research that is <u>not otherwise human subjects research</u> under 45 CFR 46. Even if the research does not require a consent form, researchers are still responsible for protecting the privacy of the research participants' information.

🖉 5-3
🖉 5-1

Applying for a Certificate of Confidentiality

For research that commenced or was ongoing on or after December 13, 2016, researchers funded by NIH need not apply for a Certificate; rather, a Certificate is issued automatically for research using identifiable, sensitive information. The applicability and requirements of the Certificate are included in the NIH Grants Policy Statement (NIH, 2019b).

For other research, researchers and IRBs still need to decide when obtaining a Certificate is an appropriate step to minimize risks to subjects. As noted, the NIH definition of "identifiable, sensitive information," is extremely broad. IRBs should consider whether a narrower definition could provide adequate protection of subjects for research that is not funded by NIH.

The NIH will issue Certificates for unfunded research and for research funded by other sources except as noted later. To obtain a Certificate, the researcher must submit an application electronically to NIH, and both the researcher and the institution must agree to manage the study data as required by 42 U.S.C. 241. For multicenter research, only one Certificate is necessary.

In cases where the researcher applies for a Certificate, IRBs will need to first approve a consent form that includes a discussion of the Certificate. NIH will not approve a Certificate without reviewing an IRB-approved consent form that discusses the Certificate. Once issued, the Certificate will apply to data collected for the IRB-approved study prior to issuance of the Certificate.

The application process is electronic and accessible through the NIH website (https://grants.nih.gov/policy/humansubjects/coc.htm). In August 2019, the NIH posted a notice in the Federal Register to solicit comments for streamlining the online system (NIH, 2019d). In anticipation of changes to the online application process, details of the current process are omitted from this chapter.

Other Agencies

The Agency for Healthcare Research and Quality (AHRQ) and the National Institute of Justice (NIJ) have their own privacy requirements for research (AHRQ, 2017; NIJ, 2007). They do not require Certificates, and NIH will not issue Certificates for AHRQ- or NIJ-funded research.

The Centers for Disease Control and Prevention (CDC) uses a similar process to NIH. The Health Resources and Services Administration (HRSA) and the Substance Abuse and Mental Health Services Administration (SAMHSA) issue Certificates for the research they fund upon application. Investigators conducting research funded by these agencies who want a Certificate should contact the certificate coordinator at the applicable funding agency.

The Food and Drug Administration (FDA) will issue Certificates upon request for research that is subject to FDA oversight but not federally funded (FDA, 2019). Requests should be made by the sponsor (i.e., the "sponsor" as defined by the FDA).

The Department of Defense (DoD) does not issue Certificates. DoD guidance instructs that researchers who have a Certificate for their research are expected to protect study information "from forced disclosures, including those that fall under the UCMJ [Uniform Code of Military Justice] or the Military Rule of Evidence" (Office of the Undersecretary of Defense, 2017). Investigators conducting research funded by the DoD who want a Certificate should contact an NIH Certificate Coordinator.

The Veterans Health Administration (VHA) does not issue Certificates (VHA, 2019). Investigators conducting research funded by VHA or conducted at VHA sites who want a Certificate should contact a certificate coordinator at the applicable funding agency or NIH if the funding agency does not issue Certificates.

Medical Record Considerations

Certificates help protect research data and research records. Certificates do not protect medical records. When clinical research is conducted in a hospital or health system, the research subjects may also be patients. Clinical research in this setting creates a combination of research data and clinical data. For example, if a clinical study requires a standard blood panel to be conducted through a hospital clinical lab, the lab results will be part of the research records and will often also be placed the patients' medical records. If the same study involves a quality-of-life (QOL) survey for study purposes, the QOL results are more likely stored only in the research records.

IRBs should also be aware of hospital policies regarding uploading signed consent forms to the medical record. Many hospitals (e.g., hospitals with Joint Commission on Accreditation of Healthcare Organizations [JCAHO] accreditation) have policies requiring that signed consent forms for any research their patients participate in be uploaded to the patients' electronic medical record. The purpose of this is to help ensure that any clinician caring for the patient has a complete picture of the treatments the patient has been receiving. Hospitals may also have policies to make exceptions to this rule for research covered by Certificates. Because the 21st Century Cures Act placed all NIH-funded clinical research under a Certificate, some hospitals have revisited their policies for research covered by a Certificate.

Neither of the previously described practices need violate the terms of a Certificate. As described earlier, disclosures are allowed for the medical treatment of the research subject with the subject's consent. This means the IRB's task when reviewing clinical research covered by a Certificate is to make sure their template consent form and/or HIPAA authorization language adequately covers the disclosures described earlier.

✎ 11-6

Conclusion

- Certificates of Confidentiality apply to all NIH-funded research involving "identifiable, sensitive information." This includes all human subjects research. It also includes research involving individual-level genomic data.
- Certificates place specific responsibilities on institutions and researchers not to release identifiable, sensitive information except in specific circumstances.
- IRBs should have template consent form language available to their researchers.
- Researchers and IRBs should contact their institutional general counsel immediately if they receive a subpoena for research records.

References

Agency for Healthcare Research and Quality (AHRQ). (2017). *AHRQ privacy program*. www.ahrq.gov/policy/privacy.html

Department of Health and Human Services (DHHS). (2013a). *Office for Civil Rights: Summary of the Health Insurance Portability and Accountability Act*. www.hhs.gov/hipaa/for-professionals/privacy/laws-regulations/index.html

Department of Health and Human Services (DHHS). (2013b). *Code of Federal Regulations. 45 CFR Part 160 - General Administrative Requirements*. www.law.cornell.edu/cfr/text/45/part-160

Food and Drug Administration (FDA). (2019). *Guidance for sponsors, sponsor-investigators, investigators, industry, and Food and Drug Administration staff: Certificates of confidentiality, draft*. www.fda.gov/regulatory-information/search-fda-guidance-documents/certificates-confidentiality

National Institutes of Health (NIH). (2019a). *What is a Certificate of Confidentiality?* grants.nih.gov/policy/humansubjects/coc/what-is.htm.

National Institutes of Health (NIH). (2019b). *NIH grants policy statement*. grants.nih.gov/policy/nihgps/index.htm

National Institutes of Health (NIH). (2019c). *Example informed consent language*. grants.nih.gov/policy/humansubjects/coc/helpful-resources/suggested-consent.htm

National Institutes of Health (NIH). (2019d). *Proposed collection; 60-day comment request; requests for NIH certificates of confidentiality*. 84 Fed. Reg. 40426. www.federalregister.gov/documents/2019/08/14/2019-17358/proposed-collection-60-day-comment-request-requests-for-nih-certificates-of-confidentiality

National Institute of Justice (NIJ). (2007). *Confidentiality and privacy protections*. nij.ojp.gov/funding/confidentiality-and-privacy-protections

Office of the Under Secretary of Defense for Personnel and Readiness Research Regulatory Oversight Office. (2017). *Guidance: Certificates of confidentiality*. health.mil/Reference-Center/Policies/2017/02/17/GD-01-001-Certificate-of-Confidentiality-Guidance-Document

U.S. Congress. (2016). Public Health Service Act, 42 U.S.C. 241, as amended by PL 114-255

Veterans Health Administration (VHA). (2019). *VHA Directive 1200.05*. www.va.gov/vhapublications/index.cfm

IRB Member and Staff Education

Mina Busch

Abigail Lowe

Abstract

The Common Rule and the Food and Drug Administration (FDA) regulations require that IRB members be qualified to do the work of review, but how board members should develop these qualifications—and what, specifically, these qualifications are—is not stipulated in the regulations. This offers a good deal of freedom to IRBs in determining how they will educate the board and staff members. Whatever the approach, a thoughtful, engaging education program can accelerate IRB members' ability to contribute to their institution and may also increase role satisfaction. This chapter covers engaging approaches and resources to consider when developing IRB education programs.

Introduction

The Common Rule and FDA regulations require that an IRB "be sufficiently qualified through the experience and expertise of its members . . . to promote respect for its advice and counsel in safeguarding the rights and welfare of human subjects" [21 CFR 56.107]. Similarly, the Office for Human Research Protections (OHRP) strongly recommends that the institution and the designated IRB establish education and oversight mechanisms (Department of Health and Human Services [DHHS], 2017a). However, the regulations are largely silent on what those mechanisms might be or how IRBs should educate IRB personnel (members and staff). While OHRP offers a wealth of educational resources online to support the development of foundational knowledge (DHHS, 2017b), institutions bear the responsibility of building their own education programs.

IRBs have a good deal of freedom in their approach to educating board and staff members. Some of the standardization that occurs in educational practice is driven by the requirements of accreditation bodies, such as the Association for the Accreditation of Human Research Protection Programs (AAHRPP, n.d.). In addition to satisfying the requirements for accreditation, the better educated

🔗 8-7

427

IRB members are, the more substantial their contributions will be on the board. When IRB members are supported in their learning with good curriculum and programs, they may become contributing members of their institution faster and may also find more satisfaction in their IRB member and staff roles.

The regulations require that the IRB "shall be able to ascertain the acceptability of proposed research in terms of institutional commitments (including policies and resources) and regulations, applicable law, and standards of professional conduct and practice. . . . If an IRB regularly reviews research that involves a category of subjects that is vulnerable to coercion or undue influence, such as children, prisoners, individuals with impaired decision-making capacity, or economically or educationally disadvantaged persons, consideration shall be given to the inclusion of one or more individuals who are knowledgeable about and experienced in working with these categories of subjects." **[45 CFR 46.107(a)]**

Building specialized knowledge within an IRB can take time and a commitment to ensuring the education provided supports thorough and thoughtful review. Consideration should be given to the best methods of initial education for novice IRB personnel, continuing education for all IRB personnel, and supplemental education for those with specialized knowledge. With this is mind, considerations for building an effective education program for IRB personnel should include (1) educating on the basics, (2) methods for IRB personnel education, and (3) advanced educational topics.

Educating on the Basics

⊘ 1-1 ⊘ 2-3

Education of IRB personnel involves introducing them to the essentials of IRB review and providing them opportunities to apply what they have learned, from the *Belmont Report* principles to local IRB standard operating procedures (SOPs). This approach is important not only for initial orientation of new IRB personnel but also for continuing education.

Educating New Personnel

⊘ 1-1 ⊘ 1-2

It is important to provide new IRB members and staff with a foundational knowledge of basic ethical principles, the historical background of human subjects research in the United States, the regulatory framework, relevant definitions, and the processes involved in participating on the IRB. Most IRBs accomplish this by providing orientation that covers these knowledge cornerstones and ensuring new personnel are equipped with critical resources. Moreover, education programs should aim to ensure that IRB personnel can effectively apply the principles and regulations when reviewing human subjects research. As such, when building an education program, one might begin by asking targeted questions to identify what IRB members and staff need to know to do the work effectively. Appropriate references to provide to new staff and board members include the following:

- *Ethical principles*: Nuremburg Code, Declaration of Helsinki, *Belmont Report*
- *Local resources*: Federalwide Assurance, IRB bylaws, institutional policies relevant to research, IRB SOPs
- *DHHS documents*: 45 CFR 46 Common Rule, National Institutes of Health Policy on Inclusion of Women and Minorities, Office for Human Research Protections (OHRP) IRB Guidebook, OHRP Expedited Review Categories (1998)
- *FDA documents*: 21 CFR 50 and 56 (basic FDA regulations), 21 CFR 312 (FDA drug regulations), 21 CFR 812 (FDA device regulations) (FDA, 2019)

Educating extensively on each item in this list may not be necessary; rather, these resources should be made readily accessible to members in the event they need a reference to support their review. Broadly speaking, orientation should provide members with a working knowledge of the critical material and show them how to access this information. Educational programs that integrate a multifaceted approach can be effective in meeting the educational needs of board members. For more information, see the later section "Methods for IRB Member Education."

Training for new IRB staff should address specific areas they may need beyond the education provided for IRB members. For example, IRB staff frequently need to know their electronic protocol systems and the regulations in much greater detail than IRB members, since they are called upon regularly by board members and the greater research community to provide direction and guidance. Similarly, IRB staff may need to know institutional procedures and SOPs in greater detail than members.

Continuing Education of the Board

One requirement of accrediting bodies, and of many IRB policies, is provision of education at board meetings or through e-learning environments, such as online courses offered by the Collaborative Institutional Training Initiative (CITI), the Protecting Human Research Participants course (PHRP), or Public Responsibility in Medicine and Research's Ethical Research Oversight Course (EROC). Independent learning, such as via online courses, can provide consistency in education to IRB personnel as well as ensure that there is documentation of education completion.

However, educating the board can take a more flexible approach, where education is provided based on the needs of the board. When education takes place during the board meetings, targeted resources can be supplied based on the knowledge gaps on the board. For instance, if a board only intermittently reviews research involving <u>humanitarian use devices</u>, educational resources can be put together to address that need. Although experienced board members may be able to step in and support the review with their expertise, educational opportunities for the board strengthen communal knowledge.

🔗 11-5

Another aspect of education is ensuring that IRB personnel have sufficient understanding of the research they are reviewing, as well as current human subject protections issues such as <u>data privacy</u>, <u>mHealth</u>, <u>genomics</u>, pay-to-play clinical trials, etc. If the board reviews research from a specific discipline in high volumes, board members may need to develop a stronger understanding of the relevant issues in order to conduct meaningful reviews. In this situation, it may be necessary to fill knowledge gaps with a consultant or focus on providing education opportunities for all IRB personnel to learn about that area of research. Some IRBs have accomplished this through bringing in a lecture series provided by faculty in that discipline or having board members visit the research department to gain a stronger understanding of their methods. Such educational opportunities ensure that board members have the basic knowledge needed to review research protocols.

🔗 12-3, 12-4 🔗 12-5 🔗 10-13

Though IRBs are likely to utilize a core amount of the same source material to train new board members, each board may require additional educational support based on the board members and the research being reviewed. While all new IRB members should familiarize themselves with resources addressing the ethical principles and basic applicable regulations governing the review of research, ongoing and supplemental education based on the unique needs of each board should be taken into consideration in the development of education programs. This can be addressed through bringing in institutional subject matter experts, as well as resources from publications such as *Retraction Watch*, *Ethics and Human Research*, and *Science* (see box, Resources for IRB Member and Staff Education).

RESOURCES FOR IRB MEMBER AND STAFF EDUCATION

- Journals and publications
  - *Ethics and Human Research*: www.thehastingscenter.org /publications-resources/ethics-human-research/
  - *Science*: www.sciencemag.org
  - *Retraction Watch*: retractionwatch.com
  - *Journal of Empirical Research on Human Research Ethics (JERHRE)*: journals.sagepub.com/home/jre
- Online courses
  - Collaborative Institutional Training Initiative (CITI): citiprogram.org
  - Ethical Research Oversight Course (EROC): primr.org/eroc/
  - Protecting Human Research Participants (PHRP): phrptraining.com/
- Narratives
  - Narrative Inquiry in Bioethics: nibjournal.org/education/narratives/
- Case studies
  - Narrative Inquiry in Bioethics: nibjournal.org/education/case-studies/
- Federal government resources
  - ORI The Lab: ori.hhs.gov/the-lab
  - OHRP educational resources for IRB administrators and staff: www .hhs.gov/ohrp/education-and-outreach/human-research-protection -program-fundamentals/resources-for-irb-administrators/index.html
  - OHRP researcher training videos: www.hhs.gov/ohrp/education-and -outreach/online-education/videos/all-videos/index.html
  - OHRP videos: www.hhs.gov/ohrp/education-and-outreach/online -education/videos/index.html
  - OHRP Luminaries Lecture Series: www.hhs.gov/ohrp/education-and -outreach/luminaries-lecture-series/index.html
  - OHRP "What Is Research?" and other participant educational videos: www.hhs.gov/ohrp/education-and-outreach/about-research -participation/informational-videos/index.html

---

Methods for IRB Member Education

While the regulations do not specify how IRB members should be trained, it is essential for their success and value as contributing members that the education they receive be effective. The previous sections have touched on many of the main elements of education; the following section will present methods and resources to support delivery of such education.

Educators have determined that most adults learn best through a blend of learning styles, which includes the following domains (Knowles, 1996):

- Cognitive (lectures, discussions, brainstorming sessions)
- Affective (group processes, consensus seeking, values clarification)
- Behavioral (role-plays, teach-back, and simulations)

When planning IRB member education, consider incorporating elements from two or more of these domains (for example, discussion and teach-back) to help increase comprehension and retention.

Static (unchanging) content, such as the regulations, is efficiently presented via online learning. There are several options available commercially, and simple "courses" can also be created in-house using readily available software such as PowerPoint. One method is to incorporate discussion of the static content as part of in-person training, to help reinforce the learning and offer the opportunity to probe more deeply the nuances of application. Using such a "blended" approach increases the efficiency of training time. For example, after new members learn about the *Belmont Report* via online learning or reading the document itself, during a meeting, discuss where and how they see the *Belmont* principles applied in the <u>criteria</u> for IRB approval of research. This application brings a richness of understanding to the content.

🖉 5-4

Another technique that has been demonstrated to affect learning is the use of narratives in education. In his paper, "Mass-audience interactive narrative ethical reasoning instruction," Mark Piper states that a considerable amount of research suggests that "humans are especially disposed to remember, enjoy, and learn from stories and narratives" (Piper, 2017). As such, IRBs should consider incorporating narrative into member education. One way to accomplish this might be to integrate videos, fiction, case studies, and/or other forms of narrative into the training in order to offer individual accounts of the experience of a research subject. Integrating an individual, humanized perspective can empower new IRB members to feel as though they are directly contributing to the protection of research subjects. Refer back to the box "Resources for IRB Member and Staff Education" for a variety of available resources to assist in developing educational programming.

Conducting the Education

How and when training occurs varies greatly across IRBs. A common approach is to allow for some dedicated training time on a regular basis during the IRB meetings. For example, some institutions plan for 15 minutes of educational content and discussion at each weekly meeting. Other institutions offer more substantial training on a quarterly basis. Still others conduct periodic conferences specific to human subject protections matters. Again, the regulations do not specify the method or schedule for training, but for those institutions accredited by AAHRPP, ongoing training is expected.

Some institutions have incorporated job aids such as placemats, bookmarks, or flow charts with information (such as the review criteria) printed on them. These tools are especially beneficial for new members to help ensure they have addressed all required elements in their reviews.

An easy approach that can be incorporated into any training program is to take advantage of occasions when the research being reviewed raises issues that are interesting, controversial, or otherwise suited for discussion. By tying the training discussion to actual scenarios (the protocols before them), it helps the training move from theoretical to actual (implementation).

Consider emailing items in advance of the meeting that members can review and come ready to discuss. Resources could be a recorded podcast, journal articles, case studies, or short videos (refer to the box for some examples of content for all of these categories).

All training, regardless of format, should be conducted in an open environment that encourages and is conducive to discussion. Discussion can be encouraged by having questions prepared in advance to stimulate conversation. Refer to the box for sources of case studies that can be utilized to generate discussion in IRB education and training.

Finally, all training should be documented, including a rough sketch of the content, the date/time delivered, who presented it, and who attended. These records should be maintained and audit-ready.

Advanced Topics

It is important to continually provide education to current IRB members. This includes having experts attend IRB meetings (or training sessions) to share their expertise on novel or cutting-edge research and science, changes to regulations, and changed practices/standards. Other topics to consider include the following:

🖉 12-2
🖉 12-1
🖉 7-6
🖉 12-6, 12-7
🖉 10-9

- Appropriate <u>participant compensation</u> and minimizing coercion
- Managing and minimizing therapeutic misconception
- Incidental findings and <u>return of results</u>
- Dealing with <u>noncompliance</u>
- <u>Conflicts of interest</u> and management of such conflicts
- Implications of research conducted <u>internationally</u>

Conclusion

Regulatory agencies and accreditation organizations require institutions to ensure that initial and continuing training are provided for IRB members, IRB staff, and any other human research protection administrators. This ongoing, effective education is beneficial and can (and should) incorporate a variety of educational resources and modalities to recognize the educational needs and learning styles of all IRB personnel. Proactive, ongoing education helps keep IRB personnel ready and able to respond to changes in the research environment.

References

Association for the Accreditation of Human Research Protection Programs (AAHRPP). (n.d.). *AAHRPP accreditation standards: Domain I: Organization.* www.aahrpp.org/apply/web-document-library/domain-i-organization

Department of Health and Human Services (DHHS). (2017a). *Assurance training.* www.hhs.gov/ohrp/education-and-outreach/human-research-protection-program-fundamentals/index.html/assurance-training

Department of Health and Human Services (DHHS). (2017b). *Educational resources for IRB administrators and staff.* www.hhs.gov/ohrp/education-and-outreach/human-research-protection-program-fundamentals/resources-for-irb-administrators/index.html

Food and Drug Administration (FDA). (2019). Code of Federal Regulations Title 21. www.accessdata.fda.gov/scripts/cdrh/cfdocs/cfcfr/cfrsearch.cfm

Knowles, M. (1996). Adult learning. In R. L. Craig (Ed.), *The ASTD training and development handbook: A guide to human resource development.* McGraw Hill.

Piper, M. (2017). Mass-audience interactive narrative ethical reasoning instruction. *International Journal of Ethics Education, 2,* 161–173.

Researcher Education and Training

Tristan McIntosh
James M. DuBois

Abstract

This chapter describes the educational responsibilities of institutions and provides an overview of evidence-informed practices for researcher ethics education. After highlighting the importance of research ethics and compliance, we discuss the need to establish appropriate educational objectives for researcher training, the role of the HRPP in fostering effective education, and strategies for developing training programs that invoke active learning and learner buy-in. We then discuss the value and mechanisms of evaluating training programs, the importance of assessing the impact of these programs, and how institutions can create an environment that facilitates the transfer of learning beyond formal education.

The Importance of Research Ethics Education

Research ethics education is a domain that includes multiple components, such as training in the responsible conduct of research (RCR), human subjects research protections, conflicts of interest, and good clinical practice. Research ethics education is an important tool for promoting the safe and ethical conduct of human subjects research.

Well-executed research ethics education addresses matters of both compliance and ethics, which are integral components to conducting quality research (Mumford et al., 2016). Compliance involves adhering to regulations, laws, and policies that operationalize and provide guidance on ethical obligations (DuBois, Chibnall, & Gibbs, 2015). Compliance and regulation systems serve multiple functions, including guiding decision making when faced with competing aims, reducing the influence of bias, and helping research professionals to achieve the goals of research (DuBois, 2004; DuBois, Chibnall, & Gibbs,

2015; Irwin, 2009; Steneck, 2007). Moreover, compliance enables appropriate oversight, helps keep research labs operating smoothly, and avoids penalties due to noncompliance.

Research ethics involves "doing good science in a good manner" and often coincides with making technical and professional decisions (DuBois, 2008; DuBois & Antes, 2017). The decisions made by researchers have considerable implications for data accuracy, collaboration quality, the protection of research subjects, and other dimensions of research ethics (Shamoo & Resnik, 2015; Steneck, 2007). When researchers make unethical or unprofessional decisions, harm to multiple stakeholders, including the researchers themselves, research subjects, collaborators, institutions, and society, can result (Olson, 2010). Therefore, it is essential that researchers are properly trained on matters of ethics, professionalism, and RCR.

IRB administrators may wonder whether research ethics education prevents or reduces unethical behavior, including research misconduct (e.g., falsification, fabrication, and plagiarism), serious noncompliance, or conflict of interest violations. Several studies have found that research ethics programs have little or no positive outcomes (Antes et al., 2009, 2016; Mozersky, 2020). However, ethics education remains important. First, a case review of researchers who were referred for remediation training found that the root cause of serious noncompliance or other lapses was a lack of knowledge. Second, ethics training can have positive effects when it is done well (Antes et al., 2009; DuBois et al., 2018).

The HRPP and Research Ethics Education

🔗 8-1

When institutions establish a <u>Federalwide Assurance (FWA)</u> with the Office for Human Research Protections (OHRP), they agree that their human research protection program will assume responsibility for:

> Educating the members of its research community in order to establish and maintain a culture of compliance with Federal regulations and institutional policies relevant to the protection of human subjects. (Department of Health and Human Services [DHHS], 2017a)

The nature of this education is not further specified in terms of who must be trained or the format, duration, frequency, content, or documentation of training.

While OHRP's training requirement may appear simple, the world of research ethics education is complex in terms of what is required and who needs to deliver and oversee it. Typically, requirements are very general (like OHRP's) and apply to institutions rather than specific offices such as the IRB. However, institutional requirements vary significantly depending on the kinds of research performed (e.g., Food and Drug Administration [FDA] requirements generally do not apply to institutions that do not research drugs or medical devices) and who funds research at the institution (e.g., National Institutes of Health [NIH] and National Science Foundation [NSF] have different requirements, foundations often have none). Accordingly, there is wide variation in how institutions structure their research ethics training programs, as well as the roles played by IRBs.

Table 8.5-1 describes some of the most common domains of training relevant to human subjects researchers who work at institutions receiving NIH funding.

Table 8.5-1 Beyond OHRP FWA Requirements: Examples of NIH Requirements in Four Domains

Education Domain	NIH Requirements
Human subject protections (NIH, 2020)	**Who**: All key personnel on grant applications to NIH, including all involved in the design or conduct of a study **Topics**: Not specified **Format**: Not specified **Frequency**: Not specified **Documentation responsibility**: Documentation required; an institutional official must verify this before funds are awarded
Financial conflicts of interest (NIH, 2019)	**Who**: Investigators responsible for the design, conduct, or reporting of research funded by Public Health Service (PHS) or proposed for such funding **Topics**: Seven suggested topics; institutions encouraged to go beyond suggestions **Format**: Unspecified **Frequency**: At least every 4 years; when onboarding; when researcher is noncompliant with financial conflicts of interest policies; when policies change **Documentation responsibility**: Not specified
Responsible conduct of research (NIH, 2009)	**Who**: All trainees (broadly defined) who receive NIH support for training, career development, research education, or dissertations. Modifications allowed for short-term trainees (e.g., summer programs) **Topics**: Nine suggested topics **Format**: Face-to-face **Frequency**: Duration of 8 hours, repeated at each training phase (e.g., predoctoral, postdoctoral, career development), and at least every 4 years **Documentation responsibility**: Institutions expected to maintain records sufficient to demonstrate that NIH-supported trainees, fellows, and scholars have received the required instruction
Good clinical practice (NIH, 2016)	**Who**: All clinical investigators and clinical trial staff who are involved in the design, conduct, oversight, or management of clinical trials **Topics**: Training to be consistent with principles of the International Council for Harmonisation (ICH) E6(R2) **Format**: Diverse formats acceptable **Frequency**: At least every 3 years **Documentation responsibility**: Recipients of training are expected to retain documentation of their training

In what follows, we briefly address some of the more common education requirements that pertain to institutions. However, these often give rise to more questions than answers, because they are so general. Just as IRBs hope that researchers will go beyond the minimum of compliance to actually care for the well-being of participants, we encourage HRPPs to go beyond the minimum educational requirements to provide the training that researchers need. After covering the basic expectations of IRBs and research institutions, we discuss the basic content that needs to be covered within three commonly mandated training areas (i.e., RCR, human subject protections, and good clinical practice), as well as training in decision-making skills and research team management and leadership practices—as these skills and practices are often essential to implementing what is learned in specific training programs.

Which Research Domains Require Education?

When researchers manifest—and reporters cover—ethical violations, a common response is to mandate training. Thus, it is not surprising that there are federal mandates for training on diverse matters of research ethics, ranging from the RCR (National Institute of Food and Agriculture, 2020; NIH, 2009; Steneck & Bulger, 2007), human subject protections (FDA, 1991; NIH, 2020; DHHS, 2017a), good clinical practice (GCP; NIH, 2016), and conflicts of interest (COI; NIH, 2019). While RCR training typically includes most elements of research ethics at a very basic level, funding agencies and oversight bodies often mandate training on specific topics as described later.

Whose Responsibility?

Championing research ethics education is not the sole responsibility of a particular individual, academic unit, or administrative unit. IRBs may be primarily responsible for training efforts on human subjects research and GCP, and perhaps COI, all of which are key elements of research ethics education. However, IRBs cannot be responsible for *all* research ethics education, which is an institution-wide responsibility involving elements of mentoring and institutional climate.

Who Needs to Receive Training?

As noted in Table 8.5-1, the question "who must receive training?" has a different answer depending on the kind of training—as well as the funding agency. Ideally, research ethics education should be required of all researchers and staff who are engaged in the relevant research activities. Providing training only to those who are federally required to take it signals that the institution views research ethics training as something that is done to "check the box" rather than something that is done because it is a priority for the institution (Kalichman, 2014). A spectrum of individuals can and should take part in research ethics education, including undergraduate and graduate students, postdoctoral scholars, faculty of all ranks, and research staff.

Although we encourage training a broad range of research personnel, it may be beneficial to tailor education to their specific needs and level of experience. For example, physicians with no research experience who plan to start conducting research may need more thorough training on the basics of research ethics education compared to seasoned research faculty who may already have received extensive training on these foundational topics. Although certain groups of individuals may need additional or more targeted research ethics education, certain domains of research ethics education are ubiquitous for all individuals who conduct research.

Educational Aims of Research Ethics Education

At the outset of designing and implementing any research ethics training, learning objectives must first be established. Learning objectives are the foundation of any training program and state what learners should be able to do or know after participating in and completing the training program (Watts et al., 2016). The learning objectives should be appropriate for the learner group and will depend on the educational focus of the given research ethics training program. Examples include increasing learner knowledge of RCR topics (Steneck, 2007; Taylor et al., 2012), professional decision-making skills (DuBois, Chibnall, Tait, et al., 2015), research leadership and management habits (Antes et al., 2019; Antes, Kuykendall, & DuBois, 2019; DuBois et al., 2018), ethical sensitivity (Clarkeburn, 2002), or improving attitudes toward compliance and research integrity (DuBois, Chibnall, & Gibbs, 2015; English et al., 2017). Once learning objectives for a research ethics training program are established, they should be used to guide instructional methods, training content, and training program evaluation (Antes & DuBois, 2014). The following sections will explore five domains of learning objectives that are essential to leading research teams with integrity.

Key Educational Domains

Five important components should be included in research ethics education for human subjects researchers.

1. **Core RCR training topics.** While there is no official mandated list of topics that must be covered during RCR training, certain topics are encouraged. The NSF leaves the focus of RCR training to the discretion of the institution so that training can be tailored to the unique needs and circumstances at the institution (NSF, 2017; NSF, 2019). The National Institute of Food and Agriculture (NIFA) requires that RCR training will at least cover the topics of authorship and plagiarism, data and research integration, and reporting misconduct but also acknowledges that additional RCR topics such as data management, human subjects research, and mentor–trainee responsibilities are suitable (NIFA, 2020). The NIH encourages certain RCR topics to be covered, as listed in the Box, The National Institutes of Health Core RCR Topics. (NIH, 2009). Each of these topics includes many different learning objectives, which may range from knowledge of regulations to navigating difficult relationships or anticipating the social consequences of novel research (DuBois & Dueker, 2009). The Office of Research Integrity (ORI) and the ORI website provide resources for teaching these core RCR topics (ORI, 2020). A variety of instructional objectives and training content can be chosen from among these resources depending on the goals of a given RCR training program. Specific objectives should reflect the unique circumstances, needs, and aptitude of learners (Antes, 2014).

> ### THE NATIONAL INSTITUTES OF HEALTH CORE RCR TOPICS
>
> 1. Conflicts of interest
> 2. Human subjects research
> 3. Animal subjects research
> 4. Mentor–trainee relationships
> 5. Collaboration
> 6. Peer review
> 7. Data management
> 8. Responding to research misconduct
> 9. Authorship
> 10. Scientists as responsible members of society
>
> Modified from Antes, A. L., & DuBois, J. M. (2014). Aligning objectives and assessment in responsible conduct of research instruction. *Journal of Microbiology and Biology Education, 15*(2), 108–116.

RCR serves as a broad rubric for education that addresses many different topics, typically at a basic level. Frequently, institutions then require additional training on specific RCR topics as they pertain to researchers' specific roles. Next we describe two specific topic areas that are relevant to human subjects researchers: human subject protections and GCP. Other special topics also apply to all researchers depending on funding sources, such as financial COI training. For example, NIH requires financial COI training every 4 years, which covers topics such as disclosure obligations

🔖 12-6

to human research participants, the need for monitoring of research by independent reviews, and options for reducing or eliminating financial COI (NIH, 2009). Such material could be covered as part of general RCR training or as a special course, as long as training is required of the full range of appropriate individuals (see Table 8.5-1).

2. **Human subjects principles and policies.** Emanuel, Wendler, and Grady (2000) developed a comprehensive framework for evaluating the ethicality of human subjects research that takes into account the myriad complexities inherent to conducting human subjects research. This framework comprises 7 requirements that can be used to evaluate the ethics of clinical research studies, which are listed in the box (Emanuel et al., 2000).

REQUIREMENTS FOR ETHICAL CLINICAL RESEARCH

1. Social or scientific value
2. Scientific validity
3. Fair subject selection
4. Favorable risk/benefit ratio
5. Independent review
6. Informed consent
7. Respect for potential and enrolled subjects

Data from Emanuel, E. J., Wendler, D., and Grady, C. (2000). What makes clinical research ethical? *Journal of the American Medical Association,* 283(20), 2701–2711.

🔖 1-2

🔖 1-1

In addition to the requirements for determining the ethics of a research trial, certain policies that regulate this domain of research should be taught when educating researchers on human subjects research. In the wake of prominent cases of unethical human subjects research (e.g., the US PHS Syphilis Study at Tuskegee), the National Commission for the Protection of Human Subjects of Biomedical and Behavioral Research produced the *Belmont Report*, which outlines key ethical principles for conducting human subjects research (National Commission, 1979). These ethical principles include beneficence, justice, and respect for persons. Beneficence includes maximizing benefits and minimizing harm to others. Justice involves establishing a fair and appropriate distribution of burden and benefits. Respect for persons encompasses treating individuals as autonomous beings by seeking informed consent to research participation and providing protection to those with limited autonomy.

Along related lines, the Code of Federal Regulations Title 45: Public Welfare, part 46 [**45 CFR 46**] was established to protect human subjects who participate in research funded by the federal government. Subpart A of 45 CFR 46 contains the Federal Policy for the Protection of Human Subjects, also known as the Common Rule, and was established to govern research involving human subjects throughout the United States (DHHS, 2017b). Researchers should also be familiar with unique considerations about additional protections put forth in subparts B, C, and D of **45 CFR 46** that are

🔖 Section 9 🔖 9-5

🔖 9-6

pertinent when research involves vulnerable populations, such as prisoners and children. Even if researchers do not conduct research with vulnerable populations, they should have a basic familiarity with all of these regulations.

3. **Good clinical practice.** NIH requires that all clinical researchers and staff are trained on GCP, which is an international standard intended to foster participant safety and scientific integrity (ICH, 2016). GCP training ensures that clinical researchers and staff have foundational knowledge

of GCP. While clinical researchers and staff should take a refresher GCP course every 3 years, there are no formal requirements for GCP training duration or format (NIH, 2016). However, eight domains of GCP competence exist that can guide the development of GCP curricula, as documented on the Joint Task Force Clinical Trial Competency infographic noted in **Figure 8.5-1** (Sonstein & Jones, 2018). Sonstein and colleagues provide a comprehensive overview and description of each competence domain, along with strategies for implementing the core competency framework (Sonstein et al., 2014).

4. **Good decision-making strategies.** Given the various decisions researchers make throughout the research process, including decisions that directly affect human subjects research participants, it is essential that professional and ethical decision-making skills are established (Antes et al., 2016). Lower scores on measures of ethical and professional decision making in research have been linked to lower knowledge of RCR and higher levels of moral disengagement, cynicism, narcissism, and exposure to unethical practices (Antes et al., 2007; Antes, et al., 2019; Mumford et al., 2007). Professional decision-making frameworks offer

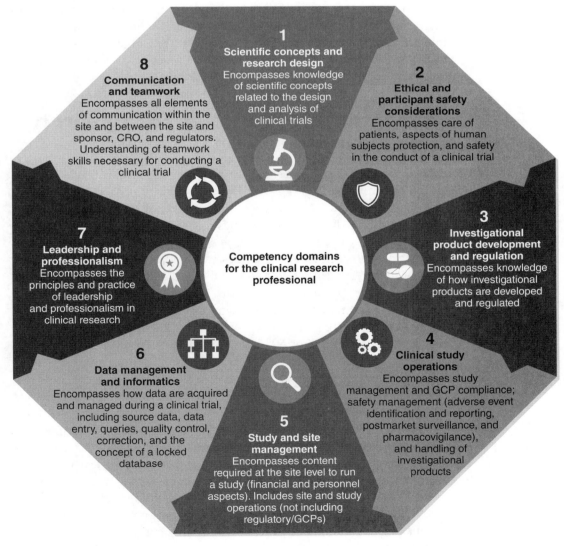

Figure 8.5-1 Joint Task Force for Clinical Trial Competency Core Competency Domains.

Sonstein, S. A., and Jones, C. T. (2018). Joint task force for clinical trial competency and clinical research professional workforce development. *Frontiers in Pharmacology*, 9, 1148.

researchers tested strategies for navigating unfamiliar situations and dealing with uncertainty, compensating for self-serving biases, and managing intense emotions such as anxiety or anger (DuBois et al., 2015; Mumford et al., 2008). Significant differences between U.S.-born and international researchers working in the United States have been observed on research decision-making measures, indicating the need for instruction to take into account cultural factors in how rules may be applied and challenging situations are navigated (Antes et al., 2018; Antes et al., 2019). Crucially, professional decision-making skills can be taught effectively in relatively brief educational interventions (English et al., 2017; McIntosh et al., 2017).

5. **Researcher leadership and management practices**. Research team leadership and management practices can affect the way research is conducted, which has direct implications for human subjects research participants. A variety of leadership and management practices may contribute to research integrity. These include holding regular meetings with research teams, examining raw data, developing standard operating procedures for matters of research compliance, stating the importance of research ethics, and training staff on matters of research ethics and compliance. Such practices are common among researchers identified as exemplars—researchers who do high-impact, federally funded research and are known for their research integrity (Antes et al., 2019; Antes, Kuykendall, & Dubois, 2019). Ongoing studies are examining the link between these practices and both the ethical culture in research teams and ethical violations.

Pedagogical Approaches to Research Ethics Training

Multiple pedagogical approaches and learning exercises are available to those teaching research ethics. Perhaps the first question to answer is whether to conduct training online, in person, or use a hybrid of both. Online training programs lend themselves well to trainings that aim to convey basic facts and knowledge related to regulations, policies, and general compliance expectations (Steele et al., 2016). For trainings with more complex aims, such as changing or improving learner attitudes, skills, and behaviors, some in-person training component appears to be necessary. The primary reason for this is because more complex training outcomes require active learning, discussion, and exchange of ideas among participants (Watts et al., 2016).

How learners learn is as important as *what* learners learn. That is, traditional didactic lectures do not fully engage learners, whereas alternate approaches that actively engage learners enable them to examine subject matter in the context of their own worldview and derive meaning from their learning (Handelsman et al., 2006). The Sidebar, Active Learning Activities presents descriptions of various active learning activities, many of which provide practice opportunities that have positive effects on learning (Miller & Tanner, 2015; Tanner, 2013; Watts et al., 2016). Engaging learners with training material via active learning serves to maximize the utility and effectiveness of their time spent in the classroom.

Careful navigation on the part of trainers is required before, during, and after active learning activities. Specifically, setting appropriate expectations up front, managing and guiding the direction of discussions, and providing clarity on issues of misunderstanding are all integral parts to conducting a successful training program. At the outset of a training program, trainers should establish expectations regarding learner participation: discussions should be conducted in a respectful manner, and learners should feel safe sharing ideas with the group (Handelsman et al., 2006). During discussions, trainers should attempt to involve all learners in participating and avoid allowing a few outspoken learners to dominate discussion in order to facilitate an inclusive learning environment. This includes keeping discussions on-topic and relevant to the training content itself. After active learning activities and discussions have taken place, trainers should take time to debrief with learners on key points to consolidate learning and clarify any areas of misunderstanding or confusion.

Learner Buy-In

Learner motivation to participate in training increases the likelihood that they will learn and apply training content (Colquitt et al., 2000). If learners are unmotivated or have negative attitudes toward the training program, learning can be inhibited. To avoid this, it is essential to garner buy-in from learners by communicating with them beforehand how the training program and its content will be useful and meaningful to their careers and how it will address many of the individual professional challenges they are likely to face throughout their careers in research (Smith-Jentsch et al., 1996). For example, a training program intended to educate researchers on professionalism and ethics in research can provide learners with strategies for effective lab management and examples of standard operating procedures that safeguard against compliance violations, both of which serve to sustain the quality and longevity of a researcher's career. Although many training programs are mandated by funding agencies or academic institutions, framing this training in terms of career development and career benefit can help inoculate against opposition to both mandated and voluntary training. After all, researchers have demanding schedules with limited free time, so demonstrating why and how research ethics training is worth the investment can help learners become motivated to take part in training, learn better, and derive meaning from training content.

Evaluating Research Ethics Training

Systematically evaluating research ethics training programs is an often overlooked, yet highly valuable and informative, step. Training program evaluation, or assessing the outcomes of training, provides information that can be used to make revisions to the training program and demonstrate its value and impact (Goldstein & Ford, 2002). Training evaluation can take place after training has occurred or before and after training has occurred by administering assessments, or tests, to learners that measure training outcomes such as learner reactions to training, changes in learner attitudes, and improvements in learner knowledge or skills (Kirkpatrick, 1983; Steele et al., 2016).

Considerable planning and resources are needed to properly design, implement, and utilize training evaluation. Although the most extensive and rigorous

---

ACTIVE LEARNING ACTIVITIES

1. *Case studies*: Present learners with scenarios that illustrate examples of key training concepts.
2. *Individual reflection*: Ask learners a question that encourages them to connect training concepts together and to their own lives.
3. *Think-pair-share*: This activity can be grouped with other activities where learners first think or write about something alone, then discuss with a neighboring learner, and finally share it with the larger group.
4. *Role plays*: Assign learners to take a role of a character in a scenario and model the character's social interactions in that scenario using a provided script.
5. *Debates*: Learners present arguments on an issue related to training content, which enhances critical thinking skills.
6. *Clickers*: Learners use devices to answer multiple choice questions that provide a summary of responses to help assess learner understanding and misperceptions.

evaluation of research ethics training is not always plausible because of time and resource constraints, evaluation should be systematic and linked directly to the learning objectives of the training program (Antes & DuBois, 2014; McIntosh et al., 2017). For example, if an objective of training is to increase learner knowledge on core RCR topics, it would be appropriate to administer an RCR knowledge assessment before and after training to determine whether learner knowledge increased as a function of taking part in training.

The next question becomes how to best utilize the data from training evaluation. At a fundamental level, this data can be used to determine whether training had the intended effect. Evaluation data can be used to identify components of the training program that are especially effective or well liked and components that are especially ineffective or disliked by learners. For example, reaction data might indicate that learners do not like a particular activity or the content of a case. In yet another example, learners may show either decreases or very small increases in ethical decision-making skills after taking a decision-making skills-based training, perhaps because of ineffective delivery of training content and instruction. This information can be used to identify and retain effective aspects of training and to revise aspects of training that are unsuccessful and ineffective in contributing to the achievement of stated learning objectives.

Systematic training evaluation is needed to obtain ongoing feedback about the quality of the training program and potential changes that need to be made to training content and processes (McIntosh et al., 2017). This feedback can also signal potential shifts in the external environment (e.g., political, social) that influence how learners interact with and respond to training content. To summarize, no training program is ever perfectly finished. Updates and improvements to training content and processes are needed to optimize the effectiveness of a training program over time, and training evaluation is an effective means of determining the efficacy of the training program and areas where modification is warranted.

Beyond Formal Research Ethics Training

Researcher education and training are not finished at the conclusion of formal research ethics training. In order for learners to be able to apply what they learned during training, their work environment needs to exhibit characteristics that facilitate this learning transfer (Broad & Newstrom, 1992). Specifically, researchers need to be provided with opportunities to practice and apply what was learned during training to their own work. Timely and behavior-specific feedback should also be provided to researchers when they integrate training into their work (Gagne & Medsker, 1996). This feedback can be informal and come from individuals in administrative positions, faculty with more senior ranking, and peers (Bell & Kozlowski, 2008; Tracey et al., 1995). Providing praise and encouragement for applying training content and rewarding researchers for this application are effective mechanisms for prompting learning transfer. Again, these observations on what helps researchers apply training to their practice reinforces the idea that effective research ethics training is a responsibility of the entire institution, not just of the IRB.

There are other steps that can be taken from an administrative standpoint, which might naturally be implemented within the human research protections program, such as by the IRB office. Updating policies and procedures to reflect and align with training content can serve to facilitate learning transfer. Providing

2-3

a "knowledge on demand" resource for researchers can promote learning transfer. A resource of this nature can take the form of a website that contains essential, easy-to-find information such as a hotline for reporting and inquiries about incidents of potential misconduct, web links to institutional policies and procedures, and a frequently asked questions webpage. Straightforward steps such as these can have a significant impact on how researchers navigate their post-RCR training work and change their research practices for the better.

Conclusion

Research ethics training is an integral component to doing rigorous high quality research that respects and protects human subjects. Simply providing, or mandating, a research ethics education program for researchers without any forethought about the content of training, evaluation of training, and execution of training is insufficient. Ensuring that a research ethics education training program is embedded thoughtfully in the broader institutional context is essential for successful researcher education and training.

References

Antes, A. L. (2014). A systematic approach to instruction in research ethics. *Accountability in Research, 21*(1), 50–67.

Antes, A. L., Brown, R. P., Murphy, S. T., Waples, E. P., Mumford, M. D., Connelly, S., & Devenport, L. D. (2007). Personality and ethical decision-making in research: The role of perceptions of self and others. *Journal of Empirical Research on Human Research Ethics, 2*(4), 15–34.

Antes, A. L., Chibnall, J. T., Baldwin, K. A., Tait, R. C., Vander Wal, J. S., & DuBois, J. M. (2016). Making professional decisions in research: Measurement and key predictors. *Accountability in Research, 23*(5), 288–308.

Antes, A. L., & DuBois, J. M. (2014). Aligning objectives and assessment in responsible conduct of research instruction. *Journal of Microbiology and Biology Education, 15*(2), 108–116.

Antes, A. L., English, T., Baldwin, K. A., & DuBois, J. M. (2018). The role of culture and acculturation in researchers' perceptions of rules in science. *Science and Engineering Ethics, 24*(2), 361–391.

Antes, A. L., English, T., Baldwin, K. A., & DuBois, J. M. (2019). What explains associations of researchers' nation of origin and scores on a measure of professional decision-making? Exploring key variables and interpretation of scores. *Science and Engineering Ethics, 25*(5), 1499–1530.

Antes, A. L., Kuykendall, A., & DuBois, J. M. (2019). Leading for research excellence and integrity: A qualitative investigation of the relationship-building practices of exemplary principal investigators. *Accountability in Research, 26*(3), 198–226.

Antes, A. L., Murphy, S. T., Waples, E. P., Mumford, M. D., Brown, R. P., Connelly, S., & Devenport, L. D. (2009). A meta-analysis of ethics instruction effectiveness in the sciences. *Ethics and Behavior, 19*(5), 379–402.

Bell, B. S., & Kozlowski, S. W. (2008). Active learning: Effects of core training design elements on self-regulatory processes, learning, and adaptability. *Journal of Applied Psychology, 93*(2), 296.

Broad, M. L., & Newstrom, J. W. (1992). *Transfer of training.* Addison-Wesley.

Clarkeburn, H. (2002). A test for ethical sensitivity in science. *Journal of Moral Education, 31*(4), 439–453.

Colquitt, J. A., LePine, J. A., & Noe, R. A. (2000). Toward an integrative theory of training motivation: a meta-analytic path analysis of 20 years of research. *Journal of Applied Psychology, 85*(5), 678–707.

Department of Health and Human Services (DHHS). (2017a). *Assurance training.* www.hhs.gov/ohrp/education-and-outreach/human-research-protection-program-fundamentals/index.html/assurance-training

Department of Health and Human Services (DHHS). (2017b). *Final revisions to the Common Rule.* www.hhs.gov/ohrp/regulations-and-policy/regulations/finalized-revisions-common-rule/index.html

DuBois, J. M. (2004). Is compliance a professional virtue of researchers? Reflections on promoting the responsible conduct of research. *Ethics and Behavior, 14*(4), 383–395.

DuBois, J. M. (2008). Solving ethical problems: Analyzing ethics cases and justifying decisions. In *Ethics in Mental Health Research* (pp. 1–12). Oxford University Press.

DuBois, J. M., & Antes, A. L. (2017). Five dimensions of research ethics: A stakeholder framework for creating a climate of research integrity. *Academic Medicine, 93*(4), 550–555.

DuBois, J. M., Chibnall, J. T., & Gibbs, J. C. (2015). Compliance disengagement in research: Development and validation of a new measure. *Science and Engineering Ethics, 22*(4), 965.

DuBois, J. M., Chibnall, J. T., Tait, R., & Vander Wal, J. S. (2018). The professionalism and integrity in research program: Description and preliminary outcomes. *Academic Medicine, 93*(4), 586–592.

DuBois, J. M., Chibnall, J. T., Tait, R. C., Vander Wal, J. S., Baldwin, K. A., Antes, A. L., & Mumford, M. D. (2015). Professional decision-making in research (PDR): The validity of a new measure. *Science and Engineering Ethics, 22*(2), 391–416.

DuBois, J. M., & Dueker, J. M. (2009). Teaching and assessing the responsible conduct of research: A Delphi consensus panel report. *Journal of Research Administration, 40*(1), 49–70.

Emanuel, E. J., Wendler, D., & Grady, C. (2000). What makes clinical research ethical? *Journal of the American Medical Association, 283*(20), 2701–2711.

English, T., Antes, A. L., Baldwin, K. A., & DuBois, J. M. (2017). Development and preliminary validation of a new measure of values in scientific work. *Science and Engineering Ethics, 24*(2), 393–418.

Food and Drug Administration (FDA). (1991). *FDA policy for the protection of human subjects.* www.fda.gov/science-research/clinical-trials-and-human-subject-protection/fda-policy-protection-human-subjects

Gagne, R. M., & Medsker, K. L. (1996). *The conditions of learning.* Harcourt-Brace.

Goldstein, I. L., & Ford, J. K. (2002). *Training in organizations: Needs assessment, development, and evaluation* (4th ed.). Wadsworth.

Handelsman, J., Miller, S., & Pfund, C. (2006). *Scientific teaching: Diversity, assessment, active learning.* W. H. Freeman and Co.

International Conference on Harmonisation (ICH). (2016). *Good Clinical Practice (ICH GCP) 1.34 Investigator.* ichgcp.net/4-investigator

Irwin, R. S. (2009). The role of conflict of interest in reporting of scientific information. *Chest, 136*(1), 253–259.

Kalichman, M. W. (2014). Rescuing responsible conduct of research (RCR) education. *Accountability in Research-Policies and Quality Assurance, 21*(1), 68–83.

Kirkpatrick, D. L. (1983). Four steps to measuring training effectiveness. *Personnel Administrator, 28*(11), 19–25.

McIntosh, T., Higgs, C., Mumford, M. D., Connelly, S., & DuBois, J. M. (2017). Continuous evaluation in ethics education: A case study. *Science and Engineering Ethics, 24*(2), 727–754.

Miller, S., & Tanner, K. D. (2015). A portal into biology education: An annotated list of commonly encountered terms. *CBE—Life Sciences Education, 14*(2), 1–14.

Mozersky, J. T., Antes, A. L., Baldwin, K., Jenkerson, M., & Dubois, J. M. (2020). How do clinical research coordinators learn Good Clinical Practice? A mixed methods study of factors that predict uptake of knowledge. *Clinical Trials, 17*(2),166–175.

Mumford, M. D., Antes, A. L., Caughron, J. J., & Friedrich, T. L. (2008). Charismatic, ideological, and pragmatic leadership: Multi-level influences on emergence and performance. *The Leadership Quarterly, 19*(2), 144–160.

Mumford, M. D., Murphy, S. T., Connelly, S., Hill, J. H., Antes, A. L., Brown, R. P., & Devenport, L. D. (2007). Environmental influences on ethical decision making: Climate and environmental predictors of research integrity. *Ethics and Behavior, 17*(4), 337–366.

Mumford, M. D., Watts, L. L., Medeiros, K. E., Mulhearn, T. J., Steele, L. M., & Connelly, S. (2016). Biomedical ethics education may benefit from integrating compliance and analysis approaches. *Nat Immunol, 17*(6), 605–608.

National Commission for the Protection of Human Subjects of Biomedical and Behavioral Research. (1979). *The Belmont Report: Ethical principles and guidelines for the protection of human subjects of research.* ohsr.od.nih.gov/guidelines/belmont.html

National Institute of Food and Agriculture (NIFA). (2020). *Responsible and ethical conduct of research.* nifa.usda.gov/responsible-and-ethical-conduct-research

National Institutes of Health (NIH). (2009). *Update on the requirement for instruction in the responsible conduct of research* (Vol. NOT-OD-10-019). National Institutes of Health.

National Institutes of Health (NIH). (2016). *Policy on good clinical practice training for NIH awardees involved in NIH-funded clinical trials.* Notice No. NOT-OD-16-148. grants.nih.gov/grants/guide/notice-files/not-od-16-148.html

National Institutes of Health (NIH). (2019). *4.1.10 Financial conflict of interest.* grants.nih.gov /grants/policy/nihgps/HTML5/section_4/4.1.10_financial_conflict_of_interest.htm?Highlight =fcoi

National Institutes of Health (NIH). (2020). *Training and resources - human subjects.* grants.nih .gov/policy/humansubjects/training-and-resources.htm

National Science Foundation (NSF). (2017). *Important Notice No. 140 training in responsible conduct of research – a reminder of the NSF requirement.* www.nsf.gov/pubs/issuances/in140.jsp

National Science Foundation (NSF). (2019). *Proposal and award policies and procedures guide 19-1 Chapter IX - Grantee standards.* www.nsf.gov/pubs/policydocs/pappg19_1/pappg_9.jsp#IXB

The Office of Research Integrity. (2020). *ORI Updates.* ori.hhs.gov

Olson, L. E. (2010). Developing a framework for assessing responsible conduct of research education programs. *Science and Engineering Ethics, 16*(1), 185–200.

Shamoo, A. E., & Resnik, D. B. (2015). *Responsible conduct of research* (3rd ed.). Oxford University Press.

Smith-Jentsch, K. A., Jentsch, F. G., Payne, S. C., & Salas, E. (1996). Can pretraining experiences explain individual differences in learning? *Journal of Applied Psychology, 81*(1), 110–116.

Sonstein, S. A., & Jones, C. T. (2018). Joint task force for clinical trial competency and clinical research professional workforce development. *Frontiers in Pharmacology, 9,* 1148.

Sonstein, S. A., Seltzer, J., Li, R., Silva, H., Jones, C. T., & Daemen, E. (2014). Moving from compliance to competency: A harmonized core competency framework for the clinical research professional. *Clinical Researcher, 28*(3), 17–23.

Steele, L. M., Mulhearn, T. J., Medeiros, K. E., Watts, L. L., Connelly, S., & Mumford, M. D. (2016). How do we know what works? A review and critique of current practices in ethics training evaluation. *Accountability in Research, 23*(6), 319–350.

Steneck, N. H. (2007). *ORI introduction to the responsible conduct of research* (Updated ed.). U.S. Government Printing Office.

Steneck, N. H., & Bulger, R. E. (2007). The history, purpose, and future of instruction in the responsible conduct of research. *Academic Medicine, 82*(9), 829–834.

Tanner, K. D. (2013). Structure matters: Twenty-one teaching strategies to promote student engagement and cultivate classroom equity. *Life Sciences Education, 12*(3), 322–331.

Taylor, H. A., Kass, N. E., Ali, J., Sisson, S., Bertram, A., & Bhan, A. (2012). Development of a research ethics knowledge and analytical skills assessment tool. *Journal of Medical Ethics, 38*(4), 236–242.

Tracey, J. B., Tannenbaum, S. I., & Kavanagh, M. J. (1995). Applying trained skills on the job: The importance of the work environment. *Journal of Applied Psychology, 80*(2), 239–252.

Watts, L. L., Medeiros, K. E., Mulhearn, T. J., Steele, L. M., Connelly, S., & Mumford, M. D. (2016). Are ethics training programs improving? A meta-analytic review of past and present ethics instruction in the sciences. *Ethics and Behavior, 27*(5), 1–34.

Preparing for a Regulatory Audit

Kristina Borror
Nancy A. Olson

Abstract

IRBs are subject to regulatory audits from many different entities. The audit may be conducted for routine monitoring, in response to a complaint or concern identified, as part of product development, or for other purposes. It may be conducted in person or remotely. It may be conducted by one or more persons. No matter the entity conducting the audit, the type of audit, or the method, preparation is key. Following best practices before, during, and after an audit will help ensure a positive, successful audit experience and outcome for all.

Types of Regulatory Audits

Food and Drug Administration

The Food and Drug Administration (FDA) conducts inspections of IRBs reviewing clinical investigations that are regulated by FDA under **21 U.S.C. 355(i)** and **21 U.S.C. 360(j)** and clinical investigations that support applications for research or marketing permits for products regulated by FDA. These inspections are conducted under the FDA Bioresearch Monitoring (BIMO) program. FDA generally does two types of IRB inspections: (1) surveillance inspections, which are recurrent, scheduled inspections to review the overall operations and procedures of the IRB; and (2) directed inspections, which are unscheduled inspections that target the IRB's review of a specific clinical trial or trials.

Office for Human Research Protections

The Office for Human Research Protections (OHRP) conducts evaluations of institutions conducting research that is supported by the U.S. Department of Health and Human Services. The institution's IRB is generally a focus of those evaluations. OHRP conducts for-cause evaluations and not-for-cause evaluations, either of which may be on site or remote (through correspondence).

Other Federal Agencies

✐ 11-8   Department of Defense (DoD) oversight of human subjects research that it conducts and supports is generally through each DoD component to ensure compliance with DoD Instruction 3216.02 and **32 CFR 219**.

✐ 11-8   The Department of Energy (DOE) Human Subjects Protection Program (HSPP) oversees research funded by DOE, conducted at DOE institutions, or performed by DOE employees or its contractors to ensure compliance with **10 CFR 745** and DOE-specific requirements, including DOE Order 443.1B. The HSPP conducts quality assurance consultations at its laboratories, both remote and in-person.

✐ 11-8   The Department of Veterans Affairs (VA) Office of Research Oversight (ORO) is the primary office within the Veterans Health Administration (VHA) responsible for providing oversight of research program compliance with **38 CFR 16**, VHA Directive 1200.05, and other federal and VHA-specific requirements. ORO conducts focused reviews and for-cause reviews both remotely and on site to target specific issues at VA research facilities determined to be of high risk. ORO also conducts combined program reviews on site to assess research programs for high-risk vulnerabilities and any noncompliance associated with the vulnerabilities.

Other Types of Audits

✐ 8-7   The most common other type of regulatory audit of IRBs is by accrediting bodies. Sponsors/funding agencies may also conduct audits of researchers and IRBs.

Always Be Prepared

Being prepared is the key to a successful audit. While your institution may receive substantial advance notice for some audits, others will be conducted with minimum, or even no notice. There will never be enough notice to allow review of your entire program and get things in order if they are not. There are many things that can be done before receiving notice of an audit that will allow your institution to be prepared when the notice comes. Preparing for a regulatory audit before receiving notice of an audit involves daily effort. Following best practices and maintaining a constant state of readiness will allow your institution to be audit ready at any time.

Files

All study and IRB files should be complete, current, and accurate. Files should be organized consistently and chronologically. This will make information easy to find. Subdividing study files by submission type, initial submission with all accompanying documents, continuing reviews/annual progress reports, amendments/modifications, unanticipated problems, and final reports, will make current information even easier to locate.

If an electronic submission system is used, file organization and ease of locating information should be carefully considered during system design. When designing an electronic submission system, design should also take into consideration access for external parties, including auditors. Creating an auditor role within the system will allow limited access to all parts of the system while maintaining confidentiality of IRB office and member informal communications. Consider maintaining hard copy files (complete, shadow, or in between) for backup and/or in the event of disaster recovery. Hard copy files will come in handy during regulatory audits or when any other third party or external entity needs access to study files. The auditors may prefer to review hard copy files. It is also less time consuming to explain file organization to the auditor or other third party than to teach the nuances of an electronic system and arrange access to a secure system.

Policies and Procedures

How your institution meets its regulatory human subjects research obligations should be documented in written <u>policies and procedures</u>. The document should be reviewed and updated as needed, but at least annually, to ensure that policies and procedures match the actual processes that are followed. When the document or individual policies within the document are updated, changes should be identified by date or a change log maintained, to show that the document is current.

🔗 2-3

Education

IRB administrative staff, IRB members, institutional leadership (including the designated Institutional Official), researchers and study staff, ancillary committees, and other offices that are part of an institution's human research protection program (HRPP) should receive initial and ongoing <u>training and education</u>. Educational efforts help ensure that those involved in and responsible for the institution's human research endeavors have appropriate understanding and expertise and that depth of knowledge is maintained. Level of knowledge and expertise is a critical part of the research review process. All should be knowledgeable about the functions of the HRPP and IRB within the organization as well as the human subjects protection regulations. During an audit, staff and/or institutional leadership may be interviewed and need to demonstrate a good understanding of the process. Ongoing education and training will ensure that they are prepared. Education and training efforts are available through many outlets, including online resources, webinars, regional and local meetings, national meetings (for example, those offered by the Association for the Accreditation of Human Research Protection Programs [AAHRPP] and Public Responsibility in Medicine and Research [PRIM&R]), and offerings from the FDA and OHRP. Education and training efforts should be documented by date, title or subject matter, and attendance.

🔗 8-4, 8-5

Quality Assurance/Quality Improvement

One way to assess audit readiness is to conduct <u>internal audits</u> on a routine schedule. The audits may be done within the IRB administrative office or by another institutional office outside of the IRB. Regardless of the office conducting the internal audit, an audit plan should be developed. This audit plan helps meet the requirements of **45 CFR 46.108(a)(3)(ii)**, regarding written procedures for "[d]etermining which projects ... need verification from sources other than the investigators that no material changes have occurred since previous IRB review." The plan should identify what is being audited, for example, the IRB or IRB records (random pull or specific number, type, or group of studies); how the audit will be done/what will be looked at; the frequency of the audits; and how and to whom results will be communicated. The audit plan should also identify steps that will be followed in the event corrective action is required to address audit findings.

🔗 2-7

Standard operating procedures (SOPs) should include ongoing quality assurance efforts. Study files should be routinely examined for completeness and accuracy. This is especially critical for hard copy files. If a recurring gap is found, identifying the root cause and addressing it will help avoid problems during an audit. Review of OHRP and FDA letters and common findings should also be part of ongoing quality assurance efforts. Common findings and warning letters that identify deficiencies allow identification of similar problems and issues at your site so that they can be addressed ahead of any audit. Review written policies and operating procedures to help ensure that they are being followed. This review will also help identify any changes that are needed.

Adequate Staffing

The ongoing, continuous efforts described will allow institutions to be as audit ready as possible at any time. These efforts cannot be done without adequate staffing. A sufficient number of qualified personnel is required to ensure that the review process meets all regulatory requirements, that appropriate and detailed documentation is maintained and up-to-date, and that the IRB is operating in compliance with all regulatory and institutional requirements.

Notification of Audit and Preparation

Timing

When notice of an audit is received, the ongoing efforts described previously will help maintain focus on the specifics of the audit. Once notice is received, establish the scope of the audit. Confirm the audit start date and time and the anticipated length of the audit, and ask if there are any specific studies, areas of concern, files or other materials that need to be available during the audit. Obtain contact information in case there are any questions prior to the audit. If institutional leadership (for example, the IRB chair or IRB director) will not be available during the scheduled audit dates, it may be possible to negotiate a slight rescheduling.

Notify Appropriate Institutional Leaders

The Institutional Official (IO), other appropriate institutional leaders, IRB and HRPP staff, IRB chairs and members, and other offices/departments involved with the HRPP (for example, legal, pre- and/or post-award, compliance, pharmacy, IT, specific researchers identified in the audit notice, as applicable) should be notified of the scheduled audit as soon as possible. These individuals should be asked to hold time on their calendars as they may need to be available for interviews during the audit, and/or for consultation with the HRPP staff during the visit. The IO, IRB chair(s) and director, and institutional leadership will also need to be available to attend the exit interview.

⌖ 2-1

⌖ 3-2

Review Auditing Body's SOPs

Familiarize yourself with the auditing body's standard audit operating procedures. This will allow your institution to know what to expect and the process that will be followed, thereby avoiding surprises along the way.

Logistics

Identify and reserve an appropriate, comfortable space for the audit. The space should be in close proximity to the IRB offices, but not within the IRB offices, to avoid unnecessary disruption of daily activities. Sufficient electrical outlets, telephone, and wifi connections will be needed. If the auditor(s) will be reviewing files electronically, they may also want a projector so that specific documents are viewable by everyone in the room. The location should also be close to conveniences such as restrooms, parking, and food. The room should be large enough to accommodate the auditor(s), interviewees, and institutional officials who will attend the exit interview, along with space for files, computers, and any other necessities. It is preferable to have the same space available for the entire audit. The space should be secure, so that materials may be kept in the room until no longer needed. Auditors will need to make copies of documents they review or have copies made for them, so access to a photocopier will be important. The IRB office will need a copy of every document the auditor(s) copy. A discussion at the beginning of the audit, or prior to, should identify who will be responsible for making copies, the IRB staff or the auditor(s). This will ensure that both the IRB office and the auditor(s) have the same documents. Having a complete file of audit documents will be vitally important in the event there are any findings or questions after the audit.

Files

If the audit notice identifies a specific study or studies to be reviewed, the sponsor/funding agency should also be notified. The applicable files should be pulled and reviewed for accuracy and completeness and be up-to-date. If documents are missing or in another location, the documents should be retrieved (or the reason they cannot be retrieved and their location should be noted). Your goal is to make it as easy as possible for the auditor(s) to find documents and information.

IRB minutes for the identified time frame (typically 1 year or more) should be pulled and organized in chronological order. Any minutes that have not yet been finalized should be clearly labeled as draft. If meeting sign-in sheets are not part of the minutes, a copy from each meeting should be provided, along with applicable membership rosters. This will help the auditor(s) verify that quorum was maintained at all times.

⊘ 2-6

Institutional documentation should be available for the auditor(s). A copy of the SOPs, organizational chart with the institutional location of the IRB clearly identified, and personnel chart for the IRB administrative staff, including reporting lines, will help the auditors familiarize themselves with the institution.

⊘ 2-2

Staffing

Plan for IRB administrative staff to be available at all times during the audit. It is likely that staff will need additional time at the beginning of each day to prepare for the day, confirm that all requested information is available, and ensure that everything is in working order. Additional time at the end of each day may also be necessary to find any additional requested information, review notes, and plan for the next day. At least one staff member should be available at all times during the audit as well, to answer administrative questions, locate information and/or people the auditor(s) wishes to interview, make copies (if this is what has been agreed to), and to help ensure a smooth flow to the day. If the auditor(s) has elected to review electronic files only, staff may need to help them locate information and documentation and orient the auditor(s) to the system. One person should be identified as the party responsible for answering questions and providing information on behalf of the institution.

Remote Audits

Audits that are conducted remotely have logistical planning needs similar to those already identified. While proximity to conveniences will not be a concern, additional planning and coordination with the institution's IT experts will be necessary. IT expertise will be needed to ensure access to information is readily available, with secure logins, and that there are no firewall issues or delays.

Investigator Audits

Researchers may also receive audit or inspection notices. These audits may be for a specific study or directed to the researcher. No matter which type of audit or what entity is conducting the audit, it is important for researchers to notify the IRB office when they receive notice of an audit or inspection. These audits are conducted similarly to IRB audits, and the IRB administrative staff can help the study team prepare. Institutional officials and applicable offices and the sponsor (unless the sponsor is conducting or overseeing the audit) should be notified. Space should be identified. Records should be reviewed for completeness and accuracy. Although the researcher's study records will include many documents that the IRB does not have access to (for example, source documents, case report forms, and signed consent documents), it is important for the IRB records to be complete and match. At least one IRB staff member should attend the audit exit interview. This ensures that the IRB has a good understanding of any issues or deficiencies identified and to assist with any corrective actions needed.

During the Audit

Documenting the Audit

Consider documenting all that takes place during the audit. This should include attendees at each session (consider using a sign-in sheet), documents provided from and to the auditor, staff interviewed at each session, questions asked by the auditor, answers provided to the auditor. If you or the auditors request an update at the end of each day, make sure to document what is said and the plans for the next day.

Review Documentation of the Auditor's Credentials

Auditors and inspectors from federal agencies should show their credentials; if they don't, ask. Ensure that anyone who is reviewing documents has the authority to do so. If there is doubt about the credentials of any federal auditor or inspector, contact the agency for verification.

Entrance Briefing/Interview

Most audits will begin with an entrance brief or interview. The auditor will generally describe the agency or organization that he or she represents and will explain the purpose of the audit and the general agenda. The signatory official

🖉 8-1

on your <u>Federalwide Assurance</u> will generally be requested to be present for any entrance briefing by a federal regulatory agency. The auditor may ask some questions during this briefing, but it is mostly an opportunity for the institutional officials to get more details about the audit plan and to ask any questions they have about process.

Document Reviews

Most regulatory audits will include a document review of IRB records, including protocol submissions, informed consent documents, IRB meeting minutes, IRB membership rosters, SOPs, and policies. The auditor will likely request specific documents and protocols in advance but may identify additional records to review while on site. If your HRPP has an electronic records system, consider giving the auditor read-only access to applicable portions of the system. Such access may even be given before the on-site portion of the audit.

Interviews

Interviews may be conducted by telephone or videoconference or on site. The auditor will name the individuals or positions that they want to interview but this usually includes the IRB chair, IRB administrator, IRB staff (with or without the administrator), IRB members (with or without the chair), and researchers. Interviews will typically be 30 to 60 minutes and will include questions about the IRB processes and the individuals' knowledge of policies and requirements. If the audit relates to a particular protocol(s) or issue(s), the interview questions will ask details about this protocol(s) or issue(s).

Observation of an IRB Meeting

Some auditors may request to observe an IRB meeting. This generally is not required, but if your IRB is having a regularly scheduled meeting while auditors are on site, it can give them an in-depth look at the operation of your review board. Auditors should just observe and not participate. Their presence should be noted in the meeting minutes. Consider asking them to sign any confidentiality agreement your IRB has regarding information that they may hear or see during the meeting.

The Exit Interview

At the end of the site visit, the auditor will generally want to have an exit briefing or interview with the principals—usually the signatory official, IRB chair, IRB administrator, and any others that the signatory official wishes to have present. The exit briefing will outline any findings or observations from the audit, any regulatory actions expected, and describe the next steps. The auditor should inform the institution if and when they can expect a formal report of the findings and how and when to respond. This is another opportunity to ask the auditor any questions about the process, as well as questions about any of the findings.

Post Audit

Audit Reports

Your institution will receive an audit report at the exit briefing (e.g., Form FDA 483) or sometime after the audit (e.g., determination letters, FDA Establishment Inspection Reports, FDA Warning Letters). This may take weeks to months. The report will contain findings of noncompliance as well as other observations; it may also contain a description of the strengths of your HRPP and suggestions for improvements (recommendations or "voluntary action indicated" for FDA inspections). Reports from regulatory agencies may include regulatory actions (e.g., suspensions of research, restrictions on your institution's assurance) and required actions that your institution must take to return to or

● 7-6
● 7-3
remain in good graces with the agency. Notify the appropriate entities (e.g., sponsor/funding agency, FDA) of any serious or continuing <u>noncompliance</u> or <u>unanticipated problems</u> involving subjects or others that are identified by the audit.

Responses to Audit Reports and Corrective Action Plans

● 7-6

● 8-5 ● 8-4

The audit report will generally include a deadline by which the institution must respond to the report. The response should be directed to the person or office indicated on the report. The regulatory agency may also begin proceedings to debar or disqualify an IRB, a researcher, or the institution if there are serious and persistent issues with <u>noncompliance</u> that adversely affect the rights or welfare of human subjects. Most reports containing findings of noncompliance will request a corrective action plan (CAP) to address the noncompliance. CAPs should be specific, include timelines for implementation, and be designed to remediate the noncompliance and prevent its reoccurrence. Examples of corrective actions include: revise particular protocols and informed consent documents; notify subjects of new risks or other information; revise written policies and procedures; and educate <u>researchers</u>, <u>IRB members</u>, or other institutional staff about particular regulatory or institutional requirements.

Continuous Improvement

The audit process can be a productive one for all. If no problems are identified during the audit, congratulations! If problems are identified, address them. In either case, once the audit is complete it is time to start preparing for the next audit. Use the audit report as a starting point to establish next steps and areas that may need additional attention. If problems identified during the audit are specific to a study, group of studies, or researcher, do not wait for similar issues to be identified during the next audit. Be proactive and look for similar issues in other studies or areas of the HRPP, and apply the audit resolution to those as well. Striving for continuous improvement in every area of the HRPP will help ensure successful audit outcomes.

Conclusion

Audits can be stressful, but with advance planning and strategic corrective actions, your institution can use the opportunity to improve your program for the protection of human subjects.

Resources

Department of Health and Human Services (DHHS). (2009). *OHRP compliance oversight procedures for evaluating institutions.* www.hhs.gov/ohrp/compliance-and-reporting/evaluating-institutions /index.html

Department of Veterans Affairs. (2019). *VA ORO site visits.* www.va.gov/ORO/ORO_site_visit _preparation.asp

Food and Drug Administration (FDA). (2006). *Information sheet: Guidance for IRBs, clinical investigators, and sponsors: FDA institutional review board inspections.* www.fda.gov/media/75192/download

Food and Drug Administration (FDA). (2018). *FDA BIMO IRB inspections.* www.fda.gov/downloads /ICECI/EnforcementActions/BioresearchMonitoring/ucm133768.pdf

Accreditation of Human Research Protection Programs

Susan S. Fish

Elyse I. Summers

Abstract

This chapter describes the rise of the concept of the human research protection program (HRPP) and, in parallel, the recognition that peer-based voluntary accreditation is a key component in helping to ensure that organizations conducting and/or overseeing human research fulfill their responsibilities to protect the human subjects involved in such research. It includes a discussion of the genesis of the notion of the HRPP as an infrastructure that includes but goes beyond the IRB in helping to ensure the protection of human research subjects. In addition, it describes some of the historical factors that gave rise to the acceptance and promotion of accreditation as a critical indicator of the quality and robustness of an HRPP.

Introduction

Since the beginning of the 21st century, there has been a growing recognition that the best way to protect human subjects in research combines two things: (1) the idea and development of HRPPs, which include but go beyond the IRB, and (2) a system of peer evaluation (accreditation) that helps organizations ensure that they are providing robust protections to research subjects. Although there have been calls for peer review of IRBs since their inception in the last third of the 20th century, accreditation of HRPPs (or IRBs) has existed for less than 20 years. This chapter discusses the history and reasons for accreditation in the human subjects protection field, describes the current status of accreditation, and discusses the implications for IRBs.

🖉 2-1

Background

Although protection of human subjects has been a keystone of clinical research for more than 50 years, thoughts of accreditation only recently reached maturity in the 21st century. However, there were calls for accreditation dating to the 1970s. In 1978, the National Commission for the Protection of Human Subjects of Biomedical and Behavioral Research did more than release the _Belmont Report,_ which provides the ethical underpinnings for the conduct of clinical research. In the report (published in 1979), the _Belmont_ authors also mention concern about requirements for the review of federally funded studies and the lack of requirements for review of all other studies (National Commission, 1979). Such a double standard might suggest that IRBs are important only for meeting federal requirements rather than because of the nature of their work. Concerned about this apparent double standard, the National Commission recommended that a program of peer-based site visits be undertaken (National Commission, 1979). They concluded that a full assessment of an IRB should be based on an examination of that IRB's performance in its particular institutional context and with its particular workload, membership, and procedures.

The National Commission disbanded after its report was issued, and the President's Commission for the Study of Ethical Problems in Medicine and Biomedical and Behavioral Research was appointed. In 1981, the President's Commission decided to explore the possible benefits of IRB site visits to assess the qualitative aspects of the functioning of IRBs, suggesting that the site visits would be collegial and more educational in orientation than is typical of inspections or investigations. Two years later, the 1983 President's Commission Report included a chapter describing a study of IRBs, with data gathered through peer-based site visits (President's Commission, 1983). The report stated that site visits and a review process stimulate improvements at the institutional level. The President's Commission's site visitors were oriented more toward the goals and purposes of IRB review than toward technical conformity with regulatory requirements. The report included 12 pages discussing an accreditation model—in 1983, more than 35 years ago.

The Need for Accreditation

Later reports from the General Accounting Office and the Department of Health and Human Services' (DHHS) Office of the Inspector General also contained references to accreditation. The General Accounting Office, in its 1996 report, "Scientific Research: Continued Vigilance Critical to Protecting Human Subjects," stated that "little data exists that directly measures the effectiveness of human subject protection regulations" (General Accounting Office, 1996). The report suggested that protection of human subjects might be more than simply abiding by the regulations. The Office of the Inspector General in 1998 issued a report entitled "Institutional Review Boards—A Time for Reform," that recommended that all IRBs under the purview of the National Institutes of Health or OPRR (the Office for Protection from Research Risks, which is now the Office for Human Research Protections [OHRP]) and the Food and Drug Administration undergo regular performance-based evaluations (Department of Health and Human Services, 1998). In addition, the evaluations were to be carried out in accordance with the federal regulations.

At the start of the 21st century, two reports issued by the Institute of Medicine (IOM) of the National Academies of Science helped jump-start in earnest calls for accreditation, "Preserving Public Trust: Accreditation and Human Research Participant Protection Programs" (2001), and "Responsible Research: A Systems Approach to Protecting Research Participants" (2002). The 2001 report articulated well how a peer system of evaluation—rather than new or greater regulation—could help preserve, and in some cases restore, public trust in our human research enterprise. And, in complementary fashion, the 2002 report laid the foundation for the recognition that the responsibility to uphold the rights and welfare of research subjects should exist in an overarching HRPP in organizations engaged in or overseeing human research. Indeed, this report posited that with the appropriate disbursement of responsibilities across an organization, the IRB itself would be free to do the ethical review of research that is its charge.

✐ 2-1

These activities did not, of course, exist in a vacuum, and the lay press had an equally important effect, continuing to highlight research activities as well as problems across the research enterprise. For example, the tragic deaths of Jesse Gelsinger in 1999 in a gene transfer study and Ellen Roche in 2001 in a healthy volunteer study garnered wide national coverage, as did government shutdowns of well-known, prestigious academic research institutions. This type of coverage in the popular press surely added to the deterioration of the public's confidence and trust in the research effort. The oversight community came to acknowledge that the public must be assured that their rights and welfare as research subjects are being protected at the same time that the development of new diagnostic and therapeutic approaches to disease is supported.

✐ 1-2
✐ 1-2

An Accreditation System

After many years of recommendations, why did accreditation move from discussion to action? There are many overlapping reasons, including the organized attention brought to the issues in the manner described earlier. Equally significant is that the protection of human subjects had grown into a recognized profession. By 2000, when accreditation really took root, Public Responsibility in Medicine and Research (PRIM&R) had been established for 36 years, encompassing a range of professional education and certification functions (i.e., the Certified IRB Professional [CIP] program). In addition, over time research had become much more complex, making it more challenging to review studies and more difficult to design studies with risks minimized. As a result, it was becoming more difficult to explain such complex studies to potential subjects and, thus, more difficult to protect them. Also, the patient empowerment movement was dramatically changing research. The genesis of this movement was in the HIV/AIDS community, where access to research was viewed as a critical right to possible survival. Cancer and other disease-specific advocacy groups learned from the leadership of the HIV/AIDS community. In some situations, subjects have become more like research partners than traditional research subjects. Finally, there was a real fear that if the community did not take ownership of policing itself through accreditation, the door would be open to greater legislation and regulation. For all of these reasons, and in order to help restore the trust of the public in the research effort, the beginning of the 21st century was the right time to develop an accreditation system for programs of protection of human research subjects.

✐ 12-9

The Accreditation Programs

When accreditation became a reality in the United States, two organizations emerged at the outset. The Partnership for Human Research Protection (PHRP) was formed when the National Committee for Quality Assurance (NCQA) joined with the Joint Commission on Accreditation of Healthcare Organizations. It was originally involved in accreditation at Department of Veterans Affairs (VA) facilities. PHRP no longer exists, and more recently, other attempts at developing U.S.-based HRPP accreditation organizations have come and gone.

The other organization, the Association for the Accreditation of Human Research Protection Programs (AAHRPP), was formed in 2000, from a beginning within PRIM&R. AAHRPP soon attracted support from seven prominent founding organizations, representing key stakeholders across the human research enterprise: the Association of American Medical Colleges, the Association of American Universities, the Association of Public and Land-grant Universities (formerly, the National Association of State University and Land-grant Colleges), the Consortium of Social Science Associations, the Federation of American Societies for Experimental Biology, the National Health Council, and PRIM&R.

AAHRPP accreditation is voluntary. Its voluntariness undergirds its philosophy that organizations take ownership of their responsibility to protect the human research subjects who make the entire enterprise possible. Its program provides an opportunity for self-assessment followed by a process of collegial peer review. AAHRPP's accreditation process is designed to be transparent and educational; the standards used to evaluate an organization are freely available to the public on the AAHRPP website. In addition, although AAHRPP's accreditation activities began in the United States, there are now AAHRPP-accredited organizations around the globe. AAHRPP's standards include a core set of requirements enhanced by country-specific addendums (posted on its website, www.aahrpp.org) that address the particularities, where they exist, of the oversight frameworks in countries outside the United States.

An important feature of the AAHRPP accreditation process is that AAHRPP is active in providing guidance for accreditation applicants and in providing education to the IRB community at large. As mentioned previously, because human subjects protection is a shared responsibility across an organization, the accreditation process focuses on the entire program of protections, beyond just the IRB's processes and responsibilities. The accreditation standards are based largely on federal regulations, although in certain areas (e.g., quality improvement) they go beyond that which regulatory frameworks typically address. The initial AAHRPP accreditation cycle is for 3 years. Thereafter, organizations up for reaccreditation are provided with a 5-year period of accreditation.

Substantively, AAHRPP accreditation is based on three domains: the overarching organizational responsibilities, the composition and processes of the IRB (or ethics committee), and the researcher's responsibilities. Each domain has elements that describe how the standard is met. Although the standards are based on federal regulations and guidance, they go beyond the requirements of the regulations to encourage the development of "best practices" in protection programs. The applicant initially completes a self-assessment, which allows an organization to identify inadequacies in its program, based on AAHRPP's standards. This allows the applicant to address inadequacies prior to application for accreditation. AAHRPP staff provide guidance during the process, even during the self-assessment exercise prior to submission of an actual application.

The application (Step 1) is submitted and reviewed in a back-and-forth process with a Step 1 peer reviewer assigned by AAHRPP, who is typically a similarly situated colleague at another AAHRPP-accredited organization. Following that, there is a second submission (Step 2 application) that provides information related to planning and implementing the site visit, an important feature of the process that allows a site team of peers to evaluate how the organization's practices actually reflect what they describe in their procedures. There are over 80 AAHRPP site visitors, who are colleagues drawn from the profession itself: IRB administrators, IRB chairs, institutional officials, and others affiliated with human subjects protection programs. The vast majority are people who work at AAHRPP-accredited organizations. When an organization achieves initial accreditation, AAHRPP works with the organization to craft a press release announcing its accomplishment, and all accredited organizations are published on AAHRPP's website. As of May 2019, there are 252 AAHRPP-accredited organizations, representing over 600 entities.

Non-U.S. Initiatives

Although the initial drive to accreditation began in the United States with AAHRPP (and the now-defunct PHRP), it has now taken on an international profile, with both transnational and country-specific programs under way, although notably, these programs focus strictly on the IRB/EC/REB (Ethics Committee/Research Ethics Board) rather than the broader HRPP. The three programs described next do not capture the universe of such activities but are merely illustrative of the heightened attention to human research protections around the globe. In 2000, the Forum for Ethical Review Committees in the Asian and Western Pacific region (FERCAP) was launched in Bangkok, Thailand. FERCAP is a project of the World Health Organization (WHO), and it exists under the umbrella of the Strategic Initiative for Developing Capacity in the Ethical Review (SIDCER). It is SIDCER, in turn, that offers a recognition program for IRBs/ECs (www.fercap-sidcer.org/recog.php). Many organizations in the Asia-Pacific region gain FERCAP-SIDCER recognition as a stepping stone to pursuing AAHRPP accreditation, given its broader substantive reach to the HRPP and its global acceptance. Similarly, although there are AAHRPP-accredited organizations in Canada and India, homegrown efforts have arisen in these countries as well. In Canada, a concerted effort to attract clinical trials led to the creation in 2012 (with support of the Ontario government) of Clinical Trials Ontario (CTO), which offers a Research Ethics Board (REB) Qualification program for organizations planning to participate in the CTO Streamlined Research Ethics Review System (www.ctoontario.ca). Importantly, this endeavor relates only to clinical research and does not touch upon research protections in the realm of nonclinical or social and behavioral research. A third non-U.S. initiative in this realm, also involving only biomedical research, was the creation in India of the National Accreditation Board for Hospitals and Healthcare Providers (NABH), with the objective of enhancing the health system and promoting continuous quality improvement and patient safety (https://nabh.co).

Potential Benefits of Accreditation

The benefits of accreditation have moved beyond the theoretical: organizations report that through the AAHRPP process, the breaking down of organizational silos and "forced" cooperation between functional units that are a part of an HRPP have brought greater efficiency to their programs. The AAHRPP accreditation process requires an organizational approach, and this

2-1

provides the IRB with opportunities to further integrate and define an institution-wide human subjects protection program. Additionally, whereas accreditation does not mean that the FDA and OHRP will not come knocking on the door, accredited organizations typically see positive outcomes related to these activities. The peer-review process will help identify areas of excellence that can make the organization more competitive in many areas, such as attracting research funding, recruiting researchers, and recruiting subjects.

⊘ Section 4   Finally, with the requirement of single IRB review of multisite studies, and the truly global nature of research, AAHRPP accreditation offers an "apples to apples" comparison and comfort level for organizations seeking partners and collaborators.

Potential Costs of Accreditation

The most obvious cost are the fees related to accreditation. The fee structure for different organizations offering accreditation varies and can be obtained by contacting the organization. The fee structure for AAHRPP accreditation (which involves both an application fee and ongoing annual fees) is available on the AAHRPP website. Less obvious, but equally significant, is the human effort necessary to embark upon and see to fruition the accreditation process. Gaining organizational buy-in for the work involved and for the dedication of human and financial resources can appropriately be viewed as the first actual accomplishment in the process—they demonstrate that the elevation of human research protections and a robust infrastructure to support it is an organizational priority. Anecdotally, accredited organizations have said, "It was worth the effort."

Conclusion

By developing a set of performance standards and making these available to IRBs and HRPPs, the intent of accreditation is to help IRBs and HRPPs improve. The accreditation process in the United States is voluntary. Self-assessment alone is a useful exercise and provides a framework to allow HRPPs to determine where their strengths and weaknesses lie. Whether the outcome of a self-assessment is positive or less than glowing, it allows an organization to gain important information that can be folded into its plan for improvement and, possibly, an application for accreditation. The subsequent application review process coupled with the site visit provides peer review and external validation of the self-assessment. In addition, the site visit affords an outside source of new ideas for improvement and referral to other resources. If accredited, the IRB and its HRPP can be identified to others as going beyond the federal regulations in protecting the rights and welfare of research subjects. This process of self-assessment and peer review, encouraged and supported by institutional officials, recognizes the organizational priority of the protection of human subjects in a visible, concrete way for everyone involved in the research process. This includes, significantly, the researchers and research staff, which is "where the rubber meets the road." Undertaking the accreditation process provides HRPP staff with an external, objective rationale for receiving the resources it requires to perform its important work.

Resources

Association for the Accreditation of Human Research Protection Programs (AAHRPP). *Our mission, vision, and values.* www.aahrpp.org/learn/about-aahrpp/our-mission

References

Department of Health and Human Services (DHHS). (1998). *Office of the Inspector General: Institutional review boards: A time for reform.* (Report No. OEI-01-97-00193). Washington, DC: Author.

General Accounting Office. (1996). *Scientific research: Continued vigilance critical to protecting human subjects.* Publication GAO/HEHS-96-72. Washington, DC: Author.

Institute of Medicine (IOM). (2001). *Preserving public trust: Accreditation and human research participant protection programs.* Washington, DC: The National Academies Press. www.nap.edu/catalog/10085/preserving-public-trust-accreditation-and-human-research-participant-protection-programs

Institute of Medicine (IOM). (2002). In Committee on Assessing the System for Protecting Human Research Participants, D. D. Federman, K. E. Hanna, & L. L. Rodriguez (Eds.), *Responsible Research: A Systems Approach to Protecting Research Participants.* Washington, DC: National Academies Press. www.nap.edu/catalog/10508/responsible-research-a-systems-approach-to-protecting-research-participants

National Commission for the Protection of Human Subjects of Biomedical and Behavioral Research (1979). *The Belmont Report: Ethical principles and guidelines for the protection of human subjects in biomedical and behavioral research.* www.hhs.gov/ohrp/regulations-and-policy/belmont-report/index.html

President's Commission for the Study of Ethical Problems in Medicine and Biomedical and Behavioral Research. (1983). Implementing human research regulations: Second biennial report on the adequacy and uniformity of federal rules and policies, and of their implementation, for the protection of human subjects. Washington, DC: Author.

Considerations Based on Study Population

Vulnerability in Research: Basic Ethical Concepts and General Approach to Review

Bruce Gordon
Robert Nobles

Abstract

The concept of vulnerability is central to the ethics of human subjects research. Humans participating in research must be offered protection from risks; vulnerable subjects require additional protections. Despite common usage of the term "vulnerability" and its centrality to "protection," the meaning and scope of the concept of vulnerability remain elusive. What, in fact, is vulnerability? Who is vulnerable, and to what? How must vulnerable persons be protected, and from what must they protected? In this chapter we will attempt to lay out a framework to help IRBs apply the concept and evaluate when potential research subjects may be vulnerable in relevant ways.

Introduction: The Concept of Vulnerability

The Common Rule requires that "when some or all of the subjects are likely to be vulnerable ... additional safeguards have been included in the study to protect the rights and welfare of these subjects" [45 CFR 46.111(b)]. This requirement is based, in part, on the _Belmont Report_ principle of respect for persons. _Belmont_ states that "persons with diminished autonomy are entitled to protection" (National Commission, 1979).

    However, neither the Common Rule nor the DHHS regulation subparts B, C, and D—which discuss research with pregnant women, fetuses, and neonates; prisoners; and children; respectively—offer any definition of vulnerability, the

🔗 1-1

🔗 9-4
🔗 9-5 🔗 9-6

characteristics that render persons vulnerable, what they may be vulnerable to, or what safeguards may be appropriate for those who are deemed vulnerable. Since *Belmont* and the publication of the Common Rule and the DHHS subparts, bioethicists and regulators have attempted to address these questions.

In their report "Research Involving Human Participants," the National Bioethics Advisory Commission (NBAC) suggests that "vulnerability, in the context of research, should be understood to be a condition, either intrinsic or situational, of some individuals that puts them at greater risk of being used in ethically inappropriate ways in research" (NBAC, 2001). The commission notes two general themes defining vulnerability: "In general, persons are vulnerable in research either because they have difficulty providing voluntary, informed consent arising from limitations in decision-making capacity ... or situational circumstances ... or because they are especially at risk for exploitation" (NBAC, 2001).

EXPLOITATION

To exploit someone is to take unfair advantage of them. It is to use another person's vulnerability for one's own benefit. (Zwolinski & Wertheimer, 2017)

The World Medical Association, in the Declaration of Helsinki, characterizes vulnerable groups and individuals as those who "may have an increased likelihood of being wronged or of incurring additional harm" (World Medical Association, 2018). Specifically, the Declaration proposes that persons are vulnerable due to a reduced ability to provide informed consent, noting that "Some research populations are particularly vulnerable and need special protection. These include those who cannot give or [cannot] refuse consent for themselves" and also those "who may be vulnerable to coercion or

✎ 12-2   <u>undue influence</u>."

Building on the Declaration of Helsinki characterization of vulnerability, the Council for International Organizations of Medical Sciences (CIOMS) notes "persons are vulnerable because they are relatively (or absolutely) incapable of protecting their own interests" or "because some feature of the circumstances (temporary or permanent) in which they live makes it less likely that others will be vigilant about, or sensitive to, their interests" (CIOMS, 2016).

One recurrent feature of a vulnerable person is the risk of some sort of harm beyond that of other persons in the same (research) situation. The nature of that additional harm is also the source of debate. It ranges from "the possibility of physical harm" (Levine et al., 2004) to "an assault [on their] respect, health, or rights" (Leavitt, 2006) to "[not] getting fair consideration in resource allocation" (Hurst, 2008). Coleman posits the potential harm is "being enrolled in research in violation of one or more of the premises of the basic 'deal' [risks are reasonable in relation to anticipated benefits; risks have been minimized; voluntary informed consent]" (Coleman, 2009).

It is critical to remember that vulnerability (of any type) is not all or nothing—a person is not "vulnerable" or "not vulnerable." Vulnerability occurs along a spectrum. A particular situation, or a particular characteristic, may place a particular person at greater risk of harm in that situation, making them, in that situation, more vulnerable. In other words, the extent of that person's vulnerability is a function of how much greater risk that person, in that situation, faces.

Approaches to Describing Vulnerability

The Categorical Approach

From a practical point of view, there are two distinct approaches to describing the features that make a person vulnerable. The first, a categorical approach, holds that membership in certain groups or populations makes a person vulnerable. This approach talks about "vulnerable populations"; vulnerable populations are those groups in society whose members share features that might make them vulnerable.

The Common Rule describes specific vulnerable groups (children, prisoners, people with impaired decision-making capacity, and economically and educationally disadvantaged persons) **[45 CFR 46.107(a)]**. The Declaration of Helsinki, CIOMS, and the International Council for Harmonisation (ICH) all provide extensive lists of the types of groups or populations that may be vulnerable (CIOMS, 2016; ICH, 2016; World Medical Association, 2018).

As noted by the Presidential Commission for the Study of Bioethical Issues (PCSBI), "the categorical approach is most applicable when all members of a particular group are vulnerable for the same reason. For example, although children vary considerably in their levels of maturity, all children are vulnerable because they lack the fully developed capacity for autonomous decision making that comes with developmental maturity" (PCSBI, 2017).

IRBs must address certain vulnerabilities using this approach: subparts B, C, and D to 45 CFR 46 assign specific protections to pregnant women, human fetuses, and neonates; prisoners; and children; respectively.

However, the categorical approach is not optimal. It is less suitable for situations where people have multiple vulnerabilities (for example, pregnant minors or cognitively impaired homeless people). Nor does it account for variation of degree of vulnerability within a group based on individual characteristics. For example, there is a wide spectrum of "economic disadvantage." A college student who needs cash because she has run out of her monthly allowance and cannot afford beer is different from a single mother without the requisite funds to feed her children. However, both situations may result in the "disadvantaged" individual making choices that they would not otherwise make if they had sufficient funds for their needs or wants.

Finally, and most limiting, the group-based characterizations of vulnerability classify certain persons as vulnerable, rather than identifying situations in which individuals, no matter which groups they belong to, might be considered vulnerable. As the NBAC notes, "vulnerability is sensitive to context, and individuals

REFRAMING THE LANGUAGE OF VULNERABILITY

Faith E. Fletcher and John A. Guidry

Some scholars argue that "labeling individuals as 'vulnerable' risks viewing vulnerable individuals as 'others' worthy of pity, a view rarely appreciated" (Ruof, 2004). While community-engaged approaches seek to empower research subjects to collaboratively address social issues relevant to their communities, relegating individuals to the status of vulnerable might lead to community disempowerment, ultimately reifying historical mistreatment and marginalization of communities we now characterize as "vulnerable." Further, labeling groups as "vulnerable" fails to acknowledge the collective resilience, assets, and unique expertise that communities bring to research interactions and that contribute to the research enterprise.

Reframing "vulnerability" language is consistent with recent shifts in terminology, from using "health disparities" to "health inequities," the latter of which gives due attention to issues of fairness and justice that must be addressed through systemic or policy-level changes (Whitehead, 1991). The field of bioethics has long been criticized for its failure to address the significant role of access, availability, and affordability of health services in health differences. Similarly, the use of vulnerability has the unintended consequence of blaming social and economic conditions and inequality on individuals and communities. A shift in language is similarly supported by the Commission on the Social Determinants of Health (CSDH) framework that highlights that individuals are differentially exposed and vulnerable to social and health-compromising conditions based on social, economic, and political mechanisms (Solar & Irvin, 2010). Thus, rather than characterizing individuals as inherently vulnerable in themselves or in specific contexts, their engagement in the research process holds out the promise of recognizing research subjects as "moral agents in their own right" (Fisher, 1998).

Fisher, C. B. (1998). Paper 3: Relational ethics and research with vulnerable populations. In National Bioethics Advisory Committee (Eds.), *Research involving persons with mental disorders that may affect decisionmaking capacity.* www.onlineethics.org/8128/mindex

Ruof, M. C. (2004). Vulnerability, vulnerable populations, and policy. *Kennedy Institute of Ethics Journal, 14,* 411–425.

Solar, O., & Irwin, A. (2010). *A conceptual framework for action on the social determinants of health. Social determinants of health discussion paper 2 (Policy and Practice).* www.who.int /sdhconference/resources/ConceptualframeworkforactiononSDH_eng.pdf

Whitehead, M. (1991). The concepts and principles of equity and health. *International Journal of Health Services, 2(3),* 429–445.

may be vulnerable in one situation but not in another" (NBAC, 2001). For example, the impoverished mother in the previous example might be at risk for exploitation in the context of a study that offers a large cash payment, but perhaps not when taking part in a short survey without compensation. An affluent, white middle-aged CEO would not usually be thought of as "vulnerable," but the same person in an emergency department with chest pain certainly would be.

The Contextual Approach

An alternate approach to characterization of vulnerability is a contextual one. NBAC defines vulnerability in terms of "situations in which individuals might be considered vulnerable" (NBAC, 2001). This approach allows for a more nuanced understanding of the nature of the specific vulnerability, and therefore a more focused approach to safeguards for addressing it. This approach broadly classifies types of vulnerability as cognitive or communicative, institutional, deferential, medical, economic, and social.

- *Cognitive or communicative vulnerability*
  This category broadly encompasses persons who have difficulty comprehending information and making decisions about participation. This would include (1) persons who lack capacity (for example, immature children or adults with cognitive impairment), (2) persons who do not lack capacity but are in situations that do not allow them to exercise their capacities effectively, such as the CEO with chest pain example, or (3) persons who cannot effectively communicate (such as a research subject who speaks a different language than does the researcher), and therefore who may be at a disadvantage with regard to receiving information or expressing their considered choices.

  🖉 6-7, 6-8

  <u>Protections</u> that might be appropriate for a person with these sorts of vulnerabilities might include use of plain-language consent forms (a laudable goal for all situations), supplementary educational measures, conversations and consent from legally authorized representatives and/or use of interpreters and translated materials. When capacity is a concern, research-

  🖉 9-7, 10-12

  ers should have a plan for objective assessment of <u>capacity</u> and the proper use of surrogates and advocates, including advance directives. The process of consent should be carefully considered and modified as needed. This might include staged consent, whereby formal consent is obtained several times during the research, to facilitate understanding by presenting manageable blocks of information. Finally, it may be appropriate to delay entry into the research until transient cognitive vulnerabilities have resolved.

- *Institutional vulnerability*
  This category includes persons who are under the formal authority of others who might have different values, goals, and priorities than those of the potential research subject. This might include <u>prisoners</u>, those in the mil-

  🖉 9-5

  itary, or any other person whose relationship with a superior might make it difficult for him to say "no." In the context of the NBAC definition of vulnerability, these persons may not be able to make a truly free decision concerning participation, and/or are at risk for exploitation.

  Protections appropriate for these persons should focus on devising a consent procedure that will adequately insulate the prospective subject from the hierarchical system. This might involve use of persons other than the researcher to approach potential subjects or to monitor the researcher's process of consent as it occurs. If this cannot be accomplished, then it might be appropriate to exclude prospective subjects if there is a concern that they cannot make a voluntary choice.

- *Deferential vulnerability*

  Like institutional vulnerability, this category includes persons who are under the authority of others. In this case, however, the authority is informal rather than hierarchical. It may be based on gender, race, or class inequalities, or on inequalities of power and knowledge (as in a doctor–patient relationship). The latter may be particularly powerful in the setting of research on medical therapies. It is worth remembering that the deference may occur as a consequence of fear of offending the authority figure and incurring retribution, or it may come from a genuine desire to please a respected other. As with institutional vulnerability, these persons may not be able to make a truly autonomous decision concerning participation and/or are at risk for exploitation. The hallmark demonstration of institutional vulnerability is the <u>Milgram Obedience Study</u> conducted between 1961 and 1963 at Yale University. In this study, the primary researcher, Stanley Milgram, sought out and was able to document the extent to which positional power could be used to coerce individuals to perform actions that they would not otherwise do.

  🔗 1-2

  Protections for these persons usually focus on the process of consent and transparency, as with institutional vulnerability. It may be useful to carry out the consent process without the presence of the party to whom the subject ordinarily defers.

- <u>*Medical*</u> *vulnerability*

  🔗 9-8

  This category includes persons who have serious health conditions for which there are no satisfactory standard treatment options. For these individuals it can be difficult to weigh the risks and potential benefits associated with the research, especially if their understanding is clouded by the misconception that the research is intended, primarily, to benefit their health situation (therapeutic misconception).

  Protections in this circumstance usually focus on the process of consent, and the efforts that should be made by the researcher and others to minimize therapeutic misconception. Kipnis also proposes that additional "protections" may be offered through modifications to the design of some <u>phase I trials</u> (where therapeutic misconception is often the most prominent) in order to actually increase the likelihood of benefit (Kipnis, 2001).

  🔗 10-15

- *Economic vulnerability*

  🔗 9-9

  This category includes people who are disadvantaged in the distribution of social goods and services such as income, housing, or health care. Monetary or other incentives (like access to otherwise unaffordable health care) might constitute inducements for such persons to participate in a research study when they otherwise would not do so. To the extent that such persons participate against their own desires or best interests because of their economic conditions, their autonomy is limited, and they are at risk for exploitation.

  Whether inducement is "due" or "undue," it is a matter of judgment and depends on context. A <u>payment</u> of \$20 for a 2-hour survey hardly seems excessive or "undue" and would be unlikely to result in causing an affluent CEO to act against their better judgment; the same could not be said about \$20 to an impoverished single mother trying to feed her children. In this case, protection for economically disadvantaged subjects may focus on limiting monetary or other compensation to avoid undue inducement to participate in the study. At the same time, as Kipnis notes, it is often hard to "discern the difference between just and unjust compensation packages. We are often inclined to honor the view that, if a bargain is satisfactory to both parties, third parties should not interfere. . . . While we do not want to see people treated unfairly, we are not very confident applying the concept of the just price" (Kipnis, 2001).

  🔗 12-2

Inducement can also be observed within a study's proposed methodology, which could unintentionally increase subjects' interest in particular studies. Consider a study designed with the intent of understanding drunk driving behaviors in order to create signage that would prevent fatal crashes related to overconsumption. Subjects who are recruited on a college campus are provided the alcohol of their choice and are asked to drink until intoxication. After the subject's blood alcohol level is confirmed to be greater than 0.08, the subjects enter a closed driving course and are subjected to various road conditions to test new safety precautions designed to reduce accidents resulting from individuals driving under the influence. For an economically disadvantaged subject, e.g. a college student, the prospect of, for instance, $20 or $40 worth of "free" alcohol might constitute an undue inducement to participate in the study. IRBs should consider whether the "interventions" provided in a study may themselves constitute an overly attractive offer for some subjects, and determine appropriate protections.

At a minimum, protections in this case should include screening procedures for potential subjects to identify and exclude subjects with a diagnosis of alcohol use disorder, a parent with alcohol use disorder, association with or experience with binge drinking (more than five drinks per day at least once per week), or who have on occasion consumed more than 15 drinks in a week and/or have past history of a mental health problem. IRBs should also consider the risks of driving under the influence, especially as it relates to the subjects' personal safety or risks to others associated with the study team. Post-intervention care for the subjects should also be taken into consideration, including, but not limited to, ensuring that the subject's blood alcohol returns to below the intoxication level, and the individual has the ability to fully recover prior to leaving the post-intervention observational activities of the study team.

IRBs should also apply a personal litmus test of whether or not they would enter the study or let someone they care deeply about participate in the study as designed and communicated. If the answer to either question is no, then IRBs have the responsibility of inquiring further and providing input on procedures that produce the best outcomes, while taking into consideration subject safety, transparency, and the spectrum of unintended consequences.

9-9 • *Social vulnerability*
This final category includes people who belong to a perceived undervalued social group. As described by NBAC, "the treatment of members of such groups is not simply attributable to their economic vulnerability, although it is true that members of undervalued groups often lack financial resources. Social vulnerability is a function of the social perception of certain groups, which includes stereotyping and can lead to discrimination. In any case, the perceptions devalue members of such groups, their interests, their welfare, or their contributions to society" (NBAC, 2001). More simply put, these individuals may be vulnerable because they are less valued and the risks they experience are considered less important, or less in need of remediation, than the same risks experienced by more valued member of society.

Protection for these persons requires recognition by researchers and IRBs of the fact that perceptions that some people are of lesser value than others exist, and that persons are vulnerable to such perceptions. NBAC suggests that "efforts should be made to allow members of such groups to participate in decision-making and oversight processes. Involving the community in the various stages of the research process, especially in study planning, can be helpful in reducing stereotyping and stigmatization" (NBAC 2001). Importantly, and in distinction to several of the other vulnerabilities, augmenting informed consent will not usefully reduce this particular vulnerability.

Basic IRB Approach

The <u>criteria for approval</u> at 45 CFR 46.111 require the IRB to determine that additional safeguards have been included in the study to protect the rights and welfare of subjects who are likely to be vulnerable. To make this determination, the IRB should consider, in sequence, two questions: is inclusion in the research necessary, and if so, are the proposed safeguards adequate?

⊘ 5-4

Is Inclusion Necessary?

It is important to recognize that the principles described in *Belmont* may be in tension with each other, and it is often a matter of balancing competing claims urged by these principles.

For example, the principle of respect for persons includes the moral requirement to protect those with diminished autonomy (including vulnerable subjects). As noted in *Belmont*, "some persons are in need of extensive protection, even to the point of excluding them from [research]" (National Commission, 1979). At the same time, the principle of beneficence includes an obligation to provide benefit to research subjects, and the principle of justice requires that researchers distribute benefits equitably and not unfairly exclude persons from those potential benefits. Thus, the IRB (and the researcher) must weigh these competing claims and determine if inclusion of vulnerable subjects is appropriate.

As part of deciding if inclusion of vulnerable subjects is scientifically (and ethically) necessary, the IRB should ask: *Are there less vulnerable persons whose participation in research could answer the same scientific questions?* Consider the situation of a phase II study of an investigational drug for depression, where the researchers choose a target population of inhabitants of a homeless shelter who have moderate to severe depression. There are certainly persons within this population who might benefit from participation (and from the downstream effect of a more effective medication for depression). However, the same societal benefit (a new effective medication) could be gained by enrolling less vulnerable people, perhaps affluent professionals whose moderate to severe depression is managed by a psychiatrist in private practice.

However, there are risks associated with limiting the involvement of vulnerable persons in research. The National Commission, in their 1977 Report on Research Involving Children, noted "The argument in favor of conducting research involving children rests on . . . the consequences of not conducting research involving children in those instances. Such consequences might include the perpetuation of harmful practices, the introduction of untested practices, and the failure to develop new treatments for diseases that affect children" (National Commission, 1977).

The case of benzyl alcohol poisoning ("gasping syndrome") in low birth weight infants is instructive on this point. Benzyl alcohol, an antimicrobial preservative that is commonly used in wide variety of parenteral medications and fluids, had been studied in adult animals of various species, but not in newborn or immature animals. Benzyl alcohol had been shown to be safe in

VOLUNTARY INFORMED CONSENT CAPACITY

In exploring whether subjects might have difficulty providing voluntary informed consent, the IRB might consider asking the following questions:

- Are there decisional issues or communication issues that might interfere with the ability of the prospective subject to understand the research or their rights, to process that information and make a reasoned choice based on their own goals and values, or to communicate their wishes?
- Are there social conditions that limit the subject's options?
- Does the subject's hope for medical benefit influence their judgment?
- Are the conditions for informed consent satisfied? That is, is information presented in an understandable manner, do the subjects comprehend the details of the research and their rights as research subjects, and is the process of consent conducive to true voluntariness?

adults. In early 1982, however, it was recognized that infusion of IV medications containing benzyl alcohol to low birth weight premature infants caused severe metabolic acidosis, encephalopathy, and respiratory depression with gasping, leading to the death of 16 infants. Benzyl alcohol is metabolized to benzoic acid and then conjugated in the liver and excreted as hippuric acid. This latter metabolic pathway is less functional in premature infants, allowing accumulation of benzoic acid with resulting toxicity. Removal of benzyl alcohol from IV medications in one NICU was associated with a decrease of mortality rate for very small infants from 81% to 46% (Hiller et al., 1986). Similar pediatric therapeutic disasters have occurred, reflecting the danger of extrapolating safety and dosage from adult studies to children (Christensen et al., 1999). These episodes clearly demonstrate the necessity of controlled testing of drugs in children before the use of these drugs, approved in adults, becomes standard practice.

If Inclusion Is Necessary, Are Safeguards Adequate (What Additional Protections Are Needed)?

Once a decision has been made that inclusion is necessary, the IRB needs to determine whether the proposed safeguards are adequate. More specifically, the IRB must identify the particular aspects of the research that place vulnerable subjects at risk and then evaluate whether the researcher has provided adequate safeguards to minimize those risks (see sidebars "Voluntary Informed Consent Capacity" and "Risk for Exploitation").

Section 6

Ultimately, the IRB needs to determine if the process of <u>informed consent</u> is designed and conducted in a manner that maximizes the ability of the subject to make an informed and voluntary decision to participate, and if not, how the consent process might be augmented to better support subject decision making. Likewise, the IRB must decide if the risks of exploitation are minimized and what structural protections might further lower those risks.

It is important to remember that informed consent, although a critical protection, is not a panacea: It is not enough to inform and ask subjects to accept a risk. That risk must be minimized to the greatest extent possible consistent with the scientific goals of the research. At the same time, "safeguards must be tailored to respond to particular types and should avoid the exclusively protectionistic attitude toward vulnerability inherent in the current regulations" (NBAC, 2001). That is to say, the safeguards can and should be more thoughtful than merely excluding potential subjects because they are "vulnerable."

We are well advised to recall the words of Henry Beecher: "the more reliable safeguard is provided by the presence of an intelligent, informed, conscientious, compassionate, responsible investigator" (Beecher, 1966).

RISK FOR EXPLOITATION

In considering whether prospective subjects are at risk for exploitation, the IRB should ask:

- How is the power differential between the subject and the researcher being addressed?
- Are there economic issues that might place the subject at risk for undue inducement?
- Are the recruitment process and payment arrangements acceptable?

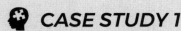 ## CASE STUDY 1

The question of inclusion often arises on college campuses as it relates to enrolling students in studies or collecting samples from students without regard to or awareness of the regulations related to human research subject protections. Consider a case in which a researcher is interested in studying mosquitoes of the *Anopheles* genus, the carrier of malaria. Undergraduate and graduate students within the laboratory are asked to provide blood samples on a routine basis to provide nourishment to the insects (study specimens). In this situation, IRBs should consider (1) the general awareness and/or campus training related to sample collection of students or laboratory employees for any purpose; (2) the sterility of the procedures for sample collection within approved research studies; (3) the rationale for inclusion of the study population versus creating a general recruitment strategy that excludes members of the laboratory and research team from participation; (4) whether or not alternative sources of materials are available to conduct research activities since human subjects are not the primary focus of the research activity; and (5) whether consenting procedures are adequate or appropriate for the study design, while taking into consideration the potential student/teacher power dynamic.

 ## CASE STUDY 2

The expectation of therapeutic benefit in the context of conducting research is a pervasive challenge that IRBs must address; they must also continue to raise their awareness regarding effective strategies to protect subjects from potential exploitation.

Consider a bariatric physician who has an interest in "curing" type 2 diabetes with an ileal interposition in a cohort of patients who do not meet the clinical criteria for the surgery.

As background, an ileal interposition is a surgical procedure that moves a significant portion of the ileum (last of three segments of the small intestine that connects directly to the large intestine) either in front of the first segment (duodenum) or in front of the second segment (jejunum). The typical clinical indication for the procedure requires the BMI to be 30 or above (among other factors), which triggers the availability of reimbursement from patient insurance. The researcher has an interest in leveraging international study findings related to the effectiveness of this bariatric procedure in individuals who are not considered obese (BMI less than 30), with the intent of increasing the patient pipeline for the surgery. The procedure typically ranges in cost from $15,000 to $30,000; the researcher has set his fees for the procedure without insurance at $20,000. In the United States this would be a proof of concept study to encourage insurance agencies to change their reimbursement practices for the procedure to cover patients with BMI of less than 30.

The researcher proposes a pilot study without an external sponsor and proposes to ask subjects to pay for half of the cost of the procedure, or $10,000. To participate, subjects must have been diagnosed with type 2 diabetes within the past 12 months and have a BMI between 20 and 29.

Most of us would agree that the researchers are being innovative in their approach to studying a novel intervention for type 2 diabetes and, if successful, reducing the burden of individuals living with type 2 diabetes. However, this case provides a good example of how exploitation can occur while designing a research study. Although the study might result in the elimination of type 2 diabetes and sustained weight loss for subjects, the case raises concerns that patients who do not meet the current clinical indication for the bariatric surgery but are eager, or even desperate, to lose weight, might be unduly induced to enroll in the study and take on the considerable risks involved in the procedure. Those risks include absorption and nutritional disorders, including the inability to maintain weight at a desired or healthy level. The challenge for IRBs is to explore (1) how subjects are being recruited for the study (including how the power differential between the subject and the researcher is being addressed, how the risks and benefits are being presented, and who is being asked to participate in the study); (2) the risks versus benefits of the study procedure (e.g., the success rate for the procedure compared to treatment options for the disease, which include modifications to diet and exercise); (3) the economic issues that might place the subject at risk for undue inducement (e.g., discounted procedure they cannot otherwise get); (4) whether the study-related costs and payment arrangements are acceptable; (5) whether the intent of the study—namely, to treat type 2 diabetes, not to induce weight loss—is appropriately communicated by the research team; and (6) whether and how long-term issues with absorption or malnutrition will be managed and corrected by the study physician.

Acknowledgment

Some of the material presented in this chapter was previously published in the Ochsner Journal (Gordon BG. (2020). Vulnerability in research: basic ethical concepts and general approach to review. Ochsner J. 20(1):34-38).

References

Beecher, H. K. (1966). Ethics and clinical research. *New England Journal of Medicine, 274*, 1354–1360.

Christensen, M. L., Helms, R. A., & Chesney, R. W. (1999). Is pediatric labeling really necessary? *Pediatrics, 104*, 593–597.

Coleman, C. (2009). Vulnerability as a regulatory category in human subject research. *Journal of Law and Medical Ethics, 37*, 12–18.

Council for International Organizations of Medical Sciences (CIOMS). (2016). *International ethical guidelines for health-related research involving humans.* cioms.ch/publications/product/international-ethical-guidelines-for-health-related-research-involving-humans/

Hiller, J. L., Benda, G. I., Rahatzad, M., Allen, J. R., Culver, D. H., Carlson, C. V., & Reynolds, J. W. (1986). Benzyl alcohol toxicity: Impact on mortality and intraventricular hemorrhage among very low birth weight infants. *Pediatrics, 77*(4), 500–506.

Hurst, S. A. (2008). Vulnerability in research and health care: Describing the elephant in the room? *Bioethics, 22*(4), 191–202.

International Conference on Harmonisation (ICH). (2016). Guideline for good clinical practice. Document E6 (R2). ichgcp.net

Kipnis, K. (2001). Vulnerability in research subjects: A bioethical taxonomy. In *Ethical and policy issues in research involving human participants: Report and recommendations of the National Bioethics Advisory Commission.* Bethesda, MD: National Bioethics Advisory Commission.

Leavitt, F. (2006). Is any medical research population not vulnerable? *Cambridge Quarterly of Healthcare Ethics, 15*, 81–88.

Levine, C., Faden, R., Grady, C., Hammerschmidt, D., Eckenwiler, L., Sugarman, J., & Consortium to Examine Clinical Research Ethics. (2004). The limitations of "vulnerability" as a protection for human research participants. *American Journal of Bioethics, 4*, 44–49.

National Bioethics Advisory Commission (NBAC). (2001). *Ethical and policy issues in research involving human participants: Report and recommendations of the National Bioethics Advisory Commission.* Bethesda, MD: Author.

National Commission for the Protection of Human Subjects of Biomedical and Behavioral Research. (1977). *Research involving children: Report and recommendations.* Bethesda, MD: Author.

National Commission for the Protection of Human Subjects of Biomedical and Behavioral Research. (1979). *The Belmont Report: Ethical principles and guidelines for the protection of human subjects in biomedical and behavioral research.* www.hhs.gov/ohrp/regulations-and-policy/belmont-report/index.html

Presidential Commission for the Study of Bioethical Issues (PCSBI). (2017). Vulnerable populations background. bioethicsarchive.georgetown.edu/pcsbi/node/4031.html

World Medical Association. (2018). *Declaration of Helsinki: Ethical principles for medical research involving human subjects.* www.wma.net/policies-post/wma-declaration-of-helsinki-ethical-principles-for-medical-research-involving-human-subjects/

Zwolinski, M., & Wertheimer, A. (2017). Exploitation. In E. Zalta (Ed.), *The Stanford Encyclopedia of Philosophy* (Summer 2017 ed.). plato.stanford.edu/archives/sum2017/entries/exploitation/Voluntary Informed Consent Capacity

Research Involving Students

Lisa Leventhal
Shannon Sewards

Abstract

Students make up an exceptionally diverse population of research subjects, from children and adolescents enrolled in K–12, to adult learners enrolled in professional development courses, to traditional and nontraditional college students. Students are recruited for studies about education and for social, behavioral, and biomedical studies that are not necessarily about education, simply because they are the most accessible population on an academic campus. Their vulnerabilities as individuals and as groups are often what makes them the focus of study; matters of literacy, language, mental or physical health, drug use, food insecurity, social identities, immigration status, and others are of interest to researchers. Those very same vulnerabilities have a direct impact on the potential risks and benefits of a given research proposal. This chapter addresses the various considerations for IRBs when reviewing research involving students and provides questions, suggestions, and resources to guide the review of studies that may be conducted inside or outside of an educational setting.

Introduction

There are many reasons to conduct research that involves students as subjects. Studies in education settings may enable researchers to gain an understanding of how children and adults learn, what makes an effective curriculum, and what role classroom dynamics play in a learner's educational experience. Academic researchers also commonly recruit college students for studies that may have little or nothing to do with the topic of education, because participation is viewed as having a positive pedagogical benefit for the students or because students are the most accessible population on an academic campus.

The purpose of this chapter is to shed light on the intricacies of conducting research with students; highlight the distinction between research and other activities; navigate the intersection of various federal regulations, state laws, and institutional policies; and define the roles and responsibilities of the IRB as distinct from those of the researchers and educational institutions.

IRB Review

Determining Whether IRB Review Is Required

Education is an area that is constantly being evaluated. Does this curriculum work? Does it work for some students but not for others? Are students meeting standard achievement levels? What should those standard achievement levels be? Is the institution meeting the needs of students? In some cases, the intent of these questions is to conduct research with human subjects, as defined by the Common Rule. In other cases, these questions are the basis for program evaluation, needs assessment, or analysis of institutional data for internal use only ("institutional research") and do not require IRB review. For example, an institution may be interested to learn trends in majors chosen by first-generation college students. The results of this inquiry will be used for internal planning and may be published on the institution's website and in annual reports.

Questions that may help an IRB determine whether a project requires IRB review can include the following:

- Is the intent to improve a specific class or program and only provide information for and about that program?
- Is the intent to decide whether a specific program should continue?
- Is the activity mandated by a program or school, thus requiring all students or teachers to participate?
- Is the intent limited to evaluating tools (e.g., workbooks, educational games, use of new technology in the classroom) or providing benchmarks for program stakeholders?

"Yes" answers to these questions would indicate that the project may not need IRB review, even if publicly posting or publishing the results is planned. However, if the intent of the project is to contribute to generalizable knowledge, IRB review will be required. Determining when an activity is intended to contribute to generalizable knowledge is a persistent challenge for IRBs. Questions that may assist an IRB in making this decision are found in the sidebar.

In education settings, it is often challenging to distinguish between research and program evaluation. A conversation with the researcher about the intent and design of the project will prove useful. To determine whether program evaluation is the intent, consider posing the following questions:

- What is the purpose of the overall project?
- Would this project happen regardless of the researcher's involvement?
- Is the intent of the project to improve a practice within the school or an aspect of the program? Or, is it to fill a gap in knowledge related to all such programs?
- Does the project involve randomization of participants?

DOES THIS MEET THE DEFINITION OF RESEARCH?

- Are the results expected to expand the knowledge base of a scientific discipline or other scholarly field of study?
- Does the project involve testing the impact of a longer recess (the experimental intervention) on classroom behavior?
- Is the intent to demonstrate a relationship or correlation between class size and student learning?
- Will the results apply to high school students beyond the site of data collection, or will the results only apply to students in that school?
- Are the results intended to be used to develop, test, or support theories, principles, and statements of relationships or to inform policy beyond the study?
- Is the project motivated in part by the professional goals of the researcher (e.g., promotion and tenure, obtaining grants, completing a thesis or dissertation)?

"Yes" answers to these questions may lead to a determination that the project meets the definition of research under the Common Rule and requires IRB review.

- Is the activity or project mandated or directed by the school or program?
- Do all of the students in the class, school, or program have to participate in the activity?
- Is the faculty member or researcher serving as a consultant by providing input on methods and design? Will they participate in other activities?
- Are they receiving data from the project? If so, might they use this data for a separate research project?
- Is there a contract in place for the services they will perform? If so, how does it describe their involvement and the purpose of the project?

Consent

Assent, Consent, Parental Permission

When research involving students is determined to need IRB review, the requirements for <u>consent</u> and approaches to obtaining the appropriate permissions can vary widely. Differences stem from which regulations apply in addition to the Common Rule, the age of the students, the nature of the education setting, the topic of the research, languages spoken, and literacy levels of the target population. While there are circumstances under which the regulations permit an IRB to <u>waive consent</u>, parental permission should not be avoided simply because parents are assumed to be disengaged or because waiting for their responses will delay data collection. Similarly, consent from college students does not become less important because the researcher already has access to their records as the course instructor.

⊘ Section 6

⊘ 6-4

Any research plan to obtain consent or provide notification to students or parents should demonstrate respect for the target population and reflect an accurate understanding of the research site; this includes knowledge of the institution or organization's policies and expectations, as well as sufficient familiarity with the languages and literacy level of the population to craft readily comprehensible written materials or verbal explanations for the subjects and, when appropriate, their parents or guardians.

Consent Versus Notification

There are two approaches to obtaining permission from students to involve them in research: consent or a notification with an opportunity to opt out.

If the research involves enrolling students who are <u>minors</u>, consent to participate must involve obtaining either verbal or written permission from one or more parents or guardians for the child to participate in the study. Verbal consent may be obtained by researchers who are meeting with parents or guardians in person when the regulatory conditions for <u>waiver</u> of signed consent are satisfied [45 CFR 46.117(c)]. Schools and structured programs for children, like 4-H, typically have a preferred method of sending written information home to parents that is then returned with signatures. *Researchers must not include students in research activities if the consent forms were returned unsigned or not returned at all.* This is in contrast to the notification process.

⊘ 9-6

⊘ 6-4

When an IRB finds that a waiver of consent or parental permission is appropriate and permissible under the regulations and state law, notification to parents that includes a reasonable opt-out period may be utilized as a means to engage parents and further safeguard children. OHRP notes that, "Even though not required by the regulations, an IRB may require that parents be given the opportunity to refuse permission even when the IRB has waived the regulatory requirement to obtain parental permission" (DHHS, 2019). It is important for IRBs to remember that receiving a notification and "opting out" (that is, when the researcher assumes that the student can participate unless the child or parent says "no") is not the same as giving consent. <u>Consent</u> is more than passively receiving information; it involves comprehension of that information and a voluntary and affirmative response. Of note, the terms "implied" and "passive" consent do not appear in the Common Rule or the *Belmont Report*. Use of an "opt-out" procedure is only permissible if the IRB has determined that the conditions for waiver of consent have been satisfied. Although parental notification does not satisfy the requirement for parental consent under the Common Rule, it is a valuable mechanism for communicating information to parents and guardians when the criteria for a waiver of consent have been met under **45 CFR 46.116** or waiver of parental permission under **45 CFR 46.408**.

6-1

Whether the subjects are minors or adult learners, the plan to obtain consent should ensure that when consent is not provided, that choice will also be honored. This can be challenging in classroom or group settings where one or more of the students (or their parents) did not agree to be part of the study. Questions that an IRB might ask when evaluating the plan for managing consent could include the following:

- Does the plan for obtaining consent ensure that any participation in research activities is voluntary? For example, if the classroom is being video recorded, will nonconsenting students be captured on video anyway? If the curriculum is experimental, are students able to withdraw from the research at any time and switch to a session teaching the traditional curriculum after the course is under way?
- Is the proposed plan for students who will not participate in research disruptive to their learning experience? For example, will nonconsenting students have to sit in the back of the classroom when they ordinarily choose to sit in the front?
- Does the plan for students who do not consent identify those students as being different, and does it disadvantage or stigmatize those students in some way? For example, if consent forms were only written in English, are children whose parents do not read English excluded from a research activity that has been described to their classmates as a game or something fun to do with visitors to their classroom?

Who Will Obtain Consent?

Students can be vulnerable to feeling pressured to participate in research, either by their peers or by the person obtaining consent. Students, and parents of students, may be concerned that choosing not to participate may jeopardize their relationship with their teacher. In order to ensure that voluntariness is emphasized, it is critical to choose the right people to obtain consent and assent.

Researchers may propose to have a member of the study team obtain assent and/or parental permission. The study team members can provide a presentation of the study in a manner that is consistent with what has been approved by the IRB, and, because they are usually not known to the child or parent, it may be less likely that they will be perceived as a person in a position of power or influence.

When a setting does not easily accommodate a researcher-led consent process, researchers may propose to rely on school personnel, program staff, or the course professor to obtain the necessary permission. As these individuals are likely to know the potential subjects, rapport has already been established, and that may bring a sense of trust and transparency that is important to the consent conversation. At the same time, parents may confuse research as having a benefit when permission to take part in a research study is sought from a school authority. Similarly, the established rapport and power structure between instructor and student may influence the decision to participate. This is not to say that school personnel should not be allowed to obtain assent or parent permission, but the IRB should take the possibility of undue influence or perceived coercion into account, as well as how potential misperceptions might be mitigated.

Although different settings may call for different individuals to conduct the consent process, the following should be considered:

- Students and/or parents may be more likely to misunderstand research as being compulsory or as having a direct benefit to the student when permission is sought from school personnel or a course instructor. What is the student and/or parent told during the initial approach and consent process to mitigate this misunderstanding?
- Researchers are motivated to enroll subjects. What strategies are in place to mitigate the potential for undue influence or the perception of pressure?
- Researchers are enthusiastic about their projects, and this can influence the way they deliver information about the potential short- and long-term benefits of their research. Does the consent form guide researchers to realistically frame potential risks and benefits?
- If recruiting from a school, are there specific requirements for an approach and/or consent process?
- What is the local context for consent? Is it permissible for the researcher to approach the student directly?

It is essential that the approach to obtaining assent, consent, and parental permission is more than just feasible; selecting the appropriate people to participate in this process is key to ensuring that potential subjects understand that participation is truly voluntary.

Risks Specific to Students

Voluntary Nature of Participation

A student must not be compelled to participate in research as part of a course requirement. The study should include a plan to ensure that students know that they may choose not to participate in the research and that their decision will not affect their grade, class standing, or relationship with any instructor.

Researchers may offer course credit or extra credit in exchange for participation. To support the voluntary nature of participation, an alternate means of earning equivalent course credit or extra credit for an equivalent commitment of time and effort should be made available for those who cannot or choose not to participate in a study. In their Informed Consent FAQs, the federal Office for Human Research Protections (OHRP) offers the following example (DHHS, 2019):

> [A]n investigator might promise psychology students extra credit if they participate in the research. If that is the only way a student can earn extra credit, then the investigator is unduly influencing potential subjects. If, however, she offers comparable non-research alternatives for earning extra credit, the possibility of undue influence is minimized.

Researchers must allow for subjects to withdraw their consent to participate at any time. A reminder of the importance of voluntary participation for the duration of a study came from OHRP in the form of a letter to Sona Systems, Ltd. (DHHS, 2010). Many entities use Sona Systems software to manage their subject pools. Originally, the software included a feature that automatically assessed penalty credits to students who failed to show up for scheduled appointments without cancelling in advance by a specified deadline. Further inquiry by OHRP resulted in the determination that use of the feature did "violate the requirements of U.S. Department of Health and Human Services (HHS) regulations at **45 CFR 46.116(a)(8)** that participation in research be voluntary and refusal to participate involve no penalty or loss of benefits to which the subject is otherwise entitled" (DHHS, 2010).

Use of Class Time

When research activities are to take place during class time, thus potentially detracting from the normal educational benefit of being in class, an IRB may ask the researcher to explain how participation in the research would be (or not be) a learning experience for the students. An alternative activity should be provided for students who choose not to participate. This is particularly important if the research is being reviewed as <u>exempt</u> under category 1, which specifically requires that the research is "not likely to adversely impact the students' opportunity to learn required education content."

🔗 5-3

Nonphysical Risks

When contemplating risk in education research, the focus is typically on risks that are not physical in nature. Examples include the following:

- Stigma or reputational harm that could result from a breach of confidentiality or accidental disclosure of sensitive, identifiable information
- Impact on students' educational experience
- Undue influence or coercion of students or parents

The nature and degree of data-related risks typically hinge on whether there are practices to protect privacy and good management plans that ensure confidentiality.

Specific Considerations for Exempt Categories With Education Research

Caveats for Using Exempt Categories

🔗 5-3

A great deal of minimal risk research with students does fall into one or more <u>exempt</u> categories. The most common exempt categories for research with students are exempt category 1 and exempt category 2.

Exempt category 1 focuses on instructional strategies, techniques, or curricula. There are specific boundaries for research to be eligible for review in this category.

1. *Educational settings.* The research must take place in established or commonly accepted educational settings. There is no OHRP guidance defining "established or commonly accepted educational settings"; however, the Secretary's Advisory Committee on Human Research Protections (SACHRP) has noted "The consistent interpretation among IRBs is that commonly

accepted educational settings can be almost anywhere as long as the setting is one where specific educational offerings normally take place or a setting where one would go in order to have an educational experience" (DHHS, 2018). Examples of settings identified by SACHRP include:

- K–12 schools and college classrooms, after-school programs, pre-schools, vocational schools, alternative education programs
- Professional development seminars for school district personnel
- Soccer practice fields
- Scout meetings
- Medical schools
- Religious education settings
- Training simulators (e.g., medical simulators, flight simulators, etc.)

2. *Normal educational practices.* The research must only involve "normal educational practices," such as research on instructional strategies. Both the procedures and the purpose of the research must be limited to normal educational practices. Again, OHRP guidance is lacking. Examples of study activities that may take place in an educational setting but would nevertheless not be considered normal educational practice include the following:

- Drug-use surveys, because "the topic/activity is not a normal educational practice" (see SACHRP Recommendations, September 18, 2008, for discussion; DHHS, 2008)
- Evaluation of a radically new instructional strategy or curriculum
- Random assignment of students to different instructional strategies or curricula for comparison

3. *Impact on learning.* The regulations specifically call out that research in an educational setting will only be eligible for exemption under this category if it is limited to "normal educational practices that are not likely to adversely impact students' opportunity to learn required educational content or the assessment of educators who provide instruction." **45 CFR 46.104(d)(1)**.

Exempt category 2 focuses on people and their individual characteristics and outcomes (e.g., Does the intervention change behavior? What is the student experience?). There are some specific boundaries with this category as well, as follows:

1. This category can only involve a task if it is part of an education assessment or other standardized assessment, as this category does not permit an "intervention" (see sidebar, Interventions Excluded from Exempt Category 2).

2. The inclusion of children is limited. While it is permissible to administer an education assessment or other standardized assessment, it is not permissible to conduct a survey or interview that is outside of "normal education practices" with children.

3. Public observation is permissible, whereas observation in a private setting is not. A public space is any area that is not considered a private residence or private workspace and where the subject does not have an expectation of privacy. Special permissions are not needed in public spaces. Note, however, that "public schools" are not public spaces.

INTERVENTIONS EXCLUDED FROM EXEMPT CATEGORY 2

Both OHRP, in the Preamble of the revision to the Common Rule (Federal Register, 2017, Preamble p. 7189) and SACHRP (DHHS, 2018) exclude interventions from exempt category 2 research. The Common Rule defines an intervention as an activity that includes both physical procedures by which information or biospecimens are gathered (e.g., venipuncture) and manipulations of the subject or the subject's environment that are performed for research purposes.

OHRP provides an example of such an intervention that is not acceptable, as well as one that is: ". . . if a research study were to randomly assign students to take an educational test in a quiet room or in a room with a moderate level of noise, or to consume a snack (or not) before taking the test, this research would not be exempt under this exemption. It should be noted, however, that educational tests may include exposing test takers to certain materials as part of the test, and that such materials do not constitute interventions distinct from the test" (Federal Register, 2017, Preamble p. 7189).

⊘ 5-3
⊘ 5-5

As with all research on human subjects, a study can only be determined to be exempt if all of the study activities fall into one or more categories of exemption. When they do not, expedited categories are the next consideration so long as the study involves no more than minimal risk.

Regulations, Laws, and Policies Beyond the Common Rule

A challenge in education research is that there are many regulations to navigate. In addition to the Common Rule, there are federal regulations such as the Family Educational Rights and Privacy Act (FERPA; see Resources), the Protection of Pupil Rights Amendment (PPRA; see Resources), and specific state laws regarding recordings and required notification. Universities, school districts, private schools, and programs may also impose specific requirements.

The difficulty is in navigating policies that are not harmonized or are even in direct conflict with each other. Identifying and separating the roles and responsibilities of the IRB, the researcher, and research site can also be a challenge.

When involving any outside entity, it is always good practice to seek permission. With some locations, it is enough to obtain permission from the local school, whereas for others it may be necessary to seek this from the school district. Very rarely it is enough to seek permission only from a teacher or course instructor. Many schools require that parents be notified of all activities taking place regardless of whether the activity is research. For example, schools routinely require parental permission for video recording that is intended solely for teaching assessments. Schools may also have requirements related to how long a research activity may take place in a classroom or with a particular group of students.

Local requirements and expectations vary greatly, and it is the researcher's responsibility to understand and comply with these requirements and obtain approval from the appropriate authority or data custodians (school districts, registrars, etc.). In K–12 settings, school district offices are excellent resources for researchers; in higher education, the office of the registrar is usually where FERPA expertise will be found, as they are usually the stewards for student data. To assist the researcher, IRB staff or members may provide tips or information about practices they have encountered.

Schools, programs, and activities receiving funding from the U.S. Department of Education (see Resources) must comply with regulations intended to protect the rights of parents and students, as well as the privacy of their information. Of note, many if not all educational institutions receive funding from the

---

FERPA AND PPRA

FERPA (20 U.S.C. § 1232g, 34 CFR Part 99). Use of education records for research purposes must comply with the Family Educational Rights and Privacy Act (FERPA). FERPA requires that schools obtain written consent from parents or students (if the student has reached 18 years of age or is attending an institution of postsecondary education) prior to release of personally identifiable information from an education record that goes beyond basic directory level information, such as name, telephone number, and dates of attendance.

PPRA (20 U.S.C. § 1232h, 34 CFR 98). The Protection of Pupil Rights Amendment (PPRA) requires that written consent be obtained from students (if adult or emancipated minor) or parents of minors before students participate in survey, analysis, or evaluation that involves one or more of the following eight topics (20 U.S.C. 1232h(b)):

1. political affiliations or beliefs of the student or the student's parent;
2. mental and psychological problems of the student or the student's family;
3. sex behavior or attitudes;
4. illegal, anti-social, self-incriminating, or demeaning behavior
5. critical appraisals of other individuals with whom respondents have close family relationships;
6. legally recognized privileged or analogous relationships, such as those of lawyers, physicians, and ministers;
7. religious practices, affiliations, or beliefs of the student or student's parent;
8. income (other than that required by law to determine eligibility for participation in a program or for receiving financial assistance under such program)

PPRA also requires schools to have policies regarding the right of parents to inspect surveys and other materials created by a third party before the survey is administered to a student.

U.S. Department of Education, either directly or indirectly. Although these rules typically apply to the school (rather than the researcher or the institution to which the researcher belongs), IRBs should be aware of these regulations, and some IRB offices may elect to notify researchers of their responsibilities and assess compliance with the relevant requirements as part of the review process.

Resources

Family Educational Rights and Privacy Act (FERPA): www2.ed.gov/policy/gen/guid/fpco/ferpa /index.html

The Protection of Pupil Rights Amendment (PPRA): www2.ed.gov/policy/gen/guid/fpco/ppra /parents.html

U.S. Department of Education: www.ed.gov

References

Department of Health and Human Services (DHHS). (2008). *Secretary's Advisory Committee on Human Research Protections. Recommendations regarding regulatory exemptions, institutional responsibilities, tribal authority, research in disaster situations, review of the human subjects protection system.* www.hhs.gov/ohrp/sachrp-committee/recommendations/2008-september-18-letter /index.html

Department of Health and Human Services (DHHS). (2010). *Use of penalties for students who fail to show up: Letter to SONA SYSTEMS (January 8, 2010).* www.hhs.gov/ohrp/regulations-and -policy/guidance/january-08-2010-letter-to-dr-justin-fidler/index.html

Department of Health and Human Services (DHHS). (2018). *Secretary's Advisory Committee on Human Research Protections. Attachment B - interpretation revised Common Rule exemptions.* www .hhs.gov/ohrp/sachrp-committee/recommendations/attachment-b-november-13-2018 /index.html

Department of Health and Human Services (DHHS). (2019). *Informed consent FAQs.* www.hhs .gov/ohrp/regulations-and-policy/guidance/faq/informed-consent/index.html

Federal Register. (2017). Vol. 82, No. 12. 45 CFR 46 and Preamble. www.govinfo.gov/content /pkg/FR-2017-01-19/pdf/2017-01058.pdf

Contraception, Pregnancy Testing, and Pregnant Partners

Marielle S. Gross
Toby Schonfeld

Abstract

The goal of this chapter is to facilitate systematic decision making by IRBs with respect to addressing reproductive risk protections in research. Specifically, we discuss risks and benefits of pregnancy testing; various forms of birth control that may be required and how to approach these requirements in the context of the study's risk profile; and considerations unique to the circumstances of pregnant partners of subjects who are enrolled in studies.

Introduction

The inclusion of pregnant women in research has been recently identified as a priority for the purpose of generating much-needed evidence for female health care (Sullivan et al., 2019). However, this development occurs within the broader context of a precautionary approach toward potential teratogenic effects on fetuses that may be conceived by female research subjects or female partners of male research subjects, especially in the setting of biomedical trials, which themselves are greater than minimal risk for subjects. In those cases, researchers often not only require confirmation that individuals are not pregnant at the time of study enrollment, but also provide strong counseling about the inadvisability of pregnancy during the course of the study and its subsequent "washout" period (the time after the study in which there is ongoing potential for study agents to have reproductive effects). Additionally, subjects are often required, as a condition of study participation, to commit to using one or more contraceptive methods during the study to help ensure that pregnancy will not inadvertently occur.

Because these contraception requirements have been identified as a barrier to research participation (Schonfeld & Gordon, 2005; Sullivan et al., 2019), there has been heightened attention to the conditions under which women of childbearing potential should be required to submit to pregnancy testing and to utilize contraception as a precondition of study participation. The focus of this discussion is on "women of childbearing potential," most broadly understood as those who are postmenarche and premenopausal. However, this general definition does not fully capture actual potential for childbearing; for example, some reproductive-aged women have had a hysterectomy. There are other categories of women, such as those who abstain from sex for personal, cultural, or religious reasons or those who are not sexually active with males, for whom "childbearing potential" may represent a technical biological possibility, though not a meaningful or realistic risk. Similarly, women who have undergone surgical sterilization have done so for the purpose of foreclosing their childbearing potential, and the extent to which contraception requirements should apply in these and other complex circumstances is not straightforward.

We recommend an approach that is sensitive to these nuances of "childbearing potential" and an understanding of contraception requirements in general as a strategy for significantly reducing, but not completely eliminating, the potential for pregnancy in a research subject or partner of a research subject. For example, consider that a woman who has only female sex partners already has a lower baseline risk of pregnancy than one who is sexually active with males and using one or more forms of contraception. Because, in terms of strict probabilities, the former case has a lower risk of potentially conceiving a fetus, requiring additional contraceptive measures for that individual may not be justified.

Contraception requirements also extend to male subjects in biomedical research studies if there is theoretical risk of study agents affecting the male reproductive system and, consequently, potential to adversely affect a fetus that they may conceive. In both cases, the personal, physical, and psychological burdens of contraceptive requirements should not be underestimated, and careful consideration should be applied as to the nature and magnitude of the prospective risks to *theoretical fetuses/potential persons,* to whom our moral obligations are small in comparison to our moral obligations to *existing persons* for whom there may be a direct benefit from study participation. In this chapter, we explore the theory and content of pregnancy testing, contraception requirements, and management of pregnant partners of research subjects for the purposes of study design and coordination.

Contraception Mandates in Research

When pregnancy is an exclusion criterion for research participation due to unacceptably high risk to a potential fetus conceived during a study, requiring prospective pregnancy testing and contraception may be justified, because it minimizes the risk of an individual's study participation resulting in potentially harmful outcomes for their offspring. The contraceptive options vary based on the sex of the subject, as discussed later. When contraception is required for female or male research subjects, or under certain circumstances, for male subjects' female partners, sponsors of the research may be responsible for providing or supporting access to contraception, for example, by offering free condoms.

When contraception is required for male subjects, options include barrier methods (male and female condoms, diaphragms, cervical caps), surgical sterilization of the participant (vasectomy) or female partner (tubal ligation, salpingectomy, or hysterectomy), or other birth control methods, including abstinence or ensuring that his female partners are using reliable contraception. This research requirement is complicated because it implies researcher responsibility for third parties (female sex partners of male study subjects), related to their partner's participation in a study to which they did not personally consent. Thus, the application of such requirements should be judicious, and theoretical risks must be sufficiently justified, for example, by a plausible underlying biomedical mechanism of harm.

Importantly, if a male research subject who is capable of fathering children is sexually active with a female of childbearing potential, researchers should discuss with him not only the prospective risks of conceiving a child during the study or washout period but also the importance of discussing these risks with his female sexual partner(s). Researchers should provide written information materials for subjects to distribute to any at-risk partners, which should include details relevant to the risks of the study agent to that individual, information and resources for accessing birth control, study protocol for following any incidental pregnancies, and contact information that female partners may use if they have further questions about theoretical risks or to follow up with study personnel in the event of pregnancy during the study or washout period.

For prospective female subjects, the contraception mandate may similarly include regular use of barriers, surgical methods, and abstinence. Unique to female subjects is the potential for hormonal birth control methods (including oral, transdermal, subcutaneous implants and intrauterine devices with or without a hormonal component). When the woman herself has enrolled in the study, requiring birth control seems ethically appropriate as long as the requirement is based on actual risk of the trial and need for it was disclosed in advance of her agreement to participate. Realistically, most commonly used forms of birth control predominantly affect women, much as pregnancy predominantly affects female bodies. This is significant because contraception mandates, particularly if they are not applied judiciously, may adversely affect recruitment and retention of women in research studies. Being proactive in these conversations is essential when birth control requirements are included in study design. Some women may embrace the context of the study as an opportunity to initiate desired birth control methods that they otherwise may have been unable to access (e.g., contraceptive methods that were not covered by insurance that will be provided by the trial or using trial participation as the justification for starting a contraceptive method that would otherwise be frowned upon by a sexual partner). Some women, by contrast, may avoid study participation because they find the contraception requirements unacceptable. The disproportionate impact routine pregnancy testing and birth control requirements have on women as prospective research subjects should be acknowledged and factored into recruitment and consent processes and, where applicable, to study design.

It is important to counsel prospective female subjects for whom pregnancy during study participation is possible. Discussions should assess whether a woman is already using a form of birth control, including her reasons for doing so, because many women who use hormonal birth control methods are not doing so for contraception but rather for menstrual control. If a woman is contemplating initiation of a new contraceptive measure in the context of the study, it is critical that she receive appropriate counseling about its use, limits of its effectiveness, side effects, etc. If a woman agrees to continue a previous form of birth control, her use of this method should be examined to ensure that her current use is safe and effective.

Of note, women enrolled in longer term studies (i.e., those taking place over many months or years), may change their mind regarding their pregnancy intentions and how contraceptive measures required for study participation fit with their life plans. Researchers involved in studies where there is serious risk of fetal harm should a woman discontinue birth control and become pregnant should regularly remind subjects of these risks. They should also provide the subject an opportunity either to withdraw from the study, to continue with updated consent appropriate for pregnancy status/intention, or to reaffirm their plan to remain on the specified birth control method for the remaining course of the study.

A further issue for contraceptive requirements relates to the varied effectiveness, reliability, and potential for user error for the various contraceptive options. In general, surgical methods and implanted devices have the greatest effectiveness, typically > 99% effective (meaning < 1 pregnancy per 100 females over 1 year). By comparison, the effectiveness of other methods decreases gradually with the greater degree of temporal proximity to individual sexual intercourse episodes that the contraceptive method must be used. (For example, the vaginal ring or the patch, changed once every week or more, is as or more effective than the daily pill, which is more effective than condoms, which are more effective than the withdrawal method.) A further ethically thorny issue relates to abstinence, which is theoretically the most effective form of contraception, although its effectiveness completely depends on its consistent use.

Whether contraception is required, if one form of contraception is adequate, or whether two or more forms should be required, should be determined relative to the degree of risk conception would present to a fetus and the relative risk of conception for a given subject. For example, it may be reasonable to require two methods if the study involves a drug that is a known teratogen. On the other hand, one method may be sufficient if the risk to a fetus is only based on a lack of evidence for safety in pregnancy, particularly if there are no animal studies or theoretical mechanisms of teratogenicity. For subjects who are sexually abstinent by lifestyle, it may be reasonable not to require any additional methods of birth control.

Lastly, the use of more than one contraceptive option may be considered in the context of a couple, as opposed to requiring one individual to use more than one method themselves. For example, if a male subject agrees to use condoms, this could be combined with his partner using oral contraceptives to count for two different methods, or a woman may use a diaphragm and her partner may have had a vasectomy. Given the > 99% effectiveness of surgical and implanted contraception, some have raised concerns that ever requiring more than one method in those cases may be overly burdensome and risky for subjects without adequate demonstration of corresponding medical necessity or marginal benefits (Frohwirth et al., 2016; Sullivan et al., 2019). If an implant or surgical method is used, it is appropriate to reserve any further contraception requirements to studies involving known teratogens or otherwise toxic agents.

Pregnancy Testing in Research

Pregnancy is a frequent exclusion criterion for drug studies, and therefore a negative pregnancy test is required for participation. This requirement is predicated on the notion that the investigational agent (or study procedures) presents sufficient risk to a pregnant woman or her fetus to justify her exclusion. The screening pregnancy test, then, protects pregnant women and fetuses from potential teratogenic exposures and protects researchers from liability for adverse pregnancy outcomes that could be related to study participation.

While common, research screening pregnancy tests should follow certain criteria in order to be ethically justified. First, as mentioned previously, the trial itself must pose possible teratogenic risk to a fetus or other harm to a pregnant woman such that enrolling her would produce an unacceptable risk/benefit ratio. Otherwise, even a relatively noninvasive test like a pregnancy test is unjustified if it is not connected to scientific risk, because it may restrict female access to research participation without ethical grounding (Schonfeld et al., 2013). Second, for trials that require contraception to ensure that subjects do not get pregnant, it is reasonable to use a negative pregnancy screen within 7 days of starting the trial as an entry requirement. If researchers are concerned that the risks to a fetus from study exposures are so high that pregnant women should not participate, then it is their responsibility to verify that females are not pregnant before they enroll. Likewise, the American College of Obstetrics and Gynecology (ACOG) recommends a negative pregnancy screen before women enroll in studies where there is greater than minimal risk to a fetus (ACOG, 2004). Finally, there is no ethical justification for conducting serum rather than urine pregnancy tests for pregnancy testing unless blood is already being drawn for other reasons. Minimizing risks to the greatest extent possible in research means, in this case of theoretical risks to fetuses, that the small increase in sensitivity of serum pregnancy testing does not outweigh the increased invasiveness or costs of serum testing when urine pregnancy is sufficient for this purpose. Similarly, although it is reasonable to confirm a report of a negative home pregnancy test with a urine screening in the clinic for enrollment in a trial that presents the possibility of greater than minimal risk to a fetus, the same is not true for enrollment in studies that present only the possibility of minimal risk to a fetus. In that case, reports of home pregnancy testing should be sufficient for enrollment.

Inconsistencies are also common in pregnancy testing practices during research trials themselves (Schonfeld et al., 2013). The frequency of pregnancy testing should be connected directly to the magnitude of expected harm to a fetus if a woman should get pregnant while on study. Additionally, pregnancy testing in research should be conducted at intervals consistent with clinical practice and not more often than monthly (Schonfeld et al., 2013). The consent process must also include careful discussion of pregnancy testing: how often testing will occur during the study, how subjects will be informed of the testing results, and the study consequences for a positive pregnancy test (i.e., whether they will be removed from the trial, if they will be asked for permission to follow the pregnancy, etc.) (Schonfeld et al., 2013). There are additional considerations related to adolescents, as described later.

Finally, as with any procedure done exclusively for research purposes, the consent process must make clear whose responsibility it will be to pay for the pregnancy test(s) (Schonfeld et al., 2013). Because there is no scientific justification to perform pregnancy tests on women who are enrolled/considering enrolling in trials that are not expected to cause fetal harm, the costs of any tests that are nevertheless required by the researchers or sponsor should be borne by the study and not the subjects themselves. Similarly, because there is no justification for pregnancy testing for women who are not of childbearing potential, they should not be charged for pregnancy tests that are required as part of a study.

Pregnancy testing results should be delivered privately to subjects, and researchers should assist subjects with finding a primary care provider for prenatal decision making if the pregnancy test is positive. Researchers should also make available study information to these providers if they received a study drug or other intervention prior to the positive pregnancy test. Even if this requires unmasking of a study arm, it is justified both by beneficence and respect for persons.

Special Populations

Adolescents

Contraception requirements and pregnancy testing present special challenges when adolescents are enrolled in research. Parents may think that pregnancy testing and contraception are unnecessary or superfluous and may demand to know the results of screening pregnancy tests. Additionally, adolescents require particularly careful contraceptive counseling to ensure adequate knowledge about the contraceptive (and reproductive biology) and to facilitate optimal contraceptive choices for their unique circumstances. Conversations about contraception and pregnancy testing should be conducted sensitively, and that often means discussing these issues with the adolescent in private, away from the parents or guardians. Additionally, given that access to contraception can be a problem for adolescents who are sexually active but concealing this from their parents, contraception required for a study should be provided directly to the adolescent through the study itself.

Results of pregnancy tests should be delivered privately to the adolescent. In states where a right to privacy is granted to pregnant minors, this information should not be disclosed to the parent. However, we advocate encouraging pregnant adolescents to discuss the pregnancy with their parents as the need for support is essential (Schonfeld & Gordon, 2005). In states without such a privacy right, however, the consent process must make clear that pregnancy test results will be shared with the parent after they are delivered privately to the adolescent. This way, an adolescent can decide if she is willing to enroll in a study where the possibility of pregnancy notification exists. Researchers should plan in advance for a course of action if the adolescent becomes pregnant while on study. In the event that she will be removed from the study, researchers must describe during the consent process what information will be shared with the pregnant adolescent's parents regarding the reason for disqualification.

Although pregnancy is only a risk for female adolescents, male adolescents who are candidates for studies where the agents may damage sperm should also be counseled sensitively about contraception. Because adherence rates to barrier contraception remain a challenge in this population, ensuring that the adolescents understand the medical reasons for the restrictions may encourage better adherence than the more common appeals to authority. Demonstrating real interest in their well-being and the welfare of their sexual partners is one way to build trust with the adolescents and increase contraceptive compliance.

Faith-Based Institutions

Faith-based institutions that conduct clinical research may object to contraception mandates in research because they are inconsistent with their values. Yet commitment to other values, such as contributing to research and scientific discourse, and giving their patients access to the opportunity to participate in potentially beneficial research, means that clinical trials are also conducted at these institutions.

Casey et al. (2012) suggest several ways to ensure that research including women of childbearing potential can proceed at faith-based institutions. Including among these principles are that ". . . potential subjects in clinical research must be given full information, including a complete description of any requirements not consistent with Catholic moral teaching" (Casey et al., 2012). Part of the justification of this requirement is respect for persons: Full information enables potential subjects to recognize the dangers of getting pregnant while on study and facilitates decision making based on this knowledge. Casey and colleagues also maintain that while Catholic institutions need not directly provide contraceptives that are contrary to their values, women who independently choose to use them should be given full information about these options and where to access them. Additionally, they advocate for a commitment to ". . . abstinence from heterosexual activity before and during the course of investigational studies" as an acceptable form of contraception for participation in studies that present the possibility of risk to a fetus (Casey et al., 2012).

Incidental Pregnancy in Partners of Research Subjects

Some research studies discourage pregnancy during a study and its washout period for both female subjects and female partners of male subjects when researchers are concerned about possible teratogenic effects of the investigational agent. When a research subject nevertheless becomes pregnant during the study, researchers will often ask for permission to collect information about the pregnancy and its outcome to learn more about possible effects of the investigational agent. Respect for persons requires that the subject be free to refuse to provide this information.

The situation is more complicated when the pregnancy occurs in a sexual partner of a research subject, but who is not herself a participant in the research, because there is no formal relationship between the researchers and the pregnant party. The researchers may still desire to collect information about the pregnancy and its outcomes to inform understanding of any potential collateral impact an investigational agent may have, but questions arise as to how best to accomplish this goal from both a regulatory and ethical perspective. Here, we discuss three options for IRBs and researchers to consider in this situation.

Option 1: Collect Deidentified Information from the Research Subject

Researchers could ask research subjects for information about the partner's pregnancy and the outcomes of the pregnancy. The IRB could facilitate the ethical collection of these data by approving the questionnaire that will be used for this purpose. Advantages of this approach are that all information gathered comes from research subjects who have provided informed consent to participate in the study and who therefore understand the nature and purpose of the research. The subject would also still be free to refuse to provide this information. This option avoids the quagmire of considering whether or not the data collection about pregnancy is human subjects research according to the federal definition and, if so, if the pregnant partner is a human subject and all that this then entails (see later). Disadvantages of this approach include that the subject may only have partial, indirect information about the pregnancy, and therefore data may be incomplete. Additionally, the information provided will be about someone else (in this case, the pregnant woman), and some would argue that it does not respect the pregnant woman as a person in her own right and perhaps is an unethical violation of privacy if the woman is not directly involved in deciding whether and what information should be provided.

Option 2: Conduct an Ethics (Nonregulatory) Review of the Data Collection Process

Even if the data collection of pregnancy outcomes does not constitute independent human subjects research according to the federal definitions promulgated by the Department of Health and Human Services (DHHS) and the Food and Drug Administration (FDA), an IRB could set institutional policy that requires researchers to describe how these data will be gathered. Setting an institutional policy would give this requirement "teeth" even in the absence of a regulatory mandate and would facilitate more consistency in approaches to this issue by researchers, which is currently mediated on a case-by-case basis. Advantages of this approach include enabling the IRB to ask questions (perhaps on an addendum application) that the researchers might not otherwise have considered. For example, there could be questions about how researchers plan to reach out to individuals whose contact information is provided by research subjects, how they expect to gather data (e.g., from the electronic health record or by questionnaire), what happens if there is misattributed paternity, what they will do if the pregnant partner is a minor, and how they will protect the partner's privacy and the confidentiality of the pregnancy data. The IRB could also establish a "pregnant partner consent document" that includes what it determines to be the ethically necessary features of the consent process and its documentation. The disadvantage of this approach is that some IRBs will be reluctant to make this a policy in the absence of regulatory requirements. If, instead, the IRB describes these concepts as "best practice," there will be no meaningful way to enforce them if researchers choose to pursue other practices. This strategy may be most appropriate if such occurrences are rare.

Option 3: Designate the Collection of Pregnancy and Pregnancy Outcome Data from Pregnant Partners to Constitute Human Subjects Research

The third option is both the most straightforward option and the one that is the most complicated, partly because there are a range of ways it might play out. An IRB could stipulate by policy that it considers the collection of identifiable information about a woman's pregnancy to be human subjects research, and then all of the policies, procedures, and regulatory criteria pertaining to human subjects research will apply. Importantly, note that the regulatory criteria at 45 CFR 46 subpart B (Additional Protections for Pregnant Females, Human Fetuses and Neonates Involved in Research) will apply. (Of course, the exemptions also apply to this subpart, so to the extent that the collection of these data fall under exemption 4 at 45 CFR 46.104(d)(4), no additional safeguards are dictated by regulation.) If the researchers want to follow pregnancy outcomes past the immediate neonate stage, the regulations at 45 CFR 46 subpart D will also apply (Additional Protections for Children Involved as Subjects in Research). The advantages of this approach are that the regulatory criteria and IRB checklists are familiar to IRB members, so they will not have to apply anything "special" for the review of this data collection. Because of the requirement of applying both the Common Rule and the additional safeguards, researchers would be expected to answer all of the application questions that are standard to research projects that involve these groups of subjects, and therefore the "special" issues outlined previously would be included as part of the process. To the extent that this data collection is part of the overall research

⊘ 9-4

⊘ 5-3

⊘ 9-6

project, then the risk level of those procedures would simply be applied here: A greater than minimal risk drug study could review everything via <u>full board review</u>, including the collection of pregnancy data. IRBs could also require a separate pregnant partner consent process that would only include information about the data collection, management, and storage of pregnancy-related data and not about the overall study. This way, potential subjects would be more likely to understand the key features of the research that would help them decide whether or not to participate, which fulfills the requirement of respect for persons. An IRB could even create a special template consent form specifically for pregnant partners of research subjects.

⊘ 5-7

However, there are several disadvantages of this approach. First, although some IRBs will see this kind of data collection as falling within the Common Rule definition of "research," it may not be consistent with FDA guidance. It is also not clear whether the consent process should be limited to the specific information relevant to the pregnant partners (and the limited risks thereof), or describe, at least superficially, the overall study to which the pregnancy data is being appended as a way of explaining to the pregnant partner why they are interested in collecting information about the pregnancy. If the latter, then the consent process and form may be burdened with significant extraneous material that may make it difficult for the pregnant partner to know what her risks will be (in this case, risks to her privacy and the confidentiality of the data).

Finally, if the data collection comes as part of a study that is greater than minimal risk to the male subject (which is likely to happen more often than not, otherwise the researchers would not be interested in the pregnancy data), the process for obtaining these data—from the identification of the pregnant partner through the return of research results—may also have to be reviewed by the full board, which may mean a delay in docketing.

If, on the other hand, the researcher submits the pregnant partner data collection as a data collection study only, it is likely that it would fall under <u>exemption</u> 4 at **45 CFR 46.104(d)(4)** if the study is a retrospective design and likely viewed as research that can be reviewed through an <u>expedited</u> process if the design is prospective. Advantages are that there would be little to no delay in data collection and, in the case of prospective data collection, the pregnant woman herself would be approached about participating and could therefore make a decision consistent with her goals, values, and priorities about providing (or not) the pregnancy and outcome data. The same disadvantages related to the inclusion of broader study information in the consent process remains for this option as well.

⊘ 5-3

⊘ 5-5

Conclusion

As with any aspect of independent oversight, IRB members should approach reproductive risk in a study systematically and scientifically. This involves only approving required protective measures and limitations on the exercise of individual autonomy to the least extent necessary to decrease risk and maximize benefit to the study subjects themselves. Excluding females of childbearing potential does not reduce their risk and fails to respect the ethical commitment to respect for persons, beneficence, and justice on which the work of independent oversight is based. Instead, we advocate a reasoned approach to concerns about reproductive risk by offering guidance for how to approach issues of contraception, pregnancy testing, and pregnant partners consistently with other aspects of the trial.

References

American College of Obstetrics and Gynecology (ACOG). (2004). Ethical considerations in research involving females. *International Journal of Gynecology and Obstetrics, 86*(1), 124–130.

Casey, M. J., O'Brien, R., Rendell, M., & Salzman, T. (2012). Ethical dilemmas of mandated contraception in pharmaceutical research at Catholic medical institutions. *American Journal of Bioethics, 12*(7), 34–37.

Frohwirth, L., Blades, N., Moore, A. M., & Wurtz, H. (2016). The complexity of multiple contraceptive method use and the anxiety that informs it: Implications for theory and practice. *Archives of Sexual Behavior, 45*(8), 2123–2135.

Schonfeld, T., & Gordon, B. (2005). Contraception in research: A policy suggestion. *IRB: Ethics and Human Research, 27*(2), 15–20.

Schonfeld, T., Schmid, K. K., Brown, J. S., Amoura, J. S., & Gordon, B. (2013). A pregnancy testing policy for females enrolled in clinical trials. *IRB: Ethics and Human Research, 35*(6), 9–15.

Sullivan, K. A., Little, M. O., Rosenberg, N. E., Zimba, C., Jaffe, E., Gilbert, S., Coleman, J. S., Hoffman, I., Mtande, T., Anderson, J., Gross, M. S., Rahangdale, L., Faden, R., & Lyerly, A. D. (2019). Women's views about contraception requirements for biomedical research participation. *PloS One, 14*(5), e0216332.

Subpart B Research: Additional Protections for Pregnant Women, Human Fetuses, and Neonates

Maggie Little

Anne Drapkin Lyerly

Abstract

It is now widely agreed that research with pregnant women is critically important and that such research must be responsibly conducted. Because research with pregnant women involves implications for potential offspring, this means added specifications for it to proceed. This chapter describes the background and key components for research with pregnant women, including an overview of the regulatory approach to such research and a discussion of the eligibility criteria for including pregnant women in research. The final section provides a brief summary of the two other, less commonly encountered, topics addressed by subpart B of the Common Rule: research on neonates born of uncertain or nonviability and research with the post-delivery placenta or a deceased fetus.

Introduction

Research with pregnant women is critically important. Pregnant women often face serious illness, ranging from immune disorders to infectious diseases to cancer and need access to effective, safe, and appropriately dosed therapeutics (Task Force on Research Specific to Pregnant Women and Lactating Women, 2018). Indeed, pregnant women are often one of the populations most in need of safe and effective therapeutics, given the increased susceptibility to illness that pregnancy can bring, as well as heightened risks when disease and pregnancy co-occur (Lyerly et al., 2008). Without pregnancy-specific research, decisions about therapeutic choice and dosing are based on assumption rather than evidence. Furthermore, evidence gaps can lead to reticence to use medications that are in fact safe and critical to preventing or managing diseases during pregnancy, leaving both pregnant women and the children they bear in harm's way. Key organizations now endorse the importance of research with pregnant women, including the American College of Obstetricians and Gynecologists (2015), the Society for Maternal-Fetal Medicine (n.d.), the Office of Women's Health of the National Institutes of Health (Foulkes et al., 2011), and a recent presidential Task Force on Research Specific to Pregnant Women and Lactating Women (2018).

Overview

Until recently, pregnant women were categorized as a "vulnerable population" in regulations governing human subjects research. Though the term did not appear in subpart B, the pre-2018 version of subpart A of the U.S. Code of Federal Regulations for the Protection of Human Subjects (the Common Rule) designated at several points pregnant women as vulnerable alongside "prisoners, children, individuals with mental disabilities, and individuals at economic or educational disadvantage"—populations that either by capacity or by context are compromised in their ability to provide valid consent to participate in research or who are at special risk of exploitation.

It was increasingly recognized that such a designation was problematic (Council for International Organizations of Medical Sciences, 2016). The term tacitly suggests that pregnancy renders women incapable of offering valid consent or that they are by nature susceptible to exploitation. Yet pregnancy does not itself limit the ability to reason, and although there are some cultures in which pregnancy meaningfully constrains women's free decision-making around matters such as research participation, the factors that lead to such constraints are highly contextual and do not redound to the category of pregnancy in its own right. Furthermore, it had become clear that the designation of pregnant women as a "vulnerable population" unintentionally had a profoundly chilling effect on the pursuit of research—even highly responsible research—into the health needs of pregnant women and the children they bear, leaving pregnant women a "therapeutic orphan" (Little et al., 2019).

The 2018 revisions to the Common Rule confirmed that "the final rule no longer includes pregnant women ... as examples of populations that are potentially vulnerable to coercion or undue influence" (Federal Register, 2017, Preamble p. 7204). Although various factors can make specific pregnant women vulnerable (e.g., being incarcerated), pregnant women as a group should not be characterized as a vulnerable population for purposes of human subjects research review.

Instead, the bioethics literature and professional guidance now frame pregnant women as a "special" or "complex" population, by virtue of both physiological differences and ethical complexities that pregnancy entails, such as the need to consider the interests of both the woman and fetus (Blehar et al., 2013; Foulkes et al., 2011). The American College of Obstetricians and Gynecologists (ACOG) has endorsed the term "scientifically complex" (encompassing both biological and ethical complexities) as a way to indicate both that pregnant women and the children they will bear need to be protected individually from research risks and also that they are protected as a population *through* the conduct of responsible research (ACOG, 2015).

Like any research involving human subjects, research with pregnant women must meet all standard research protections as <u>defined</u> in the Common Rule;

for instance, risk must be the least needed for scientific purposes, and appropriate <u>informed consent</u> must be obtained before research proceeds. Subpart B explicitly incorporates those general protections by reference. Subpart B then adds an overlay of additional requirements, on top of those specified more generally for human subjects research, laid out in **45 CFR 46.204**. These additional requirements centrally fall into three categories: (1) requirements about preliminary evidence needed before pregnant women are eligible for inclusion; (2) parameters for allowable research-related risk, especially for the fetus; and (3) questions of paternal (and, for research with pregnant adolescents, parental) consent.

✏ Section 6

It should be noted that subpart B also allows for exceptions to its requirements if the research presents an opportunity to "understand, prevent, or alleviate a serious problem" affecting pregnant women, fetuses, or neonates. Under this provision, special approval must be granted by the Secretary of the Department of Health and Human Services in consultation with an expert panel and with public commentary [**45 CFR 46.207**]. To our knowledge, this pathway has never been invoked.

Preliminary Evidence [45 CFR 46.204(a)]

Subpart B's first specific requirement for including pregnant women in research concerns the availability of preliminary evidence to inform judgments of potential research-related risks to the fetus or pregnant woman. Specifically, subpart B states: "Where scientifically appropriate, preclinical studies, including studies on pregnant animals, and clinical studies, including studies on nonpregnant women, have been conducted and provide data for assessing potential risks to pregnant women and fetuses" [**45 CFR 46.204(a)**].

The qualification "where scientifically appropriate" is not explained but is presumably meant to acknowledge that some research involves no potential for physiological risks (e.g., cohort studies) and that research that does carry such potential may have access to sufficiently rich data, apart from preclinical studies specified to inform assessment of that potential. For instance, there may be useful data from safety databases about the use of the therapeutic in nonpregnant women, observational reports on use during pregnancy, or data from unintended exposures of pregnant women in the context of research that can serve the function of providing adequate preliminary evidence even in the absence of preclinical studies involving animals or prospective studies involving nonpregnant women (Food and Drug Administration, 2018).

While subpart B itself does not provide details about which preclinical animal studies assessing risks to the fetus are adequate, it should be noted that the Food and Drug Administration (FDA) provides detailed guidance on the topic for research taking place in the <u>investigational new drug</u> (IND) space. Any research done with pregnant women in the IND space will need to conform to FDA's specific preclinical animal requirements (including female reproduction toxicity studies and the standard battery of genotoxicity tests; FDA, 2010). Furthermore, because FDA requires detailed reproductive toxicity studies (specific animal studies looking at potential fetal risks, among other things) for all applications for drug approval, any research on approved therapeutics will perforce meet subpart B's requirement regarding preliminary animal studies.

✏ 11-2

FETAL RISK CONSIDERATIONS

In establishing standards limiting allowable fetal risk, the regulations should not be seen as opining on the moral status of the fetus (Little et al., 2019). Instead, the permissible fetal risk standard is designed on the presupposition that the pregnancy will be continued. This is both because such a presupposition is empirically true of the vast majority of such research and because it serves to ensure that trials do not burden women's options around pregnancy continuation by assumption or design. This latter principle is further underscored by subpart B's direction that researchers cannot be involved in any decision making around pregnancy termination (whether, timing, method) and that no inducements, monetary or other, to terminate can be offered by researchers.

Allowable Research-Related Risk [45 CFR 46.204(b and c)]

A critical issue in conducting research with pregnant women is determining the specific standards for what research-related risk is acceptable to the fetus, which cannot consent to that risk. Allowable risk for the pregnant woman is left implicit and is hence presumably subsumed under subpart A's parameters for allowable risk in the general population.

Disjunctive Fetal Risk Standard

The standard of acceptable research-related risk depends on whether the trial in question offers the "prospect of direct benefit." Trials involving the prospect of direct benefit—sometimes called "therapeutic research"—are those in which the study intervention may provide direct individual benefit from research participation if the intervention proves successful. That is, although the overarching purpose of the research is to gather further evidence for future patient populations, the trial is at a mature enough stage that it may also carry the prospect of comparative health benefits to research subjects.

Trials with no prospect of direct benefit, in contrast, are those in which the possibility of benefit cannot reasonably be expected. For studies that have no prospect of direct benefit, enrollment is purely for the value of advancing biomedical knowledge that will potentially benefit future patients or populations. These studies include early phase trials in which researchers have intentionally minimized the study intervention dose as a strategy to answer specific questions about safety; trials marked by too little evidence to reach a threshold of any reasonable prospect of benefit (even if benefits do accrue during the study); and studies whose focus is to better understand a point of biology or physiology rather than to test a potential preventive or therapeutic intervention.

Trials Involving Prospect of Direct Benefit

For trials offering the prospect of direct benefit to the pregnant woman, the fetus, or both, subpart B is quite permissive of inclusion in research. According to subpart B, research involving the prospect of direct benefit is allowable if the risk to the fetus is "caused solely by interventions or procedures that hold out the prospect of direct benefit for the woman or the fetus" [45 CFR 46.204(b)] and the risk to fetus is the "least possible" [45 CFR 46.204(c)]. Taken literally, this provides remarkably little constraint on allowable fetal risk, because the risk to the fetus could in principle be both extremely high and disproportionate to any benefits potential to the study. However, consensus in the clinical research ethics literature finds that acceptable risk is determined by the reasonability of the relation of risk to the potential benefits offered by participation: The likelihood and importance of the potential benefits must be reasonably judged to outweigh the potential risks, and the potential risk/benefit comparison must not be worse than available alternatives.

Importantly, subpart B is silent about whether the prospect of direct benefit to the pregnant woman can justify an increment of research-related risk to the fetus. The "prospect of benefit" category is simply described as a category of potential benefit to *either* woman *or* fetus, and the standard indicates only that risks should be justified by benefits, without specificity about to whom (woman or fetus/future child) such risks and benefits apply. It is generally assumed that pregnant women may altruistically consent to some personal research-related risk for the sake of fetal/future child benefit; there is also an assumption that some degree of fetal risk can be justified by adequate potential for maternal benefit, as is true in the practice of clinical obstetric care (Little et al., 2016; Little et al., 2017). Furthermore, fetal health is often deeply linked to maternal health: If participation in a trial offers the prospect of direct medical benefit to pregnant women, very often that intervention entails specific and quantifiable medical benefits to the fetus by virtue of reducing the effects of maternal disease on neonatal health outcomes. Indeed, where pregnant women are involved in research to treat maternal illness (e.g., HIV, thyroid disease, diabetes), net benefit to the fetus/future child can often be anticipated. That said, maternal and fetal risks and benefits are not always aligned with each other, and presumably there are limits (on both sides) about when benefit to one can justify risk to the other, potentially resulting in some difficult cases for individual IRBs.

Trials Involving No Prospect of Direct Benefit

For trials that involve no prospect of direct benefit to *either* the woman *or* the fetus, research-related risks to the fetus are capped at a very low threshold. Such trials can pose no more than "minimal risk" to the fetus [45 CFR 46.204(b)]. "Minimal risk" is defined in the Common Rule as "the probability and magnitude of anticipated harms with those ordinarily encountered in daily life or during the performance of routine physical or psychological examinations or tests" [45 CFR 46.102(j)]. The "minimal risk" standard (which is also used in other arenas of the regulations), although often difficult to apply and subject to widely varying interpretations by IRBs (Shah et al., 2004; Wendler, 2005), is intended to provide a category of negligible risk. Of note, subpart B also states that the purpose of the research must be the development of important biomedical knowledge that "cannot be obtained by any other means" [45 CFR 46.204(b)].

Some have raised concerns that these requirements are problematic. The language creates an extremely low ceiling, as it may be interpreted to exclude pregnant, women from studies with negligible risk simply because they are pregnant, and to preclude gathering data in studies that may be judged to entail a very low risk that exceeds the minimal risk threshold—such as some pharmacokinetic studies—that would critically inform dosing of a drug in research or clinical contexts. Furthermore, the fetal protections outlined here are more restrictive than those outlined in the corresponding regulations for research with children. Children are allowed to participate in minimal risk studies without the added stipulations that the knowledge sought "cannot be obtained by any other means." Regulations governing research with children also allow for a "minor increase over minimal risk" for research likely to contribute generalizable knowledge of vital importance for the understanding or amelioration of the child's disorder or condition. Some, including the president's Task Force, have recommended that a revision of subpart B should include the category of "minor increase over minimal risk" parallel to what is allowed in pediatric research, so further developments on this issue are possible (Task Force on Research Specific to Pregnant Women and Lactating Women, 2018).

🔗 9-6

PATERNAL CONSENT REQUIREMENTS

In the vast majority of cases, consent of the woman alone fulfills the regulatory requirement. Maternal and fetal interests are often intertwined, and so in most research with pregnant women—even research aimed fairly narrowly at improving fetal health—a prospect of benefit to the woman can be expected. Still, serious concerns have been raised about the enduring requirement for paternal consent in cases of prospect of direct benefit to the fetus alone. Here, too, the regulation exceeds what is required in pediatric research. According to subpart D, where there is a prospect of direct benefit to a child alone, the consent of *one parent* only is sufficient. Yet before birth, the same circumstance requires the consent of *two* parents. Other concerns include that giving the father veto power does not respect a pregnant woman's autonomy; is inconsistent with standards of clinical care, in which a pregnant woman's consent for interventions to benefit the fetus alone is sufficient; may compromise the privacy or safety of a pregnant woman who may be subject to intimate partner violence; and fails to account for the range of relationships, such as same-sex partnerships and arrangements involving gamete donation. Finally, anecdotal evidence indicates that the requirement continues to operate as a barrier to inclusion of pregnant women in biomedical research. Considering these objections, the Task Force on Research Specific to Pregnant Women and Lactating Women (PRGLAC) and others have urged full removal of a paternal consent requirement from the U.S. regulations.

✐ 9-6

Additional Consent [45 CFR 46.204(d-g)]

Subpart B is clear that for most research, informed consent of the pregnant woman alone, in accordance with parameters outlined in the Common Rule, is sufficient. Identifying the rare case in which paternal consent might be required again depends on the previously noted disjunct between research with and without prospect of direct benefit. If the study holds out the prospect of direct benefit for the woman, her consent alone is sufficient, even if there is also benefit to the fetus. If the study does not hold out the prospect of direct benefit for either the woman or the fetus, then the consent of the woman alone is again sufficient, given the negligible fetal risk such research permits. Only in cases where there is the prospect of direct benefit to the fetus but not to the woman is consent of the father required, with exceptions for cases in which the pregnancy resulted from rape or incest, or the father is unavailable, incompetent, or incapacitated.

The content of consent is defined in the Common Rule [45 CFR 46.116]; subpart B also sets out the additional requirement that "each individual providing consent … is fully informed regarding the reasonably foreseeable impact of the research on the fetus or neonate" [45 CFR 46.204(f)].

Finally, children and adolescents represent a considerable proportion of the pregnant population, and their physiologies or social contexts may make them an important population for research participation (for instance, research on HIV in some communities). Subpart B specifically states that "For children … who are pregnant, assent and permission are obtained in accord with the provisions of subpart D" [45 CFR 46.204(g)].

Research Involving Neonates and Post-Delivery Research of the Placenta or a Deceased Fetus

Subpart B addresses two additional topics beyond research with pregnant women: research on neonates born of uncertain viability and nonviable neonates [45 CFR 46.205] and research involving the post-delivery placenta or a dead fetus or fetal material [45 CFR 46.206]. The latter section is very brief, centrally handing off guidance to any applicable federal, state, or local laws and regulations regarding such activities; we therefore do not discuss it in any detail here.

The section on research with neonates sets the following parameters:

1. Those conducting research may play no role in assessing or determining the neonate's viability.

2. If the neonate is determined to be nonviable, research may take place only under extremely limited conditions. The research can neither artificially maintain the neonate's vital functions nor terminate its heartbeat or respiration; the research can add *no* additional risk to the neonate; and even then can be pursued only if in service to "important biomedical knowledge that cannot be obtained by other means."

3. If the neonate is of uncertain viability, there are two different conditions under which research may be undertaken: research that carries the prospect of enhancing the probability of survival of the neonate to viability or research in service to important biomedical knowledge not otherwise obtainable and that carries *no* additional risk to the neonate.

4. Finally, if or once the neonate is determined to be viable, any proposed research is to be evaluated under <u>subpart D</u>.

⊘ 9-6

NEONATES OF UNCERTAIN VIABILITY

The inclusion of discussion regarding neonates born of uncertain viability and nonviable neonates in subpart B is in one sense surprising, because research with newborns would generally be covered under subpart D. That said, subpart D does not consider or reflect the spectrum of scenarios encountered in how and when pregnancies may end, including, for instance, a highly premature but liveborn neonate that is clearly nonviable or whose viability is profoundly unclear. At the time of the 2001 revisions to subpart B, these scenarios were a topic of extensive focus and debate, perhaps in part because they intersect with questions about the moral status of early human life (McCullough et al., 2008). Whatever the impetus, **45 CFR 46.205** encompasses extensive commentary, including detailed specifications of when one parent, both parents, or their legal representatives must be involved.

Conclusion

Overall, subpart B is permissive of research with pregnant women. Although it presents some barriers to its conduct that could be resolved through regulatory guidance, much important research can be done now, ethically and in accordance with subpart B as it currently stands. Such research is necessary and important to developing a robust evidence base that is critical to the health of women during and after pregnancy, as well as the children they bear.

References

American College of Obstetricians and Gynecologists Committee on Ethics (ACOG). (2015). Committee opinion no. 646: Ethical considerations for including women as research participants. *Obstetrics and Gynecology*, 126(5), e100–e107.

Blehar, M. C., Spong, C., Grady, C., Goldkind, S. F., Sahin, L., & Clayton, J. A. (2013). Enrolling pregnant women: Issues in clinical research. *Women's Health Issues*, 23(1), e39–e45.

Council for International Organizations of Medical Sciences. (2016). *International ethical guidelines for health-related research involving humans.* cioms.ch/wp-content/uploads/2017/01/WEB-CIOMS-EthicalGuidelines.pdf

Federal Register. (2017). Vol. 82, No. 12. 45 CFR 46 and Preamble. www.govinfo.gov/content/pkg/FR-2017-01-19/pdf/2017-01058.pdf

Food and Drug Administration (FDA). (2010). *Nonclinical safety studies for the conduct of human clinical trials and marketing authorization for pharmaceuticals: Guidance for Industry M3(R2).* www.fda.gov/regulatory-information/search-fda-guidance-documents/m3r2-nonclinical-safety-studies-conduct-human-clinical-trials-and-marketing-authorization

Food and Drug Administration (FDA). (2018). *Pregnant women: Scientific and ethical considerations for inclusion in clinical trials, draft guidance for industry.* www.fda.gov/regulatory-information/search-fda-guidance-documents/pregnant-women-scientific-and-ethical-considerations-inclusion-clinical-trials

Foulkes, M. A., Grady, C., Spong, C. Y., Bates, A., & Clayton, J. A. (2011). Clinical research enrolling pregnant women: A workshop summary. *Journal of Womens Health, 20*(10), 1429–1432.

Little, M., Lyerly, A. D., Mastroianni, A. C., & Faden, R. R. (2016). Ethics and research with pregnant women: Lessons from HIV/AIDS. In F. Baylis, A. Ballantyne (Eds.), *Clinical research involving pregnant women* (Research Ethics Forum, Vol. 3). Springer.

Little, M., Wickremsinhe, M., & Lyerly, A. (2017). Research in pregnancy: The ethics of risk-benefit tradeoffs between woman, fetus, and future child. *Obstetrics and Gynecology, 129*, 76S–77S.

Little, M., Wickremsinhe, M. N., Jaffe, E., & Lyerly, A. D. (2019). Research with pregnant women: A feminist challenge. In L. d'Agincourt-Canning, C. Ells (Eds.), *Ethical issues in women's healthcare: Practice and policy*. Oxford University Press.

Lyerly, A. D., Little, M., & Faden, R. (2008). The second wave: Toward responsible inclusion of pregnant women in research. *International Journal of Feminist Approaches to Bioethics, 1*(2), 5–22.

McCullough, L. B., & Chervenak, F. A. (2008). A critical analysis of the concept and discourse of "unborn child." *American Journal of Bioethics, 8*(7), 34–39.

Shah, S., Whittle, A., Wilfond, B., Gensler, G., & Wendler, D. (2004). How do institutional review boards apply the federal risk and benefit standards for pediatric research? *JAMA, 291*(4), 476–482.

Society for Maternal-Fetal Medicine. (n.d.). *SMFM Advocacy Agenda 2019–2020.* s3.amazonaws .com/cdn.smfm.org/media/1921/2019-2020_SMFM_Agenda.pdf

Task Force on Research Specific to Pregnant Women and Lactating Women. (2018). *Report to Secretary, Health and Human Services; Congress.* www.nichd.nih.gov/sites/default/files/2018-09 /PRGLAC_Report.pdf

Wendler, D. (2005). Protecting subjects who cannot give consent: Toward a better standard for "minimal" risks. *Hastings Center Report, 35*(5), 37–43.

Subpart C Research: Additional Protections for Prisoners

Paul P. Christopher

Julia G. Gorey

Josiah Rich

Abstract

Under the Department of Health and Human Services (DHHS) regulations, prisoners are considered a vulnerable population in need of special protections. This chapter describes the regulatory scope, interpretation, and application of 45 CFR 46 subpart C, Additional Protections for Research Involving Prisoners, to DHHS-conducted or supported research. The chapter also provides a brief history of relevant human subjects abuses and a commentary on the context of modern research involving prisoners.

Historical Overview

In 1978, thirteen years before publication of the Common Rule at 45 CFR part 46, "Additional Protections Pertaining to Biomedical and Behavioral Research Involving Prisoners as Subjects" was issued as subpart C of the Department of Health, Education and Welfare's (DHEW) human subjects regulations. The regulation was developed in response to the 1976 National Commission's *Report and Recommendations: Research Involving Prisoners* (National Commission, 1976). Two years in the making, the National Commission's report emerged as a clear repudiation of the abhorrent use of prisoners as human subjects in research that occurred in the first half of the 20th century. Prior to subpart C, the inclusion of prisoners in research, particularly in pharmaceutical testing, had been considered generally acceptable, even patriotic, through the 1960s. Research involving prisoners examined the effects of radioactive testicular injections on spermatogenesis, paralytic drugs as deterrents to antisocial behavior, testing of chemical warfare agents, evaluation of severe nutritional deficiencies, and induction of various bacterial, viral, and fungal infections (Capron, 1973; Hornblum, 1997).

By the early 1970s, however, the exposure of major research scandals focused national scrutiny on the ethical propriety of using prisoners in human subjects research. Reports emerged, such as that by *New York Times* reporter Walter Rugaber in his 1969 article, "Prison Drug and Plasma Projects Leave Fatal Trail," that prisoners were being involved in a wide range of high-risk, nontherapeutic studies (Rugaber, 1969). In some instances, prisoners were coerced into participating; in other cases, prisoners were offered a variety of inducements such as pardons, early parole, and cigarettes. Disclosure of the research procedures and study risks was largely nonexistent. Public outrage was particularly fueled by publication of Jessica Mitford's 1973 book *Kind and Usual Punishment: The Prison Business*, describing behavior modification treatments and psychosurgery techniques used on prisoners (Mitford, 1973a). Mitford's January 1973 *Atlantic Monthly* article, "Experiments Behind Bars: Doctors, Drug Companies, and Prisoners," quoted a doctor saying, "Criminals in our penitentiaries are fine experimental material—and much cheaper than chimpanzees" (Mitford, 1973b).

Due to increased public scrutiny, by 1976 eight states and the Federal Bureau of Prisons had formally moved to abandon research in prisons. After the National Commission's 1976 report, publicly funded medical research involving prisoners nearly ceased. **45 CFR part 46, subpart C**, adopted in 1978, codified stringent requirements under which prisoners could participate in DHEW (now DHHS)-sponsored research. These protections remain in effect today.

Beginning in the early 1990s, debate shifted from an almost exclusive focus on protecting prisoners from research abuses to consideration of the injustices that result from prisoners' limited access to potentially beneficial, even life-saving research. The HIV/AIDS epidemic brought these concerns into stark relief, given that prisoners suffered disproportionately from the disease, yet were excluded from even late-phase antiretroviral clinical trials. As discussed later, the central ethical question that frames modern prison research regulation emerged from this paradigm: How do we simultaneously provide adequate research protections for prisoners while ensuring their ability to participate in research to address the myriad health and social problems they face?

Scope and Application of Subpart C

The Office for Human Research Protections (OHRP) is responsible for authorizing DHHS-conducted or supported nonexempt human subjects research involving prisoners, and such research is not permitted to proceed without this authorization.

Note that current Food and Drug Administration (FDA) regulations for the protection of human subjects, codified at **21 CFR 50** and **56**, do not include additional protections for research subjects who are prisoners. The FDA does, however, consider prisoners to be a vulnerable subject population for which the IRB must include additional safeguards. In addition to subpart C, researchers and IRBs should also be aware of relevant state law affecting prisoners in research, such as the California law forbidding most biomedical research that is not in the prisoner's best medical interests (California Penal Code, 2016).

Definition of *Prisoner*

In order to successfully apply subpart C, it is important to understand how the definition of *prisoner* is interpreted. The subpart defines a prisoner as any person "involuntarily confined or detained in a penal institution" as a result of violating a criminal or civil statute, persons "detained in other facilities by virtue of states or commitment procedures which provide an alternative to criminal prosecution or incarceration in a penal institution, and individuals detained pending arraignment, trial or sentencing" [45 CFR 46.303(c)]. Although the emphasis is on custodial detention, this definition is much broader than subjects who are merely detained in a traditional jail or prison; it includes persons detained in residential treatment as a term of sentencing, persons with psychiatric illnesses who have been committed involuntarily to an institution as an alternative to a criminal prosecution or incarceration (i.e., "jail diversion"), and persons detained in accordance with this definition who may be allowed outside of the facility while wearing an electronic monitoring device. In addition, subpart C applies to the unanticipated inclusion of a prisoner in the clinical research of an institution and to subjects who become prisoners following enrollment in a study. The latter group is termed "subsequently incarcerated subjects," because they were not prisoners when they gave their informed consent to participate in the study.

The definition, however, does *not* include subjects who attend mandated treatment while residing in the community as these subjects are not "detained." Likewise, subjects who are under community-based correctional supervision (probation or parole), who voluntarily undergo substance abuse treatment, who are civilly committed, or who are merely handcuffed without any further judicial action, do not fall within the scope of subpart C.

An enrolled subject may cycle in and out of prisoner status without triggering subpart C review if all research interactions or interventions occur while the subject is outside of "prisoner" status. For example, if an enrolled subject participating in a clinical trial is arrested for driving while intoxicated and serves only a short jail term and, following release, resumes participation in the trial without any study-related activities having occurred while in jail, subpart C is not triggered.

Composition of the IRB

To better protect subjects from exploitation and coercion, subpart C review requires that the IRB membership include a prisoner representative who has "appropriate background and experience to serve in this capacity" [45 CFR 46.304(b)]. According to OHRP guidance, "In the absence of choosing someone who is a prisoner or has been a prisoner, the IRB should choose a prisoner representative who has a close working knowledge, understanding and appreciation of prison conditions from the perspective of the prisoner" (DHHS, 2003). Finding candidates to fill this role can be difficult for many institutions. In choosing a prisoner representative, it helps to consider what type of research is being reviewed by the institution and what insights the potential candidate could bring to the IRB review. A study examining drug treatment for prisoners with HIV and opioid use disorders transitioning back to the community and a study focusing on inner city youth violence ideally require different prisoner representatives with distinct backgrounds and expertise. The IRB should look to community reentry programs, social workers, medical or behavioral personnel familiar with the study's context, and of course, former prisoners, for possible recruitment as an appropriate prisoner representative. Additionally, the IRB should consider having more than one prisoner representative on its roster.

OHRP guidance also specifies that "the IRB must meet the special composition requirements of 45 CFR 46.304 for all types of review of the protocol, including initial review, continuing review, review of protocol amendments, and review of reports of unanticipated problems involving risks to subjects" (DHHS, 2003). The regulations at 45 CFR 46.304(b) state that if the research is reviewed by more than one IRB, only one IRB is required to satisfy the need for a prisoner representative; however, OHRP recommends that all reviewing IRBs include a prisoner representative. OHRP also recommends that the prisoner representative have sufficient knowledge of the prison context at each site to ensure that all IRBs will be cognizant of the potential risks and benefits of the research. An institution can rely on another IRB for subpart C review, which may be particularly useful for smaller institutions. Lastly, note that prisoner research may be expedited.

🔗 5-5

Application of Exemptions

The exemptions at 45 CFR 46.101(b) are not applicable to research involving prisoners under the pre-2018 Requirements. Under the 2018 Requirements, the exemptions are not applicable except for "research aimed at involving a broader subject population that only incidentally includes prisoners" [45 CFR 46.104(b)(2)]. A common example is the creation of a research database that seeks to include secondary data or biospecimens from other databases or from a large population; previously, under the pre-2018 Requirements, the knowing inclusion of identifiable private information about prisoners in such a database would trigger the need for subpart C review. Another example is the unforeseen inclusion of a subsequently incarcerated subject in a research study that is not intentionally seeking to enroll prisoners as subjects. In both these instances, the possibility that a subject's prisoner status could result in the subject's being coerced into study participation is extremely slight, and the application of subpart C would add little additional protection for the subject.

🔗 5-3

Subpart C Certification Process

The certification requirement is a 45 CFR 46 protection unique to subpart C. It stems from the National Commission's original reluctance to allow research involving prisoners, resulting in the creation of a subpart that allows such research only in limited circumstances. At the time of its adoption, the presumption was that research should not involve prisoners, *except for* research that: (1) fits into one of several limited categories (see later), (2) satisfies the protections found in 45 CFR 46.305, (3) has been reviewed by a properly constituted IRB with a prisoner representative, and (4) has certified the fulfillment of subpart C requirements to the Secretary of Health and Human Services, through OHRP.

When does an IRB need to review a study under subpart C and certify to the Secretary? Certainly, when the research intends to enroll prisoners and when subjects become prisoners after enrollment. In addition, an IRB should consider reviewing studies under subpart C if it can reasonably anticipate that some subjects will become prisoners over time. This may occur in some studies examining substance abuse, for instance, which do not recruit prisoners yet may have a high likelihood of subjects' becoming incarcerated before the study closes. Prospective certification allows the researcher to continue involvement with prisoner-subjects without having to stop to pursue subpart C certification. Otherwise, all research interactions or interventions with prisoners must stop until the institution has received an authorization from OHRP to proceed.

OHRP permits one exception to the requirement that subpart C review and certification precede the involvement of prisoner-subjects in research (DHHS,

2019). If the researcher deems it to be in the subject's best interests, a subject may remain in a study pending the IRB's subpart C review. In such cases, the IRB chairperson may determine that the subject may continue to participate in the research until the requirements of subpart C are satisfied, and the IRB is expected to promptly conduct additional review according to subpart C requirements.

Categories of Permitted Research

Subpart C specifies four categories of permitted research that may involve prisoners, **45 CFR 46.306(a)(2)(i)-(iv)**, with the 2003 Epidemiologic Waiver operating similarly to a fifth category of permitted research (see 68 FR 119; Federal Register, 2003). Unlike <u>subpart D</u>, these permissible categories are based on the type of research being done rather than on a risk/benefit threshold. Despite this, several of these categories reference minimal risk. Subpart C has its own definition of minimal risk and specifies that the risk of harm must be relative to the "daily lives" of "healthy persons" and not of a healthy prisoner; significant risk is often associated with a prison environment, and the authors believe a conservative interpretation of minimal risk is appropriate when reviewing research under subpart C.

⊘ 9-6

The current categories are somewhat overlapping in terms of their focus but may have different risk limitations or other requirements.

> **45 CFR 46.306(a)(2)(i)** Study of the possible causes, effects, and processes of incarceration, and of criminal behavior, provided that the study presents no more than minimal risk and no more than inconvenience to the subjects

Category (i) is limited to no more than minimal risk and is worded broadly to accommodate a wide range of research. "Causes, effects and processes of incarceration, and of criminal behavior" covers a spectrum of studies examining prisoners and largely consists of research examining varying facets of substance addiction, HIV status, homelessness, or mental illness, all conditions indicating a possible relationship with the criminal justice system. The category accommodates secondary research analyses, social-behavioral research, and longitudinal studies where recidivism is an outcome measure. The category frequently includes studies that are certified due to subjects who may be at risk of incarceration or studies that include subsequently incarcerated subjects.

> **45 CFR 46.306(a)(2)(ii)** Study of prisons as institutional structures or of prisoners as incarcerated persons, provided that the study presents no more than minimal risk and no more than inconvenience to the subjects

Category (ii) is a relatively narrow minimal risk category. Examples of authorized studies might include research examining nicotine addiction cessation programs in prisons, peer-mediated end-of-life caregiving among prisoners, cancer disparities in incarcerated men, and social determinants of HIV in an incarcerated population.

> **45 CFR 46.306(a)(2)(iii)** Research on conditions particularly affecting prisoners as a class … provided that the study may proceed only after the Secretary has consulted with appropriate experts including experts in penology, medicine, and ethics, and published notice, in the Federal Register, of his intent to approve such research

There is no ceiling on risk in category (iii), and unlike category (iv), no prospect of benefit is required; IRB approval under category (iii) triggers the need for a special expert review, known as Secretarial consultation, and a final approval determination by the Secretary. The National Commission deemed a higher level of ethical review to be an appropriate protection for prisoners involved in greater than minimal risk research not requiring a benefit to the prisoner's individual health or well-being. An example of a study that would trigger the need for a Secretarial consultation might be a greater than minimal risk study examining a novel antiretroviral therapy for HIV treatment. However, there is considerable overlap between categories (iii) and (iv), and depending on the research design and the nature of the control group, category (iii) studies may possibly be approved under category (iv) without necessitating a Secretarial consultation.

> **45 CFR 46.306(a)(2)(iv)** Research on practices, both innovative and accepted, which have the intent and reasonable probability of improving the health or well-being of the subject. In cases in which those studies require the assignment of prisoners in a manner consistent with protocols approved by the IRB to control groups which may not benefit from the research, the study may proceed only after the Secretary has consulted with appropriate experts, including experts in penology, medicine, and ethics, and published notice, in the Federal Register, of the intent to approve such research.

Category (iv) permits greater than minimal risk research; however, based on studies received by OHRP, the great majority of these studies are designated no more than minimal risk and are frequently sociobehavioral in nature (Gorey, 2019). In addition, the regulation requires that the research "have the intent and reasonable probability of improving the health and well-being of the subject." Risk level in category (iv) studies may be attributable to confidentiality concerns, as well as biomedical risk.

Category (iv) triggers the need for a Secretarial consultation only if the research assigns prisoners to a control group that may not benefit from the research. This can be problematic for studies that are greater than minimal risk and randomize subjects to a nonbeneficial control, as there is no other subpart C category to which such studies could be recategorized for approval without also triggering a Secretarial consultation. In some cases, researchers may choose to intentionally design their study to include a benefit to the control group, such as a physical or medical monitoring that they would not otherwise receive but for their research participation.

This category may include studies certified for the involvement of subjects who became prisoners *after* study enrollment, because in these instances there is no "assignment of prisoners" at the time of randomization, and the issue of the control group is not relevant.

Examples of category (iv) studies include the following:

- A comparative effectiveness study of subjects randomized to a 24-week course of buprenorphine versus extended-release naltrexone for opioid treatment.
- A study exploring the feasibility of a peer-driven intervention to improve HIV prevention among prisoners who inject drugs and who will have access to HIV and tuberculosis testing with referral to services available in the prison.
- A study examining the efficacy of an animal-assisted intervention to improve empathy skills, psychological stress symptoms, and recidivism rates in at-risk teens.

The 2003 Epidemiologic Waiver (68 Fed. Reg. 36929 ((June 20, 2003)) is a waiver under **45 CFR 46.101(i)** which functions similarly to a fifth category of permissible research for "studies that meet the following criteria: (1) In which the sole purposes are (i) To describe the prevalence or incidence of a disease by identifying all cases, or (ii) To study potential risk factor associations for a disease, and (2) Where the institution responsible for the conduct of the research certifies to the Office for Human Research Protections, DHHS, acting on behalf of the Secretary, that the IRB approved the research and fulfilled its duties under **45 CFR 46.305(a)(2)-(7)** and determined and documented that (i) The research presents no more than minimal risk and no more than inconvenience to the prisoner-subjects, and (ii) Prisoners are not a particular focus of the research." (Federal Register, 2003)

The 2003 Epidemiologic Waiver is used for a wide variety of epidemiological studies, including assay development, monitoring systems, and health registries that would otherwise not be permitted to include prisoners as subjects.

IRB Approval Criteria for Research Involving Prisoners

As with all other types of human subjects research that is regulated by DHHS, nonexempt prisoner research must comply with the requirements for IRB approval and informed consent under subpart A. In addition to these general requirements, subpart C provides specific protections for prisoners as research subjects, setting further conditions that must be satisfied before an IRB can approve a study. These seven requirements, which include appropriate categorization of the research, focus on the special circumstances of prisoners and seek to mitigate a number of ethical problems that often arise in prison research, including coercion, exploitation, and undue influence. Thus, these requirements are intended to minimize the risks to subjects, help ensure that participants are able to give valid informed consent, and assure equitable subject selection in a subpart C context. The following are the requirements specified in **45 CFR 46.305(a)**:

⌀ 5-4
⌀ Section 6

(1) The research under review represents one of the categories of research permissible under §46.306(a)(2);
(2) Any possible advantages accruing to the prisoner through his or her participation in the research, when compared to the general living conditions, medical care, quality of food, amenities, and opportunity for earnings in the prison, are not of such a magnitude that his or her ability to weigh the risks of the research against the value of such advantages in the limited choice environment of the prison is impaired;
(3) The risks involved in the research are commensurate with risks that would be accepted by nonprisoner volunteers;
(4) Procedures for the selection of subjects within the prison are fair to all prisoners and immune from arbitrary intervention by prison authorities or prisoners. Unless the principal investigator provides to the Board justification in writing for following some other procedures, control subjects must be selected randomly from the group of available prisoners who meet the characteristics needed for that particular research project;

(5) The information is presented in language which is understandable to the subject population;

(6) Adequate assurance exists that parole boards will not take into account a prisoner's participation in the research in making decisions regarding parole, and each prisoner is clearly informed in advance that participation in the research will have no effect on his or her parole; and

(7) Where the Board finds there may be a need for follow-up examination or care of participants after the end of their participation, adequate provision has been made for such examination or care, taking into account the varying lengths of individual prisoners' sentences, and for informing participants of this fact.

In some contexts, several of these requirements may not be relevant to a given subpart C study. For example, requirement (4), focusing on selection of subjects within the prison, is not relevant to a study that involves only subsequently incarcerated subjects. Likewise, not all of these requirements will be relevant to a study involving only a secondary data analysis with no active subject intervention. In such cases, the IRB should simply note for the record that the given criterion is not applicable to the study.

Requirement (7) is unclear in terms of how and to what extent the researcher, institution, or sponsor is responsible for providing care to both prisoners and parolees after their participation in research. Interpretation of this requirement is particularly problematic in clinical research on life-threatening illnesses such as cancer or AIDS, where the patient is likely to need continued treatment, perhaps for a prolonged period and at considerable expense. For example, what does "adequate provision . . . for . . . care" mean? Does it mean that the prisoner or former prisoner who participated in the research must be provided free care for as long as necessary? It seems reasonable for an IRB to ensure adequate provisions are made for the care of subjects who suffer a research-related injury but not to extend the provision for treatment of an illness that predates the beginning of the study or is unrelated to the study. In whatever form they take, these provisions (and their limitations) should be clearly communicated to prospective subjects during informed consent discussions.

Evaluation of Risk and Benefit

With regard to evaluating study risk, subpart C directs IRBs to ensure that (1) the advantages of participation do not undermine a prisoner's ability to appreciate and weigh risks of participating, and (2) the risks are commensurate with those that would be accepted by nonprisoners. Other requirements related to evaluating risk and benefit are subsumed under subpart A at **45 CFR 46.111** and merit special consideration for prisoner studies.

When executing subpart A requirements, IRBs need to consider the kinds of research risks that arise or are elevated in correctional settings. Risks to privacy and confidentiality, for example, deserve particular attention given the restricted privacy afforded to prisoners in general. The sensitive nature of much prison-based research, which may focus on mental health, trauma, substance use, and infectious disease, heightens the need to ensure adequate protections. For example, in a prison context, researchers and IRBs should be aware of the potential repercussions a positive drug test may have on the ability of a subject to remain in a given nonprison treatment setting or the implications snowball sampling (in which subjects refer other subjects) may have in locating subjects who would prefer anonymity. Researchers should address the procedures that will be used to safeguard privacy and confidentiality at each stage of a study, ranging from identification of potential subjects, informed consent discussions, follow-up assessments, and delivery of interventions. Moreover, studies that offer prisoners otherwise inaccessible treatment or provide incentives may provoke correctional staff who, at times, may actively dissuade prisoners from participating. An example might be a study that offers opioid agonist therapy to subjects in a prison that otherwise does not provide medication-based treatment for opioid use disorder; correctional staff who view the study as offering preferential treatment may dissuade prisoners from joining or remaining in the study (Christopher et al., 2017). Such influences should be evaluated when considering the risks of the study and may need to be minimized (for example through education of correctional staff) and addressed in informed consent discussions with prospective subjects.

Likewise, IRBs should consider the nature of potential study benefits to prisoners. Note that in addition to benefits directly related to a study intervention, prisoners are likely to factor nonintervention-related advantages (e.g., incentives such as cigarettes, phone cards, gift cards, or money) into their decision making. Indeed, given prisoners' limited access to a variety of social goods, these ancillary <u>incentives</u> may carry considerably more weight for prisoners than they would for nonincarcerated individuals. This heightens concern for undue influence. At the same time, inducements affect individuals differently; thus, one should not presume that all prisoners will be unduly influenced by the same incentive.

⊘ 12-2

Finally, consideration should be given to the time allotted to prisoners to ensure they have adequate opportunity to consider all study risks and benefits. In general, researchers' access to prospective prisoner subjects is quite limited as a result of strict schedules that govern prison operation. Thus, there is potential for prisoners to feel rushed to make a decision about enrollment before having adequate opportunity to make a fully informed decision. Yet prisoners are more likely to have lower levels of health literacy, general literacy, and familiarity with treatment options. In light of these disparities, researchers should allocate more time for informed consent procedures that may need to include education about illness and treatment options.

Discussion

Minimal risk studies comprise the vast majority of DHHS-conducted or supported research involving prisoners. Much of this research is sociobehavioral in nature and involves subjects who are frequently in court-mandated substance abuse treatment or other nontraditional "prison" facilities. Greater than minimal risk clinical trials targeting prisoners as a population are less commonly funded by DHHS entities and, under subpart C, are permissible only within limited circumstances. DHHS-funded research most commonly focuses on some facet of substance abuse management or treatment, often in studies in which subjects have a co-occurring condition (such as HIV or depression) and frequently examines specific racial, ethnic, or age groups (Gorey, 2019).

In one respect, subpart C has achieved its intended goal. The kinds of high-risk, nonbeneficial biomedical studies described in the beginning of this chapter that were clearly coercive and exploited prisoners are prohibited under DHHS-conducted or -supported research today. This is not to suggest that all research involving prisoners is always uniformly ethical, as the scope of subpart C is limited to research regulated by DHHS and the two federal agencies or departments that have adopted it (in 2019, the Central Intelligence Agency and the Social Security Administration). Research funded or conducted by other federal agencies, or by nongovernmental entities, is not subject to subpart C. For these investigations, broader transparency is certainly warranted.

The United States has the largest prison population in the world. Compared with the rest of Americans, prisoners are far more likely to be members of racial minorities, to face poverty, and to have poor access to health care, poor education and poor health literacy. They also have disproportionately high burdens of substance use, mental illness, infectious disease, and illness in general. Given these extraordinary disparities, it is clear that they have not benefited equally from the profound advances produced by biomedical and sociobehavioral research of the past half century. Thus, while it is important to ensure appropriate protections continue to be in place, it is imperative that funding entities, community stakeholders, and IRBs support research that has the potential to benefit this population.

Fulfilling this critical need is not an easy task. From an IRB perspective, the structure and language of subpart C can be awkward, and IRB members are advised to be aware of OHRP guidance. Moreover, the OHRP certification process, while initiated as an essential precaution to protect a vulnerable population, is now sometimes criticized as unduly burdensome and not adequately calibrated to studies that reflect a low degree of risk (Institute of Medicine, 2007). Over the years, there have been efforts to improve the subpart. At the request of the Secretary's Advisory Committee on Human Research Protections (SACHRP), in 2003, the "Subpart C Subcommittee" was formed. The group was asked to provide recommendations for improved guidance on subpart C, including changes that could be implemented without regulatory revision. The Subcommittee issued a report in 2005 which, among other points, recommended changes in the OHRP interpretation of control group in **45 CFR 46.306(a)(2)(iv)**, provided guidance on "follow-up requirements" under **45 CFR 46.305(a)(7)**, and recommended qualifications for the IRB prisoner representative (DHHS, 2005). The report requested that the National Academy of Medicine (NAM) further review the ethical framework of research involving prisoners with an eye toward possible subpart C revision.

Ethical Considerations for Research Involving Prisoners was released by NAM in 2007 and recommended that subpart C be revised to include a risk/benefit framework for categorization of studies (Institute of Medicine, 2007). It also recommended the elimination of waiver of consent for prisoners in research and elimination of the subpart C certification requirement. Several NAM recommendations were beyond the scope of OHRP to implement, such as ensuring adequate standards of care in prisons and extending the scope of subpart C beyond DHHS-conducted or funded research.

Conclusion

Although guidance responded to some of the Subcommittee and NAM recommendations, as of 2019 there has been no revision of the original 1978 subpart (there have been changes to the application of the subpart, such as the inapplicability of subpart C to the waiver of consent in emergency research; see 61 Fed. Reg. 192 (Federal Register, 1996, p. 51498). Nevertheless, much can be done to support the ethical advancement of prisoner research within the scope of these regulations. Nothing in subpart C prohibits well-crafted minimal and above minimal risk protocols that aim to address any of the profound health and social disparities prisoners face. Indeed, the strong foundation of protections afforded by subpart C can help justify and promote the expansion of such research. By working in close coordination with researchers to assist them in developing ethically sound studies, IRBs are positioned to play a major role in supporting this goal.

References

California Penal Code. (2016). *Title 2.1 Biomedical and Behavioral Research, Section 3502.* leginfo .legislature.ca.gov/faces/codes_displaySection.xhtml?lawCode=PEN&sectionNum=3502.

Capron, A. M. (1973). Medical research in prisons. *Hastings Center Report, 3*(3), 4.

Christopher, P. P., Garcia-Sampson, L. G., Stein, M., Johnson, J., Rich, J., & Lidz, C. (2017). Enrolling in clinical research while incarcerated: What influences participants' decisions? *Hastings Center Report, 47*(2), 21.

Department of Health and Human Services (DHHS). (2003). *Prisoner involvement in research.* www.hhs.gov/ohrp/regulations-and-policy/guidance/prisoner-research-ohrp-guidance -2003/index.html

Department of Health and Human Services (DHHS). (2005). *SACHRP Chair letter to HHS Secretary regarding recommendations.* www.hhs.gov/ohrp/sachrp-committee/recommendations/2005 -july-28-letter/index.html

Department of Health and Human Services (DHHS). (2019). *Prisoner research FAQs.* www.hhs .gov/ohrp/regulations-and-policy/guidance/faq/prisoner-research/index.html

Federal Register. (1996). Vol. 61, No. 192. www.govinfo.gov/content/pkg/FR-1996-10-02 /pdf/96-24967.pdf

Federal Register. (2003). Vol. 68, No. 119. Waiver of the Applicability of Certain Provisions of Department of Health and Human Services Regulations for Protection of Human Research Subjects for Department of Health and Human Services Conducted or Supported Epidemiologic Research Involving Prisoners as Subjects. www.govinfo.gov/content/pkg/FR-2003-06 -20/pdf/03-15580.pdf

Gorey, J. G. (2019). Looking through the bars: Responsible research with prisoners. *Proceedings of the public responsibility and medicine advancing ethical research conference.*

Hornblum, A. M. (1997). They were cheap and available: Prisoners as research subjects in twentieth century America. *BMJ, 315,* 1437.

Institute of Medicine. (2007). *Ethical considerations for research involving prisoners.* National Academies Press. doi:10.17226/11692

Mitford, J. (1973a). *Kind and usual punishment The prison business.* Knopf.

Mitford, J. (1973b). Experiments behind bars: Doctors, drug companies, and prisoners. *Atlantic Monthly, 76,* 64–73.

National Commission for the Protection of Human Subjects of Biomedical and Behavioral Research. (1976). *Report and Recommendations: Research Involving Prisoners* (DHEW [OS] 76-131). U.S. Government Printing Office.

Rugaber, W. (1969, July 29). Prison drug and plasma projects leave fatal trail. *New York Times.* www.nytimes.com/1969/07/29/archives/prison-drug-and-plasma-projects-leave-fatal-trail -trail-of-injury.html

Subpart D Research: Additional Protections for Children

Robert M. Nelson
Donna L. Snyder

Abstract

Children, as a vulnerable population, are afforded special protections under U.S. federal regulations when included in research. These regulations are intended to protect children from being enrolled in research that exceeds a level of justified risk without a sufficient prospect of direct clinical benefit. IRBs must have adequate expertise to ensure that research including children has both scientific merit and is ethically sound. This chapter reviews the issues that should be considered when an IRB reviews research involving children, starting with the special protections afforded to children participating in research, the composition of the IRB, the general aspects of IRB review, and requirements for parental permission and child assent.

Introduction

Research involving children requires careful attention to the additional regulatory provisions at **21 CFR 50** and **45 CFR 46** that are intended to protect children from being enrolled in research that exceeds a level of justified risk. The National Commission in the _Belmont Report_ wrote about the "special provisions" for children that respect for persons requires, including the opportunity for children to actively provide assent, honoring a child's refusal to participate unless the treatment is only available in the research setting, and seeking the permission of parents or guardians in order to protect children from harm (National Commission, 1979). In addition, the National Commission advocated for "an order of preference in the selection of classes of subjects (e.g., adults before children)" as "a matter of social justice," based on the judgment that children ought not to bear the burdens of research unless absolutely necessary (National Commission,

🔗 1-1

1979). Finally, the National Commission discussed the scope of parental authority in enrolling a child in research, arguing that such decisions may be morally justified if either the research may directly benefit the child or the risks of participation in the research are low, either "minimal risk" or no more than a "minor increase over minimal risk" (National Commission, 1978). The concepts of minimal risk, minor increase over minimal risk, prospect of direct benefit, assent, and permission are the basis for the special protections for children [21 CFR 50, 45 CFR 46]. This basis rests on the moral foundation of respect for children, beneficence, justice, and the proper scope of parental authority.

This chapter reviews the issues that should be considered when an IRB reviews research involving children, starting with the special protections afforded to children participating in research, followed by the composition of the IRB, the general aspects of IRB review, requirements for parental permission and child assent, and special scientific and regulatory considerations.

Special Protections for Children in Research

The regulations require that additional safeguards be afforded to children involved in research as they are a vulnerable population. These special protections, found in **subpart D** of **45 CFR 46** and **21 CFR 50**, apply to all children, defined as subjects "who have not attained the legal age for consent to treatments or procedures involved in the research, under the applicable law of the jurisdiction in which the research will be conducted" [45 CFR 46.402(a); 21 CFR 50.3(o)]. The safeguards of subpart D involve an additional determination by the IRB of the level of risk and the prospect of direct benefit presented by the proposed research. The IRB can approve research involving children only if it falls into one of three categories. The three categories are as follows:

1. Research not involving greater than minimal risk [21 CFR 50.51; 45 CFR 46.404]
2. Research involving greater than minimal risk but presenting the prospect of direct benefit to the individual subjects [21 CFR 50.52; 45 CFR 46.405]
3. Research involving greater than minimal risk and offering no prospect of direct benefit to individual subjects, but likely to yield generalizable knowledge about the disorder or condition. (Note that the level of risk in this section is capped at "no more than a minor increase over minimal") [21 CFR 50.53; 45 CFR 46.406]

If an IRB cannot approve the research using one or more of these three categories, it may refer the research to the Secretary of the Department of Health and Human Services (DHHS) and/or the Food and Drug Administration (FDA) Commissioner for review by a federal panel. The IRB should only refer the protocol for federal review if "the research presents a reasonable opportunity to further the understanding, prevention, or alleviation of a serious problem affecting the health or welfare of children" [21 CFR 50.54; 45 CFR 46.407]. (See additional discussion under the sections Special Considerations and Approval by Federal Review Panel).

Interpretation of Minimal Risk and Minor Increase over Minimal Risk

Key to the interpretation of subpart D is the definition of "minimal risk" and a "minor increase over minimal risk," as it establishes the level of risk to which children may be exposed through research that does not offer the prospect of direct benefit. Minimal risk is defined as "the probability and magnitude of harm or discomfort anticipated in the research are not greater in and of themselves than those ordinarily encountered in daily life or during the performance of routine physical or psychological examinations or tests" [**45 CFR 46.102(j)**; **21 CFR 56.102(i)**]. Healthy children may be exposed to interventions or procedures in research that are minimal risk.

RISK ASSESSMENT

Although the definition found in the current regulations does not include the phrase "of healthy children," the National Commission, and more recently, the IOM, recommended that minimal risk should be interpreted in relation to the experiences of average, healthy, normal children (National Commission, 1978; IOM, 2004). Even so, reasonable differences of opinion exist about the interpretation of minimal risk in the context of a healthy child. The IOM provided a table listing the risk categorization of some common medical procedures as a first step in encouraging uniformity in IRB risk assessment (see **Table 9.6-1**; IOM, 2004).

Table 9.6-1 Common Research Procedures by Category of Risk

| Procedure | Category of Risk | | |
	Minimal	Minor Increase Over Minimal	More Than a Minor Increase Over Minimal
Routine history taking	X		
Venipuncture/fingerstick/heelstick	X		
Urine collection via bag	X		
Urine collection via catheter		X	
Urine collection via suprapubic tap			X
Chest X-ray	X		
Bone density test	X		
Wrist X-ray for bone age	X		
Lumbar puncture		X	
Collection of saliva	X		
Collection of small sample of hair	X		
Vision testing	X		
Hearing testing	X		
Complete neurological exam	X		
Oral glucose tolerance test	X		
Skin punch biopsy with topical pain relief		X	
Bone marrow aspirate with topical pain relief		X	
Organ biopsy			X
Standard psychological tests	X		
Classroom observation	X		

NOTE: The category of risk is for a single procedure. Multiple or repetitive procedures are likely to affect the level of risk.

SOURCE: National Human Research Protections Advisory Committee (NHRPAC). (2002). Clarifying specific portion of 45 CFR 46 subpart D that governs children's research [online]. Accessed May 14, 2014. http://www.hhs.gov/ohrp/archive/nhrpac/documents/nhrpac16.pdf.

"Minor increase refers to a risk which, while it goes beyond the narrow boundaries of minimal risk . . . , poses no significant threat to the child's health or well-being" (Institute of Medicine, 2004; National Commission, 1978). For research where the risk might be considered a "minor increase over minimal risk," children must have a disorder or condition, and the research must be likely to yield generalizable knowledge about the subjects' disorder or condition that is of vital importance for the understanding or amelioration of the subjects' disorder or condition. Of note, having a condition may include being "at risk" for a disorder or condition. The Institute of Medicine (IOM), in their 2004 report, defined a condition as "a specific (or a set of specific) physical, psychological, neurodevelopmental, or social characteristic(s) that an established body of scientific evidence or clinical knowledge has shown to negatively affect children's health and well-being or to increase their *risk* [emphasis added] of developing a health problem in the future" (Recommendation 4.3; IOM, 2004).

Interpretation of Research That Offers a Prospect of Direct Benefit

Research that presents more than a minor increase over minimal risk must offer a prospect of direct benefit to the children in the research. Additionally, the risk must be justified by the anticipated clinical benefit, and the balance of the anticipated benefit to the risk must be at least as favorable to the child as any available alternative approaches [**45 CFR 46.405**; **21 CFR 50.52**]. A direct benefit is generally defined as the benefit to the individual child from the research intervention, and not from ancillary clinical procedures that may be included in the protocol. For example, treatment with a drug product may offer a prospect of direct benefit, but physical exams done as study assessments do not. When assessing whether an intervention offers a prospect of direct benefit, the IRB should consider whether the evidence establishing proof of concept about a potential beneficial effect is sufficient and whether the proposed dose and duration of treatment are adequate to offer a potential clinical benefit (Hume et al., 2017; King, 2000; Wendler et al., 2019).

When considering alternative approaches, there must be "research equipoise" (i.e., uncertainty) between the arm(s) of a trial and the alternatives available outside of the research. The term "research equipoise" was introduced by the National Bioethics Advisory Commission (NBAC) in their 2001 report (NBAC, 2001). The NBAC favored this term rather than "clinical equipoise" (Freedman, 1987), opining that the concept of equipoise should be broadened to include other areas of practice beyond medicine (e.g., psychology or public health). Genuine uncertainty should exist regarding whether the intervention or alternative treatment—or a control, if included—is better. Existence of research equipoise "does not require numeric equality of intervention risks or potential benefits. Rather, research equipoise requires approximate equality in the risk/potential benefit ratios of the study and control interventions" (NBAC, 2001).

Component Analysis

45 CFR 46.405 and **21 CFR 50.52** specifically state that direct benefit is assessed at the level of each *intervention or procedure* in the research protocol. Therefore, when considering research risks, the individual interventions or procedures in a protocol should be analyzed to determine whether they offer a prospect of direct benefit or they do not; this is a concept called "component analysis." Any intervention or procedure that does not offer a prospect of direct benefit must not exceed a "minor increase over minimal risk" as per **45 CFR 46.406** and **21 CFR 50.53**, unless reviewed by a federal panel [**45 CFR 46.407**; **21 CFR 50.54**]. As recommended by the IOM, "Institutional review boards should assess the potential harms and benefits of each intervention or procedure in a pediatric protocol to determine whether each conforms to the regulatory criteria for approving research involving children. When some procedures present the prospect of direct benefit and others do not, the potential benefits from one component of the research should not be held to offset or justify the risks presented by another" (IOM, 2004). Additionally, the National Commission stated that interventions or procedures in a protocol should be evaluated "individually as well as collectively, as is done in clinical practice" (National Commission, 1978).

For example, consider a bone marrow aspiration that is not needed for clinical care but is collected to obtain research information as part of an oncology treatment protocol. Consistent with subpart D, the risks and potential benefit of the bone marrow aspiration should be evaluated based on whether the procedure does or does not offer a benefit using component analysis. Since the bone marrow aspirate is not needed for clinical care, there is no direct benefit to the child. Thus, the risk of the bone marrow aspirate performed solely to answer the research question must be limited to a minor increase over minimal risk and justified in relation to the potential to generate knowledge (i.e., **45 CFR 46.406**; **21 CFR 50.53**). Of note, under **45 CFR 46.406** and **21 CFR 50.53**, one may allow a relative standard of a minor increase over minimal risk. In effect, those interventions or procedures that are reasonably commensurate with a particular child's experience in *the context of their condition or disease* could be considered as a minor increase over minimal risk. See additional information on component analysis under the subsection Choice of Control Group (Placebo Controls).

IRB Membership

Regulations require that if an IRB regularly reviews research that involves a vulnerable category of subjects, such as children, one or more individuals who are knowledgeable about and experienced in working with these subjects should be considered for inclusion on the IRB [**45 CFR 46.108(a)**; **21 CFR 56.107(a)**]. The simple addition of a single pediatrician to an

IRBs have some latitude in determining whether certain procedures might fall under the minor increase over minimal risk category. For example, FDA convened a Pediatric Ethics Subcommittee Meeting of the Pediatric Advisory Committee in March 2015 to determine if procedural sedation for nonbeneficial "research only" procedures may be considered under **21 CFR 50.53**. Although the committee was unable to reach consensus on whether one or more approaches to procedural sedation should be considered a minor increase over minimal risk, the committee did agree on several recommendations (FDA, 2015):

1. "Procedures should be performed at a high-volume center with a dedicated pediatric sedation service;
2. There should be rigorous scientific justification for the need for the nontherapeutic procedures;
3. The approach to procedural sedation and risk minimization procedures should be described in the protocol;
4. Children with chronic conditions that may place them at higher risk from procedural sedation should be carefully evaluated and potentially excluded from the protocol;
5. The nontherapeutic procedure should be terminated if complications of sedation arise or the level of sedation is inadequate as it would be inappropriate to escalate the approach to procedural sedation beyond what would be considered a minor increase over minimal risk rather than to stop the procedure;
6. If a particular procedure in a particular patient population is normally accompanied by sedation when performed for clinical reasons, sedation should not be withheld in the nontherapeutic research setting to avoid its risks and thereby enhance the procedure's approvability under federal research regulations; and
7. There should be clear communication with potential subjects (and their parents) regarding the nontherapeutic nature of the procedures and procedural sedation in child assent and parental permission documents."

IRBs are encouraged to review these recommendations to mitigate risk when making a determination for a particular protocol that includes procedural sedation for nonbeneficial, "research only" procedures (FDA, 2015).

Additionally, IRBs might consider a *single-dose* drug study conducted to collect pharmacokinetic (PK) data under **21 CFR 50.53**. Although these studies do not offer direct benefit, such studies might be considered under **21 CFR 50.53** if sufficient safety information exists to characterize the PK sampling and blood draws as no more than a minor increase over minimal risk (FDA, 2012, 2014).

adult-oriented IRB does not create an IRB capable of reviewing pediatric research. The FDA's E11 guidance document on pediatric research recommends that "there should be IRB/IEC members or experts consulted by the IRB/IEC who are knowledgeable in pediatric ethical, clinical, and psychosocial issues" (FDA, 2000). More concretely, the IOM recommends that an IRB should have at least three individuals with expertise in (1) pediatric clinical care and research, (2) the psychosocial dimensions of child and adolescent health care, and (3) the ethics of research involving children in attendance as members or alternates during the review of a research protocol involving children (IOM, 2004). The IOM also recommended that the IRB obtain, when appropriate, additional perspectives from parents, children, adolescents, and community members (Recommendation 8.3; IOM, 2004).

General Criteria for IRB Approval

The Minimization of Risk

⚓ 5-4   The general criteria for IRB approval must be considered in addition to the special protections afforded to children found in subpart D. First, the risks to children in the protocol must be minimized. The IRB should consider the risks from the perspective of a child and not simply focus on the physical and economic risks. For example, the research area should be "child friendly" with an adequate play area and space for parents to remain with the child. Study-related laboratory samples should be obtained at the time of clinical diagnostic testing whenever possible. The IRB should be familiar with the various research design methods that minimize risk to the child, such as the extrapolation of adult efficacy to children, including strategies that eliminate the need to conduct studies in the pediatric population entirely. In addition, the IRB should evaluate "only those risks and benefits that may result from the research" rather than the overall risks and benefits of therapies included in the research that the "subjects would receive even if not participating in the research." For example, using a "component analysis" of risks and benefits, a protocol that combines clinical treatment and research could be judged as "minimal risk" based on the research component alone (Wendler et al., 2019).

STRATEGY EXAMPLES

Examples of strategies that reduce the number of studies needed to be conducted in children include limiting research to the collection of pharmacokinetic (PK) data to establish pediatric dosing (i.e., matching adult exposure), or combining PK with pharmacodynamic (PD) or clinical response data (i.e., exposure/response) and safety data when extrapolation of efficacy from adults or from one pediatric population to another is appropriate (European Medicines Agency, 2018; FDA, 2018b). Other strategies include the use of PK modeling and simulation (potentially in lieu of dedicated PK studies in children), adaptive study designs, and minimizing the volume of blood withdrawn through the use of sensitive bioanalytical assays, pediatric-enabled laboratories, and population PK approaches (FDA, 2014, 2018a, 2018b).

Selection of Subjects

The IRB is required to assure that the selection of subjects is equitable, taking into account the "purposes of the research and the setting in which the research will be conducted" [45 CFR 46.111(a)(3); 21 CFR 56.111(a)(3)]. Children are at risk of being a population of convenience, especially for researchers recruiting from within their own places of employment and/or from their own colleagues. An IRB should have sufficient expertise to consider the risks of undue influence and coercion from the perspective of a child, given the setting in which recruitment takes place. Finally, children should be included in research only if their participation is necessary to answer the scientific question being investigated (National Commission, 1978; Roth-Cline & Nelson, 2014).

Expedited Review

Expedited review of research involving children can be conducted by an IRB in accord with the regulations [**45 CFR 46.110**; **21 CFR 56.110**]. Currently, the only difference between the requirements for adults and children is in category 2, concerning the volume and frequency of blood draws that can be considered under expedited review procedures.

🔗 5-5

Exempt Research

Research involving children can be considered exempt from further IRB review in accord with the pertinent regulations [**45 CFR 46.104**]. However, the exemption for "research that only includes interactions involving educational tests (cognitive, diagnostic, aptitude, achievement), survey procedures, interview procedures, or observation of public behavior" [**45 CFR 46.104(d)(2)**] cannot be used for research involving children unless the research involves only the "observation of public behavior when the investigator(s) do not participate in the activities being observed" [**45 CFR 46.104(b)(3)**]. An IRB should have a review process for determining exemptions that include individuals with sufficient expertise in pediatrics to evaluate, for example, the normal educational practices that are used in "established or commonly accepted educational settings" for children.

🔗 5-3

Permission of the Parent(s)/ Assent of the Child

Central to all four categories of research under subpart D [**21 CFR 50.51–54** and **45 CFR 46.404–407**] is a requirement to solicit the assent of the child and permission of their parent or guardian.

Parental Permission

Parental permission is treated in much the same way as informed consent, apart from some additional provisions found in **45 CFR 46.408** and **21 CFR 50.55**. A parent (defined as "a child's biological or adoptive parent") or guardian (defined as "an individual who is authorized under applicable state or local law to consent on behalf of a child to general medical care") must agree to (i.e., permit) the child's participation in research [**45 CFR 46.402**; **21 CFR 50.3**].

🔗 Section 6

For research protocols that do not involve an FDA-regulated product, all of the requirements of **45 CFR 46.116** concerning informed consent apply to parental permission, including the general and required elements. The elements of informed parental permission can be modified or waived entirely in accordance with **45 CFR 46.116(f)(3)**. The requirements for documentation of parental permission are the same as what is required for informed consent according to **45 CFR 46.117**.

🔗 6-2
🔗 6-4

For research protocols involving an FDA-regulated product, the process and documentation of parental permission must be in accordance with subparts B and D of **21 CFR 50**. Under current FDA regulations, a waiver of parental permission can be considered for emergent and life-threatening situations, either individually [**21 CFR 50.23**] or as a group [**21 CFR 50.24**]. FDA also permits a waiver of informed consent/parental permission for minimal risk clinical investigations when specific criteria are met (similar to those noted previously under **46.116(f)(3)**), and appropriate safeguards are in place (FDA, 2017b).

Of special note, the FDA did not adopt the provision under 45 CFR 46.408(c), which allows an IRB to waive parental or guardian permission if a research protocol is designed for conditions where parental permission would not be a reasonable requirement to protect children. The IRB must provide an appropriate mechanism for protecting the children who will participate in the research, and any waiver of parental permission must not be inconsistent with federal, state, or local law. Many IRBs will waive the requirement for parental permission for research using adolescent subjects that involves medical procedures and treatment that the adolescent can consent to without parental knowledge, such as the use of contraceptives, treatment of sexually transmitted disease, treatment of alcohol and drug abuse, and so forth. Such a waiver is not available under FDA regulations. However, if an IRB determines that the minor subject is not a "child" as defined by state law, these mature or "emancipated" minors can consent for themselves without the need for parental or guardian permission (FDA, 2013).

Finally, there are some additional requirements for parental permission in subpart D. Research covered by 45 CFR 46.406 and/or 21 CFR 50.53 and 45 CFR 46.407 and/or 21 CFR 50.54 requires permission to be obtained from *both* parents, "unless one parent is deceased, unknown, incompetent, or not reasonably available, or when only one parent has legal responsibility for the care and custody of the child" [45 CFR 46.408 (b)].

Child Assent

Assent is defined as "a child's affirmative agreement to participate in research" [45 CFR 46.402(b); 21 CFR 50.3(n)]. A child's mere failure to object must not be considered assent. The National Commission recommended that the assent of the children be required when they are 7 years of age or older (National Commission, 1978). However, the federal regulations do not specify any of the elements of informed assent and do not indicate an age at which assent ought to be possible. The assent process should be developmentally appropriate based on the age and capability of the child to understand the information. Children should be provided opportunities to express and discuss their willingness to participate (IOM, 2004). An IRB is granted wide discretion in determining whether a child is capable of assenting and can waive the requirement for child assent if a child is not capable of assent; if the research offers a prospect of direct benefit not available outside of the research (thus falling under the scope of parental authority in overriding a child's desires); or given the same conditions under which parental permission can be waived (as noted previously). An IRB also has wide discretion in determining whether and how a child's assent is documented (FDA, 2013). Finally, as a matter of both justice and respect for persons, if scientifically appropriate, efforts should be made to conduct research using children capable of assent before enrolling those less able to assent.

Special Considerations

Research Design

An IRB must evaluate the experimental design of a research protocol, including the sample size justification, in order to minimize risks and determine the reasonableness of the risks with respect to the knowledge to be gained. A protocol that cannot answer the research question posed should not be approved.

A sample size that exceeds the number of children necessary to answer the research question exposes additional children to unnecessary risk and should not be approved. A pediatric trial may require different efficacy endpoints than those tested in adults based on considerations of the age and development of the subjects. In addition, because children with developing organ systems may respond differently to treatments than adults, a pediatric trial should monitor for possible adverse effects that might be unique to children, such as the impact on physical and cognitive growth and development (FDA, 2000; FDA, 2018b).

Choice of Control Group (Placebo Controls)

The circumstances under which a placebo control group is appropriate are a matter of controversy. The Declaration of Helsinki states that a new intervention must be tested against the best proven intervention(s) except where no proven treatment exists, or if for compelling scientific reasons, a placebo is needed to determine the efficacy or safety of the intervention, and patients will not be exposed to serious or irreversible harm as a result of not receiving the best proven intervention (World Medical Association, 2018). The FDA document on the choice of control group (E10) states that one can use a placebo control if withholding the known effective therapy would not result in serious harm as a result of the delay or denial of treatment (FDA, 2001). The FDA E11 (FDA, 2000) and E11 R1 (FDA, 2018b) documents on pediatric trials do not discuss placebo controls. The presence of a placebo arm in a clinical trial does not preclude the research from being considered under subpart D. However, the administration of a placebo *does not* offer a prospect of direct benefit, and therefore, using a component analysis approach, a placebo arm must present *no more than minimal risk* [45 CFR 46.404; 21 CFR 50.51] or *no more than a minor increase over minimal risk* [45 CFR 46.406; 21 CFR 50.53] unless referred to a federal panel [45 CFR 46.407; 21 CFR 55.54] as discussed later (FDA, 2013). When considering the risks with use of a placebo control, the method of administration (e.g., oral, intravenous) and the risks of withholding known effective therapy, if other therapy is available, must be considered when assessing the risk.

🔗 10-11

🔗 1-1

Early Phase Pediatric Trials in Oncology

A phase 1 [use arabic numerals for phases of clinical trials throughout: phase 1, phase 2, phase 3, phase 4] pediatric oncology trial is usually considered under 21 CFR 50.52 and/or 45 CFR 46.405 when the standard alternatives for the enrolled pediatric subjects have been exhausted and the only remaining prospect for direct benefit may be the experimental intervention (FDA, 2019b). "An experimental intervention may pose greater risk to participants than accepted practice, as long as it also offers the prospect of greater direct benefit to the participant and the relation between the risks and potential benefits falls within a range of equivalency to accepted practice" (NBAC, 2001). Although a parent's decision to enroll a child in a phase 1 oncology trial is difficult, many believe the decision may be justified provided that the alternatives of no further experimental treatment and palliative care are presented. FDA offers guidance to researchers and IRBs to assess the level of evidence needed to ensure that sufficient prospect for direct clinical benefit exists before enrolling children in phase 1 studies. These guidances include recommendations on when children might be included in first-in-human (FIH) expansion cohorts, and when it is appropriate to include children and adolescents in adult oncology studies. The patient population included in these studies should be limited to patients with relapsed or refractory cancers for which no curative therapies are available. In

🔗 10-15

exceptional circumstances, nonclinical evidence of activity in tumor-derived cell lines or patient-derived xenografts may be sufficient to support initiating studies in children, but in general, preliminary activity should be established in adults prior to enrollment of children. FIH expansion cohorts should enroll adults prior to children; when early enrollment of children is considered, staged enrollment of adolescents prior to younger children is preferred to assess dosing and safety (FDA, 2018c, 2019a; King, 2000; Roth-Cline & Nelson, 2014; Wendler et al., 2019).

Approval by Federal Review Panel

Subpart D allows for the review and approval of research that is not otherwise approvable by an IRB provided that the research "presents a reasonable opportunity to further the understanding, prevention, or alleviation of a serious problem affecting the health or welfare of children" and "will be conducted in accordance with sound ethical principles" [45 CFR 46.407; 21 CFR 50.54]. An IRB may refer the protocol to the Secretary of DHHS and/or the FDA Commissioner who, after consultation with a panel of experts and after opportunity for public review and comment, may issue an approval for the research. Clearly, such a review panel can only discharge this responsibility if the referring IRB (1) has already determined that the research fails to qualify under 45 CFR 46. 404-406 and/or 21 CFR 50.51-53; (2) has determined that the research is potentially approvable under 45 CFR 46.407 and/or 21 CFR 50.54; and (3) has provided the underlying documentation and rationale for both determinations. Since 2001, a number of protocols have been reviewed under this mechanism (DHHS, 2008). In 2003, a permanent Pediatric Ethics Subcommittee of the FDA Pediatric Advisory Committee was established to review protocols referred under 21 CFR 50.54 and that involve both FDA-regulated products under 21 CFR 50.54 and research involving children as subjects that is conducted or supported by the DHHS as specified in 45 CFR 46.407 (FDA, 2003).

Federal Ethics Panel Review

In 2017, FDA conducted the first review under 21 CFR 50.54 for a commercially sponsored pediatric protocol. The IRB referral asked whether placement of a central venous catheter was acceptable for study-drug infusion (including for subjects receiving placebo) during the 96-week study period. Children in this study were having significant difficulty with peripheral venous access due to their disease. The review was completed within 10 weeks, highlighting that the 21 CFR 50.54 process can be completed in an efficient and timely manner. Transparency was promoted throughout the process, although some documents were redacted for public comment to protect commercial confidential information. Parent and patient community input were instrumental in contributing to the outcome (FDA, 2017a; Snyder et al., 2018; Snyder & Nelson, 2018).

Conclusion

This chapter reviews the existing pediatric research regulations under 45 CFR 46, subpart D, and 21 CFR 50, subpart D, and cites available guidance, publications, and resources to aid IRBs in the interpretation and implementation of these regulations. An IRB that reviews research involving children needs to be familiar with the special protections afforded pediatric research subjects by subpart D, needs to possess sufficient experience and expertise, and needs to be capable of ethical, scientific, and regulatory analysis of research trials from a pediatric perspective. Just as it is inappropriate for a researcher to conduct research involving children without sufficient pediatric expertise, an IRB that does not have the necessary knowledge and skill to analyze a pediatric research trial according to the "sound ethical principles" embodied in subpart D would not be in compliance with existing regulations.

References

Department of Health and Human Services (DHHS). (2008). *Children in research: Research proposals previously reviewed under 45 CFR 46.407.* wayback.archive-it.org/4657/20150930181816 //www.hhs.gov/ohrp/archive/children/

European Medicines Agency. (2018). *Reflection paper on the use of extrapolation in the development of medicines for paediatrics.* www.ema.europa.eu/en/documents/scientific-guideline/adopted -reflection-paper-use-extrapolation-development-medicines-paediatrics-revision-1_en.pdf

Food and Drug Administration (FDA). (2000). *Guidance for industry: E11 clinical investigation of medicinal products in the pediatric population (ICH).* www.fda.gov/regulatory-information /search-fda-guidance-documents/e11-clinical-investigation-medicinal-products-pediatric -population

Food and Drug Administration (FDA). (2001). *Guidance for industry: E10 choice of control group and related issues in clinical trials.* www.fda.gov/regulatory-information/search-fda-guidance -documents/e10-choice-control-group-and-related-issues-clinical-trials

Food and Drug Administration (FDA). (2003). *Charter of the Pediatric Advisory Committee to the Food and Drug Administration.* www.fda.gov/advisory-committees/pediatric-advisory-committee /charter-pediatric-advisory-committee-food-and-drug-administration

Food and Drug Administration (FDA). (2012). *Guidance for industry: Acute bacterial otitis media: developing drugs for treatment.* www.fda.gov/media/71197/download

Food and Drug Administration (FDA). (2013). Additional safeguards for children in clinical investigations of food and drug administration-regulated products. *Federal Register, 78*(38), 12937–12951.

Food and Drug Administration (FDA). (2014). *Guidance for industry: General clinical pharmacology considerations for pediatric studies for drugs and biological products.* www.fda.gov /regulatory-information/search-fda-guidance-documents/general-clinical-pharmacology -considerations-pediatric-studies-drugs-and-biological-products

Food and Drug Administration (FDA). (2015). *Pediatric procedural sedation. Minutes of the Pediatric Ethics Subcommittee of the Pediatric Ethics Advisory Committee.* www.fda.gov/downloads/Advisory ryCommittees/CommitteesMeetingMaterials/PediatricAdvisoryCommittee/UCM510177.pdf

Food and Drug Administration (FDA). (2017a). *FDA Determination Memo, Pediatric Advisory Committee and the Pediatric Ethics Subcommittee, May 18, 2017.* www.fda.gov/media/105555 /download

Food and Drug Administration (FDA). (2017b). *Guidance for sponsors, investigators, and institutional review boards: IRB waiver or alteration of informed consent for clinical investigations involving no more than minimal risk to human subjects.* www.fda.gov/media/106587/download

Food and Drug Administration (FDA). (2018a). *Guidance for industry: Adaptive designs for clinical trials of drugs and biologics.* www.fda.gov/downloads/drugs/guidances/ucm201790.pdf

Food and Drug Administration (FDA). (2018b). *Guidance for industry: E11 (R1) addendum: Clinical investigation of medicinal products in the pediatric population.* www.fda.gov/regulatory-information /search-fda-guidance-documents/e11r1-addendum-clinical-investigation-medicinal-products -pediatric-population

Food and Drug Administration (FDA). (2018c). *Guidance for industry: Expansion cohorts: Use in first-in-human clinical trials to expedite development of oncology drugs and biologics.* www.fda .gov/media/115172/download

Food and Drug Administration (FDA). (2019a). *Cancer clinical trial eligibility criteria: Minimum age for pediatric patients.* www.fda.gov/regulatory-information/search-fda-guidance-documents /cancer-clinical-trial-eligibility-criteria-minimum-age-pediatric-patients

Food and Drug Administration (FDA). (2019b). *Guidance for industry: Considerations for the inclusion of adolescent patients in adult oncology clinical trials.* www.fda.gov/media/113499/download

Freedman, B. (1987). Equipoise and the ethics of clinical research. *New England Journal of Medicine, 317*(3), 141–145.

Hume, M., Lewis, L. L., & Nelson, R. M. (2017). Meeting the goal of concurrent adolescent and adult licensure of HIV prevention and treatment strategies. *Journal of Medical Ethics, 43*(12), 857–860.

Institute of Medicine. (2004). *Committee on clinical research involving children, ethical conduct of clinical research involving children.* National Academies Press.

King, N. M. (2000). Defining and describing benefit appropriately in clinical trials. *Journal of Law and Medical Ethics, 28*(4), 332–343.

National Bioethics Advisory Commission. (2001). *Ethical and policy issues in research involving human participants. Vol. I. Report and recommendations.* Bethesda, MD: Author.

National Commission for the Protection of Human Subjects of Biomedical and Behavioral Research. (1978). Research involving children: Report and recommendations. *Federal Register, 43*(9), 2083–2114.

National Commission for the Protection of Human Subjects of Biomedical and Behavioral Research. (1979). *The Belmont Report: Ethical principles and guidelines for the protection of human subjects in biomedical and behavioral research.* www.hhs.gov/ohrp/regulations-and-policy/belmont-report/index.html

Roth-Cline, M., & Nelson, R. (2014). The ethical principle of scientific necessity in pediatric research. *American Journal of Bioethics, 14*(12), 14–15.

Snyder, D., Lee, C., & Nelson, R. (2018). Invasive placebos, patient burdens and community advocacy: A federal ethics panel protocol review. In E. Kodish & R. Nelson (Eds.), *Ethics and research with children, a case-based approach.* Oxford University Press.

Snyder, D., & Nelson, R. (2018). The Food and Drug Administration's federal review of a pediatric muscular dystrophy protocol. *IRB, 40*(1), 18–20.

Wendler, D., Nelson, R. M., & Lantos, J. D. (2019). The potential benefits of research may justify certain research risks. *Pediatrics, 143*(3), e20181703.

World Medical Association. (2018). *Declaration of Helsinki - Ethical principles for medical research involving human subjects.* www.wma.net/policies-post/wma-declaration-of-helsinki-ethical-principles-for-medical-research-involving-human-subjects/

Adults with Decisional Impairment in Research

Amy Ben-Arieh

Lauren Hartsmith

Abstract

The codes and laws that govern human subject protections are built upon the concept of voluntary informed consent. Questions then arise regarding whether it is possible and appropriate to include individuals with impaired decision-making capacity in ethical research or, conversely, whether it can be ethical for the decisionally impaired to be categorically excluded. Although the relevant ethical considerations have been debated extensively, the legal requirements remain minimal. Few agreed-upon ethical frameworks exist to guide IRBs in how they should approach this topic. Although there have been many calls for further guidance, no federal department or agency has issued any. This chapter grapples with this tension by defining the salient features of decisional impairment, reviewing some of the risks and ethical challenges inherent in this research, presenting the modern history of thinking on the topic, reviewing the legal requirements and impact of the 2018 Common Rule, and providing pragmatic points to consider for IRBs.

What Is Decisional Impairment?

Decisional impairment is the diminished functional ability to make choices, which results from a physical, cognitive, or psychological condition (Presidential Commission for the Study of Bioethical Issues, 2015). This section will describe key features of decisional impairment, its implications for research participation, and considerations for assessment of capacity to consent.

Key Features

Decisional capacity refers to a person's level of ability related to tasks required to make free and informed choices. From the perspective of human research subject protections, the main implication of decisional impairment relates to whether a prospective subject is capable of providing informed consent. The

1-1

Section 6

first ethical principle articulated in the *Belmont Report* is Respect for Persons (National Commission, 1979). Respect for persons explicitly encompasses both the ideas that potential research subjects' autonomy must be acknowledged and that those with diminished autonomy are entitled to protection. One way these ideas are fulfilled is by requiring *informed consent* (by the subject or someone legally authorized to provide such consent on behalf of the subject) to participate. The *Belmont Report* indicates that an effective consent process must include information, comprehension, and voluntariness (National Commission, 1979). The Common Rule codifies this by including general requirements, basic elements, and appropriate additional elements of informed consent **[45 CFR 46.116]**.

Although there is not a single, agreed-upon, comprehensive list of abilities that make up a person's ability to consent, at a minimum, a person should be able to do the following (Derenzo et al., 2019; New York State Task Force on Life and the Law, 2014; Presidential Commission, 2015):

- Absorb and understand provided information
- Comprehend its significance
- Apply that information to make a reasoned choice
- Ultimately, express that choice.

An adult with decisional impairment may have challenges with regard to any aspect of these skills, and impairments can range from mild to severe. Moreover, depending on the nature of someone's condition, capacity to consent may not be static. Because impairments may be permanent, temporary, intermittent, or progressive, capacity to consent can fluctuate over the course of a study (New York State Task Force, 2014; Presidential Commission, 2015).

NATIONAL BIOETHICS ADVISORY COMMISSION DEFINITION

As detailed in NBAC's 1998 report *Research Involving Persons with Mental Disorders That May Affect Decisionmaking Capacity*, "there are at least four types of limitations in decision-making ability [that] should be considered when planning and conducting research with [adults with impaired decision-making capacity]. First, some individuals may have fluctuating capacity, what is often called waxing and waning ability to make decisions, as in schizophrenia, bipolar disorders, depressive disorders, and some dementias. Second, decision-making deficits can be predicted in some individuals due to the course of their disease or the nature of their treatment. Although these individuals may be decisionally capable in the early stages of the disease progression, such as in Alzheimer's disease, they have prospective incapacity. Third, most persons with limited capacity are in some way still able to object or assent to research, as in the case of more advanced Alzheimer's disease. Fourth, persons who have permanently lost the ability to make nearly any decision that involves any significant degree of reflection are decisionally incapable, as in the later stages of Alzheimer's disease and profound dementia" (NBAC, 1998).

National Bioethics Advisory Commission (NBAC). (1998). *Research involving persons with mental disorders that may affect decisionmaking capacity.* https://bioethicsarchive.georgetown.edu/nbac/capacity/TOC.htm

Risk of Harm

A primary concern related to inclusion of individuals with impaired decision-making capacity in research relates to voluntariness. Due to the limited autonomy of those unable to make or express choices for themselves, there is concern that coercion or undue influence may taint the informed consent process. Additionally, there is concern that these individuals may not fully understand the information conveyed during the informed consent process.

Coercion in the context of research occurs when a threat is used in order to get a prospective subject to "agree" to participate. Undue influence occurs when an inappropriate or disproportionate incentive is offered (National Commission, 1979). This focus is the ethical legacy of studies that enrolled and abused vulnerable institutionalized persons who were unable, or otherwise not given the opportunity, to provide informed consent (Presidential Commission, 2015). Decisionally impaired subjects were enrolled to some degree for convenience—their availability, constrained mobility, and inability to refuse created opportunities for exploitation (Beecher, 1966; New York State Task Force, 2014). In other words, they were not capable of exercising free choice—a hallmark of <u>informed consent</u> (World Medical Association, 2018).

⊘ 6-1

In addition, prospective subjects with impaired decision-making capacity may not be able to absorb the salient facts of the study to make a reasoned choice regarding participation. This puts into question both the "informed" and "understanding" nature of the informed consent process. Moreover, individuals who are not in a position to fully appreciate risks or make or express an informed choice about their participation may be particularly vulnerable to other risks of the study. They may not be able to express that they are in pain, uncomfortable, or otherwise wish to stop (National Institutes of Health, 2009).

Beyond the potential for ineffective consent, the very fact of being deemed unable to provide consent for oneself may be a harm (New York State Task Force, 2014). For example, if a qualified clinician determines that someone is unable to make independent decisions, this determination could be used more broadly to determine that the individual is unable to make other healthcare choices or as evidence that they are otherwise unable to manage their affairs. These types of determinations can also impact a caregiver's perception of that person's abilities.

History

Various <u>ethical codes</u> and advisory committees have addressed the inclusion of adults with decisional impairments in research over the past 75 years. Although not legal requirements, these proposed frameworks can guide IRBs, institutions, and researchers as they develop policies and procedures for determining appropriate additional protections for this population. Thinking on this topic has evolved considerably over time.

⊘ 1-1

Nuremburg Code (1947) and the Declaration of Helsinki (1964)

"[T]he author of a memorandum to the war crimes court, from which the Nuremburg Code was derived, had originally proposed that '[i]n the case of mentally ill patients, for the purpose of experiments concerning the nature and treatment of nervous and mental illness or related subjects, such consent of the next of kin or legal guardian is required; whenever the mental state of the patient permits ... his own consent should be obtained in addition'" (National Commission, 1978). This language was not, ultimately, incorporated into the Nuremburg Code. Fifteen years later, in June 1964, the first version of the

Declaration of Helsinki was published. This statement of ethical principles did include applicable provisions, stating:

> "3a. Clinical research on a human being cannot be undertaken without his free consent after he has been informed; if he is legally incompetent, the consent of the legal guardian should be procured.
>
> 3b. The subject of clinical research should be in such a mental, physical and legal state as to be able to exercise fully his power of choice" (Declaration of Helsinki, 1964 version, World Medical Association [2018]).

National Research Act (1974)

In 1932, the United States Public Health Service (USPHS) began one of the most poignant American examples of ethically questionable human research projects: the U.S. Public Health Service Syphilis Study at Tuskegee. Knowledge of the study became widespread in July 1972 when an Associated Press reporter wrote an exposé (Heller, 1972). The public discussion around this study and the subsequent investigation were the driving forces behind the 1974 National Research Act. There were other unethical projects that caused extensive public outrage around this time. In 1963, it came to light that "[r]esearchers injected cancer cells into [22] old and debilitated patients at a Jewish Chronic Disease Hospital in the New York borough of Brooklyn" (Stobbe, 2011). From 1963 to 1966, "a controversial medical study was conducted at the Willowbrook State School for children with mental retardation. The children were intentionally given hepatitis orally and by injection to see if they could then be cured with gamma globulin" (Stobbe, 2011). It was in this context in 1973 that Congress began debating what would ultimately become the National Research Act. This Act set forth broad requirements for a research ethics system for federally supported and conducted research and established the National Commission for the Protection of Human Subjects of Biomedical and Behavioral Research. Among other things, Congress charged this commission to assess and evaluate the requirements for informed consent to participate in biomedical and behavioral research by children, prisoners, and the institutionalized mentally infirm.

🔗 1-2

🔗 9-6 🔗 9-5

Report by the National Commission for the Protection of Human Subjects of Biomedical and Behavioral Research (1978) and the Subsequent Proposed Rule (1979)

The National Commission for the Protection of Human Subjects of Biomedical and Behavioral Research (National Commission) published its report, *Research Involving Those Institutionalized as Mentally Infirm,* in 1978. It made the following recommendations:

1. No prospective subject who is institutionalized as mentally infirm should be approached to participate in research unless a person responsible for the health care of the subject has determined that participation would not interfere with such care,

2. Persons who are institutionalized as mentally infirm and cannot give informed consent must not be involved in research unless it is relevant to their condition, and

3. No one should be involved in research over their objection unless participation may benefit the subject and is specifically authorized by a court of competent jurisdiction. (National Commission, 1978)

The National Commission also proposed that IRBs overseeing such research appoint a "consent auditor" to observe the consent process, assess the capacity of prospective subjects to consent, and evaluate whether a prospective subject agreed or objected to participating in the activity (National Commission, 1978). The consent auditor would determine whether a subject should be enrolled when a subject and legally authorized representative (LAR) disagreed about participation (DHHS, 2019). The National Commission recommended that research with no prospect of direct benefit to the institutionalized mentally disabled subject would need to be approved by the Secretary of the Department of Health, Education, and Welfare (DHEW, renamed the Department of Health and Human Services in 1979) after consultation with a specialized panel of experts.

DHEW published a Notice of Proposed Rulemaking in 1979 largely adopting the specific recommendations of the National Commission, proposing to establish a subpart E for Additional Protections Pertaining to Biomedical and Behavioral Research Involving as Subjects Individuals Institutionalized as Mentally Disabled. Ultimately, this NPRM was never adopted.

National Bioethics Advisory Commission (1998) and DHHS Response (2001)

In response to a series of 1993 articles in the *Albuquerque Tribune* alleging that Americans had been injected with plutonium during the Cold War, President Clinton created the Advisory Committee on Human Radiation Experiments (ACHRE). ACHRE was charged with investigating these human radiation experiments (ACHRE, 1995). As part of its work, ACHRE also reviewed a number of ionizing radiation research protocols approved and funded from 1990 to 1993. Members of ACHRE were concerned that adults with "questionable decision-making capacity" were included in these studies (NBAC, 1998).

In response to ACHRE's final report, President Clinton established the National Bioethics Advisory Commission (NBAC) to provide recommendations related to ACHRE's findings (Executive Order, 1995). NBAC issued its report, *Research Involving Persons with Mental Disorders That May Affect Decisionmaking Capacity,* in December 1998, recommending several regulatory changes in the Common Rule, or alternatively, the creation of a new subpart, to address the unique protections that may be needed for adults with impaired decision-making capacity (NBAC, 1998). NBAC reiterated many of the same recommendations and principles as the National Commission. Similar to the National Commission's report 19 years earlier, NBAC determined that as a general matter, research protocols involving more than minimal risk and no direct benefit to the decisionally impaired adult could not be approved by an IRB. NBAC indicated this general prohibition could be overcome in two circumstances: (1) if a separate committee on research involving the decisionally impaired approved the study or (2) if a decisionally impaired subject had created a prospective authorization when they still had capacity to consent. NBAC also proposed that DHHS work with states to educate the appropriate state legislative bodies about developing legislation permitting advance directives related to research. Finally, NBAC noted the difficulties in determining who could serve as an LAR in the research context and recommended that states expand the scope of who may serve as an LAR (NBAC, 1998).

In January 2001, DHHS responded to the NBAC recommendations, agreeing with most of the areas identified by NBAC as needing additional clarification, but noting it would be more appropriately issued via guidance. DHHS disagreed with the idea of limiting the inclusion of decisionally impaired adults and with the creation of a separate committee to approve otherwise unapprovable research. DHHS took the stance that it was ethically acceptable for an LAR to consent on behalf of a decisionally impaired individual to participate in a more than minimal risk study that did not involve direct benefit to the subject. However, DHHS indicated that it would seek public comment on the NBAC proposals. Finally, DHHS noted that for NBAC's recommendations related to state laws and who could serve as an LAR in research, DHHS did not have a role beyond making states aware of NBAC's recommendations (HHS Working Group, 2001).

DHHS Advisory Committees (2002 and 2009) and OHRP Request for Information (2008)

In 2002, the National Human Research Protections Advisory Committee (NHRPAC), a DHHS advisory committee established in 2000, issued its own recommendations to the Secretary of DHHS. NHRPAC largely endorsed the NBAC report and recommended that the process to approve otherwise unapprovable research involving adults with decisional impairments mirror the 45 CFR 46.407 process under subpart D (Additional Protections for Research Involving Children; NHRPAC, 2002).

9-6

NHRPAC was replaced by the Secretary's Advisory Committee on Human Research Protections (SACHRP) in 2003. In 2007, DHHS convened the SACHRP Subcommittee for the Inclusion of Individuals with Impaired Decision-Making in Research. OHRP also issued a request for information (RFI) in 2007 to solicit public comments on the NHRPAC recommendations and NBAC proposals (Federal Register, 2007). This RFI further sought comment on whether additional protections were needed for research involving adults with impaired decision-making capacity or whether any changes were needed in the Common Rule.

Public comments on the RFI suggested that expert opinions about additional protections for adults with impaired decisional capacity had changed. Rather than endorsing a new subpart, public comments indicated that the protections in the Common Rule, and the flexibility granted to IRBs to customize protections, were sufficient. However, comments confirmed that it was often unclear who, under the Common Rule, could serve as an LAR, and requested that OHRP modify this definition.

Ultimately, SACHRP approved a set of recommendations, *Recommendation Regarding Research Involving Individuals with Impaired Decision-Making* (DHHS, 2009). The SACHRP recommendations largely outlined different points that OHRP should consider and formally requested that OHRP issue guidance for IRBs. SACHRP did recommend revising the definition of LAR to clarify who could serve as an LAR (specifically, clarifying what was meant by "applicable law" in the definition of LAR contained in the pre-2018 Requirements). SACHRP also recommended that DHHS issue a new subpart to 45 CFR part 46, but specified that this subpart should specifically define a "hierarchy of individuals who may provide consent on behalf of individuals who lack consent capacity when an LAR for research is not defined in state or local law" (DHHS, 2009).

In 2015, the Presidential Commission for the Study of Bioethical Issues recommended that federal regulatory bodies (and state legislatures) should establish "clear requirements to identify who can serve as [LAR] for individuals with impaired consent capacity to support their responsible inclusion in research" (Presidential Commission, 2015).

Protections Required Under the 2018 Common Rule for Adults with Impaired Decision-Making Capacity

Update to the Definition of Legally Authorized Representative

The definition of legally authorized representative (LAR) was updated in the 2018 Common Rule to provide clarity on how an LAR may be determined in research that is subject to that rule. Specifically, **45 CFR 46.102(i)** states "[LAR] means an individual or judicial or other body authorized under applicable law to consent on behalf of a prospective subject to the subject's participation in the procedure(s) involved in the research. If there is no applicable law addressing this issue, legally authorized representative means an individual recognized by institutional policy as acceptable for providing consent in the non-research context on behalf of the prospective subject to the subject's participation in the procedure(s) involved in the research." The first sentence of this definition is the same in both the pre-2018 Requirements and the 2018 Common Rule. The second sentence of this definition is found only in the 2018 Common Rule. Note that as of July 2020, the Food and Drug Administration (FDA) definition of LAR in **21 CFR 50.3(l)** is consistent with the pre-2018 Requirements but not the 2018 Common Rule. In the future, FDA may harmonize with the 2018 Common Rule definition of LAR.

In implementing the second sentence of this revised definition, institutions should first analyze whether they are in a jurisdiction in which legal requirements exist for who can serve as a surrogate decision maker for the specific procedures involved in the research in either the research or nonresearch context (DHHS, 2019). Note that the relevant jurisdictional law is typically state law. If the institution is not in a jurisdiction where such laws exist, then the institution (or IRB) should evaluate the institutional policies that exist in the nonresearch context for surrogate consent. Institutions are not limited in how many policies may be created to address surrogate consent in the nonresearch context.

Modernization of Terminology

References to "mentally disabled" (found in the pre-2018 Requirements at **45 CFR 46.107(a)**, **111(a)(3)**, and **111(b)**) were changed in the 2018 Common Rule to "individuals with impaired decision-making capacity" **45 CFR 46.111(b)**. According to the 2018 Common Rule preamble, this was not intended as a substantive change but rather as an update in terminology (Federal Register, 2017, Preamble p. 7170).

Considerations for IRBs—Appropriate Safeguards to Protect Rights and Welfare

The 2018 Common Rule continues to require that when some or all subjects are likely to be vulnerable to coercion or undue influence, additional safeguards be included in the study to protect their rights and welfare **[45 CFR 46.111(b)]**. Although much of the guidance and policies referenced in the history described earlier address these matters and may be deemed appropriate additional protections by an IRB, there are no specific FDA or Common Rule requirements for the following:

- Assessments of a prospective subject's capacity to consent
- Only including adults with impaired decision-making capacity in research that provides direct benefit to them or specifically applicable to the condition causing decisional impairment
- Limiting inclusion of this population to minimal risk studies and studies that are slightly above minimal risk

The human subject protections regulations leave the determination about what constitutes appropriate additional safeguards up to individual IRBs and researchers. Institutions, researchers, and IRBs have the opportunity to tailor their approach to the community they serve and to the research subject. In the absence of clear, uniform guidelines regarding how to handle studies that include such subjects, each institution should systematically address the issue and develop a framework for review. This preparatory work will help avoid uncertainty, inappropriate inclusion or exclusion, and inconsistency.

GENERAL CONSIDERATIONS FOR IRBS AND INSTITUTIONS

As a preliminary matter, IRBs and institutions may want to take into account the following when considering the inclusion of adults with impaired decision-making capacity as research subjects:

- IRBs should not assume that a particular diagnosis means that a specific prospective subject does not have the ability to provide voluntary consent for a particular study. "It is important to recognize that in some situations [conditions leading to decisional impairments] may produce substantial impairment of capacity, while in other situations, they may not affect an individual's understanding of key informed consent elements" (NIH, 2009).
- The level of capacity needed to consent to a study will vary depending on the complexity of the study and its risk level.
- Incidental inclusion of adults with decisional impairments in a research activity that will not directly benefit said individual is permissible. For example, see chapter 5 of the NBAC (1998) report, *Moving Ahead in Research Involving Persons with Mental Disorders*, Recommendation 3: "NBAC is not suggesting that individuals with mental disorders should be precluded from participating in research unrelated to their mental disorder. These same individuals, if they are able to consent, would be permitted, as any person would, to choose to enter a study unrelated to their condition" (NBAC, 1998). In other words, adults with decisional impairments do not need to be *de facto* excluded from research activities that do not target the subject's specific diagnosis.
- Although obtaining informed consent from an LAR on behalf of an adult with impaired decision-making capacity is permissible, if a subject is able to provide consent, consent should be sought from the individual.
- For minimal risk studies and studies that offer the prospect of direct benefit to the decisionally impaired adult (regardless of the risk level), the use of an LAR to provide consent on behalf of the decisionally impaired adult is appropriate in circumstances when the decisionally impaired adult cannot provide legally effective consent for themselves (DHHS, 2019). However, whether or not it is appropriate for an LAR to provide consent on behalf of the decisionally impaired adult in more than minimal risk studies where there is no prospect of direct benefit to the enrolled subject requires more thought and consideration.

- Even if a subject is deemed to be unable to provide legally effective informed consent (and thus an LAR will be used), the subject should still be asked whether or not they would like to participate (to the extent the subject's capacity permits). The subject's agreement or objection to participate should be honored. If there is ever a compelling reason to include someone despite their objection, the specifics of the situation should be reviewed by the IRB.

IRB Membership

An institution should consider whether its IRB is well constituted to make decisions impacting the decisionally impaired (DHHS, 2009, 2019). Although silent on the specifics of how to determine whether inclusion of individuals with impaired decision-making capacity is acceptable for a particular study, the Common Rule does explicitly acknowledge decisional impairment as a characteristic creating vulnerability. Decisions about appropriate <u>composition of the</u> <u>IRB</u> can vary depending on the institution and the type of research conducted. If the IRB is reviewing studies for a memory care facility, having an Alzheimer's specialist on the IRB may be appropriate. If the studies routinely take place in an outpatient facility for people with intellectual disabilities, someone who frequently serves as a guardian *ad litem* for individuals who use such facilities may be suitable. If the research will take place in an intensive care unit (ICU) or in a palliative care context, perhaps an ICU doctor and a hospital chaplain may be appropriate. If the IRB reviews such studies only infrequently, it may choose to seek a consultant on an as-needed basis (DHHS, 2019). (Note that the Common Rule specifically authorizes the use of consultants **[45 CFR 46.107(e)]**. When developing a roster that reflects the expertise necessary to review and approve research, institutions should focus on finding the expertise and perspectives needed to foster subject-centered conversations during protocol reviews (DHHS, 2009).

🔗 3-1

Acceptability of Inclusion

As described previously, neither the FDA IRB regulations, the FDA informed consent regulations, nor the Common Rule require that an IRB must prospectively determine whether or not subjects without the capacity to consent can participate in a research study. In practice, many IRBs require researchers to describe in their IRB applications whether or not adults with impaired decision-making capacity will be included in the research activity and to justify such inclusion. This practice may, however, inadvertently discourage researchers from recruiting adults with decisional impairments who also have the non-related condition being studied and who could benefit from the research. For example, a researcher studying a drug for an untreatable cancer would need to justify to the IRB why the inclusion of adults with impaired decision-making capacity would be appropriate for this study. If that justification had not been explicitly made prior to initial approval, the researcher would have to amend the study or request an exception from the IRB in order to include these individuals as subjects. Rather than go through an amendment process, the researcher may discourage participation by decisionally impaired adults. This can be avoided, to an extent, by IRBs and institutions creating clear <u>policies</u> <u>and procedures</u> on when exclusion of adults with impaired decision-making capacity is acceptable, requirements (if any) for capacity assessment, and how to identify an LAR.

🔗 2-3

A common approach is for an IRB to set risk/benefit parameters within which it will routinely consider the inclusion of individuals with impaired decision-making capacity and then either require or consider a set of safeguards for each scenario. For example, consider the framework in the regulations used for <u>children</u>. Because the concern for children relates to perceived vulnerability, a sense of duty to protect, and the lack of capacity to provide consent, it has proven to be a useful template (although not an exact parallel) for how to standardize the decision-making process around the inclusion of those with decisional impairment. Having a standard approach facilitates consistency and predictability in this otherwise fact-heavy and situation-specific decision. For this reason, many ethics bodies (such as NBAC, SACHRP, and the New York State Task Force) have recommended, and institutions have adopted, comparable frameworks tailored for the decisionally impaired. IRBs can use these recommendations to develop policies related to the types of studies where incidental inclusion of this population may not be appropriate but otherwise may presume that incidental inclusion is acceptable.

🖉 9-6

🖉 6-4

EXAMPLE OF RISK/BENEFIT PARAMETERS FOR ACCEPTABILITY OF INCLUSION OF INDIVIDUALS WITH IMPAIRED DECISION-MAKING CAPACITY: THE NEW YORK STATE TASK FORCE RECOMMENDATIONS

The New York State Task Force on Life and the Law (2014) recommended the following hierarchy of acceptability of inclusion in research of individuals with impaired decision-making capacity. Other rubrics have taken other factors into account. For example, some require that the condition of interest impact the subject's decisional capacity itself (Cooper & McNair, 2018) or that this must be a consideration (DHHS, 2009); others make special mention of appropriateness of inclusion in studies where a <u>waiver of consent</u> is warranted (NBAC, 1998) or specifically require that the research could not be conducted on those able to consent (e.g., "[t]he objectives of the trial can not be met by means of a trial in subjects who can give informed consent personally") (International Council for Harmonisation, 2016).

Risk	Possible Benefit	Approval
Minimal risk	Direct benefit	■ If risks are reasonable in relation to the benefits
Minimal risk	No direct benefit	■ If risks are reasonable in relation to the benefits ■ If important to advance the scientific knowledge of a medical condition that affects the research population, *and* ■ If the risks are reasonable in relation to such importance
Minor increase over minimal risk	Direct benefit	■ If risks are reasonable in relation to the benefits ■ If the potential benefits are similar to those available in the standard clinical or treatment setting ■ If the risk/benefit ratio is favorable to subjects

Minor increase over minimal risk	No direct benefit	■ If the research is vitally important to further the understanding of a condition that affects the research population ■ If the risks are reasonable in relation to the research's "vital importance", *and* ■ If they require mandatory rigorous procedures and oversight for enrollment and monitoring of subjects through the use of safeguards (e.g., informed consent monitors)
More than a minor increase over minimal risk	Direct benefit	■ If the risks are reasonable in relation to the prospective benefits ■ If the potential benefits are similar to those available in the standard clinical or treatment setting ■ If the risk-benefit ratio is favorable to subjects, *and* ■ If they require mandatory rigorous procedures and oversight for enrollment and monitoring of subjects through the use of safeguards
More than a minor increase over minimal risk	No direct benefit*	■ Where the potential subjects have a research advance directive (RAD), *or* ■ In special situations with notification to the department of health and use of a special review panel.

Some ethical approaches suggest that this work is not approvable (Council of Europe, 1999).
Data from Council of Europe. (1999). *Recommendation No. R (99) 4 of the Committee of Ministers to Member States on principles concerning the legal protection of incapable adults.* https://search.coe.int/cm/Pages/result_details.aspx?ObjectID=09000016805e303c

Subject Selection, Study Purpose, and Study Design

When making the decision to approve the inclusion of adults with impaired decision-making capacity in a specific study, IRBs must ask whether decisionally impaired subjects are equitably selected or inappropriately targeted (Cooper & McNair, 2018). A review strategy should be adopted that, at minimum, prompts the IRB to consider the characteristics of the study population, the nature of the research, and the setting of the research. Both the researcher and IRB should consider whether a study population is likely to include individuals with decisional impairment, how that impairment may impact them in the research context, whether inclusion in the study is necessary and desirable, how the capacity to consent to participation will be established, and what the consent process should involve (DHHS, 2009). Once this has been assessed, it is easier to focus on the type(s) of decisional impairment(s) potential subjects are most likely to have and compare these to the complexity and risks of the research, in order to ultimately determine the sufficiency of the proposed safeguards (DHHS, 2009).

SACHRP has recommended IRBs consider the following when reviewing justification for inclusion of decisionally impaired subjects (DHHS, 2009):

- The extent to which the research aims to improve the conditions that are the cause of the incapacity or related circumstances that could impact this population's well-being in the future
- Whether the research could effectively be conducted with individuals who are less burdened (i.e., are able to consent)
- Whether there is any risk that the population is being targeted solely for convenience or cost concerns
- Whether there are benefits from participation
- Whether standard care options are "ineffective, unproven, or otherwise unsatisfactory"

The SACHRP recommendations additionally state "[w]hen individuals who lack consent capacity will be incidentally included in research because they are members of a larger group of prospective research participants . . . the IRB should give careful consideration to the anticipated risks and potential benefits of the research as they might specifically affect those who lack consent capacity" (DHHS, 2009).

Consent Process

Being able to make choices is central to a person's sense of agency and voluntary informed participation a defining characteristic of ethical research. The environment in which any research occurs is complex, a space of interwoven interests and goals. In this context, even a decision that seems to be the result of free will may actually be based on manipulation, misinformation, or misunderstanding. Depending upon a prospective subject's relationship or position relative to the researcher, paternalism or coercion may impact the prospective subject's ability to make an autonomous decision. Each of these issues is compounded when decisional impairment is introduced. Therefore, developing a thoughtful consent process review strategy is critical.

🔗 Section 6   IRBs should look at whether the <u>informed consent</u> process is optimally inclusive. It is important to ensure that consent forms are clear, straightforward, and simple. People of differing abilities may need more time, different media, or further explanations or to have concepts repeated—but with these accommodations, they may have the requisite capacity to consent. The principles of health literacy should be applied to all subject-facing study materials.

Once the IRB determines that subjects without the capacity to consent may be enrolled, decisions about how to best involve LARs in the consent process must be made. Although the 2018 Common Rule has clarified who may serve in this capacity, institutions and IRBs still have a role in determining how this will be implemented at their institution (DHHS, 2019). Institutions should

🔗 2-3   have clear published <u>policies and procedures</u> in place for how to identify, verify, and document who is an appropriate LAR for research activities. Research staff should be trained on how to thoughtfully approach an LAR in a way that respects the participant and the LAR (DHHS, 2009).

IRBs should also consider whether the consent process that a researcher proposes to use is appropriate given the inclusion of adults with impaired decision-making capacity. Developing a consent process that respects a person's autonomy is a cornerstone of ethical research and in this context may require the IRB and researcher to consider and discuss challenging circumstances of the research. Ultimately, the IRB is charged with deciding upon the appropriateness of related protective measures. Examples of such circumstances and related considerations include the following:

- If a subject's condition is likely to degenerate or fluctuate, an IRB may consider adding regular capacity reassessments and engagement with an LAR as a potential safeguard to protect the rights and welfare of a subject.
- The IRB should ask researchers if consent endures beyond capacity, that is, whether past consent will serve as evidence that consent continues or whether a new formal process involving an LAR must be initiated (Dalpé et al., 2019).
- When subjects initially have the capacity to consent, their wishes on the continued participation and identity of an LAR can be obtained in advance and taken into consideration.
- Relatedly, the IRB and researcher should decide what processes ought to be followed if a subject regains the ability to consent (DHHS, 2019). Considerations include whether the IRB will require that the enrolled subject reaffirm their consent to participate and whether they should be provided the opportunity to review the research-related interventions or interactions that occurred based on an LAR's consent. When LAR consent is required, it should be thought of like any other informed consent process—as a series of interactions and exchanges rather than a signature on a page. To ensure understanding and facilitate communication, researchers should have open and ongoing conversation with involved caregivers and the LAR (NBAC, 1998).

Assessment of Capacity to Consent

A strong <u>consent process</u> confirms subject autonomy, addresses vulnerabilities, ensures all relevant and required information is shared, and ensures the potential subject understands the study and can apply the information provided to their own situation. This may mean engaging in a process that assesses whether the prospective subject has the decisional capacity and legal competence to consent to research, or, alternatively, that there is an appropriate LAR able to provide consent. An assessment of the capacity to consent is the way in which a researcher collects information to determine whether a subject has the functional capacity to consent (Dalpé et al., 2019). As part of their role in ensuring risks to subjects are minimized, IRBs often provide guidance on the assessment process, but unless an IRB determines an assessment is necessary in every instance, it is up to the researcher and research team to identify when a capacity assessment is needed (Biros, 2018). Although a formal capacity assessment can be a useful tool that researchers

---

HOW LARS MAKE THE DECISION: THE SUBSTITUTED JUDGMENT VERSUS BEST INTEREST STANDARD

LARs are asked to make challenging choices on behalf of another. How they are expected to make that choice may change depending upon the circumstances. The appropriate decision is most clear when a decisionally impaired subject has expressed clear wishes regarding their participation in research in an advance directive or is capable of clearly expressing their desires despite their impairment; however, this is often not the case. So, how should an LAR proceed?

Substituted judgment. In this approach, the LAR draws upon their knowledge of the subject—their values, choices, and beliefs—to try to make the decision.

Best interest. This approach requires that the decision be based upon what a reasonable person would choose after a thoughtful consideration of the available options, benefits, and risks.

Many states have laws that address what standard may be used by a proxy, and institutions and IRBs should ensure their policies comply.

🔗 Section 6

can use to promote inclusion of decisionally impaired adults in research, it is not required by the regulations.

Coming to a decision regarding whether someone has the ability to provide informed consent can be a challenge. It requires an evaluation not just of information retention but of all the skills required to consent in the research context (Biros, 2018). A prospective subject's decision-making capacity can be highly context and task specific and highly dependent on a specific research context (Dalpé et al., 2019). A person who has sufficient decisional capacity to make day-to-day choices about their diet and exercise does not necessarily have the decisional capacity to absorb and act on the implications of cancer trial participation (DHHS, 2009). A diagnosis or legal determination alone is insufficient to identify individuals who lack the capacity to consent, and the level of capacity necessary for an individual to make the participation decision increases with the risk and complexity of the study. Due to the highly variable nature of decisional impairment, study populations, and studies themselves, the capacity assessment must be carefully tailored (DHHS, 2009).

Researchers and IRBs should be intentional about the design and review of consent capacity assessment strategies. The first decision is generally what happens when a prospective subject does not have the capacity to consent: Will they be excluded from participation or included if an appropriate LAR is available? Once this is determined, the details of the assessment process itself can be evaluated. When deciding upon or designing an assessment, researchers should consider the likelihood of decisional impairment in the proposed study population. If it is low, a general assessment for all prospective subjects may not be necessary or appropriate. Even if a particular subject population is unlikely to include people who are decisionally impaired, either the study itself or the institution should have procedures in place for evaluating those who demonstrate a level of decisional impairment that brings consent capacity into question (New York State Task Force, 2014). When encounters are unanticipated, this initial assessment can be fairly informal (DHHS, 2009). If the likelihood of encountering decisionally impaired subjects is high, especially if impairment will increase over time or episodically, the strategies employed should specifically address continuing consent how fluctuations in capacity will be handled (DHHS, 2009).

Another important consideration is who will be performing the assessment. Does this person have a conflicting interest? For example, if an assessor is under extreme pressure to meet recruitment goals or is trying to get data from a very hard to reach subject population, their desire to enroll a specific subject has the potential to cloud their impressions. A possible alternative to consider is whether someone who is otherwise unaffiliated with the research ought to perform capacity assessment (New York State Task Force, 2014). The IRB should determine whether the assessment plan the researcher has outlined guards sufficiently against such conflicts and can mandate alternative approaches or additional protections.

As the study risk or anticipated level of decisional impairment increases, so, too, should the thoroughness of the assessment process. Are there any standardized tools or other objective measures that could enhance the assessment methodology? Although there are no perfect tools that map precisely with consent capacity, a variety of instruments are available to augment interviews (e.g., Mini-Mental State Examination, MacArthur Competence Assessment Tool), and other more subjective strategies may be incorporated in order to introduce a level of consistency and objectivity to the consent capacity assessment process (DHHS, 2009). IRBs may develop familiarity with certain commonly used measures, and researchers and expert reviewers may be able to suggest specific standard assessments for a particular patient population. Conversely, a cognitive test on its own should not be a stand-in for an expert's careful judgment (Association for the Accreditation of Human Research Protection Programs, n.d.).

Ultimately, even if an individual is determined not to have the capacity to consent, to the extent possible, they should be included in the consent process. This can include the following:

- Giving subjects the option to agree on who should serve as their LAR, with the option of rejecting any assignment
- Seeking affirmative assent and respecting dissent, with care taken to understand the many ways that these wishes can be expressed (verbal, behavioral, and emotional)
- Providing and communicating study information in such a way that they can understand to the best of their ability (New York State Task Force, 2014)

The goal of these strategies is to preserve the autonomy and self-determination of subjects to the greatest possible extent.

Additional Considerations: Other Laws That May Apply

Other authorities may impact if and how decisionally impaired individuals are included in research. There are standards that may apply depending on the funding or type of trial. For example, since 1972, research funded or supported by the <u>Department of Defense</u> may only occur when (1) the informed consent of the subject is obtained in advance; or (2) in the case of research intended to be beneficial to the subject, the informed consent of the subject or a legal representative of the subject is obtained in advance [10 U.S.C. 980]. Some state laws may be implicated by the nature of the subject population, location of the research, or type of research, as may be federal laws and regulations, such as the Disability and Rehabilitation Research Projects and Centers Program, U.S. Department of Education [34 CFR 350.4], and Americans with Disabilities Act, 42 U.S.C. 126. Institutions should develop procedures to ensure that they appropriately identify and enforce applicable requirements.

✎ 11-8

Conclusion

Both appropriately including and protecting decisionally impaired adults in human subjects research remains an ongoing challenge for the research community. Participation of this population presents a unique tension in an ethical space that prizes autonomy and voluntariness. The principle of justice makes it clear that the benefits and burdens of research ought to be equitably shared. To be categorically excluded from research means to be unrepresented in the data that ultimately informs society on how people behave, how to treat disease, and how the world works. Although there are very few regulatory requirements addressing when and how adults with impaired decision-making capacity can be included in human subjects research, historic reports and recommendations can inform how IRBs make these decisions.

References

Advisory Committee on Human Radiation Experiments (ACHRE). (1995). *Final report.* https://bioethicsarchive.georgetown.edu/achre/final/

Association for the Accreditation of Human Research Protection Programs. (n.d.). *Tip sheet 26: Reviewing research involving adult participants with diminished functional capacity to consent.* https://admin.aahrpp.org/Website%20Documents/Tip_Sheet_26_Reviewing_Research_Involving_Adult_Participants_with_Diminished_Functional_Abilities.pdf

Beecher, H. K. (1966). Ethics and clinical research. *New England Journal of Medicine, 274*(24), 1354–1360.

Biros, M. (2018). Capacity, vulnerability, and informed consent for research. *Journal of Law, Medicine & Ethics, 46*(1), 72–78.

Cooper, J., & McNair, L. (2018). A practical approach to including adults unable to consent in research. *Journal of Empirical Research on Human Research Ethics, 13*(2), 185–186.

Council of Europe. (1999). *Recommendation No. R (99) 4 of the Committee of Ministers to Member States on principles concerning the legal protection of incapable adults.* https://search.coe.int/cm/Pages/result_details.aspx?ObjectID=09000016805e303c

Dalpé, G., Thorogood, A., & Knoppers, B. M. (2019). A tale of two capacities: Including children and decisionally vulnerable adults in biomedical research. *Frontiers in Genetics, 10,* 289.

Department of Health and Human Services (DHHS). (2009). *Secretary's Advisory Committee on Human Research Protections. Attachment: Recommendations regarding research involving individuals with impaired decision-making.* www.hhs.gov/ohrp/sachrp-committee/recommendations/2009-july-15-letter-attachment/index.html

Department of Health and Human Services (DHHS). (2019). *Office for Human Research Protections. Informed consent FAQs.* www.hhs.gov/ohrp/regulations-and-policy/guidance/faq/informed-consent/index.html

Derenzo, E. G., Moss, J., & Singer, E. A. (2019). Implications of the Revised Common Rule for human participant research. *Chest, 155*(2), 272–278.

Executive Order 12975. (1995). *Protection of human research subjects and creation of National Bioethics Advisory Commission, 60 FR 52063.* www.govinfo.gov/content/pkg/FR-1995-10-05/pdf/95-24921.pdf

Federal Register. (2007). Vol. 72, No. 171. *Department of Health and Human Services. Request for information and comments on research that involves adult individuals with impaired decision-making capacity.* www.govinfo.gov/content/pkg/FR-2007-09-05/pdf/E7-17490.pdf

Federal Register. (2017). Vol. 82, No. 12. 45 CFR 46 and Preamble. www.govinfo.gov/content/pkg/FR-2017-01-19/pdf/2017-01058.pdf

Heller, J. (1972, July 26). Syphilis victims in U.S. study went untreated for 40 years. *New York Times.* www.nytimes.com/1972/07/26/archives/syphilis-victims-in-us-study-went-untreated-for-40-years-syphilis.html

HHS Working Group on the NBAC Report. (2001). *Analysis and proposed actions regarding the NBAC report: Research involving persons with mental disorders that may affect decisionmaking capacity.* https://aspe.hhs.gov/system/files/pdf/72821/nbac.pdf

International Council for Harmonisation of Technical Requirements for Pharmaceuticals for Human Use. (2016). *Integrated addendum to ICH E6(R1): Guideline for good clinical practice E6(R2).* https://database.ich.org/sites/default/files/E6_R2_Addendum.pdf

National Bioethics Advisory Commission (NBAC). (1998). *Research involving persons with mental disorders that may affect decisionmaking capacity.* https://bioethicsarchive.georgetown.edu/nbac/capacity/TOC.htm

National Commission for the Protection of Human Subjects of Biomedical and Behavioral Research. (1978). *Research involving those institutionalized as mentally infirm.* https://repository.library.georgetown.edu/bitstream/handle/10822/778715/ohrp_research_mentally_infirm_1978.pdf?sequence=1&isAllowed=y

National Commission for the Protection of Human Subjects of Biomedical and Behavioral Research. (1979). *The Belmont Report: Ethical principles and guidelines for the protection of human subjects in biomedical and behavioral research.* www.hhs.gov/ohrp/regulations-and-policy/belmont-report/index.html

National Human Research Protections Advisory Committee (NHRPAC). (2002). *Report from NHRPAC on informed consent and the decisionally impaired.* http://wayback.archive-it.org/4657/20150930183649, www.hhs.gov/ohrp/archive/nhrpac/documents/nhrpac10.pdf

National Institutes of Health. (2009). *Research involving individuals with questionable capacity to consent: Points to consider.* https://grants.nih.gov/policy/questionablecapacity.htm

New York State Task Force on Life and the Law. (2014). *Report and recommendations for research with human subjects who lack consent capacity.* www.health.ny.gov/regulations/task_force/docs /report_human_subjects_research.pdf

Presidential Commission for the Study of Bioethical Issues. (2015). *Gray matters: Topics at the intersection of neuroscience, ethics, and society* (Vol. 2). https://bioethicsarchive.georgetown.edu /pcsbi/sites/default/files/GrayMatter_V2_508.pdf

Stobbe, M. (2011, February 27). AP IMPACT: Past medical testing on humans revealed. *Washington Post.* www.washingtonpost.com/wp-dyn/content/article/2011/02/27/AR2011022700988_pf.html

World Medical Association. (2018). *Declaration of Helsinki – Ethical principles for medical research involving human subjects.* www.wma.net/policies-post/wma-declaration-of-helsinki-ethical -principles-for-medical-research-involving-human-subjects/

Medical Vulnerability

Jill Beck
Meaghann Weaver

Abstract

Research involving critically ill or terminally ill subjects presents unique ethical concerns. Subjects may have limitations in their ability to give informed consent or may be at risk for exploitation due to communicative, institutional, deferential, medical, and social vulnerabilities. The use of proxy consent, although potentially protecting subjects, raises additional concerns, including how to decide who needs a proxy, and on what basis a proxy should decide. Additional safeguards for critically ill or terminally ill subjects have been proposed and include reporting on benefit-burden scales for palliative research participation. This chapter discusses these and other issues relevant to conducting and overseeing research with individuals who are medically vulnerable.

Introduction

The concept of medical vulnerability was first noted in the National Commission's _Belmont Report_ in 1979 (National Commission, 1979; ten Have, 2015) and then expanded by Kipnis (2001) and the National Bioethics Advisory Commission. Vulnerability arises when potential research subjects have diminished ability to protect themselves due to difficulty providing voluntary, informed consent "arising from limitations in decision-making capacity . . . or situational circumstances . . . , or because they are especially at risk for exploitation (NBAC, 2001). Medical vulnerability can stem from health status, lack of capacity, and social pressures such as coercion or undue influence (Bracken-Roche et al., 2017).

⟋ 1-1

Vulnerability in the Critically Ill

Critically ill patients may have limitations in their decision-making capacity due to underlying illness, medications, medical interventions, and stress or fear. The logistics of obtaining informed consent in the setting of an urgent intervention may negatively impact thoughtful decisions. Acutely ill patients frequently undergo emergency treatments. Research on urgent interventions requires that subjects be enrolled within a short time frame and may adversely

⊘ Section 6

influence informed consent. <u>Informed consent</u> involves a thorough process of communication between a researcher and subject. The process includes an explanation of risks, benefits, and alternatives to the research that is understandable to the research subject or proxy. Effectively achieving all parts of informed consent can take a significant amount of time, which may be compromised in urgent situations.

In addition, potential subjects may be more susceptible to therapeutic misconception when critically ill. As illness becomes more severe, the scope of available treatments often narrows when standard therapies are unsuccessful, and subsequently research participation may become one of the limited available options. In these situations, subjects may not appreciate the difference between research and treatment, resulting in an unrealistic expectation of the likelihood of benefit and inaccurate understanding of the risk/benefit ratio. Finally, the power of physician endorsement of research may be exacerbated in the intensive care unit due to the close relationship between physician and patient and the patient's seeming reliance on the physician for maintaining life.

Vulnerability at End of Life

Since vulnerability occurs when at an increased risk of physical, psychological, or emotional harm, vulnerability is heightened at the end of life (Stienstra & Chochinov, 2012). This vulnerability can occur internally or due to external circumstances. Domains of vulnerability at the end of life include communicative, institutional, deferential, medical, and social (**Table 9.8-1**).

Informed Consent and Capacity

⊘ 9-7

The critically ill and dying may have <u>diminished capacity</u> to make complex decisions needed for research participation. Subjects facing the end of life may be experiencing symptom burdens such as fatigue and physical or existential pain that minimize their energy for participation. As a result, these patients rely more heavily on surrogate decision makers than many other research subjects. If a potential subject has inadequate capacity, proxy consent may be considered in order to enroll subjects in research.

Determining capacity is challenging. When developing a research design, researchers should outline a specific plan to assess the capacity of potential subjects. Assessments can consist of asking questions to evaluate a potential subject's understanding of the research involved, brief instruments (Jeste et al., 2007), or formal methods to assess capacity (Appelbaum, 2007). Clinical assessments by providers have been shown to have poor interrater reliability, whereas more structured tools require researcher training, and administration can be time consuming (Hester & Schonfeld, 2012). Regardless of the method used, care must be taken in determining capacity and whether a proxy is necessary. If capacity is underestimated, subjects can be deprived of autonomy, but if capacity is overestimated, subjects are made vulnerable to exploitation.

Selecting who can provide proxy consent depends on state laws and institutional policies. Many consider that the proxy's decision should be based first on substituted judgment, or what the patient would have wanted under the circumstances. If the potential subject's preferences are unknown, the proxy then decides based on what is best for the patient, or the best interest standard.

Any potential subject who is not fully capable of providing consent deserves the opportunity to assent, or agree to participate in the research. Dissent

Table 9.8-1 Domains of Vulnerability at the End of Life

Domain of Vulnerability*	Summary Explanation	Relevant to End-of-Life Research
Communicative vulnerability	Occurs when subjects have trouble communicating due to emotional and physical symptoms	■ Fatigue with need for energy preservation at active end of life ■ Exhaustion secondary to emotional distress or sadness ■ Preservation of time and energy for special moments together with loved ones rather than time with a researcher
Institutional vulnerability	Occurs when subjects are recruited or participate in research while under the authority of a clinician or institution; occurs when a subject's clothing, privacy, positioning, and timing of interview are at the preference of the hospital setting rather than subject's freedom of choice	■ Sensitive nature of research timed with end of life (adjusting to disease progression or relapse) ■ Perception of "medical failure" surrounding end of life
Deferential vulnerability	Occurs when subjects influenced by a particular ethnicity, economic status, or gender identity experience inequalities in ability to decline or ability to share openly and honestly	■ Setting of active end of life and dying influenced by economics and relational dynamics ■ Sense of isolation or aloneness surrounding end of life in hospital setting
Medical vulnerability	Occurs when subjects with serious medical conditions, particularly terminal conditions, grasp at participation or inclusion	■ Participation of actively dying patients out of perception of "not letting medical team down" or "remaining connected" to care team
Social vulnerability	Occurs in the context of historic injustice, current disadvantage, and risk of ongoing manipulation or misunderstanding	■ Fear of abandonment in setting of research refusal at end of life ■ Desperation to contribute to science through research at end of life ■ Altruism or sense of "duty to give back" heightened in end of life

*Domains adapted from Koffman, J., Morgan, M., Edmonds, P., Speck, P., & Higginson, I. J. (2009). Vulnerability in palliative care research: Findings from a qualitative study of black Caribbean and white British patients with advanced cancer. *Journal of Medical Ethics, 35*(7), 440–444.

should be respected. For subjects who regain decisional capacity after they were entered into a trial through proxy consent, researchers should obtain retrospective informed consent as a condition of continued participation.

A concern specific for subjects at end of life is whether dying subjects and their families are able, prior to participation, to accurately gauge the benefits and risks of their research participation to include the time, energy, and commitment involved in end-of-life research (Tomlinson et al., 2007). Insight into the potential burden of participation in research is especially relevant in end-of-life research, as subjects' and families' time is increasingly valuable due to the limited nature of time. If a dying study subject does not understand the quantified time or energy commitment required for research participation, the subject may invest an overabundance of time and energy, which are increasingly shrinking commodities.

Research subjects have also been considered vulnerable at the end of life because of their susceptibility to being coerced into research due to not wanting to disappoint their medical team or clinician influence (Hinds et al., 2007). Additionally, there may be cases when study subjects lack insight into the fact that they have a limited number of days of life left. Family members may not have been able to accept the impending death of the patient; that lack of insight may make the subject and family vulernable. (Tomlinson et al., 2007). If subjects are aware that their number of days is limited, they may prefer to spend time communicating with family and friends rather than with research teams. Even among subjects and families insightful about the end of life, there is potential for additional emotional burden associated with discussing their condition inclusive of illness, suffering, and losses (Dean & McClement, 2002).

Protections and Safeguards

In the United States, the Office for Human Research Protections and the Food and Drug Administration do not provide specific guidance on the protection of critically ill subjects and subjects at the end of life participating in research. The Common Rule **[45 CFR 46, subpart A]** directs IRBs to use safeguards to protect the "rights and welfare" of medically vulnerable research subjects but offers no details as to what constitutes adequate protection. As a result, there is significant variability among institutions regarding the need for and level of protection.

⊘ 9-6   One approach to additional protections is to utilize a framework similar to that used in the U.S. federal regulations for involvement of <u>children in research</u> **[45 CFR 46, subpart D]**. For research procedures in vulnerable populations that do not involve greater than minimal risk or involve more than minimal risk but have the prospect of direct benefit, a thoughtful approach should be taken to obtaining informed consent and determining capacity. Even when considering interventions that carry the prospect of direct benefit, the IRB must consider whether there is an upper limit of acceptable risk. For research involving no more than a minor increment above minimal risk that does not offer the prospect of direct benefit, additional "necessity" and "subject-condition" requirements (as described later) may be appropriate, due to the shift in the risk/benefit ratio (Silverman, 2011). The "necessity" requirement ensures that medically those subjects are enrolled when the desired scientific information can only be obtained by including those subjects. The "subject-condition" requirement stipulates the research involves a condition that affects the subject. For research involving greater than minimal risk that does not offer the prospect of direct benefit, the addition of an independent consent monitor may also be appropri-

⊘ 9-1   ate to minimize the risk of harm and exploitation. In addition, the <u>deferential vulnerability</u> of patients to the treating physician may influence subject participation, and therefore, physicians treating acutely ill patients should not also be responsible for obtaining informed consent from those patients.

Finally, component analysis should be utilized when assessing the risk/benefit relationship for all research and deserves special attention among subjects who are medically vulnerable. Procedures designed solely to gather data to answer a research question should be analyzed separately from procedures that have the potential to directly benefit the subject since they cannot be justified based on the prospect of direct benefit.

Inclusion of the Critically Ill in Research

Studying subjects during severe critical illness has the potential to lead to significant improvements in care. Given the complex problems and high risk of mortality for severely ill patients, clinicians and researchers are eager to improve treatments. Acutely ill patients represent a vulnerable population, however, and many interventions for critically ill patients have never been rigorously studied or proven. Critically ill patients represent an understudied group with significant opportunities for improvements in care; however, careful oversight is required to mitigate risk due to the considerable vulnerability of these subjects.

Palliative Care and End-of-Life Research

The purpose of palliative care is to provide whole-person care: physical, psychological, emotional, and spiritual support for patients when they need it most. The vulnerability of patients receiving palliative care is well recognized, but pursuing care improvement through research is important for advancing the science of palliative care to, ideally, improve patient outcomes.

Palliative and end-of-life care requires many specialized efforts and attention to accommodate patients who are inherently vulnerable due to heavy physiological and emotional symptomology (Murray et al., 2017). In order to continue providing appropriate palliative care and to improve end-of-life care efforts, research must be delicately conducted to identify the needs, wants, and experiences of subjects, even in settings of disease progression or worsened physiological outcomes (Weaver et al., 2019). Due to this subject population's inherent vulnerabilities, ethical considerations must be carefully weighed when pursuing research initiatives, particularly when discussing topics related to end of life (Koenig et al., 2003).

Some have argued that, because of the vulnerabilities of palliative populations, research should not be conducted in these groups, especially in subjects near the end of life (Lee & Kristjanson, 2003). Among the limited benefits-burdens research available, the benefits of palliative research outweigh the potential burdens for many subjects, according to self-report (Casarett et al., 2003; Emanuel et al., 2004; Fine & Peterson, 2002). Some scholars believe it is unethical to exclude palliative populations from research, since exclusion steals their right to the therapeutic and altruistic benefit that they may gain from such participation (Casarett, 1999). Although the inclusion of palliative populations among research initiatives remains controversial, evidence continues to accumulate demonstrating the importance of this work and the benefit that subjects may gain from research invitation and inclusion.

The benefits that have been described by palliative care research subjects include interpersonal and intrapersonal growth. Subjects have pointed to increased social interaction and companionship, feelings of altruism because of their contribution for future patients, and their ability to leave a legacy as benefits for themselves as well as others (Kristjanson et al., 1994; Pessin et al., 2008; Weaver et al., 2019). Research subjects have identified the opportunity to express their voice, the provocation of deeper conversation that they were unable to have with others in their life, the unloading of burden through introspection and conversation, the construction of deeper meanings, the exploration and sharing of meaningful memories, and the improved emotional stability and self-perceived dignity as personal benefits to their participation in research (Dallas et al., 2016; Fine & Peterson, 2002; Hinds et al., 2007; Jacobs et al., 2015; Scarvalone et al., 1996). Subjects perceived the benefits of research invitation and inclusion to outweigh the potential burdens experienced when participating in research and would willingly participate again if given the opportunity (Pessin et al., 2008). A summary of benefit and burden described by palliative care research subjects is presented in **Table 9.8-2**.

Table 9.8-2 Benefit-Burden Summary

Benefits	Burdens
Subject is able to express voice and personal experience	Risk of emotional and consequent physical burden due to the weight of the situation
Provokes deeper conversation for patients that they were unable to discuss elsewhere	Difficulty in discussing end of life
Altruistic service to the medical community and future patients	Participation requires time commitments and can be inconvenient
Therapeutic benefit of introspection and unloading of burden	Length of interview
Provokes construction of deeper meanings and memories for themselves	Structure of questionnaires
Increased companionship	Can be more easily coerced into research participation
Increased attention on the patient, making them feel honored	Participation occurs due to human dependency
Decreased anxiety and depression, increased relief	Invasion of privacy
Ability to leave a legacy	
Character growth personally, spiritually, and in other relationships	

Research efforts have appropriately shifted from discussion of whether the research should be done to discussion of improving the end-of-life research process in order to mitigate inconvenience and burden (Fine, 2003; Gysels et al., 2008; Hinds et al., 2007). Recommendations for minimizing research burden for palliative care research subjects include utilization of mixed-methods research protocols, in-depth evaluation by IRBs specific to the benefits and needs of the research methodologies, proper education on end-of-life care and vulnerabilities for research teams, and incorporation of large electronic data sets via healthcare record investigations to expand the sample size and foster data sharing, instead of over-approaching cohorts (Fine, 2003). Many of these efforts are already in place and should continue to evolve to meet the demands of this delicate but crucial research cohort.

Family Caregivers in Palliative Care Research

Family caregivers also experience vulnerability when their loved one develops life-limiting illnesses that result in palliative or end-of-life care services. The presence of this vulnerability requires research to be carefully evaluated to ensure it is ethically sound when including this population. Similar to patient studies, the benefits of parent and caregiver participation outweigh burdens of participation in research, according to self-report (Weaver et al., 2019; Wiener et al., 2015). Reported risks of family caregiver participation include invasion of privacy; social harm, such as feeling labeled or stigmatized in disclosing the challenges of caregiving; or psychological harm such as emotional fatigue or anxiety surrounding topic discussion. Reported benefits include feeling heard and a sense of contribution. The emotional burden among caregivers is well established, and thus participation in properly designed research studies serves a therapeutic benefit of shared narrative (Dyregrov, 2004; Michelson et al., 2006; Ullrich et al., 2017). Research with bereaved young adult siblings similarly revealed sibling perception of benefit in being included in bereavement research with appreciation for "being remembered" and "remembering the sibling" (Udo et al., 2019). Bereaved family caregivers expressed feelings of altruism for contributing to the medical community, as benefits from research participation (Hensler et al., 2013).

Conclusion

As discussed in Chapter 9-1, medical vulnerability includes persons who have serious health conditions, especially if there are no satisfactory standard treatment options. For these individuals it can be difficult to weigh the risks and potential benefits associated with the research, especially if their understanding is clouded by the misconception that the research is intended, primarily, to benefit them. Although representing different aspects of medical care and different ethical issues, the concept of medical vulnerability applies broadly to patients with acute life-threatening illness and those at the end of their lives. Recognition of the particular challenges associated with these situations and persons, and the ensuing implications for researchers interacting with them, is necessary to maximize autonomy, minimize risks, and provide appropriate protections.

References

Appelbaum, P. S. (2007). Clinical practice: Assessment of patients' competence to consent to treatment. *New England Jounal of Medicine, 357*(18), 1834–1840.

Bracken-Roche, D., Bell, E., Macdonald, M. E., & Racine, E. (2017). The concept of "vulnerability" in research ethics: An in-depth analysis of policies and guidelines. *Health Research Policy Systems, 15*(1), 8.

Casarett, D. (1999). Commentary: Looking beyond vulnerability: the ethics and science of research involving dying patients. *Journal of Pain Symptom Management, 18*(2), 144–145.

Casarett, D. J., Knebel, A., & Helmers, K. (2003). Ethical challenges of palliative care research. *Journal of Pain Symptom Management, 25*(4), S3–S5.

Dallas, R. H., Kimmel, A., Wilkins, M. L., Rana, S., Garcia, A., Cheng, Y. I., Wang, J., Lyon, M. E., & Adolescent Palliative Care Consortium. (2016). Acceptability of family-centered advanced care planning for adolescents with HIV. *Pediatrics, 138*(6), e20161854.

Dean, R. A., & McClement, S. E. (2002). Palliative care research: Methodological and ethical challenges. *International Journal of Palliative Nursing, 8*(8), 376–380.

Dyregrov, K. (2004). Bereaved parents' experience of research participation. *Social Science Medicine, 58*(2), 391–400.

Emanuel, E. J., Fairclough, D. L., Wolfe, P., & Emanuel, L. L. (2004). Talking with terminally ill patients and their caregivers about death, dying, and bereavement: Is it stressful? Is it helpful? *Archives of Internal Medicine, 164*(18), 1999–2004.

Fine, P. G. (2003). Maximizing benefits and minimizing risks in palliative care research that involves patients near the end of life. *Journal of Pain Symptom Management, 25*(4), S53–S62.

Fine, P. G., & Peterson, D. (2002). Caring about what dying patients care about caring. *Journal of Pain Symptom Management, 23*(4), 267–268.

Gysels, M., Shipman, C., & Higginson, I. J. (2008). Is the qualitative research interview an acceptable medium for research with palliative care patients and carers? *BMC Medical Ethics, 9*, 7.

Hensler, M. A., Katz, E. R., Wiener, L., Berkow, R., & Madan-Swain, A. (2013). Benefit finding in fathers of childhood cancer survivors: A retrospective pilot study. *Journal of Pediatric Oncology Nursing, 30*(3), 161–168.

Hester, D. M., & Schonfeld, T. (2012). *Guidance for healthcare ethics committees.* Cambridge University Press.

Hinds, P. S., Burghen, E. A., & Pritchard, M. (2007). Conducting end-of-life studies in pediatric oncology. *Western Journal of Nursing Research, 29*(4), 448–465.

Jacobs, S., Perez, J., Cheng, Y. I., Sill, A., Wang, J., & Lyon, M. E. (2015). Adolescent end of life preferences and congruence with their parents' preferences: Results of a survey of adolescents with cancer. *Pediatric Blood Cancer, 62*(4), 710–714.

Jeste, D. V., Palmer, B. W., Appelbaum, P. S., Golshan, S., Glorioso, D., Dunn, L. B., Kim, K., Meeks, T., & Kraemer, H. C. (2007). A new brief instrument for assessing decisional capacity for clinical research. *Archives of General Psychiatry, 64*(8), 966–974.

Kipnis, K. (2001). Vulnerability in research subjects: A bioethical taxonomy. In *Ethical and policy issues in research involving human research participants*, edited by the National Bioethics Advisory Commission, G1–G13. Bethesda, MD.

Koenig, B. A., Back, A. L., & Crawley, L. M. (2003). Qualitative methods in end-of-life research: recommendations to enhance the protection of human subjects. *Journal of Pain Symptom Management, 25*(4), S43–S52.

Koffman, J., Morgan, M., Edmonds, P., Speck, P., & Higginson, I. J. (2009). Vulnerability in palliative care research: Findings from a qualitative study of black Caribbean and white British patients with advanced cancer. *Journal of Medical Ethics, 35*(7), 440–444.

Kristjanson, L. J., Hanson, E. J., & Balneaves, L. (1994). Research in palliative care populations: Ethical issues. *Journal of Palliative Care, 10*(3), 10–15.

Lee, S., & Kristjanson, L. (2003). Human research ethics committees: Issues in palliative care research. *International Journal of Palliative Nursing, 9*(1), 13–18.

Michelson, K. N., Koogler, T. K., Skipton, K., Sullivan, C., & Frader, J. (2006). Parents' reactions to participating in interviews about end-of-life decision making. *Journal of Palliative Medicine, 9*(6), 1329–1338.

Murray, S. A., Kendall, M., Mitchell, G., Moine, S., Amblas-Novellas, J., & Boyd, K. (2017). Palliative care from diagnosis to death. *BMJ, 356*, j878.

National Bioethics Advisory Commission (NBAC). (2001). *Ethical and Policy Issues in Research Involving Human Participants. Report and Recommendations.* Bethesda, MD.

National Commission for the Protection of Human Subjects of Biomedical and Behavioral Research. (1979). *The Belmont Report: Ethical principles and guidelines for the protection of human subjects in biomedical and behavioral research.* www.hhs.gov/ohrp/regulations-and-policy/belmont-report/index.html

Pessin, H., Galietta, M., Nelson, C. J., Brescia, R., Rosenfeld, B., & Breitbart, W. (2008). Burden and benefit of psychosocial research at the end of life. *Journal of Palliative Medicine, 11*(4), 627–632.

Scarvalone, P. A., Cloitre, M., Spielman, L. A., Jacobsberg, L., Fishman, B., & Perry, S. W. (1996). Distress reduction during the structured clinical interview for DSM-III-R. *Psychiatry Research, 59*(3), 245–249.

Silverman, H. (2011). Protecting vulnerable research subjects in critical care trials: Enhancing the informed consent process and recommendations for safeguards. *Annals of Intensive Care, 1*(1), 8.

Stienstra, D., & Chochinov, H. M. (2012). Palliative care for vulnerable populations. *Palliative Support Care, 10*(1), 37–42.

ten Have, H. (2015). Respect for human vulnerability: The emergence of a new principle in bioethics. *Journal of Bioethical Inquiry, 12*(3), 395–408.

Tomlinson, D., Bartels, U., Hendershot, E., Constantin, J., Wrathall, G., & Sung, L. (2007). Challenges to participation in paediatric palliative care research: A review of the literature. *Palliative Medicine, 21*(5), 435–440.

Udo, C., Lovgren, M., Sveen, J., Bylund-Grenklo, T., Alvariza, A., & Kreicbergs, U. (2019). A nationwide study of young adults' perspectives on participation in bereavement research. *Journal of Palliative Medicine, 22*(10), 1271–1273.

Ullrich, A., Ascherfeld, L., Marx, G., Bokemeyer, C., Bergelt, C., & Oechsle, K. (2017). Quality of life, psychological burden, needs, and satisfaction during specialized inpatient palliative care in family caregivers of advanced cancer patients. *BMC Palliative Care, 16*(1), 31.

Weaver, M. S., Mooney-Doyle, K., Kelly, K. P., Montgomery, K., Newman, A. R., Fortney, C. A., Bell, C. J., Spruit, J. L., Kurtz Uveges, M., Wiener, L., Schmidt, C. M., Madrigal, V. N., & Hinds, P. S. (2019). The benefits and burdens of pediatric palliative care and end-of-life research: A systematic review. *Journal of Palliative Medicine, 22*(8), 915–926.

Wiener, L., Battles, H., Zadeh, S., & Pao, M. (2015). Is participating in psychological research a benefit, burden, or both for medically ill youth and their caregivers? *IRB, 37*(6), 1–8.

CHAPTER 9-9

Economic and Social Vulnerability

Faith E. Fletcher
John A. Guidry

Abstract

The purpose of this chapter is to discuss economic and social vulnerability within the research process. In this context, we define economic and social vulnerabilities and how they might impact research processes and the application of the *Belmont* principles in our work. We provide suggestions on how IRBs and researchers can take social and economic vulnerabilities into account to potentially mitigate their impact on subjects in research. We argue that bringing the voices of research subjects (in general and not only those who are "vulnerable") into the research process is the best available approach to address vulnerability in all phases of the research process. Models of community-engaged research have been developed over the past two decades that provide a variety of practices for integrating voices of research subjects into the design and implementation of research procedures.

Economic and Social Vulnerability

To be "vulnerable" is to be at risk of harm. In the research context, "<u>vulnerability</u>" involves any characteristic, individual or social, that (a) impairs an individual's ability to provide autonomous informed consent or (b) obscures an individual's ability to understand the risks to the individual of participating in a study; the benefits that may be gained by a study, whether to the subject or to a population more generally; or the relationship of the individual subject to the population that would benefit from the study's findings. The regulations explicitly recognize <u>pregnant women and neonates</u>, <u>prisoners</u>, and <u>children</u> as vulnerable populations with special needs in research, and Subparts B, C, and D lay out specific terms for the involvement of these populations in studies. Economic and social vulnerabilities are recognized in the regulation and supporting OHRP guidances, but interpreting and applying standards to mitigate economic and social risks are processes that each IRB must take up on its

🔗 9-1

🔗 9-4 🔗 9-5 🔗 9-6

own, given its specific context and surrounding community. In this chapter, we define economic and social vulnerabilities, provide some concrete (but not exhaustive) examples from research in the field, and recommend community engaged practices and the incorporation of qualitative, formative research into study design as ways to mitigate the risks that may come about with subjects who experience economic or social vulnerabilities.

Economic Vulnerability

Economic vulnerability in research participation is manifest in several ways—poverty, homelessness, low income, high debt, or limited access to health care due to a lack of medical insurance or low-cost policies with high deductibles and limits against long-term care or treatment. IRBs and human research protection programs (HRPPs) utilize the <u>consent</u> process and limitations on the size of incentive <u>payments</u> for participation as tools to mitigate the impact of economic vulnerability on study participation, either as a form of income or as a substitute for standard medical care. Though research and popular culture have identified some groups of individuals who utilize Phase 1 trials as a source of income (Abadie, 2010; Romm, 2015), participation in most studies (especially Phases 2 and 3, behavioral research, or evaluation) does not provide sufficient incentives to become a source of income. These incentives are frequently written into the consent forms as compensation for time and effort provided to the study.

Section 6
12-2

For persons with limited access to health care due to their lack of medical insurance or policies with few benefits, as well as those with severe illnesses that lack effective treatments (including many who are not economically vulnerable), clinical trials offer the hope of effective treatment or even a cure for illness. The tendency to approach study participation as a way to seek treatment or a cure is defined as the "therapeutic misconception," in which trial subjects conflate the purpose of research (i.e., to investigate a new therapy, device, or intervention) with the potential effect of research participation on them personally (i.e., their individualized care) (Swekoski & Barnbaum, 2013). As with individual risk and economic inducement, the consent process provides the most important way to address the therapeutic misconception. For this reason, it is standard practice in consent forms to assert that participating in the study will not necessarily result in a cure to one's condition, even if one experiences some improvement.

However, while consent forms can help to mitigate risk considerably, they are not by themselves a solution to the potential harms caused by economic vulnerability or the therapeutic misconception. The capacity of a research participant to understand consent forms is an important consideration in addressing economic and social vulnerabilities. Individuals with <u>cognitive impairments</u>, developmental disabilities, and other emotional disturbances are more likely to engage in the therapeutic misconception (Thong et al., 2016). Consent forms have grown long and complicated, and even individuals with higher levels of education may have trouble understanding what is at stake in a study. Thus, forms have been standardized around the presentation of risk, benefit, compensation, and cost to the participant, with AAHRPP <u>accreditation</u>, for example, providing concrete standards for communicating with subjects. It is now common practice to include a section on "benefits of research participation" that states that there is either "no benefit" or that one "may not benefit" from study enrollment, which is intended, among other things, to reduce the misconception that study participation will most likely lead to better health or a cure.

9-7

8-7

Social Vulnerability

Economic vulnerability may be addressed through processes such as informed consent and the limitation of payments to research subjects, which are solutions that may be implemented prior to research participation (consent forms) or during the research process (limitations on incentive payments or therapeutic potential of study participation). These methods are effective because economic vulnerability may be addressed as an individual attribute and resolved with intentional language and study processes. Social vulnerabilities, however, derive from group experience or community identity and present themselves both prior to and after the research process, particularly when findings might involve some damage to a community whether in material or reputational terms. Some well-known examples of shared experience or identities that could enhance risk due to research participation include immigration status, homelessness, indigenous community identities, LGBTQ+ identities, or stigmatized communities such as substance users (including those in recovery), people living with HIV, or individuals with mental health diagnoses.

⏣ 9-10

For example, research with undocumented immigrants on any number of topics could expose the subjects to legal and economic risk (unwanted disclosure of undocumented status, deportation, job loss, or eviction). Achkar and Macklin (2009) take up this possibility in their discussion of Achkar's earlier research on "the impact of place of birth and documentation status on the clinical presentation of pulmonary tuberculosis (TB) in patients" in New York City public hospitals (Achkar et al., 2008). The results showed that foreign-born, undocumented persons experienced significantly more aggravated symptoms and longer duration of disease, possibly related to barriers faced by undocumented persons to seeking care, leading to delayed diagnosis. In their discussion of the study's findings, Achkar and Macklin (2009) note that delayed diagnosis is a factor in elevated infection rates and therefore consider the following trade-off in publishing the findings of the 2008 study: Would the findings lead to greater services, outreach, and a reduction of barriers to seeking medical care—or could the public discussion of the findings reinforce stereotypes that immigrants are "unclean" or lend to metaphors of "infestation" that some promote in contemporary discourse on immigration? Such findings cannot be foreseen by IRBs, and OHRP Guidance (DHHS, 1993) places the consideration of harm due to long-term impact of findings beyond the purview of IRBs. In weighing the risk of stigmatization versus evidence-based support for reducing barriers to care for undocumented persons, Achkar and Macklin (2009) conclude that publishing scientific findings "should lead to an awareness that the reduction of barriers to health services for undocumented immigrants could help improve TB control in the community." Insofar as the science will provide a basis for better policy, their hope is not misplaced, and researchers generally recognize the importance of clarifying findings and correcting misinterpretations in public discourse when they occur.

Some communities are aware of their status as research subjects, both in terms of the importance of participating in clinical trials to address a common threat as well as the potential of findings to result in stigmatization. It is well documented that gay, bisexual, and other men who have sex with men (MSM) saw participation in clinical trials for HIV medications as a contribution to the difficult work of reducing the impact of HIV/AIDS in their communities and in the world more generally. At the same time, the findings of research, for example, that documents unprotected sex among MSM are routinely discussed in the queer press and blogosphere for their potential to cause harm and further HIV stigma within the LGBTQ community and reinforce HIV stigma, homophobia, and transphobia in the general population. For example, in 2013 a large Federally Qualified Health Center, that serves approximately 20,000 individuals in New York City and is well known for its HIV care and transgender medical services, published findings of a survey showing that MSM who use mobile apps for hook-up sex were more likely to have unprotected sex than those who did not use apps (Brathwaite, 2013). The survey's results were headlined in both the gay and mainstream press, but the community reaction was to push back against "Another study on our sex lives that discusses things in broad strokes" and could reinforce HIV and anti-gay stigma, including among MSM themselves (Brathwaite, 2013, reader comments). Researchers and community members following the controversy surrounding the survey's publication and other similar studies, like Achkar and Macklin (2009), tended to balance the potential policy impact of findings against the potential for miscommunication, misuse, or stigmatization in public discourse (Braithwaite, 2013). The research case for disseminating such findings, which were similarly found in other studies around the country, is that knowing that large numbers of MSM practice unprotected sex should (and ultimately did) support enhanced campaigns for the uptake of Pre-Exposure Prophylaxis (PrEP) instead of leading to greater stigma.

⊘ 9-10   For some communities, research has the potential to challenge community identity and culture in existential terms. Some of the most profound cases of this possibility are in the realm of research with <u>American Indian/Alaska Native</u> communities, as manifest in the controversy over the now well-known case of the Havasupai Navajo, whose 2004 lawsuit against Arizona State University resulted in a large payout and ban on genetic research in the tribe for over a decade (Garrison, 2013). The crux of the controversy was that blood samples collected from Havasupai members to address potential solutions to a disease common in the community were later used in another study on community genetics that (a) the original subjects had not consented to in the initial study and (b) resulted in findings about community origins that directly contradicted deeply held cultural beliefs about the community's history and traditions. Had community members and leaders known about the plan for a second study based on their samples, they would have wanted a greater voice in the study's implementation and interpretation. The case pitted local voice in the research against research prerogatives that may have been scientifically valid but required greater cultural sensitivity and humility to interpret.

The case that the benefits of research with persons experiencing social vulnerabilities outweigh the potential for group-based harm finds support among both researchers and the affected communities. As noted above, the LGBTQ+ community's support of and participation in HIV treatment trials helped to transform HIV from a death sentence into a manageable chronic condition that, with appropriate medical support, will have only a small effect on life expectancy. Flores et al. (2018) show that the growing development of research with and about transgender persons can lead to reduced stigma, though the burden remains on researchers to consider the implications of findings when designing their studies and recruiting participants for them. Other studies show how involving subjects directly in research can mitigate harm and increase the effectiveness of research on addressing health problems faced by vulnerable populations. In a 2014 study of peer-led HIV interventions with intravenous drug users (IDUs), Kostick and her colleagues found that "incorporating patient study participant feedback in the early stages" of research design to inform implementation was a "necessary step in creating supports in the intervention design that are specific and relevant to participants' experiences and concerns"

(Kostick et al., 2014). In this case, bringing participant vulnerabilities to the fore in design and addressing them resulted in beneficial impacts for subjects while also contributing to implementation science and the replicability of an effective intervention, which we will discuss further in the next section on community-engaged research.

Community-Engaged Research

Bringing research subjects and their experiences into the design and implementation of research is part of the larger practice of Community Engaged Research (CEnR). CEnR ranges from formalized Community-Based Participatory Research (CBPR; Wallerstein & Duran, 2010) processes to the implementation of formative research (e.g., focus groups or informant interviews; Bowleg, 2017) with the target population, to learn how they might experience the research process and to understand attitudes and beliefs about the research questions and their suppositions about the community (Clinical and Translational Science Awards Consortium, 2011). CEnR processes are not part of IRB activities or HRPP processes, but they are practices that IRB members can identify in study designs that recognize their subjects' experiences and attempt to mitigate potentially harmful impacts of economic and social vulnerabilities in research.

🔗 12-9

CEnR offers a useful framework to identify ethical pitfalls, classify various categories of vulnerability, and generate processes and procedures for resolving ethical problems as they arise (Fisher, 2014). Specifically, engaging communities in meaningful ways can address: "1) insensitivity to cultural concerns; 2) use of subjects from one community for research that primarily benefits individuals from other communities; 3) exploitation of vulnerable communities; and 4) in the worst of cases, outright abuse of research subjects" (Solomon, 2013). In addition to addressing potential exploitation of vulnerable communities through a CEnR approach, CEnR provides a constructive lens to understand, document, and address specific categories of vulnerability identified in the work of the National Bioethics Advisory Commission (NBAC) that alter the risk/benefit ratio of research to the detriment of subjects.

For CEnR processes to be most successful in anticipating and addressing economic or social vulnerabilities, they should be iterative and involve ongoing communication between researchers and subjects that takes into account the sociocultural context in which research is situated (Fletcher et al., 2018; Fletcher et al., 2019). Such a process redistributes power more evenly between researchers and the communities that ought to benefit from research, empowering individuals and communities to determine what constitutes acceptable research benefits and harms (Corbie-Smith et al., 2018). Qualitative Formative Research Design, Community Advisory Boards, and CBPR processes are approaches that bring the voices and experiences of subjects into the design and implementation of research and allow for risks due to social or economic vulnerabilities to be anticipated, discussed, and mitigated by mutual agreement on the appropriate safeguards to be observed during the implementation of research.

Conducting Qualitative Research to Highlight the Lived Experience of Marginalization

Community voices can be brought into the research process itself through formative research designs that use qualitative methods with target or focus populations to understand how research will be experienced by the community, how they will understand and communicate research in the community, and what elements of research design or implementation might incorporate community priorities in ways that contribute to the robustness of scientific design. Using formative qualitative research in this way not only acknowledges the importance of community concerns but also integrates these concerns into the research itself.

The earlier-referenced study of a peer-led HIV intervention with injection drug users by Kostick and her colleagues exemplifies this process and the complexities it can address (Kostick et al., 2014). The study subjects, as both peers and clients with substance use disorder diagnoses, including those in recovery, had much to lose by participating in the study, from fears of disclosure of embarrassing and illegal personal activities to the internalized burden of shame and stigma faced by substance users, MSM, and people with HIV. Like HIV, substance use is highly stigmatized in the broader society, and many persons with substance use concerns often avoid seeking help simply because of the shame they feel as substance users and the fear of being found out by family, friends, or colleagues. The intersectional combination of HIV stigma, substance use stigma, and for many the experience of discrimination as a racial or ethnic minority community member required the researchers to carefully consider how research participation could affect the subjects and the success of the research itself. By using focus groups early in the study, as well as other forms of communication between study subjects and researchers, the investigators created a study environment in which research objectives and research design reflected and addressed the concerns and vulnerabilities that subjects brought into the study.

For Spiers (2000), the complexities that surround defining vulnerability and vulnerable populations in research highlight the importance of qualitative inquiry to elicit an insider's perspective that can bring into relief the presence of factors related to economic and social vulnerabilities. Qualitative research provides a constructive lens for understanding the challenges, needs, and preferences of marginalized communities to inform the research process. Overall, the immersive approach of formative, qualitative research as a component of research design provides a structured and contextual basis for eliciting subject perspectives and recommendations to (1) inform research processes and procedures, (2) mitigate vulnerability and specific situations that give rise to vulnerability, and (3) demonstrate respect for members' values and preferences across the research continuum.

Convening Community Advisory Boards

Community advisory boards (CABs) offer another strategy to protect communities from research harms and maximize research benefits (Quinn, 2004). Funding agencies are increasingly underscoring the importance of community input to bolster research relevance and sustainability and in some cases even mandating the inclusion of community partners and perspectives into the research process through CAB implementation. According to Strauss and colleagues, CABs consist of "community members with a common identity, history, symbolism, language and culture" (Strauss et al., 2001). The various roles of CABs have been described as: "1) acting as a liaison between researchers and community; 2) representing community concerns and culture to researchers; 3) assisting in the development of study materials; 4) advocating for the rights of minority research study subjects; and 5) consulting with potential study subjects and providing recommendations about study enrollment"

(Strauss et al., 2001). Furthermore, CABs can be instrumental in shaping every aspect of the research process, including informing research questions, study design and implementation, and disseminating study results in ways that respect the preferences and values of community members.

While CABs purport to bring community voices into research, the implementation of a CAB is complicated and must be undertaken with great intentionality regarding who is represented by the CAB. It is important to recognize that CAB members might be *from* the impacted community but still fail to represent *ordinary community experience* (Lasker & Guidry, 2009). This is a particular concern when CAB members are, for example, minority scholars, community leaders, religious leaders, community-based organization stakeholders, and others who hold prominent positions in the community and may have the benefit of educational opportunities and career paths that create a palpable distance between the CAB members and ordinary community members (Fisher, 1997). Being the executive director of an organization representing the rights of homeless persons in a particular city, for example, does not necessarily result in the direct transmission of the experience of homelessness to a research team launching a study of interventions that enable individuals who are homeless to secure permanent housing.

To mitigate this concern, many research studies prioritize CABs comprising research study subjects or focus populations (and not simply leaders of movement organizations) to elicit local perspectives and recommendations on proposed study protocols and procedures, research priorities, and data quality improvement. For example, a well-established longitudinal study such as the Women's Interagency HIV Study (WIHS), a multisite prospective cohort study designed to investigate the progression of HIV in women, has relied on the input of a centralized CAB to inform all phases of the research process and promote long-term study engagement of research subjects. "The WIHS National Community Advisory Board (NCAB) is an advisory committee comprised of study subjects from each of the clinical sites, as well as a facilitator, Principal Investigator (PI), and Project Director (PD) representatives, and NIH sponsoring agency representatives" (WIHS, n.d.). Given the intersectional vulnerabilities and marginalization experienced by women living with HIV (i.e., HIV status, race, gender, poverty, and other categories; Rice et al., 2018), the NCAB seeks to provide diverse representation to: (1) shape research priorities and the national WIHS agenda; (2) develop and implement strategies to bolster recruitment and retention of subjects over time; (3) inform, educate, and support study subjects; and (4) facilitate translation of WIHS-related information to the community (WIHS, n.d.). Experienced research subjects, in particular, are an untapped resource for informing culturally responsive research ethics policies and procedures that represent the expressed needs and priorities of communities.

Community-Based Participatory Research (CBPR)

CBPR is the most enveloping research design that integrates subject voices not only through CABs or formative and qualitative research but also through the direct involvement of community members in designing studies and as members of the research team itself. In CBPR, researchers build formal structures for community participation that can endure for years. The Institute of Medicine has recognized CBPR as an essential competency for health professionals, stating that CBPR is "epidemiology enriched by contemporary social and behavioral science because it incorporates what we have learned about community processes and engagement, and the complex nature of interventions with epidemiology, in order to understand how the multiple determinants of health interact to influence health in a particular community" (Institute of Medicine, 2003).

The Family Listening Project (FLP) is an intervention that was developed in partnership between three tribal research teams (TRTs) and investigators from the University of New Mexico's Center for Participatory Research (Belone et al., 2020). The project was a 15-year process involving multiple NIH grants that resulted in the development of culturally centered curricula that provide cognitive-behavioral exercises to address health disparities and build intergenerational support for health equity in indigenous communities. The interventions account for local traditions, history, and experiences of exclusion from dominant society to address health inequities as community members experience them, providing solutions that resonate with individual and community experience. Mechanisms of participation included the TRTs; American Indian/Alaska Native researchers; multiple CABs in each community participating in the project; extensive qualitative research with American Indian/Alaska Native families; monthly meetings between the university team, the TRT, and CABs; and tribal participation in the development of dissemination and translational science to make the interventions available globally.

Conclusion

Economic and social vulnerabilities in research communities involve factors that are not addressed in detail by the regulations, OHRP, or other guidance from DHHS. Yet these vulnerabilities have impacts on individuals and communities that are well known and easy to document. Practices to address the concerns and mitigate risk engendered by economic and social vulnerability can be implemented at all phases of research—in the research design, in the writing and implementation of consent forms, in the design of research, and in research implementation and practice. Furthermore, researchers can intervene in dissemination of their findings in ways that help the public understand results and the policy implications that augur improved community and individual health and defend against using research as justification for stigma or discrimination. CEnR methods and research design provide important ways to mitigate the potential risks created by economic and social vulnerabilities. IRBs will not step outside their purview if, in the review of project protocols, they ask the researchers how the voices of vulnerable subjects are accounted for in the research design and implementation. Asking the investigators to clarify risk mitigation is an essential part of the IRB process, and it can be extended to address economic and social vulnerabilities.

References

Abadie, R. (2010). *The professional guinea pig: Big pharma and the risky world of human subjects.* Duke University Press.

Achkar JM, Sherpa T, Cohen HW, & Holzman RS. (2008). Differences in clinical presentation among persons with pulmonary tuberculosis: A comparison of documented and undocumented foreign-born versus US-born persons. Clin Infect Dis 47:1277–83.

Achkar JM, & Macklin R. (2009). Ethical Considerations about Reporting Research Results with Potential for Further Stigmatization of Undocumented Immigrants, Clinical Infectious Diseases, 48:1250–1253.

Belone L, Rae R, Hirchak KA, Cohoe-Belone B, Orosco A, Shendo K, & Wallerstein N. (2020). Dissemination of an American Indian Culturally Centered Community-Based Participatory Research Family Listening Program: Implications for Global Indigenous Well-Being. Genealogy, 4: 99.

Bowleg, L. (2017). Towards a critical health equity research stance: Why epistemology and methodology matter more than qualitative methods. *Health Education and Behavior, 44*, 677–684.

Brathwaite, L. F. (2013). *Study: Nearly 50% of gay men using hook-up apps engage in unprotected sex.* Queerty. www.queerty.com/study-50-percent-gay-men-using-hook-up-apps-have-unprotected-sex-20130122

Clinical and Translational Science Awards Consortium Community Engagement Key Function Committee Task Force. (2011). *Principles of community engagement* (2nd ed.). www.atsdr.cdc.gov/communityengagement/pdf/PCE_Report_508_FINAL.pdf

Corbie-Smith, G., Wynn, M., Richmond, A., Rennie, S., Green, M., Hoover, S. M., Watson-Hopper, S., & Nisbeth, K. S. (2018). Stakeholder-driven, consensus development methods to design an ethical framework and guidelines for engaged research. *PloS One, 13*, e0199451.

Department of Health and Human Services (DHHS). (1993). Institutional review board guidebook. http://wayback.archive-it.org/org-745/20150930181805, www.hhs.gov/ohrp/archive/irb/irb_guidebook.htm.

Fisher, C. B. (1997). A relational perspective on ethics-in-science decision-making for research with vulnerable populations. *IRB, 19*, 1–4.

Fisher, C. B. (2014). HIV prevention research ethics: An introduction to the special issue. *Journal of Empirical Research on Human Research Ethics, 9*, 1–5.

Fletcher, F. E., Fisher, C., Buchberg, M. K., Floyd, B., Hotton, A., Ehioba, A., & Donenberg, G. (2018). "Where did this [PrEP] come from?" African American mother/daughter perceptions related to adolescent preexposure prophylaxis (PrEP) utilization and clinical trial participation. *Journal of Empirical Research on Human Research Ethics, 13*, 173–184.

Fletcher, F. E., Rice, W. S., Ingram, L. A., & Fisher, C. B. (2019). Ethical challenges and lessons learned from qualitative research with low-income African American women living with HIV in the South. *Journal of Health Care for the Poor and Underserved, 30*(4S), 116–129.

Flores, A. R., Haider-Markel, D. P., Lewis, D. C., Miller, P. R., Tadlock, B. L., & Taylor, J. K. (2018). Transgender prejudice reduction and opinions on transgender rights: Results from a mediation analysis on experimental data. *Research and Politics, 5*, 1–7.

Garrison NA. Genomic Justice for Native Americans: Impact of the Havasupai Case on Genetic Research (2013). Sci Technol Human Values 38(2): 201–223.

Institute of Medicine. (2003). Who Will Keep the Public Healthy?: Educating Public Health Professionals for the 21st Century. Washington, DC: The National Academies Press.

Kostick, K. M., Weeks, M., & Mosher, H. (2014). Participant and staff experiences in a peer-delivered HIV intervention with injection drug users. *Journal of Empirical Research on Human Research Ethics, 9*(1): 6–18.

Lasker R & Guidry JA. (2009). *Engaging the Community in Decision Making.* Jefferson, NC: McFarland.

Quinn, S. C. (2004). Ethics in public health research: protecting human subjects: The role of community advisory boards. *American Journal of Public Health, 94*, 918–922.

Rice, W. S., Logie, C. H., Nápoles, T. M., Walcott, M. W., Batchelder, A. W., Kempf, M., Wingood, G. M., Konkle-Parker, D. J., Turan, B., Wilson, T. E., Johnson, M. O., Weiser, S. D., & Turan, J. M. (2018). Perceptions of intersectional stigma among diverse women living with HIV in the United States. *Social Science and Medicine, 208*, 9–17.

Romm C. (2015). "The Life of a Professional Guinea Pig," The Atlantic, 23 September 2015. www.theatlantic.com/science/archive/2015/09/life-of-a-professional-guinea-pig/406018/

Solomon, S. R. (2013). Protecting and respecting the vulnerable: Existing regulations or further protections? *Theoretical Medicine and Bioethics, 34*, 17–28.

Spiers, J. (2000). New perspectives on vulnerability using emic and etic approaches. *Journal of Advanced Nursing, 31*, 715–721.

Strauss, R. P., Sengupta, S., Quinn, S. C., Goeppinger, J., Spaulding, C., Kegeles, S. M., & Millett, G. (2001). The role of community advisory boards: Involving communities in the informed consent process. *American Journal of Public Health, 91*, 1938–1943.

Swekoski D, Barnbaum D. (2013). The gambler's fallacy, the therapeutic misconception, and unrealistic optimism. IRB. 35(2):1–6.

Thong, I. S., Foo, M. Y., Sum, M. Y., Capps, B., Lee, T. S., Ho, C., & Sim, K. (2016). Therapeutic Misconception in Psychiatry Research: A Systematic Review. Clinical psychopharmacology and neuroscience : the official scientific journal of the Korean College of Neuropsychophar-macology, 14(1), 17–25. https://doi.org/10.9758/cpn.2016.14.1.17

Wallerstein N & Duran B (2010). Community-Based Participatory Research Contributions to Intervention Research: The Intersection of Science and Practice to Improve Health Equity. Am J Public Health. 100:S40–S46.

Women's Interagency HIV Study. (n.d.). *The Women's Interagency HIV Study (WIHS) is the largest ongoing prospective cohort study of HIV among women in the U.S.* https://statepi.jhsph.edu/wihs/wordpress/ncab/

Research With American Indian and Alaska Native Individuals, Tribes, and Communities

Deana M. Around Him

Francine C. Gachupin

William L. Freeman

Abstract

Research with American Indian and Alaska Native (AI/AN) individuals, Tribes, and communities requires special considerations and processes. This chapter offers guidance to IRB and human research protection program (HRPP) personnel about reviewing such research. This chapter presents information about AI/AN peoples, Tribal sovereignty, and self-governance; reports brief histories of research that harmed or benefited them; shares best practices to minimize harms and maximize scientific and community benefits; analyzes a realistic case study; recommends shared governance and oversight for repositories; and discusses research with urban Indians. Many best practices also apply to research with other marginalized populations.

Introduction

Of the total U.S. population, an estimated 1.7%, or 5.6 million people self-identify as American Indian or Alaska Native (AI/AN) alone or in combination with one or more other races (U.S. Census Bureau, 2016). AI/AN peoples are the Indigenous peoples of North America. As of May 2020, there are 574 self-governing, federally recognized AI/AN Tribes and several state-recognized Tribes (U.S. Department of the Interior, 2020). Names of Tribes include Nations, Pueblos, Rancherias, Bands, or Villages, and each Tribe has its own culture and history. More than half of the AI/AN population lives in urban areas, most outside of federally designated tribal lands and reservations (Snipp, 2013).

> **TERMINOLOGY**
>
> This chapter uses "AI/AN Communities" to refer to Tribes, AI/AN urban communities, and Tribal-based entities (e.g., Tribal Colleges/Universities [TCUs]).

The complexity and diversity of the AI/AN population affect the ethical conduct of research with AI/AN Communities, whose experiences with and perspectives on research and research oversight processes vary widely. Although research may be with a single Tribe or geographic context (e.g., reservation, urban community), many AI/AN individuals have connections to multiple Tribes and geographic areas. For example, they may have lineage to more than one Tribe; live or work in an urban area while maintaining a close relationship to their Tribe and Tribal homeland(s) through frequent visits; live or work on a reservation different from their own; be Tribal intermarried; or self-identify as an urban Indian. Research activities or approaches thus are not completely generalizable from one AI/AN Tribe, community, or situation to another, although some general commonalities exist.

Most AI/AN Communities are underserved and experience health inequities and discrimination in general society and health care. However, many AI/AN Communities have abilities and assets to contribute to research and scholarship not recognized by outsiders. Their life experiences, values, concerns, and identified needs differ from those of many researchers and members of most IRBs. AI/AN collective history includes both positive and negative experiences with research. Their experiences offer important lessons for the ethical oversight of research with AI/AN Communities today, especially for IRBs, HRPPs, and Community Action/Advisory Boards (CABs).

The primary goals of this chapter are as follows:

- Provide historical examples of *unethical* research as well as *beneficial and ethical* research with AI/AN Communities.
- Describe the importance of Tribal sovereignty and self-governance for IRBs and HRPPs (e.g., researchers, data and safety monitoring committees, institutional officials, funders, bioethicists, lay public), especially in reference to the three principles of the *Belmont Report*.
- Outline best practices by IRBs in the ethical oversight of research involving AI/AN Communities.
- Present a case study illustrating a research plan and IRB response that implemented those best practices.
- Discuss several issues related to best practices, including shared governance and oversight of repositories, the 2018 revisions to the Common Rule, "going beyond the Common Rule," and research with AI/AN urban communities.

🖉 2-1

🖉 1-1

Brief History of Unethical Research With AI/AN Communities

Groups that suffer discrimination, experience disparities, or are disadvantaged—e.g., racial and ethnic minorities, orphans, women, or the economically disadvantaged—have often been subjects in unethical research. Instances of research injustice have important lessons for IRBs/HRPPs, and some cases have spurred improvements in research approaches and oversight. Although not as well known, the experiences of AI/AN Communities in unethical research also have important lessons for IRBs/HRPPs.

Except for the I[131] and Indian markers cases (described later), most unethical research involving AI/AN Communities has harmed primarily the *whole community*, not just the individual subjects. "[R]esearch . . . designed to study a group or that retrospectively implicates a group may . . . result in members of the group facing, among other things, stigmatization and discrimination in insurance and employment whether or not they contributed samples to the study" (National Bioethics Advisory Commission, 1999), a harm now widely recognized (Weijer, 1999; Weijer & Emanuel, 2000). Group stigmatization can even occur in meta-analyses of primary studies (Gribble & Around Him, 2014).

AI/AN Communities have experienced all six types of research harms identified by the National Bioethics Advisory Commission (NBAC) (NBAC, 2001), listed here. This chapter adds a seventh research harm: *relational*.

- *Physical*: In 1955–1956, the U.S. Air Force's Arctic Aeromedical Laboratory used radioactive iodine (I[131]) to study the thyroid function of 102 Alaska Natives from interior Alaska to see if they survived Alaska's cold by having a metabolism different from European Americans. Three of the 26 women were breastfeeding, and one was possibly pregnant (National Research Council, 1996).
- *Psychological*:
  - *Self-stigmatization by AI/AN individuals*. Researchers studied the adverse effects of alcoholism in Barrow, Alaska, and then announced the bleak results at a news conference in Pennsylvania (Klausner & Foulks, 1982; Manson, 1989). In addition to having economic implications for the town, the results of the research study produced feelings of shame and self-stigmatization among the Inupiaq people, even those living far away, which was still strongly felt decades later: "I felt that I was, and we were, bad people" (Inupiaq Elder who never drank, from a village outside Barrow, personal communication, n.d.).
  - *Disruption of the Tribe's values*. Research has made public to the outside world information that was private Tribal knowledge—a problem with some anthropological studies. Parsons, for example, observed private cultural ceremonies and subsequently published detailed accounts without authorization of the southwestern Tribe (Parsons, 1925).
- *Social*: *External stigmatization of the group*. Epidemiologists studied an outbreak of congenital syphilis in a southwestern American Indian Tribe (Gerber et al., 1989). The State Health Department publicly named the Tribe, and after local newspapers publicized it, reservation children were called derogatory names in off-reservation schools, and AI/AN people were prohibited from using restrooms in nearby gas stations (Freeman, 1998).
- *Economic*: *Loss of economic status by AI/AN Community*. See study of alcoholism in Barrow, Alaska described previously.
- *Legal*: *Public policy on genetic determinism*. A Tribal agency misappropriated an external study's results of genetic determination of "Indian markers" among Tribal members and used the results to expel members lacking those markers (study's principal investigator, personal communication, 1996). See also the proposed bill by the Vermont General Assembly Committee on Health and Welfare, "An Act Relating to DNA Testing and Native Americans" (Vermont General Assembly, 2000).

- *Dignitary:*
  - *Violation of AI/AN individual and Tribal privacy.* Researchers robbed AI/AN graves of human remains and sacred objects during the 19th and 20th centuries (Native American Graves Protection and Repatriation Act, 1990).
  - *Violation of Tribe's sovereignty and self-governance.* A researcher used DNA from a study of severe atypical arthritis among the Nuu-chah-nulth First Nations people, Canada, to conduct migration studies without their consent (Tymchuk, 2000). The dispute resulted in a code of research conduct in British Columbia, Canada (Garrison et al., 2019). See also Arizona State University (ASU) research with the Havasupai, next.
- *Relational, vis-à-vis research or health care:*
  - *Distrust of health research.* ASU researchers obtained the approval of the Tribal government to research diabetes among the Havasupai Tribe, and more than 200 Havasupai members consented and participated. Without notice, Tribal approval, or individual consent, researchers conducted unrelated studies of topics contrary to Havasupai cultural and religious beliefs—population migration, schizophrenia, and inter-relatedness—using study DNA plus data from illegal access to medical records of *all* Tribal members (Drabiak-Syed, 2010; Garrison et al., 2019).
  - *Distrust of public health activities and care.* In late spring 1993, an outbreak of an unknown illness with a high mortality rate emerged on the Navajo reservation. Intense sensationalist media coverage fostered widespread fearful shunning of Navajo people (Stumpff, 2010; Pottinger, 2005). The Centers for Disease Control and Prevention (CDC) rapidly identified the viral cause. The Navajo Nation, Navajo Nation Division of Health (NNDoH), CDC, and area State Departments of Health partnered to marshal political and public health resources, determine chain of transmission, and institute Navajo-specific and general public health education and measures to prevent more infections (Centers for Disease Control and Prevention, 1993a, 1993b). Unfortunately, that partnership was violated by the first two publications about the epidemic in prestigious scientific journals (Nichol et al., 1993; Childs et al., 1994), both of which used Navajo place names for locations of infected humans or animals despite NNDoH's explicit and repeated requests to CDC to not use them to avoid increasing the existing external stigmatization and contraventions of Navajo privacy. The two violating publications led the Navajo Nation to develop its own Research Code and establish the first Tribal IRB, the Navajo Nation Human Research Review Board (Federalwide Assurance of Compliance [FWA] number 00008894).

Brief History of Ethical Research With AI/AN Communities

AI/AN Communities have also experienced several research projects with one or more important characteristics. These projects can be characterized as follows:

- *Were innovative* in the research topic or in the strength and closeness of collaboration between academia and the AI/AN Community
- *Addressed* a high health priority
- *Directly benefited* the AI/AN Community in the research with actionable results

- *Were strengths based*
- *Incorporated the Community's values*

The examples listed are in chronological order:

- *The People Awakening Project (PAP), 1997.* Alaska Native people proposed a research project on alcoholism to Dr. Gerald Mohatt, Director of Psychology at the University of Alaska, Fairbanks (UAF). They wanted not another negative pathology study like that at Barrow but rather a partnership of AN people and UAF researchers focused on AN strengths and resilience in confronting alcoholism. Like many AI/AN Tribes, a higher percentage of AN people were abstinent from alcohol than the U.S. general population (May & Gossage, 2001), an indication of AN strengths. PAP was an AN-initiated, AN Community-Based Participatory Research (CBPR) study from its inception (Mohatt et al., 2004a) and throughout (Rasmus, 2014). It was successful scientifically (Mohatt et al., 2004b) and directly benefited the AN people by leading to an effective intervention to expand strengths and resilience against alcoholism (Allen et al., 2018).

  ⚲ 12-9

- *White Mountain Apache Tribe Suicide Surveillance and Prevention System, 2001.* Following the loss of several youth to suicide, the White Mountain Apache Tribe collaborated with researchers at the Johns Hopkins Center for American Indian Health (JHCAIH) to establish a community-based surveillance and case management system for suicide prevention (Cwik et al., 2014). One of few community-based suicide surveillance systems in the United States, the system addressed a top priority of the Tribe, was an evidence-based effective intervention for this highly sensitive and critical health disparity, and served as a mechanism to conduct important research to further refine prevention and intervention activities. The JHCAIH and Tribal community researchers continue to respectfully collaborate to contribute knowledge and skills essential for successful benefit sharing for both parties.

- *The Safe Passage Study, 2006.* The Safe Passage Study (PASS) prospectively investigated prenatal exposure to alcohol and smoking on Sudden Infant Death (SIDS). PASS enrolled almost 12,000 pregnant women in two geographic areas with high rates of prenatal drinking and SIDS; one in the Dakotas included two AI reservations, and the other in Cape Town, South Africa. Governance and oversight of PASS's science and ethics was by the participating research institutions and their IRBs, the two Tribal governments, and the Oglala Sioux Tribe Research Review Board (OSTRRB), a Tribal IRB. PASS addressed a topic that was a priority of the Tribes, yet was also psychologically sensitive and had potential stigmatizing harms. To help minimize both harms, OSTRRB required that it review and approve publications and future uses of specimens by the PASS Network (Angal et al., 2016). Results showed that exposure to smoking and alcohol together after the first trimester was associated with a 12 times higher rate of SIDS, much higher than that of smoking or

> ## THE COMMON RULE AND GROUP HARMS
>
> "The IRB should not consider possible long-range effects of applying knowledge gained in the research (e.g., the possible effects of the research on public policy) as among those research risks that fall within the purview of its responsibility" **[45 CFR 46.111(a)(2)]**. Some people believe this sentence prohibits IRBs from considering "group harms." We disagree, for three reasons. (1) NBAC (1999) did not interpret that section to prohibit consideration of group harms; (2) the Office for Human Research Protections (OHRP) has repeatedly and publicly stated that minimizing group harms can be an important part of IRB responsibility; and (3) the group harms described previously in the section Brief History of Unethical Research with AI/AN Communities occurred immediately after the research finished; i.e., they were not "long-range effects."

drinking alone (Elliott et al., 2020). These findings should lead to beneficial, community-based, public health messaging and actions.

- *American Indian and Alaska Native Head Start Family and Child Experiences Survey (AI/AN FACES), 2015.* FACES has surveyed Head Start programs annually since 1997; however, the 145 programs that served predominantly AI/AN children were not included. Instead, AI/AN FACES was conducted for them in 2015. The planning workgroup for AI/AN FACES included Tribal Head Start directors and researchers; it planned the "design, implementation, and dissemination of findings and … added questions regarding children's experience of Native language and culture" that were actionable (Administration for Children and Families, 2019). For instance, the survey found that 35% of children were in classrooms that never used the Tribe's Native language, in part due to hiring policies that disqualified Tribal members fluent in the Tribe's language. That finding led to proposals to change the policy (Sarche et al., 2020).

- *The Alaska Area Specimen Bank, 2010.* The Alaska Area Specimen Bank contains residual biological specimens from over 83,000 persons who participated in clinical testing, public health investigations, and research projects dating back to the early 1960s; about 85% of samples are from Alaska Natives. Prior to 1997, the bank was managed by the CDC and another federal agency. When Alaska Natives established responsibility for management of their healthcare system, the Bank transitioned to management by a tribal–federal partnership. That partnership developed the Bank's governance and oversight system and implemented a structure that combines the expertise of Tribal, state, and federal partners. Parkinson et al. (2013) described this innovative specimen repository with linked clinical data and included the Bank's policies and procedures in supplemental materials.

All of these examples addressed high health priorities and were guided by innovative, respectful partnerships that enabled research to directly benefit the AI/AN Communities and incorporate fundamental Community ethical values. Most examples focused on Community strengths and resilience and produced immediately actionable knowledge—all characteristics of CBPR (Wallerstein et al., 2018).

Tribal Sovereignty and "Full Scientific and Cultural Rigor"

Potential harms and benefits of any study are defined not only by researchers and IRBs, but also by the *subjects of the research*, per the Common Rule definition of "benign behavioral interventions" in which "the investigator has no reason to think the *subjects* will find the interventions offensive or embarrassing" **[45 CFR 46.104(d)(3)(ii)]**, emphasis added). Researchers and IRBs thus must include in their ethical assessments the potential harms and potential benefits as defined by the AI/AN Communities involved.

Beneficial and ethical research involving AI/AN Tribes differs from ethical research with other groups in one significant aspect: the active role of Tribal *governments* in research oversight. AI/AN Tribes reviewed and approved the ethical research listed earlier; engaged in conducting the research, from research development and modification (in the cases of the PAP and suicide prevention projects) through Tribal governance and oversight; and reviewed and approved articles that reported results. The active role of Tribal governments in overseeing research is based on *Tribal sovereignty* and *self-governance*. As self-governing, sovereign political entities, federally recognized Tribes have legal authority to permit or prohibit research and entry by researchers to/from their reservation or Tribal lands. Many Tribes have established policies and procedures to review and approve or disapprove proposed research, and some have their own IRBs (Around Him et al., 2019).

In their review, AI/AN Communities may require that research plans incorporate their own Indigenous values (National Institutes of Health [NIH], n.d.). One set of values of many Communities concerns their worldview. The AI/AN worldview varies between and within AI/AN Communities, but one aspect is common to most and is relevant to research with them: the worldview's two realms. One realm is the environment. Many AI/AN Communities consider that they are related to and accountable for the entire environment—e.g., animals, plants, land. "They are our relatives" is often expressed, and many AI/AN people feel a responsibility to respect and maintain not only the various components of the environment but also their spiritual relationships with them. In the other realm, the human realm, many AI/AN people feel accountable to past, present, and future generations. That is, they feel a responsibility to honor and respect their ancestors and their recent and current Elders ("Past"), their own generation ("Present"), and their children and grandchildren "unto the seventh generation" ("Future") (public communication, Marilyn Scott, Upper Skagit Indian Tribe Elder and leader, 2019).

Another set of values concerns the purposes of research. Many AI/AN Communities want research to have both "full scientific rigor and full cultural rigor" (A. Echo-Hawk, Director, Urban Indian Health Institute, public comment, 2019). AI/AN Communities increasingly insist that research focus on their strengths and assets that can be grown or expanded to improve the Community. AI/AN Communities want respectful <u>Community-researcher engagement</u>, in which both sides truly listen to and collaborate with each other. AI/AN Communities want to fully implement the vision of the <u>Belmont Report</u>; IRBs are essential in doing so.

✐ 12-9

✐ 1-1

Many non-AI/AN IRBs/HRPPs and researchers do not recognize or interpret potential harms or benefits in the same way that AI/AN Communities do. We recommend that those IRBs/HRPPs engage with AI/AN Communities and include one or more AI/AN persons from a nearby Community as IRB members or consultants to help the IRB more accurately assess AI/AN-specific individual *and* group harms and benefits. The AI/AN Community review systems are an important resource that can assist IRBs, HRPPs, and researchers in understanding and respecting the worldviews and values of AI/AN peoples related to research. The structures of these systems typically are the Tribal government, Tribal or AI/AN Community IRBs, and related committees and offices. The membership and procedures of these structures help ensure that the AI/AN Community's values guide its review of risks and benefits of participation, for the following reasons:

- Membership includes largely community members, often traditional healer[s] and representative[s] from the Tribal Council.
- Final Tribal approval often requires approval by both the IRB and Tribal Council/Leadership.
- *All* proposed research is reviewed from an individual, family, and community perspective when assessing potential harms and benefits.
- *All* proposed research is often reviewed by the governing body and entire IRB, irrespective of the Common Rule's categories of "<u>not research</u>," <u>exempt,</u> and <u>expedited</u>—categories that were developed without considering harms to groups/Community.

✐ 5-1

✐ 5-3 ✐ 5-5

- Abstracts, presentations, articles, and reports are also reviewed prior to dissemination to minimize harms to the AI/AN Community.
- Many Tribes require Tribal ownership and control of data access and data sharing.
- Many Tribal IRBs require that the researcher's home IRB concurrently review and approve the research.

Collectively, these structures and procedures reflect both the unique standing of Tribes as sovereign nations as well as the deeply embedded value systems present in Tribal cultures. These systems therefore are a valuable resource for non-AI/AN IRBs, HRPPs, and researchers to better understand how to minimize harms and maximize benefits of research with AI/AN Communities.

What IRBs Should Do When Research Involves AI/AN Communities

This section has recommendations to IRBs on how to strengthen their ethical oversight of research with AI/AN Communities.

- *Assist and require the researcher to engage the AI/AN Community.*
  The IRB should require that researchers who conduct research with AI/AN Communities show evidence in their IRB application that they engaged the AI/AN Community and report the results of their engagement. Such evidence may include the following (Gachupin, 2012):
  - Dates of meetings with Tribal program representatives and Committees of the Tribal government, with accomplishments
  - Letters of support from the programs and Committees showing that the study requirements, burden to community programs or services, and community involvement are understood
  - Formation of a Community Action/Advisory Board (CAB) in which the research team and community will continue to partner
  We recommend that the IRB develop a checklist and procedures, both to assist researchers in how they engage the Community and to aid the IRB

RESOURCES TO ASSIST IRBS WITH DEVELOPMENT OF AI/AN COMMUNITY ENGAGEMENT PROCEDURES

- **Collaborative Research Center for American Indian Health (CRCAIH)**, especially its IRB Toolkit and Data Management Toolkit
- **Indigenous Wellness Research Institute (IWRI)**, especially its Research Ethics Training for Health in Indigenous Communities (rETHICS) curriculum, a culturally adapted version of Collaborative Institutional Training Initiative's (CITI's) human subjects training
- **National Congress of American Indians (NCAI) Policy Research Center**, especially its *Research That Benefits Native Peoples: A Guide for Tribal Leaders* curriculum
- **Native American Cancer Prevention Center—Outreach Core Resources**, especially researcher guidelines and *How to* resources in the publications library
- **Public Responsibility in Medicine and Research (PRIM&R)**. See resources developed with the NCAI Policy Research Center, Northwest Indian College, and others, especially several free webinars (search for "Tribal" and "Indian" within past and archived webinars)
- **Urban Indian Health Institute (UIHI)**, especially support and materials for Urban Indian Programs.

in assessing applications for research with AI/AN Communities (see Box: Resources to Assist IRBs With Development of AI/AN Community Engagement Procedures).

- *Assist and require formal AI/AN Tribal-Community approval.*

  Tribes have legal authority to approve or prohibit researchers and research projects from their Tribal lands under Tribal sovereignty and self-governance. Researchers thus must obtain formal approval by the Tribal government. (TCUs are covered by the Tribe that chartered them [U.S. Court of Appeals, Ninth Circuit, 2017]: Non-Tribal urban AI/AN Communities are discussed later in this chapter.) Tribes increasingly require that the researcher's institution sign a legally binding Data and Material Sharing and Ownership Agreement (DMSOA) for control of all future uses of the research data and specimens (e.g., DNA) from their member research subjects.

  The IRB should require that researchers obtain formal AI/AN Community approval of the proposed research. IRBs can assist researchers by outlining the steps for researchers:
    - Obtain formal approval by the Community's HRPP system, e.g., its IRB/ review committee.
    - Obtain formal approval by the Tribal Council ("Tribal Council," "Business Council").
    - Offer to have the research institution and Tribe develop and sign a legally binding DMSOA. (The IRB can show researchers a prior or sample DMSOAs.)

  If more than one Community is involved, researchers should follow the steps for each entity. Around Him and colleagues (2019) present a framework for IRBs to understand the Tribal, TCU, Tribally based, and IHS IRBs. The IRB should require that the research begin only after researchers have obtained *all* required AI/AN Community approvals, a signed DMSOA if required, and of course approval by their own IRB.

- *Offer to engage with other IRBs.*

  Collaborations between Tribal IRBs and academia-based IRBs have often resulted in each IRB learning from the other and together producing more helpful, relevant, and complete reviews. For example, the potential to identify subjects in AI/AN research is much higher than in most settings due to the small size of most AI/AN Communities; collaboration of the IRBs may result in a better solution to protect identity and ensure privacy than by either IRB alone. Both IRBs often come to better understand and respect each other and to share their respective skills.

- *Engage their institution's HRPP.*

  IRBs can assist their HRPP to issue an effective policy that respects Tribal sovereignty. IRBs can then implement the policy by widespread and recurrent dissemination, education, oversight, correction, and enforcement as part of those activities to implement the Common Rule. The HRPP must clearly support the IRB's efforts.

🧠 Case Study: A Collaborative Project

This case study is a composite of several research projects the authors have been part of or observed over more than a decade. It illustrates that AI/AN Community research can truly maximize benefits and minimize harms by collaborative planning.

A multidisciplinary research team applies to its IRB for an ethnographic, behavioral, pathophysiologic, and genomic study of emotional stress among the AI of a reservation, with the goal to reduce debilitating chronic stress. The researcher had conducted her doctoral dissertation there 27 years earlier. The reservation has two population centers: one more "traditional" in the reservation's western hills, the other more "acculturated" in its eastern plains.

Research methods include qualitative ethnography, quantitative surveys of current stressors and prior related factors (e.g., childhood sexual/physical abuse), and measurements of stress hormones and genetic variants associated with chronic emotional stress. Research hypotheses are (1) self-reported stresses, related factors, and stress hormones will be higher in the "more traditional" population, but (2) the prevalence of genes associated with stress will be similar in both. The study will return all clinically meaningful results to subjects as required by state law.

The university IRB's policy is that research with Tribes must be approved by the Tribal government and by the Tribal IRB with which it collaborates closely. The Tribal IRB notes six serious potential harms not minimized or addressed and two conditions always required for this type of research as follows:

- Results could disrupt intra-tribal relationships between the two populations.
- Self-stigmatization by individuals interpreting their genetic results as "defective."
- No plan to manage rare but expected adverse reactions to survey questions on sensitive topics.
- No plans and written agreement[s] with the Tribe's Counseling Service for emergency response to subjects with acute psychological reactions.
- Some questions from standard surveys have ethnocentric terms unfamiliar to many Tribal members.
- Consent document is too long and complex.
- In all "multicenter research," each center chooses its experts for the research team—the Tribe's choices include spiritual leaders and Elders widely respected in the Tribe.
- The Tribe requires a legal DMSOA signed by Tribe and university that the Tribe controls all use of specimens and data from its members.

Concurrently, the university IRB requires that the researcher do the following:

- Show how she engaged with the Tribe.
- Answer all concerns by the Tribal IRB and gain its approval.
- Sign a legal agreement not to identify any research subject, subject's relative, or their genome by any means, e.g., social media (Gymrek et al., 2013).
- When returning results of tests to individuals, minimize potential harms by providing the university's telemedicine genetic counseling service if requested by any subject, subject's family, researcher, or Tribal clinician.

The university IRB also gives the researcher its handout "Engaging with AI/AN Communities in Research."

The collaborating IRBs learn from one another as follows:

- The university IRB learns that intra-community conflict is a potential harm, behavioral counseling services are scarce on this reservation, and concrete plans and agreements are needed to respond to adverse events.
- The Tribal IRB learns that identification of individuals using multiple databases and social media is a potential risk and genetic counseling can be provided by telemedicine.

After 7 months of intense respectful engagement, the researcher answers all concerns of both IRBs, with one exception. She acknowledges that the Tribe and its approval of research had changed from 27 years ago and admits that the research plan now is scientifically and culturally much improved, will be more beneficial to the Tribe, and is more likely to achieve its purpose. The unanswered issue is the DMSOA. The Tribe and university agree on its terms, but the funder requires all data and specimens be deposited in a large national repository named Research in Environmental and Genomic Interactions For new Therapies (REGIFT).

REGIFT aims to have specimens and linked clinical data of more than 100,000 subjects age 18+ years from the research studies contributing to it. Its purpose is to develop new preventive and treatment interventions by discovering previously unknown genetic–disease interactions. REGIFT hopes to receive an oversample of Tribal and racial/ethnic minority populations to find genetic–disease interactions more common among them.

REGIFT has a 10-member single IRB with four lay members whose primary education and expertise are nonscientific, two of whom are people of color. REGIFT's Scientific Review Board (SRB) is composed entirely of scientists respected by the U.S. scientific community. The SRB governs the scientific uses of the repository; it approves/disapproves all applicant researchers and their proposed projects. REGIFT has no procedure for a nonscientist Tribal government or any donor population/stakeholder to participate in the governance and oversight of the scientific uses of the repository.

The inability of the Tribal government to control the future use of data and specimens from its members in REGIFT is unacceptable to the Tribe. The Tribe asserts that Tribal sovereignty and self-governance mean that it controls uses of its members' data and specimens. The university agrees with the Tribe. The study is at an impasse.

The two IRBs together propose a solution that draws on the agreement by the Navajo Nation and NIH for the "Environmental influences on Child Health Outcomes (ECHO)" project (NIH, 2019) and elements of the NIH All of Us Program's Tribal Consultation Report Draft (NIH, 2020). ECHO is a large multicenter, NIH-funded NIH-cooperative study, a network of 71 centers conducting long-term research in children's health outcomes. One center is the "Navajo Birth Cohort Study" (Hunter et al., 2015). In the Navajo-ECHO agreement, the Navajo Nation has shared governance and oversight of future uses of the Navajo Birth Cohort data it contributes to the ECHO data repository. If the Navajo Nation sees that a proposed study is unacceptable and the study does not change to make it acceptable, the Nation can exclude its data from that study. The Navajo-ECHO agreement concerned only data; therefore, the two IRBs additionally propose a "shared governance and oversight" system to the funder and REGIFT for the Tribe's specimens similar to that outlined in the NIH All of Us Program's Tribal Consultation Report Draft (NIH, 2020). All of Us, a research program that aims to collect data, including biospecimens, from one million or more people living in the U.S., specifies that it intends to reflect the diversity of its participants in the program's governance bodies. As such, All of Us has AI/AN representation on its IRB, Resource Access Board and Biospecimen Access Policy Task Force.

Shared Governance and Oversight of Repositories

Although genomic science has greatly advanced technologically, federal regulations and the ethical, legal, and social implications (ELSI) lag (Gachupin & Freeman, 2015). Some researchers continue to share with others or use Tribal data and <u>biospecimens</u> for unapproved research and deposit them in public-use <u>repositories</u>—without Tribal knowledge or approval (Garrison et al., 2019). IRB oversight may not apply when biospecimens are deidentified or are from people now deceased, according to **45 CFR 46**.

🔗 10-10
🔗 12-3

Many experts and international associations emphasize the importance of a repository's governance and oversight processes to maintain both the public's trust and its willingness to donate data and biospecimens to repositories (Bledsoe, 2018; Cicek, 2018; Fullerton et al., 2010; International Society for Biological and Environmental Repositories, 2018). Accordingly, some repositories involve the general public or donors of data and biospecimens in their *nonscientific* governance and oversight. For example, each location of the Mayo Clinic has a local CAB, and the Marshfield Clinic's repository has a CAB (McCarty et al., 2011; Olson et al., 2019). Those CABs advise the repository about the general use of biospecimens and/or researchers about how to report results in ways that are understandable and relevant to the patient/donor population.

Many repositories have *scientific* governance and oversight systems that decide which research projects are approved to use their data and biospecimens. CABs generally do not participate in the scientific governance and oversight of the repository, i.e., scientific review of applications to approve access to the repository's data and biospecimens for specific research projects.

Like many Indigenous communities worldwide, most AI/AN Communities will agree to donate their data and specimens to a repository only if the repository includes them in a shared or participatory governance and oversight system that determines the scientific uses of the repository's data and specimens (Angal et al., 2016; Hudson et al., 2020). The participation desired is more than solely to approve/disapprove a research project's application to use data and biospecimens from the AI/AN Community. Another important purpose of shared governance and oversight is to improve projects by increasing "benefit sharing"—that is, maximizing the likelihood of obtaining results that can directly benefit the Community by helping plan the project's methods and analyses.

To include AI/AN Communities in shared governance and oversight of the repository's scientific uses may appear to counter the principle of unrestricted open scientific access to the data and biospecimens of repositories (Johnson et al., 2020; Wright et al., 2019). Yet lay involvement in the scientific governance and oversight of repositories has a long history, starting in 1995; it was and remains highly acceptable to the leaders, scientists, and funders of NIH and others. The first repository with strong participatory governance and oversight was by PXE, International, self-organized by parents of, and people affected with, the rare genetic-recessive metabolic disorder, pseudoxanthoma elasticum. They did the following:

- Donated their own biospecimens and clinical data to their repository
- Carefully attended to ELSI issues
- Obtained funding for research
- Invited researchers to conduct studies using the repository with the proviso that PXE, International lay leaders were full members of the research team
- Discovered the gene
- Made all results public—thus speeding up scientific progress on the disease (Terry & Boyd, 2001)

Other advocacy groups for rare genetic diseases and consortia of groups (e.g., Genetic Alliance Registry and Biobank, Parents Like Me, Registries For All), followed (Workman, 2013). They continue to be active, make discoveries, and receive funding from NIH and others.

These "patient-powered registries and research networks" (Workman, 2013) are models for "AI/AN-powered" and "Indigenous-powered" registries and research networks with participatory governance and oversight systems, as are the Alaska Area Specimen Bank, agreement by the Navajo Nation and NIH for the ECHO project, and procedures presented in the Tribal Consultation Report Draft by the NIH All of Us Program (NIH, 2020). We propose that Tribes, other AI/AN Communities, non-AI/AN researchers, IRBs, HRPPs, and funders consider these models of participatory or shared governance and oversight as they propose, partner in, review, initiate, conduct, and publish genomic research.

The 2018 Common Rule and AI/AN Communities

The 2018 Common Rule contains two changes that benefit AI/AN Tribes:

- It recognizes Tribal authority over research [45 CFR 46.101(f), 45 CFR 46.102(k), 45 CFR 46.116(i), 45 CFR 46.116(j)]. Tribal sovereignty applied to the equivalent subsections in the pre-2018 Requirements but was not explicitly stated.
- It has an exemption process for Tribes within the single IRB review system [45 CFR 46.114(b)(2)(i)] based on Tribal sovereignty. Tribes can make sure that mandated single IRB research has minimized harm and maximized benefit to them by themselves reviewing the research.

⊘ Section 4

The 2018 Common Rule thus helps raise awareness about Tribal sovereignty among IRBs, researchers, and HRPPs.

The 2018 Common Rule, however, may also harm AI/AN Communities by its expansion of activities "deemed not to be research" [45 CFR 46.102(l)] to include "oral history" and "[p]ublic health surveillance activities." Many oral histories of AI/AN individuals make general statements about their Community (see Left Handed, 2018). The report of the public health investigation detailing an outbreak of congenital syphilis, described previously, harmed that Tribe. For those reasons and others already discussed, many AI/AN IRBs "go beyond the Common Rule." For Federalwide Assurance (FWA) IRBs to "go beyond the Common Rule," the OHRP recommends that the IRB's institution include in its IRB policy that the IRB is to minimize harms to and maximize benefits for AI/AN Communities (DHHS, 2012, 2017).

⊘ 5-1

⊘ 8-1

Research With Urban Indians

AI/AN research frequently involves non-Tribal AI/AN Communities, i.e., urban Indians who constitute more than half of all AI/AN, many in larger cities (Snipp, 2013). Some IRBs and researchers believe they need not engage approval processes when research involves urban Indians, because they do not have the same legal status as do sovereign Tribal governments. Yet urban AI/AN Communities are disadvantaged and marginalized like Tribal Communities and have related life experiences, values, strengths, concerns, and identified needs.

Many large urban areas have Urban Indian Programs (UIPs), some related to health (e.g., clinics serving AI/AN people) and some nonhealth (e.g., providing social services). In many ways, their role is like that of a Tribe vis-à-vis their AI/AN population: as an interface trusted by the AI/AN urban Community regarding researchers and research. Moreover, many health-related UIPs conduct research, have a structure to engage and actively partner with researchers, have IRBs, and review and approve proposed research much like Tribes (Dominguez & James, 2018).

We therefore encourage IRBs, researchers, and HRPPs to do the following:

- Consider and relate to UIPs as similar to Tribes.
- Assist and require that researchers engage UIPs, especially health-related UIPs.
- Seek and obtain formal UIP approval of the research and a legal DMSOA if indicated.
- Have a policy that all research with urban Indians follow equivalent procedures of engagement as with Tribes.

Conclusion

When reviewing research involving AI/AN individuals, Tribes, and communities, IRBs and HRPPs should consider potential harms and benefits of the research in the contexts of the Community's values, concerns, and traditions. IRBs can, and should, promote and lead researchers to properly engage the AI/AN Community(ies) in the proposed research. IRBs can also lead their HRPP to implement the procedure recommended by OHRP that enables the FWA IRB to go beyond the Common Rule (see The 2018 Common Rule and AI/AN Communities earlier) and thus to honor Tribal sovereignty and self-governance, minimize harms, and maximize benefits in AI/AN research. The best practices of AI/AN Community-engaged research are also applicable to research with other marginalized populations.

Acknowledgments

We acknowledge the many AI/AN individuals, Tribes, and Urban Indian Programs that endeavor to improve research for their Communities and for all peoples. We thank those who planned and took part in highly important and beneficial research with and for AI/AN Communities; we are grateful for their participation and willingness to share their experiences to protect, benefit, and strengthen AI/AN participation in future research. We also thank IRB members who have advocated for protections of AI/AN peoples. We acknowledge most of all our ancestors, Elders, parents, and spouses/partners to whom we are deeply indebted for the knowledge shared and support of our work in this space. Gachupin was supported by the National Cancer Institute of the NIH under the award for the Partnership of Native American Cancer Prevention U54CA143924 (UACC). Freeman was supported by the National Institute of General Medical Sciences (NIGMS) and National Institute of Drug Abuse (NIDA) under the award for the American Indian Wellness through Research Engagement (AIWRE) 5S06GM123552 and by the Department of Education under the award for American Indian Tribally Controlled Colleges and Universities Title III Part F P031D150020.

References

Administration for Children and Families. (2019). *Home and community Native language and cultural experiences among AI/AN children in Region XI Head Start: Findings from the American Indian and Alaska Native Head Start Family and Child Experiences Survey 2015*. Office of Planning, Research and Evaluation, OPRE Report #2019-87. www.acf.hhs.gov/opre/resource /home-and-community-native-language-and-cultural-experiences-among-ai-an-children-in -region-xi-head-start

Allen, J., Rasmus, S. M., Fok, C. C. T., Charles, B., Henry, D., & Qungasvik Team. (2018). Multi-level cultural intervention for the prevention of suicide and alcohol use risk with Alaska Native youth: A non-randomized comparison of treatment intensity. *Preventive Science, 19*(2), 174–185.

Angal, J., Petersen, J. M., Tobacco, D., Elliott, A. J., & Prenatal Alcohol in SIDS and Stillbirth Network. (2016). Ethics review for a multi-site project involving Tribal Nations in the Northern Plains. *Journal of Empirical Research on Human Research Ethics, 11*(2), 91–96.

Around Him, D., Andalcio T. A., Frederick, A., Larsen, H., Seiber, M., & Angal, J. (2019). Tribal IRBs: A framework for understanding research oversight in American Indian and Alaska Native Communities. *American Indian and Alaska Native Mental Health Research, 26*(2), 71–95.

Bledsoe, M. (2018). Custodianship, commercial use, and benefit sharing. In *Biobanking in an era of precision medicine research: Approaches to the ethical, regulatory, and practical challenges.*

Preconference workshop presented at Public Responsibility in Medicine and Research Advancing Ethical Research conference, San Diego, CA.

Centers for Disease Control and Prevention (CDC). (1993a). Hantavirus disease – Southwestern United States, 1993. *Morbidity and Mortality Weekly Report.* www.cdc.gov/mmwr/preview/mmwrhtml/00021294.htm

Centers for Disease Control and Prevention (CDC). (1993b). Hantavirus infection – Southwestern United States: Interim recommendations for risk reduction. *Morbidity and Mortality Weekly Report.* www.cdc.gov/mmwr/preview/mmwrhtml/00030643.htm

Childs, J. E., Ksiazek, T. G., Spiropoulou, C. F., Krebs, J. W., Morzunov, S., Maupin, G. O., Gage, K. L., Rollin, P. E., Sarisky, J., & Enscore, R. E. (1994). Serologic and genetic identification of *Peromyscus maniculatus* as the primary rodent reservoir for a new hantavirus in the southwestern United States. *Journal of Infectious Disease, 169*(6), 1271–1280.

Cicek, M. (2018). *Stakeholder engagement.* Workshop presented at Public Responsibility in Medicine and Research Advancing Ethical Research conference, San Diego, CA.

Cwik, M. F., Barlow, A., Goklish, N., Larzelere-Hinton, F., Tingey, L., Craig, M., Lupe, R., & Walkup, J. (2014). Community-based surveillance and case management for suicide prevention: An American Indian tribally initiated system. *American Journal of Public Health, 104*(S3), 18–23.

Department of Health and Human Services (DHHS). (2012). When PIs come a'knockin: Everything investigators want to know but are afraid to ask [OHRP Webinar]. www.hhs.gov/ohrp/sites/default/files/ohrp/education/training/piswebinartranscript.pdf (Source courtesy of Lauren Hartsmith, Division of Policy and Assurances, OHRP).

Department of Health and Human Services (DHHS). (2017). *Federalwide Assurance (FWA) for the Protection of Human Subjects.* www.hhs.gov/ohrp/register-irbs-and-obtain-fwas/fwas/fwa-protection-of-human-subjecct/index.html (Source courtesy of Lauren Hartsmith, Division of Policy and Assurances, OHRP).

Dominguez, A., & James, R. (2018). Rethinking our approach for urban Indian research. Washington State Public Health Association [Blog post, July 1]. www.wspha.org/blog-rethinking-our-approach-for-urban-indian-research

Drabiak-Syed, K. (2010). Lessons from Havasupai Tribe v. Arizona State University Board of Regents: Recognizing group, cultural, and dignitary harms as legitimate risks warranting integration into research practice. *Journal of Health and Biomedical Law, 6,* 175–225.

Elliott, A. J., Kinney, H. C., Haynes, R. L., Dempers, J. D., Wright, C., Fifer, W. P., Angal, J., Boyd, T. K., Burd, L., Burger, E., Folkerth, R. D., Groenewald, C., Hankins, G., Hereld, D., Hoffman, H. J., Holm, I. A., Myers, M. M., Nelsen, L. L., Odendaal, H. J., … Dukes, K. A. (2020). Concurrent prenatal drinking and smoking increases risk for SIDS: Safe passage study report. *EClinicalMedicine, 19,* 100247.

Freeman, W. L. (1998). The role of community in research with stored tissue samples. In R. F. Weir (Ed.), *Stored tissue samples: Ethical, legal, and public policy implications* (pp. 267–301). University of Iowa Press.

Fullerton, S. M., Anderson, N. R., Guzauskas, G., Freeman, D., & Fryer-Edwards, K. (2010). Meeting the governance challenges of next-generation biorepository research. *Science Translational Medicine, 2*(15), 15cm3.

Gachupin, F. C. (2012). Protections to consider when engaging American Indians/Alaska Natives in human subjects research. In J. R. Joe & F. C. Gachupin (Eds.), *Health and social issues of Native American women* (pp. 237–264). Praeger Publishers.

Gachupin, F. C., & Freeman, W. L. (2015). Ethics of biospecimen research. In T. Solomon & L. Randall (Eds.), *Conducting health research with Native American communities* (pp. 197–210). American Public Health Association.

Garrison, N. A., Hudson, M., Ballantyne, L. L., Garba, I., Martinez, A., Taualii, M., Arbour, L., Caron, N. R., & Rainie, S. C. (2019). Genomic research through an Indigenous lens: Understanding the expectations. *Annual Review of Genomics and Human Genetics, 20*(1), 495–517. https://doi.org/10.1146/annurev-genom-083118-015434

Gerber, A. R., King, L. C., Dunleavy, G. J., & Novick, L. F. (1989). An outbreak of syphilis on an Indian reservation: Descriptive epidemiology and disease-control measures. *American Journal of Public Health, 79*(1), 83–85.

Gribble, M. O., & Around Him, D. (2014). Ethics and community involvement in syntheses concerning American Indian, Alaska Native, or Native Hawaiian Health: A systematic review. *AJOB Empirical Bioethics, 5*(2), 1–24.

Gymrek, M., McGuire, A. L., Golan, D., Halperin E., & Erlich, Y. (2013). Identifying personal genomes by surname inference. *Science, 339*(6117), 321–324.

Hudson, M., Garrison, N. A., Sterling, R., Caron, N. R., Fox, K., Yracheta J., Anderson, J., Wilcox, P., Arbour, L., Brown, A., Taualii, M., Kukutai, T., Haring, R., Te Aika, B., Baynam, G. S., Dearden, P. K., Chagné, D., Malhi, R. S., Garba, I., & Carroll, S. R. (2020). Rights, interests, expectations: Indigenous perspectives on unrestricted access to genomic data. *Nature Reviews Genetics, 21,* 377–384. (See especially Table 1.)

Hunter, C. M., Lewis, J., Peter, D., Begay, M. G., & Ragin-Wilson, A. (2015). The Navajo Birth Cohort Study. *Journal of Environmental Health, 78*(2), 42–45.

International Society for Biological and Environmental Repositories. (2018). *ISBER best practices: Recommendations for repositories* (4th ed.). ISBER; pp. 8–9, 77, 87–88.

Johnson, S. B., Slade, I., Giubilini, A., & Graham, M. (2020). Rethinking the ethical principles of genomic medicine services. *European Journal of Human Genetics, 28,* 147–154.

Klausner, S., & Foulks, E. (1982). *Eskimo capitalists: Oil, alcohol and social change.* Allenheld and Osmun.

Left Handed. (2018). Left Handed, son of Old Man Hat: A Navajo autobiography [recorded by W. Dyk; foreword by E. Sapir; introduction by J. Denetdale]. University of Nebraska. (Original work published 1938.)

Manson, S. M. (Ed.). (1989). Special issue on the Barrow Alcohol Study. *American Indian and Alaska Native Mental Health Research, 2*(3), 5–90.

May, P. A., & Gossage, P. (2001). New data on the epidemiology of adult drinking and substance use among American Indians of the northern states: Male and female data on prevalence, patterns, and consequences. *American Indian and Alaska Native Mental Health Research, 10*(2), 1–26.

McCarty, C. A., Garber, A., Reeser, J. C., Fost, N. C., & Personalized Medicine Research Project Community Advisory Group and Ethics and Security Advisory Board. (2011). Study newsletters, community and ethics advisory boards, and focus group discussions provide ongoing feedback for a large biobank. *American Journal of Medical Genetics, 155A*(4), 737–741.

Mohatt, G. V., Hazel, K. L., Allen, J., Stachelrodt, M., Hensel, C., & Fath, R. (2004a). Unheard Alaska: Culturally anchored participatory action research on sobriety with Alaska Natives. *American Journal of Community Psychology, 33*(3–4), 263–273.

Mohatt, G. V., Rasmus, S. M., Thomas, L., Allen, J., Hazel, K., & Hensel, C. (2004b). Tied together like a woven hat: Protective pathways to sobriety for Alaska Natives. *Harm Reduction Journal, 1*(10).

National Bioethics Advisory Commission. (1999). Ethical perspectives on the research use of human biological materials. In *Research involving human biological materials: Ethical issues and policy guidance* (Vol. 1, pp. 41–54). National Bioethics Advisory Commission. repository.library.georgetown.edu/handle/10822/559356

National Bioethics Advisory Commission. (2001). Assessing risks and potential benefits and evaluating vulnerability. In *Ethical and policy issues in research involving human participants* (Vol. 1, pp. 69–96). National Bioethics Advisory Commission. repository.library.georgetown .edu/handle/10822/559360

National Institutes of Health (NIH). (n.d.). *American Indian and Alaska Native research in the health sciences: Critical considerations for review of research applications.* https://dpcpsi.nih.gov/sites /default/files/Critical_Considerations_for_Reviewing_AIAN_Research_508.pdf

National Institutes of Health (NIH). (2019). *NIH facilitates first Tribal data-sharing agreement with Navajo Nation: Navajo Birth Cohort Study will share participant data as part of major NIH research initiative.* www.nih.gov/news-events/news-releases/nih-facilitates-first-tribal-data -sharing-agreement-navajo-nation

National Institutes of Health (NIH). (2020). *All of Us Research Program Tribal consultation report draft.* allofus.nih.gov/sites/default/files/draft-tribal-consultation-report.pdf

National Research Council Committee on Evaluation of 1950s Air Force Human Health Testing in Alaska Using Iodine-131. (1996). *The Arctic Aeromedical Laboratory's thyroid function study: A radiological risk and ethical analysis.* National Academies Press.

Native American Graves Protection and Repatriation Act (NAGPRA). (1990). 25 U.S.C. 3001-3013, 43 CFR Part 10.

Nichol, S. T., Spiropoulou, C. F., Morzunov, S., Rollin, P. E., Ksiazek, T. G., Feldmann, H., Sanchez, A., Childs, J., Zaki, S., & Peters, C. J. (1993). Genetic identification of a hantavirus associated with an outbreak of acute respiratory illness. *Science, 262*(5135), 914–917.

Olson, J. E., Ryu, E., Hathcock, M. A., Gupta, R., Bublitz, J. T., Takahashi, P. Y., Bielinski, S. J., St Sauver, J. L., Meagher, K., Sharp, R. R., Thibodeau, S. N., Cicek, M., & Cerhan, J. R. (2019). Characteristics and utilisation of the Mayo Clinic Biobank, a clinic-based prospective collection in the USA: Cohort profile. *BMJ Open, 9*(11), e032707.

Parkinson, A. J., Hennessy, T., Bulkow, L., Smith, H. S., & Alaska Area Specimen Bank Working Group. (2013). The Alaska Area Specimen Bank: A Tribal-federal partnership to maintain and manage a resource for health research. *International Journal of Circumpolar Health, 72*(1).

Parsons, E. C. (1925). *The Pueblo of Jemez.* Yale University Press.

Pottinger, R. (2005). Hantavirus in Indian Country: The first decade in review. *American Indian Culture and Research Journal, 29*(2), 25–56.

Rasmus, S. (2014). Indigenizing CBPR: Evaluation of a community-based and participatory research process implementation of *Elluam Tungiiun* (Towards Wellness) Program in Alaska. *American Journal of Community Psychology, 54*(0), 170–179.

Sarche, M., Dobrec, A., Barnes-Najor, J., Cameron, A., & Verdugo, M. C. (2020). American Indian and Alaska Native Head Start. In J. B. Benson (Ed.), *Encyclopedia of infant and early childhood development* (2nd ed., pp. 31–44). Elsevier.

Snipp, C. M. (2013). American Indians and Alaska Natives in urban environments. In E. Peters & C. Andersen (Eds.). *Indigenous in the city: Contemporary identities and cultural innovation.* University of British Columbia Press.

Stumpff, L. M. (2010). *Hantavirus and the Navajo Nation: A double jeopardy disease.* nativecases .evergreen.edu/collection/cases/hantavirus-navajo

Terry, S. F., & Boyd, C. D. (2001). Researching the biology of PXE: Partnering in the process. *American Journal of Medical Genetics, 106*(3), 177–184.

Tymchuk, M. (2000, October 7). *Bad blood.* Quirks and Quarks, CBC Radio.

U.S. Census Bureau. (2016). *Table S0201: Selected population profile in the United States, 2016 American Community Survey 1-year estimates.* factfinder2.census.gov

U.S. Court of Appeals, Ninth Circuit. (2017). United States *ex rel.* Cain v. Salish Kootenai College, Inc. 862 F.3d 939–945.

U.S. Department of the Interior, Bureau of Indian Affairs. (2020). *Indian entities recognized and eligible to receive services from the United States Bureau of Indian Affairs.* Federal Register, Vol. 85, No. 20. www.govinfo.gov/content/pkg/FR-2020-01-30/pdf/2020-01707.pdf

Vermont General Assembly Committee on Health and Welfare. (2000). An act relating to DNA testing and Native Americans. Proposed bill H-809.

Wallerstein, N., Duran, B., Oetzel, J., & Minkler, M. (2018). *Community-based participatory research for health: Advancing social and health equity* (3rd ed.). Jossey-Bass.

Weijer, C. (1999). Protecting communities in research: Philosophical and pragmatic challenges. *Cambridge Quarterly of Healthcare Ethics, 8*(4), 501–513.

Weijer, C., & Emanuel, E. J. (2000). Protecting communities in biomedical research. *Science, 289*(5482), 1142–1144.

Workman, T. A. (2013). *Engaging patients in information sharing and data collection: The role of patient-powered registries and research networks.* Report No. AHRQ 13-EHC124-EF. Agency for Healthcare Research and Quality. www.ncbi.nlm.nih.gov/books/NBK164513/pdf /Bookshelf_NBK164513.pdf

Wright, C. F., Ware, J. S., Lucassen, A. M., Hall, A., Middleton, A., Rahman, N., Ellard, S., & Firth, H. V. (2019). Genomic variant sharing: A position statement. *Wellcome Open Research, 4*(22).

Issues Based on Study Design or Category

Overview of Qualitative Research

Kathleen E. Murphy

Julie F. Simpson

Abstract

This chapter will review research paradigms with a focus on qualitative research. Understanding the nature of qualitative inquiry is important to understanding the issues that it may raise. Ethical issues that qualitative inquiry may raise will be identified, and strategies for minimizing harm to subjects[1] will be discussed. Some of the ethical issues are not unique to this type of inquiry, but how they present themselves and the ways in which researchers address them may differ from similar issues in quantitative inquiry. Finally, this chapter will suggest ways that IRBs and researchers can assist each other in facilitating IRB review and approval of studies involving qualitative inquiry.

History of Qualitative Inquiry

Qualitative inquiry studies phenomena in context to understand them and has its roots in anthropology, philosophy, and sociology. It started in an unstructured form in the 1800s with early ethnographers (primarily Western researchers) traveling to distant places to study "primitive societies." The 1950s–1970s, often called the Golden Age of qualitative inquiry, saw a backlash against more quantitative methods to study social issues and the development of rigor in qualitative inquiry. Since the 1960s it has experienced steady growth, with the emergence of different approaches and an increase in the number of disciplines adopting and adapting it to meet their needs. Journals focused on qualitative

---

1 For consistency with the rest of this book, we use the term "subject" throughout this chapter to reference the people who are participating in research. However, the term "participant" is preferred in social and behavioral research, particularly in ethnography; participatory action and community engaged research; and other social science methodologies that emphasize empowerment and collaboration between researchers and participants, and in qualitative inquiry more broadly. For more on this distinction, please see the Preface.

inquiry appeared in the 1970s and 1980s, and theoretical perspectives, data collection methods, data analysis techniques, and strategies for reporting research findings expanded. Many disciplines now employ qualitative inquiry, including health sciences (e.g., nursing, occupational therapy), social work, psychology, communication, and political science (Denzin, 2008; Lockyer, 2008).

Examining Research Paradigms

Before discussing the specifics of qualitative inquiry as it exists today, it is important to have a basic understanding about the differences among research paradigms in order to understand the philosophical underpinnings for qualitative inquiry and to identify related ethical considerations. A research paradigm is a framework rather than a set of methods/techniques. The appropriateness of the structure of the inquiry (i.e., question, methodology, methods) is based on the nature of the phenomenon being studied and what the researcher is interested in discovering (Leavy, 2014; Morgan & Smircich, 1980).

When conducting research, a variety of factors influence a researcher's approach, which may contribute to how a study is conceptualized and carried out. A researcher's *ontology* is their beliefs about being, existence, and reality—what they believe can be known and how. A researcher's *epistemology* is their understanding of what knowledge is and how it can be acquired. For example, if the researcher holds an objectivist epistemology, they believe that reality exists independently of the knower and that they can measure or determine it. A researcher with a subjectivist epistemology, however, believes that they construct reality and view it through their own lens such that meaning is imposed on the object by the researcher. A *theoretical perspective* is a set of assumptions about reality that underlies the questions asked and the kinds of answers that result. Positivism, critical inquiry, feminism, and postmodernism are different theoretical perspectives. *Methodology* is a systematic way to solve a problem; it is how researchers go about their work of describing, explaining, and predicting phenomena. Examples of qualitative methodology include experimental research, phenomenology, ethnography, grounded theory, case study, and discourse analysis. Finally, *methods* include the more specific tools used to collect data such as interview, survey, observation, behavioral analysis, data mining, and so forth (Creswell, 2013; Hesse-Biber, 2016; Lichtman, 2014; Morgan & Smircich, 1980; Schram, 2006).

Resulting from these factors of ontology, epistemology, theory, methodology, and methods are general characteristics of *subjectivist* and *objectivist* research paradigms (**Table 10.1-1**). These characteristics are meant to be broad and illustrative of fundamental differences between the two paradigms (Leavy, 2014; Morgan & Smircich, 1980).

Qualitative inquiry is an approach whose appropriateness depends on the nature and type of research question or problem, the epistemology and theoretical stance of the researcher, and the appropriate methods. **Table 10.1-2** presents a side-by-side view of the characteristics of qualitative and quantitative inquiry, using broad terms to demonstrate fundamental differences between the two (Lichtman, 2014).

Qualitative and quantitative inquiry may differ in practice. Consider the following examples:

- To study instructor effectiveness, a qualitative inquiry might involve observing class, experiencing the learning environment, and interviewing

Table 10.1-1 General Characteristics of Subjectivist and Objectivist Research Paradigms

Characteristic	Subjectivist Paradigm	Objectivist Paradigm
Epistemology	Realities are multiple, constructed by knowers	Social world is a reality independent of knower
Relationship between researcher and what is being studied	Interdependence between scientist and knowing subjects	Scientist detached from object of knowledge
Approach to inquiry	Theories emerge from data gathered (inductive process)	Theories and hypotheses tested, often by controlled experiments (deductive process)
How findings may be applied	Findings are descriptive; may be transferable	Findings ideally are generalizable
Type of representation	Provides situated, interpretative portrayal of phenomenon	Provides objective, value-neutral portrayal of phenomenon
Data collection method	Uses primarily qualitative methods	Uses primarily quantitative methods

Data from Morgan, G., & Smircich, L. (1980). The case for qualitative research. *The Academy of Management Review, 4*, 491–500.

Table 10.1-2 Characteristics of Qualitative and Quantitative Inquiry

Characteristic	Qualitative Inquiry	Quantitative Inquiry
Purpose of study	Understand phenomena	Measure/quantify phenomena or explain causes
Approach to study	Study phenomena in context	Isolate phenomena from context
Approach to inquiry	Generate hypotheses/theory/principles	Test hypotheses/theory
Focus of data collection	Describe/explain properties	Measure properties
Final knowledge product or outcome	Detailed descriptions of phenomena which may be transferable to like situations	Generalizable knowledge

Data from Lichtman, M. (2014). *Qualitative research for the social sciences.* Sage Publications.

students and the instructor; a quantitative inquiry might involve surveying students, collecting student grades or evaluations, and measuring time lecturing versus questioning.

- In studying disease in a community, a qualitative inquiry might involve interviews or focus groups of patients or providers, subject observation in various settings, and documenting media coverage. A quantitative inquiry might involve surveying community members, analyzing medical records, and collecting community-level data.

There are myriad examples where similar research questions posed from different paradigms can result in very different scientific inquiry. Understanding the basics of research paradigms and the differences between qualitative and quantitative inquiry allows for thorough consideration of the ethical conduct of such research.

Basics of Qualitative Inquiry

🔗 10-2

Today, there are various labels for qualitative inquiry, including ethnography, grounded theory, and phenomenology, to name a few. _Ethnography_ is a methodology developed by cultural anthropologists that aims to depict and understand cultural behavior. It involves fieldwork and often many different types of data collection methods. _Grounded theory_ is a methodology that involves a systematic set of procedures for developing substantive theory grounded in data. _Phenomenology_ is a methodology focused on the study of lived experience from the perspective of the individual (Creswell, 2013; Schram, 2006; Schwandt, 2015).

Data collection methods commonly used in qualitative inquiry include study of artifacts/documents; observation and subject observation; various types of interviews, such as informal, unstructured, or structured; content and discourse analysis; focus groups; video or audio recording or photography; and open-ended questionnaires or surveys, in-person and online. _Subject observation_ is a data collection strategy inherited from ethnography. It consists of the dual roles of participation and observation, best understood as a continuum from mostly observer to mostly subject, and all combinations in between.

In practice, researchers conducting qualitative inquiry immerse themselves in the natural setting of the people (subjects) whom they are studying, getting direct personal experience in real-world settings. _Fieldwork_ is a term that describes activities that take place in the field, including observing, listening, talking, recording, and interpreting (Schwandt, 2015). This type of inquiry is context bounded, and researchers must be context-sensitive. Data has primacy, and principles, relationships and/or theory are derived from the data. The inquiry is not looking for simple one-to-one relationships but seeks many viewpoints and facets of the social context and embraces complexity. The inquiry is emergent in that it unfolds as the study progresses, both in terms of what researchers learn and what happens in the study site; that is, not everything that will happen is known in advance. The researcher seeks to access and understand people's experiences and perceptions and how they make sense of themselves, their lives, and their social environment. The researcher is the data collection instrument; the researcher's beliefs, values, and predispositions knowingly (and by design) influence the research process. Accordingly, researchers must make their biases explicit and share their motivations. Finally, qualitative inquiry is often nonlinear; although researchers develop an initial plan, it may unravel in an organized and systematic way. They often need to go back and forth, use different methods concurrently, and adapt to changes in the environment (Creswell, 2013; Schram, 2006).

Ethical Issues for IRBs

Study Design

In addressing study design and data collection methods, we focus on the appropriateness of the design as well as the methods in relation to ethical issues, rather than on only methodological issues.

Regarding the appropriateness of study design, consider an example of an individual who is a facilitator of a domestic abuse support group who proposes to conduct research with group members by observing meetings and interviewing members. The researcher is not going to cofacilitate at sessions when they conduct their research but rather observe and take notes and conduct follow-up questioning with group members who are the subjects of the research. They propose that members who do not participate in the study attend a different session if they feel uncomfortable with the research taking place. Issues that this study raises include the following:

- Potential undue coercion, in that clients may feel that they have to participate in the research to continue in the support group or to maintain their relationship with the researcher in the facilitator role once the study ends.
- The role conflict of facilitator versus researcher. Will group members who participate in the research have difficulty understanding how the person they know as their facilitator is taking on a different role within the group as researcher? What does that mean for these group members in terms of the information shared within the support group context? These concerns are exacerbated by the fact that these individuals are vulnerable and come to a support group to seek help.
- This support group provides critical services to a vulnerable population. The research agenda introduces the possibility of altering the group dynamics that may negatively affect delivery of a critical service.
- The fact that the researcher proposes that group members who are uncomfortable with the research sign up for a different session appears to be a high cost for the participants, particularly since they are a vulnerable population, and due to the role and function of the support group in their lives. This may pose an unfair burden on support group members who do not want to participate in the research, because a different group session could present scheduling problems or impose other costs, such as transportation difficulties.

The researcher could have proposed to observe a group where they were not a facilitator and where they had no prior relationships with subjects. In this case, the concerns for IRBs and researchers remain about altering group dynamics, the efficacy of the group as a support group, and the opportunity costs to group members who do not want to participate. Another option would have been to conduct one-on-one interviews or focus groups with members outside the context of the support group.

The second issue is the appropriateness of certain methods for collecting data. For example, is it ever appropriate to use focus groups to discuss issues such as illegal behavior or sensitive topics? Concerns center on sharing sensitive information in settings where subjects know each other's identity and possible sharing of sensitive information outside the group setting. If there is no way to ensure privacy and confidentiality, is it ever appropriate to propose a research method that places subjects at risk of reputational, social, legal, or economic harm? Here, IRBs need to inform researchers about these concerns and work together to address them in order to minimize harm to subjects. In this example, a solution might be to suggest one-on-one interviews, which could decrease the likelihood of disclosure.

Effect of Research Participation on Subjects' Lives

Many field researchers leave their location at the end of the study period, whether that is 2 months or 2 years, and then publish the results of the study. However, the people who were the focus of the research remain in place going about their daily lives. Does participating in the research affect subjects' lives, and if so, how? What are the social, group, or community harms that can result from the research (see Ellis, 1995)? In international research or research in areas where the population is not mainstream or is disenfranchised for some reason, although research may be useful, it can also have negative effects on the community (see, for example, Sterling, 2011).

🖉 10-9

⊘ Section 9

By introducing themselves into a new setting or taking on a research role in an existing setting, researchers need to be cognizant of how they may affect individuals' lives, particularly <u>vulnerable populations</u>. The IRB must ask whether the potential effects pose risks and/or present benefits. If the former, how will those risks be minimized? Researchers need to recognize how inserting themselves into a place may impact subjects (and even nonparticipants), particularly in terms of presenting harm, and explain to the IRB how they are going to disengage from the study site and the lives of the community members to minimize the risk of harm. Similarly, researchers also need to explain their plan for the dissemination of information if the findings could be negative or have a negative effect on individuals or the community. Just because researchers can study a community, does not mean it is the right thing to do. Similarly, just because research can do good does not mean it cannot also do harm. The IRB has to engage with the researcher around the issue of harm as a larger construct, rather than focusing solely on the impact on the individual.

The IRB also needs to confirm that researchers have the expertise and the cultural awareness to conduct the research as proposed. In that regard, Hook et al. (2013) frame cultural humility as the "ability to maintain an interpersonal stance that is other-oriented (or open to the other) in relation to aspects of cultural identity that are most important to the [person]." The authors found that there was consistent reporting of the importance of cultural humility with therapists, and it stands to reason that this would be the case also with researchers who are embedded in communities for extended periods of time. Cultural humility is an important construct to impress upon researchers in the exercise of

⊘ 12-9

<u>community engaged</u> scholarship.

Emergent Nature

Events may happen unexpectedly that materially influence the research and require the researcher to alter the study design in response. World events, such as natural disasters, epidemics, or political upheaval, may significantly alter the research location and require changes in research plans. Contingency plans are extremely useful, although some events cannot be anticipated. Although some changes may not present ethical issues, others may. What are a researcher's professional obligations, and what does that mean regarding specific situations? Consider the following examples of contingency planning in research:

- Houghton, a nurse researcher, and colleagues (2010) reported on a study of student nurses that included a clinical setting. Houghton developed a written list of situations when she would have to intervene in patient care; that is, step out of the researcher role. These were primarily emergency situations, such as life-threatening events and a risk of physical harm.
- For her book, Nathan (2005), a professor, lived as a first-year student at her university. She reported giving formal notice to her institution that she would relinquish her role as an officer of the institution and let the university know she would not record names nor report any violation of university policy or public law.

Other examples that raise questions about research obligations include the following:

- In an online survey assessing depression with no identifiers, what is the ethical obligation if, someone reports that they want to commit suicide?
- What does a researcher do if, on a home visit with families with children with special needs, they view behavior that indicates neglect or abuse?

- What does a student research assistant do about a student athlete who shows up for a lab visit so intoxicated that they cannot provide reliable data? It is easy to not collect any data at that visit or to collect it and discard it, but what are the ethical responsibilities for the researcher? Should they report the intoxicated underage student or ensure the student returns to the dorm safely?

Researchers need to think about and plan for the myriad scenarios of what can go wrong with the research and provide information as part of their IRB application regarding how they will respond. IRBs need to consider whether a researcher's contingency planning has been comprehensive enough in anticipating what could happen and whether the plans are realistic and adequate. In these cases, seeking advice from experts outside the IRB can be helpful.

Assessing risk to subjects may be quite difficult due to the emergent nature of much qualitative inquiry. Many factors may be involved, including the nature of the research, what is being studied, the type of risk, and how the research may impact subjects. The existing literature may provide insight in some disciplines (such as nursing) where such issues have been explored indepth. Also, the literature of confessional tales (e.g., Ellis, 1995; Van Maanen, 1988) where researchers recount what actually occurred in the field and afterward, "warts and all," may provide a window into this area, particularly regarding publishing information about people's lives (making the private public).

As with other approaches, primary risks raised by qualitative inquiry may include loss of confidentiality and loss of privacy. Confidentiality pertains to the treatment of information/data disclosed in a trust relationship, whereas privacy pertains to a person's control over sharing aspects of themselves with others. Another risk may be related to negative impact on daily life. This is illustrated in the domestic abuse support group study described earlier, where there was the potential harm to subjects and nonparticipants alike from not receiving adequate services. Thus, as qualitative inquiry takes place in a naturalistic setting and also may have consequences for nonparticipants, researchers should look broadly at potential community-level harms: could nonparticipants be harmed by the nature of what is revealed and/or how the research tangentially affects their lives? Similarly, in <u>international research</u>, understanding cultural issues may also be critical in the risk assessment. Furthermore, risk may differ for subjects depending on their level of involvement in a study.

🔗 10-9

As with quantitative inquiry, researchers have to anticipate risks and explain to the IRB how they will minimize harms and maximize benefits. But with qualitative inquiry, they also need to think more broadly, related to the naturalistic setting and emergent nature, about what issues may arise in subjects' lives and in the community that may present risks relative to the study. Again, a thorough literature review will aid in this task, and researchers should also consult with gatekeepers about potential risk, if appropriate.

Recruitment

Ethical issues regarding recruitment often relate to the population involved and the nature of the research. How do researchers plan to access subjects? Is it through an existing role where access is privileged, or is the location accessible to anyone? Is there a gatekeeper, and what role will that gatekeeper play in allowing the study to take place or in the study itself? Principals or superintendents are powerful gatekeepers to conducting research in most <u>K–12 schools</u>; the moderator of an online support group is also a

🔗 9-2

gatekeeper. Researchers need to explain in their IRB application the path or process through which they are accessing a location that is not publicly accessible and the role of any gatekeepers. If this information is missing, the IRB should inquire to ensure that subjects' privacy is protected and that the gatekeeper role is appropriate, particularly in terms of coercion or undue influence.

Another issue related to recruitment is the researcher's relationship with subjects. This is an area in which qualitative inquiry differs from quantitative research; in much qualitative inquiry, researchers are expected to develop relationships with subjects in order to gain subjects' perspectives and to understand meaning in the setting. This is a critical step in a research study, particularly in subject observation. It is often referred to in the literature as building rapport. These relationships are often complex, emotional, and personal and thus ripe for ethical concerns. Issues include the following:

- Are the relationships being developed solely for the purpose of the study, or does the researcher have existing relationships with subjects in some other role (e.g., an educator or a coach)? If a new relationship, under what pretext is it being built?

⊘ Section 6

- When will <u>consent</u> be administered? How is the relationship itself described in the consent form (if at all)?

- If there is an existing relationship, how will the research role be explained to subjects? How will the researcher ascertain which role they will play, and when? How will subjects know when information is being gathered? How will the researcher minimize confusion for subjects in terms of which role they are playing? Researchers ideally want subjects to forget their research role and to see them only in their other role, but how does this align with informed consent? (For additional information, see de Laine, 2000.) Depending on the nature of the study, should researchers set boundaries around when they are collecting data? Are there times when they are not in their researcher role (e.g., when talking in the bathroom or when going out to dinner)?

- What information do researchers share with subjects about themselves in the development of a relationship, and when is not sharing such information considered incomplete disclosure or <u>deception</u>?

⊘ 10-3

The questions posed here are ones that researchers need to consider in the development of their study and where applicable, address in IRB applications. Such relationships have a huge potential for misinterpretation/misunderstanding by subjects, particularly when they do not understand the concept of research. This is exacerbated when researchers add to the confusion by misrepresenting their purpose and role in the setting to further their research. (For additional information, see Fine, 1993.)

It is often argued that researchers have more power than subjects in research studies due to their knowledge of what is being studied and their level of expertise, such as when the researcher is a psychotherapist. In qualitative inquiry, however, the argument has been made that subjects may have more power than researchers because subjects are the experts on their own lives. There are anecdotes of naïve researchers being led astray by "wily" subjects. Again, the actual situation will depend on the specifics of the study. For example, in a scenario where doctoral students are interviewing former senators and diplomats, the latter have extensive knowledge and are likely very politically savvy compared with the students.

Informed Consent

The ethical issues concerning <u>consent</u> are not unique to qualitative inquiry, but in qualitative inquiry they may take on a different flavor. Subjects' understanding of research is of particular concern in qualitative inquiry because it involves (1) subject relationships with researchers for research purposes and (2) research about subjects' everyday lives.

🔗 Section 6

A particularly complicated issue arises when thinking broadly about qualitative inquiry methods and consent. In studies involving observation and participation observation in public places, who needs to give consent and in what form? Houghton and colleagues (2010) discuss this in terms of consent taking place in a public clinic waiting room. Should consent for observation be sought from everyone in the waiting room or just for individuals who are primary study subjects? If so, should consent be oral or written? Written consent was initially sought from patients in the study; the researchers reported favorable reaction from patients until they were asked to sign a form, when they became apprehensive. The researchers then moved to obtaining oral consent. Patients who were deemed not to have the <u>capacity to consent</u> (too ill or cognitively impaired) were not included in the observations. Researchers and IRBs need to consider when literacy may be an issue and support use of oral consent if it might save someone from being embarrassed that they cannot read. IRBs need to consider what spaces are public and what are private in discussions about consent. To complicate matters, the definition of whether <u>online spaces</u> are considered public or private is constantly evolving, as are ethical issues in such research, particularly in qualitative inquiry (a further discussion of research in online environments is provided later).

🔗 9-7

🔗 10-5

Although ensuring informed consent may be difficult in studies that are more linear, the emergent nature of qualitative inquiry compounds problems. How do the researcher and the IRB ensure adequacy of information about things that can only be anticipated conceptually (and those that cannot), while not scaring off subjects? If the research agenda is altered in response to an event or the discovery of new information, how will subjects be informed about a change in focus? How are subject relationships with researchers addressed? Such issues speak to the need for informed consent as a process rather than an event, where the researcher can update subjects on the progress of the study and how things may be changing in response to environmental factors. Qualitative inquiry researchers ideally want to become part of subjects' lives, so they become part of the scene and their research role forgotten. But researchers' desire to become transparent conflicts with the concept of informed consent as a process. Should researchers continually remind subjects about the study, particularly if there is any risk associated with participation? If researchers are looking into issues where informing subjects ahead of time may result in the researcher being excluded or subjects changing their behavior (e.g., illegal or deviant), the challenge of deception arises. IRBs need to work with researchers to balance their needs with those of subjects and to use the flexibility in the regulations vis-à-vis consent, such as waiving the requirement of obtaining signatures on forms.

Similarly, researchers and IRBs need to consider when seeking re-consent is the ethically right action to take. With mildly cognitively impaired individuals or people in early to middle stages of dementia, <u>capacity to consent</u> may be transient, and what someone agreed to last week may not still stand at the second visit. It is a sensitive issue for subjects, and the study team and the IRB

🔗 9-7

need to work together to come to a mutually acceptable, compliant way to respectfully make sure someone is still competent to provide informed consent to participate in research. For studies involving <u>minors</u>, researchers should obtain informed consent from them if they reach the age of majority during their participation in the study.

9-6

Privacy and Confidentiality

In the area of privacy and confidentiality, again there are similarities with studies involving quantitative methods, but also unique challenges.

Being in a field site may make protecting the confidentiality of raw data more challenging, particularly if facilities for safe storage are scarce. Researchers need to ensure that digital devices are safely secured and that data transferred via a portable device are encrypted where possible because such devices are easily lost. In that regard, researchers should consult with information technology professionals to verify methods of encryption and to secure data once it is collected, including where it can be stored if there is, or is not, access to the internet. Researchers need to ensure that they do not make promises that they cannot keep, such as keeping all data collected confidential when they are a mandated reporter or not sharing data with anyone when a sponsor requires data be submitted to a repository. This is of particular concern in light of the emergent nature of qualitative inquiry. It speaks to anticipating issues and contingency planning and to ensuring that consent information reflects such issues. A related, but not ethical, issue arises when researchers make promises that they later regret because the promise limits their research. A common example is promising not to share data but later on finding it would have been useful in a collaborative study. An IRB can help in both these instances by providing sample language.

Another consideration for confidentiality is the fact that keeping track of multiple individuals over a long period of time necessitates including identifiers in field notes and recordings. These should be kept to a minimum and replaced at the earliest possible convenience with codes or pseudonyms. The list of identifier and associated codes or pseudonyms should be kept separately or erased. Not identifying subjects may be challenging due to detailed descriptions used in reporting outcomes. It may pertain not only to individual subjects but also to communities and sites. The use of quotations can be a powerful tool when reporting findings and generating detailed descriptions, but this can be problematic if subjects can be identified by what they say. It is a balancing act to keep true to the meaning of the quote, without revealing who said it (or who it was about), if subjects' identity is being masked. Similarly, problems may arise in concealing the identity of unique individuals, particularly when reporting characteristics that are key to the study and when using small samples (especially bounded samples).

When deciding whether to use pseudonyms versus identifying subjects, do subjects understand any ramifications if they choose to be identified? What does it mean for subjects to be identified in the context of the results of the study; that is, what will be revealed about them? Choices need to be made up front about whether subjects and/or the field site will be identified in reporting. That decision may depend in part on the nature of the study and the theoretical perspective employed. Some perspectives actively encourage identification to empower subjects or communities.

In qualitative inquiry, the bottom line is that the researcher is being trusted with personal and often private information, observations of unguarded behavior, and with shining a light on the phenomenon under study. Therefore, what should be disclosed, at what costs, and for what audiences needs to be carefully thought through by the IRB and the researcher, in the interest of protecting subjects from harm and maximizing the benefits of the research for the greater good.

Online Spaces

The issues described previously are common to many studies involving qualitative inquiry. Conducting qualitative research in <u>online spaces</u> may raise additional questions (Convery & Cox, 2012; Gerber et al., 2017; Im & Chee, 2006). Although there is a great deal of diversity in such studies, common ethical questions include the following:

🔗 10-5

- Is the online space public or private? What are the terms of service (TOS) online? What are the expectations of the individuals using that space? If people use an online "public" space as a "private" space, what is the researcher's ethical responsibility?
- If a researcher obtains permission and gains entry to an online space, what is their ethical responsibility to the other people in the space?
- How does a researcher authenticate the person on the other end? Is an avatar a "person" in the IRB sense of the term? Is virtual reality a "place"?
- How can researchers ascertain the integrity of the data collected?
- Do researchers need to obtain informed consent from users? If so, how can they do so practically?
- How can researchers protect the confidentiality of data collected through online spaces when it is relatively easy to find the source of verbatim quotes via search engines?
- How should researchers "interpret" emotion/text/words/jargon? Reading text is not the same as face-to-face communication.
- Particularly with <u>vulnerable populations</u>, what responsibility do researchers have to intervene with subjects during a study, if necessary, and how might they accomplish this?

🔗 Section 9

- Who owns the information presented on a website, including data posted by users? Is "text" in a chat room or online forum in the public domain?

Conclusion

Qualitative inquiry is not one-size-fits-all. The ethical, moral, and oversight issues found in the context of one study can often yield different ethical dilemmas for researchers and for IRBs to consider in another. Recommendations for researchers conducting qualitative inquiry and for IRBs reviewing such research are summarized in the boxes that follow.

STRATEGIES FOR RESEARCHERS TO MINIMIZE HARM AND MAXIMIZE BENEFITS

- Read the literature thoroughly.
- Plan for contingencies.
- Set boundaries for data collection.
- Minimize subject confusion about research and role conflicts.
- Have different requirements for consent for different levels of participation.
- Operationalize consent as a process.
- Use one-on-one methods for sensitive data collection.
- Develop a robust data management and data security plan.

- Be reflective throughout study.
- Do not make promises that cannot be kept.
- Plan for leaving the study location and preparing subjects at the conclusion of the study.
- Be realistic about impacts of making the private public.
- Have a plan for reporting to the IRB when something goes awry on the study.

🖉 1-1
- Adhere to the principles in the _Belmont Report_.

GUIDANCE FOR IRBS THAT REVIEW QUALITATIVE INQUIRY

- Have at least one qualitative researcher on each IRB.
- Have at least one staff member in the IRB office trained in qualitative research design.
- Given the rapid changes in research methodologies, keep current with the qualitative research literature.
- Request a consult with an expert for novel methodologies or special populations.
- Ensure that researchers:
  - Identify potential issues with their methodology and the risks/harms to the subjects and provide adequate plans for mitigating risk.
  - Set boundaries on sample size and for data collection; the methods have to match the study questions.
  - Explain how they will minimize subject confusion about research and role conflicts.
  - Use one-on-one methods for sensitive data collection.
  - Develop a robust data management and data security plan.
  - Plan for leaving the study location and preparing subjects for the conclusion of the study.
- Have different requirements for consent for different levels of participation and for different subjects in a study.
- Require consent as an ongoing process.

References

Convery, I., & Cox, D. (2012). A review of research ethics in internet-based research. _Practitioner Research in Higher Education, 6_(1), 50–57.

Creswell, J. W. (2013). _Qualitative inquiry & research design_ (3rd ed.). Sage Publications.

de Laine, M. (2000). Fieldwork, participation and practice: Ethics and dilemmas in qualitative research. Sage Publications.

Denzin, N. K. (2008). Evolution of qualitative research. In L. M. Given (Ed.), _The SAGE encyclopedia of qualitative research methods_. Sage Publications.

Ellis, C. (1995). Emotional and ethical quagmires in returning to the field. _Journal of Contemporary Ethnography, 24_, 68–98.

Fine, G. A. (1993). Ten lies of ethnography: Moral dilemmas of field research. _Journal of Contemporary Ethnography, 22_, 267.

Gerber, H. R., Abrams, S. S., Curwood, J. S., & Magnifico, A. M. (2017). _Conducting qualitative research of learning in online spaces_. Sage Publications.

Hesse-Biber, S. J. (2016). _The practice of qualitative research: Engaging students in the research process_ (3rd ed.). Sage Publications.

Hook, J. N., Davis, D. E., Owen, J., Worthington Jr., E. L., & Utsey, S. O. (2013). Cultural humility: Measuring openness to culturally diverse clients. _Journal of Counseling Psychology, 60_(3), 353–366.

Houghton, C. E., Casey, D., Shaw, D., & Murphy, K. (2010). Ethical challenges in qualitative research: Examples from practice. _Nurse Researcher, 18_(1), 15–58.

Im, E., & Chee, W. (2006). An online forum as a qualitative research method: Practical issues. *Nurse Researcher, 55*(4), 267–273.

Leavy, P. (2014). Introduction. In P. Leavy (Ed.), *The Oxford handbook of qualitative research.* Oxford University Press.

Lichtman, M. (2014). *Qualitative research for the social sciences.* Sage Publications.

Lockyer, S. (2008). Qualitative research, history of. In L. M. Given (Ed.), *The SAGE encyclopedia of qualitative research methods.* Sage Publications.

Morgan, G., & Smircich, L. (1980). The case for qualitative research. *The Academy of Management Review, 4,* 491–500.

Nathan, R. (2005). *My freshman year: What a professor learned by becoming a student.* Cornell University Press.

Schram, T. H. (2006). *Conceptualizing and proposing qualitative research: Mindwork for fieldwork in education and the social sciences* (2nd ed.). Pearson Education.

Schwandt, T. A. (2015). *The Sage dictionary of qualitative inquiry* (4th ed.). Sage Publications.

Sterling, R. L. (2011). Genetic research among the Havasupai: A cautionary tale. *American Medical Association Journal of Ethics Virtual Mentor, 13*(2), 113–117.

Van Maanen, J. (1988). *Tales of the field.* University of Chicago Press.

Ethnographic and Observational Research

Kathleen E. Murphy

Julie F. Simpson

Abstract

This chapter reviews two qualitative research methodologies—ethnography and observational research. Ethnography is a unique, complex research methodology that raises specific challenges for researchers and IRBs. In order for these challenges to be addressed during IRB oversight without substantially affecting the implementation of the study, it is important for IRBs to understand ethnography. Observational research, although less complex in nature, also requires a working understanding in order to knowledgeably review it for ethical issues. Some ethical challenges raised by these methodologies are covered in the previous chapter. This chapter focuses on the issues specific to the qualitative methodologies of ethnography and observation. It also briefly explores how ethnography has changed in its recent history, including moving into online spaces. This chapter builds on the recommendations identified for IRBs in the previous chapter. Additionally, this chapter concludes with recommendations that are specific to reviewing ethnographic and observational research.

Introduction

Ethnography is a qualitative research methodology this is primarily field based. It started in social anthropology in an unstructured form in the 1800s, when early ethnographers (primarily Western researchers) travelled to distant locations to study "primitive societies." Since that time, researchers across a broad range of disciplines, including sociology, education, communication, health sciences, and organizational behavior, have employed ethnography to study an extensive range of groups and topics in a variety of settings, including on the internet (Denzin, 2008; Lockyer, 2008). Observation is a method of data collection that is commonly used in ethnography but also is used as part of other research designs. (Readers new to qualitative inquiry should read the <u>previous chapter</u> in order to better understand the fundamentals of

🖉 10-1

qualitative research, in which ethnography and observational research are grounded. Furthermore, the previous chapter examines ethical issues raised by qualitative methods in general and provides recommendations, some of which pertain to ethnographic and observational research and which are not addressed again here.)

What Is Ethnography?

Ethnography is a qualitative research methodology that aims to depict and understand cultural behavior and social interactions. Ethnographers conduct fieldwork, often involving multiple data collection methods, including participant observation, informal or formal/structured interviews, surveys, video/audio recording, photography, document/artifact analysis, and online/digital communications. *Fieldwork* is a term that describes data collection activities that take place in the location of interest, which include observing, listening, talking, recording, following online, and interpreting (Schwandt, 2015). Using these data collection methods in a mixed method format, ethnographers generally study a single community (e.g., a town, an online cancer support group), a group of individuals (e.g., the Ku Klux Klan, a specific street market), an organization (e.g., a prison, a start-up company), or a culture (e.g., orthodox Jews living in a specific suburb). Conducting ethnography requires researchers to immerse themselves in the natural setting (including online) and daily lives of the people (subjects)[1] whom they are studying. Through fieldwork, ethnographers study people's behavior (language, culture, values, etc.) in those individuals' everyday social contexts. As such, ethnography is an *inductive approach* to research, whereby researchers generate a theory about human behavior or culture from the descriptive data collected in the field, rather than developing a theory first and collecting data in a contrived context in order to test it (*deductive approach*). Accordingly, ethnography is framed and conducted in a manner that differs from most experimental research, wherein researchers construct situations in controlled environments (e.g., a laboratory) and study human behavior in such environments for causal phenomena, as well as from large-scale surveys in which researchers look for factors common or constant in a representative sample of the general population (Iphofen, 2015).

Observational research involves collecting data via observation. The data collection can be structured or unstructured, and researchers can have varying levels of integration into the setting in which they are conducting their observations.

Participant Observation

While many of ethnography's data collection methods are commonly employed in other research methodologies, participant observation, for the most part, is unique to ethnography. In participant observation, researchers take part in the lives of groups of people to learn about their activities of daily living and to gain understanding of social life processes. They do so by being in settings for extended periods of time and actively participating in the routine and extraordinary activities of the people in those settings (DeWalt, 2002). Participant

---

1 For consistency with the rest of this book, we use the term "subject" throughout this chapter to reference the people who are participating in research. However, the term "participant" is preferred in ethnographic and observational research. For more on this distinction, please see the Preface.

observation is often described as "hanging out," due to the inordinate amount of time researchers spend informally observing and participating in activities of daily life in settings (Simpson, 2007). Researchers gather data through observation and gain understanding through relationships with subjects (Sanders, 1980). Although traditionally participant observation occurs in physical settings, the multifaceted nature of people's modern lives often necessitates incorporating data collection in online spaces when conducting ethnography on many contemporary topics (Hallett & Barber, 2014).

Participant observers have a dual purpose in research settings: first, to engage in the activities of the setting, and second, to observe as much as possible what occurs (Spradley, 1980). Thus, researchers must become involved with both the people and their activities, yet retain enough distance to be able to observe and document. Fox describes this ongoing balance as "a dynamic equilibrium between participation and observation—a continuous balancing and rebalancing of involvement and detachment" (Fox, 2004). Several commentators have proposed typologies to help understand participant/observation orientations in different settings (**Table 10.2-1**). Although these schemas differ somewhat, they all address the degree of participation in settings. In reality, the degree of observation and participation moves along a continuum as researchers enter settings, spend time participating, experience life as it unfolds, and then eventually leave. For example, Gans describes how, throughout his study of Levittown, he went from total participant when participating in the Saturday morning "bull sessions" with neighbors while mowing their lawns, to researcher participant while attending parties where he could steer conversations to his topics of interest, to total researcher when he attended a public meeting (Gans, 1982; Simpson, 2007).

The need for researchers to actively participate in settings, rather than conduct their studies as detached observers watching from afar or in

Table 10.2-1 Typologies of Participant/Observation Orientations

Author	Typology of Different Participant/Observation Orientations
Gold (1958)	Complete observer Observer as participant Participant as observer Complete participant (covert research)
Freilich (1970)	Zero participant Privileged stranger Marginal native Make-believe native Temporary native
Spradley (1980)	Nonparticipation Active participation Complete participation
Gans (1982)	Total participant Researcher participant Total researcher
Adler and Adler (1987)	Peripheral membership Active membership Complete membership

contrived settings, in order to test specific hypotheses raises unique practical and ethical issues. These include setting boundaries for behaviors they will engage in and data they will collect while in the setting, playing different roles in the setting (discussed later), developing relationships with subjects, and responding to naturally occurring events as they unfold (emergent nature). The <u>previous chapter</u> addresses the last two topics. This chapter examines the first two, along with other ethical issues presented by ethnographic and observational research, followed by a brief discussion of ethnography in online spaces.

🔗 10-1

Ethical Issues for IRBs

There is a consistent body of literature on the ethical issues presented to IRBs by ethnography (Beauchamp, 1982; Bell, 2018; Fine, 1993; Iphofen, 2015). In addition, there is a body of literature on the discontent and aggravation that social scientists have experienced with the IRB review process (AAUP, 2000; Bell, 2018; Lewis & Russell, 2011; Newmahr & Hannem, 2018). These critiques frequently dismiss IRB review of ethnography, perceiving the IRB as trying to impose a biomedical, quantitative research model on a methodology that is qualitative, reflective, and emergent rather than hypothesis testing. Anthropologists and sociologists, among others, have been outspoken about the barriers to research posed by IRB review, arguing that it interferes with the methodology as it is intended to be implemented. IRBs often expect that research must be presented as a chronology of events; there is a Step 1, Step 2, and Step 3, and in Step 1 there will be a survey, in Step 2 there will be interviews with individuals, and in Step 3 there will be a follow-up focus group. However, that is not how ethnography typically happens. IRBs often misunderstand the emergent nature of ethnography and that ethnography is by design exploratory, multilayered, and multifaceted: Interviews may be interspersed with observations, and the researcher may be in a home, a school, or a tent interacting with one person or a multigenerational family, or cooking dinner or hanging out on the street corner. Ethnography is neither linear nor chronological in the traditional sense of an inductive research design and so can seem chaotic and "messy" for IRBs. To obtain some control over the research, IRBs often react based on what they know and attempt to impose standard rules of engagement and informed consent, privacy, and confidentiality. How researchers engage with subjects, the importance of informed consent, and the protection of privacy do not change as values in ethnography; however, these factors must be implemented in a way that is sensitive to the methodology, without twisting the methodology to fit what IRBs know how to do.

In an attempt to ameliorate some of the tension between researchers and IRBs, the remainder of this chapter identifies key ethical challenges and explains where IRB review might clash with ethnographic methodology. It also presents practical guidance for how IRB staff and reviewers can collaborate with ethnographers and their research in ways that are congruent with applicable ethical principles and the regulatory requirements that are designed to protect the people who participate in ethnographic research.

As previously stated, the primary methodology of ethnography and participant observation rests on the relationship between the researcher and the people participating in the research. This methodological approach raises three central, interrelated issues for the IRB: transparency; roles and boundaries; and community engagement, recruitment, and informed consent.

Transparency

Transparency is an overarching concern for establishing the quality of qualitative research and relates to both the researcher's relationship with subjects during the research as well as the dissemination of the research findings to the outside world. Both have implications for IRB review.

1. *Transparency with subjects in the research*

   Ethnographic inquiry is the study of people in their own environment. As outlined previously, the study design may use multiple methods, such as surveys and interviews, as well as different forms of participant observation. There typically will be a "sampling" of people and events over time—usually months, sometimes years. In addition, "reflexivity," which refers to the researcher's use of their self-awareness to inform and refine the research design over time, is a hallmark of ethnography. Inherent in ethnography is the use of the researcher's presence as part of the research dynamic, in which relationships with subjects emerge over time. In order to blend in with the community, the researcher must establish one or more roles in the setting that are acceptable to the study community and adaptable to the needs of the research. It is because of this dynamic nature of ethnography—the use of mixed methods, coupled with self-reflection, the use of different roles, and its evolving nature—that ethnography presents challenges for the usual IRB review.

   Ethnographers need to develop relationships with people in their own environment in a way that gives researchers access to the "inside" of the social environment being studied. In his seminal article, Fine writes about what is needed to establish that rapport: ". . . illusions that are necessary for professional survival" (Fine, 1993). Among other attributes, the ethnographer has to present as a kind, friendly, honest, and interested person, or they will not be allowed into the inner circle of the community being studied. Indeed, researchers must present as having the best interest of the individuals and the community at the center of the research, even when this may be contrary to their personal and professional beliefs. Although the knowledge gained by in-depth understanding of challenging social behavior such as child abuse, pedophilia, gang life, or addiction is valuable, it may require researchers to gain access to the group or community being studied by presenting themselves in ways that are disingenuous or deceptive. From an IRB perspective, the use of incomplete disclosure or <u>deception</u> in the conduct of research will therefore be an important point of discussion. The issue of transparency, in light of the methodology necessitating incomplete disclosure or deception, has been a point of tension between ethnographers and IRBs because ethnographers may need to be less than fully transparent in order to engage people. This challenges the IRB to figure out how to make sure that the use of incomplete disclosure or deception is consistent with ethical guidelines and regulatory requirements.

   🔖 10-3

2. *Transparency in dissemination*

   Closely related to the concerns about deception are questions regarding where and how collected data are reported, with what specificity, and to whom. The social sciences have sometimes struggled with how to deal with pressure, across the research enterprise, for replicability and sharing of raw data. Ethnography takes place in natural settings and in the context of those settings as a whole, and events and observations that take place organically in such settings are difficult to reproduce. Furthermore, ethnography is commonly practiced as a solitary endeavor over a long period of time; thus the researcher may spend months (sometimes years) collecting large quantities of qualitative data. This data is often the kind of information that is not practical to share, because it cannot be deidentified. Furthermore, it may not be desirable to share simply because one could never replicate the presence of that researcher in that community, in that time and context. The information is not just facts—it consists of reflections, experiences, thoughts, and notes about those thoughts. It is as personal as any research could ever be, and thus ethnographers are not used to sharing their data (Reyes, 2018). Nonetheless, <u>data sharing</u> is an important consideration for researchers and IRBs.

⌀ 12-3

Roles and Boundaries

Roles and boundaries are two attributes of ethnographic methodology that are complex in nature and thus can be difficult to understand. These attributes affect researchers, the people participating in the research, and the research itself and are often central to the ethical and practical issues that arise in ethnography. To that end, it is important for IRBs when reviewing ethnographic studies to understand the importance of roles and boundaries and how they intersect.

Roles are how researchers present themselves to subjects in the setting. Boundaries concern what a researcher will and will not do in those roles in the context of the research. Boundaries should be set by the researcher ahead of time in order to minimize ethical dilemmas and prevent harm to subjects. The more a researcher participates with a group, the more they will have to confront problems of roles possibly conflicting with boundaries. Luvaas states: "Ethnography, more than any other social scientific method, requires its practitioners to transform who they are. To do participant-observation, the cornerstone of ethnography, we often have to learn a new language, a new lifestyle, and a new way of behaving and interacting with others" (Luvaas, 2017). For example, a researcher who is in the role of a person interested and amenable to understanding and learning about gang culture will set a boundary about not participating in a robbery. Within their roles, researchers must be clear and thoughtful about defining the limits of their involvement (boundaries) to protect both their subjects and themselves from harm.

Playing multiple roles in a setting is a function of the need of ethnographers to participate in the daily life of settings. Although roles are part of every person's life, studying in settings requires researchers to take on additional roles, formal and informal, implicit and explicit, specific to their research activities, including those that link them into a variety of relationships (de Laine, 2000). These may include roles such as volunteer, coach, church member, or friend. Rarely are researchers afforded the opportunity to choose their roles in settings; their roles are influenced by a variety of factors, including the setting, the initial status in the setting, personal characteristics (e.g., age, gender), the subjects themselves, the level of participation/involvement in the setting, and focus and context of the study (Simpson, 2007). Furthermore, researchers who conduct studies in settings they frequent (e.g., a researcher studying life at a nursing home where their parent resides) face different challenges explaining their new role within the setting and addressing any subsequent potential role confusion or ambiguity for their subjects (see, for example, Davis, 2001; Goodwin et al., 2003).

Researchers' roles may change as relationships with their subjects develop and circumstances change, although boundaries, arguably, should remain stable. Researchers commonly balance and carry out many roles simultaneously, and some may result in ethical and practical dilemmas, especially where roles overlap or conflict (e.g., being a researcher as well as a friend to a subject and witnessing them abuse a spouse; de Laine, 2000). As a result of multiple roles, there are multiple opportunities where the researcher needs to establish boundaries around what they will do with and for subjects while in their roles. Will the researcher just observe spousal abuse or will the researcher intervene? When the researcher is at a birthday party late at night observing but also participating in the celebration, will they drink with the partygoers? Or go joy riding with the young people who asked the researcher to help them get alcohol? Or babysit for the mother who needs to go to work and does not have child care? What researchers will or will not do in their roles as a researcher and a temporary community member is important, because a blurring of boundaries can result in harm to the people participating in the research. There is a power differential in the relationship between the researcher and the people being studied, and the maintenance of boundaries is the responsibility of the researcher. It is not up to subjects to refrain from asking for favors or special attention from researchers, but rather it is up to researchers to maintain a boundary around the role of researcher.

In that regard, after a number of years working as part of an academic social and behavioral IRB and consulting with ethnographers in the field, one of the authors (Murphy) observes that the inherent power differential between researcher and the researched is an initial "barrier" that researchers try to minimize by becoming more like the people being studied. As time progresses, the researcher needs more information and depends on deeper continued engagement with subjects; the people being studied thereby gain more actual power in the relationship. The researcher needs something from them, and if the subjects opted to leave, months of work would disappear. As the power differential between researcher and subject shifts, the boundaries, in terms of what the researcher is willing to do, may start to shift and can become problematic. The researcher who, for example, in the beginning may only have coffee with a subject might in a few months start driving that person to appointments or helping to pay for groceries. When roles begin to change and boundaries begin to shift, it is harder to reestablish the boundaries set at the beginning of the research. For example, we can see this dynamic in anticipating leave taking. The people who opened their lives to the researcher can feel shut out at the end of the research as their "friend" leaves, and the researcher can feel a sense of both guilt and sadness at leaving. This is but one example of the importance of maintaining boundaries, as the blurring of boundaries or boundary violations can result in harm to subjects.

IRBs can help researchers anticipate role conflict and boundary issues that can arise and the associated harms to subjects—including, for example, identifying the practical limits to confidentiality raised by mandatory reporting requirements. IRBs should ask researchers to describe in as much detail as they can the activities in which they anticipate engaging, so they can help researchers identify when they might have to step out of their role and respond (e.g., situations involving trauma, the witnessing of child abuse or neglect, or imminent harm to self or others) and create a plan for responding. The description should include situations in which researchers will collect data as well as those in which they will not collect data; this exercise helps researchers consider what aspects of a relationship will not become part of the study (e.g., discussions in a bathroom, behaviors when someone is intoxicated) and what the researcher will or will not do in the context of maintaining boundaries in the research. Furthermore, because of these complexities around roles and boundaries, IRBs should ensure that researchers have adequate expertise to conduct ethnographic research and that novice ethnographers have an adequate plan for supervision or consultation with a senior researcher during field work, all with the goal of minimizing risk to subjects.

Community Engagement, Recruitment, and Informed Consent

🖉 12-9
🖉 Section 6

Community engagement and recruitment are the essential precursors to informed consent. Engaging the community is a concrete means of showing respect for the structure and the functioning of the community, and it is necessary to have an in-depth understanding of the gatekeepers of the community. Gatekeepers are the leaders of a community who provide for the protection of the members of that community. These gatekeepers could be the village chief or queen, the tribal council, the leader of a team, a well-known activist, or the head of a gang. IRBs should help researchers identify the gatekeeper by role and function in order to ensure that researchers have appropriate permission to conduct a study within a setting. IRBs should also support researchers in mapping out an appropriate plan for soliciting community engagement in the study, recruiting individual subjects, and obtaining informed consent. Although in ethnography recruitment of individuals will generally occur by word of mouth, in field studies researchers need to do more work identifying and then engaging key informants for access to the community. IRBs need to ensure that researchers have done this in a manner that is thoughtful and ethical with regard to the community and the individuals.

Relationships between researcher and subjects in ethnography will vary in duration, intensity, tone, and depth. Requiring a comprehensive written, signed, and (in most cases) independently witnessed consent document is often seen by the IRB as evidence that the important process of informed consent was appropriately carried out, and subjects' rights and interests have been respected. Whereas such a formalized requirement seems sensible for some kinds of research, such as biomedical research in which there are a number of procedures and risks to be communicated, in field research that is for the most part minimal risk, the requirement to adhere to only one standard way to recruit, engage, or obtain informed consent can seem unreasonable. Imposing a standard process may be antithetical to the flow of the research in the way it is intended to be conducted and incompatible with different levels of participation by subjects. Furthermore, such a process may not actually protect anyone's rights or welfare, especially when such formality is culturally anathema to subjects who might be wary of "contracts" or who might fear that the researcher is a representative of the government or other authority.

Of course, to conduct research "upon" people without their agreement is contrary to ethical practice as well as to the regulations, so as with all research, ethnography requires some sort of consent process. However, given the different data collection methods that may be used, informed consent can take many different forms. Generally, consent should be a process that is related to the information needed to protect the people being studied, based on an in-depth understanding of what is happening in the study, how and where it is being conducted, and by (or with) whom. An appropriate process will enable subjects to understand what they are being asked to do and how it will affect their lives, and give them an opportunity to agree or decline. But it must also meet the needs of this multimodal, multimethod research methodology. To that end, to facilitate consent, IRBs should educate themselves about the ethnographic methodology being used in any given study and consider what approach to consent would be appropriate for that study, being flexible regarding issues such as what information is provided, how it is conveyed, to whom and in what format. There are ethical and regulatory reasons for a standard consent process, but there are also ethical and regulatory reasons for considering oral consent as an alternative, as well as alterations of consent content based on risk of participation, that provide enough information to subjects without being overwhelming. IRBs need to work with researchers to determine the most effective and efficient consent process that protects the rights and welfare of the people participating in the research, rather than requiring a uniform consent process for everyone participating in the study, because levels of participation among subjects may vary. Flexibility, including taking advantage of waivers of consent <u>documentation</u> and using an information sheet or script instead of a formal consent document, is not a compromise or inferior way of making sure people know what is going on in the research in which they are being asked to participate. The IRB can support ethnographers by helping to identify informed consent processes that are appropriate for the study and subject population.

🔗 6-5

In cases of embedded researchers collecting information about individual, family, and community functioning for months at a time, IRBs may want to know how often the individual, the social group, or the community will be reminded about being a research subject. Will consent be sought only for formal interviews? If the researcher is observing a group during activities that occur in public, such as a community gathering for sports or worship, is that different from wanting to observe activities that occur in private, such as family gatherings for birthday, wedding or other "by invitation only" events? Should researchers be required to obtain formal consent to observe cultural events that may involve illegal activity? These are all questions that the IRB has to grapple with, and their answers will depend in large part on the potential risks to the people participating in the research and to the larger community. IRBs can be creative in helping researchers figure out an appropriate way to make sure people participating in the research know what is happening and why, without it being unduly burdensome for either subjects or researchers.

Online Spaces

The questions raised in the previous chapter regarding qualitative inquiry moving into <u>online spaces</u> apply to ethnographic research. Hallett and Barber argue that conducting contemporary ethnography requires following subjects online, because life online and off-line overlap (Hallett & Barber, 2014). In some cases, the research topic will result in an ethnography where the lives examined are exclusively online (e.g., studies of online gambling websites, support groups, role-playing games). Different styles of such studies include cyber-ethnography; virtual, digital, or internet ethnography; netnography; expanded ethnography; or ethnography of virtual worlds (Caliandro, 2018). Using online spaces in ethnography may require researchers to follow subjects through a variety of online contexts (personal webpages, blogs, YouTube, Twitter, Facebook, Instagram, etc.). Doing this can be challenging, particularly methodologically, as subjects present different aspects of themselves in different spaces, often depending on the structure of the space (Hallett & Barber, 2014). The range of ethical issues that may arise also presents challenges, particularly in the realm of the <u>public versus private nature</u> of individuals' interactions and their expectations (if any)

🔗 10-5

🔗 10-1

of privacy online. While conducting ethnography off-line requires researchers to make decisions about how to present themselves before entering the field, collecting data in online spaces, particularly as an observer, does not in most cases require researchers to announce their presence or explain themselves; they can frequently "lurk" in a space without anyone knowing they are there. Whether they should do this is an ethical question, not only in terms of obtaining informed consent, but also in terms of subjects' privacy expectations.

IRBs should ensure that researchers who employ online spaces for data collection understand the applicable ethical considerations for such activities, including the range of spaces they anticipate entering, the level of privacy that users of those spaces expect, and the appropriate permissions to enter private spaces (e.g., closed chat rooms) and have an informed consent process for subjects in those spaces. As explained earlier, IRBs need to understand what is involved for individuals participating in a study and work with researchers to design an appropriate consent process based on the levels of participation and the risk that participation presents to individuals. Furthermore, whereas an IRB needs to understand the privacy limitations of whatever platform is being studied, it is worth noting that a lot of information online is publicly available, and thus its use in a study would likely present no more than minimal risk. Finally, questions remain about the validity of findings from studies of constructed online communities versus from studies of nonvirtual communities, which could result in harm to the former, particularly if the findings are undesirable (Chandler et al., 2019). Studying human behavior and social and cultural context online is not necessarily methodologically or ethically unsound, but the implications are certainly not yet fully understood. Accordingly, IRBs should determine whether researchers have adequate training to understand and handle the ". . . unique methodological and ethical issues that accompany this sort of work . . ." (Hallett & Barber, 2014, p. 325).

A Note on Illegal Behavior and IRB Review of Studies of Unsavory Characters

Ethnographic research that involves people engaging in illegal behavior may present ethical challenges for IRBs, given their mission to protect research subjects. IRBs are cautioned to approach these projects as they do other research proposals, and IRB review should always include an analysis of the probability and magnitude of harm to subjects. In ethnography, assessing and weighing the risks faced by subjects can be complicated. For example, when studying drug-using behavior, actual drug use can certainly cause harm, but if something happens in the study and the drug user is apprehended as a result of study participation, not having access to the addictive substance also can cause harm. When studying gangs, if it becomes known to other gang members that someone is talking to a researcher, contrary to gang norms, that person could be killed. It is important to remember that although the data collection procedures in a study may not in and of themselves present risk (e.g., interviews), the context of some research may create its own risk for subjects. IRBs must consider all of those risks.

In addition, exposure to illegal activity in the course of research also may expose researchers to personal dangers, both physical and emotional. Developing a relationship with a subject that leads to attempts to advise or counsel the person to get out of the illegal activity also further blurs boundaries (see, for example, Goffman, 2014). Some researchers may even believe they have a moral duty to help subjects change their behavior. While it is not an IRB's primary responsibility to protect researchers, IRBs need to be cognizant of what can go wrong when studying illegal activity and help researchers, particularly novice ethnographers, to anticipate their own risks when studying illegal behavior.

A related issue for IRB reviewers that is not unique to ethnography but is often present in ethnographic studies is the reviewers' own personal biases and reactions to applying the ethical principles of the <u>Belmont Report</u> to the protection of unsavory subjects. It can be all too easy for IRB reviewers to "throw the book" at a research project in which they find the people being studied unworthy of the usual ethical considerations and protections. For example, IRBs may find it challenging to protect the privacy and confidentiality of a study population recruited because they have an expressed interest in sex with children, who engage in human trafficking, or any number of other abhorrent behaviors. However, there is social good in understanding behaviors such as pedophilia and domestic violence, and although it can be very difficult, IRBs have a responsibility to facilitate the ethical study of perpetrators as well as victims, even when it may feel anathema to apply "respect for persons" to those who harm and degrade others.

🔗 1-1

Recommendations and Conclusion

Qualitative inquiry comes in many shapes and sizes, and so do the ethical and oversight issues raised by this type of research. These issues include the appropriateness of study design and data collection methods; the emergent nature of ethnography; the need for researchers to occupy multiple roles; and challenges surrounding setting boundaries, recruitment, informed consent, privacy and confidentiality, transparency, and leaving the setting. Based on years of experience with IRB review of ethnography and participant observation, the authors recommend the following guidelines for IRBs (which supplement the recommendations in the previous <u>chapter</u>).

🔗 10-1

- Collaboration between the IRB and ethnographers is key. Most IRB professionals and reviewers are not ethnographers and are not trained in this methodology. It is a different way of learning and conducting research and deserves informed review. Ideally, there should be an <u>expert</u> in ethnography on the board whom the IRB can consult about the nuances of the methodology and ethical conduct of a study. There are subtle differences between domestic and <u>international</u> research, so finding a board member or consultant who can do both is desirable.

🔗 3-1

🔗 10-9

- Competence to conduct ethnography is extremely important for the protection of human subjects as well as to the success of the study. Competence is not just education and training or even previous research experience; competence is a demonstrated ability to make ethical decisions in the field. Field research does not take place in a controlled environment such as a lab or office, and all kinds of things that were not anticipated can occur (in part due to the emergent nature of ethnographic research). Because novice researchers have less experience making quick decisions in the field, IRBs should not only evaluate whether researchers can follow the protocol but also whether they demonstrate an understanding of what can go wrong and how they should respond in such situations. This is particularly crucial in terms of anticipating and minimizing harm to subjects if something

9-1

unexpected happens. Ethnography is a complex research methodology. IRBs should ensure that researchers, particularly students, are well prepared, particularly if subjects are <u>vulnerable</u>.

- An important ability related to competence is understanding that there is an inherent tendency to overidentify with the people being studied, especially if they are people in need. Less experienced researchers can lose objectivity, get overinvolved, and develop dual relationships that compromise subjects and the research. There is a body of qualitative research literature addressing when researchers go astray in the field, including having sexual relationships with subjects, committing illegal acts, and having subjects

10-1

become dependent upon them (as explained in the <u>previous chapter</u>). IRBs need to ask researchers to address this specific issue if their research proposal indicates full participation/immersion in settings and how they are going to prevent themselves from "going native." This is particularly important if subjects are vulnerable or the researcher is a novice; for the latter, the IRB should require a specific plan for ongoing consultation with a senior researcher who is not in the field and who understands the challenges of field work.

- Finally, the authors highly recommend the Iphofen report, "Research Ethics in Ethnography/Anthropology," as a resource for any IRB that reviews studies using ethnography as a primary method (Iphofen, 2015). The report's primary audience is ethics review committees who might not be familiar with the methods regularly adopted by ethnographers. The report is available online.

Ethnography and observation are labor intensive and time-consuming methods of research that can provide a depth and breadth of information that adds astounding color and valence to understanding human behavior and the social environment. IRBs can work collaboratively with these dedicated researchers so that the oversight review process adds value to their research and is not unduly burdensome.

References

Adler, P. A., & Adler, P. (1987). *Membership roles in field research.* Sage Publications.

American Association of University Professors (AAUP). (2000). *Institutional review boards and social science research: A report on protecting human beings.* www.aaup.org/AAUP/comm/rep/A/protecting.htm

Beauchamp, T. L. (1982). *Ethical issues in social science research.* Johns Hopkins University Press.

Bell, K. (2018). The "problem" of undesigned relationality: Ethnographic fieldwork, dual roles and research ethics. *Ethnography, 20*(1), 8–26.

Caliandro, A. (2018). Digital methods: Analytical concepts for ethnographers exploring social media environments. *Journal of Contemporary Ethnography, 47*(5), 551–578.

Chandler, J., Rosenzweig, C., Moss, A. J., Robinson, J., & Litman, L. (2019). Online panels in social science research: Expanding sampling methods beyond Mechanical Turk. *Behavior Research Methods, 51*(5), 2022–2038.

Davis, H. (2001). The management of self: Practical and emotional implications of ethnographic work in a public hospital setting. In K. R. Gilbert (Ed.), *The emotional nature of qualitative research* (pp. 37–61). CRC Press.

de Laine, M. (2000). *Fieldwork, participation and practice: Ethics and dilemmas in qualitative research.* Sage Publications.

Denzin, N. K. (2008). Evolution of qualitative research. In L. M. Given (Ed.), *The SAGE encyclopedia of qualitative research methods.* Sage Publications.

DeWalt, K. M., & DeWalt, B. R. (2002). *Participant observation: A guide for fieldworkers.* AltaMira Press.

Fine, G. 1993. Ten lies of ethnography: Moral dilemmas of field research. *Journal of Contemporary Ethnography, 22*(3), 267–294.

Fox, R. C. (2004). Observations and reflections of a perpetual fieldworker. *Annals of the Academy of Political and Social Science, 595*, 309–326.

Freilich, M. (1970). Toward a formalization of field work. In M. Freilich (Ed.), *Marginal natives: Anthropologists at work* (pp. 485–585). Harper and Row Publishers.

Gans, H. J. (1982). The participant observer as a human being: Observations on the personal aspects of fieldwork. In R. G. Burgess (Ed.), *Field research: A sourcebook and field manual* (pp. 53–61). George Allen and Unwin (Publishers).

Goffman, A. (2014). *On the run: Fugitive life in an American city*. Picador/Farrar, Straus and Giroux.

Gold, R. L. (1958). Roles in sociological field observations. *Social Forces, 36*, 217–223.

Goodwin, D., Pope, C., Mort, M., & Smith, A. (2003). Ethics and ethnography: An experiential account. *Qualitative Health Research, 13*, 567–577.

Hallett, R. E., & Barber, K. (2014). Ethnographic research in a cyber era. *Journal of Contemporary Ethnography, 43*(3), 306–330.

Iphofen, R. (2015). *Research ethics in ethnography/anthropology*. European Commission, Directorate General for Research and Innovation. http://ec.europa.eu/research/participants/data/ref/h2020/other/hi/ethics-guide-ethnog-anthrop_en.pdf

Lewis, S., & Russell, A. (2011). Being embedded: A way forward for ethnographic research. *Ethnography, 12*(3), 398–416.

Lockyer, S. (2008). Qualitative research, history of. In L. M. Given (Ed.), *The SAGE encyclopedia of qualitative research methods*. Sage Publications.

Luvaas, B. (2017). Unbecoming: The aftereffects of autoethnography. *Ethnography, 20*(2), 245–262.

Newmahr, S., & Hannem, S. (2018). Surrogate ethnography: Fieldwork, the academy, and resisting the IRB. *Journal of Contemporary Ethnography, 47*(1), 3–27.

Reyes, V. (2018). Three models of transparency in ethnographic research: Naming places, naming people, and sharing data. *Ethnography, 19*(2), 204–226.

Sanders, C. R. (1980). Rope burns: Impediments to the achievement of basic comfort early in the field research experience. In W. B. Shaffir, R. A. Stebbins, & A. Turowetz (Eds.), *Fieldwork experience: Qualitative approaches to social research*. St. Martin's Press.

Schwandt, T. A. (2015). *The Sage dictionary of qualitative inquiry* (4th ed.). Sage Publications.

Simpson, J. F. (2007). More than simply "hanging out": The nature of participant observation and research relationships [Unpublished doctoral dissertation]. Durham, NH: University of New Hampshire.

Spradley, J. P. (1980). *Participant observation*. Holt, Rinehart and Winston.

Research Involving Deception

Melissa Abraham
Ivor Pritchard

Abstract

Deception is a common research technique in studies examining human behavior. This chapter discusses research where subjects are intentionally deceived about the research. Deception is generally acceptable in studies where the deception cannot be avoided, the knowledge to be gained is seen as meaningful, and the harms of participation, including those of the deception itself, are seen as minimal. When deception is used, the researchers should justify why it is necessary to accomplish their aims and how they plan to conduct the study. The aim of this chapter is to outline how to evaluate the use of deception and related research methods when reviewing research studies.

Background

If people know what is expected of them or that their behavior is being judged, they may act differently than they would otherwise. To observe and understand how people behave or respond to certain conditions, researchers may need to disguise their observation or lead people to believe something that has been fabricated or is untrue. Research should be scientifically valid, and certain studies of behavior will be scientifically valid only if the subjects are led to believe something false.

Researchers have used deception in research involving humans for over a century (Korn, 1997). Social psychology studies have frequently used deception to answer questions of how and why people behave in certain scenarios. More recently, neuroscience, biomedical, and health services researchers have been borrowing methods from social and psychological research and using them in new areas that IRBs can find novel and challenging to review.

At the same time, withholding truth or misleading individuals, however benign, goes against an essential principle of ethical research: Respect for persons normally requires the informed consent of individuals to participate in research, which implies that they are fully aware of the actual purpose and procedures of study participation. Because of this, the use of deception has been debated extensively.

What Is Deception?

There is some variation regarding how the term *deception* is used and to what it applies. Joan Sieber, an influential psychologist in the field, defines deception as

> research in which subjects are purposely allowed to or caused to have false beliefs or assumptions or to accept as false that which is true, and in which the researcher studies their reactions; the reactions and the study of those reactions are made possible by the incorrect beliefs of the subject. (Sieber, 1983)

Deception in the strict sense entails deceit, i.e., lying or otherwise manipulating someone's beliefs, such as providing false feedback or using research associates (actors) to contrive situations that are misperceived by the subject. Methods that are also sometimes called "deception" but are somewhat different include intentionally withholding aspects of the study purpose or procedures (incomplete disclosure), "authorized deception" (telling someone they will not be told about some aspect of the study purpose or procedure), and observing people who are not aware their behavior is being observed. Although the ethical concerns are different when subjects are not told lies, compared to when they are truly deceived, within the context of IRB review and application of regulations, the use of these methods is often grouped with actual deception, because they all preclude obtaining informed consent as prescribed by the regulations 45 CFR 46.116(a-c).

It is important that the IRB reviewers and researchers have a good understanding of the concept of deception being used and that they be able to interpret properly how the deception might be experienced by the research subject. Reviewers and researchers should assess the use of deception and interpret its risks and benefits.

For the purposes of discussion, the following are four general categories of use of deception and related methods in human subjects research:

1. *Outright deception.* Misleading people who are aware of their participation in research, but not of the deception
2. *Covert deception.* Having people participate in research without being aware of their participation
3. *Incomplete disclosure.* Withholding significant information from people who knowingly participate in the research
4. *Authorized deception.* Withholding information or misleading people who agree to being ignorant or deceived

Outright Deception

In studies involving outright deception, a subject enrolls in a study and provides informed consent that involves deception. This is probably the type of deception that has attracted the most attention.

In some classic studies in the 1950s, Solomon Asch used outright deception to conduct studies on conformity (Asch, 1955) to see whether people would agree with others' judgments even though those judgments were clearly incorrect. In his experiments, a group of individuals were put together and asked to compare the length of a line on one card to the length of three different lines on another card and to indicate which of the three lines was the same length as the line on the first card. This task was repeated for a series of card pairs. Only one of the individuals was actually a research subject, while the others were research associates pretending to be subjects. For some card pairs, the associates all agreed on a wrong answer about the length of lines, prior to the real subject being asked to make a judgment. The studies showed that most people resisted the group pressure, but some conformed and answered incorrectly like the research associates (Asch, 1955).

Some of the subjects became worried, surprised, and paused before answering, and often showed embarrassment. At the time, concern for the experience of the subjects in such experiments, such as might be raised by IRBs now, was uncommon to nonexistent. Some of the subjects did feel some distress, but this was largely thought to be small enough to be acceptable because the study resulted in important findings that might benefit society.

Stanley Milgram's studies of obedience from 1960 to 1963 triggered widespread debate about the ethics of the use of deception. Milgram's studies are considered some of the most impressive and informative experiments in psychology. Residents of New Haven and Bridgeport, Connecticut, were asked to participate in a study examining learning, where one subject would be the "teacher," and a second subject would be the "learner." The teacher would give the learner a word pairing task, and whenever the learner gave an incorrect answer, the teacher was instructed to administer an electrical shock to the learner, using what appeared to be an electrical shock machine. The machine was fake, and the person who was assigned to be the "learner" was actually a research associate who deliberately made mistakes and pretended to be shocked. The machine indicated that shocks ranged from "slight shock" to "Danger—severe shock," followed by "XXX" (Milgram, 1974).

The real purpose of the study, hidden by the research associates, was to study obedience to authority. Many ingenious details went into this design to create a very convincing atmosphere so that the subjects believed the deception, including the electric shocks, were real. However, the true purpose of the study was to examine what people would do when they were directed to inflict pain on another person for no good reason, and what their behavior would be when an authority figure directed them to continue despite protests of discomfort or great pain by the "learner." Before the studies began, most people believed that others would always stop before the painful shock level. No one predicted that even when the "learner" pounded on the wall, yelling in pain, about 65% of subjects did not stop using the shock machine. They administered the highest levels of shock, with the authority figure providing encouragement with statements such as, "It is absolutely essential that you continue" (Milgram, 1974). However, Milgram reported that even though they kept giving the shocks, many of the "teachers" became quite upset. Many have since pointed out how these studies produced important knowledge (without the "learner" experiencing any true physical pain or harm) that would not have been able to be obtained otherwise. Milgram believed they shed light on how ordinary people would follow orders and could commit atrocities such as the Holocaust (Milgram, 1974).

Another example of outright deception is the use of the "placebo run-in" used in clinical trial designs. In some trials, there is a substantial likelihood that there will be placebo responders, subjects who might report an improvement or worsening of symptoms or side effects when they are given what they think

🖉 1-2

is a medication, based on their own unconscious expectations. In an attempt to exclude placebo responders from trials of medications where the experience and reporting of symptoms could be influenced by this "expectancy effect," some researchers will use a "placebo run-in" design, where the subject is led to believe the pill they take is active medication, when it is actually a substance without any active ingredients. This method has been called into question as to whether it causes bias toward active treatment in clinical trials (e.g., Senn, 1997), but it is sometimes used as an acceptable method when it is thought to be effective and important in excluding subjects with this tendency, so that the "true effect" of the medication could be studied.

Covert Deception

In the preceding examples, the subject is told something false about the study purpose or procedures. In other studies involving deception, subjects are unaware they are in a study, but their environment has been manipulated so that a false belief or assumption is allowed to occur. This deception is typically temporary and frequently involves a research associate who does not reveal their researcher identity. In such cases, *disclosure and consent are absent* at the start of the study procedures.

For example, in research on bystander behavior, people are not told that a research study is being conducted and are exposed to a controlled situation or experience in which their responses and reactions are being observed covertly by researchers. For example, a research associate may act as if they are experiencing a medical emergency on the subway platform to learn how people will respond. The research associate may be a white or black man or woman, dressed in a suit or in dirty clothing, in order to examine how race, gender/sex, and appearance play a role in the response of the bystanders. Latané and Darley (1969) staged emergencies to examine responses and found that if other bystanders were present, the rate of someone stepping forward to help a person in distress fell to 40%, compared to 70% when there was no other bystander. This was considered important knowledge about human behavior, and to many, well worth the temporary distress of the subject during the study. Many elaborate and similar studies were conducted in this vein. In 1965, Humphreys began what became a controversial study involving deception, in which he covertly observed men having sex with men in a public bathroom. Humphreys subsequently interviewed the subjects to obtain background information about them, having used their car license numbers to identify them and then posed as a health services surveyor to obtain their cooperation for the interviews (Humphreys, 1970). In recent decades, ethical concerns for the discomfort of subjects in these situations has led to a decline in such covert research.

A more recent example of covert deception is studies involving "secret shoppers" (Rhodes & Miller, 2012). For example, a research associate acting as a "patient" calls an insurance company to sign up for an individual coverage plan. They use a script in which the demographic information supplied to the insurance representative varies by race, age, and other traits, to examine aspects of discrimination in applying for coverage. Typically, in this type of study, debriefing of the insurance representative on the phone would not occur if adequate protections of confidentiality are in place.

There is no satisfactory alternative to deception in order to conduct these types of studies; for example, if you ask someone to imagine how they will react in this situation, they may tell you what they think they would do, but you will not be able to observe their actual reactions. And the situation must be realistic to enable to researcher to evaluate the person being observed. Studies in general on bystanders, along with other topics social psychologists study, such as aggression, motivation, attitude, and behavior research, all may require concealing a truth from their subjects in order to examine that truth. However, although these types of studies may reveal important societal truths about bias or discrimination, the experience of the subject during and after the study procedures should still be carefully considered.

Incomplete Disclosure

Some studies use incomplete disclosure, in which the study's purpose or reason for procedures is withheld from the subjects. For example, subjects are told they are taking a test as part of a research study to examine how well they do on a timed reading comprehension test. In reality, the temperature in the room is being manipulated to see how it affects performance on the test (but the researcher does not mention this). There is nothing "untrue" in what the researcher discloses, but the full purpose of the study has intentionally been omitted from the consent information.

Authorized Deception

In authorized deception or "disclosed concealment" studies, the researcher specifically informs subjects that they will be participating in a research study in which some information about the purpose or procedures in the study will be withheld or will be misrepresented, and the subject consents to being misled (Miller et al., 2005). For example, subjects might be told during the consent process that they are in a study examining how well they do on an intelligence test but that there are some things about the study that they cannot be told until afterward. In truth, the study examines the effect of receiving false feedback about the results of the test on the subjects' self-perception. (The study includes debriefing the subjects when they complete their participation.)

Arguments for and Against Deception

Is deception research wrong? It may be helpful to keep in mind that deception comes in many forms and practices in modern society, some of which are considered unethical, some of which are not, and some of which are controversial (Benham, 2008). Many people think politicians and used car salespeople who try to deceive others are wrong. On the other hand, deception is an integral part of magic shows, card games, theatrical performances, and many sports, such as football, baseball, basketball, and tennis. Many people approve of these activities and admire those who participate in them who are good at deception. Covert observation is acceptable in many circumstances, such as unmarked police cars, traffic cameras, and surveillance cameras. In the activities that society considers acceptable, the individuals who are deceived understand and accept that they may be deceived, and that the deception is an inherent part of the activity. The activity in which there is deception or covert observation is valued because of the enjoyment or benefits it provides.

The same thinking can be applied to deception in research: if the research findings are valuable in some way, and deception is accepted as an integral part of the research, then the research may be ethical. To the degree that the subjects can accept the possibility of deception, this is more consistent with respect for persons, because the subjects are making an autonomous choice. Authorized deception and incomplete disclosure are easier to justify on this basis than outright deception or covert observation. Arguably, outright deception is easier to justify than covert deception, because at least the subject is aware that they are participating in research. Deception may be unethical, on the other hand, if the person who is deceived has not accepted the possibility of deception and may be harmed or wronged through participation in research.

Potential Discomforts, Harms, and Other Drawbacks

The research ethics literature includes many examples in which deception has been used to answer questions of varying scientific value and contains diverse commentary on the potential harms of research involving deception. Debates about the harms of deception grew after the Milgram studies, despite the fascination and excitement about the study findings at the time. Some have claimed the harms to the Milgram study subjects were underreported (Baumrind, 1964, 1985; Kelman, 1972). Debate continues to this day about the role of deception in research and how it should or should not be utilized in experimental designs. Some have argued that the use of deception is wrong, even when one has permission from an individual to deceive them under specified circumstances. In addition, it has been proposed that engaging in deception as a researcher erodes one's own ethical sensibilities (Baumrind, 1985). On the other side, the use of deception in research might be justified as part of the larger argument that there is a general obligation for people to contribute to the advancement of science, because of the social benefits that scientific advances make possible (Faden et al., 2013).

What are the potential individual harms and discomforts? Are there potential harms to the research enterprise when deception is utilized? Kelman (1972) stated that deception was harmful to subjects, the profession of psychology, and to society in general. He highlighted the unequal power relationship in the research situation but concluded that, if the study is "very important and no alternative methods are available," then very mild forms of deception might be justified. Baumrind (1964) wrote that researchers should avoid research procedures that may "involve loss of dignity, self-esteem, and trust in rational authority." For a subject, finding out that they were misled by a researcher could lead to anger, feeling offended, and feeling used. In this view, deception itself (even if socially acceptable), makes people feel exploited and diminished, resulting in a general harm of making people more suspicious of each other and less willing to participate in research. At the same time, in some studies there is no meaningful harm or invasion of privacy, for example, seeing if people who are near a nice-smelling bakery in a mall are more likely to offer money to a stranger (Baron, 1997).

Deception can have negative consequences when people are put into an uncomfortable situation they might have avoided if they had known what was going to be done to them. Researchers often want to gain a better understanding of the types of human behavior that people are not especially proud of. Deception can lead to harm or discomfort when subjects are unwittingly put into a position where the research procedure or intervention makes them feel embarrassed, ashamed, guilty, frightened, or angry. Deception could also lead to an invasion of privacy that a knowing subject would have refused to allow. Christensen (1988) found that people were more concerned about the use of deception when it invaded privacy than when nonprivate behavior was observed. At the end of study participation, subjects may learn something about themselves that might bring about shame or discomfort, sometimes called "in-flicted insight," as illustrated by the Milgram studies. Even if this information is kept confidential from others, the potential negative experience of this new awareness should be considered and mitigated.

In general, withholding aspects of the purpose or nature of a study while obtaining consent to participate is of less concern to autonomy and respect than not informing people they are part of a research study at all, because at least they have some awareness of their participation in the practice of research. Deception becomes more difficult to justify if the research is likely to result in harm to the subjects: The American Psychological Association's guidelines state that "Psychologists do not deceive prospective participants about research that is reasonably expected to cause physical pain or severe emotional distress" (American Psychological Association, 2017). Yet some have argued in favor of research studies in which there is no consent, on the grounds that the society of today has benefitted from the knowledge gained in earlier research studies involving human subjects, and therefore they have inherited a reciprocal obligation to participate themselves for the public good (Schaefer, 2009). This could sometimes include deception research, especially given the expanding scope of deception research in different areas, but this argument does rely on the critical significance of the research. However, some question this argument based on concerns about the obligatory nature of research and power dynamics (Rennie, 2011).

It may be crucial to the approval of a study that findings about individuals' behaviors in deception studies are kept anonymous, so that the subject understands they cannot be linked to the specific behaviors they had shown, and if anonymity is not possible, that confidentiality is strictly preserved. In some cases, when findings might cause shame, some advocate for the importance of offering people the opportunity to withdraw their data from use, for example, if it involved a recording of their behavior.

Role Conflict

When deception research is conducted in a medical or clinical setting, there is another layer that IRBs should consider: If an individual is misled, even in a benign fashion, by their own doctor or therapist or another person in whom they are otherwise putting great trust (e.g., a child's doctor or care provider, teacher, etc.), the simple fact of having been told an untruth or "not the whole truth" can have effects that go beyond the study. If the research is done in a setting (such as their church or school) where the subject is deceived by people they entrust with material, emotional, or other valuables, they can similarly feel negative repercussions beyond the study that affect their relationship with these people or entities. It is important that the IRB think through these layers and consider the internal reactions that subjects might have to being recruited, participating in, and being debriefed about research involving deception or incomplete disclosure. At times this may involve obtaining input from patients, students, or others who would be in their shoes or from those who have clinical or other relevant experience that could help assess the potential for harm in these areas.

Research Involving Children

Studies involving deception with <u>children</u> add a set of developmental considerations. For example, conducting a study to examine children's responses to

📎 9-6

peer rejection may have important scientific or educational value, yet the question about whether debriefing is an adequate remedy to the risks should be raised. After being deceived, a child might believe that "adults lie"; their parent may feel the child was used as a "guinea pig"; or the child may not believe the debriefing. The child might be left with knowledge about themselves and how they reacted that they may not be prepared to absorb, resulting in greater harm compared to that experienced by a more psychologically mature adult population (Fisher, 2005). Studies that involve injury to self-esteem or negative feelings warrant a close look and careful determination that the risk is indeed minimal.

Regulatory Issues for IRBs

Review and approval of deception research requires that the proposed research study be acceptable, in the necessary absence of fully informed consent, on the condition that <u>waiver</u> or alteration of consent is acceptable. In nonexempt studies regulated under the Common Rule, deception research must satisfy the other regulatory criteria for the approval of research, in particular the criteria that "risks to subjects are minimized" [45 CFR 46.111(a)(1)] and "risks to subjects are reasonable in relation to anticipated benefits, if any, to the subjects, and the importance of the knowledge that may reasonably be expected to result" [45 CFR 46.111(a)(2)]. As discussed earlier, it is arguable that some deception studies cannot be approved and/or should not be carried out.

6-4

The 2018 Common Rule identifies five criteria to apply to proposed non-exempt research where informed consent will be waived or altered [45 CFR 46.116(f)]. Four of these criteria pertain to deception research, and these will be addressed next. (The fifth criterion, which is new to the regulations, pertains to the secondary research use of biospecimens or data). The IRB can only approve studies with a waiver or alteration of informed consent if the criteria are met.

- The research has to be *impracticable without the waiver or alteration of informed consent* [45 CFR 46.116(f)(3)(ii)].

  Typically, deception research proposals claim that the research cannot be done if there is informed consent. As described previously, informing the subjects beforehand of what the research is about, or even letting them know that research is being conducted, is expected to influence the subjects' behavior in such a way as to prevent the researchers from finding out what they want to know. However, this does not always mean that informed consent should be discarded entirely; often it is true that the prospective subjects can know that they are being asked to participate in research and can be given some relevant information about the research and the opportunity to decide whether to participate. Prospective subjects in psychology experiments involving deception often understand that they will be participating in research and can be given information that may influence their decisions (e.g., how long the research will take to carry out), without invalidating the scientific design. When this is true, informed consent may be either altered or waived.

  6-2

  If alteration of informed consent is considered, the regulatory provision that allows alteration states that the <u>general requirements</u> for informed consent, some of which are new in the 2018 Common Rule, cannot be altered and therefore still apply to the informed consent [45 CFR 46.116(f)(2) and 45 CFR 46.116(a)]. The general requirements include having to give prospective subjects information about the reasons why one might or might not want to participate in the research. Any information that would have been included in the standard (unaltered) informed consent can only be omitted from the altered informed consent if the informed consent will still satisfy those requirements.

For example, if knowing the purposes of the research would not be likely to change prospective subjects' willingness to participate, then those purposes would not need to be disclosed to prospective subjects. If, on the other hand, it would be reasonable to think that the information about the purposes of the research could influence prospective subjects' decision to participate, then alteration of consent would not be allowable. Imagine a deception research study in which investigators want to compare subjects' prejudices about people of different religions; disclosing this purpose would probably affect the subjects' responses, and it would also be reasonable to think that knowing this purpose might affect someone's willingness to participate in the research. If this is true, alteration of consent would not be approvable. The IRB could still approve a waiver of consent for such a study, provided that the criteria for waiver of consent are satisfied. In addition, when waiving consent, the IRB could also approve as a condition of the research that prospective subjects be given information about the study before they participate in the study, e.g., information about the procedures of the study, a statement that they can stop participating at any time, etc.

- *The research must involve no more than minimal risk* **[45 CFR 46.116(f)(3)(i)]**. The principle here is that people should not be exposed to considerable risk of harm if they have not made an informed decision to participate. According to the federal regulations, "*Minimal risk* means that the probability and magnitude of harm or discomfort anticipated in the research are not greater in and of themselves than those ordinarily encountered in daily life or during the performance of routine physical or psychological examinations or tests" **[45 CFR 46.102(j)]**. Historically, the minimal risk standard has been difficult to apply in some instances, and different IRBs presented with the same study have disagreed about whether it is minimal risk or more than that (Shah et al., 2004). IRB members often rely on their intuitive reactions in applying the minimal risk standard, and it is likely that these intuitions may be subject to various biases, such as whether the considered discomfort is familiar or not. If possible, it may be worthwhile to consider whether other similar studies have already been conducted, and whether evidence is available about how much or how frequently subjects experienced negative reactions.

The regulatory requirements actually contain two standards, either one of which may be employed in a particular case, depending on the particular study: (1) the probability and magnitude of harm or discomfort ordinarily encountered in daily life or (2) the probability and magnitude of discomfort encountered during the performance of routine physical or psychological examinations or tests. If a research study involves the possibility of the harm or discomfort of something that is actually part of daily life, such as being required to wait for 5 minutes with nothing to do, the daily life standard would be appropriate; likewise, if the research involves the administration of a routine psychological test, e.g., the Rorschach or the Thematic Apperception Test (TAT), the routine physical or psychological test standard could be utilized. At the same time, it should be noted that the possible harm or discomfort of participating in a research study does not have to be the same as those of daily life or examinations or tests, but rather only no greater in probability and/or magnitude combined; a research study could involve a completely contrived harm or discomfort never experienced in daily life or used in examinations or tests, so long as the risk of the harm or discomfort is small and unlikely enough.

- *The research cannot adversely affect the rights and welfare of the subjects* [45 CFR 46.116(f)(3)(iv)].

  In addressing the rights of the subjects, this regulatory standard cannot be referring to a right of informed consent to research, since this would mean that waivers could never be permitted. Rather, it means that there must not be some other right—such as the right to agree to or refuse medical treatment—that would be negatively affected by the waiver and associated research study. Welfare is not defined or explained in the regulation, and it is a fairly general term; however, the term is commonly used to refer to the more positive features of people's lives and circumstances, rather than the negative ones. As such, the regulation should probably be interpreted to include not having a negative impact on the positive aspects of subjects' lives, such as their sense of security, contentment, or opportunities, and not just avoiding actual negative consequences such as pain, impairment, shame, or loss.

- *The subjects must be provided with additional pertinent information after participation, whenever it is appropriate* [45 CFR 46.116(f)(3)(v)].

  This standard seems to directly address deception research specifically. As discussed earlier, the justification for deception research often involves the notion that the subject would otherwise be entitled to be informed about the research, but for the fact that having that information could invalidate the research. Once the research is over, that justification for withholding information or misleading subjects no longer holds. Respect for the subject would seem to dictate that, if possible, subjects deserve to be told afterward what happened to them in the research study or the true purpose of the study. Debriefing may also serve to uphold subjects' autonomy by including the opportunity to withdraw the subject's data from the study, although this is not always an option. Furthermore, debriefing is considered to serve as a way of ameliorating some negative effects of participation in a research study; for example, if a research study was designed to find out if an intervention caused the subject to believe something false about themselves, debriefing could be used to relieve the subject of that misperception, which might also eliminate a potential harm. Additionally, debriefing is often offered as part of the justification for including undergraduate students in research studies; the educational gains of participation in research would ostensibly be heightened if the subjects are presented with an explanation of how they were involved in research and why deception was required.

  There are some arguments against debriefing or about how debriefing may fall short. In some cases, such as staged experiments in natural environments where the subjects do not know they are participating in research, it is sometimes impracticable to debrief the subjects. For studies recruiting undergraduate students from an organized student subject pool, researchers might not want to debrief subjects because of a concern that debriefed subjects will inform other prospective subjects about the true nature of the research study, and thereby "contaminate" those prospective subjects. One way to address this problem might be to delay debriefing until all the subjects have participated. Another problem is whether the debriefing actually accomplishes its purpose: In a recent study addressing the lack of research attention to this question, researchers found that various debriefing strategies did not fully relieve the subjects of the negative feelings they experienced through participation in the research study (Miketta & Friese, 2019). This would seem to put the onus on the field to develop more effective debriefing procedures for researchers whose research involves deliberately inducing negative experiences in their subjects (Smith & Richardson, 1983). Something similar may be said about participation and debriefing as an educational tool: There is scant evidence to show that the experience of participating as a subject in a research study provides a meaningful learning experience. Similarly, the "antidote" to the damage that might have been temporarily experienced during some studies with deception is not fully understood.

🖋 5-3

The federal regulations include an <u>exemption</u> (new in the 2018 regulations) for research involving benign behavioral interventions, which may include a kind of deception [**45 CFR 46.104(d)(3)**]. The exemption requires the "prospective agreement" of the subject, and so this exemption does not cover deception research where the subjects are completely unaware of being involved in research. Prospective agreement is not necessarily the same as informed consent, however, but rather just requires that the subject is aware of and agrees to participate in research and has been made aware of the intervention and information collection [**45 CFR 46.104(d) (3)(i)**]. This awareness does not need to include specific disclosure of exactly what the research question is, and so deception may be part of one of these exempt studies. If the research involves deception regarding the nature or purposes of the research, the prospective agreement must include being told that the subject will be unaware of or misled regarding the nature or purposes of the research [**45 CFR 46.104(d)(3)(iii)**]. The exemption does limit the kinds of research studies that may be included, because the exemption only covers studies where the interventions are "… brief in duration, harmless, painless, not physically invasive, not likely to have a significant adverse lasting impact on the subjects, and the investigator has no reason to think the subjects will find the interventions offensive or embarrassing" [**45 CFR 46.104(d)(3)(ii)**]. Here again, for some studies it will be quite obvious whether they fit the exemption, whereas others are questionable. For the latter, there may be other studies already conducted where there was evidence related to subject discomfort or the absence thereof. Another option might be to describe the study to some number of individuals from the target subject population and ask them how they think they would react. Unlike research involving fully informed consent, prospective agreement to deception research may leave out information that would enable the prospective subjects to anticipate that they might find the research uncomfortable, embarrassing, or offensive.

Ethical Issues

The use of deception has been treated variably by IRBs, from restricting to banning the practice (Boynton et al., 2013). The preceding discussion has identified a number of ethical issues as being pertinent when considering research involving some type of deception (see box, Ethical Issues in Deception Research).

ETHICAL ISSUES IN DECEPTION RESEARCH

- The validity of the study design and the potential importance of the study findings, in terms of the contribution to scientific knowledge, social policy, or social improvement
- The degree to which the lack or incompleteness of informed consent required by the study limits or eliminates the autonomy of the subjects
- Potential harms to individual subjects, including negative emotional impact on mood or self-esteem, shame, or embarrassment
- Potential harms to individual subjects or others who may be affected by actions taken by people who are unaware that the situation has been "staged" for research purposes
- The possibility of inflicted insight for individual subjects who may learn something about themselves that they might not wish to know
- Respecting the privacy of individual subjects
- Whether and when debriefing of subjects will occur, and the quality and effectiveness of debriefing in terms of remediating harms, correcting false information, and providing educational value
- Potential damage to the reputation of the research enterprise or to professional researchers who routinely conduct deception research
- Whether the researcher also occupies another role in relation to the individual subjects, e.g., care provider, teacher, or authority figure, such that carrying out the research study may have an impact on the quality of this other relationship

Guidelines and Implementation

As described in this chapter, there is considerable variety in the ethical propriety and value of deception research studies, and deception research proposals should be evaluated carefully. Although some deception research studies would clearly be unethical, it is hard to justify an across-the-board prohibition of its use. It is important that IRBs not see deception as a "dirty word," as it can be justified by scientific value. However, this value should not be determined by a researcher in isolation (National Research Council, 2003). The primary interest of the researcher is to pursue scientific knowledge, whereas the IRB may be in a better position to consider the ethical interests of all parties concerned. It is important to see the IRB as being in a position to improve the conduct of a study involving deception and ensuring that ethical issues have been appropriately attended to, rather than simply blocking the use of deception. In order to perform this function, an IRB should obtain information about the proposed research study and its justification from the researcher, so that it can perform an informed evaluation of the study and consider whether revisions would improve its ethical status The researcher should provide convincing evidence to the IRB that the research is sufficiently important to warrant the deception and demonstrate that the study design and methods are scientifically sound, in order to justify as an ethical matter a waiver or alteration in the standard informed consent process for research. The researcher should provide the IRB with information that addresses the guidelines that an IRB should consider in its decision making (see box, General Guidelines for IRB Review).

GENERAL GUIDELINES FOR IRB REVIEW

1. The value of the study should be sufficient to warrant waiving some aspects of the requirement for full disclosure in the informed consent process.
2. There should be no feasible alternative to the use of deception/incomplete disclosure for addressing the scientific question in a valid manner. The researcher should be able to justify the proposed methods by providing a scientific rationale and by verifying that there are no comparable alternatives to the design to achieve the goals.
3. When appropriate, subjects could be informed prospectively of the use of deception/incomplete disclosure and consent to its use, for example:

   "In some research studies, the investigators cannot tell you exactly what the study is about before you participate in the study. We will describe the tasks in the study in a general way, but we can't explain the real purpose of the study until after you complete these tasks. When you are done, we will explain why we are doing this study, what we are looking at, and any other information you should know about this study. You will also be able to ask any questions you might have about the study's purpose and the tasks you did. Though we may not be able to explain the real purpose of the study until after you complete the tasks, there are no additional risks to those that have been described in this consent form."

4. Studies in which the deception would likely affect individuals' willingness to participate should be justified by a compelling rationale.
5. Deception research should not cause significant harms to the welfare of the subjects and should incur no more than minimal risk.
6. Debriefing is done, when appropriate, using methods likely to remediate harms, reestablish trust, and provide educational benefits. If applicable, there should be a description of the methods to be used for prompt disclosure and debriefing of each subject as soon as possible after their participation is complete. This description should explain how the debriefing will ensure that the subjects leave the research setting with a clear and accurate understanding of the deception/incomplete disclosure. If appropriate, the statement should describe how subjects may withdraw their data if they wish. A script or written statement of the debriefing should be included, if feasible. If immediate or delayed debriefing is not planned, this should be justified.

References

American Psychological Association. (2017). *Ethical principles of psychologists and code of conduct: Section 8.07 on deception in research.* www.apa.org/ethics/code/

Asch, S. (1955). Opinions and social pressure. *Scientific American, 193*(5), 31–35.

Baron, R. A. (1997). The sweet smell of ... helping: Effects of pleasant ambient fragrance on prosocial behavior in shopping malls. *Personality & Social Psychology Bulletin 23*(5), 498–503.

Baumrind, D. (1964). Some thoughts on ethics of research: After reading Milgram's "Behavioral Study of Obedience." *American Psychologist, 19*(6), 421–423.

Baumrind, D. (1985). Research using intentional deception: Ethical issues revisited. *American Psychologist, 40*(2), 165–174.

Benham, B. (2008). The ubiquity of deception and the ethics of deceptive research. *Bioethics, 22*(3), 147–156.

Boynton, M. H., Portnoy, D. B., & Johnson, B. T. (2013). Exploring the ethics and psychological impact of deception in psychological research. *IRB, 35*(2), 7–13.

Christensen, L. (1988). Deception in psychological research: When is its use justified? *Personality and Social Psychology Bulletin, 14*(4), 664–675.

Faden, R. R., Kass, N. E., Goodman, S. N., Pronovost, P., Tunis, S., & Beauchamp, T. L. (2013). An ethics framework for a learning health care system: a departure from traditional research ethics and clinical ethics, ethical oversight of learning health care systems. *Hastings Center Report, 43*(Suppl 1), S16–S27. https://doi.org/10.1002/hast.134

Fisher, C. B. (2005). Deception research involving children: Ethical practices and paradoxes. *Ethics & Behavior, 15*(3), 271–287.

Humphreys, L. (1970). *Tearoom trade: Impersonal sex in public places*. Aldine Transaction.

Kelman, H. C. (1972). The rights of the subject in social research: An analysis in terms of relative power and legitimacy. *American Psychologist, 27*(11), 989–1016.

Korn, J. H. (1997). *Illusions of reality: A history of deception in social psychology*. State University of New York Press.

Latané, B., & Darley, J. (1969). Bystander "apathy." *American Scientist, 57*(2), 244–268.

Miketta, S., & Friese, M. (2019). Debriefed but still troubled? About the (in)effectiveness of post-experimental debriefings after ego threat. *Journal of Personality and Social Psychology, 117*(2), 282–309.

Milgram, S. (1974). *Obedience to authority: An experimental view*. Harper and Row.

Miller, F. G., Wendler, D., & Swartzman, L. C. (2005). Deception in research on the placebo effect. *PLoS Med, 2*(9), e262.

National Research Council. (2003). *Protecting participants and facilitating social and behavioral sciences research*. The National Academies Press. https://doi.org/10.17226/10638.

Rennie, S. (2011). Viewing research participation as a moral obligation: In whose interests? *Hastings Center Report, 41*(2), 40–47.

Rhodes, K. V., & Miller, F. G. (2012). Simulated patient studies: An ethical analysis. *Milbank Quarterly, 90*(4), 706–724.

Schaefer, G. O., Emanuel, E. J., & Wertheimer, A. (2009). The obligation to participate in biomedical research. *JAMA, 302*(1), 67–72.

Senn, S. (1997). Are placebo run-ins justified? *British Journal of Medicine, 314*, 1191–1193.

Shah, S., Whittle, A., Wilfond, B., Gensler, G., & Wendler, D. (2004). How do institutional review boards apply the federal risk and benefit standards for pediatric research? *JAMA, 291*(4), 476–482.

Sieber, J. E. (1983). Deception in social research II: Evaluation the potential for harm or wrong. *IRB, 5*(1), 1–6.

Smith, S. S., & Richardson, D. (1983). Amelioration of deception and harm in psychological research: The important role of debriefing. *Journal of Personality and Social Psychology, 44*(5), 1075–1082.

Survey Research

Cecilia Brooke Cholka

Dean Gallant

Abstract

Survey research is a common human subjects research method and is used in a variety of research areas. Both ethical and regulatory considerations apply to the review of survey research. Additionally, there are a variety of issues that may affect the risk of harm for subjects of survey research, including subject characteristics, study design, privacy and confidentiality, and the mere fact of participation. This chapter discusses various components that should be considered when reviewing survey research and offers examples to highlight some nuances of survey research.

Defining Survey Research

Survey research is a popular method because it captures a wide variety of information through relatively quick and easy processes. The flexibility of the method means that researchers from various disciplines and with different levels of expertise utilize surveys in their research and that the topics covered and populations used in survey research can vary widely. The *Sage Handbook of Survey Methodology* discusses several definitions of survey research and defines survey research as an examination of units (i.e., people) through a systematic method of gathering information through asking questions (Joye et al., 2017). Survey research can be done via paper and pencil, online, telephone, or in-person verbal interactions. Survey research excludes other methods such as interviews, focus groups, observations, or content analysis of existing data.

Surveying is a common human subjects research method, but just because a survey is being used does not mean that the activity always requires IRB review; some surveys, such as opinion polling and program evaluation, <u>may not meet the definition of research involving human subjects</u> and would thus not need IRB review. Some surveys may be validated measures that have been developed and statistically tested, whereas other surveys may be designed by researchers for use with their specific study without validation. Validated surveys are not inherently better or worse than nonvalidated surveys, and the expectation for validation varies among disciples. This chapter will discuss reviewing

🔗 5-1

survey research through ethical and regulatory lenses and will highlight issues that might impact the risk of harm to people who participate in survey research studies.

Ethical Review

The Common Rule is usually considered the framework to use for review of survey research. However, many survey research studies do not receive federal funding, are reviewed using regulatory flexibility, or are determined to be exempt. However, even when Common Rule regulatory requirements do not apply, the ethical principles of the *Belmont Report* are still relevant (National Commission, 1979). Student researchers and others who are learning how to conduct human subjects research often start with simple survey studies; in these instances, the regulations may not be applicable, but ethical concerns still need to be considered. *Belmont* provides a foundation for consideration of ethical issues in survey research.

Applying *Belmont* Principles to Survey Research

The *Belmont Report* defines three guiding ethical principles: respect for persons, beneficence, and justice (National Commission, 1979). The first principle, respect for persons, has two implications: people should be treated as autonomous agents, and those with diminished autonomy deserve special protections. Treating people as autonomous agents implies that the survey researcher will provide sufficient information for people to make an informed and uncoerced decision about their participation. This is accomplished through the informed consent process. Although an exempt or non-federally funded survey need not adhere to the specific informed consent requirements set forth in the federal regulations, that does not mean that informed consent should be abandoned. Subjects ought to understand the nature of the survey, that their participation is voluntary, and that the data collected will be used for research. Additional information (how long the survey may take to complete, the extent to which their responses will be kept confidential, whether there is compensation for participation, whether their responses will be correlated with other data, and the availability of relevant resources) should also be provided when appropriate. This information can be presented in a separate screen at the start of an online survey, at the beginning of a paper and pencil survey, or in the introductory discussion of a telephone or in-person survey. In such cases, a signed consent form will not be necessary, particularly if subjects' identity need not be recorded or associated with their responses.

In some instances, a more robust consent process may be warranted. For example, surveys that involve individuals with diminished autonomy (e.g., children, prisoners, individuals suffering from dementia) present more complex consent issues, because those subjects may not fully understand the presentation, content, or potential risks of the survey. In research with these populations, consent may include procedures for written parental or proxy consent and/or institutional authorization, and additional requirements of subparts C or D may apply.

The second *Belmont* principle, beneficence, states that researchers should do no harm and should strive to maximize benefits while minimizing the risk of harm. The latter is often referred to as the "risk/benefit balance" or "risk/benefit ratio." Typically, survey research does not present the likelihood of benefit to subjects (beyond the satisfaction of a possible contribution to the goals of the research), and therefore the risks to subjects should be minimal. However, surveys on some topics may be more sensitive in nature, such as drug use or criminal behavior, and present some risks to subjects. In these instances, procedures to minimize the risks of harm to subjects should be implemented (these might include not collecting identifiers, encrypting data, and monitoring responses, among others). If surveys are designed to probe sensitive aspects of subjects' own experiences or behavior (e.g., self-harm, suicidality, abuse or neglect, legal status), the researcher may need to monitor the data and take steps to offer resources or to facilitate connection of subjects with counseling or medical or legal assistance. The risks of participation and minimization of those risks are dependent on the particulars of an individual study, including the content of the survey, the setting, and the population.

The third *Belmont* principle, justice, says that the selection of subjects should be equitable, and any risks and benefits should be shared among those likely to be affected by the conduct and the results of the research. Thus, subjects in survey research should be recruited because they represent the relevant population, not simply because they are readily available to the researcher. For example, a teacher surveying students about their experience with a new curriculum that is in use across a school district should take steps to recruit from multiple classrooms, not just their own.

The *Belmont* principles provide a useful lens for examination of all research and can help IRBs and survey researchers ensure that research is conducted responsibly and ethically.

Common Rule Review of Survey Research

The principles and ethical considerations in the *Belmont Report* serve as the foundation for the Common Rule. Federally funded survey research regulated by the Common Rule can be reviewed through exempt, expedited, or full board mechanisms, but typically falls under exempt or expedited review. Each review type has specific concerns that determine the appropriate review mechanism.

Exemption Categories and Survey Research

There are several categories of <u>exemption</u> **[45 CFR 46.104]** that may apply to survey research; these are listed in the box.

🖉 5-3

EXEMPTION CATEGORIES IN SURVEY RESEARCH

- *Category 1*: Research conducted in established or commonly accepted educational settings that specifically involves normal educational practices that are not likely to adversely impact students' opportunity to learn required educational content or the assessment of educators who provide instruction.
- *Category 2*: Research that only includes interactions involving educational tests (cognitive, diagnostic, aptitude, achievement), survey procedures, interview procedures, or observation of public behavior (including visual or audio recording) when certain criteria are met.
- *Category 3*: Research involving benign behavioral interventions, in conjunction with the collection of information from an adult subject through verbal or written responses or audiovisual recording, if the subject

prospectively agrees to the intervention and information collection and certain criteria are met.

- *Category 5*: Research and demonstration projects that are conducted or supported by a federal department or agency, or otherwise subject to the approval of department or agency heads, and that are designed to study, evaluate, improve, or otherwise examine public benefit or service programs.

Department of Health and Human Services (DHHS). (1998). *OHRP expedited review categories (1998). Categories of research that may be reviewed by the institutional review board (IRB) through an expedited review procedure.* www.hhs.gov/ohrp/regulations-and-policy/guidance/categories-of-research-expedited-review-procedure-1998/index.html

Surveys are often used as a data collection method for research that would be reviewed under one of these categories. For example,

⊘ 9-2

- *Exempt category 1* research, on effectiveness or comparison of educational practices, would typically involve surveys to determine <u>students'</u> and/or teachers' perspectives on educational practices, curricula, or management methods. The important aspect of this category is that the focus of the research is on *normal educational practices*, so general surveying of students and/or teachers on other issues would not be considered exempt from the requirements of the regulations under this category.
- *Exempt category 2* encompasses much survey research. Important components of this category are the three considerations specified in the exemption regarding collection of identifiers: (1) not recording identifiers, (2) limitations on risks related to breach of confidentiality, and (3) collection of identifiers with appropriate safeguards for privacy and confidentiality.
- *Exempt category 3* research may include surveys as a way to collect information through verbal or written responses. The inclusion of a benign behavioral intervention in addition to surveying would move research from category 2 to category 3.
- *Exempt category 5* research may include surveys as part of a larger project to examine a federally supported program.

When reviewing survey research using the Common Rule, often there is a question of whether the study would fall under one of these exempt categories or, alternatively, should be reviewed under expedited category 7 (discussed later). Considerations, such as the content of the survey or additional procedures included with the survey, may push a study out of an exempt category and into the domain of expedited review.

When a study falls under exempt review, institutional policy indicates who conducts the review and what ethical considerations are included in that review. Just because a study meets the exemption criteria does not mean that the IRB cannot review it or that ethical components like informed consent are not important. Some survey research designs might pose risks for some subjects; for example, a mailed questionnaire with a return address including "AIDS Patient Study" or "Recidivism Project" could link subjects with sensitive information about themselves. Reviewing to ensure that appropriate privacy and confidentiality concerns

⊘ 5-6

are addressed by the researcher is reasonable and, in the case of <u>limited IRB review</u>, required. Much survey research that is regulated by the Common Rule will meet the criteria for exemption, but if not, expedited review can be used.

Expedited Review

In some instances, the IRB may determine that a study is not eligible for exemption due to the sensitivity of the data or for other reasons. In those cases,

the study would most likely be reviewed using <u>expedited procedures</u>. In order   ✎ 5-5
to be reviewed using expedited procedures, the research must involve no more
than minimal risk and use only procedures included in the expedited review
categories **[45 CFR 46.110(a)]**. An important consideration is that expedited
review can only be used when identification of the subject would not "reasonably place them at risk of criminal or civil liability or be damaging to the
subjects' financial standing, employability, insurability, reputation, or be stigmatizing" unless appropriate protections for privacy and confidentiality are implemented, such that those risks are no greater than minimal (OHRP Expedited
Review Categories, C; Department of Health and Human Services [DHHS],
1998). The expedited category that would be used for survey research is described in OHRP Expedited Review Categories, 7 (DHHS 1998):

> Research on individual or group characteristics or behavior (including, but not limited to, research on perception, cognition, motivation,
> identity, language, communication, cultural beliefs or practices, and
> social behavior) or research employing survey, interview, oral history,
> focus group, program evaluation, human factors evaluation, or quality
> assurance methodologies.

This category is similar to exempt category 2 discussed previously, and
decisions regarding whether a study would be reviewed using exempt or expedited procedures would depend on the specific circumstances of the study
(e.g., population, risks, sensitivity of the data). For example, a study that asked
about attitudes toward illicit drugs and drug use might be considered exempt,
but a study that asks about personal history of illicit drug use might be reviewed through expedited procedures, including consideration of whether subjects' responses were considered identifiable.

Full Board Review

In some (likely rare) instances, survey research might be reviewed using <u>full board</u>   ✎ 5-7
<u>review</u> procedures. This can occur when the survey research does not meet the requirement for expedited review because of criminal or civil liability, as discussed
previously (OHRP Expedited Review Categories, C; DHHS 1998). An example
of a survey research study that would potentially be reviewed by the full board
is a study that collects identifiable drug use data from people who are on probation for drug-related crimes. In this instance, the IRB would need to determine
whether the collection of that information would reach a threshold where disclosure of the data would put individuals at risk beyond those of daily life, considering the consequences for drug use in that population. Given appropriate privacy
and confidentiality protections, like obtaining a <u>certificate of confidentiality</u> and   ✎ 8-3
robust data encryption, perhaps the study in this example could be reviewed
using expedited procedures. Studies reviewed using expedited or full board procedures, and that include pregnant women, prisoners, or children, will also need
to comply with subparts <u>B</u>, <u>C</u>, and <u>D</u> (respectively) of 45 CFR 46. In reviewing   ✎ 9-4 ✎ 9-5 ✎ 9-6
survey research in these populations, it is important to consider the content and
delivery modality of the surveys to ensure appropriate safeguards.

Risks to Subjects in Survey Research

Due to the utility and flexibility of survey research and the broad use of surveys,
it is important to consider the circumstances of survey research studies to ensure appropriate protections. For example, surveys about breakfast foods and

habits in a general population might have no known risks, whereas surveys about breakfast foods and habits in a population of people seeking treatment for eating disorders could have significantly different risks and require plans for minimizing those risks. Most survey research presents only minimal risk; however, certain circumstances, such as subject characteristics, study design, privacy and confidentiality concerns, and even the mere fact of participation, can present risks to subjects.

Subject Characteristics

Questions that appear innocuous for most individuals could expose some subjects to risk if their responses became known outside the study, depending on the characteristics of those subjects. For example, subjects who may be legally undocumented or who may be involved in activities that could present legal jeopardy or be stigmatizing are likely to be at greater risk (compared to subjects without those characteristics) when asked questions such as, "How long have you lived at your current address/where did you live prior to moving here?" or "Have you ever been arrested?" or "Have you used any of the following [illegal drugs]?" Similarly, questions that are appropriate for adults may be inappropriate for minors. Researchers should be aware of the range of individuals who might participate and should consider the possible characteristics of respondents to ensure that proper precautions are taken to minimize the risks of harm. Surveys on private or sensitive issues can present special risks for some subjects. Individuals with a history (or current experience) of physical assault, sexual abuse, or other trauma may find some questions on those topics disturbing or offensive. While this does not mean that such surveys are inappropriate, researchers should consider the experience of participation from the subjects' point of view—with assistance from counselors or other professionals in the field—to ensure proper respect for subjects whose personal experiences may render them disproportionately at risk of harm in research involving certain lines of inquiry.

 Survey Research Example 1

A university faculty member proposes to email all female students and staff at her institution with an invitation to participate in a study about body image and eating habits. The email will contain a unique personalized link to a web-based survey. General demographic information (race, age range, family constellation, socioeconomic status, home zip code) will be collected. Other questions will deal with dieting history, body mass index, and history of eating disorders. The researcher wants to assign each subject a code number that will in turn be linked, in a separate file, to an email address for possible (yet unspecified) follow-up.

Questions for consideration include the following:

- Does institutional policy permit "broadcast" emails to solicit research participation?
- Information is sensitive and potentially stigmatizing; are data security arrangements (including coding of subjects) adequate? Will minors be involved? If so, what protections are needed for stigmatizing information about those minors?
- Is there a way to correlate follow-up responses with original data without retaining email addresses—perhaps by using a non-obvious user-generated code?
- What information is appropriate for the informed consent document?

Study Design

In addition to the subject characteristics, it is important to consider the design of survey research to ensure that risks are minimized. Some formats of questionnaires (e.g., "checklists" of recreational drugs, deviant behaviors, or methods of self-harm) are used because they are often easier for the researcher to code compared to open-ended questions. However, the format of these questionnaires may not be appropriate for surveying minors, because in some cases such questions could be viewed as suggesting, or even tacitly condoning, the listed behaviors. Additionally, the distribution of these surveys might put subjects at risk if others can easily see subject responses.

Some common survey research designs may have unique considerations needed to evaluate and minimize risk, such as subject pools and Amazon Mechanical Turk (often referred to as mTurk). Many researchers favor these survey distribution modalities because of the access to large numbers of potential subjects; however, both subject pools and mTurk require special consideration. In subject pools, students in certain classes may be required as part of a class to participate in studies. Ethical issues that arise when using subject pools include ensuring that participation in research is voluntary; the availability of an alternate activity equal to the time and effort investment of participating in research is an important protection for this population. Research using mTurk also needs special considerations regarding the design of the research. mTurk is similar to online subject pools, but instead of students, mTurk is a pool of people who sign up online to be workers. Some issues include the use of automated software, or bots, to complete tasks; the potential for negative impact on subjects who do not complete surveys (a "rejected hit") and consequently receive a downgrade in reputation in the mTurk system; and other realities specific to this unique space. In both modalities, it is important for researchers and reviewers to be familiar with the setting of the research to ensure that necessary precautions are taken.

Another issue in survey research design is data authenticity and the interaction between the value of the research and risks to subjects. For example, in the case of online surveys, particularly those that offer compensation for participation, some subjects may be tempted to participate more than once. Others may

 ## Survey Research Example 2

A state-funded survey on suicidal ideation among municipal public employees (police, fire, EMTs) is proposed in a large metropolitan area. Questions will include experience with thoughts of and/or attempts of suicide and gun ownership. Results are intended to inform establishment of proactive employee mental health service programs. Subjects are told that their data will be confidential and individual responses will not be shared with supervisors. Researchers wish to retain identifiers for future correlation with actual behavior.

Questions for consideration include the following:

- If the survey will occur during work hours, how will voluntariness of participation be ensured? Can a (non-onerous) activity be available as an alternative?
- If subjects will complete the survey online from home or on a portable device, will the connection to the survey server be private and secure?
- How will identifiable data be stored? Who will have access? How will summary data be reported to administrative authorities?
- What action (if any) will be taken if a subject's responses indicate they are at serious risk? Are confidential resources available for such individuals?

misrepresent their age or other eligibility criteria in order to participate. Some subjects or bots may submit inaccurate or bogus responses. If there is reasonable cause to question the authenticity of data, then the value of the research is reduced, perhaps significantly. Asking subjects to participate in research that cannot possibly yield accurate findings is, at a minimum, a waste of subjects' time and, depending on the nature and sensitivity of the research, can expose subjects to unnecessary risk. When considering survey research study design, especially of online surveys, it may be important to consider strategies for enhancing data authenticity, such as monitoring device IP addresses and time stamps, monitoring response times, and inclusion of open-ended questions, among others. These strategies may complicate the identifiability of survey responses and so should be evaluated in combination with the other aspects of the study, such as sensitivity of the data being collected.

An important aspect of research design that requires consideration to ensure the minimization of risks to subjects in survey research includes instances when researchers perform multiple roles with the subjects. Common examples include teachers surveying their students, medical providers surveying their patients, or employers surveying their employees. In these cases, the voluntary nature and purpose of the research may be obscured due to the power dynamics between teachers and students, providers and patients, or employers and employees. When reviewing research that includes these power dynamics, it is important to consider ways that the study design can mediate the power differential, such as having someone other than the teacher or practitioner obtain subjects' consent. Because other survey research study design issues (in addition to the ones mentioned in this section) may arise that might impact the risk to subjects, each study should be evaluated to assess its unique circumstances.

Privacy and Confidentiality Issues

The most common risks of harm to subjects in survey research are related to loss of privacy and breach of confidentiality. Survey questions about illegal or immoral activities, drug use, self-injurious behaviors, or suicidality can elicit responses that may threaten subjects' legal or social status, reputation,

 Survey Research Example 3

A researcher has received funding from the National Institute of Child Health and Human Development to study the etiology of internet sexual predation. Data collection would consist of surveys of perpetrators with prior convictions. Topics would include how victims are identified and contacted (e.g., email, chat rooms, instant messaging), what approach is used in the communications (e.g., whether the perpetrator poses as a teen or child), what the underlying motivators are, effectiveness of treatment programs, and related topics. Potential subjects will be recruited through internet sex offender treatment programs.

Questions for consideration include the following:

- Subjects' responses are likely to include sensitive and stigmatizing information. Is it necessary to retain identifiers? If so, can a CoC be obtained?
- Are any subjects prisoners? If yes, what additional protections are needed for prisoners?
- Should the officials of the treatment program know who is and is not participating in the study? If so, might subjects feel coerced into participating?
- Are members of the research team mandated reporters? What if they learn details of previously unknown crimes? How should researchers explain this to subjects?

or employability if responses become known outside the research context. In studies that include these topics, special attention should be paid to the identifiability of data. Mere separation of name or other obvious identifiers from responses may not ensure protection of subjects' identities, particularly if the survey collects other demographic information or is focused on a limited population. Obvious identifiers are not the only concern; common demographic characteristics, in concert with publicly available databases, can pinpoint an individual. In a classic case, the "anonymized" medical claims records of William Weld, then governor of Massachusetts, were identified by comparing date of birth, ZIP code, and gender with local voter registration records (Sweeney, 1997). More recently, it has been shown that even current standards for deidentifying data sets may not prevent reidentification (Rocher et al., 2019). Identifiers should be collected only if they are essential for the research, and any link between responses and identifiers should be severed as soon as possible. Additionally, appropriate confidentiality protections for studies that collect identifiable sensitive or criminal data may include obtaining a <u>certificate of confidentiality</u> (CoC). CoCs protect data by prohibiting disclosure of identifiable sensitive research information to anyone not connected to the research, such as disclosure in a court of law. And, as a best practice, identifiable research data should always be encrypted.

🔗 8-3

Special care should be taken when a survey collects identifiable data and deals with activities that could necessitate reporting to authorities by the researcher, such as child or elder abuse or neglect. Mandated reporting laws differ by state, but in most jurisdictions a researcher has an obligation to report suspected maltreatment to appropriate authorities. Assurances of absolute confidentiality of survey responses should not be made or should include an appropriate caveat when surveys may elicit identifiable information about reportable offenses. If survey questions include areas where details of such behavior may be discussed, the subject should be reminded of the researcher's obligation to report.

Mere Fact of Participation

In some cases the simple fact of participation in survey research could present an element of risk. In-person surveys of undocumented individuals conducted outside a legal aid office by a researcher whose area of interest is known to Immigration and Customs Enforcement (ICE) officials could alert ICE to subjects' legal status. Surveys distributed by employers at a workplace that ask for critiques of policies or other employees may reflect on the subjects who are completing the surveys. The preamble to the 2018 Common Rule acknowledges such possibilities:

> Concerns have also been raised about psychological risks of participating in surveys or interviews, and of situational risks where the simple awareness that someone was surveyed or interviewed poses a risk. We recognize that this is possible, but believe that this is rare enough that it does not warrant adding additional conditions to the exemption category. (Federal Register, 2017, Preamble pp. 7189–7190)

The regulators chose to allow these concerns to be addressed as a matter of institutional policy rather than in the regulations. While the regulations do not provide direction in these instances, the ethical principles do address the need to minimize risk of harm to subjects, and IRBs should expect researchers to be knowledgeable and thoughtful of the research topic, population, and survey content to ensure the ethical conduct of survey research.

References

Department of Health and Human Services (DHHS). (1998). *OHRP expedited review categories (1998). Categories of research that may be reviewed by the institutional review board (IRB) through an expedited review procedure.* www.hhs.gov/ohrp/regulations-and-policy/guidance/categories-of-research-expedited-review-procedure-1998/index.html

Federal Register. (2017). Vol. 82, No. 12. 45 CFR 46 and Preamble. www.govinfo.gov/content/pkg/FR-2017-01-19/pdf/2017-01058.pdf

Joye, D., Wolf, C., Smith, T. W., & Fu, Y. (2017). Survey methodology: Challenges and principles. In C. Wolf, D. Joye, T. W. Smith, & Y. Fu (Eds.), *The SAGE Handbook of Survey Methodology*. Sage.

National Commission for the Protection of Human Subjects of Biomedical and Behavioral Research. (1979). *The Belmont Report: Ethical principles and guidelines for the protection of human subjects of research.* www.hhs.gov/ohrp/regulations-and-policy/belmont-report/read-the-belmont-report/index.html

Rocher, L., Hendrickx, J. M., & de Montjoye, Y. (2019). Estimating the success of re-identifications in incomplete datasets using generative models. *Nature Communications, 10*, 3069.

Sweeney, L. (1997). Weaving technology and policy together to maintain confidentiality. *Journal of Law, Medicine, and Ethics, 25*, 98–110.

Internet Research

Elizabeth A. Buchanan

Abstract

Today's internet is complex, ubiquitous, and powerful. Researchers across disciplines have found enormous potential in websites, chat rooms, gaming environments, and more, and with the potential for novel forms of investigation, traditional and new ethical concerns have emerged. Even as the research oversight field starts to define best practices for recruitment, informed consent, privacy and confidentiality, and data security, emerging issues are challenging IRBs in the areas of machine learning, artificial intelligence, and data analytics. These newer techniques are confounding the very notions of human subjects research and instead pushing the discourse toward a "data subjects" approach. IRBs and researchers must continually review their best practices in light of changing and developing research technologies, methods, and ethics. This chapter provides an overview of salient issues related to internet research.

Introduction

The origins of today's internet date to the 1960s ARPANET project; this network looked and behaved radically differently from what we experience today. It is hard to imagine how a network that started out with only two nodes evolved through the World Wide Web (WWW) of the 1990s into today's global presence, used by 4.57 billion people worldwide (Internet World Stats, 2020), over half of the world's population. Today's internet is complex, ubiquitous, and powerful. A tool or set of tools for global business, banking, medicine, entertainment—and research—the internet is almost taken for granted, as it seamlessly resides in and on all forms of devices, from smartphones to wearables. Researchers across disciplines have found enormous potential in websites, chat rooms, gaming environments, and more, over the years, and with the potential for novel forms of investigation, traditional and new ethical concerns have emerged. While IRBs/research ethics boards (REBs) were brought into the internet research conversation as early as 1995, the expansion of research uses of the internet continues to create challenges for research oversight.

Background: The Rise of Internet Research

While the original ARPANET was built to facilitate research communications between and among universities and research labs, today's internet is used across disciplines and domains for a variety of research purposes. Early internet studies scholars in the late 1990s called attention to the ways in which the internet can serve as a tool or a medium of/for research, for example, as a search engine or a network to collect and transmit data, or as a site or locale of research, such as an online community or patient group. This early dichotomy between being a tool to conduct research and a site of research itself started to break down in the face of the rise of social media and big data. Buchanan (2017b) has suggested that internet research has progressed through identifiable phases along a continuum of development, as described later.

Internet research is an umbrella term, encompassing a range of activities. Two different professional bodies have offered definitions, showing the scope and range of activities under this umbrella term (see box, Definitions of Internet Research).

DEFINITIONS OF INTERNET RESEARCH

Secretary's Advisory Committee on Human Research Protections (SACHRP) definitions (SACHRP, 2013):

- Research studying information that is already available on or via the internet without direct interaction with human subjects (harvesting, mining, profiling, scraping—observation or recording of otherwise-existing data sets, chat room interactions, blogs, social media postings, etc.)
- Research that uses the internet as a vehicle for recruiting or interacting, directly or indirectly, with subjects (self-testing websites, survey tools, Amazon Mechanical Turk®, etc.)
- Research about the internet itself and its effects (use patterns or effects of social media, search engines, email, etc.; evolution of privacy issues; information contagion; etc.)
- Research about internet users—what they do, and how the internet affects individuals and their behaviors
- Research that utilizes the internet as an interventional tool, for example, interventions that influence subjects' behavior
- Others (emerging and cross-platform types of research and methods, including m-research (mobile)
- Recruitment in or through internet locales or tools, for example social media, push technologies.

Association of Internet Researchers definitions (Markham & Buchanan, 2012): Internet research encompasses inquiry that:
(a) Utilizes the internet to collect data or information, e.g., through online interviews, surveys, archiving, or automated means of data scraping
(b) Studies how people use the internet, e.g., through collecting and observing activities or participating on social network sites, listservs, web sites, blogs, gaming, or other online environments or contexts
(c) Utilizes or engages in data processing, analysis, or storage of datasets, databanks, and/or repositories available via the internet
(d) Studies software, code, and internet technologies
(e) Examines the design of systems, interfaces, pages, and elements
(f) Analyzes visual and textual content of sites, including websites and internet-facilitated images, writings, and media forms
(g) Studies large scale production, use, and regulation of the internet by governments, industries, corporations, and military forces.

Early internet research (phase one) circa the 1990s often involved researchers interacting with or observing online communities, and communications were often in simple displays and formats such as text/script, email, and listservs (see, for example, Ess, 2002). With the development and quick adoption of the graphical WWW, researchers found greater opportunity to engage in virtual settings and environments such as multiuser dungeons or domains. Some years later, a number of computer science students at Harvard were experimenting with their internal network, eventually launching it as "The Facebook" in 2004, the same year as the launch of the file-sharing service Napster. This "social era" of the internet (phase two) changed everything for researchers, as it involved the production of seemingly infinite amounts of data appearing as available to anyone for marketing and research purposes. Social networking enabled researchers to look not only at individuals and their behaviors, patterns, and beliefs as expressed through postings and shares but also at the interconnections across individuals' communities.

The ease with which social media facilitated the creation and sharing of mass amounts of data, coupled with tremendous growth in computing power, fed directly into the phase of <u>big data</u> research, what Buchanan refers to as phase three, where extremely large data sets could be created, parsed, and analyzed (Buchanan, 2017a). Big data refers, in part, to the plethora of sources that are combined into vast data sets; these data come from chatter from social networks, web server logs, traffic flow sensors, satellite imagery, broadcast audio streams, banking transactions, the content of web pages, scans of government documents, GPS trails, telemetry from automobiles, financial market data, and more (Dumbill, 2012). Big data, sometimes referred to as "real-world data," exploded into vast industries by the early 2010s. Concurrently, the rise of artificial intelligence and machine learning (AI/ML) has pushed "internet research" into its next phase (phase four), realizing these phases are not discrete but represent development and change across a continuum (**Figure 10.5-1**).

🖉 12-4

Throughout this evolution, scholars and researchers have been asking questions about the ethics and norms around internet research as they relate to traditional research ethics principles (**Table 10.5-1**). Specifically, concerns about privacy, ownership of data, consent of subjects, positionality of researcher or relationship to subjects, identity, and age verification were identified. Basic ethical principles were tested in these new domains, with SACHRP asserting that "Investigators and IRBs should remember that the *Belmont* principles . . . are as applicable to Internet research as they are to any other form of human subjects research. Regardless of how the regulations may be interpreted in individual studies, adherence to these fundamental principles is important to encouraging public trust in the ethical conduct of Internet research" (SACHRP, 2013).

In 1999, Frankel and Siang's landmark American Association for the Advancement of Science (AAAS) report defined human subjects concerns and considerations in relation to internet research (Frankel & Siang, 1999). This report was followed by the Association of Internet Researchers (AoIR, 2002), the

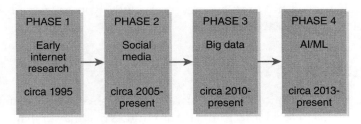

Figure 10.5-1 Phases of internet research.

Table 10.5-1 **Ethical Reconsiderations**

Traditional Research Ethics Principles	Emergent Ethical Considerations
Ethical research is that which seeks to do no harm.	Harms may occur "downstream," not immediately foreseeable to the researcher or subjects due to the malleability and reuses of data.
The greater the vulnerability of the subject, the greater the obligation to protect.	Vulnerabilities may not be evident; data sets might further marginalize individuals or communities, or, conversely, fail to represent individuals or communities.
Sound methods and ethics produce sound research.	Common practices may be compromised, including verification of subjects; data integrity, data privacy, and confidentiality are often beyond the control of the researcher.

Norwegian National Research Ethics Committees (NESH, 2002), and Buchanan (2002, 2003), all of which raised additional internet research ethics concerns. By 2005, IRBs in the United States were more regularly considering the implications of internet research and the interplay with human subjects regulations. The first empirical study conducted on internet research and IRBs in the United States (Buchanan & Ess, 2009) resulted in the development of numerous guidelines and best practices for IRBs to use when reviewing internet research. In 2011, SACHRP first took on the topic of internet research, releasing draft recommendations in 2013, articulating the following rationale: "Current human subjects regulations, originally written over thirty years ago, do not address many issues raised by the unique characteristics of Internet research" (SACHRP, 2013). Buchanan and Zimmer documented internet research concerns in a 2012 *Stanford Encyclopedia of Philosophy* entry, later updated in 2016 (Buchanan & Zimmer, 2012). That same year, AoIR revised its "Ethical Decision Making and Internet Research" to reflect the many technological changes around social media that had occurred since its 2002 version (Markham & Buchanan, 2012), with AoIR's 2019 version looking more directly at big data, industry data, and overall challenges in human/data subjects protections in a data-intensive environment (frankze et al., 2020). The preamble to the 2018 Common Rule speaks directly to technical, social, and methodological developments and their impact on human subjects research and IRB review: "This final rule recognizes that in the past two decades a paradigm shift has occurred in how research is conducted. Evolving technologies—including imaging, mobile technologies, and the growth in computing power—have changed the scale and nature of information collected in many disciplines" (Federal Register, 2017, Preamble p. 7151).

The Common Rule does not address internet research concerns directly, but the 2018 revisions were certainly influenced by developments in the scale and scope of data-intensive research in both social-behavioral as well as biomedical domains. Major areas of IRB concern in internet research mirror traditional research environments to some degree. There are nuances and particularities that ground internet research. The remainder of this chapter will focus on areas that have challenged IRB practices, and it concludes with suggested strategies for regulatory and ethical compliance.

Recruitment

As reflected in the definitions of internet research given earlier, researchers can use the internet as a tool for recruitment into studies that may or may not themselves be internet based (**Figure 10.5-2**).

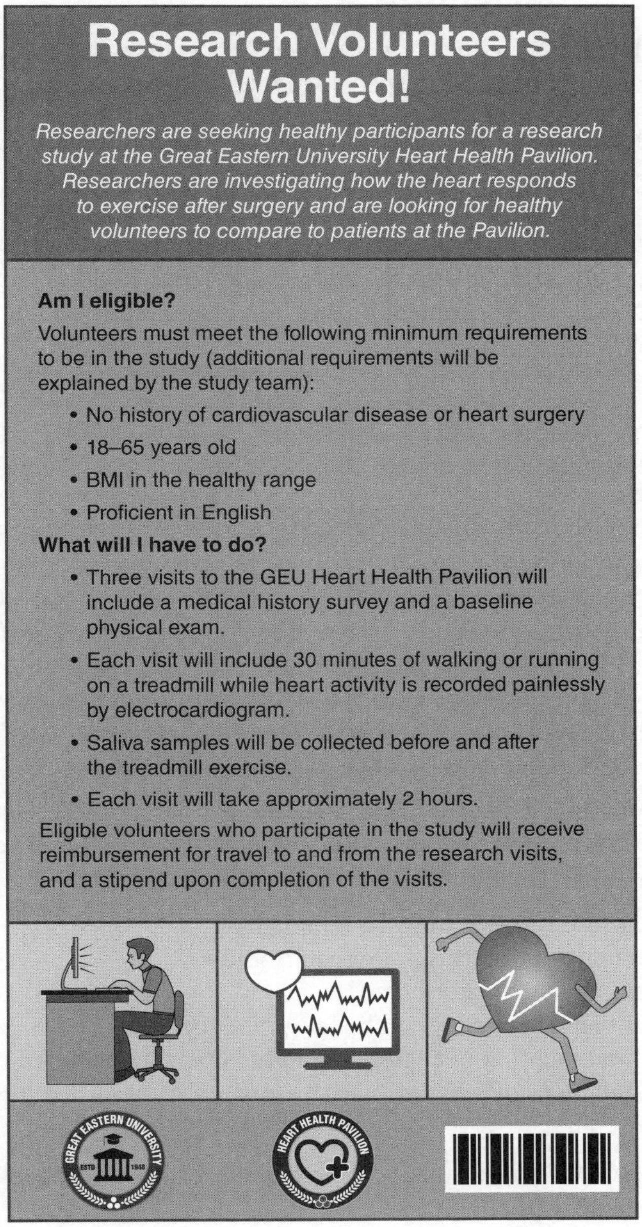

Research Volunteers Wanted!

Researchers are seeking healthy participants for a research study at the Great Eastern University Heart Health Pavilion. Researchers are investigating how the heart responds to exercise after surgery and are looking for healthy volunteers to compare to patients at the Pavilion.

Am I eligible?

Volunteers must meet the following minimum requirements to be in the study (additional requirements will be explained by the study team):

- No history of cardiovascular disease or heart surgery
- 18–65 years old
- BMI in the healthy range
- Proficient in English

What will I have to do?

- Three visits to the GEU Heart Health Pavilion will include a medical history survey and a baseline physical exam.
- Each visit will include 30 minutes of walking or running on a treadmill while heart activity is recorded painlessly by electrocardiogram.
- Saliva samples will be collected before and after the treadmill exercise.
- Each visit will take approximately 2 hours.

Eligible volunteers who participate in the study will receive reimbursement for travel to and from the research visits, and a stipend upon completion of the visits.

Figure 10.5-2 Example of internet advertisement for research subject recruitment.

Depending on the type of research and specificity of the research questions, there is a range of possible recruitment methods in internet research. IRBs should review the recruitment plan to ensure it is fair, that there is an equitable distribution of risks and benefits across all subjects, and that the means of recruiting do not themselves put subjects in harm's way. While these principles are the same as those that apply to any recruitment method, there are considerations unique to an online environment: It may be difficult to ascertain the exact population or sample; it may be unclear if an online community or space requires membership to study or use content as part of an analysis; and, depending on the site, research recruitment may be in violation of end-user license agreements or terms of service. Gelinas and colleagues distinguish between active and passive recruitment:

Passive recruitment involves distributing recruitment materials (ads, posters, flyers) with the aim of attracting potential participants to contact the research team for more information and for consideration of enrollment. By contrast, *active recruitment* occurs when research staff approach and interact with specific individuals with the aim of enrolling them in research, usually on the basis of knowledge of characteristics that would make them suitable candidates for particular trials. (Gelinas et al., 2017).

IRBs should assess both approaches in their considerations, paying particular attention to the ethics of direct targeting and predictive analytical activities. Common methods of recruitment include the following:

- Postings on social media sites
- Email
- Web pages
- Text messaging
- Registries
- Using big data and data analytics to target subjects. For example, ads for studies can be targeted to appear in potential subjects' newsfeeds, or AI applications can be utilized that use deep learning and natural language processing to automate clinical trial matching by directly partnering with health institutions (Varadharajan & Lee, n.d.). An example is the Autism & Beyond app, developed by Duke University and Apple, using Apple's ResearchKit researchers, that used iPhone video technology to analyze children's behavior and emotion (Egger et al., 2018).

As with any protocol, the IRB should review any recruitment text, advertisements, or postings as part of their considerations, and the required components of a recruitment document must include:

- The study title and IRB study number
- A clear statement that this is a research study
- The principal investigator's name
- A contact name with either a phone number or email address
- At least brief mention of eligibility criteria, if applicable
- A clear statement of whether participants will be paid for their time and effort

Gelinas et al. (2017) have suggested best practices for recruiting participants via internet/social media:

1. Provide the IRB with a statement describing the proposed social media recruitment techniques, including:
   - A list of the sites to be used.
   - A description of whether recruitment will be passive and/or active.
   - If utilizing active recruitment, a description of how potential participants will be identified and approached, and their privacy maintained.
2. Ensure that the social media recruitment strategy complies with applicable federal and state laws.
3. Provide the IRB with a statement certifying compliance (or lack of noncompliance) with the policies and terms of use of relevant websites, OR if proposed techniques conflict with relevant website policies and Terms of Use:
   - Seek an exception from the website to its terms of use; provide the IRB with written documentation of the exception, if granted.

- Depending on IRB policy, in compelling circumstances make the case that the recruitment strategy should be allowed to proceed in the absence of an exception from the site.

4. Ensure that the proposed recruitment strategy respects all relevant ethical norms, including:
   - Proposed recruitment does not involve deception or fabrication of online identities.
   - Trials are accurately represented in recruitment overtures.
   - Proposed recruitment does not involve members of research team 'lurking' or 'creeping' [on] social media sites in ways members are unaware of.
   - Recruitment will not involve advancements or contact that could embarrass or stigmatize potential participants.

5. If the research team intends to recruit from the online networks of current or potential study participants:
   - Provide the IRB with a statement explaining this approach and describing plans to obtain consent and documentation of consent from participants before approaching members of their online networks or to invite the individual themselves to approach members of their network on the research team's behalf.

6. Consider whether a formal communication plan is needed for managing social media activities among enrolled participants, including:
   - Steps to educate participants about the importance of blinding and how certain communications can jeopardize the scientific validity of a study (e.g., a section in the orientation or consent form)
   - Triggers for intervention from the research team (e.g., misinformation or speculation among participants on social media that could lead to un-blinding)
   - Interventions from the research team (e.g., corrections of misinformation or reminders about importance of blinding on social media)

Consent

A large majority of internet research will meet the criteria for <u>exemption</u> from the human subjects regulations and, thus, will not require informed consent. However, best ethical practices dictate that informational documents or the equivalent of a <u>short form consent</u> be included for subjects at the outset of the research, through email, consent portals, or screen pop-ups. The information sheet provided to the subjects should include elements such as contact information for the study and IRB contact, the study procedures, the purpose of the research, confidentiality/anonymity issues, etc.

Specific types of internet research that typically do not require consent include uses of, or analyses involving, public information or data (data on open internet spaces that do not require any membership or login/password criteria) and data in which the research topic does not exceed minimal risk. Many IRBs classify data according to tiers, which can help in determining the necessity of a consent process (**Figure 10.5-3**).

🔗 5-3

🔗 6-8

RESTRICTED
Information that, if disclosed, would cause severe harm to individuals or the institution.

- Data stored in a high security environment such as a "clean room" or "air gapped" computing environment
- Data are subject to legal or regulatory requirements
- Data use could result in criminal or civil liability and access may require additional institutional or legal permissions

HIGH
Information that, if disclosed, would likely cause serious or significant harm to individuals or the institution.

- Data with personally identifiable information, such as personal, financial, medical, or criminal information
- Disclosure could result in criminal and/or civil liability

MODERATE
Information that, if disclosed, could cause moderate or limited harm to individuals or the institution.

- Information protected under state privacy laws, such as employment records
- Information that could be confidential and/or proprietary

LOW
Information that is publicly available or that poses little to no risk of harm to individuals or the institution.

- Published data such as course catalogs
- Institutional or organizational affiliation is not a requirement for access
- Data accessible by anyone, such as public property registries

Figure 10.5-3 Data tier model.

🔗 10-4

For internet research that requires consent, there are a range of consent options. Online surveys, which make up a large majority of internet research, frequently use consent portals, web pages that describe the survey and include language such as "By clicking the submit button to enter the survey, you acknowledge that you have read and understand the above consent form, that you are 18 years old or older, and indicate your willingness to voluntarily take part in the study" (Buchanan & Hvizdak, 2009; Buchanan & Samuel, 2019). It is helpful to remind subjects to print or retain a copy of the document, as it will have study-specific information and contact information. When a signature is required, alternatives such as electronic signatures or stamps can be used.

Other processes for consent include establishing study-specific chat rooms, where individuals can virtually meet with a study team member, review the consent form in a document viewer, and ask questions via a chat or phone line. In their first virtual clinical trial, for example, Pfizer utilized video and multimedia modalities and employed an online consent "test" to ensure participants understood the study. More recently, in the National Institutes of Health's All of Us project, consent information is presented in short videos, with text alternatives.

Given the frequent use of terms of service (TOS) agreements and/or end-user license agreements (EULAs) across internet spaces, tools, and services, researchers and IRBs should carefully consider whether their consent document stands in contrast to, or contradicts, the TOS/EULA. For example, a researcher may use language about maintaining confidentiality, or state that no one besides the researcher will have access to the research data, but this may be in direct opposition to common terms of service, which often state:

> Your personal data is kept on secure servers. Information that is gathered from visitors in common with other websites, log files are stored on the web server saving details such as the visitor's IP address, browser type, referring page and time of visit. Cookies may be used to remember visitor preferences when interacting with the website. Where registration is required, the visitor's email and a username will be stored on the server. The information is used to enhance the visitor's experience when using the website to display personalised content and possibly advertising . . . . (Terms Feed, 2020)

In addition to reviewing for contradictions to TOS/EULAs, informed consent forms or informational documents should include language such as the following:

> "Participation in this research is distinct from your use or membership on X platform. Third-party actors may have access to your data."

> "Your participation in this online survey involves risks similar to a person's everyday use of the internet. There are no additional risks to individuals participating in this research beyond those that exist in daily life."

> "Your confidentiality will be maintained to the degree permitted by the technology used. Specifically, no guarantees can be made regarding the interception of data sent via the internet by any third parties."

Privacy/Confidentiality/Anonymity

Internet research has long raised difficult questions about what should count as "public" or "private" data, and there is still no clear consensus. Early internet research scholars thought of internet spaces along two continua: public to private and sensitive to nonsensitive (Sveningsson, 2003). This is still a helpful heuristic in making determinations about the nature of personal data, since the Common Rule at 45 CFR 46.111 requires that IRBs review the provisions for protecting privacy and maintaining confidentiality. The IRB should consider the privacy of individuals throughout the research process from data collection to transmission to archiving and deletion; the provisions in place to protect the data during use and storage; the individuals who will have access to any identifiable data; and plans for deidentification, storage, and destruction. Furthermore, the Common Rule at 45 CFR 46.102(e) notes that obtaining identifiable private information or identifiable specimens for research purposes constitutes human subjects research. Obtaining identifiable private information or identifiable specimens, in turn, includes, but is not limited to, the following:

- Using, studying, or analyzing for research purposes identifiable private information or identifiable specimens that have been provided to researchers from any source
- Using, studying, or analyzing for research purposes identifiable private information or identifiable specimens that were already in the possession of the researcher

It is notable, too, that the Common Rule has a provision that requires agencies to regularly reexamine the meanings of "identifiable private information" and "identifiable biospecimen" and technologies and techniques that could generate them [45 CFR 46.102(e)(7)].

DEFINITIONS

Confidentiality. Pertains to the treatment of information that an individual has disclosed in a relationship of trust and with the expectation that it will not be divulged without permission to others in ways that are inconsistent with the understanding of the original disclosure.

Privacy. Pertains to having control over the extent, timing, and circumstances of sharing oneself (physically, behaviorally, or intellectually) or information about oneself, with others.

Private information. Information about behavior that occurs in a context in which an individual can reasonably expect that no observation or recording is taking place; information which has been provided for specific purposes by an individual and which the individual can reasonably expect will not be made public.

Publicly available. Data that the public can obtain and is readily available to anyone (without special permission/application) regardless of occupation, purpose, or affiliation.

In evaluating the public or private nature of the data, basic considerations such as the following are helpful:

- What are the current cultural expectations for privacy?
- Are there any restrictions on use/access of data, imposed by the researcher, sponsor, or funder of the research that generated the data? What sorts of restrictions? For example, see the Inter-university Consortium for Political and Social Research (ICPSR) policy on restricted access data (ICPSR, n.d.).
- Are there policies in place that dictate the nature of the site/space? Are there distinct norms regarding privacy? For example, is the site/space considered by its users or membership to be open or private? Or is access to the site/space governed by particular requirements?
- Will the research involve merging any of the data sets in such a way that individuals might be identified?
- Will the researcher enhance public data sets with identifiable or potentially identifiable data?

In addition to these considerations, Markham and Buchanan (2012) and SACHRP's recommendations (questions 3, 4, 6, 7, specifically) provide exhaustive questions for researchers and IRBs to consider in determining the public/private nature of data (SACHRP, 2013).

Data Security

Data security has been a long standing area of concern for IRBs, and traditionally, IRBs encouraged researchers to keep their data in a "locked filing cabinet in an undisclosed location." In the era of dispersed and cloud computing, data security is no longer this simple. For best practices, IRBs should consider data in its various stages: during collection, at rest, in transmission, and at deletion. Many

IRBs have taken a tiered approach to data security, and often IRBs work directly with their institutional information technology departments. Harvard has a useful data classification system (Harvard University, n.d.), which differentiates data as follows:

Level 5: Extremely sensitive information

Level 4: Very sensitive information

Level 3: Sensitive or confidential information

Level 2: Benign information to be held confidentially

Level 1: Nonconfidential research information

For institutions whose researchers engage in large amounts of data-intensive research, it is advisable to have a computer scientist or security expert on the board.

IRBs should consider the following when assessing data security:

- The nature of the identifiers associated with the data
- The justification for needing identifiers in order to conduct the research
- Characteristics of the study population
- The proposed use of the information
- The overall sensitivity of the data
- Persons or groups who will have access to study data
- The process used to share the data
- The likely retention period for identifiable data
- The security controls in place, such as

  - Physical safeguards for paper records
  - Technical safeguards for electronic records
  - Secure sharing or transfer of data outside the institution, if applicable

- The potential risk for harm that would occur if the security of the data was compromised

Additionally, researchers and IRBs should be aware of current industry standards for data security, as well as their institutional policies regarding data maintenance. For example, current best practices include the following:

- Ensure data is securely stored.
  - Use institutional resources for data storage, such as secure department server, institution-approved cloud/server (e.g., Box, REDCap), locked campus office.
  - Only use approved portable devices for temporary storage.
    - Move data to more secure location as soon as reasonably possible, and delete data on portable device.
  - Level of sensitivity of information should guide level of security required for storage.
    - If protected health information (PHI) is collected, storage location *must* be HIPAA compliant.
    - Sensitive/identifiable information should be stored separately from remainder of data.
    - Use encrypted files or clean/cold room servers when necessary.

Readers will find the Johns Hopkins "Risk/Controls Assessment" (it.john shopkins.edu/policies/risk.html) valuable when considering data security measures in relation to human subjects research; additional resources are listed later.

Conclusion

This chapter has provided readers with an overview of salient issues related to internet research. With technological developments, internet research continues to evolve, and different ethical and regulatory considerations arise. Even as the research oversight field starts to define best practices for recruitment, informed consent, privacy and confidentiality, and data security, as outlined in this chapter, emerging issues are again challenging IRBs in the areas of machine learning, artificial intelligence, and data analytics. These newer techniques are confounding the very notions of human subjects research and instead pushing the discourse toward a "data subjects" approach. This concept has emerged in various contexts, ranging from the EU's General Data Protections Regulations, in which a "data subject" is simply any person about which personal data is being collected, held, or processed; to more philosophical questions around the rights of data subjects vis-à-vis human subjects protections (see, for example, Buchanan, 2017b). The 2018 Common Rule gestured toward such technologies but stopped short of providing any regulatory guidance on IRB review of research using them. As with early internet research, social media, and big data research, IRBs and the research community will learn from each other and from their shared experiences with these new domains. Predictions for the data-intensive landscape suggest that reliance on data will only increase as the second decade of the 20th century begins. The regulated research community shares a large piece of this landscape with industry, market researchers, and countless other stakeholders who use data in myriad ways. IRBs and researchers must continually review their best practices in light of changing and developing research technologies, methods, and ethics.

Recommended Reading

Buchanan, E. A., & Zimmer, M. (2018). Internet research ethics. In E. N. Zalta (Ed.), *The Stanford encyclopedia of philosophy* (Winter 2018 Edition). plato.stanford.edu/archives/win2018/entries/ethics-internet-research

Secretary's Advisory Committee for Human Research Protections. (2013). *Considerations and recommendations concerning internet research and human subjects research regulations, with revisions.* www.hhs.gov/ohrp/sites/default/files/ohrp/sachrp/mtgings/2013%20March%20Mtg/internet_research.pdf

Secretary's Advisory Committee for Human Research Protections. (2016). *Human subjects research implications of big data.* www.hhs.gov/ohrp/sachrp-committee/recommendations/2015-april-24-attachment-a/index.html

Resources

Association of Internet Researchers: Ethics Guidelines (2002, 2012, 2019)
http://aoir.org/ethics/

Johns Hopkins: Risk/Control Assessment
https://it.johnshopkins.edu/policies/risk.html

Secretary's Advisory Committee for Human Research Protections (SACHRP). (2016). *Human subjects research implications of big data.* www.hhs.gov/ohrp/sachrp-committee/recommendations/2015-april-24-attachment-a/index.html

Sample IRB Guidelines

Rutgers University
https://orra.rutgers.edu/internet-research

University of California-Berkeley
https://cphs.berkeley.edu/internet_research.pdf

University of Georgia
https://research.uga.edu/docs/policies/compliance/hso/IRB-Internet-Research.pdf

University of Pittsburgh Data Security
www.irb.pitt.edu/electronic-data-security

University of Wisconsin
https://kb.wisc.edu/sbsedirbs/page.php?id=42376

References

Association of Internet Researchers (AoIR). (2002). Ethical decision-making and Internet research: Recommendations from the AoIR ethics working committee. https://aoir.org/reports/ethics.pdf

Buchanan, E. (2002). Internet research ethics and institutional review board policy: New challenges, new opportunities. *Advances in Library Organization and Management, 19*, 85–100.

Buchanan, E. (Ed.). (2003). *Readings in virtual research ethics: Issues and controversies.* Idea Group.

Buchanan, E. (2017a). Considering the ethics of big data research: A case of Twitter and ISIS/ISIL. *PLoS ONE, 12*(12), e0187155.

Buchanan, E. (2017b). Internet research ethics: Twenty years later. In M. Zimmer & K. Kinder-Kurlanda (Eds.), *Internet research ethics for the social age: New challenges, cases, and contexts.* Peter Lang Publishers.

Buchanan, E., & Ess, C. M. (2009). Internet research ethics and the institutional review board: Current practices and issues. *Computers and Society, 39*(3), 43–49.

Buchanan, E. A., & Hvizdak, E. E. (2009). Online survey tools: Ethical and methodological concerns of human research ethics committees. *Journal of Empirical Research on Human Research Ethics, 4*(2), 37–48.

Buchanan, E., & Samuel, G. (Eds.). (2019). Ethical issues in social media research. *Journal of Empirical Research and Human Research Ethics, 15*, 1–2.

Buchanan, E. A., & Zimmer, M. (2012). Internet research ethics. In E. N. Zalta (Ed.), *The Stanford encyclopedia of philosophy.* plato.stanford.edu/entries/ethics-internet-research/

Dumbill, E. (2012). What is big data? An introduction to the big data landscape. http://radar.oreilly.com/2012/01/what-is-big-data.html?

Ess, C., & AoIR Ethics Working Committee. (2002). *Ethical decision-making and Internet research: Recommendation from the AoIR Ethics Working Committee.* Association of Internet Researchers. aoir.org/reports/ethics.pdf

Federal Register. (2017). Vol. 82, No. 12. 45 CFR 46 and Preamble. www.govinfo.gov/content/pkg/FR-2017-01-19/pdf/2017-01058.pdf

Frankel, M. S., & Siang, S. (1999). *Ethical and legal aspects of human subjects research on the Internet.* research.utexas.edu/wp-content/uploads/sites/3/2015/10/report_internet_research.pdf

franzke, a. s., Bechmann, A., Zimmer, M., Ess, C., and the Association of Internet Researchers (2020). Internet research: Ethical guidelines 3.0. https://aoir.org/reports/ethics3.pdf

Gelinas, L., Pierce, R., Winkler, S., Cohen, I., Lynch, H., & Bierer, B. (2017). Using social media as a research recruitment tool: Ethical issues and recommendations. *American Journal of Bioethics, 17*(3), 3–14.

Harvard University. (n.d.). *Information security policy: By data security level.* https://policy.security.harvard.edu/view-data-security-level

Inter-university Consortium for Political and Social Research (ICPSR). (n.d.). *Accessing restricted data at ICPSR.* www.icpsr.umich.edu/icpsrweb/content/ICPSR/access/restricted/

Internet World Stats. (2020). Usage and population statistics. www.internetworldstats.com/stats.htm

Markham, A., & Buchanan, E. (2012). *Ethical decision-making and internet research: Recommendations from the AoIR Ethics Working Committee* (Version 2.0). Association of Internet Researchers. aoir.org/reports/ethics2.pdf

The National Committee for Research Ethics in the Social Sciences and the Humanities (NESH). (2002). Samisk forskning og forskningsetikk. Seminarrapport [Sami research and research ethics. Seminar Report]. Olso: De nasjonale forskningsetiske komiteer [The Norwegian National Research Ethics Committees].

Secretary's Advisory Committee for Human Research Protections (SACHRP). (2013). *Considerations and recommendations concerning internet research and human subjects research regulations, with revisions.* www.hhs.gov/ohrp/sites/default/files/ohrp/sachrp/mtgings/2013%20 March%20Mtg/internet_research.pdf

Sveningsson, M. (2003). Ethics in internet ethnography. In Buchanan, E.A. (Ed.). *Virtual research ethics: Issues and controversies.* Idea Group Publishing.

Terms Feed. (2020). *Sample terms of service template.* www.termsfeed.com/blog/sample-terms-of -service-template/

Varadharajan, D., & Lee, J. (n.d.). *AI in healthcare: The future of clinical trials.* CBINSIGHTS. www .cbinsights.com/research/briefing/ai-in-healthcare-future-clinical-trial/

Epidemiology and Public Health Research

Laura Youngblood

Abstract

Public health research spans the spectrum of scientific study. The same ethical principles and regulatory framework that apply to other fields of study apply to public health research. Although it involves information about individuals, the focus of inquiry in public health research is the population, which presents unique challenges in the interpretation and application of ethical standards and regulatory requirements. This chapter discusses the ethical and regulatory considerations that are unique to public health research, including the Common Rule's exclusion of certain public health surveillance activities, the Health Insurance Portability and Accountability Act (HIPAA) exception for disclosure of protected health information for public health activities, and the Secretarial waiver for the incidental inclusion of prisoners in epidemiological research.

Introduction

Public health research spans the spectrum of scientific study. It includes scientific questions directed at understanding biological processes, behaviors, and social interactions, as well as a wide range of interventions to improve the health of the population. The methods used in public health research are as varied as the research questions that are addressed.

As a scientific discipline, epidemiology is the systematic study of the frequency and patterns of health-related outcomes in specified populations. This includes the study of the causes and risk factors influencing such outcomes and the application of findings to the control of public health problems (Porta, 2014). Epidemiological methods are the cornerstone of public health, and these methods are used in both research and nonresearch settings.

Although public health research involves information about individuals, the focus of inquiry is the population or community. The public health mission to protect the health and well-being of the population is recognized as a public good (Federal Register, 2017, Preamble). It is generally agreed that the _Belmont principles_ of respect for persons, beneficence, and justice (National Commission,

🔗 1-1

1979) have equal moral force across the range of human studies. However in the context of public health, these principles may be expressed differently, and the individual principles may carry different moral weight (Council for International Organizations of Medical Sciences [CIOMS], 2009). There is often tension between autonomy and the protection of public health. Communitarian and utilitarian perspectives favoring the good of the community may be afforded greater weight in the context of public health (Coughlin, 2006).

Many of the ethical issues of concern to IRBs regarding specific methods, such as surveys or the use of existing data or biospecimens, are covered in other chapters (see sidebar, Chapters that Address Issues Relevant to Public Health Research). The focus here is on a few key issues of importance to IRBs when they consider public health research, specifically epidemiological research.

Defining Public Health Research

The Common Rule defines research as "a systematic investigation, including research development, testing, and evaluation, designed to develop or contribute to generalizable knowledge" [45 CFR 46.102(l)]. In the context of public health, determining whether

🔗 5-1   activities constitute research is important for both practical and ethical reasons. From a practical standpoint, activities that do not meet the definition of research do not require application of the administrative and review requirements of the Common Rule. This frees IRBs to focus their resources on those activities that are subject to regulatory oversight. From an ethical standpoint, applying the regulatory framework of the Common Rule when it is not required may unduly impede a public health authority's ability to accomplish its mandated mission to protect and maintain health and welfare (Federal Register, 2017, Preamble).

DEFINITION OF PUBLIC HEALTH AUTHORITY

Public health authority means an agency or authority of the United States, a state, a territory, a political subdivision of a state or territory, an Indian tribe, or a foreign government, or a person or entity acting under a grant of authority from or contract with such public agency, including the employees or agents of such public agency or its contractors or persons or entities to whom it has granted authority, that is responsible for public health matters as part of its official mandate. (Common Rule, **45 CFR 46.102(k)**)

Public health authority means an agency or authority of the United States, a State, a territory, a political subdivision of a State or territory, or an Indian tribe, or a person or entity acting under a grant of authority from or contract with such public agency, including the employees or agents of such public agency or its contractors or persons or entities to whom it has granted authority, that is responsible for public health matters as part of its official mandate. (HIPAA, **45 CFR 164.501**)

Note: The only distinction between the Common Rule and HIPAA definitions is that the Common Rule includes foreign governments.

The Common Rule does not prescribe any particular mechanism by which a research determination must be made, but it is recommended that such determinations be thoughtful and deliberate. Such determinations do not require review by an IRB. However, finding that an activity does not meet the definition of research does not excuse it from the ethical obligation to adhere to principles articulated in the *Belmont Report*. Such activities are often subject to other systems of protection (e.g., state laws regarding confidentiality protection or informed consent). Even in the absence of such systems, consideration of the *Belmont* principles should be part of the deliberation.

There are three key considerations in determining whether any activity is research under the Common Rule:

1. Whether it is within the scope of activities deemed not to be research under the Common Rule, including *public health surveillance*
2. Whether it is a *systematic investigation*
3. Whether it is *designed* to develop or contribute to *generalizable knowledge*

Public Health Surveillance

The Common Rule has explicitly deemed four categories of activities <u>not to be research</u> (see sidebar, Categories of Activities Deemed Not to be Research), including certain public health surveillance activities. Specifically, the Common Rule excludes from its definition of research:

🔗 5-1

> Public health surveillance activities, including the collection and testing of information or biospecimens, conducted, supported, requested, ordered, required, or authorized by a public health authority. Such activities are limited to those necessary to allow a public health authority to identify, monitor, assess, or investigate potential public health signals, onsets of disease outbreaks, or conditions of public health importance (including trends, signals, risk factors, patterns in diseases, or increases in injuries from using consumer products). Such activities include those associated with providing timely situational awareness and priority setting during the course of an event or crisis that threatens public health (including natural or man-made disasters). [45 CFR 46.102(l)(2)]

Activities meeting the criteria of this exclusion, by definition, are not research, even when the methods are systematic or when the findings may be generalizable. Furthermore, the four exclusions are not exhaustive. Public health activities that do not meet the criteria for exclusion might still be classified as nonresearch, through application of the core definition of research: "a systematic investigation, including research development, testing, and evaluation, designed to develop or contribute to generalizable knowledge" [45 CFR 46.102(l)].

Systematic Investigation

Activities are generally considered to be systematic investigations when there is a plan for carrying out the orderly collection and analysis of information using scientific procedures and methods, reflecting generally accepted norms of scientific or academic inquiry

CATEGORIES OF ACTIVITIES DEEMED NOT TO BE RESEARCH [45 CFR 46.102(*l*)]

- Scholarly and journalistic activities (e.g., oral history, journalism, biography, literary criticism, legal research, and historical scholarship), including the collection and use of information, that focus directly on the specific individuals about whom the information is collected
- Public health surveillance activities, including the collection and testing of information or biospecimens, meeting specified criteria
- Collection and analysis of information, biospecimens, or records by or for a criminal justice agency for activities authorized by law or court order solely for criminal justice or criminal investigative purposes
- Authorized operational activities (as determined by each agency) in support of intelligence, homeland security, defense, or other national security missions

(Pritchard & Olson, 2012). In the context of public health, looking at methods or data collection techniques is often not useful for distinguishing between research and nonresearch, because both rely on the use of the same epidemiological methods. For example, a case-control design is frequently used to determine the risk factors in an outbreak investigation for the purpose of bringing the disease under control; in this context, the design is not research. Yet, the case-control design is also routinely used in public health for research purposes, such as to study disease etiology.

Designed to Develop or Contribute to Generalizable Knowledge

Because the "systematic investigation" element of the definition is often not useful for distinguishing between research and nonresearch in the context of public health, one must consider the purpose for conducting the activity and the underlying objectives. When an activity has one or more *a priori* objectives to make progress toward generalizable knowledge, it is generally considered to meet the definition of research, unless otherwise excluded. "Generalizable knowledge" refers to information that is both generalizable, in the sense that information about some people is used to draw conclusions about other people, and that this improves the scientific or academic understanding of the topic under study (Pritchard & Olson, 2012).

Public health practice activities that are carried out for the purpose of preventing or controlling disease or injury, improving health, or improving a public health program or service, frequently lead to generalizable knowledge. It is often difficult to distinguish between activities that *happen to* contribute to generalizable knowledge and those that are *designed for* such a purpose. However, careful review of the background information, justification, rationale, and intended use for a proposed activity may provide clues to the underlying purpose, beyond what is articulated in the objectives. For instance, activities that emphasize gaps in general knowledge, development of new insights, or unique learning opportunities are often research.

Explicit acknowledgment that an activity is intended to generate new knowledge that will contribute to the scientific literature (i.e., that revises or improves on an existing principle, theory, or knowledge), in the absence of a clearly identified plan for timely dissemination of results to prompt public health action or decision, is generally an indication that an activity is designed to develop or contribute to generalizable knowledge.

Intention to publish or present results is not an indication that an activity is research (Department of Health and Human Services [DHHS], 2008a). As part of their civic responsibilities, federal, state, or local government officials are obligated to publish results in government documents or share findings with other public officials. In addition, people seek to publish descriptions of nonresearch activities for a variety of reasons, because even in the absence of generalizable knowledge, the scientific findings of nonresearch activities are often useful to others in the field of public health. Conversely, a public health activity may involve research even if there is no intent to publish the results.

Reviewing Public Health Research

Nonexempt public health research involving human subjects requires IRB review under the Common Rule. Considerations about whether research involves human subjects and whether research qualifies for <u>exemption</u> from IRB review

5-3

are the same for public health as for other disciplines and thus are not covered in this chapter. This section addresses IRB review considerations that are specific to public health research.

Benefits and Risks

A key consideration for IRBs is to ensure that the "risks to subjects are reasonable in relation to anticipated benefits, if any to subjects, and the importance of the knowledge to be gained" [45 CFR 46.111(a)(2)]. With many public health research studies, however, the distribution of risks and potential benefits may involve individual subjects, populations, and nonsubjects, making the risk/benefit calculation more difficult. In reviewing public health research, IRBs must consider who the expected beneficiaries are, who bears the risk, and how to weigh these various and possibly competing interests.

- **Benefits**. Individuals may benefit directly from public health research activities, such as the opportunity to participate in a program. However, much of public health research involves use of data or biospecimens for the purpose of understanding and reducing health risks, and it often does not confer any direct benefit on the individual subjects. In these cases, subjects benefit indirectly, through improvements in public health that may be relevant to specific communities or to broader populations.

- **Risks**. Most public health activities, including epidemiological research, involve minimal physical risk, if any. The physical risks encountered in public health are typically associated with the collection of <u>biospecimens</u>, and they are usually limited to noninvasive procedures that are commensurate with the nature and types of biospecimens that are collected during a routine physical exam. The collection and use of <u>data</u>, however, can lead to psychosocial harms to individuals or communities, such as psychological harm through the collection of sensitive information, affronts to personal dignity through the loss of privacy, and social harms resulting from breaches in confidentiality or the dissemination of research results.

🖉 10-10

🖉 12-3, 12-4

Direct collection of new data from subjects, e.g., through interviews, surveys, or focus groups, may cause psychological distress or embarrassment if the topic is sensitive. When research involves a sensitive issue, IRBs and others should consider how to minimize the risk, such as ensuring interviewers have appropriate training and whether subjects may be particularly vulnerable in relation to the issue being investigated.

Privacy and Confidentiality

Although often used interchangeably, the terms *privacy* and *confidentiality* represent distinct concepts. Privacy refers to an individual's right to control access to, and use of, their information. Confidentiality refers to the expectation that private information will not be disclosed (Office for Protection from Research Risks, *IRB Guidebook*, 1993, as quoted in Forster, 2006). Breaches in confidentiality, whether through failure to maintain confidentiality or through unauthorized disclosure, undermine individuals' right to privacy. Potential harms that may result include discrimination, stigmatization, or economic loss. Common Rule requirements regarding privacy and confidentiality are limited to the directive that IRBs may approve a research study only when they have judged that the study contains adequate protections for privacy and maintenance of confidentiality [45 CFR 46.111(a)(7)].

Specific methods for protecting privacy and maintaining confidentiality are not unique to public health, and relevant issues are discussed in many chapters throughout this book. Similarly, state and federal protections apply to public health research the same way they apply to other human subjects research disciplines. For example, certificate of confidentiality protections are applicable to all research conducted or supported by the U.S. Public Health Service in which identifiable sensitive information is obtained.

🖉 8-3

One notable exception is the HIPAA Privacy Rule (Privacy of Individually Identifiable Health Information, 2016), which includes specific provisions permitting covered entities to use or disclose protected health information (PHI) to public health authorities for legitimate public health purposes, without individual patient authorization (Refer to box "Definition of Public Health Authority" in Centers for Disease Control and Prevention, 2003). Permitted public health disclosures include, but are not limited to, public health surveillance, public health investigations, and public health interventions. However, this provision does not apply to public health *research*. Disclosure for research purposes, even in the context of public health, is subject to the same restrictions and requirements as other types of research. It should also be noted that many public health authorities are not "covered entities" under HIPAA; specific protections afforded to patients under HIPAA are no longer applicable to PHI after it has been disclosed to a noncovered public health authority.

🖉 11-6

Equitable Selection

🖉 5-4

Although the Common Rule generally requires that subject selection be equitable, there are a few aspects of equitable selection and justice that are unique to public health research. Public health research is often carried out in settings and populations that are affected by the condition under study, e.g., a population suffering from an infectious disease outbreak or recovering from a natural disaster. IRBs and other reviewers should be mindful of overburdening the populations under study and, to the extent possible, conduct research and other activities in populations that are likely to benefit from the findings.

Incidental Inclusion of Vulnerable Populations

As a population-based science, it is often necessary for the sake of scientific validity to include all eligible people within a defined population of interest. The inclusion, even incidentally, of pregnant women, prisoners, or children requires IRB review and approval under 45 CFR 46, subparts B, C, and D, respectively, if the research is conducted or supported by DHHS. These populations should not be systematically excluded from public health research without careful consideration of the ethical and scientific implications. Excluding vulnerable populations may unfairly deprive individuals of direct benefits or deprive a segment of the population from the benefits of the knowledge to be gained. Additionally, systematic exclusion may bias study results and undermine the benefits to be derived from the study's findings.

🖉 9-4 🖉 9-5 🖉 9-6

Special Considerations for the Inclusion of Prisoners in Epidemiological Research

Studies designed to describe the prevalence or incidence of disease, as well as research designed to study potential risk factor associations for a disease or condition, are common in public health. Due to the population-based methodologies used in epidemiology, <u>prisoners</u> may be included incidentally in the study population. There are four categories for permissible research involving prisoners, which generally limit research involving prisoners to studies that directly target prisoners as a class or prisons as institutional structures. Studies focusing on a condition or disease that might affect prisoners in the same way that it would any other member of the general population do not meet any of the four categories of permissible research under subpart C of 45 CFR 46.

🔗 9-5

In 2003, the Secretary of DHHS waived the applicability of certain provisions of subpart C for epidemiological research meeting certain criteria, hereafter referred to as the *Secretarial waiver* (DHHS, 2003). The Secretarial waiver allows IRBs to approve studies that do not meet any of the four categories of permissible research with prisoners, if certain criteria are met. Specifically, the only purpose of the research must be either to describe the prevalence or incidence of a disease by identifying all cases or to study potential risk factor associations for a disease. In addition, the research must present no more than minimal risk and no more than inconvenience to the prisoner-subjects, and prisoners must not be a particular focus of the research.

The Secretarial waiver does not waive the applicability of subpart C in its entirety; it only waives the requirement that the research satisfy one or more of the four categories of permissible research. All other requirements under subpart C, including requirements to include a prisoner or prisoner representative on the IRB, and to certify to the Secretary that the duties of the IRB have been fulfilled, apply to research that is approved under the Secretarial waiver. The Secretarial waiver, in effect, serves as a fifth category of permissible research under subpart C (DHHS, 2008b).

Informed Consent

As with other types of research, obtaining the <u>informed consent</u> of subjects remains an important mechanism for respecting their autonomy. Public health research may be conducted in a broad range of settings and under a broad range of scientific disciplines (e.g., clinical, behavioral, and molecular research). This section will focus on the special issues and considerations related to informed consent that are unique to public health research.

🔗 Section 6

Waiving Informed Consent

The Common Rule specifies a number of criteria under which informed consent may be <u>waived</u>. Public health research frequently involves the <u>secondary use</u> of existing data or biospecimens collected in the context of clinical care, surveillance, or other settings in which formal written consent is not typically obtained. IRBs often face challenges when reviewing requests to waive informed consent requirements in the absence of subjects' express approval to store data and biospecimens for future research.

🔗 6-4 🔗 12-3

When considering whether waiving consent would adversely affect subjects' rights or welfare [45 CFR 46.116(f)(3)(iv)], IRBs may take a number of factors into account:

- For what purpose were the data and/or biospecimens originally collected?
- Does the proposed research address a topic that is relevant to the purpose for which the data and/or biospecimens were originally collected?

- Does the research address a topic that is sensitive in nature? For example, does it involve HIV or genetic testing or otherwise address a topic that subjects might reasonably find objectionable?

Taken together, these attributes may be useful in determining whether the requested waiver presents an undue affront to subjects' autonomy or personal dignity.

IRBs also struggle with the assessment of whether research could practicably be conducted without waiving consent [45 CFR 46.116(f)(ii)]. In making this assessment, IRBs may consider the feasibility of locating and contacting subjects or whether contacting subjects might, in itself, introduce risks related to privacy and confidentiality. In addition, because of the population-based nature of epidemiology, consideration of scientific validity may also be relevant. The inability to locate, contact, and obtain consent from all identified cases, for example, may lead to underrepresentation of disease estimates. Additionally, unmeasurable differences between locatable and nonlocatable subjects may introduce biases that undermine the validity of study findings.

While most IRBs waive consent requirements under paragraph (f) of 45 CFR 46.116, it should be noted that paragraph (e) of that section, which allows IRBs to waive consent requirements for research involving state or local public benefit or service programs, may be applicable to public health research as an alternative to paragraph (f). This provision similarly requires a finding that the research could not practicably be conducted without a waiver, but it does not require a finding that the waiver would not adversely affect subjects' rights or welfare.

Consent in the Context of Community-Level Interventions

Public health research may also involve the implementation and evaluation of community-level interventions, in which it is often not practicable to get individual consent from every community member impacted by the intervention. Examples of such interventions might include the following:

- Implementing vector control programs in communities with mosquito-borne disease transmission
- Treating community point-of-use water sources
- Implementing hospital-wide decolonization procedures

Because the Common Rule applies only to individuals about whom information or biospecimens are obtained, members of the community whose information or biospecimens are not obtained fall outside the scope of the regulation. However, researchers' and institutions' duty to adhere to the *Belmont* principles of respect, beneficence, and justice remains, and they should be encouraged to engage with communities affected by the research.

Cultural Considerations

12-9

9-10

6-4

Public health research is often conducted in <u>communities</u> that require the permission of a community leader, council, or other designated authority. Such communities include villages, <u>tribes</u>, and institutions, such as schools or prisons. The permission of a community leader, however, does not take the place of individual consent (CIOMS, 2009). Individual consent must always be obtained unless the requirement has been <u>waived</u>.

Additionally, public health research may involve distinct cultural groups for which the signing of documents is not the norm. In these cases, IRBs may consider waiving the requirement to <u>document informed consent</u> **[45 CFR 46.117(c)(1)(iii)]**.

IRBs have considerable flexibility within the confines of the Common Rule to consider <u>alternative approaches</u> to obtaining and documenting informed consent. In keeping with the *Belmont* principle of respect for persons (National Commission, 1979), reviewers should be encouraged to exercise such flexibility, when applicable, to accommodate the cultural norms of the communities under study.

🔗 6-5

🔗 Section 6

Consent for Nonresearch Public Health Activities

The Common Rule applies only to activities that meet the regulatory definition of research **[45 CFR 46.102(l)]**. Thus, the general requirements to obtain and document informed consent do not apply to nonresearch public health surveillance or other epidemiological studies outside the scope of research. However, as previously described, researchers' and institutions' ethical duty to adhere to the *Belmont* principles remains, even outside the scope of the Common Rule. Individuals or entities tasked with determining whether an activity is or is not research should consider whether, in the case of a nonresearch determination, consent remains a reasonable requirement.

Conclusion

Public health research can raise some special issues for IRBs. Distinguishing between public health practice and public health research is challenging. Institutions that conduct public health studies should develop processes for identifying public health activities that are not subject to the regulatory requirements of the Common Rule.

Because of the unique issues that IRBs face in the interpretation and application of ethical standards and regulatory requirements in the context of public health, IRBs that review a substantial amount of public health research should consider having one or more public health professionals as members. It may also be useful to the IRB to have a member from either the state or local health department or to build a relationship with the health department for consultative purposes.

Acknowledgment

The author wishes to thank Nancy Ondrusek for contributing to this chapter.

References

Centers for Disease Control and Prevention. (2003). HIPAA Privacy Rule and public health: Guidance from CDC and the US Department of Health and Human Services. *Morbidity and Mortality Weekly Report, 52*, 1–12. www.cdc.gov/mmwr/preview/mmwrhtml/m2e411a1.htm

Coughlin, S. S. (2006). Ethical issues in epidemiologic research and public health practice. *Emerging Themes in Epidemiology, 3*, 16.

Council for International Organizations of Medical Sciences (CIOMS). (2009). *International ethical guidelines for epidemiological studies*. World Health Organization.

Department of Health and Human Services (DHHS). (2003). *Waiver of the applicability of certain provisions of Department of Health and Human Services regulations for protection of human research subjects for Department of Health and Human Services conducted or supported epidemiologic research involving prisoners as subjects.* 68 Fed. Reg. 36929.

Department of Health and Human Services (DHHS). (2008a). *Quality improvement activities FAQs.* www.hhs.gov/ohrp/regulations-and-policy/guidance/faq/quality-improvement-activities/index.html

Department of Health and Human Services (DHHS). (2008b). *Prisoner research FAQs.* www.hhs.gov/ohrp/regulations-and-policy/guidance/faq/prisoner-research/index.html

Federal Register. (2017). Vol. 82, No. 12. 45 CFR 46 and Preamble. www.govinfo.gov/content/pkg/FR-2017-01-19/pdf/2017-01058.pdf

Forster, D. G. (2006). Privacy and confidentiality. In E. A. Bankert & R. J. Amdur (Eds.), *Institutional review board management and function* (2nd ed.). Jones & Bartlett.

National Commission for the Protection of Human Subjects of Biomedical and Behavioral Research. (1979). *The Belmont Report: Ethical principles and guidelines for the protection of human subjects of biomedical and behavioral research.* www.hhs.gov/ohrp/regulations-and-policy/belmont-report/read-the-belmont-report/index.html

Porta, M. (2014). *A dictionary of epidemiology* (6th ed., p. 95). Oxford University Press.

Pritchard, I., & Olson, N. (2012). *You'll know it when you see it: Defining "human subjects research" under the DHHS regulations* [Presentation]. Advancing Ethical Research Conference, Public Responsibility in Medicine & Research (C20). San Diego.

Privacy of Individually Identifiable Health Information. (2016). Department of Health and Human Services. 45 CFR 164, subpart E.

Disaster and Emergency-Related Public Health Research

Christopher J. Kratochvil

Abigail Lowe

Julia Slutsman

Abstract

During public health emergencies, potential treatments and relief efforts must be studied in a timely manner, while maintaining protections for research subjects and compliance with regulations and frameworks governing the ethical review of the research. To support robust and timely human subject protections review of public health emergency (PHE) research, IRBs should be aware of the range of topic areas considered PHE research, the kinds of research ethics issues associated with such studies, and approaches for enhancing efficient review of these studies. This chapter will provide an overview of considerations for IRB review of PHE research and share case studies illustrating how institutions and IRBs have approached review of a variety of PHE studies.

Background

The need for the conduct of research during and following disasters has received increased attention and funding since the World Trade Center attacks in 2001 (Packenham, 2017). Multiple federal agencies have committed funds to study the impact of disasters as well as public health emergencies in order to enhance preparedness and response efforts and to identify which healthcare interventions can help mitigate adverse health effects (Substance Abuse and Mental Health Services Administration [SAMHSA], 2016). To support robust and timely human subject protections review of such research, IRBs should be aware of common topic areas for PHE research, common research ethics issues associated with such studies, and approaches for enhancing efficiency of review for these time-sensitive studies. This chapter will provide an overview of considerations for IRB review of such research and share case studies illustrating how institutions and IRBs have approached review of PHE protocols.

PHE research spans a wide range of areas and includes studies related to preparedness, response, recovery, and effects of natural or manmade disasters, as well as response and containment related to infectious disease outbreaks and biochemical threats (Packenham et al., 2017). Studies can include biomedical as well as sociobehavioral approaches and range in design from randomized trials, to case control trials, to observational studies, to chart reviews. Subjects in such studies can include victims immediately affected, as well as responders, aid workers, and healthcare or other service providers. Due to the nature of research in emergency situations, there will typically be a limited window of time for launching and conducting the research during or shortly after the occurrence of a PHE. This time pressure is often combined with increased uncertainty associated with conducting research involving an unplanned event in an uncontrolled environment.

Review and consideration of such research therefore requires interpretation of ethical and regulatory requirements within these constraints. Despite such challenges, there are multiple examples of successful and robust review of PHE research by IRBs across multiple settings. Although in this chapter we focus on examples of minimal risk and greater than minimal risk research, some research related to PHEs may be exempt, considered as part of public health surveillance activities, or not considered to be human subjects research. IRB staff should ensure that the appropriate and least burdensome review pathway is utilized. Although IRBs must, of course, apply relevant regulatory requirements and analyze these studies through the lens of well-established research ethics frameworks (such as Emanuel et al., 2008), there are a number of considerations particular to PHE research that IRBs should take into consideration when reviewing and analyzing such studies and consulting with researchers on the design and conduct of possible studies.

5-3
5-1

Human Subject Protections Review Considerations

There is a growing literature identifying examples of research conducted during or subsequent to a disaster, with attention to ethical considerations relevant to human subject protections as well as approaches to facilitating the IRB review process. There has also been limited empirical work, bringing together IRB leaders, researchers, and other stakeholders with experience in IRB review or study design, to identify strategies that may be useful in the review of future studies (Packenham et al., 2017; Taylor, 2016).

Drawing on this work is helpful in identifying the kinds of research ethics issues that IRBs should pay particular attention to when reviewing PHE protocols. A list of key considerations for IRBs is below. This is not intended to be an exhaustive list but rather a list of key critical considerations that will apply to the review of most PHE research protocols.

Uncertainty About Specific Risks and Benefits

While IRBs routinely consider how best to balance risks and benefits in the face of uncertain risk/benefit profiles, certain PHE studies, for instance, those studying treatment of emerging infectious diseases, may include substantial uncertainties to which IRBs are not typically accustomed. Although oncology research may involve early phase 1 studies based on limited prior human data,

10-15

trials in PHE can include multiple layers of uncertainty. Outbreaks of emerging infectious diseases may involve unknown trajectories in the progression of the epidemic on top of an unknown risk/benefit profile of investigational interventions and a lack of certainty about production and ongoing availability of an interventional product (Alirol et al., 2017). IRBs will need to grapple with such uncertainties about the relative risks and benefits of research participation during deliberations to ensure that they can be expressed as clearly as possible in informed consent materials.

Characteristics of Research Design Affecting Risk/Benefit Ratio

Recent outbreaks of Ebola virus disease (EVD) in Africa have spurred discussions of a variety of novel research designs, such as adaptive trial designs that pit various medical countermeasures against each other in a flexible, randomized approach. PHE research may take place in communities that have damage to infrastructure, state and local services, and availability of healthcare services, or that have limitations in resources to begin with. IRBs should ensure that the study design has a plan for referral and facilitating access to necessary services that are viable, given the realities of what is available in the community. Additionally, IRBs should ensure that researchers can provide sufficient assurance that research participation will not adversely affect subjects' access to any services or benefits offered to them as part of the response efforts (Collogan et al., 2004; Taylor, 2016).

Equitable Subject Selection

IRBs need to ensure that robust efforts are made to include and recruit all appropriate populations, including those historically underrepresented in research. Should exclusion criteria specify that certain groups be excluded from the research due to unacceptable risks, a compelling justification must accompany that decision.

The push to be broadly inclusive may run contrary to typical study designs of certain higher risk novel therapies, where initial safety and efficacy studies with healthy individuals are often done prior to studies with those who are most likely to use the intervention being studied, if shown successful. However, given that a promising standard of care may not be available or feasible in the case of emerging outbreaks or biological/chemical disasters, IRBs need to ensure that an appropriate and justifiable risk/benefit balance exists in the context of disaster research. For instance, in some of the interventional studies conducted during the Ebola outbreak in West Africa, the World Health Organization's ethics review committee recognized that mortality rates were highest in children under 4 years old and that maternal and newborn mortality rates were extremely high as well (Alirol et al., 2017). For a number of studies, the ethics review committee requested that these groups be included in the study to provide them access to a potentially beneficial intervention (Alirol et al., 2017). This, in turn, would also help to ensure that appropriate data on use were collected.

Subject Vulnerability

Victims of a disaster or PHE can be subject to substantial vulnerabilities. The loss of resources and support systems, coupled with possible relocation, can strain an individual's ability to make a decision, and this could make them

🔗 Section 9

feel beholden to caregivers to agree to requests to participate in research. The subject may assume that the researcher is acting in their best interest and thus make a decision without truly weighing the risks and benefits of participation. Additionally, a long-standing concern about research involving communities in the wake of a disaster is that the event itself can reduce an individual's ability to cope with stressors. Some have suggested that populations of individuals who have survived a disaster should inherently be considered vulnerable (Ferreira et al., 2015; Fleishman & Wood, 2002). Although more data on the effects of participating in PHE research is needed, recent empirical work has found that serious distress due to retelling of individuals' experiences of going through a disaster does not generally exacerbate the harm or distress stemming from the initial trauma (Legerski & Bunnell, 2010).

⊘ 7-2 Some IRBs have asked researchers to include items asking about distress associated with participation in the research as part of the study and report back to the IRB at the time of <u>continuing review</u> (Taylor, 2016). Some IRBs have developed standard consent language with contact information for mental health counseling services targeted to disaster survivors (Quick, 1998). Studies have found that vulnerable populations tend to experience greater health consequences in the wake of disasters, so the need for inclusion of such populations in research is key to improving health outcomes and addressing existing disparities (Packenham, 2017).

Finally, it is incumbent on research teams to describe to the IRBs the context and conditions in the community so that the IRB can identify whether there is potential for undue influence and ensure that it is minimized.

Study Conduct and Subject Recruitment

IRBs should ensure that research activities conducted during a PHE are designed in such a way as to minimize the potential for the research activity to interfere with or be inappropriately perceived as part of a response activity. ⊘ Section 6 The <u>informed consent process</u> should make explicit when the activity taking place is research and not part of response efforts. Researchers' questions may be similar to those asked by individuals conducting needs assessments as part of organized disaster response. Therefore, it is incumbent on research teams to make clear that they are conducting research and not providing support services (Collogan et al., 2004; Taylor, 2016).

⊘ 12-2 In considering <u>remuneration or incentives</u> to research subjects, IRBs should be attuned to the potential for undue influence in the recruitment and consent process if disasters have created resource scarcities (Knack et al., 2006). Some authors have suggested that it is preferable to provide items that support survivors' basic needs in lieu of monetary incentives, or to donate their time to recovery efforts (Knack et al., 2006; Lavin et al., 2012). IRBs need to review the context of a disaster and the condition and needs of the ⊘ 12-9 community, ideally with feedback and representation from <u>community stakeholders</u>, when considering the appropriateness of incentives for participation in disaster research.

IRBs may rely on research teams to provide this context and may also consider inviting a member of the public health response effort or a community leader involved in the response effort to serve as an ad hoc consultant to the IRB to help inform the board's review and deliberations (Packenham, 2017). Drawing on the knowledge base of a community leader familiar with the disaster's effects and response can also help IRBs maintain awareness of the overall burden of research for a given community. Although IRBs typically review studies on a protocol-by-protocol basis, IRBs reviewing multiple studies related to a single disaster may be asked to play a role in ensuring that the research is not unduly burdensome to the communities under study (Lavin et al., 2012). This could be particularly important in austere or resource-limited settings, where conducting research may draw down limited resources and infrastructure.

While the IRB's focus is on the protection of study subjects, disaster research may place a burden on, elicit distress in, or compromise the physical safety of the research team (Knack et al., 2006). Some have suggested that IRBs ask research teams about whether any resources are in place to support the study team should this be needed or that study teams consider identifying professional facilitators or mental health professionals, if they are not included on the study team, to conduct interviews with research subjects to identify and minimize distress (Collogan et al., 2004; Taylor, 2016).

Informed Consent

Obtaining valid <u>informed consent</u> during a disaster or in the midst of an infectious disease outbreak can be particularly challenging. In these circumstances, IRBs could consider requiring monitoring of the informed consent process, as well as monitoring during recruitment of subjects in disaster studies. For <u>critically ill patients</u> and, specifically, those for whom there are no approved or alternative treatment options, it can be difficult to limit susceptibility to undue inducement and therapeutic misconception. The difficulty of obtaining informed consent may increase in circumstances when the patient has been transported long distances on an emergency basis, is <u>cognitively impaired</u>, or has few or no family members immediately present to give proxy consent (Kraft et al., 2019). In such situations, it is important to bear in mind that consent is a process, and encouraging involvement of family or other social support structures in the process may be particularly important.

🔗 Section 6

🔗 9-8

🔗 9-7

In disaster studies, research teams should consider establishing a standard approach for determining the decision-making ability of disaster-affected research subjects to provide informed consent (e.g., this may include a capacity or competence assessment screening questionnaire). As a precaution to eliminate confusion concerning the exchange of disaster aid for participating in research, consent forms may include a section requiring the subjects to initial to indicate that they understand that they are participating in research and that their participation in the study is independent of disaster aid administered by local, state, or federal agencies or other entities (Packenham, 2017). Even under optimal conditions, additional issues related to risk and benefit, innovative study design, subject privacy, and evolving regulations present challenges for IRBs.

Approaches to Creating Efficiency in IRB Review During Public Health Emergencies

Challenges are inherent to PHE research, including operational considerations for IRB review. PHEs are by their very nature unpredictable, and when they occur, efforts to engage in "response research" must occur immediately, activating processes and resources proactively established well before the event. PHE studies should be reviewed first to identify whether the submission is

⊘ 5-1 ⊘ 5-3

⊘ 5-5, 5-6, and 5-7

⊘ 10-6

research with human subjects, whether it falls into exempt categories, and if it is determined nonexempt, to identify the most appropriate and efficient review pathway. The Common Rule designates certain surveillance activities performed under the auspices of a public health authority not to be research [45 CFR 46.102(l)]. Accordingly, close attention to the role of a public health authority in a PHE project is important to identifying whether a PHE study should be considered research.

⊘ 2-3

Optimizing data collection and introducing experimental interventions in a disaster setting may require a compressed timeline for regulatory approval. Importantly, past PHEs have offered data essential to ongoing efforts to improve preparedness and response (Lurie et al., 2013). Emerging disease outbreaks may not provide much warning or lead time to initiate research, placing strain and setting unrealistic expectations upon ill-prepared research support systems. Conducting research under these circumstances is an operational challenge. Institutional human research protection programs should consider developing standard operating procedures describing the IRB review process and timeline for review of public health preparedness research activities and communicate these to the research community to help support timely review of research when disasters occur (Saxena, 2019).

In the midst of the H1N1 pandemic, the National Heart, Lung, and Blood Institute provided funding to the Acute Respiratory Distress Syndrome Network (ARDSNet) for protocol modification and rapid analysis of clinical data from critically ill patients. The results offered important information; however, at some participating sites, IRBs were not able to approve changes to the data collection protocol during the pandemic, demonstrating the strain placed on IRBs attempting to operate in step with response efforts (Lurie et al., 2013). This is not surprising, given the organization and infrastructure at many human research protection programs does not always lend itself to rapid review.

⊘ Section 4

With the Common Rule mandate for single IRB (sIRB) review of cooperative research as well as the Final NIH Policy on the Use of a Single Institutional Review Board for Multi-Site Research policy in effect, institutions will be required to take part in sIRB review for studies meeting one or both requirements. In instances where neither the Common Rule nor the NIH sIRB policy applies, institutions can consider voluntarily entering into cooperative review to help streamline the review process for collaborative research and may seek out an IRB experienced in reviewing PHE studies to serve as the sIRB of record. In point of fact, one of the stated goals of the NIH sIRB policy is to "enhance and streamline IRB review for multi-site research," and multisite PHE studies may be a good example of content areas utilizing an sIRB in order to streamline review and rely on institutions with expertise in PHE research review (NIH, 2016).

Preapproved Templates

⊘ 5-5 ⊘ 5-7

The use of generic preapproved protocol templates and template language as well as preapproved survey tools useful in PHE studies is an effective strategy for facilitating efficient expedited and full board review in the contexts of both pandemics and natural disasters. For example, research on the 2010 Deepwater Horizon environmental disaster leveraged preapproved protocol templates and questionnaires that can be tailored to specific research studies (Miller et al., 2019).

Médecins Sans Frontières (MSF) has also utilized preapproved templates for several research studies (MSF, 2019). The MSF Ethics Review Board encourages submission of generic protocols, which can be rapidly adapted to a specific context. Once a disease outbreak emerges, the final protocol can be submitted for expedited review. Full ethics approval can only be granted once the context is known and the generic protocol has been contextualized for the specific location and community. That said, the preestablished foundation of the research has the potential to shorten the IRB approval period during an outbreak. One of the challenges with preapproved templates, however, is adequately anticipating enough generalizable aspects of the next PHE to make the prior work useful, while not making erroneous assumptions. Even with a template, final details critical to ethics review may still cause delays prior to initiating research.

A Rapid Response IRB

A rapid response IRB can be convened quickly and utilized to provide convened board review in the case of a PHE, which is especially useful for the review of clinical protocols on a compressed timeline. Rapid response IRBs may achieve this through a number of mechanisms that accelerate the process of a thorough review. For example, leveraging the expertise of the IRB staff through extensive prereview of protocols and developing consent documents in an iterative process that involves close collaboration with the researchers and can optimize human subject protections during traumatic times while shortening timelines. A key aspect is establishing the IRB composition, infrastructure, and processes in advance.

Some institutions form a rapid response IRB *ad hoc* from an existing board or boards, whereas others may <u>constitute</u> a board specifically for times when a protocol review is needed for an urgent issue. A rapid response IRB must meet all membership requirements as stated in **45 CFR 46.107(f)**.

🔗 3-1

A rapid response IRB is intended to provide more timely full board review for studies that require it, where otherwise an institution might decline to be involved in the research because it is not feasible given time limitations, or decide that an intervention can be used as an emergency treatment but data cannot be collected for research. When forming a rapid response IRB, experience in reviewing PHE research is key, as PHE research requires a sophisticated understanding of the circumstances of crisis, as well as susceptibility of the population. Members of a rapid response IRB should receive education in the characteristics and review of PHE research and the kind of review considerations described in this chapter (Kraft et al., 2019). A rapid response board that is set up to review PHE research should understand the pressures and constraints of conducting research in the context of a PHE and be supported by

A RAPID RESPONSE IRB AT THE UNIVERSITY OF NEBRASKA MEDICAL CENTER

The University of Nebraska Medical Center (UNMC) established a rapid response IRB to provide a mechanism for review of human subjects research when insufficient time was available for the standard review schedule. It is a fully constituted and registered IRB, composed of eight members, including a nonscientist, a member not otherwise affiliated with the institution, and a prisoner representative. It also includes a diverse membership representing a variety of colleges, departments, and medical disciplines, including but not limited to the college of public health, infectious disease, pharmacy, and ethics. This rapid response IRB was activated repeatedly during the 2014–2016 Ebola outbreak, in order to review investigational therapies for those patients who were repatriated by the State Department from West Africa to the United States.

INVESTIGATIONAL DRUGS, EMERGENCY USE, AND EXPANDED ACCESS

In PHE research, at times there is a need for unapproved therapeutics that may be subject to FDA regulations. One approach for researchers to consider is to utilize one of FDA's allowed expanded access mechanisms that offer a pathway for one or more patients to gain access to an investigational intervention for treatment outside of clinical trials when no comparable or satisfactory alternative therapy options are available.

adequate information technology (IT), communications infrastructure, and staff to conduct review and reach out to research teams in real time as questions arise during a quick review process.

Leveraging Single IRB Mechanisms

Consistent with revisions to the Common Rule and the Final NIH Policy on the Use of a Single Institutional Review Board for Multi-Site Research (NIH, 2016), the designation and use of single IRBs for multisite studies has become routine. Numerous institutions, such as those designated as NIH Clinical and Translational Science Awards (CTSA) Program Trial Innovation Centers (TICs), are developing the capacity to serve as sIRBs, whereas other institutions are choosing to rely on sIRBs and not act in this capacity. To prepare to review multisite PHE research, institutions should have clear policies in effect for operationalizing the Common Rule and NIH requirements. They should formulate their position on whether they will cede review to an sIRB in a PHE and maximize their ability to rely on sIRBs through participation in reliance agreements such as the SMART IRB platform. Establishing relationships and communication pathways with IRBs that have the capacity to serve as sIRBs can be a helpful approach to institutions that do not develop this capacity.

⊘ Section 4

An early example of consolidating both scientific and human subject protections review in a single institution and sIRB is the research that followed in the wake of the 1995 Oklahoma City bombing. Then governor Keating requested that all human subjects research be reviewed through the University of Oklahoma IRB. The mission of the University of Oklahoma IRB was to guarantee consistency in quality of research; ensure sensitivity and compassion in the conduct of each study; protect the confidentiality of the victims, their families, and rescue workers; and monitor the quantity of research conducted with these potential subjects (Quick, 1998).

In 2011, the National Preparedness and Response Science Board (NPRSB) called for the creation of a specialized IRB capable of rapidly convening to assess research protocols while maintaining robust protections for human subjects. The Public Health Emergency Research Review Board (PHERRB) was subsequently established to review multisite protocols (or other studies that would require review by multiple IRBs) that are conducted, supported, or regulated by DHHS and subject to **45 CFR 46** and, as applicable, **21 CFR 50 and 56** (IOM, 2015; Lurie et al., 2013).

The PHERRB was established in 2012 by DHHS and is maintained by NIH. The PHERRB leverages the existing NIH intramural IRB system and the expertise of its members to allow for high-quality and efficient review of PHE research across a wide range of scientific areas and designs. The PHERRB is a national resource, and review can be requested by contacting the NIH Office of Human Subjects Research Protections (OHSRP) via PHERRB@mail.NIH.gov.

Lessons Learned From Previous Public Health Emergencies

The Ebola outbreak of 2014–2016 infected more than 28,000 individuals with EVD, and more 11,000 people lost their lives to the disease (CDC, 2016). In 2015, several clinical trials were launched in the affected countries of Guinea, Liberia, and Sierra Leone. Although there were several trials ultimately initiated in West Africa, a variety of factors led to delayed starts, ultimately leading to these studies being launched too late to be completed within the window of the outbreak. This was not simply a challenge for the West African sites; the United States and Europe similarly lacked the infrastructure and capacity to launch an organized and coordinated research response (Presidential Commission, 2015). By the end of the epidemic, only a single patient with EVD, cared for in the United States or Europe, was enrolled in a randomized controlled trial (PREVAIL II et al., 2016).

A Need for Standardization of Protocols and Supporting Materials

The 2014–2016 EVD epidemic revealed the difficulty of rapidly initiating research across multiple sites, with multiple independent protocols running in parallel to one another at various academic health centers. This highlighted the need to move to a standardized centralized approach, especially in guiding the administration of medical countermeasures (MCMs), as well as in prospectively collecting clinical data during the course of a patient's illness (Kraft et al., 2019). The lack of coordinated clinical research efforts and protocols during the EVD outbreak led to the use of a wide variety of investigational MCMs, often lacking in coordination, rather than a cohesive and more focused approach, which could better lead to generation of useful data. Even in resource-rich environments such as the United States and Europe, a multitude of MCMs, typically in combination, were generally given under compassionate use, with no consistent or coordinated approach (Kraft et al., 2019).

In 2016, the DHHS Office of the Assistant Secretary for Preparedness and Response (ASPR) provided funding to the National Ebola Training and Education Center (NETEC) to develop research capabilities (CDC, 2016). The Special Pathogens Research Network (SPRN) was initiated as a resource under NETEC, to support research infrastructure at the 10 regional treatment centers in the United States (NETEC, 2017). This funding included the development of a central rapid response IRB (Kratochvil et al., 2017). SPRN was established to efficiently and systematically operationalize the conduct of research and data collection. The SPRN central IRB is acutely aware of special considerations affecting patients hospitalized in biocontainment units and the constraints of conducting research in this unique setting. Obtaining <u>valid informed consent</u> is particularly challenging in the context of serious medical illness due to the accompanying fear of death and the lack of approved or alternative treatment options (Kraft et al., 2019).

& 9-8

In the realm of environmental health disasters and man-made disasters, the NIH has had an ongoing effort, Rapid Acquisition of Pre- and Post-Incident Disaster Data (RAPIDD), to develop standardized protocol templates and materials to help advance efficient IRB review and protocol development (Miller et al., 2016). Materials from this initiative are publicly available (dr2.nlm.nih.gov).

A Need for Training and Infrastructure

Incorporating healthcare workers who are highly skilled at relief efforts and critical care into a research response can be a challenge. Healthcare workers without prior research experience may lack the skills to effectively support the conduct of the research, although their participation may be critical to gathering the data needed for research. Initial and ongoing training, communication strategies, and clear standard operating procedures may be required in order to ensure that physicians and nurses understand the role and responsibilities of participating in the conduct of research. Researchers who plan to conduct PHE research should engage with local emergency response resources to create relationships and channels for communication that could be mobilized in the event of a PHE, in order to facilitate coordination across research and response efforts (Miller et al., 2016).

A Need for Preparedness

Drills and table-top exercises in emergency preparedness are common and highly effective in national preparedness, since they facilitate community stakeholders' testing and validation of plans. Exercises help identify capability gaps in order to create plans for improvement in the areas tested (Vasa et al., 2019). A well-designed exercise provides a low-risk environment to test plans, familiarize personnel with their roles and responsibilities, and foster meaningful interactions and communication, especially between disparate groups (Department of Homeland Security, 2013).

NETEC and SPRN collaborated with DHHS/ASPR, Mapp Biopharmaceutical, Inc., and the Regional Ebola and Other Special Pathogen Treatment Centers (RESPTCs) in a full-scale, 4-day table-top exercise, Tranquil Terminus. This national exercise was funded and coordinated by DHHS/ASPR. The exercise tested the ability of multiple states to move patients with EVD and other special pathogens safely and securely from diverse domestic healthcare facilities to specialized centers throughout the United States. It involved more than 50 local, state, regional, federal, private sector, and nongovernmental organizations. Importantly, the exercise incorporated the use of <u>investigational therapeutics</u> in the treatment of patients with EVD (Vasa et al., 2019).

🖉 11-2

The infrastructure for a central IRB system with a rapid response capability is important in order to be able to efficiently activate a clinical trial network in response to a PHE such as an outbreak. At the time of the Tranquil Terminus exercise, the central IRB had already reviewed and approved the main study protocol for ZMapp. According to the exercise plans, one of the four sites chose to activate its own rapid response IRB in order to test capacity to do single site review outside of the central IRB in the event of an emergency (Vasa et al., 2019).

As expected, given the complicated nature of executing reliance agreements, institutional variation with respect to institutional processes and requirements was observed (Vasa et al., 2019). This variation further illustrates the importance of IRBs working in a closely coordinated manner within networks specialized in PHE research.

The uncertainties of PHE require development of mechanisms to effectively support research in a PHE. The ability to quickly activate a network study using a central IRB is critical to administering and studying investigational drugs and products as well as to conducting other kinds of important research in the context of a PHE. However, we need to consider mechanisms that allow for greater flexibility and closer coordination without undermining conscientious, thoughtful review.

Lessons Learned

To protect the welfare of future research subjects who have experienced PHEs and to maximize the knowledge that can be gained from studying PHEs and responses to them, it is important that IRBs prepare to conduct a prompt review that considers issues particular to PHE research response. We have explored key considerations for human subject protections review in the context of PHEs to help IRBs identify how issues related to equitable selection of subjects, identification and communication of risk and benefit, considerations of vulnerability, and administration of informed consent might be considered in the context of a PHE. Additionally, we discussed concerns about safety and roles of research teams specific to the PHE context.

Like all domains of preparedness, human subject protections review is optimized when developed and tested outside of an actual disaster. This increases the likelihood of efficiencies and effectiveness in an emergency setting. A variety of current models for IRB review of PHE research have been highlighted to enhance learning from IRBs' experience in recent PHEs. Throughout this chapter, we have provided examples of past, current, and ongoing efforts by IRBs to address the challenges of human subjects research in disaster and outbreak settings.

Finally, table-top exercises can test human research protection programs and engage researchers, other key institutional offices, and community partners, providing important lessons for future disasters and public health emergencies. Similar to table-top exercises used to help prepare and identify workflows and challenges for disaster response efforts, institutions and IRBs can create a simulated submission of a PHE protocol to test the capacity of the human research protection program to provide an efficient review (or to rely on an sIRB). This kind of teaching exercise helps identify strengths, weaknesses, and bottlenecks to improve operations in advance of an actual need for IRB review of a PHE study.

References

Alirol, E., Kuesel, A. C., Guraiib, M. M., Fuente-Núñez, V. D. L., Saxena, A., & Gomes, M. F. (2017). Ethics review of studies during public health emergencies - the experience of the WHO ethics review committee during the Ebola virus disease epidemic. *BMC Medical Ethics*, *18*(1), 43.

Centers for Disease Control and Prevention (CDC). (2016). *2014–2016 Ebola outbreak in West Africa*. www.cdc.gov/vhf/ebola/outbreaks/2014-west-africa/index.html

Collogan, L. K., Tuma, F., Dolan-Sewell, R., Borja, S., & Fleischman, A. R. (2004). Ethical issues pertaining to research in the aftermath of disaster. *Journal of Traumatic Stress*, *17*(5), 363–372.

Department of Homeland Security. (2013). *Homeland Security Exercise and Evaluation Program (HSEEP)*. www.fema.gov/media-library-data/20130726-1914-25045-8890/hseep_apr13_.pdf

Emanuel, E. J., Wendler, D., & Grady, C. (2008). An ethical framework for biomedical research. In E. J. Emanuel, C. C. Grady, R. A. Crouch, R. K. Lie, F. G. Miller, & D. D. Wendler (Eds.), *The Oxford textbook of clinical research ethics* (pp. 123–135). Oxford University Press.

Ferreira, R., Buttell, F., & Ferreira, S. (2015). Ethical considerations for conducting disaster research with vulnerable populations. *Journal of Social Work Values and Ethics*, *12*(1), 29–40.

Fleischman, A. R., & Wood, E. B. (2002). Ethical issues in research involving victims of terror. *Journal of Urban Health*, *79*(3), 315–321.

Institute of Medicine (IOM). (2015). Enabling rapid and sustainable public health research during disasters: Summary of a joint workshop by the Institute of Medicine and the U.S. Department of Health and Human Services. The National Academies Press.

Knack, J. M., Chen, Z., Williams, K. D., & Jensen-Campbell, L. A. (2006). Opportunities and challenges for studying disaster survivors. *Analyses of Social Issues and Public Policy*, *6*(1), 175–189.

Kraft, C. S., Kortepeter, M. G., Gordon, B., Sauer, L. M., Shenoy, E. S., Eiras, D. P., Larson, L. A., Garland, J. A., Mehta, A. K., Barrett, K., Price, C. S., Croyle, C., West, L. R., Noren, B., Kline, S., Arguinchona, C., Arguinchona, H., Grein, J. D., Connally, C., ..., Kratochvil, C. J. (2019). The Special Pathogens Research Network: Enabling research readiness. *Health Security*, *17*(1), 35–45.

Kratochvil, C. J., Evans, L., Ribner, B. S., Lowe, J. J., Harvey, M. C., Hunt, R. C., Tumpey, A. J., Fagan, R. P., Schwedhelm, M. M., Bell, S., Maher, J., Kraft, C. S., Cagliuso, N. V., Sr., Vanairsdale, S., Vasa, A., & Smith, P. W. (2017). The National Ebola Training and Education Center: Preparing the United States for Ebola and other special pathogens. *Health Security, 15*(3), 253–260.

Lavin, R. P., Schemmel-Rettenmeier, L., & Frommelt-Kuhle, M. (2012). Conducting research during disasters. *Annual Review of Nursing Research, 30*(1), 1–19.

Legerski, J. P., & Bunnell, S. L. (2010). The risks, benefits, and ethics of trauma-focused research participation. *Ethics & Behavior, 20*(6), 429–442.

Lurie, N., Manolio, T., Patterson, A. P., Collins, F., & Frieden, T. (2013). Research as a part of public health emergency response. *New England Journal of Medicine, 368*, 1251–1255.

Médecins Sans Frontières (MSF). (2019). *Reviewing the ethical acceptability of MSF research.* www .msf.org/msf-ethics-review-board

Miller, A., Yaskey, K., Garantziotis, S., Arnesen, S., Bennett, A., O'Fallon, L., Thompson, C., Reinlib, L., Masten, S., Remington, J., Love, C., Ramsey, S., Rosselli, R., Galluzzo, B., Lee, J., Kwok, R., & Hughes, J. (2016). Integrating health research into disaster response: The new NIH Disaster Research Response Program. *International Journal of Environment Research and Public Health, 13*(7), 676.

National Ebola Training and Education Center (NETEC). (2017). *About NETEC.* http://netec.org /about/

National Institutes of Health (NIH). (2016). *Final NIH policy on the use of a single institutional review board for multi-site research.* grants.nih.gov/grants/guide/notice-files/not-od-16-094.html

Packenham, J. P., Rosselli, R. T., Ramsey, S. K., Taylor, H. A., Fothergill, A., Slutsman, J., & Miller, A. (2017). Conducting science in disasters: Recommendations from the NIEHS Working Group for Special IRB Considerations in the Review of Disaster Related Research. *Environmental Health Perspectives, 125*(9), 094503.

Presidential Commission for the Study of Bioethical Issues. (2015). *Bioethics Commission: Ebola teaches us public health preparedness requires ethics preparedness.* bioethicsarchive.georgetown .edu/pcsbi/node/4632.html

PREVAIL II Writing Group, Multi-National PREVAIL II Study Team, Davey, R. T., Jr., Dodd, L., Proschan, M. A., Neaton, J., Neuhaus Nordwall, J., Koopmeiners, J. S., Beigel, J., Tierney, J., Lane, H. C., Fauci, A. S., Massaquoi, M., Sahr, F., & Malvy, D. (2016). Multi-National PREVAIL II Study Team: A randomized, controlled trial of ZMapp for Ebola virus infection. *New England Journal of Medicine, 375*(15), 1448–1456.

Quick, G. (1998). A paradigm for multidisciplinary disease research: The Oklahoma City Experience. *Journal of Emergency Medicine, 16*(4), 621–630.

Saxena, A., Horby, P., Amuasi, J., Aagaard, N., Köhler, J., Gooshki, E. S., Denis, E., Reis, A. A., ALERRT-WHO Workshop, & Ravinetto, R. (2019). Ethics preparedness: facilitating ethics review during outbreaks - recommendations from an expert panel. BMC medical ethics, 20(1), 29

Substance Abuse and Mental Health Services Administration (SAMHSA). (2016). *Disaster technical assistance center supplemental research bulletin. Challenges and considerations in disaster research.* www.samhsa.gov/sites/default/files/dtac/supplemental-research-bulletin -jan-2016.pdf

Taylor, H. A. (2016). Review and conduct of human subjects research after a natural or man-made disaster: Findings from a pilot study. *Narrative Inquiry in Bioethics, 6*(3), 211–222.

Vasa, A., Madad, S., Larson, L., Kraft, C. S., Vanairsdale, S., Grein, J. D., Garland, J., Butterworth, V. M., & Kratochvil, C. J. (2019). A novel approach to infectious disease preparedness: Incorporating investigational therapeutics and research objectives into full-scale exercises. *Health Security, 17*(1), 54–61.

Pragmatic Clinical Trials and Comparative Effectiveness Research

Judith Carrithers

Stephanie Morain

Abstract

This chapter introduces pragmatic clinical trials (PCTs) and comparative effectiveness research (CER) and discusses the ethical issues that arise within the PCT/CER context. PCTs and CER have gained attention as efficient means to provide evidence to support healthcare decisions, capitalizing on novel techniques and evolving data analytics capabilities to conduct research more rapidly and at far lower cost than traditional research. These advantages notwithstanding, PCT/CER may also present ethical and regulatory challenges. This chapter defines PCT and CER and briefly outlines the features of the healthcare system driving their use. It then discusses challenges related to determining when and what form of individual consent is required, evaluating what constitutes minimal risk, proposed alternative consent models, privacy and confidentiality, quality improvement and PCT/CER, and harmonization and streamlining research oversight.

Definition of PCT and CER

Pragmatic clinical trials (PCTs) are "[d]esigned for the primary purpose of informing decision-makers regarding the comparative balance of benefits, burdens and risks of a biomedical or behavioral health intervention at the individual or population level" (Califf & Sugarman, 2015). They can be distinguished from more traditional explanatory trials by three attributes. First, unlike explanatory trials that evaluate a biological or social mechanism, PCTs aim to inform decision making by healthcare stakeholders. Examples include trials comparing clinically relevant alternative interventions to one another (Califf & Sugarman, 2015; Tunis et al., 2003). Second, PCTs enroll a population that is representative of and relevant to the clinical settings for which the decision regarding the intervention is relevant (Califf & Sugarman, 2015). Third, the study design either (a) collects data on a broad range of outcomes or (b) streamlines procedures and data collection to enable larger sample sizes and sufficient power to detect what are likely modest treatment effects of the clinical or policy decisions targeted by the trial (Califf & Sugarman, 2015; Yusuf et al., 1984).

DEFINITION: PRAGMATIC CLINICAL TRIALS

Pragmatic clinical trials are "[d]esigned for the primary purpose of informing decision-makers regarding the comparative balance of benefits, burdens, and risks of a biomedical or behavioral health intervention at the individual or population level." (Califf & Sugarman, 2015)

Reproduced from Califf R.M., and Sugarman J. (2015). Exploring the ethical and regulatory issues in pragmatic clinical trials. Clinical Trials 12(5): 436-441. Reprinted by Permission of SAGE Publications, Ltd

Comparative effectiveness research (CER), as defined by the National Institutes of Health (NIH), is research "comparing the benefits and harms of different existing interventions and strategies to prevent, diagnose, treat, and monitor health conditions in 'real world' settings . . . CER can be performed using a variety of methods, including prospective observational studies, clinical trials, or structured evaluation of existing evidence from registries, electronic health records, or other databases" (NIH, 2019). The primary distinguishing feature of a CER as compared to traditional or "explanatory" research is that CER compares two or more approved or standard therapies, whereas traditional trials examine investigational products, often in comparison to approved therapies. While CER can be done on a small scale, many studies will, like PCTs, be conducted in the context of large, multisite trials.

DEFINITION: COMPARATIVE EFFECTIVENESS RESEARCH

Comparative effectiveness research, as defined by the National Institutes of Health, is research "comparing the benefits and harms of different existing interventions and strategies to prevent, diagnose, treat, and monitor health conditions in 'real world' settings." (NIH, 2019)

National Institutes of Health (2019) Comparative Effectiveness Research in Clinical Neurosciences. https://grants.nih.gov/grants/guide/pa-files/ PAR-19-171.html

Both large-scale CER and PCT have gained attention in recent decades as strategies by which to improve the relevance and efficiency of knowledge generation, which in turn can advance the health of individuals and populations. Consequently, national funding agencies, including the Patient-Centered Outcomes Research Institute (PCORI) and the NIH have made considerable investments into these types of trials. This chapter will focus on the issues arising in the context of large-scale settings.

Numerous stakeholders have promoted PCT/CER as a means to address various shortcomings in the U.S. healthcare system. Notably, many critical health decisions, such as the choice between therapies, lack rigorous evidence to guide patients, clinicians, and other stakeholders. Furthermore, traditional research studies may have limited applicability to the real-world needs of decision makers due to a variety of factors, including study aims that explore biological mechanisms rather than real-world outcomes, exclusion criteria that lead to enrollment that does not match the underlying patient population in need of treatment, and sample sizes that are underpowered to detect clinically relevant differences. PCT/CER are designed to address these gaps, capitalizing on expanding data and analytic capabilities and embedding research into usual care settings to increase both the relevance and efficiency of research.

Why PCT/CER Are Ethically Complex

By embedding trials into settings in which clinical care is routinely delivered, PCT/CER offers the promise of generating evidence to inform important health-care decisions, and doing so far more efficiently than traditional explanatory trials. Yet PCT/CER may also present ethical and regulatory challenges. One key issue is whether and how existing regulatory and ethical frameworks, premised on the view that research and clinical care are distinct activities and thus merit different oversight, are capable of overseeing the ethical challenges arising from research that deliberately integrates these activities (Califf & Sugarman, 2015; Kass et al., 2013). Specifically, traditional framings of research ethics and regulatory oversight rest upon a sharp delineation between clinical care and research. Clinical care is understood as having a primary moral commitment to the medical best interests of each individual patient, whereas the primary moral commitment of clinical research is to the generation of knowledge to benefit future patients. However, several commentators have criticized these distinctions in the context of PCT/CER, which deliberately integrate research and usual clinical care (Faden et al., 2014; Kass et al., 2013; Selker et al., 2011).

Additional challenges are presented by the diversity of PCT/CER, both with respect to the type of intervention (medical, behavioral, or technological) and the target of the intervention (patients, clinicians, and/or system processes). For example, a PCT targeting patients might compare the effects of two or more commonly used medications, diet, or exercise regimens. A PCT targeting clinician practices might explore whether introducing epidemiological benchmark information into lumbar spine imaging reports ordered by primary care physicians impacted subsequent spine-related interventions (Ali et al., 2015; Jarvik et al., 2015). Finally, a PCT targeting health systems might compare different dialysis session durations to assess their impact on mortality, hospitalizations, and quality of life (Dember et al., 2016).

The previous examples suggest a related challenge. Specifically, as the constituency served by PCTs is broader than that of explanatory trials, PCTs may have both direct and indirect targets. This variety in both the interventions and stakeholders in PCTs increases the potential for these trials to generate wide-ranging benefits, advantages, harms, and burdens (Ali et al., 2015).

Ethical Challenges Arising Within PCT/CER

Several specific ethical challenges presented by PCT/CER are described later. This list is not intended to be exhaustive, but rather it is intended to introduce those involved in the oversight of human subjects research to key issues likely to be encountered in the review of individual PCTs.

When and What Form of Individual Consent Is Required?

One ethical challenge presented by PCT/CER is determining when and what form of individual <u>consent</u> should be required—and from whom it should be solicited. The proposal that some trials, such as those that compare widely used standard therapies, may permissibly be conducted without traditional written consent was first introduced to the literature nearly two decades ago (Truog et al., 1999). Support for this view has reemerged in the context of PCT/CER, although there is substantial disagreement regarding the precise conditions under which informed consent could ethically be <u>waived</u> and whether or when other forms of patient authorization, such as a streamlined consent process, should be employed (Faden et al., 2014; Grady, 2015; Kim & Miller, 2014; Largent et al., 2011; Menikoff, 2013; Truog et al., 1999). For example, the "integrated consent" model has been proposed for PCT/CER comparing treatments commonly used in routine practice and which in clinical practice require only verbal consent. In the integrated consent model, the patient's treating physician discusses the rationale for, alternatives to, and potential harms and benefits of the compared treatments, as they would typically do in the context of clinical care. However, the physician would also discuss that the choice between treatments would be made by randomization. If a patient chooses to enroll in the trial, the physician would document the interaction in the electronic health record, including that they discussed the rationale and risks and benefits of both options, that a treatment was chosen, and that it was chosen through random selection. The physician would also check a box for the patient's outcomes to be included in the trial database (Kalkman et al., 2017; Kim & Miller, 2014).

Empirical research exploring stakeholder views regarding consent in the context of research comparing widely used treatments involving low risk and for which patients are unlikely to have meaningful preferences among treatments (e.g., comparing two or more medications for hypertension) suggests that majorities of patients and members of the general public would find it permissible for such trials to be conducted without traditional written consent (Cho et al., 2015; Kass et al., 2016; Weinfurt et al., 2017). However, others have expressed skepticism about whether it is ever ethically acceptable to conduct randomized comparative effectiveness studies without written informed consent (Kim & Miller, 2014).

This debate over the appropriate use of <u>altered informed consent</u> in the context of PCT/CER has critical practical implications. Requiring researchers to obtain "traditional" informed consent can pose substantial barriers for the conduct of PCT research (McKinney et al., 2015). For example, although both clinicians and patients may be amenable to participating in research comparing different beta blockers for patients receiving dialysis, they are unlikely to devote time during the clinical visit to a lengthy research consent form, particularly when the research examines low-risk treatments that are widely used in clinical care. This may be due to a range of factors, including concerns about practicability, given the short length of clinical visits and competing time pressures on clinicians, as well as the fact that clinical staff may lack the appropriate training in obtaining research consent (Department of Health and Human Services [DHHS], 2018). In some cases, the inability to use an altered consent process may prevent some studies from being conducted altogether. Such challenges have the potential to harm future patients by limiting the generation of needed evidence to guide them and their treating clinicians in making informed decisions.

Currently, researchers proposing an alternate consent procedure must meet the same requirements as those seeking to <u>waive consent</u> altogether (McKinney et al., 2015). As stated in **45 CFR 46.116(f)(3)**, an IRB can approve a waiver or alteration of consent only if all five of the following conditions are met:

(i) The research involves no more than minimal risk to the subjects; (ii) The research could not practicably be carried out without the requested waiver or alteration; (iii) If the research involves using identifiable private information or identifiable biospecimens, the research could not practicably be carried out without using such information or biospecimens in an identifiable format; (iv) The waiver or alteration will not adversely affect the rights and welfare of subjects; and (v) Whenever appropriate, the subjects or legally authorized representatives will be provided with additional pertinent information after participation.

Applying these criteria to the context of PCT/CER presents several challenges. Assessing the nature and extent of risks in PCT/CER involves determining which risks should be considered when evaluating therapies widely used in regular clinical practice—those of the underlying treatments themselves or only those introduced by study participation? This challenge is described in further detail in the following section. In addition, assessment of a trial's impact on the rights and welfare of research subjects turns upon which rights are considered relevant (McKinney et al., 2015). For example, if one believes that an individual has an absolute right regarding decisions about their medical care, then waivers or alterations of consent might be viewed as violating this right. Furthermore, assessments about practicability present IRBs with wide latitude with respect to burdens on the research process. While the Secretary's Advisory Committee on Human Research Protections (SACHRP) has advised that "Practicability should not be determined solely based upon considerations of convenience, cost, or speed," these conditions nevertheless may be relevant for determinations of the practicability of obtaining consent (DHHS, 2008). Thus, as McKinney and colleagues have argued, when study risks are low, it may be appropriate to consider cost and related burdens when assessing possible alterations to the consent process (McKinney et al., 2015).

What Constitutes Minimal Risk?

A related type of challenge relates to determining what constitutes minimal risk in the context of PCT/CER. In overseeing individual research proposals, IRBs must classify the riskiness of proposed research according to the Common Rule **[45 CFR 46, subpart A]** and related regulations governing the Food and Drug Administration (FDA) codified in **21 CFR 50** (Lantos et al., 2015). An IRB determination of "minimal risk" carries several practical implications, including making the research eligible to be carried out with certain <u>vulnerable populations</u>, to be reviewed using an <u>expedited</u> process, and/or for the IRB to allow a waiver or alteration of the informed consent process. Determination of risk also has important implications for how researchers should describe the study to prospective subjects through the consent process (Joffe & Wertheimer, 2014).

Determining what should constitute "minimal risk" in the context of PCT/CER raises several questions. For example, in trials comparing treatments that are in widespread use, should IRBs consider the risks of the treatments themselves or only the "incremental risks" associated with enrollment into research? One argument is that only those risks associated with enrollment in research should be considered research risks. Those risks associated with a person's disease or the risks associated with the treatments being studied for that disease should be disclosed as part of the informed consent for treatment but should not be considered as research risks, and therefore should not be included in research informed consent (Lantos et al., 2015). Support for this view is offered by the Common Rule, which states: "**In evaluating risks and benefits, the IRB should consider only those risks and benefits that may**

🔗 Section 9
🔗 5-5

result from the research (as distinguished from risks and benefits of therapies subjects would receive even if not participating in the research)" [45 CFR 46.111(a)(2)]. Thus, as the standard therapies being compared by the PCT/CER represent usual therapy outside the trial, they are the baseline against which the risks of the trial intervention should be evaluated (Joffe & Wertheimer, 2014).

However, evidence suggests that IRBs do not consistently apply this standard, and several bioethicists have objected to this view (Polito et al., 2014). If, instead, all of the risks of treatments being studied in a PCT must be considered as research risks, then only studies involving treatments that are themselves minimal risk could be considered minimal risk—a standard very few PCTs are likely to meet (Lantos et al., 2015).

Determination of minimal risk is particularly important in cluster randomized trials (CRTs), in which it may not be feasible to seek informed consent from individual subjects. For example, interventions in a CRT might be environmental or might be delivered at the unit or hospital level. However, a waiver of consent is only permitted if the IRB has determined that the trial involves no more than minimal risk (Joffe & Wertheimer, 2014).

DEFINITION: CLUSTER RANDOMIZED TRIAL

A *cluster randomized trial* (CRT) is one in which "the unit of randomization is something other than an individual participant or patient," such as a hospital ward or an entire outpatient clinic. CRTs are well-suited to testing different methods or approaches to patient care (DeLong, 2020).

DeLong E.R. (2020) Experimental Designs and Randomization Schemes: Cluster Randomized Trials. In: Rethinking Clinical Trials: A Living Textbook of Pragmatic Clinical Trials. Bethesda, MD: NIH Health Care Systems Research Collaboratory. https://rethinkingclinicaltrials.org/chapters/design/experimental-designs-randomization-schemes-top/cluster-randomized-trials/.

Alternative Consent Models for PCT/CER

6-4   For PCT/CER that meets the "minimal risk" requirement for a <u>waiver</u> or alteration of consent, various alternative consent models have been proposed. These models focus on PCT/CER where individual consent is not a viable option and a waiver or alteration is allowable under the applicable regulations. Some alternative approaches focus on streamlining the consent process, such as the "integrated consent" approach discussed previously. Other models are focused on the context of CRT. For example, consider a situation in which all patients at a particular hospital (Hospital A) will be assigned to an intervention (e.g., use of specific antibacterial agent for bathing) while the other hospital (Hospital B) will follow routine bathing policy. In this scenario, obtaining individual consent is logistically challenging because it is the choice of hospital that determines whether patients will receive the intervention or not; patients in Hospital A receive a minimal risk intervention that is different from standard care while patients in Hospital B receive standard care. In addition, there are no burdens or risks related to data collection because these data are collected as part of routine care. Although a waiver or alteration of consent may be allowable for this type of trial, there continues to be debate over whether written consent should be obtained and, if not, what type of waiver or alteration may be acceptable (Nayak et al., 2015).

One model suggested for research conducted with a waiver of consent is called "broadcast notification," which involves placing notices about the research in prominent locations in the facility. These notices inform patients that they could be part of research, allow them to ask questions, and advise them that they can decide to seek care in another facility if they do not want to participate (if there is no opt-out option at the facility). The type and amount of information provided in the notices is dependent on the type of study (McKinney et al., 2015). Although this model does not provide all of the research information that would be included in a traditional written consent form, it does serve the purpose of notification and provides contact information for patients who have questions. Providing this information about the research respects the individuals from whom data were collected and provides transparency about the research.

A second model is a modified "opt out," in which subjects are notified of the research after it has been conducted and are given the option of declining to have their data used in the research. For example, in the antibacterial agent for bathing study discussed previously, patients would be informed of the research at discharge and have the option to decline having their data used. This model is also focused on PCT/CER in a setting where individual consent is not practicable (for example, when all patients in the facility will receive the intervention) and risks are minimal.

Privacy and Confidentiality

Respect for persons participating in research includes protecting their privacy and ensuring the confidentiality of their data. Traditionally, the research policies governing privacy and confidentiality rest on seeking an individual's consent to use their identifiable data (and describing in that consent how the data will be safeguarded) or on removing personally identifiable information from the data. The Common Rule, FDA regulations, and the Health Insurance Portability and Accountability Act (HIPAA; DHHS, 2013) generally require express consent or authorization of an individual for the use of identifiable data, except for some minimal risk research as described earlier.

But signing a written consent form that includes information about privacy and confidentiality of data does not ensure that a subject understands the risks associated with providing the identifiable data that will be used in the research. The privacy and confidentiality provisions typically appear at the end of a long and complex consent form, and subjects (and researchers obtaining consent) are often more focused on the study procedures and health risks and potential benefits than risks associated with the subject's data. And, as discussed earlier, the type of consent that may work best in a PCT/CER may not be a written consent form with a full description of how data will be safeguarded.

Although removing personally identifiable information from the data addresses many of the concerns about ensuring privacy and confidentiality, it is only applicable to a limited subset of research where collection and retention of identifiable data are not critical to the study. For example, survey research may not require collection of identifiable information about subjects because the study purpose is to identify group trends/responses. However, in a drug or device trial, retention of each subject's identifiable data for a period of time is required for data analysis and also required under both Office for Human Research Protections (OHRP) and FDA regulations governing research data retention.

Respect for persons demands that sharing private health information occur only under appropriate conditions, to appropriate parties, and for appropriate reasons (McGraw et al., 2015). Subjects should be able to control who has access to their data, or, at minimum, be informed about who will have access and under what circumstances. There are real and tangible risks associated with the inappropriate release of health information—it could impact an individual's employment, insurance, reputation, or other areas of their life. These concerns may be exacerbated in PCT/CER because of the large numbers of potential subjects—although the individual harm remains the same, the number of people who may be affected in an inappropriate release or breach requires continuing attention in this type of research.

Overlap Between PCT and Quality Improvement (QI)

The increasing use of pragmatic research in routine care settings, juxtaposed with increasingly extensive and sophisticated QI activities, has made the boundary between QI and research less distinct (Finkelstein et al., 2015). As described in this chapter, PCTs often compare medical interventions to improve healthcare delivery within and across healthcare systems. QI has been defined as "systematic, data-guided activities designed to bring about *immediate improvements* in health care delivery in particular settings" (emphasis added; Lynn et al., 2007). Although sometimes hard to distinguish, traditional QI looks at how to improve processes in a particular healthcare organization and is not intended to be generalizable to other settings, whereas PCTs examine healthcare delivery and systems in a broader setting.

🖉 5-1   Making this distinction is important for determining what type of ethical oversight is required for the activity in question. Activities that clearly fall within the QI realm generally do not require IRB oversight but may require authorization or oversight by local administration/department heads (depending on institutional policies). However, QI activities that are more than minimal risk and "could result in substantial changes to care and/or include the possibility of additional risks and burdens to patients should have independent review to assess if they are research or QI" (Finkelstein et al., 2015). This independent review could be conducted by an administrative committee, the IRB, or another mechanism for review; if the QI project is determined to be research, it requires IRB review.

IRBs frequently have difficulty determining whether a project is QI or research, a problem that is exacerbated in the case of PCT/CER. By definition, PCT/CER is research that requires IRB review and oversight, but correctly identifying the type of project that is being conducted may require close attention to the details of the project.

Streamlining IRB Review for PCT/CER

A critical issue emerging with the growth of PCT/CER is the need for a streamlined research oversight process. With multiple sites, institutions, and healthcare delivery systems involved in a single PCT/CER, multiple IRBs may be required to review the research. Each of these IRBs is likely to have its own submission system, processes, and requirements, and submitting the PCT/CER for review at each site IRB may cause significant delays in approval and initiation of the research. In addition, "[d]ata regarding variability in decision-making and interpretation of the regulations across IRBs have led to a perception that variability among institutional review boards is a primary contributor to the problems with review of multisite research" (O'Rourke et al., 2015).

For several years, many stakeholders have called for the use of a single
🖉 Section 4   IRB of record to streamline and harmonize the IRB review process and provide

overall research oversight. Many institutions and their IRBs have resisted this call for a variety of reasons: the institutional concern about retaining local oversight of research conducted within their facilities; the IRB's role in coordination of multiple non-IRB institutional reviews (e.g., grants/contracts, radiation safety committee, pharmacy, conflict of interest); and the local IRB's knowledge of the local community, the institution's policies and practices, and the researchers. However, under recent NIH and Common Rule mandates, use of an sIRB is no longer optional for many multisite studies (NIH, 2016). Use of an sIRB for PCT/CER should streamline the review process and enhance consistency across the research sites.

Conclusion

PCTs and CER have become increasingly important in bringing research into real-world settings. PCTs test what works in daily clinical practice and provide results that may be generalized and applied to a broader population. CER also looks to real-world settings to compare the benefits and harms of existing interventions. Both PCTs and CER raise regulatory and ethical challenges related to conducting research in this setting, including obtaining consent without affecting clinic functioning, assessing whether an altered consent process is allowed under the regulations and appropriate for the research, and determining how to notify subjects of the research if traditional written consent is not obtained. Various alternative consent models are still being explored and developed, and we can expect this to continue to evolve in the future. Methods of respecting privacy and protecting confidentiality of data in the PCT/CER setting continue to be discussed and developed and may vary with the nature of the research and type of consent. In addition, harmonizing and streamlining IRB review through use of an sIRB, as required under NIH and the revised Common Rule, will provide for more efficient and consistent review of PCTs and CER.

References

Ali, J., Andrews, J. E., Somkin, C. P., & Rabinovich, C. E. (2015). Harms, benefits, and the nature of interventions in pragmatic clinical trials. *Clinical Trials, 12*(5), 467–475.

Califf, R. M., & Sugarman, J. (2015). Exploring the ethical and regulatory issues in pragmatic clinical trials. *Clinical Trials, 12*(5), 436–441.

Cho, M. K., Magnus, D., Constantine, M., Lee, S. S., Kelley, M., Alessi, S., Korngiebel, D., James, C., Kuwana, E., Gallagher, T. H., Diekema, D., Capron, A. M., Joffe, S., & Wilfond, B. S. (2015). Attitudes toward risk and informed consent for research on medical practices: A cross-sectional survey. *Annals of Internal Medicine*, *162*(10), 690–696.

DeLong, E. R. (2020). Experimental designs and randomization schemes: Cluster randomized trials. In *Rethinking clinical trials: A living textbook of pragmatic clinical trials*. NIH Health Care Systems Research Collaboratory. https://rethinkingclinicaltrials.org/chapters/design/experimental-designs-randomization-schemes-top/cluster-randomized-trials/

Dember, L. M., Archdeacon, P., Krishnan, M., Lacson, E., Jr., Ling, S. M., Roy-Chaudhury, P., Smith, K. A., & Flessner, M. F. (2016). Pragmatic trials in maintenance dialysis: Perspectives from the Kidney Health Initiative. *Journal of the American Society of Nephrology, 27*(10), 2955–2963.

Department of Health and Human Services (DHHS). (2008). *January 31, 2008 SACHRP letter to HHS Secretary: Recommendations related to waiver of informed consent and interpretation of "minimal risk."* www.hhs.gov/ohrp/sachrp-committee/recommendations/2008-january-31-letter/index.html

Department of Health and Human Services (DHHS). (2013). *Office for Civil Rights summary of the Health Insurance Portability and Accountability Act.* www.hhs.gov/hipaa/for-professionals /privacy/laws-regulations/index.html

Department of Health and Human Services (DHHS). (2018). *Meeting new challenges in informed consent in clinical research: An exploratory workshop.* Sponsored by the Office of Human Research Protections, Department of Health and Human Services. September 7, 2018. www .hhs.gov/ohrp/sites/default/files/meeting-new-challenges.pdf

Faden, R. R., Beauchamp, T. L., & Kass, N. E. (2014). Informed consent, comparative effectiveness, and learning health care. *New England Journal of Medicine, 370*(8), 766–768.

Finkelstein, J., Brickman, A., & Capron, A. (2015). Oversight on the borderline: Quality improvement and pragmatic research. *Clinical Trials, 12*(5), 457–466.

Grady, C. (2015). Enduring and emerging challenges of informed consent. *New England Journal of Medicine, 372,* 855–862.

Jarvik, J. G., Comstock, B. A., James, K. T., Avins, A. L., Bresnahan, B. W., Deyo, R. A., Luetmer, P. H., Friedly, J. L., Meier, E. N., Cherkin, D. C., Gold, L. S., Rundell, S. D., Halabi, S. S., Kallmes, D. F., Tan, K. W., Turner, J. A., Kessler, L. G., Lavallee, D. C., Stephens, K. A., & Heagerty, P. J. (2015). Lumbar imaging with reporting of epidemiology (LIRE)—Protocol for a pragmatic cluster randomized trial. *Contemporary Clinical Trials, 45*(Pt B), 157–163.

Joffe, S., & Wertheimer, A. (2014). Determining minimal risk for comparative effectiveness research. *IRB: Ethics & Human Research, 36*(3), 16–18. www.thehastingscenter.org/irb_article /determining-minimal-risk-for-comparative-effectiveness-research/

Kalkman, S., van Thiel, G., & Zuidgeest, M. (2017). Series: Pragmatic trials and real world evidence. Paper 4: Informed consent. *Journal of Clinical Epidemiology, 89,* 181–187.

Kass, N. E., Faden, R. R., Fabi, R. E., Morain, S., Hallez, K., Whicher, D., Tunis, S., Moloney, R., Messner, D., & Pitcavage, J. (2016). Alternative consent models for comparative effectiveness studies: Views of patients from two institutions. *AJOB Empirical Bioethics, 7*(2), 92–105.

Kass, N., Faden, R. R., Goodman, S. N., Pronovost, P., Tunis, S., & Beauchamp, T. L. (2013). The research-treatment distinction: A problematic approach for determining which activities should have ethical oversight. *Hastings Center Report, 43*(Suppl 1), S4–S15.

Kim, S. Y. H., & Miller, F. G. (2014). Informed consent for pragmatic trials—the integrated consent model. *New England Journal of Medicine, 370*(8), 769–772.

Lantos, J., Wendler, D., Septimus, E., Wahba, S., Madigan, R., & Bliss, G. (2015). Considerations in the evaluation and determination of minimal risk in pragmatic clinical trials. *Clinical Trials, 12*(5), 485–493.

Largent, E. A., Joffe, S., & Miller, F. G. (2011). Can research and care be ethically integrated? *Hastings Center Report, 41,* 37–46.

Lynn, J., Baily, M. A., Bottrell, M., Jennings, B., Levine, R. J., Davidoff, F., Casarett, D., Corrigan, J., Fox, E., Wynia, M. K., Agich, G. J., O'Kane, M., Speroff, T., Schyve, P., Batalden, P., Tunis, S., Berlinger, N., Cronewett, L., Fitzmaurice, J. M., ..., James, B. (2007). The ethics of using quality improvement methods in health care. *Annals of Internal Medicine, 146*(9), 666–673.

McGraw, D., Greene, S. M., Miner, C. S., Staman, K. L., Welch, M. J., & Alan Rubel, A. (2015). Privacy and confidentiality in pragmatic clinical trials. *Clinical Trials, 12*(5), 520–529.

McKinney, R. E., Beskow, L. M., Ford, D. E., Lantos, J. D., McCall, J., Patrick-Lake, B., Pletcher, M. J., Rath, B., Schmidt, H., & Weinfurt, K. (2015). Use of altered informed consent in pragmatic clinical research. *Clinical Trials, 12*(5), 494–502.

Menikoff, J. (2013). The unbelievable rightness of being in clinical trials. *Hastings Center Report, 43,* S30–S31.

National Institutes of Health (NIH). (2016). *Final NIH policy on the use of a single institutional review board for multi-site research.* Notice Number: NOT-OD-16-094. https://grants.nih.gov /grants/guide/notice-files/not-od-16-094.html

National Institutes of Health (NIH). (2019). *Comparative effectiveness research in clinical neurosciences.* https://grants.nih.gov/grants/guide/pa-files/PAR-19-171.html

Nayak, R. K., Wendler, D., Miller, F. G., & Kim, S. Y. H. (2015). Pragmatic randomized trials without standard informed consent?: A national survey. *Annals of Internal Medicine, 163*(5), 356–364.

O'Rourke, P., Carrithers, J., Patrick-Lake, B., Rice, T. W., Corsmo, J., Hart, R., Drezner, M. K., & Lantoset, J. D. (2015). Harmonization and streamlining of research oversight for pragmatic clinical trials. *Clinical Trials, 12*(5), 449–456.

Polito, C. C., Cribbs, S. K., & Martin, G. S. (2014). Navigating the institutional review board approval process in a multicenter observational critical care study. *Critical Care Medicine, 42,* 1105–1109.

Selker, H., Grossman, C., Adams, A., Goldmann, D., Dezii, C., Meyer, G., Roger, V., Savitz, L., & Platt, R. (2011). The Common Rule and continuous improvement in health care: A learning health system perspective. *NAM Perspectives.* [Discussion Paper]. National Academy of Medicine. https://doi.org/10.31478/201110a

Tunis, S. R., Stryer, D. B., & Clancy, C. M. (2003). Practical clinical trials: Increasing the value of clinical research for decision making in clinical and health policy. *JAMA, 290,* 1624–1632.

Truog, R. D., Robinson, W., Randolph, A., & Morris, A. (1999). Is informed consent always necessary for randomized, controlled trials? *New England Journal of Medicine, 340*(10), 804–807.

Weinfurt, K. P., Bollinger, J. M., Brelsford, K. M., Bresciani, M., Lampron, Z., Lin, L., Topazian, R. J., & Sugarman, J. (2017). Comparison of approaches for notification and authorization in pragmatic clinical research evaluating commonly used medical practices. *Medical Care, 55*(11), 970–978.

Yusuf, S., Collins, R., & Peto, R. (1984). Why do we need some large, simple randomized trials? *Statistics in Medicine, 3,* 409–422.

CHAPTER 10-9

International Research

Delia Wolf Christiani
Kelly O'Keefe

Abstract

As the landscape of human subjects research broadens, so does the geographical span of the locations in which it takes place (Alfano, 2013; Glickman et al., 2009; Rowland, 2004; Thiers et al., 2008). Efforts to promote globalization in disciplines aside from human research have resulted in a vastly expanded social, cultural, economic, and geopolitical context where researchers can test hypotheses (Ali et al., 2012; Glickman et al., 2009; Rowland, 2004). U.S.-based academic research centers have seen a dramatic increase in the number of studies taking place outside of U.S. borders. According to one estimate, the number of studies regulated by the U.S. Food and Drug Administration, but conducted outside of the United States, has grown at an annual rate of 15% since 2002 (Glickman et al., 2009). As of August 2019, more than 50% of all clinical trials registered with ClinicalTrials.gov are conducted in countries other than the United States, according to the National Library of Medicine (2020). The ever-increasing quantity of human research performed in international settings calls for a commensurate rise in awareness of variations in regulatory requirements in different countries and regions, and the challenges in conducting IRB review of international research. This chapter is intended to guide IRBs through the process of review, approval, and oversight of international research.

Introduction

Although the basic ethical principles of respecting and protecting individuals participating in research described in the <u>Declaration of Helsinki</u> can be regarded as universal, there is no set of universal regulations that apply to human research conducted around the world. In fact, most countries have country-specific rules, regulations, and requirements. Because these rules, regulations, and requirements are often different, conducting research internationally and applying regulatory requirements, especially those promulgated by the U.S. government, can impose unique challenges and create obstacles in reviewing and overseeing human subjects research. Special attention should be given to local requirements, culture, and customs, as well as scientific and ethical review infrastructures.

🔗 1-1

Prereview Information Gathering

When an IRB receives an international research proposal, certain information needs to be gathered prior to review of the proposal itself. The following questions will help to determine whether review by the U.S. IRB is required, and if so, what relevant U.S. and local regulations, guidelines, and requirements need to be followed and/or taken into consideration.

Is the U.S. Institution Engaged in Human Subjects Research?

Institutions may not be considered to be engaged in human subjects research if all study-related procedures are to be conducted outside the United States and the U.S. researchers' role is limited to study design and/or data analysis of deidentified data. In other words, if the U.S. institution's employees or agents do not enroll subjects or obtain informed consent, neither are they responsible for overseeing study-related activities. If a U.S. institution is not engaged in human subjects research, review and approval from the U.S. IRB are not required.

Is the Study Funded or Conducted by U.S. Department of Health and Human Services (DHHS)?

If the answer is yes, the non-U.S. institution involved must obtain a Federalwide Assurance (FWA) for the protection of human subjects and must comply with the requirements stated in **45 CFR 46** according to the Department of Health and Human Services, Protection of Human Subjects: Interpretation of Assurance Requirements (DHHS, 2006). The Office for Human Research Protections (OHRP) provides instructions for registering IRBs and obtaining FWAs on its website (DHHS, 2016).

What Are Relevant Country-Specific Laws, Regulations, and Guidelines?

In addition to relevant U.S. regulations, the U.S. IRB should be familiar with specific in-country laws, regulations, and guidelines governing human subjects research. OHRP's *International Compilation of Human Research Standards* is a listing of over 1,000 laws, regulations, and guidelines on human subject protections in more than 130 countries and from many international organizations (DHHS, 2019). Increasingly, various standards and specific guidelines governing social-behavioral research have been developed and implemented in many countries, either as part of a larger document or as free-standing regulations or guidelines (DHHS, 2018). Some countries also require permits/licenses from national government agencies to conduct research, in addition to ethics review. It is important to distinguish laws and regulations from guidelines, because mixing them may result in increasing regulatory burden by overregulating.

Is There a Local IRB to Review the Proposed Research?

In general, if study-related activities are to be conducted at sites outside the United States, review and approval by a local IRB or equivalent committee such as research ethics committee (REC) is required, either by the U.S. institution's policy or host county's laws and/or regulations. The researcher who submits the proposal to the U.S. IRB should provide information on the local review committee. If a site does not have a local reviewing body, the IRB may require establishing a community advisory board (CAB) at the site to provide local context review for the proposed research. A CAB may include a minimum of three members who are independent of study staff to avoid any perceived, potential, or actual conflict of interest. The members should include one lay, nonscientist, member but otherwise include members with appropriate experience/expertise based on personal or professional qualifications. At a minimum, the CAB should review the recruitment/consent process and materials, study procedures, and dissemination of study results, if applicable.

Does the U.S. IRB Have Appropriate Expertise and Knowledge?

When reviewing international research, the U.S. IRB is expected to obtain and demonstrate sufficient knowledge of the local context where the research will take place, including relevant laws and regulations, the scientific and ethical review infrastructure, and local community and culture.

Although it is common for countries across the globe to maintain requirements for scientific and ethical review, not all countries are alike. For example, some countries require regional and national ethics committee review in addition to institutional review. In other countries, letters of support from local authorities must be gathered prior to submission to the local reviewing board. In many countries, there are no specific exemption categories in their regulations; therefore, studies that can be <u>exempt</u> under U.S. regulations may require review and approval by the local ethics committee.

⊘ 5-3

In addition to understanding local review requirements, the U.S. IRB must have appropriate knowledge of the local community, including subject population, standard care, health needs, literacy level, and native language(s); as well as local culture, including status of women, status of children, and community leaders' role in recruitment and informed consent processes.

To ensure appropriate and sufficient expertise in reviewing international research, U.S. IRBs are encouraged to use alternate members and/or consultants who are familiar with local context. IRBs may also consider direct communication with local ethics review committees. Direct communication provides an opportunity to understand each institution's review requirements and to resolve any inconsistencies in institutional policies. This communication can be established by reaching out through information provided publicly and/or by connections through researchers at collaborating institutions.

Is Ceding Review to a Local Ethics Review Committee Appropriate?

The U.S. regulations allow for institutions engaged in research to rely on another institution's IRB to review research studies, provided an agreement is put in place outlining each institutions' roles and responsibilities and the REC is registered with OHRP. U.S. IRBs may consider relying partially or fully on local REC review in one of two ways:

1. Because the review of consent documents and the <u>informed consent</u> process require a deep understanding of the local environment (including study population, culture, language, and current political context), IRBs

⊘ Section 6

> may consider relying on a local REC to review and approve the consent documents and informed consent process.

2. In order to reduce the burden on institutions and researchers, U.S. IRBs may consider ceding review to the local REC if certain criteria are met. Criteria to cede review may include that the local institution's policies and procedures are in compliance with the U.S. regulations, the U.S. researcher's role does not include interaction or intervention with subjects, and all study procedures are conducted at the local site.

IRB Review and Approval: Points to Consider

Researcher Qualifications

When U.S.-based researchers propose to conduct international research, specific qualifications and experience may be necessary. The IRB may require information, such as years of direct experience in conducting research at the proposed study site, speaking/understanding the local language, familiarity with local culture, and an established relationship with the local collaborator (coinvestigators). In addition, the U.S. IRB should establish mechanisms to assess the qualifications and experience of local researchers and research staff. Relevant information to be gathered in assessing qualifications includes local licensure/certification in conducting human research, clinical/research workload, financial or other conflicts of interest, and training in research ethics, including human subject protections.

Documenting and Understanding Local Context

U.S. IRBs may rely on researchers to provide essential information about the local research context. Protocol templates should request information to better understand the political, legal, and cultural considerations specific to the study under review. Researchers can rely on peer review articles, personal expertise, local experts, and documented policies and laws to explain the local context.

Political. IRBs should seek to understand how the macro and micro politics of the locality could impact research. For example, political instability could impact recruitment, or subjects' legal status could impact risks related to participation. Political pressures may impact the use of identifiable data, particularly if the study population is vulnerable or the research topic is sensitive.

Legal. A host of laws and legal requirements may impact study design, implementation, and analysis. IRBs should focus on understanding those legal requirements that pertain specifically to the study's population, health area, or type of data collected. For example, age of majority and the legal status of married minors may differ among countries, and this may impact recruitment and the consent process. Legal requirements for mandatory reporting of health data (i.e., HIV status) must be documented in the study design and well explained in the consent process. Privacy and data use laws must also be understood, including but not limited to a country's laws to bring identifying data or specimens out of the country and region-specific laws such as the General Data Protection Regulation (GDPR).

Cultural. When research takes place outside of the familiar context of the United States, reviewing boards must take time to understand the culture context in which the research takes place. For example, researchers must document knowledge of the languages used by the participant population and how literacy levels could impact recruitment materials and consent processes. Understanding how an at-risk population navigates daily life can inform recruitment and participation. Pervasive social stigma of a specific health condition may impact recruitment, study participation, and documentation of informed consent. Also, appropriate levels and types of subject compensation can only be determined once the cultural context is understood.

Avoiding Overregulating

Because country-specific laws and regulations governing human research vary, compliance with the regulatory requirements of different countries can be challenging. Identifying relevant regulations is critical, since overregulating may not only delay IRB review and approval but also lead to noncompliance. In order to avoid overregulating, it is important to distinguish laws and regulations from guidelines. For example, if back-translation of consent documents is not mandated by any participating country regulations, it may be eliminated. Also, although U.S. regulations permit <u>waiver</u> or alteration of the informed consent process when the proposed research meets specific criteria, such specific provisions do not exist in all countries' laws or regulations. If there are no specific provisions against a waiver or alteration, the U.S. IRB should exercise a certain degree of flexibility, based on local context, with regard to a waiver or alteration of the consent process, as well as documentation of consent.

🔗 6-4

Compensation to Subjects

<u>Paying research subjects</u> for their time and effort in participating in a research study is a common and, in general, acceptable practice in the United States. When a proposed research study offers monetary and/or in-kind compensation to research subjects, the IRB should be careful to avoid any undue influence. The IRB should consider the amount of payment to research subjects according to the host country's social and economic status, as well as local culture and tradition. For example, in some countries, providing monetary compensation for studies involving blood draws is offensive and insulting. The IRB should also keep in mind that compensation to subjects may be prohibited in certain institutions.

🔗 12-2

Determining Vulnerability of a Study Population Beyond the U.S. Regulations

Vulnerable populations include those defined in 45 CFR 46 subparts **B** (<u>pregnant women</u>), **C** (<u>prisoners</u>), and **D** (<u>children</u>) and those mentioned in 45 CFR 46.111(b), namely individuals with <u>impaired decision-making capacity</u>, or <u>economically</u> or educationally disadvantaged persons. Vulnerability in research is often regarded as a diminished capability to make autonomous decisions in one's own interest, and individuals are considered <u>vulnerable</u> when their voluntariness to participate in research is compromised. Because the causes of potential research subjects' diminished capacity can be both physical/mental and situational/positional, depending on the social, economic, or cultural context where the research will be conducted, it is possible for a U.S. IRB to determine that a specific study population is "vulnerable" beyond those groups defined in the U.S. regulations, requiring additional protections.

The identification of a particular study population as "vulnerable" and in need of specific ancillary considerations and augmented protections requires a

🔗 9-4 🔗 9-5 🔗 9-6
🔗 9-7
🔗 9-9

🔗 9-1

deep knowledge of local context, the study population, and the requirements of study participation. For example, in some countries, premarital sex remains highly stigmatized and even illegal. Adult women from these countries who are asked to provide information relating to their premarital sexual behavior assume much higher risks than those from countries where premarital sex is not punishable. As a result, the IRB may consider this group of women vulnerable, and additional protections would be necessary to minimize or eliminate coercion and undue influence, in order to ensure voluntary participation and safeguard the safety and welfare of these subjects.

Post-Approval Monitoring, Auditing, and Training

⚫ 7-4

Because the U.S. IRB is responsible for overseeing research after its approval, some monitoring activities are necessary to fulfill its responsibility. Although conducting post-approval monitoring and auditing of international study sites in the form of onsite review would be an effective way of ensuring compliance, it can be costly. Remote audit, also known as e-audit, of study records via electronic communication platforms, such as interactive video and audio chat or secure file sharing, may be an effective alternative.

⚫ 7-3

Increasingly, different forms of remote monitoring/auditing have been used to review study records, from simple sharing of nonconfidential files via email to utilizing sophisticated virtual communication tools that permit web-based user access, data sharing and communication among users, audit trails, and data security. Remote auditing facilitates real-time evaluation of study status, data quality, and timely reporting of adverse events and unanticipated problems involving risks to subjects and others. No matter what forms of remote auditing are used, timely communication about findings and following up on resolutions to corrective actions is key.

In addition to monitoring compliance, electronic communication platforms also enable the U.S. IRB and local REC, as well as the study site, to effectively communicate with each other and offer training opportunities (possibly based on audit findings) to local study staff and researchers.

Conclusion

⚫ 2-3

Review, approval, and oversight of human research conducted internationally can be challenging for U.S. IRBs, not only because of the lack of a set of universal regulations and standards but also due to variations and inconsistencies in regulatory requirements among different countries. Current U.S. regulations allow for OHRP to determine whether another country's guidelines provide protections for research subjects that are equivalent to those provided by the U.S. regulations, but OHRP has not provided criteria for determining what constitutes equivalent protections. To that end, it is critical for U.S. IRBs to establish institutional policies and procedures for reviewing international research. Although it may be impractical and sometimes inappropriate to strictly follow U.S. regulations in other countries and cultural settings, understanding the applicable laws, regulations, and guidelines, as well as local context, including culture and custom, would enable U.S. IRBs to assert flexibility in applying relevant legal/regulatory requirements and avoid overregulating. Establishing direct communication with local RECs can promote and facilitate the harmonization of institutional requirements, in addition to regulatory policies and procedures, among all collaborating institutions. Finally, using technology to oversee international research by conducting remote monitoring, auditing, and training can enable both IRBs and researchers to ensure compliance and improve performance.

References

Alfano, S. L. (2013). Conducting research with human subjects in international settings: Ethical considerations. *Yale Journal of Biology and Medicine, 86*(3), 315–321.

Ali, J., Hyder, A. A., & Kass, N. E. (2012). Research ethics capacity development in Africa: Exploring a model for individual success. *Developing World Bioethics, 12*(2), 55–62.

Department of Health and Human Services (DHHS). (2006). *Protection of human subjects: Interpretation of assurance requirements.* www.govinfo.gov/content/pkg/FR-2006-07-07/html/E6-10511.htm

Department of Health and Human Services (DHHS). (2016). *Register IRBs & obtain FWAs.* www.hhs.gov/ohrp/register-irbs-and-obtain-fwas/index.html

Department of Health and Human Services (DHHS). (2018). *Listing of social-behavioral research standards.* www.hhs.gov/ohrp/international/social-behavioral-research-standards/index.html

Department of Health and Human Services (DHHS). (2019). *International compilation of human research standards.* www.hhs.gov/ohrp/sites/default/files/2019-International-Compilation-of-Human-Research-Standards.pdf

Glickman, S. W., McHutchison, J. G., Peterson, E. D., Cairns, C. B., Harrington, R. A., Califf, R. M., & Schulman, K. A. (2009). Ethical and scientific implications of the globalization of clinical research. *New England Journal of Medicine, 360*(8), 816–823.

National Library of Medicine. (2020). *ClinicalTrials.gov. Trends, charts, and maps.* www.clinicaltrials.gov/ct2/resources/trends

Rowland, C. (2004). Clinical trials seen shifting overseas. *International Journal of Health Services: Planning, Administration, Evaluation, 34*(3), 555–556.

Thiers, F. A., Sinske, A. J., & Berndt, E. R. (2008). Trends in the globalization of clinical trials. *Nature Reviews Drug Discovery, 7*, 13–14.

Research Involving Human Biospecimens

Marianna J. Bledsoe, Sara F. Goldkind*

Susannah M. Logsdon

William E. Grizzle

Abstract

Biospecimens are extremely valuable for research. Although the risks of such research are often considered low, the use of biospecimens in research raises a number of ethical, policy, and regulatory issues that need to be considered. Regulatory approaches for the use of biospecimens in research are complex, and governmental regulations and guidelines may be confusing and sometimes contradictory. This chapter describes how biospecimens are collected, stored, and used in research and considers some of the ethical, policy, and regulatory issues relating to IRB review of research involving biospecimens. These issues include considerations of whether the collection, storage, and/or use of the biospecimens falls under federal regulations and involves human subjects research, what the appropriate informed consent procedures are for the research, and whether the research qualifies for exemptions from the Common Rule or for a limited IRB review. This chapter also includes some important special topics related to the collection, storage, distribution, and use of biospecimens.

Introduction

The uses of biospecimens are almost unlimited in their impact on biomedical research, and they have contributed greatly to major advances in science and medical care. The term "biospecimens" includes a wide range of human biological materials (International Society for Biological and Environmental Repositories, 2018; National Cancer Institute, n.d.; National Institutes of Health, 2019a). The International Society for Biological and Environmental Repositories (ISBER) defines a specimen/biospecimen as follows: "In a clinical context, a specimen is specific tissue, blood, urine, or other material collected for analysis or a small fragment of tissue for microscopic study, taken from a single subject

*Co-first authors.

or donor at a specific time" (ISBER, 2018). By this definition, biospecimens include not only solid tissues but also blood (e.g., whole blood, serum, plasma, buffy coat), urine (e.g., whole urine, pellet, and supernatant), saliva/sputum, and other bodily fluids (e.g., joint fluids) as well as cellular preparations (e.g., fine needle aspirates). They also include cellular derivatives, such as DNA and RNA, as well as immortalized cell lines, organoids, and patient-derived xenografts.

Biospecimens have contributed to the understanding of normal and disease processes and the development, evaluation, and understanding of new advances in medical care. Almost all experimental techniques in biology and medicine have utilized biospecimens and associated data to characterize the biology and pathobiology of disease such as cancer. Research using biospecimens has been critical in the evolution of precision medicine. An example of this is the identification of three primary molecular targets that are used to treat specific subtypes of breast carcinoma (Waks & Winer, 2019). Moreover, biospecimen research may support Food and Drug Administration (FDA) applications of new products, including development of in vitro diagnostic tests and clinical trials of therapeutic drugs and medical devices.

The use of biospecimens in research has also contributed significantly to the development of immunotherapy approaches for the treatment of subsets of melanomas, lung adenocarcinomas, and other cancers (Dougan et al., 2019). Research is frequently initiated in cell lines or using animals. However, promising results usually must be confirmed in additional studies with human biospecimens and, ultimately, in clinical trials (Hall & Traystman, 2009).

Biospecimens obtained from pathology archives have been used for much important research (Gaffney et al., 2018). According to the College of American Pathologists (CAP), biospecimens collected solely for clinical purposes must be maintained for a minimum of 10 years to aid in future diagnostic questions concerning the patient as well as to address new molecular issues such as the presence of therapeutic molecular targets in the tissue. If there is more than adequate tissue stored, some aliquots can be used to support biomedical research provided this use is approved by the department of pathology. Thus, aliquots of small biopsies, including needle biopsies, may not be available for use in research. It should be stressed that 10 years is a minimum. As the uses of precision medicine accelerate, this minimum may increase.

Applicable Regulations, Guidelines, and Policies

Biospecimen research may be governed by a variety of different laws, regulations, international norms, guidelines, court decisions, and institutional policies. There are three main sets of federal regulations in the United States that IRBs must consider that are related to biospecimen research (in addition to state and local laws).

- The Federal Policy for the Protection of Human Subjects (Common Rule), codified by the Department of Health and Human Services (DHHS), at **45 CFR Part 46 subpart A**.
- FDA regulations that govern research involving drugs, devices, or biologics, **21 CFR Parts 50** (informed consent) and **56** (IRB); **21 CFR Part 312** (investigational new drugs) and **21 CFR Part 812** (investigational devices).
- The Health Insurance Portability and Accountability Act (HIPAA) Privacy Rule at **45 CFR Part 160** and **subparts A** and **E** of **Part 164**.

🖉 11-2 🖉 11-3

The Common Rule applies to human subjects research that is conducted or supported by one of the federal agencies that have adopted the Federal Policy for the Protection of Human Subjects. FDA regulations apply to all clinical investigations that are regulated by FDA under certain sections of the Federal Food, Drug, and Cosmetic Act, as well as clinical investigations that support applications for research or marketing permits for products regulated by FDA. The <u>HIPAA Privacy Rule</u>, although it does not apply to biospecimens per se, applies to the use and disclosure of protected health information that may be associated with biospecimens from HIPAA "covered entities" (DHHS, 2013). Additionally, there may be other federal regulations and/or laws, as well as state laws (e.g., regarding genetic testing, ownership of DNA, privacy, etc.), and court decisions that apply. These may be more restrictive or have additional requirements that go beyond the federal regulations and/or laws. Finally, funding agencies, such as the National Institutes of Health (NIH), may have their own policies that apply to biospecimen research, such as the NIH policy for genome sequencing studies (NIH, 2014).

⊘ 11-6

When <u>international</u> collaborations are involved, IRBs should consider the laws of other countries and jurisdictions. For example, the European Union General Data Protection Regulation (GDPR) governs the use and transfer of personal data that may apply under certain circumstances (European Commission, n.d.). Some countries, such as China and India, have laws governing the export of biospecimens and associated data. IRBs should be aware of any relevant regulatory requirements and whether there will be local ethics review. Furthermore, IRBs should document any division of responsibilities for review and oversight. IRBs should also consider any relevant institutional policies and whether other institutional committees may also need to be involved (e.g., export control committees). Finally, ethical oversight of biospecimen research may be informed by recommendations, guidelines, best practices, and other nonbinding statements.

⊘ 10-9

Collection, Storage, and Use of Biospecimens

Biospecimens may be obtained from patients diagnosed with a disease or condition and/or from individuals serving as controls. They may be collected as part of a research study (e.g., basic, translational, or clinical research), clinical care (e.g., during surgery), or at autopsy or from cadaveric donors. They may be collected, stored, maintained, and, ultimately, used for a known research study or used later for <u>secondary research</u> that may or may not be related to the purpose of the initial collection.

⊘ 12-3

A biospecimen may be in the form of excess material (i.e., remnants) obtained for clinical purposes or may represent material purposefully obtained for research through another intervention (e.g., additional blood draws or biopsies). Some researchers may establish formalized collections of biospecimens for use by one or more researchers within a single institution, or they may be distributed to other researchers outside the institution or the country for appropriate research purposes (Grizzle et al., 2010, 2019).

Regardless of the purpose for which the biospecimens are collected (fulfillment of specific research aims or creation of a biobank), biospecimens used to support research fall into five categories that have different ethical and regulatory considerations:

1. Pathology clinical archives. Biospecimens that were collected for clinical purposes only and stored in the pathology archives (e.g., microscopic

slides and paraffin blocks) may be used for research purposes as long as the use will not impact future clinical care of the patient. In this scenario, research use may not have been anticipated at the time the clinical biospecimens were collected, and therefore, consent for research may not have been obtained.

2. Remnant biospecimens are those left over after all standard clinical care (i.e., diagnosis and/or treatment) testing has been completed. Any biospecimens that a pathologist or designee has determined are not needed for patient care would ordinarily be discarded and not incorporated into pathology clinical archives. These biospecimens can be provided for research with appropriate institutional oversight. If it is known at the time a biospecimen is collected for clinical care that a portion of the residual biospecimen may be used for research, <u>informed consent</u> is generally required unless the IRB has determined that a <u>waiver</u> of consent can be granted. Sending remnant biospecimens primarily intended for research use to the pathology archives in order to avoid regulatory requirements of the Common Rule is inappropriate.

    ⊘ Section 6
    ⊘ 6-4

3. Biospecimens collected by doing a procedure solely for research purposes. Biospecimens may be collected and used for a research study that requires specific interventions or procedures such as a blood draw, oral swab, urine collection, or biopsies. When biospecimens from patients are obtained specifically for research, these biospecimens are not sent to pathology, and pathology department approval is not required. Informed consent for research would generally be required.

4. Biospecimens collected for research purposes during a clinically indicated procedure or a clinical protocol. Biospecimens, for example, extra biopsy samples, needed for research purposes may be collected at the same time as a clinically indicated procedure. In this case, informed consent for research would generally be required in addition to the clinical informed consent.

5. Biospecimens can be collected for research from autopsies or cadaveric donors or from tissues that were initially obtained for transplant that could not be utilized. Under the Common Rule and by FDA policy, a research subject must be living; thus, research on biospecimens obtained at autopsy is not considered human subjects research. However, the <u>HIPAA Privacy Rule</u> must be considered because it applies to deceased individuals under certain circumstances. Performance of autopsies typically is controlled by state laws as well as institutional policies. Applicable laws often vary with respect to the types of permissions that are required and from whom. Institutions in which autopsy biospecimens are being collected and used for research should be aware of the applicable laws of the jurisdiction, how they apply to such research, and how oversight will be provided.

    ⊘ 11-6

6. Some research studies involve collecting identifiable information from living research subjects prior to their death and obtaining informed consent that would allow their tissues to be collected and used for research after their death. In this case, IRB review and informed consent would be required under the relevant Common Rule and/or FDA regulations for activities prior to the subject's death. Compliance with HIPAA and any relevant state laws and institutional policies may also be required.

    ⊘ 12-3

Once collected, biospecimens may be stored in biobanks for <u>future use</u> in research. The terms *biobank*, *biorepository*, or *bioresource*, etc. are often used synonymously to refer to the collection, processing, storage, and distribution of biospecimens for use in future unspecified research or scientific inquiry. Although the term *biobank/bioresource* has been used in a variety of different ways, there is no commonly accepted definition (Hewitt & Watson, 2013). ISBER defines a biobank as "[a]n entity that receives, stores, processes, and/or distributes specimens, as needed. It encompasses the physical location as well as the full range of activities associated with its operation" (ISBER, 2018). A biobank is distinct from a registry; registries may be associated with a biobank, but registries contain only data and do not typically include biospecimens or biospecimen-derived data.

Biobanks may vary in many ways. They may vary in the types of biospecimens and associated data that are collected (discussed previously) and in how biospecimens and the associated data are processed, stored, and distributed. Biobanks may also vary in the data that are associated with the biospecimens, including subject identifiers. Biobanks may be established at a single site, such as an academic institution, hospital, or commercial organization or may include multiple sites, sometimes within different countries.

Some researchers or biobanks may interact directly with subjects and obtain <u>informed consent</u> for collecting a subject's biospecimens and associated data to support biomedical research. Other biobanks/researchers may have no direct interaction with subjects and instead obtain remnant aliquots from archival biospecimens to support research. Other biobanks may only serve as storage facilities and store biospecimens controlled by others outside the biobank (Grizzle et al., 2019).

🔗 Section 6

Of note, some biobanks receive biospecimens that are identifiable to the biobank, but ultimately, before leaving the biobank, the biospecimens and associated data are coded and provided to researchers without direct identifiers. The creation of such a biobank generally requires consent or a <u>waiver</u> of consent for the creation of the biobank.

🔗 6-4

There are several major types of collecting activities/biobanking models (Grizzle et al., 2019). These models may differ with regard to the extent of their interactions with subjects and their ethical and regulatory considerations. As a result of this significant variability, a "one size fits all" approach to policy requirements for biobanks is not feasible.

Biospecimens are often used in "secondary research." <u>Secondary research</u> refers to the subsequent research use of biospecimens and associated data that are collected for purposes other than the proposed research, such as other distinctly separate research studies, or biospecimens that are collected for nonresearch purposes, such as biospecimens that are left over from routine clinical care. As discussed later in this chapter and summarized in the box, Secondary Research on Identifiable Biospecimens, identifiable biospecimens

🔗 12-3

SECONDARY RESEARCH ON IDENTIFIABLE BIOSPECIMENS

Under the Common Rule, secondary research on identifiable biospecimens can be performed in one of the following ways:

- Study-specific consent with IRB review
- Broad consent and limited IRB review (under Exemption 7 and/or 8)
- Waiver of consent with IRB review
- Other exemptions (e.g., Exemption 4)
- Deidentification of the biospecimens such that the activity no longer meets the definition of human subjects research

can be used for secondary research under the Common Rule in a variety of different ways.

Ethical, Social, and Cultural Considerations

In their review of research involving human biospecimens, it is important that IRBs consider not only human subject protections as required in the regulations, but also ethical, social, and cultural considerations. Critically, these include consideration of the ethical principles of respect, beneficence, and justice as articulated in the *Belmont Report*. When applying the principles, the IRB should include in its considerations:

🔗 1-1

- Whether the effort is of sufficient scientific value
- How to adequately protect individual rights
- How to assure that the risks are minimized and justified by the benefits of the research either to the individual or society
- How to assure that there is equitable distribution of burdens and benefits to avoid inappropriately targeting disadvantaged groups or discriminating against groups as a result of the research
- Whether cultural or community values will be respected

During the review and oversight of biospecimen research, it is particularly important for IRBs to be mindful of social and cultural considerations of the subject population. Biospecimens may have intrinsic meaning to certain individuals or groups (Kowal, 2015; Lee et al., 2019). For example, indigenous populations and some ethnic and religious groups may have beliefs regarding the types of research that are acceptable to them, such as research on diseases that may be more prevalent in their groups, and those that are not, such as ancestry studies or studies of potentially stigmatizing conditions. Some groups may also have requirements for the disposition of their unused biospecimens and/or their return to the individual or tribe. Under certain circumstances, it may be appropriate to engage communities, their representatives, or their appointed oversight bodies (e.g., tribal authorities or council) in the design, conduct, or oversight of research.

🔗 9-10

Even when biospecimens have been deidentified, the results of some types of research have the potential to induce stigma or dignitary harms to the group (see Sidebar, The Havasupai Case) or to contribute to discriminatory health policies. Such social and cultural considerations and the potential for group and dignitary harms should be kept in mind in the review and oversight of biospecimen research.

Ethical, social, and cultural considerations regarding human biospecimens research have received considerable attention in the media. In addition to the Havasupai case, examples include the Henrietta Lacks case (Beskow, 2016; Skloot, 2010, 2013; see Sidebar, The Henrietta Lacks Case), and the newborn dried bloodspot cases in Texas and Minnesota (Grody & Howell, 2010).

THE HAVASUPAI CASE

In the Havasupai case, researchers obtained more than 200 blood samples from members of the Havasupai tribe located in Northern Arizona. Although the consent form described the research as studying the causes of behavioral/medical disorders, communications with tribal leaders before the study centered on diabetes (Mello & and Wolf, 2010). The biospecimens were subsequently used for research other than diabetes that the tribe found objectionable, including studies of schizophrenia, inbreeding, and population migration that challenged the tribe's beliefs about the tribe's origins. This led to legal claims that the researchers improperly used tribe members' blood samples in genetic research. The lawsuits were settled with a monetary payment of $700,000 and return of the biospecimens to the tribe (Assche et al., 2013; Mello & Wolf, 2010). This case illustrates the importance of considering cultural sensitivities in biospecimen research, the potential for group harms even when biospecimens are used without direct identifiers, and the importance of informed consent as a process and not just a form.

IRB Review Considerations

There are many complex considerations that may directly affect IRB deliberations and determinations regarding research involving the collection, processing, storage, distribution, and/or use of biospecimens. These include, but may not be limited to, determining (1) whether a particular activity is human subjects research; (2) what type of review (if any) is necessary (exemption from the 2018 Common Rule or required review by either by the convened IRB or through expedited review procedures); and (3) if the activity is human subjects research, whether informed consent is required, or whether it qualifies for a waiver of informed consent.

Common Rule

In determining whether an activity involving biospecimens falls under IRB oversight, an IRB should consider the following three questions, in order:

1. Is the activity research?
2. If so, does the research involve human subjects?
3. If the research involves human subjects, does it qualify for an exemption to the Common Rule?

THE HENRIETTA LACKS CASE

The daughter of an African American tobacco farmer, Henrietta Lacks was diagnosed in 1951 with a highly aggressive form of cervical cancer. As was common practice at the time, biospecimens were taken during the course of her diagnosis and treatment and used for research without her knowledge and permission (Beskow, 2016). Her cells, labeled "HeLa" based on her initials, were found to be able to survive and grow in culture indefinitely and were used to develop commercially available cell lines. The cells were widely distributed and used in laboratories around the world for a wide variety of research, leading to many important discoveries (Skloot, 2010). Later, the genomic sequence of Henrietta Lacks was posted on a publicly available website without the consent of the Lacks family and was afterward withdrawn (Skloot, 2013). In an agreement with the Lacks family, NIH established a process whereby researchers are expected to deposit HeLa sequence data in a controlled access database with requests for access to the data being reviewed by a committee that includes Lacks family members. This case brought much attention to issues related to informed consent and commercial use of specimens and led to many of the changes related to biospecimen research in the Common Rule. Beskow published a comprehensive discussion of the policy issues raised by this case (Beskow, 2016).

Is the Activity Research?

The Common Rule at **45 CFR 46.102(l)** defines research as, "a systematic investigation, including research development, testing, and evaluation, designed to develop or contribute to generalizable knowledge." Some activities involving the collection or use of identifiable biospecimens are excluded from this definition, including the collection or use of biospecimens for public health surveillance activities or for criminal justice or criminal investigative purposes. Other activities involving the collection of biospecimens, such as routine clinical care and blood donation, are not explicitly excluded from the regulation but are commonly accepted as nonresearch. The use of biospecimens solely for quality control or for teaching and education is generally considered to be outside the scope of research.

5-1

Importantly, the Office for Protection from Research Risks (OPRR, precursor office to the Office for Human Research Protections [OHRP]) issued guidance in 1997 clarifying that the collection of biospecimens specifically for the purpose of establishing (or for inclusion in) a biobank for research purposes is considered a research activity.

Does the Research Involve Human Subjects?

A human subject under **45 CFR 46.102(e)** is "a living individual about whom an investigator conducting research: 1) obtains information or biospecimens through intervention or interaction with the individual, and uses, studies, or analyzes the information or biospecimens; or 2) obtains, uses, studies, analyzes, or generates identifiable private information or identifiable biospecimens." Under the Common Rule at **45 CFR 46.102(e)(6)**, an identifiable biospecimen is a "biospecimen for which the identity of the subject is or may readily be ascertained by the investigator or associated with the biospecimen." See box, Terminology Related to Identifiability, for definitions of other terms used in this chapter.

TERMINOLOGY RELATED TO IDENTIFIABILITY

Identifiable. Under the Common Rule at **45 CFR 46.102(f)**, an identifiable biospecimen is "a biospecimen for which the identity of the subject is or may readily be ascertained by the investigator or associated with the biospecimen." (Note that the definition of *identifiable* is slightly different under HIPAA).

Deidentified. Deidentified biospecimens are those for which direct and indirect personal identifiers have been removed. Under HIPAA, this would include the removal of the 18 HIPAA identifiers specified in the HIPAA Privacy Rule and meeting the other requirements of the Rule at **45 CFR 164.514(a)(2)**.

Anonymous. Anonymous biospecimens and associated data are those that were collected without identifiers and are not traceable back to the subject. Coded biospecimens are not anonymous.

Anonymized. Anonymized biospecimens are those that were previously identifiable for which identifiers have been removed and for which a code or other link to subject identities no longer exists. They are not traceable back to the subject.

The collection, storage, distribution, and/or use of biospecimens for research is considered to be human subjects research (as defined in the Common Rule) when it involves either an interaction or intervention with a living individual for the purposes of research or identifiable biospecimens and/or associated identifiable information from a living individual.

In contrast, the creation of a biobank would not be considered to involve human subjects when the following conditions are met:

- The biospecimens are collected for purposes other than the biobank (e.g., the material was collected solely for clinical purposes or comprises residual biospecimens from an unrelated research protocol).
- The biospecimens are submitted to the biobank without any identifiable private data or information that would allow the biobank to readily ascertain the identities of the living individuals from whom the biospecimens are obtained.

Secondary Use of Biospecimens from a Biobank

Coded biospecimens (i.e., biospecimens for which the direct identifiers have been replaced by an alphanumeric code and for which there exists a key linking the codes to identifiers) are considered identifiable under the Common Rule. However, OHRP issued guidance in 2008 specifying certain conditions under which research using coded biospecimens would not be considered to involve human subjects (DHHS, 2008; see box, Excerpts from the 2008 OHRP Guidance on Coded Biospecimens).

EXCERPTS FROM THE 2008 OHRP GUIDANCE ON CODED BIOSPECIMENS

Coded means that (DHHS, 2008):

1. Identifying information (such as name or social security number) that would enable the investigator to readily ascertain the identity of the individual to whom the private information or specimens pertain has been replaced with a number, letter, symbol, or combination thereof (i.e., the code).
2. A key to decipher the code exists, enabling linkage of the identifying information to the private information or specimens.

In general, OHRP considers private information or specimens to be individually identifiable as defined at **45 CFR 46.102(e)** when they can be linked to specific individuals by the investigator(s) either directly or indirectly through coding systems.

Conversely, OHRP considers private information or specimens not to be individually identifiable when they cannot be linked to specific individuals by the investigator(s) either directly or indirectly through coding systems. For example, OHRP does not consider research involving *only* coded private information or specimens to involve human subjects as defined under **45 CFR 46.102(e)** if the following conditions are both met:

1. The private information or specimens were not collected specifically for the currently proposed research project through an interaction or intervention with living individuals.
2. The investigator(s) cannot readily ascertain the identity of the individual(s) to whom the coded private information or specimens pertain because, for example:

   a. The investigators and the holder of the key enter into an agreement prohibiting the release of the key to the investigators under any circumstances, until the individuals are deceased (note that DHHS regulations do not require the IRB to review and approve this agreement).
   b. There are IRB-approved written policies and operating procedures for a repository or data management center that prohibit the release of the key to the investigators under any circumstances, until the individuals are deceased.
   c. There are other legal requirements prohibiting the release of the key to the investigators, until the individuals are deceased.

When making a determination that the research using coded biospecimens from a biobank does not involve human subjects (under the OHRP coded specimens guidance; DHHS, 2008), it should be should confirmed that the biobank is:

1. Not collecting the biospecimens and/or associated data specifically for the research study through an interaction/intervention.
2. An agreement, policy, or applicable law expressly prohibits the release of the key to the researcher.
3. The researcher will not attempt to identify the subjects from whom the biospecimens were collected.

OHRP took the position that the mere act of providing coded biospecimens from a biobank does not make the biobank involved in the conduct of the secondary research using the biobank biospecimens (DHHS, 2008). However, if the biobank is functioning in any other capacity and collaborating in the secondary research (e.g., the analysis of study data) the biobank would be involved in the secondary research.

If the research involves biospecimens that are completely anonymous or anonymized (i.e., there is no link to identities), the research would not be considered to involve human subjects.

It should be noted that the interpretation of what constitutes identifiable private information or biospecimens may evolve with advances in science and technology. The Common Rule stipulates that these terms will be reassessed periodically and guidance issued as needed [45 CFR 46.102(e)(7)(i)]. This is particularly relevant for biospecimen research. As discussed later (see section, Special Topics), advancements in genome sequencing technology and accessibility to genomic data have the potential to impact whether an individual's identity is "readily ascertainable." IRBs should be mindful of this important point and periodically seek updated information regarding current interpretive guidance related to this definition.

Does the Research Qualify for Exemption from the Common Rule?

5-3

The exemptions from the 2018 Common Rule at 45 CFR 46.104(d)(4) and (d)(7-8), hereafter referred to as "Exemptions 4, 7, and 8," are of particular relevance to biobanking activities and biospecimen research, specifically, secondary research on biospecimens.

As outlined in the Common Rule, secondary research uses of biospecimens may qualify for Exemption 4 if one of three conditions is met:

1. The biospecimens are publicly available. For example, biospecimens are obtained from a commercial source that is available to the public without restrictions or special permissions.
2. The information associated with the biospecimens is recorded by the investigator in such a way that the identity of the subject cannot be readily ascertained, the investigator does not contact the subjects, and the investigator will not attempt to reidentify subjects.
3. The research is conducted under 45 CFR Parts 160 and 164 for the purposes of healthcare operations or public health activities.

6-9
5-6

The Common Rule allows for institutions to determine whether or not to utilize two new (in the 2018 Requirements) exemption categories, 7 and 8, that pertain to the storage and secondary use of identifiable biospecimens and associated data. The use of both exemptions requires broad consent under 45 CFR 46.116(d), as well as limited IRB review. Broad consent under 45 CFR 46.116(d) refers to the consent for storage, maintenance, and secondary research use of identifiable private information and identifiable specimens. Generally speaking, broad consent is optional. It is only considered to be required in the context of applying Exemptions 7 and 8.

Exemption 7 applies specifically to the storage or maintenance of identifiable biospecimens for secondary research. As described previously in this chapter, secondary research is research with biospecimens originally obtained for nonresearch purposes or for research other than the current research proposal. The exemption can only be used when there is broad consent under 45 CFR 46.116(d) from the subjects for the storage, maintenance, and secondary research use of their identifiable biospecimens. For the use of Exemption 7, an IRB performs a limited review to make the determinations described in 45 CFR 46.111(a)(8), which relate to protections for privacy and confidentiality and broad consent.

Exemption 8 at **45 CFR 46.104(d)(8)** covers the secondary research use of identifiable biospecimens originally obtained for nonresearch purposes or for research other than the current proposal. For the use of this exemption, four requirements, described at **45 CFR 46.104(d)(8)(i)-(iv)**, must be met: (1) broad consent at **45 CFR 46.116(d)** must be obtained from the subjects for the secondary research use of their identifiable materials, (2) documentation or <u>waiver of documentation</u> of informed consent must be obtained, (3) an IRB must conduct a limited review to make certain determinations described at **45 CFR 46.111(a)(7)** relating to privacy and confidentiality protections and broad consent, and (4) investigators cannot include the return of individual research results to subjects in the study plan.

🖉 6-5

For Exemption 8, the IRB conducts a <u>limited review</u> to determine whether the following criteria are met: (1) there are adequate privacy and confidentiality protections as required under **45 CFR 46.111(a)(7)** and (2) the research to be conducted is within the scope of the broad consent.

🖉 5-6

For a useful discussion of the application of these exemptions, please see the Secretary's Advisory Committee on Human Research Protections (SACHRP) guidance (DHHS, 2018a, 2018b).

FDA

FDA-regulated clinical investigations of investigational products require IRB review either by a <u>convened IRB</u> or by <u>expedited</u> review procedures, if permissible. Although FDA regulations do not specifically address the collection, storage, maintenance, and use of biospecimens, IRB review of FDA-regulated research involving biospecimens to support a marketing application is generally subject to **21 CFR Parts 50** and **56** and any other applicable FDA regulations (e.g., **21 CFR Parts 312** or **812**). IRBs must consider the same <u>criteria</u> for IRB approval under **21 CFR 56.111** and requirements for informed consent under **21 CFR 50.25** as for any other FDA-regulated research.

🖉 5-5 🖉 5-7

🖉 5-4

As of 2019, there are several areas worth noting where the Common Rule and FDA regulations have <u>not been harmonized</u>. First, FDA device regulations at **21 CFR Part 812** consider a human subject to include any individual on whose specimen an <u>investigational device</u> is used, even when they are not identifiable. Second, FDA's regulations do not have any exemptions from IRB review for biospecimen research. Third, all FDA-regulated clinical investigations involving biospecimens from living individuals must undergo IRB review, even if they are outside the scope of the Common Rule. Fourth, as discussed later, FDA and OHRP differ in their policies regarding retention of data upon withdrawal of consent.

🖉 11-1

🖉 11-3

HIPAA

Although the <u>HIPAA Privacy Rule</u> does not explicitly apply to biospecimens directly, it may apply to the health information associated with the biospecimens. This would affect biospecimen research at covered entities or business associates of covered entities, as human biospecimens are often accompanied by protected health information (PHI; National Cancer Institute, 2016). The use and disclosure of PHI by a covered entity for research purposes generally requires the written authorization of the patient. However, there are mechanisms to disclose PHI without written authorization,

🖉 11-6

including the waiver of HIPAA authorization or use of a limited data set with a signed data use agreement (DUA) that complies with the requirements in **45 CFR 164.514(e)(4)**.

IRBs may be delegated the responsibility of serving as a HIPAA Privacy Board. With respect to HIPAA, the Privacy Board's authority is limited to acting on requests for a waiver or an alteration of the Privacy Rule's authorization requirement, such as with the creation of a biobank for which the IRB has waived the requirement for informed consent. IRBs may be delegated additional responsibilities as a matter of institutional policy. For example, IRBs may be asked to determine whether information constitutes a "limited data set" and to review associated DUAs.

IRB Review of Nonexempt Research

Nonexempt research involving biospecimens must be reviewed by the IRB at a convened meeting or by an expedited review procedure. Expedited review may be conducted if the research is considered to be no more than minimal risk and if it falls into the list of expedited review categories approved by the Secretary of DHHS and/or FDA. Some of these relate specifically to biospecimens.

As for all research, IRBs reviewing biospecimen research must find that the applicable approval criteria under **45 CFR 46.111** and/or **21 CFR 56.111** have been satisfied. In addition, the IRB should carefully consider the ethical, social, and cultural considerations of using biospecimens in research discussed earlier. The next section focuses on risks and benefits and privacy and confidentiality as they relate to biospecimen research in more detail.

Risks and Benefits

The benefits of biospecimen research are primarily societal, although rapid advances in precision medicine may translate the benefits from research with a patient's biospecimen to their effective medical care. While IRBs may not consider the indirect benefits to research subjects in their assessment of risks and benefits, subjects may derive some personal benefit from the altruism associated with contributing to a worthwhile research study.

The risks of biospecimen research are generally low. The risks may include physical harms/discomfort if there is an additional intervention or procedure to obtain a biospecimen specifically for research (e.g., blood draw or additional biopsy). Biospecimen research also includes informational risks related to loss of privacy and confidentiality or potential dignitary harms to individuals and/or groups. Resultant harms from such disclosures may include discrimination, embarrassment or stigmatization, or potentially, the loss of healthcare benefits or employment. In assessing potential dignitary harms, it is important that the IRB consider the source of the biospecimens and the identifiable information that will be retained and/or used, as well as the circumstances under which the biospecimens were collected and for what purpose(s). IRBs must determine whether these risks have been minimized and whether they are reasonable in relation to the anticipated benefits of the research.

Privacy and Confidentiality

A number of methods can be used to maintain privacy and confidentiality and minimize the risks of reidentification in biospecimen research. Appropriate risk minimization includes establishing and implementing procedures to protect privacy and confidentiality. These include coding, restricting access to identifying information, using secure information technology (IT) systems and honest brokers (Vaught & Lockhart, 2012), and reviewing requests for access to biospecimens and associated data and their release to qualified researchers. They also may include collecting and maintaining only those data necessary for current or anticipated <u>future research uses</u>. Researchers should provide a justification for why identifiable information is being retained and with whom it might be shared. Material transfer agreements (MTAs) and good biobank governance and appropriate access procedures and policies can further help mitigate the risks of reidentification and loss of confidentiality (see the section, Special Topics). <u>Certificates of confidentiality</u> (CoC) may also help mitigate the risk of disclosure of identifying information in such studies (NIH, 2019b). Finally, good institutional policies and procedures for maintaining the privacy of research subjects and the confidentiality of their data are absolutely essential. Institutional policies should include approaches for dealing with researchers who may attempt to breach subject privacy and confidentiality.

⌗ 12-3

⌗ 8-3

Informed Consent

As with all nonexempt research, IRBs reviewing biospecimen research must assess whether the research complies with the <u>consent</u> requirements under **45 CFR 46.116** and/or **21 CFR 50.25**, as applicable.

⌗ Section 6

As mentioned previously, when biospecimens are collected prospectively for research purposes, including those that are collected in a clinical setting, informed consent is generally required. IRBs must confirm whether the general regulatory requirements are met. There are a number of different consent models that may be used for the collection and storage of identifiable biospecimens under the Common Rule. These include standard consent under **45 CFR 46.116(b)** and (c) (and/or **21 CFR 50.25** if FDA regulated) and <u>broad consent</u> at **45 CFR 46.116(d)**.

⌗ 6-9

Consent considerations may vary depending on how the biospecimens were collected (see the previous discussion of the five categories of biospecimens). Collecting and storing residual clinical or diagnostic biospecimens for future research use may occur in a context in which consent cannot be obtained. This is discussed in the next section on waiver of consent.

IRBs reviewing research involving the secondary use of stored identifiable biospecimens must determine whether informed consent has been obtained, and if so, is the proposed <u>secondary use</u> consistent with any previous informed consent? In addition, unless the biospecimens were originally obtained under broad consent at **45 CFR 46.116(d)**, it must be determined whether the secondary research use requires additional consent or qualifies for a <u>waiver</u> of informed consent. The box, Consent for Secondary Use of Identifiable Biospecimens, describes some useful considerations when making these determinations.

⌗ 12-3

⌗ 6-4

Standard Consent Content

The requirements of standard consent are described at **45 CFR 46.116(b)** and **(c)** (and/or **21 CFR 50.25** if FDA regulated). Besides the basic and additional <u>elements</u> of informed consent that are regulatory requirements, the consent process and form for the collection and/or storage of biospecimens should include a clear explanation of the type of potential research (e.g., cancer research)

⌗ 6-2

CONSENT FOR SECONDARY USE OF IDENTIFIABLE BIOSPECIMENS

In assessing whether an existing consent for the use of identifiable biospecimens is sufficient for use in secondary research (either a broad consent or a consent previously obtained for another research study), SACHRP acknowledged that such determinations are generally context specific based on a number of considerations. These include the nature of the proposed secondary research, whether it could reasonably be understood to fall within the scope of research that was described in the original consent form, whether the secondary research use imposes new or significantly greater risks (including privacy risks) than what was described in the initial consent form, and whether it is known that the proposed secondary use raises concerns for the study population(s). SACHRP further noted that if the original consent form specifically excluded or prohibited the proposed use, it is presumed the use would not be permissible (DHHS, 2018a).

that could be conducted using the biospecimens, with whom the biospecimens may be shared (e.g., researchers at external institutions or for-profit companies), and a general description of the biospecimens and the PHI or other information that may be collected, stored, and/or distributed with the biospecimens. The consent process and form should clearly describe the extent to which subjects can withdraw their identifiable biospecimens and associated information, and, as applicable, what this means in the context of biobanking (e.g., that it may not be possible to discontinue further research use of their biospecimens and data once biospecimens have been distributed for research or once the biospecimens and associated data have been anonymized).

It is important to note that the withdrawal of biospecimens and associated data raises some ethical and practical implementation issues. IRBs should consider whether the procedures for the withdrawal of a subject's biospecimens and associated data are reasonable and appropriate (e.g., destroying or anonymizing biospecimens and associated data). It is important to note that FDA requires that all data collected on a subject to the point of withdrawal must remain part of the study database when a subject chooses to withdraw from an FDA-regulated study. OHRP, however, in consultation with the funding agency, may permit the destruction of a subject's data upon withdrawal of that subject from the research (DHHS, 2010; FDA, 2008).

Specifically, the Common Rule includes several required basic and additional elements that explicitly address research that involves the collection of identifiable private information or identifiable biospecimens. The Common Rule requires that all consent documents include a disclosure about the extent to which biospecimens might be deidentified and shared with other researchers without additional informed consent. It also requires, as appropriate, an acknowledgment that biospecimens might be used for commercial purposes and whether the subject will share in any profits, the extent to which clinically relevant results will be disclosed to subjects and under what conditions and whether the research might include whole genome sequencing.

IRBs should keep in mind that funding agencies or sponsors may have specific consent requirements. For example, whole genome sequencing studies conducted or supported by NIH are required to have language that covers the broad sharing of genotypic and phenotypic data. In addition, for biospecimen research covered by an NIH-issued <u>CoC</u>, IRBs should ensure that the consent form includes language that describes the additional protections offered by the CoC.   🖈 8-3

A number of different approaches exist for implementing consent for biobanking. These include tiered consent, which offers choices for subjects in the ways their biospecimens may be used, or dynamic consent, which allows ongoing communication with research subjects through IT approaches (Kaye et al., 2012). In such cases, an IRB may need to consider whether the biobank has the necessary infrastructure to make sure that a subject's choices are honored. **Table 10.10-1** summarizes the advantages and disadvantages of various consent models for biobanking.

Broad Consent

As referenced earlier, the Common Rule provides the option of using <u>broad consent</u> for secondary uses as an alternative to the informed consent requirements specified in **45 CFR 46.116(b)** and **(c)**. The stated goal of broad consent   🖈 6-9

Table 10.10-1 Informed Consent Models for the Collection, Storage, Distribution, and Use of Biospecimens for Research

Type of Consent	Description	Advantages	Disadvantages
Study-specific consent	A consent approach that is limited to a specific research study	Provides the most specific information to biospecimen donors May be the most acceptable form of consent in some study populations	Limits downstream secondary use of biospecimens for other research studies
Tiered consent	A consent approach that allows subjects/donors to choose among various types of research or types of biospecimens they wish to donate	Provides greater choices to subjects than general consent for future use of biospecimens Biospecimens can be used for a wider array of types of research than a study-specific consent	Choices require rigorous tracking systems to ensure that subject choices are honored Decisions must be made about whether a future use fits within the type of research category to which the subject has agreed
General consent for future use of biospecimens	A consent approach that describes the general types of research for which the biospecimens will be used	Allows maximum flexibility for a wide array of downstream future research uses and facilitates optimal biospecimen utilization	May not be acceptable in some jurisdictions or study populations
Dynamic consent (Kaye et al., 2012)	A consent approach that uses IT to permit an ongoing discourse and negotiation between researchers and subjects/donors to decide whether they wish to consent broadly to future uses or to each subsequent future research study	Provides the greatest choice to subjects/donors Enables ongoing engagement of subjects/donors	Requires considerable infrastructure and resources to implement (e.g., time, money, expertise) May work better for certain types of studies and study populations than others

Data from Bledsoe, M. J., & Sexton, K. C. (2019). Ensuring effective utilization of biospecimens: Design, marketing, and other important approaches. *Biopreservation and Biobanking, 17*(3), 248–257.

under the Common Rule is to give subjects greater choice in how their biospecimens will be utilized while increasing the flexibility for researchers concerning how the biospecimens are used in the future. The consent form can either apply to a specific type of future research (e.g., diabetes research) or can be written in a broader sense (e.g., biomedical research). Broad consent obtained in accordance with **45 CFR 46.116(d)** serves as legally effective consent for subsequent research uses that are consistent with the uses described in the broad consent; broad consent obviates the need to obtain standard consent or for an IRB to consider a waiver of consent for secondary uses of identifiable biospecimens.

Broad consent includes required elements that are in addition to the nine required elements under **45 CFR 46.116(d)**. These additional elements include the following [**45 CFR 46.116(d)(2)-(7)**]:

2. A general description of the types of research that may be conducted with the identifiable private information or identifiable biospecimens. This description must include sufficient information such that a reasonable person would expect that the broad consent would permit the types of research conducted;

3. A description of the identifiable private information or identifiable biospecimens that might be used in research, whether sharing of identifiable private information or identifiable biospecimens might occur, and the types of institutions or researchers that might conduct research with the identifiable private information or identifiable biospecimens;

4. A description of the period of time that the identifiable private information or identifiable biospecimens may be stored and maintained (which period of time could be indefinite), and a description of the period of time that the identifiable private information or identifiable biospecimens may be used for research purposes (which period of time could be indefinite);

5. Unless the subject or legally authorized representative will be provided details about specific research studies, a statement that they will not be informed of the details of any specific research studies that might be conducted using the subject's identifiable private information or identifiable biospecimens, including the purposes of the research, and that they might have chosen not to consent to some of those specific research studies;

6. Unless it is known that clinically relevant research results, including individual research results, will be disclosed to the subject in all circumstances, a statement that such results may not be disclosed to the subject; and

7. An explanation of whom to contact for answers to questions about the subject's rights and about storage and use of the subject's identifiable private information or identifiable biospecimens, and whom to contact in the event of a research-related harm.

Use of broad consent described at **45 CFR 46.116(d)** comes with one very important limitation: An IRB may not waive or alter consent when an individual has refused to provide broad consent. Thus, entities that use broad consent need to have systems to track refusals of consent. It is important to emphasize that the use of a broad consent is not mandatory. Other options exist for obtaining consent for the collection, storage, and use of identifiable biospecimens for research.

For example, researchers have long relied on consent for future uses of biospecimens for the collection, storage, and use of subject data and leftover biospecimens for future research. Under the 2018 Common Rule, a consent for future research using identifiable biospecimens should be analyzed to make sure that the consent has sufficiently described the future uses, even if the consent does not meet the requirements for a broad consent for the purposes of Exemptions 7 and 8 (DHHS, 2017). In order to rely on such a consent, an IRB would need to determine that the <u>requirements</u> of a traditional consent at **45 CFR 46.116(c)** have been met.

✎ 6-2

Combined Consent

In general, an informed consent process for the collection and future use of biospecimens in research may be combined with other types of informed consent (e.g., consent for clinical treatment) in appropriate and carefully defined circumstances. The consent process should provide prospective subjects with sufficient opportunity to discuss and consider whether or not to participate in the research involving the biospecimens. The process should clearly be voluntary and not be coercive or unduly influential, and this should be clearly explained during the consent process, such that patients understand their clinical treatment will not be affected by their decision to participate or not in the biospecimen research. Furthermore, IRBs should consider the timing and circumstances regarding when consent will be obtained. For example, if consent for biospecimen collection will be obtained at the time of surgery, IRBs should consider whether patients will have considerable anxiety at that time and how this may affect their ability to provide consent.

When combining a consent for research use of biospecimens with a surgical consent, all of the required elements for a valid research consent must be present. For example, statements indicating that a patient's remnant biospecimens may be collected, stored, and used in research sometimes may be added to a surgical or other consent form that is not primarily focused on biospecimens. The IRB should consider whether this approach meets all the requirements of a valid research consent, is fully informative about the research, and is not coercive.

Waiving Consent

The Common Rule allows for the <u>waiver</u> or alteration of informed consent if specific criteria are satisfied. Under the Common Rule, an IRB may waive the requirement for informed consent if it finds the following **[45 CFR 46.116(f)(3)(i)-(v)]**:

✎ 6-4

i. The research involves no more than minimal risk to the subjects;
ii. The research could not practicably be carried out without the requested waiver or alteration;
iii. If the research involves using identifiable private information or identifiable biospecimens, the research could not practicably be carried out without using such information or biospecimens in an identifiable format;
iv. The waiver or alteration will not adversely affect the rights and welfare of the subjects; and
v. Whenever appropriate, the subjects or legally authorized representatives will be provided with additional pertinent information after participation.

At the time of this writing, FDA regulations do not contain provisions allowing the waiver or alteration of informed consent except under emergency conditions (**21 CFR 50.23** and **21 CFR 50.24**). However, FDA has issued two enforcement guidances that permit the waiver of informed consent under limited circumstances. The two guidance documents that permit FDA-regulated clinical investigations to be conducted without informed consent are: (1) "Informed Consent for In Vitro Diagnostic Device Studies Using Leftover Human Specimens that are Not Individually Identifiable" (FDA, 2006). This guidance permits the use of remnant biospecimens collected for routine clinical care to be used in clinical investigations if seven conditions are met; and (2) "IRB Waiver or Alteration of Informed Consent for Clinical Investigations Involving No More Than Minimal Risk to Human Subjects" (FDA, 2017). As a result of the statutory changes made to the Federal Food, Drug, and Cosmetic Act (FD&C Act) by section 3024 of the Cures Act (Pub. L. 114-255), FDA issued this guidance in 2017, which allows IRBs to waive consent for minimal risk clinical research under the same criteria as the pre-2018 Common Rule. At the time of this writing (2019), FDA regulations at **21 CFR Part 50** are under revision to incorporate the waiver of informed consent as described in its Code of Federal Regulations.

Waivers of informed consent may be necessary for the research to be conducted, particularly when the biospecimens are obtained from pathology archives. When biospecimens are collected specifically for research, or when it is known at the time of collection that clinically obtained biospecimens will be used for research, consent generally should be obtained at the time the biospecimens are collected. However, this is usually not the case when biospecimens needed for research are obtained from clinical (pathology) archives. In most cases, it is unknown whether or not tissues will be used in research when biospecimens are added to a clinical archive, so informed consent typically is not obtained for use of these biospecimens in research due to the extensive resources required to consent all such patients. Moreover, obtaining consent after a patient has left a medical center is challenging. Experience shows that once a patient leaves a medical facility, it is difficult to obtain informed consent for research use of biospecimens collected at that facility because patients may be difficult to locate. In addition, communicating with patients who have not provided consent for further contact may not be acceptable to the local IRB or to the medical facility. The use of such biospecimens, when identifiable, are often eligible for a waiver of informed consent.

When considering whether a biospecimen research activity meets the criteria for a waiver of informed consent, SACHRP recommended considering the following factors: the nature of the research, privacy and confidentiality protections, the ability to locate or contact subjects, the length of time since the biospecimens were first collected, and the likelihood that subjects would object to the proposed secondary use based on the nature of the original collection (DHHS, 2018a, FAQ #5).

Special Topics

Children

Parental permission and assent (when in the judgment of the IRB, children are capable of providing assent) are required for biospecimen research involving children. These requirements are described at **45 CFR 46.408** (for research

9-6

supported or conducted by DHHS.), and **21 CFR 50.55** (for FDA-regulated research). When the biobank includes the collection, storage, distribution, and use of identifiable biospecimens from children, the biobank should consider how to address the transition of minors to adults; that is, whether to obtain consent when the child subject reaches the age of majority or whether the requirements for a waiver of informed consent can be met.

The IRB as Gatekeeper

IRBs are often tasked to be the "gatekeepers" to ensure that other institutional requirements for biospecimen research are met. These may include, but are not limited to, approvals from other internal committees (e.g., scientific review committee, investigational device committee) and/or the execution of contractual agreements such as MTAs (see discussion later). Furthermore, when biospecimens are received from an external institution (even if they are deidentified), it may be the IRB's responsibility to verify that the biospecimens were obtained in accordance with relevant regulations and good ethical practice.

Biobank Governance

As noted and discussed by numerous groups and in international guidelines (Bledsoe, 2017), governance and oversight systems are important for ensuring that the biospecimens and associated data managed by biobanks are used in ways that are scientifically sound and ethically appropriate. However, governance systems may vary considerably depending on the purpose and nature of the biobank and the biospecimens that they manage and distribute.

Biobank governance systems may contain multiple components with responsibilities for oversight shared among multiple stakeholders. For example, the biobank manager may be responsible for developing biobanking operating procedures and policies to ensure human subject protections and ethical handling of biospecimens as well as day-to-day oversight of regulatory compliance, ethical conduct, and scientific best practices. The IRB is responsible for overseeing compliance with regulations and good ethical conduct and reviewing the biobanking protocol and informed consent. In addition, the IRB may review protocols for <u>secondary use</u> of identifiable biospecimens.

⚙ 12-3

Biobanking governance committees may also play an important role in the oversight of biobanks. Because the biospecimens and associated data that are distributed for research are often deidentified, secondary uses of biospecimens may be reviewed by a biospecimen utilization committee established by the biobank. These committees typically review requests for biospecimens and data from the biobank to ensure that they are an appropriate use of the resource. Additionally, they may review requests for uses of biospecimens to ensure that they are ethically appropriate and fall within the scope of the general consent under which the biospecimens may have been obtained. Other components of a biobank governance system may sometimes include other committees such as executive committees, scientific advisory boards, ethics advisory boards, or community advisory boards, as appropriate. Some biobanks have included research subjects in the governance and oversight of biobanks to help shape biobank policy (McCarty et al., 2008). Although biobank governance systems play an important role, the biobank governance system should not unnecessarily restrict access from qualified researchers for valid research studies or become so labor intensive that the functions of the biobank to support biomedical research are impeded.

Access Policies and Procedures

An important part of biobank governance is having well-documented policies and procedures for access to biospecimens and the review of biospecimen requests. The process for reviewing requests for biospecimens and associated data should address a number of issues, including ethical, legal, and social considerations, as appropriate. These are further described in several best practice documents for biobanks (ISBER, 2018; NCI, 2016).

Appropriate procedures for the distribution of biospecimens and data are another important part of biobank governance. In order to protect privacy and confidentiality, in general, biobanks should distribute materials in a deidentified manner or in a coded manner, with written agreements prohibiting the release of the identifying key. Biobanks operated by covered entities may choose to incorporate the elements required for a DUA into an MTA or utilize a separate DUA. MTAs and DUAs are important ways of controlling downstream uses of biospecimens. These agreements document the obligations of the recipient researcher, including, for example, obligations to protect the privacy of research subjects and the confidentiality of their data, use the biospecimens only for approved uses consistent with any consent, and not share the biospecimens and associated data with third parties without prior approval of the biobank (ISBER, 2018; NCI, 2016).

In summary, good governance and oversight are essential to biobank operations. Biobank governance is critical to protect research subjects and respect their autonomy, maintain their trust and the trust of funding agencies and the public, promote biobank sustainability, ensure future research participation, and promote research progress. Because of the great variability in the nature, purpose, and design of biobanks, a "one size fits all" approach is not often appropriate.

Commercial Use of Biospecimens

The use of biospecimens by commercial for-profit companies such as pharmaceutical companies has been essential for major advancements in modern medical care. If biospecimens were not provided to commercial entities, the development of new drugs and medical devices would be greatly reduced. However, numerous studies have shown that research subjects may be less willing to share their biospecimens with for-profit entities than with researchers in academia or government (Garrison, 2015). For this reason, a new additional element of consent was added to the Common Rule to address commercial use of biospecimens. As mentioned earlier, this element requires, as appropriate, a statement that the subject's biospecimens may be used for commercial profit and an indication of whether the subject will or will not share in this commercial profit.

It may be reasonable and appropriate to compensate people for the time and effort involved in providing biospecimens, such as blood or urine, for a research study. However, it may be very difficult to <u>pay</u> subjects, and it can be argued that it may even be inappropriate to pay subjects for discoveries made from their biospecimens for several reasons. Biospecimens are only one of many factors that make research discoveries possible. Research often requires significant resources, intellectual input, and effort by many researchers, institutions, and companies, often over many years and involving biospecimens from hundreds or thousands of individuals to support the development of a profitable product. Individual biospecimens are of little commercial value without the scientific effort that goes into using them for organized research.

It is extraordinarily rare for a single individual's biospecimens to result in a profitable product or discovery. Furthermore, no single biospecimen is usually more useful or valuable than another biospecimen. Thus, it would be difficult to assign a value to any one individual's contributions, and it would be ethically problematic to pay only some of the people who have provided biospecimens for discoveries made possible from their biospecimens.

Ownership/Custodianship

Although at the time of writing (2019), there is no U.S. federal law addressing the ownership of human biospecimens, there are several examples in the case law that address this issue. These include Moore v. Regents of the University of California (1990), the Canavan case (Greenberg v. Miami Children's Hospital Research Institute, 2003), and Washington University v. Catalona (2006, 2007). These cases involved lawsuits related to claims of private ownership of human biospecimens used in research. In each of these cases, the courts found that research subjects did not have any ownership rights to their biospecimens; however, they noted the importance of obtaining informed consent for their use.

The concept of custodianship has been proposed as a framework to govern the ethical management of biospecimens in biobanks. In the custodianship model, biobank managers adopt the role as "caretakers" rather than owners of the biospecimens (NCI, 2016). This responsibility extends from collection through research use and includes ensuring long-term physical quality of the biospecimens, the integrity of associated data, the privacy of human subjects, the confidentiality of their data, and appropriate use of the biospecimens and data.

Custodianship plans are an essential part of the responsibility of biobanks. These plans should address the handling and disposition of biospecimens and associated data at the end of the study period, when there is a loss of management or termination of funding, when the research objectives have been accomplished, when the biospecimens have been depleted, or when participation in the research has been discontinued by human research subjects (NCI, 2016). It is particularly important for such plans to address what will happen to the biospecimen collection when the researcher or biobank manager leaves the institution and to affirm that this plan is agreed upon by appropriate institutional officials.

Biospecimen Underutilization

Biospecimen underutilization has been identified as an important ethical issue (Cadigan et al., 2014). Research subjects who provide their biospecimens for research expect their biospecimens to be well utilized and contribute to the advancement of science and medicine. However, a number of recent surveys of biobankers in the United States and globally indicate that they have major concerns about underutilization of biospecimens in their collections (Cadigan et al., 2013, Henderson et al., 2013; iSpecimen, 2018). Underutilization may be affected by a number of factors, including the design of the biobank and choice of biobanking model; identification of a scientific need; strategic planning, marketing, informed consent considerations; and access policies and procedures (Bledsoe & Sexton, 2019). These issues should be given serious consideration in the design, planning, and continued operations to ensure optimal biospecimen utilization. Optimal biospecimen utilization is critical to maintain the trust of research subjects and for sustainability of biobanking operations. IRBs should keep these ethical issues in mind when reviewing bio-banking protocols as they may affect decisions about the risks versus benefits of the research activity.

Return of Research Results

⊘ 12-1 The return of research results from biobanks received inadequate attention until around 2012, when a special issue of *Genetics in Medicine* published a series of articles devoted specifically to this topic (Wolf et al., 2012). Context is critical with regard to return of individual research results, particularly for biobanking because of the wide variation in types of biobanks and the relationships of research subjects with the biobank and the researchers (Beskow, 2016). Context affects not only the ethical obligations but also considerations related to practical implementation, feasibility, and costs of returning research results (Bledsoe et al., 2012a; Bledsoe et al., 2012b). For example, in some cases a researcher may have direct interaction and an ongoing relationship with subjects to obtain the biospecimens and use them for their own research. In this case, it might be relatively straightforward to return individual research results. However, in a biobanking context, the biobank may not have any direct interaction or ongoing relationship with the subjects from whom the biospecimens are obtained and may distribute thousands of biospecimens to many secondary researchers that may generate a wide range of different kinds of findings, some of which may be wrong, making return of findings impracticable. IRBs should give careful consideration to these issues in evaluating plans for return of individual research results from biobanks.

In summary, the wide variation in types of biobanks, biobank and researcher relationships to subjects, and types of studies being performed makes it difficult for a "one size fits all" policy to be developed for the return of individual research results from biobanks. However, whatever policies are decided upon should be ethically appropriate and defensible and based on risks versus benefits (individuals and societal).

Identifiability of Biospecimens

Because genomic data are unique to an individual, concerns have been expressed about the identifiability of biospecimens and associated data (Weil et al., 2013). For example, some studies have demonstrated the ability to identify ⊘ 10-13 the subjects of anonymous DNA donors in genomic research studies by matching their DNA to publicly available databases containing the donor identities (Gymrek et al., 2013). These developments have raised questions about the inherent identifiability of biospecimens and have led to a number of key policy changes, including changes to the Common Rule and other regulations. The identifiability of biospecimens, even when all direct identifiers have been removed, is contextual. At the time this chapter was written (2019) it is not possible to readily ascertain the identity of an individual from their biospecimen alone, without access to other identifying or potentially identifying information. This may change over time, however, with further advancements in science and technology and the proliferation of genetic and genomic databases and other large data sets containing extensive clinical and other information.

Living Biobanks

An expanded approach to biobanking is the development of a "living biobank" that will distribute viable biospecimens to researchers. This approach might include cell lines, organoids, patient-derived xenografts, and other viable cellular preparations. These preparations are immortal and renewable. Hence, such biospecimens would have different ethical consequences than other biospecimens that are nonrenewable, especially if they were widely distributed to many researchers, including those at international laboratories. Moreover, it would be difficult to withdraw and discontinue use of such biospecimens.

Conclusion

As discussed in this chapter, human biospecimens are critical for scientific discovery, medical advancements, and diagnostic and therapeutic innovations. While the risks to subjects from use of their biospecimens are generally considered to be relatively low, a number of legal, ethical, regulatory, and social issues must be considered. These include federal, state, and local regulatory requirements and policies; cultural considerations; privacy and confidentiality; identifiability; appropriate consent approaches; secondary use of biospecimen; and return of research results. Carefully addressing these issues is essential for maintaining the trust of individuals, the public-at-large, and other stakeholders, thereby ensuring participation in research and continued research progress.

Resources

Council for International Organizations of Medical Sciences. (2016). *International ethical guidelines for health-related research involving humans.* cioms.ch/shop/product/international -ethical-guidelines-for-health-related-research-involving-humans/

Council of Europe. (2016). *Recommendations on research on biological materials of human origin.* search.coe.int/cm/Pages/result_details.aspx?ObjectId=090000168064e8ff

International Society for Biological and Environmental Repositories. (2018). *ISBER best practices: Recommendations for repositories* (4th ed.). www.isber.org/page/BPDownload4ed

National Cancer Institute. (2016). *NCI best practices for biospecimen resources.* biospecimens.cancer .gov/bestpractices/2016-NCIBestPractices.pdf

National Institutes of Health. (2019). *Office of intramural research: Guidelines for human biospecimen storage, tracking, sharing, and disposal within the NIH intramural research program.* oir .nih.gov/sites/default/files/uploads/sourcebook/documents/ethical_conduct/guidelines -biospecimen.pdf

Organisation for Economic Co-operation and Development. (2009). *Guidelines for human biobanks and genetic research databases (HBGRDs).* www.oecd.org/sti/emerging-tech/guidelines-for -human-biobanks-and-genetic-research-databases.htm

World Medical Association. (2016). *WMA declaration of Taipei on ethical considerations regarding health databases and biobanks.* www.wma.net/policies-post/wma-declaration-of-taipei-on-ethical -considerations-regarding-health-databases-and-biobanks/

References

Assche, K. V., Gutwirth, S., & Sterckx, S. (2013). Protecting dignitary interests of biobank research participants: Lessons from Havasupai Tribe v Arizona Board of Regents. *Law, Innovation and Technology, 5*(1), 54–84.

Beskow, L. M. (2016). Lessons from HeLa cells: The ethics and policy of biospecimens. *Annual Review of Genomics and Human Genetics, 17,* 395–417.

Bledsoe, M. J. (2017). Ethical legal and social issues of biobanking: Past, present, and future. *Biopreservation and Biobanking, 15*(2), 142–147.

Bledsoe, M. J., Clayton, E. W., Mcguire, A. L., Grizzle, W. E., O'Rourke, P. P., & Zeps, N. (2012a). Return of research results from genomic biobanks: Cost matters. *Genetics in Medicine, 15*(2), 103–105.

Bledsoe, M. J., Grizzle, W. E., Clark, B. J., & Zeps, N. (2012b). Practical implementation issues and challenges for biobanks in the return of individual research results. *Genetics in Medicine, 14*(4), 478–483.

Bledsoe, M. J., & Sexton, K. C. (2019). Ensuring effective utilization of biospecimens: Design, marketing, and other important approaches. *Biopreservation and Biobanking, 17*(3), 248–257.

Cadigan, R. J., Lassiter, D., Haldeman, K., Conlon, I., Reavely, E., & Henderson, G. E. (2013). Neglected ethical issues in biobank management: Results from a U.S. study. *Life Sciences, Society and Policy, 9*(1), 1.

Cadigan, R. J., Juengst, E., Davis, A., & Henderson, G. (2014). Underutilization of specimens in biobanks: An ethical as well as a practical concern? *Genetics in Medicine, 16*(10), 738–740.

Department of Health and Human Services (DHHS). (2008). *Office for Human Research Protections. Coded private information or specimens use in research, 2008.* www.hhs.gov/ohrp/regulations -and-policy/guidance/research-involving-coded-private-information/index.html

Department of Health and Human Services (DHHS). (2010). *Office for Human Research Protections. Withdrawal of subjects from research guidance.* www.hhs.gov/ohrp/regulations-and-policy /guidance/guidance-on-withdrawal-of-subject/index.html

Department of Health and Human Services (DHHS). (2013). *Office for Civil Rights. Summary of the Health Insurance Portability and Accountability Act.* www.hhs.gov/hipaa/for-professionals /privacy/laws-regulations/index.html

Department of Health and Human Services (DHHS). (2017). *Secretary's Advisory Committee on Human Research Protections. Attachment C - Recommendations for broad consent guidance.* www.hhs .gov/ohrp/sachrp-committee/recommendations/attachment-c-august-2-2017/index.html

Department of Health and Human Services (DHHS). (2018a). *Secretary's Advisory Committee on Human Research Protections. Attachment C - Updated FAQs on informed consent for use of biospecimens and data.* www.hhs.gov/ohrp/sachrp-committee/recommendations/attachment -c-faqs-recommendations-and-glossary-informed-consent-and-research-use-of-biospecimens -and-associated-data/index.html

Department of Health and Human Services (DHHS). (2018b). *Secretary's Advisory Committee on Human Research Protections. Attachment A - FAQs relating to recommendations on broad consent.* www.hhs.gov/ohrp/sachrp-committee/recommendations/attachment-a-faqs-relating-to -recommendations-on-broad-consent/index.html

Dougan, M., Dranoff, G., & Dougan, S. K. (2019). Cancer immunotherapy: Beyond checkpoint blockade. *Annual Review of Cancer Biology, 3*, 55–75.

European Commission. (n.d.). *Data protection in the EU.* ec.europa.eu/info/law/law-topic /data-protection/data-protection-eu_en

Food and Drug Administration (FDA). (2006). *Guidance on informed consent for in vitro diagnostic device studies using leftover human specimens that are not individually identifiable.* www.fda.gov /media/122648/download

Food and Drug Administration (FDA). (2008). *Data retention when subjects withdraw from FDA-regulated clinical trials. guidance for sponsors, clinical investigators, and IRBs.* www.fda .gov/regulatory-information/search-fda-guidance-documents/data-retention-when-subjects -withdraw-fda-regulated-clinical-trials

Food and Drug Administration (FDA). (2017). *IRB waiver or alteration of informed consent for clinical investigations involving no more than minimal risk to human subjects.* www.fda.gov /media/106587/download

Gaffney, E., Riegman, P., Grizzle, W., & Watson, P. (2018). Factors that drive the increasing use of FFPE tissue in basic and translational cancer research. *Biotechnic & Histochemistry, 93*(5), 373–386.

Garrison, N. A., Sathe, N. A., Antommaria, A. H. M., Holm, I. A., Sanderson, S. C., Smith, M. E., McPheeters, M. L., & Clayton, E. W. (2015). A systematic literature review of individuals' perspectives on broad consent and data sharing in the United States. *Genetics in Medicine, 18*(7), 663–671.

Greenberg v. Miami Children's Hospital Research Institute. (2003). 264 F.Supp. 2d 1064 (S.D. Fla. 2003).

Grizzle, W. E., Bell, W. C., & Sexton, K. C. (2010). Issues in collecting, processing and storing human tissues and associated information to support biomedical research. *Cancer Biomarkers, 9*(1–6), 531–549.

Grizzle, W. E., Bledsoe, M. J., Diffalha, S. A., Otali, D., & Sexton, K. C. (2019). The utilization of biospecimens: Impact of the choice of biobanking model. *Biopreservation and Biobanking, 17*(3), 230–242.

Grody, W. W., & Howell, R. R. (2010). The fate of newborn screening blood spots. *Pediatric Research, 67*(3), 237–237.

Gymrek, M., McGuire, A. L., Golan, D., Halperin, E., & Erlich, Y. (2013) Identifying personal genomes by surname inference. *Science, 339*, 321–324.

Hall, E. D., & Traystman, R. J. (2009). Role of animal studies in the design of clinical trials. *Frontiers of Neurology and Neuroscience, 25*, 10–33.

Henderson, G. E., Cadigan, R. J., Edwards, T. P., Conlon, I., Nelson, A. G., Evans, J. P., & Weiner, B. J. (2013). Characterizing biobank organizations in the U.S.: Results from a national survey. *Genome Medicine, 5*(1), 3.

Hewitt, R., & Watson, P. (2013). Defining biobank. *Biopreservation and Biobanking, 11*(5), 309–315.

International Society for Biological and Environmental Repositories. (2018). *ISBER best practices: Recommendations for repositories* (4th ed.). www.isber.org/page/BPDownload4ed

iSpecimen, Inc. (2018). *A worldwide study of the factors affecting sustainable biobanking operations and technology-based approaches to increase utilization rates: An independent survey.* pages.ispecimen.com/Worldwide-Biobanking-Survey-Download.html

Kaye, J., Curren, L., Anderson, N., Edwards, K., Fullerton, S. M., Kanellopoulou, N., Lund, D., MacArthur, D. G., Mascalzoni, D., Shepherd, J., Taylor, P. L., Terry, S. F., & Winter, S. F. (2012). From patients to partners: Participant-centric initiatives in biomedical research. *Nature Reviews Genetics, 13*(5), 371–376.

Kowal, E. E. (2015). Genetics and indigenous communities: Ethical issues. In J. D. Wright (Ed.), *International encyclopedia of the social & behavioral sciences* (2nd ed., pp. 962–968). Elsevier.

Lee, S. S. J., Cho, M. K., Kraft, S. A., Varsava, N., Gillespie, K., Ormond, K. E., Wilfond, B. S., & Magnus, D. (2019). "I don't want to be Henrietta Lacks": Diverse patient perspectives on donating biospecimens for precision medicine research. *Genetics in Medicine, 21*(1), 107–113.

McCarty, C. A., Chapman-Stone, D., Derfus, T., Giampietro, P. F., & Fost, N. (2008). Community consultation and communication for a population-based DNA biobank: The Marshfield clinic personalized medicine research project. *American Journal of Medical Genetics, 146A*(23), 3026–3033.

Mello, M. M., & Wolf, L. E. (2010). The Havasupai Indian tribe case — lessons for research involving stored biologic samples. *New England Journal of Medicine, 363*(3), 204–207.

Moore v. Regents of the University of California. (1990). 51 Cal.3d 120. 271 Cal. Rptr. 146. 793 P.2d 479.

National Cancer Institute (NCI). (n.d.). *NCI dictionary of cancer terms.* www.cancer.gov /publications/dictionaries/cancer-terms/def/biospecimen

National Cancer Institute (NCI). (2016). *NCI best practices for biospecimen resources.* biospecimens.cancer.gov/bestpractices/2016-NCIBestPractices.pdf

National Institutes of Health (NIH). (2014). *Final NIH genomic data sharing policy. 79 FR 51345.* www.federalregister.gov/documents/2014/08/28/2014-20385/final-nih-genomic -data-sharing-policy

National Institutes of Health (NIH). (2019a). *Office of Intramural Research. Guidelines for human biospecimen storage, tracking, sharing, and disposal within the NIH intramural research program.* oir.nih.gov/sites/default/files/uploads/sourcebook/documents/ethical_conduct/guidelines -biospecimen.pdf

National Institutes of Health (NIH). (2019b). *Certificates of Confidentiality (CoC) - Human subjects.* grants.nih.gov/policy/humansubjects/coc.htm

Skloot, R. (2010). *The immortal life of Henrietta Lacks.* Crown Publishing, Random House.

Skloot, R. (2013, March 23). The immortal life of Henrietta Lacks, the sequel. *The New York Times.* www.nytimes.com/2013/03/24/opinion/sunday/the-immortal-life-of-henrietta-lacks-the -sequel.html

Vaught, J., & Lockhart, N. C. (2012). The evolution of biobanking best practices. *Clinica Chimica Acta, 413*(19–20), 1569–1575.

Waks, A. G., & Winer, E. P. (2019). Breast cancer treatment: A review. *JAMA, 321*, 288–300.

Washington University v. Catalona. (2006). 437 F.Supp. 2d 985, 1002 (E.D. Mo. 2006).

Washington University v. Catalona. (2007). 490 F.3d 667 (8th Cir. (Mo.) 2007).

Weil, C. J., Mechanic, L. E., Green, T., Kinsinger, C., Lockhart, N. C., Nelson, S. A., Rodriguez, L. L., & Buccini, L. D. (2013). NCI think tank concerning the identifiability of biospecimens and "omic" data. *Genetics in Medicine, 15*(12), 997–1003.

Wolf, S. M., Crock, B. N., Van Ness, B., Lawrenz, F., Kahn, J. P., Beskow, L. M., Cho, M. K., Christman, M. F., Green, R. C., Hall, R., Illes, J., Keane, M., Knoppers, B. M., Koenig, B. A., Kohane, I. S., Leroy, B., Maschke, K. J., McGeveran, W., Ossorio, P., Parker, L. S., . . . , Wolf, W. A. (2012). Managing incidental findings and research results in genomic research involving biobanks and archived data sets. *Genetics in Medicine, 14*(4), 361–384.

The Placebo-Controlled Clinical Trial

Melissa A. Epstein

Charles B. Hall

Stefanie E. Juell

Gabriella Weston

Abstract

Thr placebo-controlled clinical trial is considered the gold standard for studies that seek to determine the effectiveness of health-related interventions. Careful review by the IRB is required to ensure that the trial will produce scientifically valid results, thus not causing undue harm to subjects. Justification, design, and implementation plan are important aspects to consider in the review of placebo-controlled trials. The use of a placebo must be justified through evidence of equipoise between proposed study arms. Randomization of subjects into study arms reduces the chance that findings are due to confounding variables and eliminates selection bias. To ensure that subjects contribute to generating meaningful results toward scientific progress, the trial should also have adequate sample size. Regulatory criteria required for approval protects human subjects by ensuring that risks and benefits are balanced, potential subjects will be adequately informed of the risks and benefits of participation, and a safety monitoring plan is in place.

Introduction

Placebo-controlled clinical trials present challenges from both a regulatory and ethical standpoint. This chapter will define what is a clinical trial and what is a placebo control. This is followed by a discussion of some important study design issues, randomization, size of study, and statistical power. Finally, the important ethical issue of equipoise is addressed, and a regulatory framework for the review of placebo-controlled clinical trials is presented.

Clinical Trial

The U.S. National Institutes of Health (NIH) defines a clinical trial as follows:

> A research study in which one or more human subjects are prospectively assigned to one or more interventions (which may include placebo or other control) to evaluate the effects of those interventions on health-related biomedical or behavioral outcomes. (NIH, 2017a)

NIH further defines the following terms:

> The term "prospectively assigned" refers to a pre-defined process (e.g., randomization) specified in an approved protocol that stipulates the assignment of research subjects (individually or in clusters) to one or more arms (e.g., intervention, placebo, or other control) of a clinical trial.
>
> An "intervention" is defined as a manipulation of the subject or subject's environment for the purpose of modifying one or more health-related biomedical or behavioral processes and/or endpoints. Examples include: drugs/small molecules/compounds; biologics; devices; procedures (e.g., surgical techniques); delivery systems (e.g., telemedicine, face-to-face interviews); strategies to change health-related behavior (e.g., diet, cognitive therapy, exercise, development of new habits); treatment strategies; prevention strategies; and diagnostic strategies.
>
> A "health-related biomedical or behavioral outcome" is defined as the pre-specified goal(s) or condition(s) that reflect the effect of one or more interventions on human subjects' biomedical or behavioral status or quality of life. Examples include: positive or negative changes to physiological or biological parameters (e.g., improvement of lung capacity, gene expression); positive or negative changes to psychological or neurodevelopmental parameters (e.g., mood management intervention for smokers; reading comprehension and/or information retention); positive or negative changes to disease processes; positive or negative changes to health-related behaviors; and, positive or negative changes to quality of life. (NIH, 2017a)

Note that there is no requirement for there to be a placebo or any comparison group, and there is no requirement for randomization. Nonmedical behavioral outcomes are also included within the scope of the definition.

NIH offers four simple questions to determine whether a research study falls under its definition of a clinical trial (NIH, 2017b):

1. Does the study involve human participants?
2. Are the participants prospectively assigned to an intervention?
3. Is the study designed to evaluate the effect of the intervention on the participants?
4. Is the effect being evaluated a health-related biomedical or behavioral outcome?

If the answer to *all* four questions is yes, the research study is a clinical trial for NIH purposes. The International Committee of Medical Journal Editors (ICMJE) and World Health Organization (WHO) have similar definitions (ICMJE, 2020; WHO, 2020). The U.S. Food and Drug Administration (FDA) has somewhat less broad definitions (ClinicalTrials.gov, 2019). However, any research that fits the broader NIH definition could safely be considered a clinical trial.

Placebo

The term *placebo* is from a Latin root meaning, roughly, "I will please." Remedies thought to have no curative effect were often used in premodern medicine, and by the end of the 18th century the term "placebo" was used to describe such treatments that, whether biologically active or inert, were given as a way to reduce patient distress (Kerr et al., 2008).

By the mid 20th century, the term referred to an inert substance given as a comparison to an active drug, such as in the study of streptomycin for tuberculosis mentioned later. While these inert substances would have no biological effect on the disease being studied, at times positive effects of placebos do occur, particularly for pain and nausea or for outcomes that are measured only subjectively (Hrobjartsson & Gotzsche, 2010). Where such potential for placebo effects exist, care must be taken in the study design to address those effects.

Randomization

Almost all placebo-controlled clinical trials today randomly assign patients to receive active intervention or the placebo. There is a long history of studying health outcomes in groups of individuals receiving different exposures. The first modern example, what we would call today a nonrandomized clinical trial, was conducted by the famous Scottish physician James Lind to prove that scurvy could be prevented by diet (Lind, 1753). Randomization was pioneered in agricultural experiments by Sir Ronald Fisher (Fisher, 1926), and the assignment of human study subjects to different treatments through a formal random allocation was first used by Sir Austin Bradford Hill in the famous study of streptomycin for treatment of tuberculosis (Daniels & Hill, 1952). Within a few years, hundreds of thousands of children would be randomized to treatment or placebo in the Salk polio vaccine trial (Meldrum, 1998), and the randomized clinical trial became the gold standard for all clinical medical research (Armitage, 1982).

For large studies, randomization makes treatment groups likely to be comparable not only for measured covariates (measures associated with treatment success) but also for unmeasured covariates and factors unknown to the researcher. This is a strong argument for the use of randomization, because it reduces the likelihood that findings from the study are due to confounding. The simplest randomization would be a 1:1 randomization with two arms, where every study subject has an equal probability of being assigned to one arm or the other. A straightforward extension is to design a study with multiple interventions or multiple doses being compared to placebo, with equal numbers in each arm. Because of considerations involving cost or logistics, it could be appropriate for the sizes of the arms to not be equal, and appropriate adjustments would be made to the randomization probabilities.

In small studies with simple randomization, it is likely that there will be differences among intervention groups purely due to chance, and therefore more sophisticated randomization methods are now commonly used. Typically, the potential study population is stratified by factors known or suspected to be associated with the disease outcome, and separate randomizations are done within those strata. In addition, in multicenter studies where individual sites will recruit from different populations, it would be appropriate to stratify recruitment within each site. Obviously, there is a limit to the number of factors for which there can be stratification, and too many stratifications can make recruitment more difficult.

Another important reason to randomize study subjects is to avoid the selection bias that comes from providers nonrandomly assigning certain patients to the intervention that the provider believes would be most likely to benefit that particular patient. Whether randomization is implemented using prepared assignment cards in opaque sealed envelopes, hard copy lists of sequential assignments, or computer generated assignments, it is essential that providers who have contact with study subjects not know and be unable to determine to which arm the next subject will be assigned. This is known as allocation concealment. The staff member of the institution who is responsible for determining the assignment should have no contact with potential study subjects.

Similarly, it is important to mask study subjects and, where possible, the study researchers, to the assignment after randomization. For pharmaceuticals, the appearance of the study drug and the placebo should not reveal the identity of the arm.

In recent years a number of innovative "adaptive" study designs have been implemented that can potentially increase the power of the study and result in fewer subjects receiving less effective or less safe interventions as the study progresses. In these designs, the probability of assignment to an intervention arm is adjusted during the course of the study to reflect early results from the study. This can be done continuously, or at fixed landmarks during the progression of the study. It is even more critical that the integrity of the randomization process be maintained in these studies. However, these designs also present far more logistical and statistical challenges than do parallel arm designs (Chow, 2014).

Size of Study and Statistical Power

In order to provide benefit in terms of increased scientific knowledge, a study must be large enough to make it at least somewhat unlikely that the results observed will be due to chance. The probability that a study will correctly show that an intervention is better (or worse) than a placebo is called statistical power and increases with sample size. In order to properly estimate statistical power, one must make some assumptions regarding the likely occurrence of the endpoint(s) of interest in each arm. For example, based on preliminary data, one might know that the incidence of a primary outcome is 40% and that there is evidence that the intervention might reduce this to 30%. For this example, 355 study subjects in each of the two arms results in an 80% power that the study will find a statistically significant difference between intervention groups, and 475 study subjects result in approximately 90% power. Larger sample sizes also result in narrower confidence intervals and thus more precise estimates of the effects of the intervention. A pilot study will need to be sufficiently large so that its preliminary findings will be useful to the design of a future confirmatory study.

Equipoise

In the context of human subjects research, equipoise means that there is an equal chance that any arm of a randomized clinical trial will be just as effective as any of the other arms. Thus, for a well-designed and ethically justified trial, there must exist genuine uncertainty regarding which treatment modality is most effective and least harmful to study subjects. Despite some philosophical disagreement regarding various types of equipoise and how equipoise is actually maintained throughout the course of a clinical trial, the research community and IRBs have generally accepted the concept of *clinical equipoise* as the standard in the conduct of the placebo-controlled randomized clinical trial (Gifford, 2007). Clinical equipoise means that *clinicians*, who are experts in the particular disease or condition being treated, disagree as to the appropriate course of treatment.

In order to determine that clinical equipoise exists for a particular protocol, IRBs review the study justification, including relevant literature, and may consult with experts as needed (Weijer & Miller, 2004). It is also important for the IRB to carefully consider not only the risks and benefits of the overall trial but also the separate risks and benefits of each arm. Placebo comparison groups are not appropriate for all studies. If there is clear evidence that one arm is preferable to another, the trial may be ethically problematic and unapprovable by an IRB. Much literature exists as to the appropriateness of placebos in different types of situations (e.g., Freedman, 1990).

There is widespread agreement that placebo controls are appropriate when there is no standard therapy for a condition, when the standard therapy is known not to be better than placebo, or (rarely) standard therapy *is* a placebo. Cases where there is doubt regarding net therapeutic advantage of standard therapy over placebo may also justify the need to conduct a placebo-controlled trial. For example, standard therapy might have some efficacy advantage over placebo but at the cost of higher adverse event rates, or studies comparing standard therapy to placebo might be limited and/or inconclusive. Another example of this would be a study involving an investigational drug that utilizes a novel mechanism. In such a trial, the net therapeutic advantage of the placebo arm may actually be greater than the net therapeutic advantage of the experimental arm because the risks of the novel mechanism may be unknown or may outweigh the benefits.

A more difficult situation would be one in which effective standard treatment may exist but is unavailable to the population that is the intervention target for the proposed research. These cases would warrant an ethical discussion regarding the appropriateness of conducting that particular trial (with or without placebo) involving that population.

Regulatory Framework

In the IRB's review of a placebo-controlled clinical trial, consideration of three Common Rule <u>criteria</u> may be particularly relevant: (1) Risks to subjects are minimized [45 CFR 46.111(a)(1)]; (2) Risks to subjects are reasonable in relation to anticipated benefits, if any, to subjects, and the importance of the knowledge that may reasonably be expected to result [45 CFR 46.111(a)(2)]; and (6) When appropriate, the research plan makes adequate provision for monitoring the data collected to ensure the safety of subjects [45 CFR 46.111(a)(6)].

🔗 5-4

Criteria (1) and (2) are attained by sound study design. For criterion (2), important knowledge may only be obtained in a trial that is feasible and conducted and analyzed in a scientifically valid manner (Zarin et al., 2019).

Criterion (6) is the basis for the requirement for a data and safety monitoring plan. Depending on the complexity of the trial, the risks of the intervention, and the number of sites, data and safety monitoring may be overseen by the local principal investigator (PI), a local committee, or an external board. The data and safety monitoring plan may also require a plan for an interim analysis; this can help to reduce the number of patients who are assigned to inferior intervention.

Both the Common Rule and FDA regulations require a statement of risks and potential benefits in the process of consent and in the consent documents [**45 CFR 46.116(b)(2)** and **(3)**; **21 CFR 50.25(2)** and **(3)**].

✎ 6-3

The Common Rule also requires "a concise and focused presentation of the key information" [45 CFR 46.116(a)(5)(i)]. This section is an opportunity to require researchers to further digest for subjects the pros and cons of participating in a placebo-controlled clinical trial. In the Albert Einstein College of Medicine Key Information template,[1] we require researchers to answer the following questions:

- What is the study about, and how long will it last?
- What are the key reasons you might choose to volunteer for this study?
- What are they key reasons you might choose not to volunteer for this study?

In the context of a theoretical placebo-controlled clinical trial of a drug to treat arthritis, we might encourage researchers as follows. Note that the "key reasons to volunteer" and the "key reasons not to volunteer" roughly correspond to the benefits and risks sections of the consent document.

EXAMPLE: KEY INFORMATION PRESENTATION

What Is the Study About, and How Long Will It Last?

The purpose of this study is to compare the effects, good and/or bad, of StudyDrug with a placebo (an inactive pill). The Food and Drug Administration (FDA) has approved StudyDrug to treat some conditions, but not for the treatment of arthritis.

If you are eligible for the study, we will use a computer program to place you in one of the two groups. The group the computer picks is by chance, like a flip of a coin. You will have an equal chance of getting in either group. The test group will take StudyDrug. The placebo group will take an inactive pill. Neither you nor the study staff will know which pill you get. They both look the same. Participants in both groups will have monthly research study visits for one year. See Appendix A for the study visit schedule.

What Are Key Reasons You Might Choose to Volunteer for This Study?

Some doctors have noticed an improvement in arthritis on patients taking StudyDrug. While on the study, we will monitor your arthritis. If your arthritis worsens, the study doctor may take you off the study so that your personal doctor may treat you.

What Are Key Reasons You Might ChooseNot to Volunteer for This Study?

You should not participate in this study if you do not want to leave the choice of medicine you take for arthritis up to chance. The study computer picks which medicine and dose you receive instead of you and your doctor choosing. Half the people who participate in this study will not receive StudyDrug.

You may have side effects while on the study. The most serious effect that has happened in one percent of people who have taken StudyDrug is shortness of breath. The researchers do not know all of the side effects that could happen. For a complete description of risks, refer to the Consent Document below.

---

1 We would like to thank the Office of Research Integrity at the University of Kentucky for generously sharing their Key Information templates and samples with us. This example is based on a sample from the University of Kentucky.

Checklist

Here is a brief checklist for the evaluation of a placebo-controlled clinical trial.

- Ethics
  - Does this study have equipoise?
- Feasibility
  - Can the placebo be managed by the local PI and/or the institution (e.g., the pharmacy)?
  - Can the randomization be managed?
  - Can the blinding be managed?
- Sound design
  - Does this study have adequate power?
  - Do you have enough potential subjects?
- Consent
  - Does the consent document adequately address randomization and placebo?

Conclusion

Placebo-controlled clinical trials are an important and necessary tool in our evaluation of novel treatments. They are the gold standard for research into the efficacy of interventions. The use of a placebo, however, requires that IRBs pay particular attention to the feasibility and design of the study and whether or not the study meets the requirements for equipoise. Often, an IRB will need outside expert guidance in assessing these sometimes difficult issues. With care taken in all these issues, the IRB will succeed in protecting the interests of subjects while supporting scientific progress.

References

Armitage, P. (1982). The role of randomization in clinical trials. *Statistics in Medicine, 1*(4), 345–352.

Chow, S. C. (2014). Adaptive clinical trial design. *Annual Review of Medicine, 65,* 405–415.

ClinicalTrials.gov. (2019). *FDAAA 801 and the final rule.* https://clinicaltrials.gov/ct2/manage-recs/fdaaa

Daniels, M., & Hill, A. B. (1952). Chemotherapy of pulmonary tuberculosis in young adults: An analysis of the combined results of three Medical Research Council trials. *BMJ, 1*(4769), 1162–1168.

Fisher, R. A. (1926). The arrangement of field experiments. *Journal of the Ministry of Agriculture of Great Britain, 33,* 503–513.

Freedman, B. (1990). Placebo-controlled trials and the logic of clinical purpose. *IRB, 12*(6), 1–6.

Gifford, F. (2007). Taking equipoise seriously: The failure of clinical or community equipoise to resolve the ethical dilemmas in randomized clinical trials. *Philosophy and Medicine, 90,* 215–233.

Hrobjartsson, A., & Gotzsche, P. C. (2010). Placebo interventions for all clinical conditions. *Cochrane Database of Systematic Reviews, 2010*(1), CD003974.

International Committee of Medical Journal Editors. (2020). *Clinical trials.* www.icmje.org/recommendations/browse/publishing-and-editorial-issues/clinical-trial-registration.html

Kerr, C. E., Milne, I., & Kaptchuk, T. J. (2008). William Cullen and a missing mind-body link in the early history of placebos. *Journal of the Royal Society of Medicine, 101*(2), 89–92.

Lind, J. (1753). *A treatise of the scurvy in three parts. containing an inquiry into the nature, causes, and cure, of that disease; together with a critical and chronological view of what has been published on the subject.* A. Kincaid and A. Donaldson.

Meldrum, M. (1998). "A calculated risk": The Salk polio vaccine field trials of 1954. *BMJ, 317*(7167), 1233–1236.

National Institutes of Health (NIH). (2017a). *NIH's definition of a clinical trial.* https://grants.nih .gov/policy/clinical-trials/definition.htm

National Institutes of Health (NIH). (2017b). *Decision tree for NIH clinical trial definition.* https:// grants.nih.gov/policy/clinical-trials/CT-decision-tree.pdf

Weijer, C., & Miller, P. (2004). When are research risks reasonable in relationship to anticipated benefits? *Nature Medicine, 10*(6), 570–573.

World Health Organization (WHO). (2020). *Clinical trials.* www.who.int/health-topics/clinical-trials/

Zarin, D. A., Goodman, S. N., & Kimmelman, J. (2019). Harms from uninformative clinical trials. *JAMA, 322*(9), 813–814.

Anticipating and Mitigating Risk in Research on Mental Illness

David H. Strauss

Abstract

This chapter offers both practical and conceptual approaches to IRB review of research involving individuals with mental illness. Mental illnesses comprise a heterogeneous group of conditions affecting individuals across the life span and varying widely in course of illness and associated emotional, behavioral, and cognitive features. As a group, mental illnesses are highly prevalent; however, they remain incompletely understood, undertreated, and subject to considerable stigma. This chapter will emphasize research with adults with serious mental illness (SMI; National Institute of Mental Health, 2019), defined as individuals who experience substantial functional limitation or impairment. The application of the *Belmont* principles (National Commission, 1979) and federal regulation to research on SMI requires an appreciation of the manner in which these disorders affect decision making and confer increased susceptibility to risk. The thoughtful anticipation and mitigation of risk during IRB review is necessary to advance research that is ultimately aimed at improving treatment of mental illness.

Introduction

Mental Illness, Serious Mental Illness, and Comorbidity

Although a detailed description of mental illness is beyond the scope of this chapter (for further information, see National Alliance on Mental Illness [NAMI], n.d.; Roberts, 2019), specific clinical features will be referenced when relevant to IRB considerations. Mental illness is common, with approximately half of all Americans diagnosed with a mental illness during their lifetime (Centers for Disease Control and Prevention [CDC], 2018a). SMI, defined as a mental, behavioral, or emotional disorder that substantially interferes with or limits one or more major life activities, affects 4.5% of adults (Substance Abuse and Mental Health Services Administration [SAMHSA], 2018). SMI includes schizophrenia, bipolar disorder, major depressive disorder, and obsessive–compulsive disorder.

Mental illness represents a major risk factor for suicide (CDC, 2018b), which is the 10th leading cause of death in the United States and the second leading cause of death for those between ages 10 and 34 (CDC, 2020). Approximately 48,000 Americans died by suicide in 2018, nearly 1 million die annually by suicide worldwide (World Health Organization, 2018), and the rates are increasing. The inclusion in research of individuals at risk for suicide is essential to efforts to predict and prevent suicide. IRB strategies to effectively balance subject protections while advancing suicide research are addressed next.

Comorbidity in mental illness is common, and the careful assessment of co-occurring psychiatric, substance use, and medical disorders is important when evaluating study methods and inclusion and exclusion criteria and in determining how associated disorders may confound outcome measures or contribute to risk. For example, the prevalence of substance dependence or abuse in the prior year for individuals with SMI was 36.8% in the 18- to 25-year-old group, 21.1% among those aged 26 to 49, and 13.1% in individuals aged 50 or older (SAMHSA, 2012).

Similarly, medical comorbidity frequently occurs. For example, smoking and obesity are highly prevalent among people with schizophrenia, with estimates of nicotine dependence ranging from 58% to 90%, and obesity, hyperlipidemia, hyperglycemia, and hypertension (metabolic syndrome) present in 40%. For individuals with SMI, life expectancy is estimated at 56 years, with 25 years of premature mortality resulting from cardiopulmonary disease or other chronic medical conditions (Olfson et al., 2015). Therefore, researchers and IRBs must be cognizant of the likelihood of comorbidity in these populations and carefully weigh the scientific and risk-related implications of including or excluding comorbid conditions in studies of SMI.

Historical Context: Vulnerability to Coercion and Undue Influence

1-2 The history of human experimentation is replete with examples of exploitation of those described in the National Research Act of 1974 as mentally infirm ("individuals who are mentally ill, mentally retarded, emotionally disturbed, psychotic, or senile, who have other impairments of a similar nature and who reside as patients in an institution"; quoted in Federal Register (1978, p. 11330; National Research Act, 1974). By and large, such research in the early and mid-20th century sought answers to scientific questions of little or no relevance to the health or well-being of those individuals; their inclusion in research can be explained only by their ease of availability, captivity, and incompetence (Rothman, 1992). Some were recruited as a matter of convenience rather than because of scientific relevance or the possibility that the subject might directly benefit. Others were included because the setting (e.g., the institutional context, such as prisons) deprived them of any meaningful notion of freedom or volun-
9-7 tariness in decision making. Still others who became subjects were unable to understand or process information relevant to a decision to take part in research. Specific examples can be found in descriptions of Noguchi's research efforts to develop a skin test for the diagnosis of syphilis (Lederer, 1985), Krugman's studies of hepatitis at the Willowbrook State School (Krugman, 1971), and the U.S. Public Health Service studies of sexually transmitted diseases in Guatemala (Presidential Commission for the Study of Bioethical Issues, 2011).

In response to the National Research Act, the National Commission issued a 1978 report and recommendations entitled "Research Involving Those Institutionalized as Mentally Infirm" (National Commission, 1978). Unlike the Commission's reports on the research with children, prisoners, and fetuses, this set of recommendations did not find its way into a subpart of the federal regulations governing human subjects research. Instead, the pre-2018 Common Rule included only broad reference to a category of subjects "likely to be vulnerable to coercion or undue influence" appearing in sections **45 CFR 46.107** on IRB membership, and **45 CFR 46.111** on IRB approval of research and, with regard to avoidance of coercion or undue influence, in **45 CFR 46.116**, General Requirements for Consent. "Mentally disabled persons" are included in the listing of such "vulnerable" subjects, but the term is not defined in regulation or regulatory guidance. The 2018 Common Rule replaces the term "mentally disabled" with "individuals with impaired decision-making" **[45 CFR 46.111(b)]**. As with its predecessor, the 2018 Rule requires "additional safeguards to be included in the study to protect the rights and welfare of these subjects" **[45 CFR 46.111(b)]**. However, neither regulation nor formal guidance defines <u>impaired decision making</u> or what is expected by way of "additional safeguards." An important question is whether this void in specific regulatory direction has left such subjects underprotected in research or has resulted in their unjustified exclusion from research (National Institutes of Health [NIH], 2009). In the absence of a regulatory subpart specifically addressing subject selection and risk/benefit considerations for this population, the field's focus has been solely on consent and on vulnerability in relation to coercion or undue influence.

9-7

Mental Illness and Impaired Decision Making

Many, if not most, patients with SMI demonstrate the capacity to make consent decisions (Carpenter et al., 2000). Some demonstrate impairment only at some points in time. An individual seen in the emergency department with psychotic disorganization may be unable to understand the information provided during a consent procedure, appreciate its implications, or make a choice, but that individual may have the ability to do those same things once treated.

Decision-making ability is best understood as occurring along a continuum of impairment and must be assessed in relation to specific tasks. An individual with cognitive impairment may demonstrate the capacity to consent to a study involving familiar procedures, such as a blood test and interview, but not to a more complex intervention. Capacity is also calibrated in relation to risk and benefit; the threshold for capacity to make a decision in higher risk studies and studies with less direct benefit would be set higher than that for a minimal risk intervention.

In practice, the language of the Common Rule is typically understood by IRBs to require a categorical determination: Is vulnerability to coercion or undue influence likely or not? When likely, the "additional safeguards" required in subpart A most commonly take the form of additional protections in consent, and most often, these are instituted only at the time of the consent decision. An approach to vulnerability that is only applied with regard to consent fails to capture the ethical demands of research protections for the mentally ill. Some mentally ill individuals may have emotional, behavioral, or cognitive impairments such that they are unlikely to be able to look after their best interests at the time of consent and *throughout their research participation*. For them, the

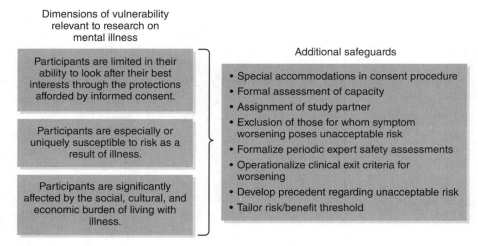

Figure 10.12-1 Dimensions of vulnerability relevant to research on mental illness.

protections available to healthy individuals may not be available—for example, the ability to anticipate, recognize, or express concerns about relapse or other deterioration in functioning. Mental illness confers "vulnerability" in ways that extend beyond the consent decision, and a broader framework for safeguards in research on SMI is warranted (**Figure 10.12-1**).

At the same time, it is essential for IRBs to appreciate that many individuals with SMI live in the community; effectively manage the demands of independent living, work, school, and family; and make all categories of decisions in their daily lives, including those related to their health care. Any broad assumption that such individuals are unable to make a decision with regard to research can introduce an unnecessary impediment to inclusion and to research itself (see **Case Study 10.12-1**).

 CASE STUDY 10.12-1

An IRB that primarily reviews investigational drug studies has a written policy for all studies involving people with psychotic disorders, which requires a formal assessment of capacity to consent by a licensed psychologist or psychiatrist who is not a member of the research team. A new study proposes to collect information from outpatients in a community mental health center on the acceptability of an evidence-based cognitive remediation software program administered online. Each subject will complete a 45-minute computer-based module on three occasions using a secure online portal, an hour-long set of cognitive measures before and after the cognitive remediation, and a survey of attitudes and satisfaction with the methods.

The IRB took the following actions:

1. Recognized that a requirement for a formal capacity assessment for a study otherwise conducted remotely would not be feasible. Furthermore, the procedures were determined to be no more than minimal risk. Finally, given the general level of functioning of the clinic patients, their ability to understand the nature of the research and make a decision about participation were not in question.
2. Waived the policy requirement in order to better calibrate additional safeguards with the study and study population.
3. Stipulated that clinic staff familiar with the patient confirm that their participation in the research was clinically appropriate.

Susceptibility to Risk

The suicide in 1991 of a subject in a longitudinal study of individuals with schizophrenia drew national attention to the risks associated with drug discontinuation research in the seriously mentally ill (*Los Angeles Times*, 1994). Patients with SMI may be especially susceptible to study risk, and these research risks relate not simply to the effects of experimental treatments but to the effects of the research protocol on the underlying disorder. For example, in patients with SMI, psychotic disorders, and mood disorders such as depression and bipolar disorder, relapse or symptomatic worsening as a result of a study-related delay to effective treatment can have acute, significant, and irreversible consequences. A patient with major depression for whom the investigational therapy is ineffective may be increasingly unable to perform at work, fail to meet other personal and financial obligations, or may experience a worsening of suicidal ideation or behavior. Ensuring that the anticipated consequences of research participation are listed in the consent procedure and understood by the subject is essential, and unreasonable risk must be defined and prevented to the extent possible. Some individuals are susceptible to risk or its consequences because their impairment affects their ability to recognize, report, or seek help for symptomatic worsening (Amador et al., 1994; see **Case Study 10.12-2**). The implications for ongoing assessment, safety monitoring, and study dropout are discussed later in this chapter.

 ## CASE STUDY 10.12-2

Deborah, a 31-year-old woman with schizophrenia who works part time in a bookstore, agrees to participate in a comparative effectiveness study of two currently marketed antipsychotic medications; both she and her psychiatrist believe a change in her current medication regimen is in order. On study day 4, the subject's mother, with whom Deborah lives, calls the study team and reports that her daughter is refusing to eat and is not willing to leave her room.

Although Deborah was symptomatically stable and judged to have capacity to consent to research at baseline, within days of initiation of the study treatment she experienced a return of psychotic symptoms, including the delusion that her food is poisoned.

The study protocol anticipated that some subjects would be unable to tolerate or would not respond to the study treatments, and the associated risks could range from subjective distress to self-injurious or aggressive behavior. The study team also recognized that some patients with schizophrenia, even while able to provide consent when stable, may be unlikely to recognize or report a worsening of symptoms.

The IRB protocol was as follows:

1. Stipulated that only individuals who, in consultation with their psychiatrist, were viewed as requiring a change in medication would be considered for enrollment.
2. Stipulated that the protocol be initiated on an inpatient unit for any patient with a history of suicidal or violent behavior.
3. Stipulated that patients will be excluded from the study if judged by a qualified and licensed clinician to be at significant risk for suicidal or violent behavior or otherwise judged to be unlikely to tolerate medication discontinuation or crossover to the study treatment.
4. Stipulated that outpatient study subjects were required to have a study partner—a family member or friend who would monitor the subject's well-being during the study.
5. Stipulated that a clinician be available around the clock to reply to calls or queries from subjects or study partners.

Finally, negative public attitudes regarding mental illness require special attention to privacy protections to ensure that "[a]ny disclosure of the human subjects' responses outside the research would not reasonably place the subjects at risk of criminal or civil liability or be damaging to the subjects' financial standing, employability, educational advancement, or reputation" (**45 CFR 46.104(d)(2)(ii)**).

Burden of Illness, Socioeconomic Disadvantage, and Access to Care

As described, vulnerability can be understood within the regulatory context of capacity to consent. Susceptibility to research risks captures a second meaning of vulnerability of great importance for the IRB review of research on mental illness. A third dimension of vulnerability that warrants consideration is the social, cultural, and economic burden of living with SMI. People with mental illness experience significant barriers in access to affordable mental health care. Mental illness is underdiagnosed and undertreated in adults and children in the United States (NAMI, 2017). In one recent study, only 29% of adults diagnosed with depression received treatment for the disorder in the prior 12-month period (Olfson et al., 2016). Startling evidence of early morbidity in people with SMI speaks to inadequate access to quality primary care (Olfson et al., 2015). Stigma is known to have a negative impact on access to employment, housing, and health care (Link, 2006). Socioeconomic disadvantage associated with SMI has implications for the consent process, susceptibility to risk, and what constitutes reasonable or acceptable risk. For example, the effects of a study subject's inability to access or afford care and treatment following research participation or in the event of an adverse medical event, or to sustain employment or housing in the face of functional impairment, are among important considerations for the IRB in its assessment of the risks of study involvement.

Anticipating and Mitigating Risk

⬩ 3-1 IRB Membership

The work of anticipating and mitigating risk requires an understanding of the clinical features of the mental illness being studied. Similarly, aspects of study design and methodology bear importantly on risk. For these reasons, it is usually necessary for the IRB to include those with clinical and scientific expertise with these disorders and with the study design and methodology commonly employed in these types of studies. Alternatively, the IRB may make use of consultants with this expertise. Preferably, IRB deliberations will also be informed by an IRB member or consultant who can offer the perspective of a patient, family member, or advocacy group.

Treatment Setting

A careful assessment of the nature and the phase of the illness under study can determine whether the research can safely be conducted in the clinic or community or whether it requires a hospital (or research unit) stay for observation and assessment. A safety and efficacy trial for acutely manic patients will pose significantly different risk considerations than a study of persistent and treatment-resistant depression in bipolar patients. In each instance, the research proposal should define the characteristics of the study population (are manic and psychotic patients included? Are patients judged to be at acute risk for suicide included?). Similarly, the IRB should assess whether the proposed setting is safe, staff are appropriately trained, and a higher level of care is available when necessary.

Duration of Study Interventions and Delay to Effective Treatment

In order to anticipate and minimize risk while preserving sound research design, the IRB should understand the rationale for the proposed duration of any period when the subject will receive an investigational therapy or be left untreated. Research examining the pathophysiology of psychiatric disorders, such as a study involving imaging of brain neurotransmitter systems, commonly requires a subject to be off medication, often for weeks. Other clinical research examines strategies for drug discontinuation itself. Of course, even a research intervention that is of "known efficacy" may be ineffective for the individual subject. For example, only approximately half of patients with depression will experience symptomatic improvement following treatment with an antidepressant, and only 50% to 70% of these will achieve symptom remission (Rush et al., 2003). Therefore, the IRB must always consider the duration of the treatment component and the anticipated consequences of ineffective treatment or no treatment on the subject.

In general, a guiding principle regarding risk minimization is that for any risk to be ethically acceptable, it must be scientifically necessary. Furthermore, whereas such a scientific rationale may be necessary, it is not sufficient. A 3-week drug washout may be scientifically necessary prior to a receptor-binding study using positron emission tomography, but the IRB may determine that considerable symptomatic worsening or a heightened risk of self-injury is not acceptable. Therefore, the IRB should first evaluate the scientific rationale for the proposed duration of study interventions and the delay to effective treatment. If scientifically appropriate, the board must then determine whether the risks associated are reasonable and whether they can be further mitigated. For example, if the IRB determines that a 6- to 8-week placebo-controlled clinical trial is required for the approval of a new investigational drug, the protocol must be written to specify exclusion criteria, periodic safety assessment, and forced dropout criteria to protect subjects from unreasonable risk related to assignment to placebo. Active efforts to identify and manage risk permit the use of scientifically important research designs, such as drug washout and placebo controls. These approaches are described in the sections that follow.

✐ 10-11

Delay to Treatment and Discontinuation of Treatment

Delay to treatment associated with scheduled screening and baseline assessment procedures, drug washout, and drug titration are common in research. The transition from an investigational treatment to ordinary care at the conclusion of research also defines a period of risk. IRBs should collaborate with researchers to minimize administrative delays in initiation of treatment, seek to exclude subjects unlikely to tolerate delay, and ensure that the postprotocol transition of care is carefully managed.

Research Procedures Inappropriate for the Developmental Phase of the Research and Research Aims

An IRB can consider whether the proposed research design is consistent with the study aims or whether it introduces unnecessary risk. For example, a small early study of a new approach to psychotherapy for obsessive–compulsive disorder aims only to demonstrate whether research therapists can adhere to the therapy guidelines specified in the treatment manual. The study randomizes subjects to the therapy or an 8-week wait-list control and prohibits use of sleep aids by the subjects. The withholding of concurrent treatment (medication during a psychotherapy trial) or concomitant medication (sleep aids during an investigational drug trial) is often necessary in controlled studies to limit confounding factors and mitigate risk associated with drug interactions. In this case, the 8-week delay, like the restrictions on sleep medication, imposes a scientifically unnecessary set of risks. Neither element is consistent with the study aim, and an IRB should evaluate its necessity.

Diagnosis and Assessment

Clinical evaluation alone is generally considered inadequately rigorous and unreliable in the diagnosis of mental disorders and the assessment of psychiatric symptoms. Instead, diagnosis is typically made by research staff using well-validated and highly reliable structured diagnostic interviews (see, for example, First et al., 2015). Similarly, the evaluation of response or nonresponse to treatment and treatment-emergent side effects requires the use of formal and disorder-specific symptom inventories and rating scales. Structured tools and interviews are now routinely employed in the assessment of suicide risk in clinical and research settings (Posner et al., 2011). The quality of these assessments and therefore of the overall data will depend on the extent that validated instruments are used and whether staff are properly credentialed, trained, observed, and supervised. Raters are ordinarily not those involved in providing care and are masked (blinded) with regard to treatment assignment in order to minimize bias.

Furthermore, an IRB or institution might require specific methods or credentials for specific tasks. For example, an IRB might permit a research assistant with a bachelor's degree to collect some forms of data but require a licensed clinical social worker, psychologist, or psychiatrist to evaluate treatment response in significantly depressed patients undergoing a delay to treatment and during the treatment phase of the study.

Frequency of Assessment

The frequency with which research staff monitor subjects for symptomatic change should be appropriate to the nature, phase, and severity of illness in the context of the research intervention. In general, whether the subject is likely to report a change in status will vary depending on the disorder, nature of impairment, and instructions from the research team.

Dropout Criteria

Typically, in clinical trials, criteria for study exit, or dropout, are limited to the occurrence of a <u>serious adverse event</u>, evidence of nonadherence to study procedures, or subject request. Dropout criteria can also be employed to reevaluate

7-3

the appropriateness of a subject's continued participation in cases where symptoms worsen or the subject does not respond. These circumstances can prompt a reassessment of consent provided by subjects with diminished autonomy. Because researchers have incentives to retain subjects in research, the use of an operationalized measure with specified thresholds for action (drop from study, seek-consent again, reevaluate in 1 week) lessens conflict. An IRB, in collaboration with the study team, can specify criteria, the time point(s) at which they are evaluated, and required action. For example, a Clinical Global Impression scale can be used to rate and track the subjects' change from baseline in an investigational, placebo-controlled trial (Guy, 1976). Dropout criteria may be applied so that subjects who are rated as "very much worse" by a specified time point are dropped from the research. Subjects who have evidenced no improvement at a time point in which some improvement is expected may be reassessed in a week and then dropped if not showing improvement. In this way, the clinical research team individualizes treatment decisions as they might be individualized in clinical care.

Inclusion and Exclusion Criteria

Limiting risk through the informed and cautious application of inclusion and exclusion criteria is an effective approach to risk mitigation in research on mental illness. One might ask whether it is scientifically necessary to include the most severely ill patients in an early stage study of a new therapy or in a study involving a medication-free period. On one hand, this adapts the principle of studying the less vulnerable (less susceptible to risk) individuals before the more vulnerable and does not preclude inclusion of the more severely ill at a later stage of investigation. Similarly, subjects at significant risk for self-injury or aggressive behavior may be excluded when the risks associated with their inclusion are judged to outweigh the direct benefits of their participation, even when the scientifically important A criterion may read, "exclude subjects who, based on clinical history and current assessment, are judged unlikely to be able to tolerate a 7-day drug washout." The IRB, however, must be cautious not to favor risk reduction at the expense of necessary science. Excluding all patients at risk for suicide from a clinical trial might mean not learning whether a particular medication is effective in treating the subset of patients with a particular disorder who also have suicidal ideation. The balance between protection and inclusion requires careful analysis.

As stated earlier, mental illnesses frequently co-occur with other mental, substance use, and medical disorders. From the perspective of risk reduction, it is necessary to identify and characterize the study population and evaluate the impact of study procedures and treatments on the comorbid condition. Consider a treatment study of posttraumatic stress disorder (PTSD). Depression and alcohol use disorders are common in PTSD. Will treatments for the comorbid condition be allowed during the study? It is reasonable to discontinue the treatments? Should patients with comorbid depression and alcohol use be excluded? Here the IRB must balance risk reduction (and a homogeneous PTSD-only sample) with the merits of a more inclusive (and real-world) study population. As with the considerations of severity of illness, a study of a less at-risk population can be conducted first. With evidence of efficacy, a more complex trial can be undertaken subsequently.

The decision by the IRB to modify its view of what constitutes "reasonable risk" for vulnerable populations favors paternalism (protectionism) over the prospective subjects' autonomy interests. Given the many dimensions of

🔗 9-1 vulnerability that characterize some individuals with mental illness, an IRB may choose to exclude such subjects from a research study, although it would permit a less vulnerable population to consider participating in that same research. For example, an IRB may exclude individuals with severe mental illness who have never previously been treated with known, effective therapies from participation in a placebo controlled clinical trial of an investigational agent, when populations who are not vulnerable in the same ways (also not previously treated) might be appropriately enrolled. An IRB can also exclude prospective subjects who are stable and tolerating current treatment and for whom the risks of an investigational study are not clinically justifiable. The exclusion of subjects at risk may be necessary but may also have considerable impact on the individual subject (who will be denied access) and on the knowledge base derived from the research. Thoughtful approaches to risk minimization by the IRB often permit the safe and ethical inclusion of such subjects.

Consent and Key Information

🔗 Section 6 🔗 9-7 The topics of consent and research with individuals with impaired decision making are covered elsewhere in this volume, but some discussion of consent as it relates to risk mitigation is indicated.

As previously noted, discussion of the risks of research tends to emphasize anticipated adverse effects of the investigational treatment itself. In research with the SMI, risks related to delay of treatment or failure to treat the underlying illness are equally important. Therefore, consent should include and
🔗 6-2 personalize this information, and the key information section should serve to emphasize it.

Because research interventions typically offer short-term treatments for what are typically chronic conditions, the research protocol (and consent) should emphasize how poststudy treatment and transition to poststudy treatment are provided to avoid symptomatic worsening. Will the study treatment be available after the study ends? Will subjects learn what treatment they received so that this information may be of use to them in the future?

The tendency in the research and research protections community is to
🔗 9-7 emphasize the impact of impaired decision making as it relates to consent at the time of study enrollment. Although procedures to enhance the consent process and accommodate individuals with impairment are important, it is equally important to ensure that subjects with impairment are capable of communicating their needs and wishes during the course of research. The assumption that an individual who is doing poorly or having difficulty tolerating treatment will express interest in discontinuing the research may not apply for certain individuals with mental illness. The formal and informal engagement of friends, family members, and other caregivers as study partners to the research subject serves to protect subjects, enhance communication with the study team, and allow early identification of emerging risk (NIH, 2009).

Conclusion

Mental illness is common, poorly understand, and contributes to disability and suffering on a large scale. The effective review of research involving subjects with mental illness requires an appreciation of the importance of advancing relevant research on neurobiology, treatment, services, and policy. To do so, the IRB must anticipate risk by understanding features of mental illness that give rise to vulnerability in all its dimensions. Risk mitigation is accomplished through the revision of inclusion and exclusion criteria, refinement of the study procedures, application of operationalized dropout criteria, requirements for frequent and expert symptom assessment, and adapting notions of reasonable risk for the population under study. IRB review of research on mental illness is informed by the principles that risk that is scientifically unnecessary is ethically unacceptable, that the less vulnerable should be studied before the more vulnerable, and that "some persons are in need of extensive protection, even to the point of excluding them from activities which may harm them" (National Commission, 1979).

References

Amador, X. F., Flaum, M., Andreasen, N. C., Strauss, D. H., Yale, S. A., Clark, S. C., & Gorman, J. M. (1994). Awareness of illness in schizophrenia and schizoaffective and mood disorders. *Archives of General Psychiatry, 51*(10), 826–836.

Carpenter, W. T., Jr., Gold, J. M., Lahti, A. C., Queern, C. A., Conley, R. R., Bartko, J. J., Kovnick, J., & Appelbaum, P. S. (2000). Decisional capacity for informed consent in schizophrenia research. *JAMA Psychiatry, 57*(6), 533–538.

Centers for Disease Control and Prevention (CDC). (2018a). *Mental health: Data and publications.* www.cdc.gov/mentalhealth/data_publications/index.htm

Centers for Disease Control and Prevention (CDC). (2018b). *Suicide rising across the US: More than a mental health concern.* www.cdc.gov/vitalsigns/suicide/

Centers for Disease Control and Prevention (CDC). (2020). *Preventing suicide: How big is the problem?* www.cdc.gov/violenceprevention/suicide/fastfact.html

Federal Register. (1978). Vol. 43, No. 53. *Research involving those institutionalized as mentally infirm: Report and recommendation.* Office of the Federal Register, National Archives and Records Service, General Services Administration.

Federal Register. (2017). Vol. 82, No. 12. 45 CFR 46 and Preamble. www.govinfo.gov/content/pkg/FR-2017-01-19/pdf/2017-01058.pdf

First, M. B., Reed, G. M., Hyman, S. E., & Saxena, S. (2015). The development of the ICD-11 clinical descriptions and diagnostic guidelines for mental and behavioural disorders. *World Psychiatry, 14*(1), 82–90.

Guy, W. (1976). *ECDEU Assessment Manual for Psychopharmacology—Revised* (DHHS Pub. No. ADM 91–338). U.S. Department of Health and Human Services, pp. 218–222.

Krugman, S. (1971). Experiments at the Willowbrook State School. *Lancet, 1*(7706), 966–967.

Lederer, S. E. (1985). Hideyo Noguchi's luetin experiment and the antivivisectionists. *Isis, 76*(281), 31–48

Link, B. (2005). Stigma and its public health implications. *Lancet, 367,* 528–529.

Los Angeles Times. (1994, March 11). When the patient is also an experiment: Feds find fault with UCLA schizophrenia study [Editorial]. www.latimes.com/archives/la-xpm-1994-03-11-me-32605-story.html

National Alliance on Mental Illness (NAMI). (n.d.). *About mental illness: Mental health conditions.* https://nami.org/About-Mental-Illness

National Alliance on Mental Illness (NAMI). (2017). *The doctor is out: Continuing disparities in access to mental and physical health care.* www.nami.org/Support-Education/Publications-Reports/Public-Policy-Reports/The-Doctor-is-Out/DoctorIsOut

National Commission for the Protection of Human Subjects of Biomedical and Behavioral Research. (1978). *Research involving those institutionalized as mentally infirm: Report and recommendations.* https://repository.library.georgetown.edu/handle/10822/778715

National Commission for the Protection of Human Subjects of Biomedical and Behavioral Research. (1979). *The Belmont Report: Ethical principles and guidelines for the protection of human subjects in biomedical and behavioral research.* www.hhs.gov/ohrp/regulations-and-policy/belmont-report/index.html

National Institute of Mental Health. (2019). *Mental illness: Definitions.* www.nimh.nih.gov/health/statistics/mental-illness.shtml

National Institutes of Health (NIH). (2009). *Secretary's Advisory Committee on Human Research Protections: Recommendations regarding research involving individuals with impaired decision-making.* www.hhs.gov/ohrp/sachrp-committee/recommendations/2009-july-15-letter/index.html

National Research Act. (1974). Public Law 93-348. https://history.nih.gov/download/attachments/1016866/PL93-348.pdf

Olfson, M., Gerhard, T., Huang, C., Crystal, S., & Stroup, T. (2015). Premature mortality among adults with schizophrenia in the United States. *JAMA Psychiatry, 72*(12), 1172–1181.

Olfson, M., Blanco, C., & Marcus, S. C. (2016). Treatment of adult depression in the United States. *JAMA Intern Med, 176*(10), 1482–1491.

Posner, K., Brown G. K., Stanley, B., Brent, D. A., Yershova, K. V., Oquendo, M. A., Currier, G. W., Melvin, G. A., Greenhill, L., Shen, S., & Mann, J. J. (2011). The Columbia-Suicide Severity Rating Scale: Initial validity and internal consistency findings from three multisite studies with adolescents and adults. *American Journal of Psychiatry, 168*(12), 1266–1277.

Presidential Commission for the Study of Bioethical Issues. (2011). *"Ethically impossible" STD research in Guatemala from 1946 to 1948.* https://bioethicsarchive.georgetown.edu/pcsbi/node/654.html

Roberts, L. W. (Ed.). (2019). *The American Psychiatric Association Publishing textbook of psychiatry* (7th ed.). American Psychiatric Association Publishing.

Rothman, D. J. (1992). *Strangers at the bedside: A history of how law and bioethics transformed medical decision making.* Basic Books.

Rush, J. A., Trivedi, M., & Fava, M. (2003). Depression, IV: STAR*D treatment trial for depression. *American Journal of Psychiatry, 160*(2), 237.

Substance Abuse and Mental Health Services Administration (SAMHSA). (2012). *Results from the 2011 Survey on Drug Use and Health: Mental health findings* (HHS Publication No. SMA 12-4725, NSDUH Series H-45). www.samhsa.gov/data/sites/default/files/NSDUHmhfr2011/NSDUHmhfr2011.htm#ch4

Substance Abuse and Mental Health Services Administration (SAMHSA). (2018). *Key substance use and mental health indicators in the United States: Results from the 2017 National Survey on Drug Use and Health* (HHS Publication No. SMA 18-5068, NSUDH Series H-53). www.samhsa.gov/data/sites/default/files/cbhsq-reports/NSDUHFFR2017/NSDUHFFR2017.pdf

World Health Organization (WHO). (2018). *World health statistics data visualization dashboard: Suicide.* https://apps.who.int/gho/data/node.sdg.3-4-viz-2?lang=en

IRB Review of Genomic Research

Stacey Donnelly

Carol Weil

Abstract

This chapter will discuss genetic research and the related technologies involved in genomic research, including next-generation sequencing, such as whole genome and whole exome, as well as the special considerations IRBs may want to consider in reviewing such research. Those considerations include (1) the collection of samples from genomic research subjects, (2) informed consent, (3) the secondary use of collected biospecimens in genomic research, and (4) the return of genomic information or results to research subjects.

Introduction

This chapter is designed to introduce four main topics related to the review of genomic research: (1) basic concepts and definitions of genomic research, (2) important issues regarding consenting for genomic research, (3) ensuring data protections while promoting data sharing, and (4) patient engagement in research and the return of genetic/genomic results.

Basic Concepts and Definitions

Terminology

In order to review studies that involve genomic research, it is very useful to understand some basic terms (see Box, Common Terms Used in Genomic Research). The terms and definitions, with some adaptation, were obtained from a more extensive list created by the National Human Genome Research Institute (NHGRI, 2014).

COMMON TERMS USED IN GENOMIC RESEARCH

Basics

Exome. The set of protein-coding segments of DNA (called exons), that constitutes 1-2% of the human genome.

Genome. The genome is the entire set of genetic instructions found in a cell. In humans, the genome consists of 23 pairs of chromosomes, found in the nucleus, as well as a small chromosome found in the cells' mitochondria. Each set of 23 chromosomes contains approximately 3.1 billion bases of DNA sequence.

Genotype. A genotype is an individual's collection of genes. The term also can refer to the two alleles inherited for a particular gene. The genotype is expressed when the information encoded in the genes' DNA is used to make protein and RNA molecules. The expression of the genotype contributes to the individual's observable traits, called the phenotype.

Germline. A germline is the sex cells (eggs and sperm) that are used by sexually reproducing organisms to pass on genes from generation to generation. Egg and sperm cells are called germ cells, in contrast to the other cells of the body that are called somatic cells.

Phenotype. A phenotype is an individual's observable traits, such as height, eye color, and blood type. The genetic contribution to the phenotype is called the genotype. Some traits are largely determined by the genotype, while other traits are largely determined by environmental factors.

Somatic cell. A somatic cell is any cell of the body except sperm and egg cells. Somatic cells are diploid, meaning that they contain two sets of chromosomes, one inherited from each parent. Mutations in somatic cells can affect the individual, but they are not passed on to offspring.

Components of DNA

Allele. An allele is one of two or more versions of a gene. An individual inherits two alleles for each gene, one from each parent. If the two alleles are the same, the individual is homozygous for that gene. If the alleles are different, the individual is heterozygous. Though the term allele was originally used to describe variation among genes, it now also refers to variation among non-coding DNA sequences.

Gene. The gene is the basic physical unit of inheritance. Genes are passed from parents to offspring and contain the information needed to specify traits. Genes are arranged, one after another, on structures called chromosomes. A chromosome contains a single long DNA molecule, only a portion of which corresponds to a single gene. Humans have approximately 20,000 genes arranged on their chromosomes.

Nucleotide. A nucleotide is the basic building block of nucleic acids. RNA and DNA are polymers made of long chains of nucleotides. A nucleotide consists of a sugar molecule (either ribose in RNA or deoxyribose in DNA) attached to a phosphate group and a nitrogen-containing base. The bases used in DNA are adenine (A), cytosine (C), guanine (G), and thymine (T). In RNA, the base uracil (U) takes the place of thymine.

Oncogene. An oncogene is a mutated gene that contributes to the development of a cancer. In their normal unmutated state, onocgenes are called proto-oncogenes, and they play roles in the regulation of cell division. Some oncogenes work like putting your foot down on the accelerator of a car, pushing a cell to divide. Other oncogenes work like removing your foot from the brake while parked on a hill, also causing the cell to divide.

Single-nucleotide polymorphisms (SNPs). Single nucleotide polymorphisms (SNPs) are a type of polymorphism involving variation of a single base pair. Scientists are studying how single nucleotide polymorphisms, or SNPs (pronounced "snips"), in the human genome correlate with disease, drug response, and other phenotypes.

Explaining Genetic Differences

Candidate gene. A candidate gene is a gene whose chromosomal location is associated with a particular disease or other phenotype. Because of its location, the gene is suspected of causing the disease or other phenotype.

Mapping. Mapping is the process of making a representative diagram cataloging the genes and other features of a chromosome and showing their relative locations. Cytogenetic maps are made using photomicrographs of chromosomes stained to reveal structural variations. Genetic maps use the idea of linkage to estimate the relative locations of genes. Physical maps, made using recombinant DNA (rDNA) technology, show the actual physical locations of landmarks along a chromosome.

Marker. A marker is a DNA sequence with a known physical location on a chromosome. Markers can help link an inherited disease with the responsible genes. DNA segments close to each other on a chromosome tend to be inherited together. Markers are used to track the inheritance of a nearby gene that has not yet been identified but whose approximate location is known. The marker itself may be a part of a gene or may have no known function.

Polymorphism. Polymorphism involves one of two or more variants of a particular DNA sequence. The most common type of polymorphism involves variation at a single base pair. Polymorphisms can also be much larger in size and involve long stretches of DNA. Called a single nucleotide polymorphism, or SNP (pronounced "snip"), scientists are studying how SNPs in the human genome correlate with disease, drug response, and other phenotypes.

Population genomics. Population genomics is the application of genomic technologies to understand populations of organisms. In humans, population genomics typically refers to applying technology in the quest to understand how genes contribute to our health and well-being.

Proband. A proband is an individual being studied or reported on. A proband is usually the first affected individual in a family who brings a genetic disorder to the attention of the medical community.

These definitions, and more, can be found in the National Human Genome Research Institute. (2014). Talking glossary of genetic terms. www.genome.gov/genetics-glossary

Genomic Testing in Research

Researchers conduct genomic testing to understand the relationship between genomic variation and disease. Their work is best advanced when data are aggregated and harmonized from a wide variety of large-scale sequencing projects, making summary data broadly available. IRBs may be asked to review studies that involve genomic data derived from open access databases (such as ClinVar, a public archive reporting relationships among human variation and observed health status, and gnomAD, a resource of exome and whole genome sequences derived from disease-specific as well as population genetic studies). Currently, the data used in such studies do not require IRB review because the data are considered deidentified, and therefore the study is not considered to involve "human subjects" as defined in the Common Rule [45 CFR 46.102(e)]; von Thenen, 2019). However, many have questioned the merits of this view, given institutions' declining ability to protect individual identity when massively parallel sequencing technologies, including whole genome sequencing, are employed. The Common Rule at 45 CFR 46.102(e)(7)(ii), however, requires periodic reassessment of whether there are analytic technologies or techniques that should be considered to generate identifiable information or biospecimens. Whole genome sequencing and whole exome sequencing are likely candidates for such consideration, given reported instances of reidentification from such data (von Thenen, 2019; Weil, 2013).

When genetic testing is conducted in the course of clinical research, questions arise for IRBs regarding whether the testing is conducted in a lab certified under rules implementing the Clinical Laboratory Improvement Amendments of 1988 (CLIA; **42 CFR part 493**) to test human specimens for the purpose of diagnosis, health assessment, or prevention or treatment of disease. CLIA was designed to ensure that lab results disclosed for patient care are analytically validated and reproducible, with the requisite attention to quality and rigor befitting a medical-grade test. Thus, CLIA prohibits the disclosure for clinical use of test results conducted in a non–CLIA-certified research lab. But the CLIA regulations arguably conflict with different Department of Health and Human Services (DHHS) regulations promulgated under the Health Insurance Portability and Accountability Act of 1996 (HIPAA), which grant individuals a right of access to their laboratory results regardless of whether they were generated in a CLIA-certified laboratory (DHHS, 2013). In a September 28, 2015, letter, the Secretary's Advisory Committee on Human Research Protections (SACHRP) noted DHHS's statement that the expanded access rights enshrined in HIPAA were intended to facilitate individuals' being "more proactive and more informed with regard to their health" (DHHS, 2015). SACHRP suggested that concerns about emotional distress or other harms resulting from the return of research-grade test information, such as the possibility that people might make medical decisions based on insufficient or inaccurate data, should not diminish these access rights.

🔖 11-6

IRBs sometimes require retesting in a CLIA-certified laboratory of any genomic testing results to be returned to subjects in clinical studies. For example, researchers conducting genome sequencing in a research laboratory to identify a new variant associated with pancreatic cancer may also identify a clinically relevant variant that has a known association with a completely different condition, such as cardiomyopathy. If the IRB believes that the cardiomyopathy variant finding should be disclosed because it is potentially clinically actionable, the result should either (1) be retested in a CLIA laboratory as part of the protocol or (2) returned with a clear communication that this is a research result and should not be used for clinical decision making without further evaluation by a treating physician and confirmatory testing in a clinical lab.

🔖 12-1

Consent for Genomic Research

Consent Requirements at 45 CFR 46.116

Research institutions, including biobanks, that collect tissue as part of clinical research that includes a genomic component or that access archived tissue for secondary research must state in the informed consent whether the research "will (if known) or might include whole genome sequencing (i.e., sequencing of a human germline or somatic specimen with the intent to generate the genome or exome sequence of that specimen)" [45 CFR 46.116(c)(9)]. As a best practice, IRBs should advise researchers to mention the possibility of genomic research whenever they collect or access research tissue for possible sequencing now or in the future. This avoids the need to re-contact individuals, a process that may inconvenience or distress patients and adds to the burdens of research staff. Tissue donors can also become lost to follow-up, potentially precluding future research.

🔖 6-2

Additional elements of informed consent likely to be relevant to genomic research covered in **45 CFR 46.116 (c)** include "(7) A statement that the subject's biospecimens (even if identifiers are removed) may be used for commercial profit and whether the subject will or will not share in this commercial profit;

(8) A statement regarding whether clinically relevant research results, including individual research results, will be disclosed to subjects, and if so, under what conditions" [**45 CFR 46.116(c)(7 and 8)**]. The elements of informed consent may additionally include a "statement that identifiers might be removed from the identifiable private information or identifiable biospecimens and that, after such removal, the information or biospecimens could be used for future research studies or distributed to another investigator for future research studies without additional informed consent" [**45 CFR 46.116(b)(9)(i)**].

In the era of personalized medicine, some researchers are interested in hypothesis-generating research where they assemble disease or population cohorts and broadly collect individuals' molecular data to determine possible phenotype-genotype associations. Such research can involve ongoing interaction with engaged subjects and an iterative or dynamic approach to informed consent as scientific understanding deepens (Biesecker, 2013; Weil, 2013). For example, biobank donors may consent to one or more research uses of their biological samples initially, but later be contacted for permission to expand these uses to new research activities not foreseen in the original consent (such as broader data sharing or the return of incidental research findings; Budin-Ljosne et al., 2017).

GENOMICS RESEARCH AND THE DECEASED

Although deceased individuals are not considered to be research subjects under the Common Rule, there are consent-relevant considerations related to the ongoing use of samples and data from deceased participants. Because the Health Insurance Portability and Accountability Act (HIPAA) protects confidentiality for 50 years after death, use of a deceased individual's identifiable data for research would require next-of-kin authorization for any information covered by HIPAA. The results of post-mortem genomics research analyses may be clinically relevant to surviving family members, raising questions about whether those family members should be informed that the research on their deceased relative's samples, genomic data, and health information is ongoing, whether they should be informed of these results, and when an individual's confidentiality should be protected after his or her death. If appropriate to the study, recruited participants can be asked explicitly at the time of informed consent whether, and with whom, their post-mortem results of clinical relevance should be shared, and any authorization to disclose protected health information should be documented according to HIPAA requirements. (DHHS, 2019).

Informed Consent for Incidental Findings

As genomic technologies have advanced and their cost has dramatically decreased (NHGRI, 2019a), it has become feasible to produce more and more genomic research data. The greater volume of genomic data available to researchers makes the discovery of incidental research findings (i.e., findings not related directly to the purpose of the research) more likely. To maximize utility, genomic research data is often <u>made available</u>, with appropriate subject privacy protections, to the broader scientific community. As the data is analyzed for different scientific purposes, additional incidental findings will surface. Increasingly, researchers are <u>returning results</u> from genomic research to study subjects, but there is still debate about when it is appropriate to return such results (including variants of unknown significance), what types of results should be returned (using an objective standard of clinical significance, or a subjective standard of participant utility), and how to return results (genetic counseling, etc.).

🔗 12-3

🔗 12-1

Laws and Policies Regarding Consent

- Broad consent
  As progress in medical research and precision medicine advances, there has been an increase in the establishment of <u>biobanks</u> for genomic studies around the globe. One example of this is the National Institutes of Health (NIH)-funded Human Heredity and Health in Africa Initiative (H3Africa; https://h3africa.org/) which has established biobanks in Africa to facilitate future indigenous genomic studies. For biobanks collecting genetic and genomic data for future research, the concept of "<u>broad consent</u>" has been

🔗 10-10, 12-3

🔗 6-9

proposed as a mechanism to enable potential research subjects in biobanks to give permission for their samples to be used in future, currently unknowable, studies.

Broad consent maximizes the utility and scientific value of collected biospecimens and data and is therefore the preferred approach to obtaining consent in studies involving genomic research. Genomic studies thus often contain provisions for the storage and future research use of collected biospecimens and associated data, including when there are plans to deidentify the specimens and information. IRBs and ethicists have long used the phrase "broad consent" to describe these provisions (Grady et al., 2015; Warner et al., 2018). The 2018 Common Rule uses the phrase "broad consent" to describe an optional regulatory pathway establishing two new exemption categories for the storage, maintenance, and research use of identifiable—but not deidentified—data and biospecimens, which can supplant traditional informed consent [45 CFR 46.104(d)]. The exemptions permit biological specimens and data to be collected and used or banked for future use, as long as the IRB conducts a "limited" review to ensure that consent and documentation requirements have been met.

🔗 5-6

- Waiver of consent

🔗 6-4

Under the Common Rule at 45 CFR 46.116(f), in order for an IRB to waive or alter consent for research involving the use of identifiable information or biospecimens, it must determine that the research could not practicably be carried out with deidentified data or biospecimens. Thus, to approve any genomics studies under the Common Rule that use identifiable tissue, IRBs must consider whether the research could be conducted with deidentified tissue instead.

The broad consent pathway at 45 CFR 46.116(d) includes a significant limitation on IRBs' ability to waive informed consent. If broad consent is refused by a research subject, then consent cannot be waived for *any* future research uses of the identifiable data and biospecimens for which broad consent was refused, including specific uses that involve no appreciable risks of harm. This constraint makes the broad consent pathway an unwieldy, complicated choice for research institutions by diminishing the future value of collected specimens and data and imposing burdensome oversight responsibilities for broad consent refusals.

- Screening, recruiting, and determining eligibility for genomics research
Under the Common Rule at 45 CFR 46.116(g), IRBs may approve researchers obtaining biospecimens or data for the purpose of screening, recruiting, or determining eligibility of prospective subjects without their informed consent by accessing stored records or biospecimens or if the information is obtained from oral or written communication with the prospective subjects.

Recruitment within families is a special hallmark of genomics research. Researchers may ask subjects for family histories containing the names and contact information of eligible family members, a practice that raises ethical issues. IRBs must consider how researchers can recruit within families while minimizing undesired outreach and undue pressures to enroll. The IRB should determine the appropriateness of the recruitment plan and decisions about the timing of informed consent for family members.

Ontology

As discussed earlier, many clinical and research subjects consent to either (1) broad research use (may be used for any future research) or (2) more narrow uses for their biological specimens. Having a common ontology, or a formal way of naming and defining categories of consent, is important to ensure public trust. For research subjects and IRBs, understanding how a biological sample and the subsequent data may be used is critical to the decision making and review processes. While the regulations permit use of deidentified biospecimens for genetics research without subject consent (i.e., secondary use), this approach is considered ethically suspect, particularly for controversial research technologies (cloning stem cells, for example). IRBs often refrain from approving the use of samples without consent due to the possibility of reidentification of living subjects, the potential for erosion of public trust, and NIH as well as publication requirements prohibiting the use of nonconsented samples. In some cases, however, there may be compelling scientific reasons for IRBs to approve research using samples collected without express consent, such as rare disease studies. For research involving rare diseases, if the study cohort involves individuals who donated tissue for research previously but are now lost to follow-up, the regulatory criteria for waiver of informed consent are met because such studies cannot practically be conducted if consent is required and consent cannot practically be obtained from the cohort.

🔗 12-3

🔗 6-4

As production of genetic data continues to accelerate exponentially, the ability to standardize, streamline, and automate the ethical use and disclosure of this data will be critical. To ensure that researchers can honor the consents of future subjects, it is important to have a shared ontology where terms have universal meaning. An example of inexact ontology would be if a patient consented to their biospecimens and data being used for "diabetes research and research related to diabetes"; this statement is ambiguous due to the fact that many diseases could be related to diabetes. It would be far better to either change the consent to ask for permission for all biomedical research or name the additional related diseases that would be allowed (heart disease, autoimmune disease, etc.).

It also important to provide research subjects with examples to better understand the research for which their sample might be used. The difference between *general research use* and *biomedical research use* may not be obvious to a layperson. An informed consent document should use examples a layperson can readily understand. For example: "We would like to use your biospecimen for *any type of research* which includes disease research (biomedical) as well as ancestry research, research on origin and migratory and populations patterns, and other social behavioral research." Some researchers now provide specific examples of social behavioral or population pattern research to help the subjects decide if they want to consent to participate in that type of study.

The best ontology will be fully understood by researchers for their use in consents and by the research subjects, allowing them to provide unambiguous informed consent. It would allow the automation of this type of research as the explosion of data available will necessitate that data can be accessed in an automated fashion. The ontology should also be clear about what types of researchers or research organizations may

GUIDANCE FOR DRAFTING DATA USE LIMITATION STATEMENTS

The Global Alliance for Genomics and Health has developed a set of "data use" categories attempting to "bucket" many consents into common consent codes (Dyke et al., 2016). The list is broken down into primary and secondary uses, and includes additional requirements that may be layered into a consent. The chart can be found at Global Alliance for Genomics and Health (2016). Although organizations may not parse consent documents in the exact same manner (for example, an organization may not see any difference between "no restrictions" and "general research use and clinical care"), it is a useful table and, conceptually, a systematic way in which to categorize genetic data.

Another useful resource for IRBs and researchers is the NIH's "Points to Consider in Drafting Effective Data Use Limitation Statements" (NIH, 2015). This document contains helpful information for writing consent form statements and accurately conveying potential data uses and sharing.

THE NIH GENOMIC DATA SHARING POLICY

For NIH-funded genomic studies initiated after January 25, 2015 (the effective date of the NIH Genomic Data Sharing (GDS) Policy; gds.nih.gov), NIH expects researchers to obtain subjects' explicit consent for sharing their genomic and phenotypic data (which may include some clinical information) to be used for future research purposes and to be shared broadly with scientific databases and biorepositories. The informed consent process should include: (1) information on the types of genomic samples and data that will (or may in the future) be shared, individually or as part of summary results; (2) whether the sharing will involve identifiable or deidentified material; (3) the nature of the access (public/unrestricted access or controlled access via committee) and implications for protecting subject privacy and confidentiality, including whether recontact for additional information or requests to participate in other studies are anticipated. If samples will be used to create cell lines that will keep reproducing and can be used long term for currently unanticipated uses, that should be highlighted (NHGRI, 2019b).

access the data. Information such as use by for-profit companies versus academic or nonprofit institutions should be clear. If use is not prohibited, it should be explicitly allowed, and this factor should be taken into account when both developing and reviewing consent forms.

Promoting the Twin Goals of Data Sharing and Data Protection

In reviewing research involving genomics, IRBs must balance two competing ethical-legal mandates—the need to share subjects' data broadly to maximize its value and the need to protect subjects' privacy. Data security is particularly challenging with genomics research because genetic data is never completely anonymous. Genomic reidentification strategies can, for example, determine people's names based solely on their DNA and trace amounts of associated meta-data potentially available in public databases (Gymrek et al., 2013; Phillips, 2018). Moreover, genomic data sets that have been coded can be susceptible to reidentification, even when they are considered deidentified under the HIPAA Privacy Rule. However, in the era of precision medicine, broad data sharing is favored as a public policy, which furthers medical progress by facilitating greater understanding of how genomic variation influences disease (Raza & Hall, 2017; Siu et al., 2016).

🖊 12-3

Privacy is of particular concern in research involving genomics, as genetic information can be stigmatizing, especially for members of an identifiable population at high risk for a variant associated with a devastating disease or condition. DNA testing without the knowledge or permission of the person being tested (e.g., when researchers wish to link ancestry to their scientific inquiry into disease or to determine family history of disease) is another potential threat to individual privacy. In 2008, Congress passed the Genetic Information Nondiscrimination Act (GINA) to restrict the access of health insurers and employers to individuals' genetic information (NHGRI, 2020). Many states have passed laws as well, including some that prohibit genetic discrimination by disability insurers and life insurers (American Civil Liberties Union, 2020).

Publishing Findings

Although not necessarily directly in the purview of the IRB, it is everyone's desire that important scientific findings are made publicly available. Many of the leading scientific journals (e.g., *Nature, Cell, Science*) require that the underlying data must be submitted to a public repository (such as the Database of Genotypes and Phenotypes, dbGaP) prior to publication and may require accession numbers as proof. Because dbGaP is the most commonly used controlled-access repository in the United States, consents must meet the standards set out by NIH before dbGaP will allow that deposition (National Center for Biotechnology Information, n.d.).

Patient Engagement/ Patients as Partners

One of the key duties of an IRB is to protect the rights and welfare of research subjects. However, IRB review also provides the community with a voice, one of the reasons every IRB must have a nonaffiliated community member. It is critically important that the community member feels fully empowered to contribute to the discussion and decisions of the IRB.

In past decades there has been an increasing desire for public and patient engagement in medical research. A significant turning point was during the AIDS crisis, when the patient community became their own advocacy group (National Research Council, 1993). That community of patients illustrated how to advocate for themselves and led to other patient advocacy groups finding their voices. Patient engagement is also a hallmark of NIH-funded research initiatives such as the National Cancer Institute (NCI) Cancer Moonshot, whose Blue Ribbon Panel made the establishment of a network for direct patient engagement a key recommendation (NCI, 2017).

One excellent example of patient engagement was the first project undertaken by Count Me In, a collaborative organization led by "Emerson Collective, a California-based social change organization; the Broad Institute of MIT and Harvard, a leading nonprofit biomedical research institution; the Biden Cancer Initiative, an independent nonprofit organization that builds on the federal government's Cancer Moonshot; and the Dana-Farber Cancer Institute, a leading cancer hospital" (Broad Institute, 2020). The first Count Me In initiative was a successful "direct to patient" research study of metastatic breast cancer. Prior to its launch, the researchers spent months engaged with numerous breast cancer support groups and individual patients. Although the process took many months and posed logistical challenges, the enrollment rates were much higher than expected and the community continues to be key partners in all aspects of the study (Broad Institute, 2020). Although researchers may be concerned that this type of community outreach is too time consuming, it can actually improve research outcomes in the long run by streamlining data collection and promoting higher recruitment.

The Patient-Centered Outcomes Research Institute (PCORI) was mandated as part of the Affordable Care Act (ACA) passed by Congress in 2010 (PCORI, n.d.). PCORI funds research "that can help patients and those who care for them make better-informed healthcare choices" (PCORI, n.d.). A major goal of PCORI research is to determine what works

RETURNING RESULTS TO SUBJECTS

(See Chapter 12-1 for more in-depth information on this topic.)

- Individual results
  Under the 2018 Common Rule, informed consent must include a statement regarding whether, and under what conditions, clinically relevant research results will be disclosed to subjects **[45 CFR 46.116 (c)(8)]**. This requirement reflects the increasing consensus that communication of research results is a critical component of subject engagement and an ethical mandate when subjects' health is implicated (Multi-Regional Clinical Trials Center, 2017a). Genomics research studies often offer to disclose research findings that are personally meaningful to subjects, even if the information is not clinically actionable or even medically significant (Thorogood et al., 2019).

  When individual genomic research results are returned as part of a study, subjects effectively become gatekeepers for information involving their biologically related family members. Learning about a relative's variants could influence someone's decision to undergo genetic testing or impact reproductive decision making. Genomic research results may also reveal unexpected information about family relationships, such as misattributed paternity or unknown adoptive relationships. Researchers should plan how to manage such information, and subjects should be informed about the circumstances under which such information would and would not be disclosed to them or to family members.

- Summary results
  Clinical research subjects are increasingly interested in plain language summaries of study results, in order to understand the value of their contribution to science and public health. Disclosing aggregate results to research subjects promotes transparency and communicates respect and appreciation for donors' contributions. There is no one method or approach for returning study results, because the process will depend upon the type and size of study and the roles of researchers (academic, sponsor, government) involved (Multi-Regional Clinical Trials Center, 2017b).

  The informed consent for studies generating genomic data should include notice that deidentified summary results may be shared through open access database resources as well as in the scientific literature. As of November 1, 2018, NIH enables unrestricted access to genomic summary results (GSR) from nonsensitive genomic studies, in order to further medical advances (NIH, 2018).

well in various communities and learn from best practices. The ACA contains a principle that health care and research become more "patient centered," and many agreed with the goal. The article "The PCORI Engagement Rubric: Promising Practices for Partnering in Research" proposes a number of "engagement principles" that are well aligned with those of Count Me In and that may be useful for IRBs that want to ensure patient engagement in the proposed research (Sheridan et al., 2017).

References

American Civil Liberties Union. (2020). *Summary of laws regarding genetic discrimination.* www.aclu.org/other/summary-laws-regarding-genetic-discrimination

Biesecker, L. (2013). Hypothesis-generating research and predictive medicine. *Cold Spring Harbor Laboratory Press, 23,* 1051–1053. ISSN: 1088-9051/13

Broad Institute. (2020). *Count me in.* www.broadinstitute.org/count-me-in

Budin-Ljosne, I., Teare, H. J. A., Kaye, J., Beck, S., Bentzen, H. B., Caenazzo, L., Collett, C., D'Abramo, F., Felzmann, H., Finlay, T., Javaid, M. K., Jones, E., Katic, V., Simpson, A., & Mascalzoni, D. (2017). Dynamic consent: a potential solution to some of the challenges of modern biomedical research. *BMC Medical Ethics, 18,* 4.

Department of Health and Human Services (DHHS). (2013). *Office for Civil Rights: Summary of the Health Insurance Portability and Accountability Act.* www.hhs.gov/hipaa/for-professionals /privacy/laws-regulations/index.html

Department of Health and Human Services (DHHS). (2015). *Secretary's Advisory Committee on Human Research Protections. Attachment C: Return of individual results and special consideration of issues arising from amendments of HIPAA and CLIA.* www.hhs.gov/ohrp/sachrp-committee /recommendations/2015-september-28-attachment-c/index.html

Department of Health and Human Services (DHHS). (2019). *Special Considerations for Genomics Research.* www.hhs.gov/guidance/document/special-considerations-genomics-research

Dyke, S. O., Philippakis, A. A., Rambla De Argila, J., Paltoo, D. N., Luetkemeier, E. S., Knoppers, B. M., Brookes, A. J., Spalding, J. D., Thompson, M., Roos, M., Boycott, K. M., Brudno, M., Hurles, M., Rehm, H. L., Matern, A., Fiume, M., & Sherry, S. T. (2016). Consent codes: Upholding standard data use conditions. *PLoS Genetics, 12*(1), e1005772.

Global Alliance for Genomics and Health. (2016). *Consent codes.* www.ga4gh.org/wp-content /uploads/DataUseBeacon_160209_tab_0.pdf

Glossary of genomics terms. (2013). *JAMA, 309*(14), 1533–1535. doi:10.1001/jama.2013.2950

Grady, C., Eckstein, L., Berkman, B., Brock, D., Cook-Deegan, R., Fullerston, S., Greely, H., Hansson, M., Hull, S., Kim, S., Lo, B., Pentz, R., Rodriguez, L., Weil, C., Wilfond, B., & Wendler, D. (2015). Broad consent for research with biological samples: Workshop conclusions. *American Journal of Bioethics, 15*(9), 34–42.

Gymrek, M., Mcguire, A. M., Golan, D., Halperin, E., & Erlich, Y. (2013). Identifying personal genomes by surname inference. *Science, 339,* 321–324.

Multi-Regional Clinical Trials Center. (2017a). *Return of individual results to participants: Principles.* https://mrctcenter.org/wp-content/uploads/2017/02/2017-02-15-MRCT-Individual-Return -of-Results-Principles.pdf

Multi-Regional Clinical Trials Center. (2017b). *MRCT return of aggregate results guidance document.* https://mrctcenter.org/wp-content/uploads/2017/03/2017-03-20-MRCT-Return-of-Aggregate -Results-Guidance-Document-3.0.pdf

National Cancer Institute (NCI). (2017). *Cancer Moonshot Blue Ribbon Panel.* www.cancer.gov /research/key-initiatives/moonshot-cancer-initiative/blue-ribbon-panel

National Center for Biotechnology Information. (n.d.). *dbGaP.* www.ncbi.nlm.nih.gov/gap/

National Human Genome Research Institute. (2014). Talking glossary of genetic terms. www.genome.gov/genetics-glossary

National Human Genome Research Institute. (2019a). *The cost of sequencing a human genome.* www.genome.gov/about-genomics/fact-sheets/Sequencing-Human-Genome-cost

National Human Genome Research Institute. (2019b). *Special considerations for genomics research.* www.genome.gov/about-genomics/policy-issues/Informed-Consent-for-Genomics-Research /Special-Considerations-for-Genome-Research

National Human Genome Research Institute. (2020). *Genetic discrimination.* www.genome.gov /about-genomics/policy-issues/Genetic-Discrimination#gina

National Institutes of Health (NIH). (2015). *Points to consider in developing effective data use limitation statements.* https://osp.od.nih.gov/wp-content/uploads/NIH_PTC_in_Developing_DUL _Statements.pdf

National Institutes of Health (NIH). (2018). *Update to NIH management of genomic summary results access.* https://grants.nih.gov/grants/guide/notice-files/NOT-OD-19-023.html

National Research Council Panel on Monitoring the Social Impact of the AIDS Epidemic. (1993). *The social impact of AIDS in the United States.* A. R. Jonsen & J. Stryker (Eds.). National Academies Press.

Patient-Centered Outcomes Research Institute (PCORI). (n.d.). *Improving outcomes important to patients* [Home page]. www.pcori.org

Phillips, M. (2018). *Can genomic data be anonymised?* Global Alliance for Genomics and Health. www.ga4gh.org/news/can-genomic-data-be-anonymised/

Raza, S., & Hall, A. (2017). Genomic medicine and data sharing. *British Medical Bulletin, 123,* 35–45.

Sheridan, S., Schrandt, S., Forsythe, L., Hilliard, T. S., Paez, K. A., & Advisory Panel on Patient Engagement (2013 inaugural panel). (2017). The PCORI engagement rubric: Promising practices for partnering in research. *Annals of Family Medicine, 15*(2), 165–170.

Siu, L., Lawler, M., Haussler, D., Knoppers, B., Lewin, J., Vis, D., Liao, R., Andre, F., Andre, F., Banks, I., Barrett, C. J., Caldas, C., Camargo, A. A., Fitzgerald, R., Mao, M., Mattison, J. E., Pao, W., Sellers, W., Sullivan, P., The, B. T., Ward, R., Zen Klusen, J. C., Sawyers, C., & Voest, E. (2016). Facilitating a culture of responsible and effective sharing of cancer genome data. *Nature Medicine, 22,* 464–471.

Thorogood, A., Dalpe, G., & Knoppers, B. (2019). Return of individual genomic research results: Are laws and policies keeping step? *European Journal of Human Genetics, 27,* 535–546.

von Thenen, N., Ayday, E., & Cicek, A. E. (2019). Re-identification of individuals in genomic data-sharing beacons via allele inference. *Bioinformatics, 35*(3), 365–371.

Warner, T., Weil, C., Degenholtz, H., Perker, L., Carithers, L., Feige, M., Wendler, D., & Pentz, R. (2018). Broad consent for research on biospecimens: The views of actual donors at four U.S. medical centers. *Journal of Empirical Research on Human Research Ethics, 13*(2), 115–124.

Weil, C., Mechanic, L., Green, T. C., Lockhart, N., Nelson, S., Rodriguez, L., & Buccini, L. (2013). NCI think tank concerning the identifiability of biospecimens and "-omic" data. *Genetics in Medicine, 15*(12), 997–1003.

Gene Transfer, Stem Cells, and Embryo Research

J. Graham Sharp

Sharon P. Shriver

Abstract

In biomedicine, there is arguably no field more dynamic or that holds more promise and peril than gene editing and therapy. Similarly, work with human stem cells has the potential to create unprecedented treatments and cures, while vastly expanding our understanding of human cellular development. These fields are evolving so rapidly, however, that guidelines and regulations lag behind scientific advances, and the ethical and social issues surrounding this research are intense and challenging. This chapter will provide an overview of the historical and scientific background and summarize the current regulatory landscape relevant to research using gene transfer and gene editing techniques, stem cells, and human embryos.

Gene Transfer and Gene Editing

Introduction

The gene therapy era, where the notion that missing or nonfunctional genes leading to disease could be repaired by transfer of a normal gene, opened with great promise (Wirth et al., 2013). However, many unanticipated challenges have arisen, and while many of them have been overcome, progress toward the widespread use of gene therapy has been delayed (Kaemmerer, 2018). Many of these obstacles have involved the choice of vector needed to carry the gene to be transferred into the tissues or cells (Cipolla et al., 2000; Dismuke et al., 2013; **Figure 10.14-1**).

Other challenges relate to the ability to target specific cells or tissues, qualities related to the target cells, and the reactions of the recipient's natural immune system to the gene transfer (Bessis et al., 2004; Zhang et al., 2019). A gene therapy protocol that generated a significant inflammatory response led to the death of a teenager, Jesse Gelsinger (R. F. Wilson, 2010; Yarborough & Sharp, 2009). An attempt to replace a nonfunctional gene that causes

⬿ 1-2

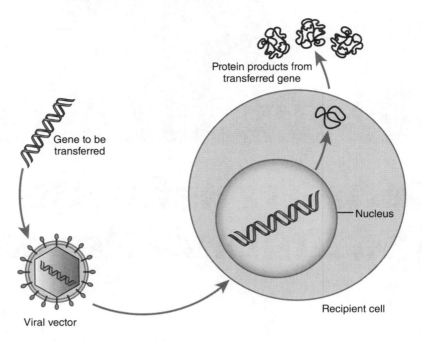

Figure 10.14-1 Gene transfer diagram.

immunodeficiency led to rare natural killer cell (NK) leukemias in the first subjects enrolled, who were children (Hacien-Bey-Albina et al., 2003; Nam & Rabbitts, 2006). Subsequently, a successful protocol was developed and approved (Ferrua & Aiuti, 2017; Mamcarz et al., 2019).

One way to categorize gene transfer studies is by likely short-term and long-term risks. Examples of relatively short-term risks are development of inflammatory or immune responses to cellular targets of the gene therapy vector and/or development of malignancy due to potential sites of integration. Longer term risks could also include later-developing malignancy or could arise from gene manipulations that involve heritable DNA changes in sperm, eggs, or embryos, which could affect subsequent generations (Caplan, 2019; Straiton, 2019).

Regulation of Recombinant DNA

Originally, because of concerns regarding the safety of research involving recombinant DNA, federally funded protocols were regulated by a National Institutes of Health (NIH)-organized Recombinant DNA Advisory Committee (RAC) that followed extensive guidelines originally issued June 14, 1977 (Piana, 2019; Wivel, 2014). Because of significant progress in the field and the assumption of regulatory roles by institutions, in 2019 the RAC was refocused to address new and emerging technologies (NIH, 2019a). At the same time, techniques of gene editing continue to evolve rapidly. Recent approaches, such as CRISPR/Cas9 (clustered regularly interspaced short palindromic repeats/CRISPR-associated protein 9), allow precise editing of specific DNA sequences (Vassena et al., 2016). This approach is likely to increase in importance and applicability for treating and potentially curing diseases, including the potential modification of the genome of embryos prior to implantation. In response to these developments, researchers and ethicists in 2018 expressed concerns over germline modification research, and a World Health Organization (WHO) advisory committee proposed that the WHO create a global registry of such studies (Brokowski, 2018; Reardon, 2019a). NIH supports a moratorium (Wolinetz & Collins, 2019). A summary of ethical statements from multiple countries concerning germline gene editing has been provided by Brokowski (2018), and *The CRISPR Journal* has an issue on "The Ethics of Human Genome Editing" (Chan & Sternberg, 2019). To address the lack of international consensus, the U.S. National Academy of Medicine (NAM), the U.S. National Academy of Sciences (NAS), and the UK Royal Society have joined with science and medical academies worldwide to convene an international commission to address germline genome editing (National Academies, n.d.).

IRB Review of Gene Transfer and Gene Editing Studies

According to NIH guidelines, the institutional biosafety committee (IBC) initially reviews, approves, and oversees research involving recombinant/synthetic DNA/RNA (as well as studies involving other biohazardous agents). Institutions may also have an embryonic stem cell research oversight (ESCRO) committee or scientific research oversight committee (SROC) with broader responsibilities that include fetal tissue use, as well as potentially other controversial procedures such as gene editing, according to International Society for Stem Cell Research (ISSCR) guidelines (2016). Alternatively, institutions may decide to form an ad hoc subcommittee to review studies requiring specific scientific and/or ethical knowledge. If the study has any components that meet the definition of human subjects research, it will require additional review and approval by the IRB. The efficiency and effectiveness of IRB review of studies utilizing gene transfer and editing can be

🔗 3-1 enhanced by ensuring that these committees <u>include members</u> with expertise in molecular genetics and other topics related to these areas, that institutional guidelines and procedures are in place to facilitate engagement and communication among appropriate committees, and that the IRB review incorporates the findings of these committees when reviewing gene modification studies.

It may be helpful for IRBs to consider the following proposed categories of gene transfer:

(i) Situations where human cells are employed in vitro for gene transfer with no intent to transfer them back to a human subject. This would be very low risk.

Category (i) studies should be reviewed and administered according to guidelines applicable to other research.

GENE TRANSFER TERMS AND DEFINITIONS

DNA. Deoxyribonucleic acid (DNA) is the chemical structure making up the genome of higher organisms. It consists of four molecular subunits (bases), known as A, G, T, and C. These bases form chains that are paired to make a double-stranded molecule that takes the shape of a helix. The base pairing allows for DNA replication during cell division, and thus DNA serves as the means of transmitting information from cell to cell during development and reproduction (heredity). Most adult cells ae diploid, meaning they contain two full copies of the organism's DNA.

Gamete. The germ cell of an organism (sperm in human males, eggs or ova in human females). Gametes are haploid, containing half the full number of chromosomes needed to form a functional cell.

Gene. A segment of DNA, located on a chromosome, that directs cellular functions, ultimately contributing to physical traits, and is the basic unit of heredity.

Gene transfer. The process of introducing a gene into a cell, either a gene isolated or copied from a host cell, or created or altered in the lab. Gene transfer requires identification and isolation (or creation) of the gene in question, incorporating it into a vector to allow entry into the recipient cell, and (if used in vivo) a means of targeting the recipient cell. Sometimes this is referred to as horizontal gene transfer, to distinguish it from vertical gene transfer, or the transmission of genes from parent to offspring.

Gene editing. The process of mechanically altering a gene (or the genome, if the alteration is heritable) of a living organism.

Genome. The entire genetic material of an organism, found in each cell and gamete of an organism. The human genome comprises more than 3 billion base pairs of DNA.

Germline. Pertaining to the germ cells (gametes) of an organism. Genes (natural or altered) in the germline are transmitted to offspring during reproduction. Nongermline cells are known as somatic cells.

In vivo. Occurring within a living organism.

In vitro. Literally, "in glass." Occurring in a laboratory setting, in a petri dish, or otherwise outside a living organism.

Recombinant DNA. DNA which has been altered using biotechnology, most often used to refer to a DNA segment or gene that has been inserted into a vector prior to gene transfer.

Somatic. Cells of the organism that are not part of the germline.

Vector. DNA that is used as a carrier for gene transfer, often constructed in the lab from viral or bacterial segments of DNA that have natural abilities to enter cells. A vector combined with DNA for transfer is known as recombinant DNA.

CHIMERIC ANTIGEN RECEPTOR T CELL (CAR-T) THERAPY

CAR-T immunotherapy is used to treat recurring malignant cancer. In this approach, a patient's own T cells (immune system cells) are harvested and engineered to express a tumor cell–targeting receptor (Gomes-Silva & Ramos, 2018; Tariq et al., 2018). These constructs are referred to as "chimeric" to reflect the fact that the hybrid antigen receptors produced are derived from a variety of DNA segments spliced together. When reinfused, the chimeric-receptor T cells can then attack and eliminate residual tumor cells. The IRB may be concerned with possible subsequent toxicities, such as cytokine release syndrome and potential autoimmune attack of normal issues, which, although severe, generally can be managed (Liu et al., 2017). FDA has approved the use of several CAR-T therapeutic protocols (Liu et al., 2017; Zheng et al., 2018).

(ii) Studies in which the subjects' cells are harvested, undergo in vitro gene transfer and selection, and are then returned to the subject. This is low risk from a gene transfer perspective (i.e., independent of other risks, such as from the procedures involved in cell harvesting).

For category (ii) studies, the IRB should ask researchers to provide evidence that the vector is safe and effective and that procedures manipulating the human cells meet Food and Drug Administration (FDA) cell processing regulations (e.g., good manufacturing procedure requirements). In circumstances where there may be concerns that cells could transform, or become tumorigenic when returned in vivo, a suicide vector (one that cannot replicate after transfer to the host) could potentially be employed to counter the risk. The therapeutic use of these cells should be for a condition that is serious and cannot be adequately treated by an alternative approach (see sidebar Chimeric Antigen Receptor T Cell (Car-T) Therapy, for example).

(iii) Studies that deliver a gene transfer vector in vivo to a subject. Based on past research, this is most likely a moderate risk situation.

For category (iii) studies, in order to demonstrate safety and efficiency of the vector, it is recommended that large animal model or prior human use studies demonstrate that the vector-transduced cells do not cause life-threatening inflammatory/immune reactions or off-target effects and that the risk of subsequent malignancy is very low. The target disease should be very serious, with no alternative therapies, and a safety monitoring program should be in place. Examples of this type of research are ongoing studies of somatic gene therapy for sickle cell disease (Ribeil et al., 2017); hemophilia (Nathwani et al., 2017; Pipe, 2018); beta-hemoglobinopathies (Cavazzana et al., 2017; Karponi & Zogas, 2019); and other nonmalignant hematological diseases (Beck, 2019).

(iv) Germline gene manipulation. Because of currently unknown long-term risks, this is a very high-risk procedure and currently would be considered very controversial. Such research should not be undertaken without careful review of any applicable current regulations, guidance, and debate on this topic.

Any consideration of a category (iv) study to manipulate germline DNA in vivo should be approached with utmost caution and with reference to any federal, state, or other regulations or rules. See previous section on Regulation of Recombinant DNA for references to current and forthcoming international guidance.

CATEGORIES OF GENE TRANSFER RESEARCH

Risk estimates for gene transfer research based on prior research and trial outcomes:

(i) Situations where human cells are employed in vitro for gene transfer with no intent to transfer them back to a human subject: Low risk.

(ii) Studies in which the subject's cells are harvested, undergo in vitro gene transfer and selection, and are then returned to the subject: Low risk.

(iii) Studies that deliver a gene transfer vector in vivo to a subject: Moderate risk.

(iv) Germline gene manipulation: High risk.

Stem Cells

Introduction

Stem cells (see Box, Stem Cells Concepts and Terms) are of great interest for research and development of potential therapies, both because of their ability to renew and their ability to give rise to different specialized cells and tissues (Dulak et al., 2015; Eaves, 2015). Research with human (and other mammalian) stem cells holds promise for many disorders previously thought untreatable, such as neurological injury or illness affecting the brain and spinal cord (Assinck et al., 2017; Cox, 2018). However, because these cells and their derivative cell lines often originate in embryonic or fetal tissue, their use is controversial and the regulatory landscape surrounding this research is dynamic. This section begins with a general overview of the relevant scientific background and terms, followed by separate sections addressing issues unique to research with adult stem cells, fetal tissue–derived cells, embryonic stem cells, and induced pluripotent stem cells.

Regulation and Guidelines

In the United States and internationally, laws and regulations governing the isolation and uses of these cells and their derivative cell lines vary from place to place and over time. In general, three organizations have created guidelines for appropriate research use of embryonic stem cells: The National Institutes of Health (NIH), the National Academy of Sciences (NAS), and the International Society for Stem Cell Research (ISSCR). NAS has recommended forming an institutional ESCRO committee to review and monitor the creation and use of embryonic stem cells (ESCs) in research (Institute of Medicine and National Research Council [IOM & NRC], 2010). In 2019, there are no corresponding guidelines or regulations regarding stem cells of nonembryonic origin, although there are national accrediting bodies that oversee nonembryonic stem cell harvest, production, processing, and use. In the United States, this oversight is maintained by the Foundation for the Accreditation of Cellular Therapies (see FACT-JACIE, 2018); there are similar bodies in Europe and Australia. In reviewing any protocols utilizing stem cells, it is critical to consult current guidelines from any relevant organizations, as well as current local and federal regulations and guidance.

STEM CELL CONCEPTS AND TERMS

- *Differentiation and potency.* The process by which a single fertilized egg (a zygote) becomes an embryo, a fetus, and eventually a complex, multicellular adult organism, is one of cell proliferation (by division) and differentiation. The most undifferentiated cell type is the single-cell zygote, which has the ability to generate all the specialized cell types in the mature body. The potential to give rise to various specialized cell types is referred to as potency, and the zygote, which can divide to generate all the cells of the embryo as well as the placenta, is considered totipotent. Once the zygote begins to divide, its offspring begin to differentiate, so that cells further along the developmental pathway have more limited potency. Embryonic stem cells (ESCs) can be harvested from human embryos approximately 5 days after fertilization, and are pluripotent, since they can give rise to all cell types of the body except the placenta.

Other types of stem cells isolated from various stages of differentiated tissue may be pluripotent, or may be able to give rise to a more limited variety of differentiated cell types (multipotent), or they may be terminally differentiated.

■ The zygote is a stem cell, since when it divides it not only creates daughter cells that go on to differentiate, but it renews itself. In humans, stem cells (of various potency, but not totipotent) are also found in the fetus, the bone marrow, and in a limited number of adult tissues. Human ESCs can be isolated from excess embryos previously created by in vitro fertilization (IVF) for reproduction and designated for research. Stem cells for research purposes can also be created in vitro, either by IVF or by somatic cell nuclear transfer (SCNT; also known as research, therapeutic, or reproductive cloning). In some cases, specialized cells can be induced in vitro to dedifferentiate (or be "reprogrammed") into a state of greater potency (induced human pluripotent stem [iPS] cells).

■ *Sources and types of stem cells.* The source of stem cells is important not only for scientific reasons, but because there are a number of ethical and political issues surrounding this work. Historically, pluripotent stem cells could only be obtained from an embryo or from the germline of a fetus. Some object to these sources, because harvesting these cells necessarily destroys the embryo or fetus. Excess embryos from IVF procedures may be designated for research purposes, but some find this objectionable, just as some find the creation of embryos specifically for research purposes to be unacceptable.

Stem Cells: Adult Stem Cells

Introduction

Most human stem cell studies have employed "adult stem cells," which exclude stem cells of fetal or embryonic origin but include stem cells harvested from children and umbilical cord blood (Dulak, 2015). Although there are some differences in the consent and harvesting of adult, child, and cord blood stem cells, their uses are well developed, very similar, and generally noncontroversial (with some relatively rare religious objections). Transplantation of hematopoietic (blood-forming) stem cells in the treatment of cancers such as leukemia and lymphoma is a well-established use of adult stem cells (Thomas, 1999).

Significant challenges in stem cell transplantation can arise from tissue antigen mismatches (Petersdorf, 2017). Human leukocyte antigen (HLA) proteins are normally expressed on the surface of cells, and each individual's HLA profile is recognized by their immune system. When stem cells or other tissues are transplanted from one host to another, an HLA (or "histocompatibility") mismatch can trigger attack by host immune cells (Dupont, 1997). Thus, tissue typing and HLA matching of donor stem cells to the recipient is important, and (often) treatment of the recipient is required to reduce rejection. If the tissue match is imperfect and immunosuppression of the recipient inadequate, the grafted (transplanted) stem cells may be rejected by the host (Ozdemir & Civriz Bozdaq, 2018).

In extreme cases, the opposite situation can occur, in which immune cells in the graft may recognize the host as foreign and react against their tissues. This is known as graft versus host disease (GVHD), which can be serious or fatal (Ghimire et al., 2017). Methods to eliminate, reduce, or treat GVHD are active topics of research reviewed by the IRB.

IRB Review of Studies Involving Adult Stem Cells

Stem cell treatments and research are novel, evolving, and unique in their use in extremely ill subjects and healthy donors. Consequently, IRBs reviewing such studies should include clinicians/scientists with experience relevant to such situations and should be aware of the following issues:

- *Multicenter research.* Frequently, in order to enroll a sufficient number of subjects (especially for rare conditions), research studies and trials will be multisite and may involve <u>international collaborations</u>. A potential issue in such studies, from an IRB perspective, is the standardization of risk/benefit analyses across multiple IRBs in a number of countries. Increasingly, there may be merit in employing a <u>single overarching IRB</u>. Another issue concerns controversies that have arisen regarding fast tracking of approvals (for example, of regenerative medicine procedures in Japan; Cyranoski, 2019a).   🔗 10-9   🔗 Section 4

- *Consent and assent.* The subjects of these studies and trials may be critically ill <u>pediatric</u> patients; the subjects and their parents need to fully understand complicated, technically novel procedures in order to <u>consent</u> or provide assent.   🔗 9-6   🔗 Section 6

- *Donors.* Often, these protocols involve invasive procedures on healthy donors, including children.

- *Privacy.* There may be serious <u>privacy concerns</u> raised by tissue typing. For example, many subjects may not have the parents they think they have (Bellis et al., 2005).   🔗 12-1

- *Toxicity.* Stem cell studies involve treatment of subjects who have serious, life-threating disease. Potential complications of stem cell use include serious toxicity, which may be life threatening. Consequently, an accurate, documented benefit/risk analysis is key to effective IRB review of such proposals.

Although these discussions focus largely on hematopoietic stem cell transplantation, research on the broader use of stem cells is also growing rapidly (Trounson & McDonald, 2015). Attempts are being made to isolate cells with stem cell-like features from other tissues such as fat (adipose/mesenchymal tissue; Mushahary et al., 2018; A. Wilson et al., 2019) and placental tissue (Parolini et al., 2008). Clinical trials using various cell types have been initiated to treat myocardial infarcts and heart failure (Michler, 2018; Yu et al., 2017); to treat eye diseases (Mead et al., 2015; Park et al., 2017; Tang et al., 2017); to repair damaged cartilage in joints (McIntyre et al., 2018); to treat brain and spinal cord injuries (Kamelska-Sadoweska et al., 2019); and to reverse GVHD (Zhao et al., 2019). IRBs should be prepared to carefully and critically review research protocols that might address the application of a wide range of human adult stem cell types for a variety of clinical applications.

Nonapproved Uses of Stem Cells

Excitement surrounding the potential uses of stem cell therapies is being exploited by some practitioners, at a significant cost to patients, in procedures that have not been approved by FDA (Fu et al., 2019). IRBs should be aware of the proliferation of unregulated clinics that offer stem cell therapies for profit (Cyranoski, 2019b; Turner & Knoepfler, 2016). A review by Knoepfler (2018) identified over 500 such clinics in the United States in 2018; this information was updated in 2019 (Knoepfler, 2019). A wide range of conditions are advertised as treatable, including knee pain, neuropathy, back pain, joint pain, osteoarthritis, retinal degeneration, and autism. In 2019, FDA began enforcement actions to close a "stem cell center" in Florida where clients who had poor vision were blinded after bilateral injection of stem cells into their eyes (Kuriyan et al., 2017; Rodriguez, 2017). Treatments for back and joint pain at similar facilities in Texas, Arizona, and Florida were associated with the development of severe bacterial infections in over a dozen clients injected with a stem cell product (Taylor, 2018). In all of these cases there is little or no evidence of efficacy, and neither the procedures nor the products used had FDA approval. IRBs should be aware of similar activities in their region and potential involvement by practitioners that they regulate. In early 2019, Kaiser Health News noted that some major health centers, citing FDA exceptions, were promoting such therapies (Szabo, 2019).

Stem Cells: Fetal Tissue Stem Cells

Introduction

Fetal tissue stem cell research is currently a limited niche activity. An important rationale for this area of research is that some tissue stem cell populations only appear to be present in the fetus. An example is brain microglia, which cannot be derived from adult hematopoietic stem cells or cord blood stem cells; their origins are unique to fetal tissue. Similarly, primordial germ cells are only found in fetal tissue (De Miguel et al., 2009). A major challenge to this work is obtaining fetal tissues in a charged and changing political environment, where there may be federal and state initiatives to prevent fetal tissue research or a ban on funding for it (Frieden, 2018; Leask, 2017; Reardon, 2019b).

IRB Review of Studies Involving Fetal Tissue Stem Cells

⊘ Section 6

On receipt of a proposal to perform research utilizing human fetal tissue, IRB administrators should verify that the cells or tissue were obtained with appropriate <u>informed consent</u> and without inappropriate financial incentives or payments. Restrictions on the use of human fetal tissue obtained from elective abortions may apply to federally funded research (NIH, 2019b). In some cases, fetal tissue or cells can be obtained from commercial suppliers, which may or may not have obtained (or be distributing) the material appropriately.

🧠 CASE STUDY: CELLS AS THERAPY

A research protocol was submitted to an IRB proposing to evaluate a new drug therapy. An alert member of the IRB noted that the drug was, in fact, a fetal neuronal precursor cell. In some circumstances (for example, if such a cell secretes a therapeutic product) FDA permits classification of the cell as a drug. The protocol sponsor obtained the fetal cells from a commercial source. The IRB asked the supplier to provide evidence of consent (which was provided) together with a summary of fees charged. In addition to fees for processing and distribution (which are legitimate) there was a fee for "tissue acquisition." When the IRB asked for details on this point, they were informed that this information was proprietary. Consequently, the IRB could not be sure that the acquisition of these cells met appropriate regulations and, ultimately, the protocol was not approved and was subsequently withdrawn.

IRB administrators may wish to be proactive and identify approvable fetal tissue suppliers in advance of receiving any proposals and make this information available to their researchers. When reviewing submitted protocols that utilize an approvable supplier, the IRB will need to ensure that the funding source permits fetal tissue research and any state restrictions are met. Once those criteria are met, then standard IRB review may take place prior to approval.

Stem Cells: Embryonic Stem Cells

Introduction

Embryonic stem cells are derived primarily from the inner cell mass of the blastocyst stage embryo (**Figure 10.14-2**), approximately 4 to 5 days after fertilization of the oocyte (Pera et al., 2000; Yee, 2010). Other methods of derivation include somatic cell nuclear transfer (Markoulaki et al., 2008) or activation of cell division of oocytes without fertilization (parthenogenesis; Brevini & Gandolfi, 2008). Mouse embryonic stem cells were first derived in the early 1980s; these cells have become critical tools to study embryonic development and cell biology (Saunders, 2020). These developments led to the production of transgenic and gene knockout mice, which are important tools to devise new therapeutic approaches to treatment of diseases. More recently, these technologies have been extended to pigs (Xu et al., 2019) and primates (Thomson et al., 1995).

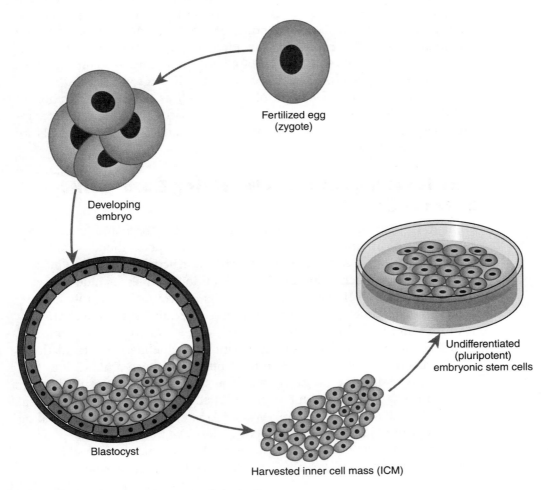

Figure 10.14-2 Embryonic stem cell derivation.

It was technologically challenging to replicate these studies using human cells, but in 1998, researchers at the University of Wisconsin (using excess embryos from in vitro fertilization procedures and at Johns Hopkins University (using discarded fetal tissue) were able to develop human embryonic stem cell (hESC) lines (Shamblott et al., 1998; Thomson et al., 1998). Subsequently, many hESC lines have been developed by other investigators. Culture procedures have been developed that permit these cells to proliferate (self-renew) so that they maintain their ability to generate all tissue types of the embryo without differentiation. When hESC lines are maintained in this undifferentiated state, the cells can be manipulated in a variety of ways, such as the application of various cell differentiation signals or by gene editing. This permits analysis of the roles of various signals and genes in maintenance of the undifferentiated state, or, if the line is allowed or induced to differentiate, developmental pathways can be investigated. Cell lines that represent disease states can be employed to evaluate the effectiveness of gene replacement or other potentially therapeutic options and can potentially be used for diseased cell replacement (Ilic & Ogilvie, 2017).

Embryonic Stem Cell Derivation

Human ESC lines are primarily derived from excess blastocyst-stage embryos created for in vitro fertilization procedures (see Figure 10.14-2). These embryos can be donated for research with written informed consent from the parents, as long as no reimbursement or financial incentive is provided for donation (IOM & NRC, 2010). Generally, the attending physician obtaining consent should be independent of the researcher proposing to use the donated cells. The cells should be identified by an anonymized (coded) identifier to protect the identity of the donor. Additional recommendations are outlined in appendix C of the NAS report (IOM & NRC, 2010). There are other methods of generation of hESC, such as SCNT or activation of cell division in oocytes without fertilization (parthenogenesis). These approaches are less commonly employed, but generally, the same regulatory requirements apply.

IRB Review of Studies Involving Embryonic Stem Cells

From an IRB perspective, a major issue is that the embryo and fetus cannot give informed consent. Individuals who believe that personhood is conferred at conception or those uncomfortable with destruction of human embryos may object to the derivation of hESCs. Additional issues include concerns that the use of fetal tissues for research might encourage or justify elective abortions. Consequently, research with these cells and tissues is a controversial topic, and IRB administrators need to be aware of community concerns as well as local, regional, state, and national guidelines and regulations. Within this framework, research in the United States using hESC lines that are on an NIH-approved registry (see details later) and that meets all other

🖉 5-4   IRB approval criteria can be approved and is eligible for funding from federal sources. Note that the U.S. Dickey-Wicker Amendment bans federal funding of research in which a human embryo is destroyed (with the exception of the approved cell lines mentioned previously), and some nonfederal funding sources exclude research on hESC. See later for further details on regulatory issues.

When the IRB receives a protocol proposing research involving hESCs, it is recommended that the following checklist be consulted. The rationale for these guidelines is described in more detail in subsequent sections.

(i)   Check that the researchers have the appropriate skills and training (such as that provided by a relevant online course) to conduct hESC research.

(ii)   Review federal law and regulations governing hESC research.

This includes consulting the NIH website (nih.gov) to determine if the hESC line(s) to be employed are listed as approved. This is especially relevant if the research proposal is associated with federal government funding sources such as NIH or the Department of Defense. Research that involves human embryonic stem cells or cell lines not listed on the NIH registry may not be approvable (e.g., documentation of consent might not be available or sufficient; it may not be possible to confirm the lack of financial incentives). In addition, nonregistered cell lines may not qualify for use in projects supported by federal funds or be used in laboratories with equipment purchased using federal funds (or certain other funding sources). Note also that although federal regulations have largely been stable over the decade from 2009 to 2019, this is a dynamic and politically charged topic, so it is important to confirm the current regulations and guidance.

(iii)   Check whether a materials transfer agreement (MTA) is required for the hESC line(s) and (if, according to institutional policy, review of MTAs is the IRB's responsibility) whether limitations of use are cited or annual reports of use are required (see Davey et al., 2015).

(iv)   Check that the proposed hESC use also meets state and institutional laws/regulations. Although the majority of institutions follow federal regulations, some states and institutional governing bodies have additional laws and/or regulations.

(v)   For approved hESC lines, the general principles of IRB review (including risk/benefit analyses, confidentiality, etc.) apply.

(vi)   Potentially, the proposed research might employ a newly developed hESC line. For example, an hESC line may have been derived to represent a specific disease genotype or phenotype, and such a cell line might not yet have been registered with NIH.

In this situation, research employing this cell line might be approvable, but the approval process would have to ensure that development of the line followed appropriate procedures. Minimally, this includes voluntary donation with informed consent and an absence of financial incentives. It should be recommended that the investigators seek federal registration; this is a requirement for the use of federal funds for this research.

(vii)   Implantation of hESCs into animals other than humans or primates (for example, immunodeficient mice, in order to study cell differentiation), requires additional review (likely in concert with Institutional Animal Care and Use Committee [IACUC] review). No animal into which hESCs have been introduced should be allowed to breed (IOM & NRC, 2010).

(viii)   If the proposal includes using hESC lines for creation of cells for potential transplantation to human subjects, additional careful and thorough review is required.

Such uses pose significant challenges and concerns regarding issues such as histocompatibility matching of cells to potential recipients and risks of tumorigenesis of cells derived from hESC (Blum & Benvenisty, 2008). Although hESC cells that have differentiated can no longer self-renew, it is possible that a tumor could develop from a single cell retaining this ability. To overcome some of these problems, interest has shifted toward the use of induced pluripotent stem cells (iPSC) for research leading to transplantation into human subjects (see the section, Stem Cells: Induced Pluripotent Stem Cells, later).

(ix)   hESC research in which hESC are introduced into nonhuman primate blastocysts or a human blastocyst may be subject to additional regulation (in 2019, these projects should not be permitted or approved; IOM & NRC, 2010; ISSCR, 2016). Japan allows hybrid human-animal embryo research (Cyranoski, 2019c).

CHECKLIST FOR IRB REVIEW OF RESEARCH INVOLVING HUMAN EMBRYONIC STEM CELLS*

(i)   Check that the researchers have the appropriate skills and training to conduct hESC research.
(ii)   Review federal law and regulations governing hESC research, and ensure that any acquisition of embryos/embryonic stem cells meets guidelines for donation of embryos.
(iii)   Check whether a MTA is required for the hESC line(s) and whether limitations of use are cited or annual reports of use are required.
(iv)   Check that the proposed hESC use meets state and institutional laws/regulations.
(v)   For approved hESC lines, apply general principles of IRB review (including risk/benefit analyses, confidentiality, etc.).
(vi)   For proposed research that employs a newly developed hESC line, check that appropriate procedures were followed.
(vii)   For implantation of hESC into animals other than humans or primates, ensure appropriate additional reviews (likely in concert with IACUC review).
(viii) For research proposals that include using hESC lines for creation of cells for potential transplantation to human subjects, conduct additional careful and thorough review.
(ix)   For research in which hESC are introduced into nonhuman primate blastocysts or a human blastocyst, consult any applicable additional regulations.

*Note that some of these items may fall outside of the IRB's responsibility, depending on institutional policy.

Stem Cells: Induced Pluripotent Cells

Introduction

In 2006, Shinya Yamanaka and colleagues discovered that transferring just four growth-regulating genes to adult somatic cells such as fibroblasts could reprogram those cells to exhibit embryonic stem cell–like properties, including the potential to differentiate (under defined circumstances) to all types of cells of the body (Takahashi et al., 2007; Yamanaka, 2008). They called these "dedifferentiated" cells induced pluripotent stem cells (iPSCs).

Reprogramming of adult somatic cells to iPSCs not only avoids the controversies of using embryonic or fetal tissues, but also potentially bypasses the challenges of the need for histocompatibility matching of donor cells for therapy, because the donor can be autologous (i.e., the recipient donates their own cells). It does not obviate the challenges of correcting a genetic defect, because the iPSC will carry this defect. However, if combined with gene transfer/gene editing, this technology offers a new therapeutic avenue for subjects with serious diseases and has become an important component of regenerative medicine research. It is likely that IRBs will see an increasing number of such projects in years to come.

IRB Review of Research with Induced Pluripotent Cells

iPSC research is not subject to many of the regulatory aspects (or controversies) of hESC research; however, the risks for human subjects fall into similar categories.

For example, since iPSCs are not terminally differentiated, they have the potential to form a type of tumor called a teratoma when transplanted in vivo (Fong et al., 2010; Peterson et al., 2012; Simonson et al., 2015). These tumors carry similar risks to tumors arising from hESC transfer. Therefore, the same four categories of risk/benefit evaluation proposed for hESC research are recommended for iPSC review (in 2019), and similar cautions about germline transfer in animals and humans apply. As this technology advances, built-in safety elements may alleviate or minimize risks; conversely, new discoveries may present new risks.

CATEGORIES OF GENE TRANSFER RESEARCH USING IPSC

Risk estimates for gene transfer research using iPSC based on prior research and trial outcomes:

(i)   Situations where human cells are employed in vitro for gene transfer with no intent to transfer them back to a human subject: Low risk.

(ii) Studies in which the subject's cells are harvested, undergo in vitro gene transfer and selection, and are then returned to the subject: Low risk.

(iii) Studies that deliver a gene transfer vector in vivo to a subject: Moderate risk.

(iv) Germline gene manipulation: High risk.

Human Embryo Research

Introduction

As noted previously, any research involving human embryos is controversial for a variety of reasons, including the fact that the embryo cannot consent to be a research subject. However, donors of eggs and sperm provided for in vitro fertilization can donate embryos that are determined to be in excess (or abnormal) under carefully designated circumstances. Guidelines issued in 1994 by the Human Embryo Research Panel convened by NIH recommended permitting the creation of embryos for research (rather than for reproduction) under restricted circumstances. However, subsequent regulatory actions have limited this activity (see Sidebar, Regulation, Registry, and Guidance for hESC Research).

REGULATION, REGISTRY, AND GUIDANCE FOR hESC RESEARCH

Regulations governing the development and federal funding of hESC lines have changed several times since their original derivation in 1998. Consequently, IRB administrators should be aware of a brief history of the regulations for use of hESC lines, so that they can prepare to respond to changes that may arise. Alternatively, they might delegate this responsibility to the chair of their ESCRO/SROC committees.

On August 9, 2001, U.S. President Bush announced a policy that restricted funding of research to the use of existing hESC lines and banned (in the United States) federal support for derivation of new hESC lines.

In the early 2000s, there was considerable growth in stem cell research and in the understanding and treatment of human disease. ISSCR was formed, and became a "clearinghouse" for stem cell research topics and terminology. Concerns arose regarding the validity of informed consent for some of the hESC lines included in President Bush's executive order and about the appropriateness of some proposed research procedures, such as human reproductive cloning. Consequently, ISSCR convened a task force that issued "Guidelines for the Conduct of Human Embryonic Stem Cell Research, Version 1" on December 21, 2006. This document, and the "Guidelines for Human Embryonic Stem Cell Research" issued in 2005 from the National Academy of Sciences, were widely adopted as an effective set of guidelines by most stem cell scientists worldwide.

On March 9, 2009, President Obama issued a new executive order (E013505) "Removing Barriers to Responsible Scientific Research Involving Human Stem Cells." This rescinded the prior restrictions issued by President Bush, but left in place the Dickey-Wicker Amendment that prohibits the use of federal funds to derive new hESC lines (although other sources of funds could be used).

The 2009 executive order directed NIH to review its guidelines and the updated "National Institutes of Health Guidelines for Human Stem Cell Research" were issued on July 7, 2009. This led to the creation of a new registry of hESC lines eligible for NIH funding that is updated regularly. Note that this registry does not include some of the earlier cell lines for which concerns were raised or which could not be routinely maintained in culture or had other abnormalities.

In 2010, NAS updated its 2005 Guidelines and issued the "Final Report of the National Academies' Human Embryonic Stem Cell Research Advisory Committee and 2010 Amendments to the National Academies' Guidelines for Human Embryonic Stem Cell Research" (https://nas-sites.org/stemcells/national-academies-guidelines). These guidelines, which include the recommendation for ESCRO committees to supplement IRB reviews of hESC research, have been adopted by most major research institutions in the United States.

In 2016, ISSCR released a broader document on stem cell research, "Guidelines for Stem Cell Research and Clinical Translation" (www.isscr.org/policy/guidelines-for-stem-cell-research-and-clinical-translation). It includes sections on pluripotent stem cell lines, stem cell repositories, animal models, clinical translation of stem cell-based research, stem cell manufacturing, chemical trials, off-label uses of stem cell-based interventions, and marketing of unproven stem cell therapies.

Examples of Potentially Controversial Research

IRB administrators should be aware that some areas of human embryo research are especially controversial, whereas other activities are more accepted by the public. In conjunction with in vitro fertilization procedures, the use of preimplantation genetic diagnosis of embryos, in which a single cell of the blastocyst is removed and evaluated for genetic evidence of a serious disease, has become common for couples where the risk of such a disease in their offspring is high (Imudia & Plosker, 2016). If the genetic defect involves a single gene, the selection of a healthy embryo for implantation (discarding embryos that will be affected) has led to successful outcomes. More recently, attempts to extend such procedures to screen embryos for implantation on the basis of risks or traits other than serious disease are more controversial (LeMieux, 2019).

Many disorders and traits (such as diabetes or obesity) involve the interaction of multiple genes. In theory, this information can be obtained by genome analysis and converted into a "risk score" (Loos & Janssens, 2017). Additionally—and also, in theory—genomic information could be used to predict specific traits, such as intelligence, in embryos. The science behind such predictions is not yet valid or robust, and many ethicists and investigators are uncomfortable with this approach, especially as a basis for embryo selection (Karavani et al., 2019). This is an illustration of one of the many future challenges with which IRBs will need to wrestle, and for which guidelines issued at a national (or international) level may be needed.

A variation on somatic cell nuclear transfer, mitochondrial replacement therapy, involves the creation of triparental embryos for the purposes of (healthy) reproduction. In this process, nuclear DNA from the mother's egg is transferred to an unaffected surrogate's egg from which the nucleus was removed. The resulting oocyte (containing the mother's nuclear DNA, and the surrogate's mitochondria) is fertilized with the father's sperm. Because the sperm contribute negligible mitochondrial DNA to the zygote, the resulting embryo has the mother's and father's nuclear DNA and the surrogate's mitochondrial DNA (Mullen, 2019a). In 2015, the UK Fertilisation and Embryology Authority approved the creation of triparental embryos for situations where the mother might pass on a mitochondrial genetic defect (Grant, 2015; UK Draft Statutory Instruments, 2015). Other recent uses of the technique in the Ukraine and Greece have shown promise as an infertility treatment, especially for older women (Mullen, 2019a). In the United States, research on this procedure would be ineligible for federal funding because of the Dickey-Wicker Amendment and may be prohibited by state or local regulations. Moreover, use of the technique for treatment of mitochondrial disease in the United States is prevented by a 2015 provision in the annual federal appropriations law that prohibits FDA from accepting applications for clinical research using mitochondrial replacement therapy (FDA, 2018). This provision is the target of protests and planned appeals to Congress for clearer interpretation (Mullen, 2019b). If this technology were to become the clinical standard of care, however, rather than a research procedure, it might be approvable in certain U.S. jurisdictions, even where this could not be approved by the IRB as a research protocol.

IRB Review of Human Embryo Research

Research involving human embryos may be approved by IRBs, provided that such research is approved by an appropriately constituted ESCRO committee (see guidelines, IOM & NRC, 2010; ISSCR, 2016). Note that state or local regulations may not permit some research procedures that are allowed under ISSCR guidelines, so these regulations must also be followed. Restrictions on associating human and nonhuman blastocysts and breeding animals with human germline contributions would apply in all jurisdictions. IRB administrators would need to research the specific regulations that apply to human embryo research at the locale of the proposed research.

🧠 CASE STUDY: STATE-SPECIFIC REGULATIONS

The National Academy of Sciences Advisory Committee (2010) recommendations (Appendix C) section 1.3 notes that "research involving *in vitro* culture of any intact human embryo, regardless of derivation method, for longer than 14 days or until formation of the primitive streak begins, whichever occurs first" should not be permitted. Cultures and embryos, under these guidelines, must be terminated by this time. However, the state of Nebraska, by law (LB 606) does not permit the destruction of embryos for research or their creation by somatic cell nuclear transfer. Therefore, the NAS Committee recommendations would conflict with Nebraska state law, so an IRB in Nebraska could not approve such research. However, such research may be legal in other states/jurisdictions. It is important to note that some state laws might impact human embryo research, even if that is not the primary focus of the law. For example, laws that confer personhood on the embryo are likely to conflict with more permissible regulations and guidelines.

Acknowledgments

JGS acknowledges the advice and input over many years from multiple members of the UNMC ESCRO, now SROC, especially representatives of the community and religious organizations and its administrator, Susannah Logsdon. Support of research from the State of Nebraska to the Pediatric Cancer Research Group (Director D. Coulter, MD) of the Child Health Research institute of UNMC/Children's Hospital is gratefully acknowledged.

References

Assinck, P., Duncan, G. J., Hilton, B. J., Plemel, J. R., & Tetzlaff, W. (2017). Cell transplantation therapy for spinal cord injury. *Nat Neurosci, 20*(5), 637–647.

Beck, D. L. (2019). What does the future hold for gene therapy in nonmalignant hematology? *Focus on Classical Hematology, 5*(12.1), 11–13. www.ashclinicalnews.org/spotlight/future-hold-gene-therapy-nonmalignant-hematology/

Bellis, M. A., Hughes, K., Hughes, S., & Ashton, J. R. (2005). Measuring paternal discrepancy and its public health consequences. *J Epidemiol Community Health, 59*(9), 749–754.

Bessis, N., Garcia-Cozar, F. J., & Boissier, M. C. (2004). Immune responses to gene therapy vectors: Influence on vector function and effector mechanisms. *Gene Ther, 11*(Suppl 1), S10–S17.

Blum, B., & Benvenisty, N. (2008). The tumorigenicity of human embryonic stem cells. *Adv Cancer Res, 100*, 133–158.

Brevini, T. A., & Gandolfi, F. (2008). Parthenotes as a source of embryonic stem cells. *Cell Prolif, 41*(Suppl 1), 20–30.

Brokowski, C., (2018). Do CRISPR germline ethics statements cut it? *The CRISPR Journal, 1*(2), 115–125. https://doi.org/10.1089/crispr.2017.0024

Caplan, A. (2019). Getting serious about the challenge of regulating germline gene therapy. *PLoS Biology, 17*(4), e3000223.

Cavazzana, M., Antoniani, C., & Miccio, A. (2017). Gene therapy for b-hemoglobinopathies. *Mol Ther, 25*(5), 1142–1154.

Chan, S., & Sternberg, S. (Eds.). (2019). The ethics of human genome editing. *The CRISPR Journal, 2*(5), 247–330. https://home.liebertpub.com/publications/the-crispr-journal/642

Cipolla, D. C., Gonda, I., Shak, S., Kovesdi, I., Crystal, R., & Sweeney, T. D. (2000). Coarse spray delivery to a localized region of the pulmonary airways for gene therapy. *Hum Gene Ther, 11*(2), 361–371.

Cox, C. S. (2018). Cellular therapy for traumatic neurological injury. *Pediatr Res, 83*(1–2), 325–332.

Cyranoski, D. (2019a). The potent effects of Japan's stem-cell policies. *Nature, 573*, 482–485.

Cyranoski, D. (2019b). Chinese hospitals set to sell experimental cell therapies. *Nature, 569*, 170–171.

Cyranoski, D. (2019c, 26 July). Japan approves first human-animal embryo experiments. *Nature.* www.nature.com/articles/d41586-019-02275-3

Davey, S., Davey, N., Gu, Q., Xu, N., Vatsa, R., Devalaraja, S., Harris, P., Gannavaram, S., Dave, R., & Chakrabarty, A. (2015). Interfacing of science, medicine and law: The stem cell patent controversy in the United States and the European Union. *Front Cell Dev Biol 3*, 71.

De Miguel, M. P., Arnalich Montiel, F., Lopez Iglesias, P., Blazquez Martinez, A., & Nistal, M. (2009). Epiblast-derived stem cells in embryonic and adult tissues. *Int J Dev Biol, 53*(8–10), 1529–1540.

Dismuke, D. J., Tenenbaum, L., & Samulski, R. J. (2013). Biosafety of recombinant adeno-associated virus vectors. *Curr Gene Ther, 13*(6), 434–452.

Dulak, J., Szade, K., Szade, A., Nowak, W., & Józkowicz, A. (2015). Adult stem cells: Hopes and hypes of regenerative medicine. *Acta Biochim Pol, 62*(3), 329–337.

Dupont, B. (1997). Immunology of hematopoietic stem cell transplantation: A brief review of its history. *Immunol Rev, 157*, 5–12.

Eaves, C. J. (2015). Hematopoietic stem cells: Concepts, definitions and the new reality. *Blood, 125*(17), 2605–2613.

FACT-JACIE. (2018). *FACT-JACIE international standards for hematopoietic cellular therapy product collection, processing and administration* (7th ed.). Foundation for the Accreditation of Cellular Therapy and the Joint Accreditation Committee. www.factweb.org

Ferrua, F., & Aiuti, A. (2017). Twenty-five years of gene therapy for ADA-SCID: From bubble babies to an approved drug. *Hum Gene Ther, 28*(11), 972–981.

Fong, C. Y., Gauthaman, K., & Bongso, A. (2010). Teratomas from pluripotent stem cells: A clinical hurdle. *J Cell Biochem, 111*(4), 769–781.

Food and Drug Administration (FDA). (2018). Advisory on legal restrictions on the use of mitochondrial replacement techniques to introduce donor mitochondria into reproductive cells intended for transfer into a human recipient. www.fda.gov/vaccines-blood-biologics/cellular -gene-therapy-products/advisory-legal-restrictions-use-mitochondrial-replacement-techniques -introduce-donor-mitochondria

Frieden, J. (2018, Dec. 13). House members wrangle over fetal tissue research. *MedPage Today.* www.medpagetoday.com

Fu, W., Smith, C., Turner, L., Fojtik, J., Pacyna, J. E., & Master, Z. (2019). Characteristics and scope of training of clinicians participating in the US direct-to-consumer marketplace for unproven stem cell interventions. *JAMA, 321*(24), 2463–2464.

Ghimire, S., Weber, D., Mavin, E., Wang, X. N., Dickinson, A. M., & Holler, E. (2017). Pathophysiology of GvHD and other HSCT-related major complications. *Front Immunol, 8*, 79.

Gomes-Silva, D., & Ramos, C. A. (2018). Cancer immunotherapy using CAR-T cells: From the research bench to the assembly line. *Biotechnology Journal, 13*(2), 1700097. doi:10.1002 /biot.201700097

Grant, B. (2015, Feb. 25). UK OKs three-parent IVF. *The Scientist.* www.the-scientist.com/the -nutshell/uk-oks-three-parent-ivf-35882

Hacein-Bey-Abina, S., Von Kalle, C., Schmidt, M., McCormack, M. P., Wulffraat, N., Leboulch, P., Lim, A., Osborne, C. S., Pawliuk, R., Morillon, E., Sorensen, R., Forster, A., Fraser, P., Cohen, J. I., de Saint Basile, G., Alexander, I., Wintergerst, U., Frebourg, T., Aurias, A., Stoppa-Lyonnet, D., …, Cavazzana-Calvo, M. (2003). LMO2-associated clonal T cell proliferation in two patients after gene therapy for SCID-X1. *Science, 302*(5644), 415–419.

Ilic, D., & Ogilvie, C. (2017). Concise review: Human embryonic stem cells—What have we done? What are we doing? Where are we going? *Stem Cells, 35*(1), 17–25.

Imudia, A. N., & Plosker, S. (2016). The past, present and future of preimplantation genetic testing. *Clin Lab Med, 36*(2), 385–399.

Institute of Medicine and National Research Council (IOM & NRC). (2010). Final report of the National Academies' Human Embryonic Stem Cell Research Advisory Committee and 2010 amendments to the National Academies' Guidelines for Human Embryonic Stem Cell Research. The National Academies Press. https://doi.org/10.17226/12923

International Society for Stem Cell Research (ISSCR). (2016). *Guidelines for stem cell research and clinical translation.* www.isscr.org/policy/guidelines-for-stem-cell-research-and-clinical-translation

Kaemmerer, W. F. (2018). How will the field of gene therapy survive its success? *Bioeng Transl Med, 3*(2), 166–177.

Kamelska-Sadowska, A. M., Wojtkiewicz, J., & Kowalski, I. M. (2019). Review of the current knowledge on the role of stem cell transplantation in neurorehabilitation. *Biomed Res Int, 2019*, 3290894.

Karavani, E., Zuk, O., Zeevi, D., Barzilai, N., Stefanis, N. C., Hatzimanolis, A., Smyrnis, N., Avramopoulos, D., Kruglyak, L., Atzmon, G., Lam, M., Lencz, T., & Carmi, S. (2019). Screening human embryos for polygenic traits has limited utility. *Cell, 179*(6), 1424–1435.

Karponi, G., & Zogas, N. (2019). Gene therapy for beta-thalassemia: Updated perspectives. *Appl Clin Genet, 12*, 167–180.

Knoepfler, P. S. (2018). Too much carrot and not enough stick in new stem cell oversight trends. *Cell Stem Cell, 23*, 18–20.

Knoepfler, P. S. (2019). Rapid change of a cohort of 570 unproven stem cell clinics in the USA over 3 years. *Regen Med, 14*(8), 735–740.

Kuriyan, A. E., Albini, T. A., Townsend, J. H., Rodriguez, M., Pandya, H. K., Leonard, R. E., 2nd, Parrott, M. B., Rosenfeld, P. J., Flynn, H. W., Jr., & Goldberg, J. L. (2017). Vision loss after intravitreal injection of autologous "stem cells" for AMD. *New England Journal of Medicine, 376*(11), 1047–1053.

Leask, F. (2017). *ISSCR releases statement opposing possible U.S. ban on federal funding for fetal tissue research.* www.regmednet.com/channels/195-ethics-policy/posts/18545-isscr-releases-statement-opposing-possible-u-s-ban-on-federal-funding-for-fetal-tissue-research

LeMieux, J. (2019). The risky business of embryo selection. *Gen Eng Biotech News, 39*(4). www.genengnews.com/topics/omics/the-risky-business-of-embryo-selection/

Liu, Y., Chen, X., Han, W., & Zhang, Y. (2017). Tisagenlecleucel, an approved anti-CD19 chimeric antigen receptor T-cell therapy for the treatment of leukemia. *Drugs Today, 53*(11), 597–608.

Loos, R. J. F., & Janssens, C. J. W. (2017). Predicting polygenic obesity using genetic information. *Cell Metab, 25*(3), 535–543.

Mamcarz, E., Zhou, S., Lockey, T., Abdelsamed, H., Cross, S. J., Kang, G., Ma, Z., Condori, J., Dowdy, J., Triplett, B., Li, C., Maron, G., Aldave Becerra, J. C., Church, J. A., Dokmeci, E., Love, J. T., da Matta Ain, A. C., van der Watt, H., Tang, X., Janssen, W., …, Sorrentino, B. P. (2019). Lentiviral gene therapy combined with low-dose busulfan in infants with SCID-X1. *New England Journal of Medicine, 380*(16), 1525–1534.

Markoulaki, S., Meissner, A., & Jaenisch, R. (2008). Somatic cell nuclear transfer and derivation of embryonic stem cells in the mouse. *Methods, 445*(2), 101–114.

McIntyre, J. A., Jones, I. A., Han, B., & Vangsness, C. T. (2018). Intra-articular mesenchymal stem cell therapy for the human joint: A systemic review. *Am J Sports Med, 46*(14), 3550–3563.

Mead, B., Berry, M., Logan, A., Scott, R. A., Leadbeater, W., & Scheven, B. A. (2015). Stem cell treatment of degenerative eye disease. *Stem Cell Research, 14*(3), 243–257.

Michler, R. E. (2018). The current status of stem cell therapy in ischemic heart disease. *J Card Surg, 33*(9), 520–531.

Mullen, E. (2019a, January 24). Pregnancy reported in the first known trial of "three-person IVF" for infertility. *STAT.* www.statnews.com/2019/01/24/first-trial-of-three-person-ivf-for-infertility/

Mullen, E. (2019b, April 16). Patient advocates and scientists launch push to lift ban on "three-parent IVF." *STAT.* www.statnews.com/2019/04/16/mitochondrial-replacement-three-parent-ivf-ban/

Mushahary, D., Spittler, A., Kasper, C., Weber, V., & Charwat, V. (2018). Isolation, cultivation and characterization of human mesenchymal stem cells. *Cytometry A, 93*(1), 19–31.

Nam, C., & Rabbitts, T. H. (2006). The role of LMO2 in development and in T cell leukemia after chromosomal translocation or retroviral insertion. *Mol Ther, 13*(1), 15–25.

Nathwani, A. C., Davidoff, A. M., & Tuddenham, E. G. D. (2017). Gene therapy for hemophilia. *Hematol Oncol Clin North Am, 31*(5), 853–868.

National Academies. (n.d.). *International Commission on the Clinical Use of Human Germline Genome Editing.* www.nationalacademies.org/our-work/international-commission-on-the-clinical-use-of-human-germline-genome-editing

National Institutes of Health (NIH). (2019a). *Office of Science Policy. Introducing the NExTRAC.* https://osp.od.nih.gov/2019/04/24/introducing-the-nextrac/

National Institutes of Health (NIH). (2019b). *Changes to NIH requirements regarding proposed human fetal tissue research.* https://grants.nih.gov/grants/guide/notice-files/NOT-OD-19-128.html

Ozdemir, Z. N., & Civriz Bozdag, S. (2018). Graft failure after allogeneic hematopoietic stem cell transplantation. *Transfus Apher Sci, 57*(2), 163–167.

Park, S. S., Moisseiev, E., Bauer, G., Anderson, J. D., Grant, M. B., Zam, A., Zawadzki, R. J., Werner, J. S., & Nolta, J. A. (2017). Advances in bone marrow stem cell therapy for retinal dysfunction. *Prog Retin Eye Res, 56*, 148–165.

Parolini, O., Alviano, F., Bagnara, G. P., Bilic, G., Bühring, H. J., Evangelista, M., Hennerbichler, S., Liu, B., Magatti, M., Mao, N., Miki, T., Marongiu, F., Nakajima, H., Nikaido, T., Portmann-Lanz, C. B., Sankar, V., Soncini, M., Stadler, G., Surbek, D., Takahashi, T. A., …, Strom, S. C. (2008). Concise review: Isolation and characterization of cells from human term placenta: Outcome of the first International Workshop on Placenta Derived Stem Cells. *Stem Cells, 26*(2), 300–311.

Pera, M. F., Reubinoff, B., & Trounson, A. (2000). Human embryonic stem cells. *J Cell Sci, 113*(1), 5–10.

Petersdorf, E. W. (2017). Which factors influence the development of GVHD in HLA-matched or mismatched transplants? *Best Pract Res Clin Haematol, 30*(4), 333–335.

Peterson, C. M., Buckley, C., Holley, S., & Menias, C. O. (2012). Teratomas: A multimodality review. *Curr Probl Diagn Radiol, 41*(6), 210–219.

Piana, R. (2019, April 10). Human gene therapy, progress and oversight. *The ASCO Post.* www.ascopost.com/issues/april-10-2019/human-gene-therapy-progress-and-oversight.

Pipe, S. W. (2018). Gene therapy for hemophilia. *Pediatric Blood Cancer, 65*(2), e26865. https://doi.org/10.1002/pbc.26865

Reardon, S. (2019a). World Health Organization panel weighs in on CRISPR-babies debate. *Nature, 567*, 444–445.

Reardon, S. (2019b). Trump administration halts fetal-tissue research by government scientists. *Nature, 570*, 148.

Ribeil, J. A., Hacein-Bey-Abina, S., Payen, E., Magnani, A., Semeraro, M., Magrin, E., Caccavelli, L., Neven, B., Bourget, P., El Nemer, W., Bartolucci, P., Weber, L., Puy, H., Meritet, J. F., Grevent, D., Beuzard, Y., Chrétien, S., Lefebvre, T., Ross, R. W., Negre, O., …, Cavazzana, M. (2017). Gene therapy in a patient with sickle cell disease. *New England Journal of Medicine, 376*, 848–855.

Rodriguez, C. H. (2017, March 15). Experimental stem cell treatment leaves three women blind. *Kaiser Health News.* https://khn.org/news/experimental-stem-cell-treatment-leaves-3-women-blind/

Saunders, T. L. (2020). The history of transgenesis. In M. Larson (Ed.), *Transgenic mouse: Methods in molecular biology* (Vol. 2066). Humana.

Shamblott, M. J., Axelman, J., Wang, S., Bugg, E. M., Littlefield, J. W., Donovan, P. J., Blumenthal, P. D., Huggins, G. R., & Gearhart, J. D. (1998). Derivation of pluripotent stem cells from cultured human primordial germ cells. *Proceedings of the National Academy of Sciences, 95*, 13726–13731.

Simonson, O. E., Domogatskaya, A., Volchkov, P., & Rodin, S. (2015). The safety of human pluripotent stem cells in clinical treatment. *Annals of Medicine, 47*(5), 370–380.

Straiton, J. (2019). Genetically modified humans: The X-men of scientific research. *BioTechniques, 66*(6), 249–252.

Szabo, L. (2019). Elite hospitals plunge into unproven stem cell treatments. *Kaiser Health News.* https://khn.org/news/elite-hospitals-plunge-into-unproven-stem-cell-treatments/

Takahashi, K., Tanabe, K., Ohnuki, M., Narita, M., Ichisaka, T., Tomoda, K., & Yamanaka, S. (2007). Induction of pluripotent stem cells from adult human fibroblasts by defined factors. *Cell, 131*, 861–872.

Tang, Z., Zhang, Y., Wang, Y., Zhang, D., Shen, B., Luo, M., & Gu, P. (2017). Progress of stem/progenitor cell-bases therapy for retinal degeneration. *J Transl Med, 15*(1), 99.

Tariq, S. M., Haider, S. A., Hasan, M., Tahir, A., Khan, M., Rehan, A., & Kamal, A. (2018). Chimeric antigen receptor T-cell therapy: A beacon of hope in the fight against cancer. *Cureus, 10*(10), e3486.

Taylor, A. P. (2018, Dec 21). FDA cracks down on purveyors of stem cell treatments. *The Scientist.* www.the-scientist.com/news-opinion/fda-cracks-down-on-purveyors-of-stem-cell-treatments-65268

Thomas, E. D. (1999). A history of haemopoietic cell transplantation. *J Haematol, 105*(2), 330–339.

Thomson, J. A., Itskovitz-Eldor, J., Shapiro, S. S., Waknitz, M. A., Swiergiel, J. J., Marshall, V. S., & Jones, J. M. (1998). Embryonic stem cell lines derived from human blastocysts. *Science, 282*, 1145–1147.

Thomson, J. A., Kalishman, J., Golos, T. G., Durning, M., Harris, C. P., Becker, R. A., & Hearn, J. P. (1995). Isolation of a primate embryonic stem cell line. *Proceedings of the National Academy of Sciences, 92*, 7844–7848.

Trounson, A., & McDonald C. (2015). Stem cell therapies in clinical trials: Progress and challenges. *Cell Stem Cell, 17*(1), 11–22

Turner, L., & Knoepfler, P. (2016). Selling stem cells in the USA: Assessing the direct-to-consumer industry. *Cell Stem Cell, 19*(2), 154–157.

UK Draft Statutory Instruments. (2015). *The human fertilisation and embryology (mitochondrial donation) regulations 2015.* www.legislation.gov.uk/ukdsi/2015/9780111125816

Vassena, R., Heindryckx, B., Peco, R., Pennings, G., Raya, A., Sermon, K., & Veiga, A. (2016). Genome engineering through CRISPR/Cas9 technology in the human germline and pluripotent stem cells. *Hum Reprod Update, 22*(4), 411–419.

Wilson, A., Chee, M., Butler, P., & Boyd, A. S. (2019). Isolation and characterization of human adipose-derived stem cells. *Methods Mol Biol, 1899,* 3–3.

Wilson, R. F. (2010). The death of Jesse Gelsinger: New evidence of the influence of money and prestige in human research. *Am J Law Med, 36*(2–3), 295–325.

Wirth, T., Parker, N., & Yia-Herttuala, S. (2013). History of gene therapy. *Gene, 525*(2), 162–169.

Wivel, N. A. (2014). Historical perspectives pertaining to the NIH Recombinant DNA Advisory Committee. *Human Gene Therapy, 25*(1), 19–24.

Wolinetz, C. D., & Collins, F. S. (2019). NIH supports call for moratorium on clinical uses of germline gene editing. *Nature, 567,* 175.

Xu, J., Yu, L., Guo, J., Xiang, J., Zheng, Z., Gao, D., Shi, B., Hao, H., Jiao, D., Zhong, L., Wang, Y., Wu, J., Wei, H., & Han, J. (2019). Generation of pig induced pluripotent stem cells using an extended pluripotent stem cell culture system. *Stem Cell Res Ther, 10*(1), 193.

Yamanaka, S. (2008). Induction of pluripotent stem cells from mouse fibroblasts by four transcription factors. *Cell Prolif, 41*(Suppl 1), 51–56.

Yarborough, M., & Sharp, R. R. (2009). Public trust and research a decade later: What have we learned since Jesse Gelsinger's death? *Mol Genet Metab, 97*(1), 4–5.

Yee, J. (2010). Turning somatic cells into pluripotent stem cells. *Nature Education, 3*(9), 25.

Yu, H., Lu, K., Zhu, J., & Wang, J. (2017). Stem cell therapy for ischemic heart diseases. *Br Med Bull, 121*(1), 135–154.

Zhang, X. P., Zhang, W.T., Qiu, Y., Ju, M. J., Tu, G. W., & Luo, Z. (2019). Understanding gene therapy in acute respiratory distress syndrome. *Curr Gene Ther, 19*(2), 93–99.

Zhao, L., Chen, S., Yang, P., Cao, H., & Li, L. (2019). The role of mesenchymal stem cells in hematopoietic stem cell transplantation: Prevention and treatment of graft-versus-host disease. *Stem Cell Res Ther, 10*(1), 182.

Zheng, P. P., Kros, J. M., & Li, J. (2018). Approved CAR T cell therapies: Ice bucket challenges on glaring safety risks and long-term impacts. *Drug Discovery Today, 23*(6), 1175–1182.

Phase 1 and First-in-Human Studies

Stacey L. Berg

Abstract

Phase 1 and first-in-human studies involve the earliest uses of new agents in humans. The IRB's review of these studies will be aided by an understanding of the late phases of preclinical drug development and the Food and Drug Administration (FDA) investigational new drug (IND) application process. While phase 1 and first-in-human studies do not face special requirements for IRB review, the IRB may focus especially on the potential risks and benefits (including potential social and scientific value in addition to any individual benefits), as well as on accurate description of these in the informed consent. This chapter will discuss important IRB considerations regarding early phase studies.

Types of Early Phase Studies

In the classical paradigm, new drug development is divided into three phases of active clinical research that occur before a drug is marketed for an indication, and a fourth phase of surveillance that occurs post marketing (**Figure 10.15-1**). This chapter will discuss the earliest phases of new drug studies in humans, with a focus on potential risk, benefit, and informed consent issues that the IRB should consider during the initial and continuing review process.

PHASES OF AN INVESTIGATION

An Investigational New Drug (IND) Application may be submitted for one or more phases of an investigation (FDA, 2018c). The clinical investigation of a previously untested drug is generally divided into three phases. Although in general the phases are conducted sequentially, they may overlap. These three phases of an investigation are as follows:

- Phase 1.
  - Includes the initial introduction of an investigational new drug into humans. Phase 1 studies are typically closely monitored and may be

🔗 11-2

conducted in patients or normal volunteer subjects. These studies are designed to determine the metabolism and pharmacological actions of the drug in humans, the side effects associated with increasing doses, and, if possible, to gain early evidence on effectiveness. During phase 1, sufficient information about the drug's pharmacokinetics and pharmacological effects should be obtained to permit the design of well-controlled, scientifically valid, phase 2 studies. The total number of subjects and patients included in phase 1 studies varies with the drug, but is generally in the range of 20 to 80.

- Phase 1 studies also include studies of drug metabolism, structure-activity relationships, and mechanism of action in humans, as well as studies in which investigational drugs are used as research tools to explore biological phenomena or disease processes.

■ Phase 2. Includes controlled clinical studies conducted to evaluate the effectiveness of the drug for a particular indication or indications in patients with the disease or condition under study and to determine the common short-term side effects and risks associated with the drug. Phase 2 studies are typically well controlled, closely monitored, and conducted in a relatively small number of patients, usually involving no more than several hundred subjects.

■ Phase 3. Are expanded controlled and uncontrolled trials. They are performed after preliminary evidence suggesting effectiveness of the drug has been obtained, and are intended to gather the additional information about effectiveness and safety that is needed to evaluate the overall benefit/risk relationship of the drug and to provide an adequate basis for physician labeling. Phase 3 studies usually include from several hundred to several thousand subjects.

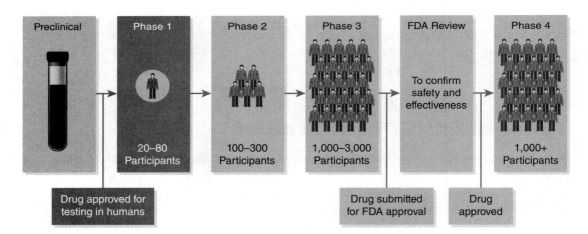

Figure 10.15-1 Clinical trials.

HIV/AIDS Glossary, Phase 1 Trial, retrieved from https://aidsinfo.nih.gov/understanding-hiv-aids/glossary/568/phase-1-trial

Phase 1 studies involve the earliest uses of new agents in humans. These studies are typically small, involving fewer than 100 subjects, and are designed primarily to determine the frequency and severity of adverse events at escalating doses, as well as to obtain preliminary information regarding pharmacokinetics (PK) and pharmacodynamics (PD) (see box, Pharmacokinetics and Pharmacodynamics). The exact endpoints will vary based on mechanism of action of the drug and anticipated biological effects. Most nononcology phase 1 studies are conducted in healthy individuals, who by definition have no prospect of benefitting directly from the research. The use of healthy individuals permits faster accrual and evaluation of drug effects without the confounding issues of preexisting conditions (Karakunnel et al., 2018). In this case, the benefits of the study are to society—from its contribution to scientific knowledge. In contrast, studies of potentially toxic agents like anticancer drugs are more likely to be conducted in patients. When patients are the subjects, the studies may offer the potential for direct benefit to the individual subject in addition to contributing to generalizable knowledge. Such studies often have assessment of the drug's activity against a disease as a secondary goal.

PHARMACOKINETICS AND PHARMACODYNAMICS

Pharmacokinetics is the study of how drug is absorbed, distributed, metabolized, and eliminated from the body. In early phase studies, blood samples are usually obtained over a period of hours to days after the first dose, then periodically through the first few weeks in the case of multiple dosing. Other samples, such as urine or cerebrospinal fluid, may also be obtained.

Pharmacodynamics is the study of the effect of the drug on targets in the body. For example, blood samples may be obtained to see whether the agent has the intended effect of inhibiting a target enzyme in white blood cells. More invasive sampling, such as tumor biopsy, may be scientifically desirable, as the activity of the drug against the actual target may not be assessable on more easily obtained samples.

Exploratory IND studies (sometimes called *phase 0* studies) are also conducted early in drug development and may be viewed as a specialized subset of phase 1. This phase is not required and is often not conducted. Like many noncancer phase 1 studies, phase 0 studies have no therapeutic or diagnostic intent; they are usually conducted in healthy individuals receiving small drug doses for a short time and are intended to provide biological information about the mechanism of action of a drug (such as effect of drug on a target biomarker) or to provide early PK data to guide more traditional phase 1 studies (FDA, 2006). Together, phase 1 and exploratory IND studies are often referred to as first-in-human (FIH) studies.

These early phase studies form the bridge between preclinical development of a drug and human testing, with the intent to establish the agent's place in the treatment of a disease or condition. From the regulatory perspective, there are no separate requirements for IRB review of FIH studies, and the criteria for approval at **45 CFR 46.111** apply as they do to any other type of research. Perhaps the most important duty of the IRB in the FIH setting is to evaluate the risks and potential benefits of the research and to ensure the adequacy of the informed consent process. Especially with respect to evaluating risks, it may be helpful for IRBs to have a general understanding of the steps involved in preclinical development of a new agent for FIH studies.

🔗 5-4

🔗 Section 6

Food and Drug Administration Oversight

Before a new agent can be administered to humans, FDA must approve the IND application as detailed in **21 CFR part 312** (FDA, 2018b). The IND application documents the preclinical development of the agent, including the

🔗 11-2

manufacturing process, animal toxicology and pharmacology studies, and a description of the anticipated potential risks to humans based on the preclinical studies. The IND application, in addition to detailing the preclinical information about the agent, also includes the human research protocol(s) that will be used for the FIH study, as well as the plan for monitoring the safety of human subjects.

Both the FDA and the IRB review the proposed human study, and there is no regulatory requirement regarding which entity must perform the review first. The IRB may want to know whether a particular early phase protocol is part of an IND that has already received FDA approval (as is usual when the study is sponsored by a pharmaceutical company, sometimes called a "commercial IND"), or whether the protocol is being submitted by a sponsor-investigator for IRB review prior to IND submission. The latter path is advantageous for sponsor-investigators because they can benefit from the IRB's scientific and ethical review before submitting the protocol to FDA, and it is likely easier for them to amend the protocol with the IRB if FDA asks for changes than to amend a previously submitted IND if the IRB asks for changes. However, the IRB-first path may mean that there has been less scientific review of the proposed research prior to the IRB review. Regardless of the path, the IRB should not grant final approval to the study until the researcher confirms that the 30-day period for FDA review has passed without notification that FDA has placed the study on clinical hold. Of note, FDA does not necessarily provide documentation of approval. Rather, if FDA does not notify the sponsor of further review requirements within 30 days of IND submission, the human investigation may proceed.

Because of the rigorous requirements for preclinical testing before human drug administration at the time of FIH testing, at least some data will be available to predict adverse events and to plan the appropriate starting dose and drug administration schedule. This information should be presented to the IRB in the protocol itself or in the investigator's brochure (International Council for Harmonisation, 2016), which summarizes the chemistry, toxicology, and PK/PD data from nonclinical development, as well as any safety and efficacy information known from human studies to date. Preclinical models are not perfect, however, so no FIH study is entirely without risk.

IRB Assessment of Risks and Benefits

An investigator's brochure (IB) is required for commercial sponsors but not for sponsor-investigators (FDA, 2015). Importantly for the IRB, the IB will likely contain information regarding the established no observed adverse event level, as well as a human equivalent dose or other discussion of how the recommended starting dose for the study was derived (FDA, 2010). There may also be information available regarding the risks and benefits of similar agents in humans or regarding the current agent in other diseases or conditions. Nonetheless, there will be at least some uncertainty regarding dosing and potential toxicity in every FIH trial. Therefore, the IRB may wish to pay particular attention to how many subjects will be exposed to the investigational agent at the same time and how long each subject or group of subjects will be observed for adverse events before subsequent subjects can be enrolled or doses escalated (see sidebar, The Lessons of TGN1412). In addition, the IRB should examine the eligibility criteria to ensure that the subject population is appropriate for the study and that subjects who are at special risk for known or predicted adverse events are excluded. At the same time, however, the IRB should consider the balance between subject safety and the importance of obtaining information that will be relevant to the patient population in which the drug will actually be used. Important safety signals may be missed if the study population is much healthier than the intended patient population. Therefore, eligibility criteria should be as reasonably broad within the constraints of safety, and exclusion of large groups of patients, such as those with HIV or mild organ dysfunction, should not occur without good scientific justification (FDA, 2019).

The IRB should also consider risks of the research beyond adverse events associated with the agent itself. Virtually all investigational drug studies include some aspect of <u>biospecimen</u> acquisition. In healthy volunteer studies, the samples obtained are often limited to blood, urine, skin, or other tissues that can be obtained without undue risk to the subject. In some populations, such as cancer patients, the agents may be administered in a "window of opportunity" prior to a planned surgery where tissues are going to be sampled for a clinical reason, and some of the tissue can be used for study purposes. As with any study, the IRB should consider the potential risks of procedures being performed strictly for research, and the study design should seek to minimize risk by taking advantage of planned clinical procedures whenever possible.

🔗 10-10

In order to comply with **45 CFR 46.111(a)(2)**, "Risks to subjects are reasonable in relation to anticipated benefits, if any, to subjects, and the importance of the knowledge that may reasonably be expected to result," the IRB must also evaluate the potential for benefit to both the individual subject and to society. In phase 0 studies, individuals receiving the agent cannot benefit directly because the dosing and administration of the agent are generally too low and short term to be therapeutic. In order for the IRB to approve the research, it should be clear that the study will provide answers to important questions; if it will not, then the risk/benefit ratio is unlikely to be favorable, even if the risks are quite low. One key factor is adequacy of the statistical design, since a study that fails to answer the research question will not have benefits to offset potential risks.

In the past, some have argued that because the primary objective of a phase 1 trial is related to tolerability rather than efficacy, the trial should be interpreted as having no potential for direct benefit to the individual subject (Joffe & Miller, 2006). This argument has been prominent with regard to oncology drugs, because the overall response rate to new anticancer drugs reported for phase 1 studies of cytotoxic drugs in the past was often less than 10% (Estey et al., 1986; Horstmann et al., 2005; Roberts et al., 2004; Smith et al., 1996; Von Hoff & Turner, 1991). However, especially in the era of molecularly targeted anticancer agents, the response rate can be significant, even approaching 100% as seen in the phase 1 study of imatinib in chronic myeloid leukemia (Baselga et al., 2002; Brahmer et al., 2012; Druker et al., 2001; Maude et al., 2014; Mosse et al., 2013). This data clearly demonstrates that there is a potential for direct benefit to subjects in phase 1 oncology studies. Unfortunately, it is difficult or impossible to estimate in advance whether a particular agent is likely to be active, although some information may be gleaned from the agent's clinical trial "portfolio" if prior studies have been performed (Kimmelman et al., 2017). Although the researcher and IRB may not be able to quantify

THE LESSONS OF TGN1412

TGN1412 is a "superagonist" monoclonal antibody that binds to CD28 and directly stimulates T cells. In 2006, eight healthy individuals were enrolled the same day in a phase 1, placebo-controlled study. The six individuals who received the study agent felt ill within minutes and were all critically ill within hours (Suntharalingam et al., 2006). Subsequent evaluations identified that the subjects were suffering from severe cytokine release syndrome—now a known effect of T-cell activating therapies, but not predicted by the preclinical models in use at the time (Hunig, 2012). Among the lessons learned from the study is to consider requiring the first dose of a new agent to be given to a single subject who is monitored for adverse effects before subsequent subjects are enrolled (European Medicines Agency, 2017).

the likelihood of direct benefit for an individual subject, there is no regulatory threshold that the probability of benefit must cross for the IRB to determine that it may exist.

Phase 1 Studies in Children

⊘ 9-6

Pediatric FIH or phase 1 trials present special concerns for the IRB because of the additional protections required for this vulnerable population. The IRB can approve studies with minimal risk, and some phase 0 trials could fall into this category. IRBs may also find that phase 1 trials represent greater than minimal risk with the prospect of direct benefit to the individual subjects [45 CFR 46.405] or greater than minimal risk and no prospect of direct benefit to individual subjects, but likely to yield generalizable knowledge about the subject's disorder or condition [45 CFR 46.406]. Some authors argue that phase 1 trials are so risky and inherently without the potential for direct benefit to the subject that pediatric patients should not be entered into them (Oberman & Frader, 2003) or that new criteria for IRB approval should be developed for them (Kimmelman et al., 2019; Ross, 2006). As mentioned previously, however, numerous phase 1 studies, including pediatric studies, have resulted in clinical responses in children with cancer (DuBois et al., 2018; Maude et al., 2014; Mosse et al., 2013), demonstrating that there is indeed the potential for individual benefit. It is therefore reasonable for IRBs to approve pediatric phase 1 studies if they meet the relevant criteria.

Informed Consent

⊘ 6-2

As with other aspects of IRB review, there are no special requirements for review of FIH studies other than that some of the "additional elements of informed consent" are likely to be required (FDA, 2018a) (see box, Additional Elements of Informed Consent). Key issues in the informed consent for an early phase study include the description of potential risks and benefits in the context of an agent that is relatively new in human use. In some FIH studies, subjects may

⊘ 12-2

be compensated for their time and inconvenience. This compensation should not be regarded as a benefit when evaluating the risk/benefit profile of the trial, and the IRB should consider whether the compensation amount or schedule of payment might unduly influence a subject to enroll or remain in a study despite a desire to withdraw. There is also debate about whether paying healthy volunteers to participate in phase 1 studies has the potential to disproportionately burden participants of lower socioeconomic status, who might rely on research compensation as an important source of income (Chen et al., 2017; Elliott, 2017; Grady, 2017; Grady et al., 2017).

ADDITIONAL ELEMENTS OF INFORMED CONSENT

45 CFR 46.116

(c) Additional elements of informed consent. One or more of the following elements of information, when appropriate, shall also be provided to each subject or the legally authorized representative:

1. A statement that the particular treatment or procedure may involve risks to the subject (or to the embryo or fetus, if the subject is or may become pregnant) that are currently unforeseeable;

2. Anticipated circumstances under which the subject's participation may be terminated by the investigator without regard to the subject's or the legally authorized representative's consent;

3. Any additional costs to the subject that may result from participation in the research;

4. The consequences of a subject's decision to withdraw from the research and procedures for orderly termination of participation by the subject;

5. A statement that significant new findings developed during the course of the research that may relate to the subject's willingness to continue participation will be provided to the subject;

6. The approximate number of subjects involved in the study;

7. A statement that the subject's biospecimens (even if identifiers are removed) may be used for commercial profit and whether the subject will or will not share in this commercial profit;

8. A statement regarding whether clinically relevant research results, including individual research results, will be disclosed to subjects, and if so, under what conditions; and

9. For research involving biospecimens, whether the research will (if known) or might include whole genome sequencing (i.e., sequencing of a human germline or somatic specimen with the intent to generate the genome or exome sequence of that specimen).

As discussed earlier, there may be some potential for individual benefit, and there should be potential for benefit to society in an early phase study. However, these benefits, especially the potential for personal benefit to the subject, should not be overstated in the consent (Abdoler et al., 2008). This is especially important when the subjects are patients who may not have nonstudy treatment options available. For these patient/subjects, the potential for "therapeutic misconception" is high. Therapeutic misconception originally referred to a subject's misunderstanding that the research interventions were designed for their benefit (Appelbaum et al., 1982). However, the term is now often used to reflect a subject's misunderstanding about whether the trial is likely to represent effective therapy for their condition. The IRB should review the consent language regarding benefit and the plans for the consent process in general to minimize the likelihood of such a misunderstanding.

Occasionally an agent being tested in early phase trials produces such dramatic responses that physicians and patients hope for access to the agent through trial participation. In this circumstance, the IRB should review the consent documents to be sure that potential benefits are not overstated and that options to obtain the agent outside the trial, if any, are clearly delineated. Although all studies will include in the consent that subjects have the option not to participate, IRBs may wish to consider how this option is conveyed to participants who have limited other therapeutic choices. For example, options such as symptom-directed care, beyond merely nonparticipation, are appropriate to include in phase 1 cancer study consents.

Similarly, the potential risks should not be downplayed. While some early phase studies, especially FIH studies in healthy volunteers, may use such a small drug dose that adverse events are highly unlikely, others, such as dose escalation studies in cancer patients, may expose the subject to substantial risks. The informed consent should clearly describe this possibility. For dose escalation studies, the IRB may also consider whether information about a decreased chance of benefit at lower doses and an increased chance of adverse events at higher doses should be provided.

When new information about the investigational agent is obtained, the IRB will need to reevaluate the risks and benefits of the agent and determine whether risks remain reasonable in relation to potential benefits. Particularly for new risks or adverse events, the informed consent document may need to be amended to include the new information, and the IRB will also need to determine whether subjects currently on the study should be provided with the new information and asked whether they consent to continued participation.

References

Abdoler, E., Taylor, H., & Wendler, D. (2008). The ethics of phase 0 oncology trials. *Clinical Cancer Research, 14*(12), 3692–3697.

Appelbaum, P. S., Roth, L. H., & Lidz, C. (1982). The therapeutic misconception: Informed consent in psychiatric research. *International Journal of Law and Psychiatry, 5*(3–4), 319–329.

Baselga, J., Rischin, D., Ranson, M., Calvert, H., Raymond, E., Kieback, D. G., Kaye, S. B., Gianni, L., Harris, A., Bjork, T., Averbuch, S. D., Feyereislova, A., Swaisland, H., Rojo, F., & Albanell, J. (2002). Phase 1 safety, pharmacokinetic, and pharmacodynamic trial of ZD1839, a selective oral epidermal growth factor receptor tyrosine kinase inhibitor, in patients with five selected solid tumor types. *Journal of Clinical Oncology, 20*(21), 4292–4302.

Brahmer, J. R., Tykodi, S. S., Chow, L. Q., Hwu, W. J., Topalian, S. L., Hwu, P., Drake, C. G., Camacho, L. H., Kauh, J., Odunsi, K., Pitot, H. C., Hamid, O., Bhatia, S., Martins, R., Eaton, K., Chen, S., Salay, T. M., Alaparthy, S., Grosso, J. F., Korman, A. J., …, Wigginton, J. M. (2012). Safety and activity of anti-PD-L1 antibody in patients with advanced cancer. *New England Journal of Medicine, 366*(26), 2455–2465.

Chen, S. C., Sinaii, N., Bedarida, G., Gregorio, M. A., Emanuel, E., & Grady, C. (2017). Phase 1 healthy volunteer willingness to participate and enrollment preferences. *Clinical Trials, 14*(5), 537–546.

Druker, B. J., Talpaz, M., Resta, D. J., Peng, B., Buchdunger, E., Ford, J. M., Lydon, N. B., Kantarjian, H., Capdeville, R., Ohno-Jones, S., & Sawyers, C. L. (2001). Efficacy and safety of a specific inhibitor of the BCR-ABL tyrosine kinase in chronic myeloid leukemia. *New England Journal of Medicine, 344*(14), 1031–1037.

DuBois, S. G., Laetsch, T. W., Federman, N., Turpin, B. K., Albert, C. M., Nagasubramanian, R., Anderson, M. E., Davis, J. L., Qamoos, H. E., Reynolds, M. E., Cruickshank, S., Cox, M. C., Hawkins, D. S., Mascarenhas, L., & Pappo, A. S. (2018). The use of neoadjuvant larotrectinib in the management of children with locally advanced TRK fusion sarcomas. *Cancer, 124*(21), 4241–4247.

Elliott, C. (2017). Commentary on Grady et al.: Using poor, uninsured minorities to test the safety of experimental drugs. *Clinical Trials, 14*(5), 547–550.

Estey, E., Hoth, D., Simon, R., Marsoni, S., Leyland-Jones, B., & Wittes, R. (1986). Therapeutic response in phase 1 trials of antineoplastic agents. *Cancer Treatment Report, 70*(9), 1105–1115.

European Medicines Agency. (2017). *Guideline on strategies to identify and mitigate risks for first-in-human and early clinical trials with investigational medicinal products.* www.ema.europa .eu/en/documents/scientific-guideline/guideline-strategies-identify-mitigate-risks-first -human-early-clinical-trials-investigational_en.pdf

Food and Drug Administration (FDA). (2006). *Guidance for industry, investigators, and reviewers: Exploratory IND studies.* www.fda.gov/media/72325/download

Food and Drug Administration (FDA). (2010). *Guidance for industry. M3(R2) nonclinical safety studies for the conduct of human clinical trials and marketing authorization for pharmaceuticals.* www.fda.gov/media/71542/download

Food and Drug Administration (FDA). (2015). *Investigational new drug applications prepared and submitted by sponsor-investigators.* www.fda.gov/media/92604/download

Food and Drug Administration (FDA). (2018a). *Informed consent for clinical trials.* www.fda.gov /patients/clinical-trials-what-patients-need-know/informed-consent-clinical-trials

Food and Drug Administration (FDA). (2018b). *Investigational new drug application 21 CFR 312 Food and Drug Administration.* www.govinfo.gov/app/collection/cfr/2018/title21/chapterI /subchapterD/part312/subpartB/Section§312.21

Food and Drug Administration (FDA). (2018c). *Phases of an investigation 21 CFR 312.21.* www .ecfr.gov/cgi-bin/text-idx?SID=f32baf97aa80b6ce02d5f15026200967&mc=true&node=s e21.5.312_121&rgn=div8

Food and Drug Administration (FDA). (2019). *Enhancing the diversity of clinical trial populations — eligibility criteria, enrollment practices, and trial designs guidance for industry.* www.fda.gov/media/127712/download

Grady, C. (2017). Response. *Clinical Trials, 14*(5), 551–552.

Grady, C., Bedarida, G., Sinaii, N., Gregorio, M. A., & Emanuel, E. J. (2017). Motivations, enrollment decisions, and socio-demographic characteristics of healthy volunteers in phase 1 research. *Clinical Trials, 14*(5), 526–536.

Horstmann, E., McCabe, M. S., Grochow, L., Yamamoto, S., Rubinstein, L., Budd, T., Shoemaker, D., Emanuel, E. J., & Grady, C. (2005). Risks and benefits of phase 1 oncology trials, 1991 through 2002. *New England Journal of Medicine, 352*(9), 895–904.

Hunig, T. (2012). The storm has cleared: Lessons from the CD28 superagonist TGN1412 trial. *Nature Reviews Immunology, 12*(5), 317–318.

International Council for Harmonisation of Technical Requirements for Pharmaceuticals for Human Use. (2016). *Integrated addendum to ICH E6(R1): Guideline for good clinical practice E6(R2).* database.ich.org/sites/default/files/E6_R2_Addendum.pdf

Joffe, S., & Miller, F. G. (2006). Rethinking risk-benefit assessment for phase 1 cancer trials. *Journal of Clinical Oncology, 24*(19), 2987–2990.

Karakunnel, J. J., Bui, N., Palaniappan, L., Schmidt, K. T., Mahaffey, K. W., Morrison, B., Figg, W. D., & Kummar, S. (2018). Reviewing the role of healthy volunteer studies in drug development. *Journal of Translational Medicine, 16*(1), 336.

Kimmelman, J., Carlisle, B., & Gonen, M. (2017). Drug development at the portfolio level is important for policy, care decisions and human protections. *JAMA, 318*(11), 1003–1004.

Kimmelman, J., Waligora, M., & Lynch, H. F. (2019). Participant protection in phase 1 pediatric cancer trials. *JAMA Pediatrics, 173*(1), 8–9.

Maude, S. L., Frey, N., Shaw, P. A., Aplenc, R., Barrett, D. M., Bunin, N. J., . . ., Grupp, S. A. (2014). Chimeric antigen receptor T cells for sustained remissions in leukemia. *New England Journal of Medicine, 371*(16), 1507–1517.

Mossé, Y. P., Lim, M. S., Voss, S. D., Wilner, K., Ruffner, K., Laliberte, J., Rolland, D., Balis, F. M., Maris, J. M., Weigel, B. J., Ingle, A. M., Ahern, C., Adamson, P. C., & Blaney, S. M. (2013). Safety and activity of crizotinib for paediatric patients with refractory solid tumours or anaplastic large-cell lymphoma: A Children's Oncology Group phase 1 consortium study. *Lancet Oncology, 14*(6), 472–480.

Oberman, M., & Frader, J. (2003). Dying children and medical research: Access to clinical trials as benefit and burden. *American Journal of International Law, 29*(2–3), 301–317.

Roberts, T. G., Jr., Goulart, B. H., Squitieri, L., Stallings, S. C., Halpern, E. F., Chabner, B. A., Gazelle, G. S., Finkelstein, S. N., & Clark, J. W. (2004). Trends in the risks and benefits to patients with cancer participating in phase 1 clinical trials. *JAMA, 292*(17), 2130–2140.

Ross, L. (2006). Phase 1 research and the meaning of direct benefit. *Journal of Pediatrics, 149*(1 Suppl), S20–S24.

Smith, T. L., Lee, J. J., Kantarjian, H. M., Legha, S. S., & Raber, M. N. (1996). Design and results of phase 1 cancer clinical trials: Three-year experience at M.D. Anderson Cancer Center. *Journal of Clinical Oncology, 14*(1), 287–295.

Suntharalingam, G., Perry, M. R., Ward, S., Brett, S. J., Castello-Cortes, A., Brunner, M. D., & Panoskaltsis, N. (2006). Cytokine storm in a phase 1 trial of the anti-CD28 monoclonal antibody TGN1412. *New England Journal of Medicine, 355*(10), 1018–1028.

Von Hoff, D. D., & Turner, J. (1991). Response rates, duration of response, and dose response effects in phase 1 studies of antineoplastics. *Investigational New Drugs, 9*(1), 115–122.

Research Regulated by FDA and Other Agencies

Differences Between the Common Rule and FDA Regulations

David Forster

Abstract

The Food and Drug Administration (FDA) has regulations related to research involving human subjects that are separate and different from the Common Rule. From the standpoint of IRB policy and procedure, the two sets of regulations are similar in many ways, but they also have some significant differences with which the IRB needs to be familiar. This chapter will highlight those differences.

Introduction

The Food and Drug Administration has regulations that are distinct from the DHHS Regulations that have been adopted as the Common Rule. From the standpoint of IRB policy and procedure, the two sets of regulations are similar in many ways, but they also have some significant differences with which the IRB needs to be familiar. The Common Rule was updated effective July 19, 2018, and as a result the differences between the Common Rule and FDA regulations are more pronounced than they were prior to that date. However, FDA is working on a revised version of FDA regulations, with the goal of harmonizing FDA regulations to the Common Rule to the extent possible. Such modifications would, of course, affect the conclusions noted in this chapter.

Institutions that review both Common Rule agency-funded and FDA-regulated research must ensure that their registration on the Office for Human Research Protections (OHRP) website includes both OHRP and FDA. When an institution conducts research that is subject to both the Common Rule and FDA regulations, the process of IRB review must comply with both sets of regulations.

Differences Between the Common Rule and FDA Regulations

The first significant difference between the Common Rule and FDA regulations is their jurisdiction. The Common Rule applies "to all research involving human subjects conducted, supported, or otherwise subject to regulation by any Federal department or agency that takes appropriate administrative action to make the policy applicable to such research" [45 CFR 46.101(a)]. The application is not affected by the subject matter of the research, just the involvement of DHHS or another Common Rule agency in conducting or supporting the research. In contrast, FDA regulations apply to clinical investigations that support applications for research or marketing permits for products regulated by FDA, such as drugs, biologics, and medical devices. The source of the funding or support for the study is not relevant in establishing the jurisdiction of FDA regulations.

There are also several differences in the definitions in the two sets of regulations. Most important, the Common Rule uses the term "research" while FDA regulations use the term "clinical investigation." Research under the Common Rule is "a systematic investigation, including research development, testing, and evaluation, designed to develop or contribute to generalizable knowledge" [45 CFR 46.102(l)]. In contrast, a clinical investigation under FDA regulations is "any experiment that involves a test article and one or more human subjects" [21 CFR 50.3(c)]. Note there are also distinct definitions of "clinical investigation" at 21 CFR 812.3(h) and 21 CFR 312.3(b). Furthermore, the two sets of regulations have distinct definitions of "human subject." Under the Common Rule, human subject "means a living individual about whom an investigator (whether professional or student) conducting research (i) Obtains information or biospecimens through intervention or interaction with the individual, and uses, studies, or analyzes the information or biospecimens; or (ii) Obtains, uses, studies, analyzes or generates identifiable private information or identifiable biospecimens" [45 CFR 46.102(e)]. In contrast, under FDA regulations, the term "human subject" "means an individual who is or becomes a participant in research, either as a recipient of the test article or as a control. A subject may be either a healthy individual or a patient" [21 CFR 50.3(g)]. IRB staff and members must be aware of these differences in order to appropriately determine when the Common Rule and FDA regulations apply to a given research project.

🔗 5-3

Another area of significant difference between the two sets of regulations is the types of research that are <u>exempt</u> from IRB review. The Common Rule has eight categories of exempt research, at 45 CFR 46.104, whereas FDA regulations have only four at 21 CFR 56.104. There is only one overlapping exemption between the two sets of regulations, which involves certain taste and food quality evaluation and consumer acceptance studies [45 CFR 46.104(b)(6); 21 CFR 56.104(d)]. Therefore, there is unlikely to be much confusion about the application of the distinct sets of exempt categories.

🔗 Section 4

Beginning January 2020, the Common Rule regulations required use of a <u>single IRB</u> for multisite research conducted in the United States, with some minor exceptions [45 CFR 46.114(b)]. FDA currently allows single IRB review for FDA-regulated research, although it is not required. Therefore, this difference in the regulations is unlikely to have any impact in practical terms, because single IRB review can occur under both sets of regulations.

The Common Rule requires several <u>elements of consent</u> that are not in the current FDA regulations. These include a requirement that the informed consent must begin with a concise and focused presentation of <u>key information</u>, and the informed consent as a whole must be presented in a way that facilitates the prospective subject's or legally authorized representative's understanding of the reasons why one might or might not want to participate [45 CFR 46.116(a)(5)]. Another element of consent in the Common Rule but not the FDA regulations is a statement indicating whether or not "identifiers might be removed from the identifiable private information or identifiable biospecimens and that, after such removal, the information or biospecimens could be used for future research studies or distributed to another investigator for future research studies without additional informed consent" [45 CFR 46.116(b)(9)]. Three additional elements of consent, to be included when appropriate, were also added to the Common Rule in 2018 45 CFR 46(c)(7), (8), and (9) but do not appear in the FDA regulations: "(7) a statement that the subject's biospecimens (even if identifiers are removed) may be used for commercial profit and whether the subject will or will not share in this commercial profit; (8) a statement regarding whether clinically relevant research results, including individual research results, will be disclosed to subjects, and if so, under what conditions; and (9) for research involving biospecimens, whether the research will (if known) or might include whole genome sequencing (i.e., sequencing of a human germline or somatic specimen with the intent to generate the genome or exome sequence of that specimen)."

⊘ 6-2

⊘ 6-3

The Common Rule defines a category of <u>broad consent</u>, with distinct elements of consent, for the storage, maintenance, and secondary research use of identifiable private information or identifiable <u>biospecimens</u>. Because there is no equivalent in the current FDA regulations, these broad consent provisions are not applicable to FDA-regulated research.

⊘ 6-9

⊘ 10-10

The Common Rule also has a requirement that an IRB-approved informed consent form used to enroll subjects must be posted by the awardee or the federal department or agency component conducting the trial on a publicly available federal website that will be established as a repository for such informed consent forms. There is no corollary requirement in FDA regulations.

There is one element of consent that always has been and continues to be distinct between the two sets of regulations. FDA regulations require that the consent form must note the possibility that the Food and Drug Administration may inspect the records [21 CFR 50.25(a)(5)]. The Common Rule does not have an analogous obligation.

There are some differences in the ability to <u>waive</u> consent between the two sets of regulations as well. The Common Rule allows a waiver of consent for "research involving public benefit and service programs conducted by or subject to the approval of state or local officials" [45 CFR 46. 116(e)]. However, this type of research is highly unlikely to fall under the jurisdiction of FDA regulations, so this difference is not important. FDA also has three waivers of consent that are not found in the Common Rule, including a (1) waiver of consent for emergency use of a test article [21 CFR 50.23(a)-(c)], (2) waiver of consent "for the administration of an investigational new drug to a member of the armed forces in connection with the member's participation in a particular military operation" [21 CFR 50.23(d)], and (3) waiver of consent for "investigational in vitro diagnostic devices used to identify chemical, biological, radiological, or nuclear agents . . . that would suggest a terrorism event or other public health emergency" [21 CFR 50.23(e)].

⊘ 6-4

Another distinction between the two sets of regulations is that FDA requires IRB review for expanded access to investigational drugs [21 CFR 312, subpart I] and devices for individuals or groups of individuals (FDA, 2019). The Common Rule does not consider these activities to be research, through long standing guidance (DHHS, 1991). For both drugs and devices, review by an IRB chair is sufficient in lieu of review at a convened IRB.

🔗 3-2 🔗 5-7

Conclusion

🔗 2-3

To the extent that an IRB reviews research under both the Common Rule and the FDA regulations, it should have written procedures that capture the differences between the two for IRB staff and board members.

References

Department of Health and Human Services (DHHS). (1991). *Emergency medical care and research: OPRR letter (1991)*. www.hhs.gov/ohrp/regulations-and-policy/guidance/emergency-medical -care-and-research/index.html

Food and Drug Administration (FDA). (2019). *Expanded access for medical devices*. www.fda.gov /medical-devices/investigational-device-exemption-ide/expanded-access-medical-devices

Research Involving Investigational Drugs: IRB Review and the FDA'S IND Process

Jacqueline Corrigan-Curay

Lauren C. Milner

Walter Straus

Abstract

The Food and Drug Administration's Investigational New Drug Application (IND) regulations outline the regulatory process by which FDA oversees the clinical testing of the safety and efficacy of investigational medical products. This chapter provides an overview of the IND process, as well as selected regulatory and scientific issues that may influence the drug review process. This chapter also provides information on the roles and responsibilities of the parties engaged in clinical research involving an FDA-regulated drug.

Introduction

The Food and Drug Administration is responsible for protecting public health through, among other activities, the regulation and oversight of human drug and biological products. As part of its public health mission, FDA helps advance the availability of innovative therapies while ensuring that they are safe and effective for their intended use.

FDA reviews marketing applications for new medical products and approves those determined by the agency to be safe and effective, i.e., have an appropriate risk/benefit profile. For drugs,[1] a multistage process, often referred

---

1 For the purposes of this chapter, unless otherwise noted, the term "drug" refers both to a drug approved under section 505(c) of the Federal Food, Drug, and Cosmetic Act (FD&C Act) and to a biological product licensed under section 351 of the Public Health Service Act (PHS Act) 42 U.S.C. 262.

to as "drug development," generates and collects the evidence provided to FDA, allowing the agency to reach the regulatory determinations required. Drug development generally involves five steps that are sequenced in a manner intended to minimize risks to human research subjects as efficacy, safety, and tolerability are assessed:

1. Drug discovery, where promising candidates are identified and tested in animals or in vitro models for general features (e.g., drug absorption and distribution, mechanism of action)
2. Preclinical research, using in vitro and in vivo models, to determine if the drug is toxic or has other properties rendering it unsuitable for human use
3. Clinical research, where the drug is tested in humans to determine its safety and efficacy for its intended use
4. FDA review and decision whether to approve the drug for marketing, based on whether (a) substantial evidence of effectiveness exists for the intended use, as shown in adequate and well-controlled clinical investigations; and (b) evidence exists that the benefits outweigh the risks for such use
5. Post-market activities, which include monitoring marketed drugs for safety, review of additional studies for new indications, and FDA's oversight of drug advertising and promotion

The process of bringing a product to market is often costly and time consuming, with one calculation of the average capitalized cost to bring each conventional drug to market (including the cost of related failures) estimated at $1.3 billion (DiMasi et al., 2016; Kaitin et al., 2010; Moore et al., 2018).

Regulatory guidance is important throughout drug development, but oversight largely begins when a research activity involving human research subjects commences. For drugs and biologics, the regulatory process generally begins when an IND is submitted to FDA, although FDA will provide solicited advice to sponsors in advance of an IND submission.

Purpose of the IND

Federal law requires that a drug be FDA approved (or "licensed" if a biological product) before it is transported or distributed across state lines for commercial use. The IND provides an exemption to this requirement for the purpose of research [21 U.S.C. 355(i)]. After an IND is in effect, the IND sponsor and individual(s) conducting the research (i.e., investigator) are subject to IND regulations that, among other intended purposes, are designed to safeguard the rights and welfare of the human research subjects participating in a clinical investigation and enhance the quality of evidence intended to support an FDA marketing application (note that for this chapter, the terms *clinical investigation*, *study*, *clinical trial*, and *trial* are used interchangeably).

For INDs submitted to pursue commercial interests, the sponsor is usually a company, although an IND sponsor can also be an academic or research institution or an individual investigator. In the latter case, the investigator is often referred to as a sponsor-investigator and must fulfill the roles of both the sponsor and the investigator.

Overview of the IND Process

The IND process begins when a sponsor of a new drug (or marketed drug) considers its product ready to be tested in human research subjects for a particular indication. The sponsor will submit an IND, and if allowed to proceed, the IND will remain in effect until the sponsor withdraws it, or in rare cases, FDA terminates the IND. FDA termination may be based on deficiencies in an IND or in the conduct of an investigation under an IND **[21 CFR 312.44]**. FDA may also place an IND on inactive status if "no subjects are entered into clinical studies for a period of 2 years or more under an IND, or if all the investigations under the IND remain on clinical hold for 1 year or more" **[21 CFR 312.45]**.

Preclinical Phase and IND Submission Requirements

After a drug candidate is discovered (usually through lab "bench" research), a series of nonclinical studies are performed to determine if the candidate warrants pursuit of commercial development. This "preclinical phase" of development generally involves in vitro studies to characterize the potential medicinal properties of the candidate and in vivo studies to examine the safety of the candidate in specific laboratory animal models. The information provided by these studies will inform whether an IND for the candidate should be submitted (i.e., to allow the drug to be tested in humans).

An IND typically contains information in three areas: (1) animal pharmacology and toxicology studies (which, in this case, allow FDA to assess whether a molecule is sufficiently safe for initial testing in humans); (2) manufacturing information (to ensure that the drug manufacturer has demonstrated the ability to produce and supply consistent batches of the drug for clinical research); and (3) clinical protocols and supporting documentation (which provide information needed to determine whether the proposed studies are scientifically appropriate to address the proposed research questions, as well as to assure the protection of human research subjects). The application must also include information about the qualifications of, and commitments from, sponsors and investigators, including commitments to obtain IRB review and informed consent from human research subjects, as appropriate.

Clinical Investigation Phases

During the period when an IND is in effect, clinical trials are generally conducted in successive phases to provide information about a drug's safety and efficacy in a manner that minimizes risks to human research subjects, while progressively informing safety and efficacy for the proposed indication (FDA, 2018a):

- *Phase 1 trials* are generally conducted in a small group of people, usually representing the first human exposure. Such trials are designed to assess the treatment's short-term safety, determine a safe dosage range, and identify acute side effects. Pharmacokinetic (absorption, distribution, metabolism, and excretion of a drug) and pharmacodynamic (physical, biochemical, and molecular effects of the drug upon the organism) data may be obtained. Phase 1 trials are closely monitored by both sponsors and FDA and are usually conducted in a small number (around 20–100) of either healthy subjects or patients with the disease. Approximately 70% of Phase 1 trials are followed by a Phase 2 clinical trial.   ✐ 10-15

- *Phase 2 trials* are generally conducted in a few hundred human research subjects who have been diagnosed with the disease targeted by the drug and are usually controlled trials with short-term clinical or pharmacological endpoints. Phase 2 trials can be "adequate and well-controlled" studies that support a finding of effectiveness for a particular indication. Currently, about one-third of Phase 2 trials lead to Phase 3 clinical trials.

- *Phase 3 trials* are designed to obtain the additional evidence of effectiveness and safety information that is needed to support drug approval. The sample size and duration of Phase 3 trials vary considerably, depending on the disease targeted by the drug and the size of the drug's effect. Phase 3 trials for drugs developed for acute conditions are usually smaller than those targeting long-term outcomes for chronic diseases, especially when outcomes are relatively infrequent, e.g., studies intended to show a reduction in an uncommon outcome, such as a heart attack or stroke.

- *Phase 4 trials* are carried out after the drug has been approved by FDA, during post-market safety monitoring and may include thousands of people. Given that clinical trial designs rely on clinical assessment in a smaller, and often more homogeneous, population than those who are likely to use the drug following approval, information gaps often arise that can be addressed following approval. These gaps may include further refining the drug's benefit/risk profile under conditions of clinical practice or characterization of the safety profile in populations that may not have been studied in clinical development (e.g., pediatric and geriatric populations). Additionally, Phase 4 trials may be required to further characterize the effectiveness of drugs that have been approved through accelerated approval mechanisms (discussed later).

The description of clinical trial phases provided previously outlines the general sequence of activities for IND processes; in certain cases, particularly for rare diseases or other serious or life-threatening diseases or conditions associated with unmet need, these phases may be compressed depending on the evidence. For example, the first one or two well-controlled studies (Phase 2) may provide sufficient support for a marketing application (a new drug application [NDA] or equivalent biologics license application [BLA]).

Submission of Data for FDA Review

Generally, the sponsor continues to perform clinical trials under the IND until sufficient data to support an NDA are obtained or until a drug fails to demonstrate safety or efficacy (e.g., if the trial does not meet its planned endpoint or shows unacceptable toxicity). The information provided to FDA in an NDA must demonstrate that the drug is safe and effective for its intended use. A sponsor must provide "substantial evidence" of effectiveness—the statutory standard, which also states that the source of such evidence must be "adequate and well-controlled investigations, including clinical investigations" [21 U.S.C. 355(d)]. This regulation has generally been interpreted as calling for two randomized controlled clinical trials. However, FDA can determine that there is substantial evidence of effectiveness based on one adequate and well-controlled clinical trial and confirmatory evidence [21 U.S.C. 355(d)]. In addition, in certain circumstances, "historically controlled" trials may be adequate in lieu of concurrent controls [21 CFR 314.126].

Drug approvals are limited to a specific indication(s); this information is provided in the "drug label," which also provides a summary of the essential prescribing information needed by clinicians.

Expedited Development Programs for Serious Conditions

When reviewing drugs that are being developed to treat life-threatening and severely debilitating diseases, especially "where no satisfactory alternative therapy exists" **[21 CFR 312.80–312.84]**, the clinical trial phases can be compressed and/or the sequence can be flexible, and the amount of data needed is subject to interpretation. Specifically, FDA's regulations at **21 CFR 312 subpart E** allow flexibility in applying the statutory standards, while preserving appropriate guarantees for safety and effectiveness.

In addition, FDA has several distinct programs (collectively referred to as expedited programs) designed to facilitate and expedite the development and review of drugs for serious conditions for which there is an unmet medical need (FDA, 2014; Woodcock and Marks, 2019):

- *Fast track designation* (FTD) may be given to an investigational drug(s) that provides evidence demonstrating its potential to address an unmet medical need based on nonclinical data and/or clinical data—for example, a drug that shows early promise based on preclinical data or in an initial trial. Sponsors of investigational drugs with FTDs receive additional opportunities to engage with FDA to seek clarity on requirements for drug approval with the goal of enhancing the efficiency of investigational drug development for those drugs.

- *Breakthrough therapy designation* (BTD) may be granted for an investigational drug that provides preliminary clinical evidence demonstrating that the drug may provide substantial improvement over available therapy on a clinically significant endpoint(s); for example, a drug may be shown in early-phase clinical trials to be more effective at reducing relapses of multiple sclerosis than standard therapies. BTD differs from FTD in both the type and level of evidence required. First, unlike an FTD, which can be submitted using nonclinical data, a BTD requires submission of clinical data. Second, FTDs require the applicant to show "potential" of a drug to address an unmet medical need, whereas BTD applicants must provide preliminary evidence of a substantial benefit above available therapy on a clinical endpoint. BTD includes similar features as FTD but provides additional opportunities for communication with FDA and increased coordination of cross-disciplinary review between FDA review staff and oversight by senior FDA management.

- *Regenerative medicine advanced therapy* (RMAT) designation may be granted for a regenerative medicine therapy (defined as a cell therapy, therapeutic tissue engineering product, a human cell and tissue product, or any combination product using such therapies or products) that shows preliminary evidence that the therapy will address an unmet need, for example, a cell therapy associated with rapid and substantial wound reepithelialization of deep partial thickness burns. RMAT designations have the same benefits as FTDs and BTDs, including early interactions with FDA to discuss potential surrogate or immediate endpoints that may qualify the RMAT for accelerated approval (described later).

- *Priority review* may be given to an investigational drug showing potential for significant improvement in the safety or effectiveness of a treatment or diagnosis, or prevention of a serious disease, at the time a marketing application is submitted. FDA's goal in priority review is to complete review and act on a new drug application within 6 months rather than the 10 months for standard review of new drug applications. Any drug, including those that have received an FTD or BTD, can be granted priority review if the relevant criteria are met. Receiving an FTD or BTD does not automatically confer priority review, as priority review is based on the results contained in the marketing application (which are not known at the time that the FTD or BTD is granted).

The programs described previously do not alter the traditional route to marketing approval, which is based on showing that the drug affects a clinical endpoint(s) that measures how a patient survives, feels, or functions. Clinical endpoint(s) can take many years to manifest. In some cases, a "validated surrogate endpoint"—where there is extensive clinical evidence demonstrating that a change in the surrogate endpoint is predictive of clinical benefit—may be used in lieu of a clinical endpoint to support drug approval. For example, blood pressure is a validated surrogate endpoint used to support drug approvals, given that many studies have documented the relationship between reduction in blood pressure and reduction in rates of stroke, myocardial infarction, and mortality. Similarly, lowering low-density lipids (LDL) has been shown to reduce the risk of cardiovascular events in those who have had a cardiovascular event in a number of studies, so sponsors may use LDL as validated surrogate endpoint instead of a cardiovascular clinical endpoint in their drug marketing application.

Data may be available to support a relationship between a "surrogate endpoint" and a clinical endpoint (e.g., laboratory measurement, radiographic image, physical sign, or other clinical measure), but the data may not be sufficiently strong to make it a "validated surrogate endpoint" for a clinical outcome. For example, a surrogate endpoint of clearance of bacteria from the bloodstream, as evidenced by a laboratory-based assessment of bacteria in the blood, has been considered reasonably likely to predict the clinical resolution of infection, but lacks the clinical evidence needed to confirm this association. Surrogate endpoints that are not considered sufficient to support traditional drug approval, but evidence that the surrogate endpoint that is "reasonably likely" to predict clinical benefit may support drug approval under the accelerated approval (AA) program. To qualify for approval under AA, the drug must be intended to diagnose, treat, or prevent a serious disease for which there is an unmet medical need.

AA has been used primarily in settings in which the disease course is long and an extended period of time would be required to measure the intended clinical benefit of a drug. Drugs granted AA must meet the same statutory standards for safety and effectiveness as those granted traditional approval, but substantial evidence of effectiveness is based on adequate and well-controlled clinical investigations for which the drug is shown to have an effect on the surrogate endpoint rather than a clinical endpoint. For safety, the standard is having sufficient information to determine whether the drug is safe for use under conditions prescribed, recommended, or suggested in the proposed labeling. If approved under AA, FDA requires that the sponsor conduct additional studies to confirm the drug's clinical benefit after the drug is approved for marketing.

In summary, expedited programs are intended to promote the drug development and review process, but the evidence supporting drugs reviewed under these programs must meet the same scientific and clinical standards as the evidence supporting drugs undergoing traditional FDA review. Although these programs are the main mechanisms to expedite drug development for promising therapies, there are additional programs that provide incentives for the development of certain types of medical products (e.g., Generating Antibiotic Incentives Now [GAIN; **21 U.S.C. 355f**] provides incentives for the development of antibacterial and antifungal drugs for human use intended to treat serious and life-threatening infections).

Clinical Holds and Investigator Disqualification

Circumstances occasionally occur that require FDA to delay, interrupt, or terminate research conducted under an IND. FDA has the authority to place a "clinical hold" on a trial, either before the trial begins or during the course of the trial. A sponsor may also choose to withdraw an IND for any reason. When an IND is withdrawn, sponsors are responsible for ensuring that all trials under the IND stop and that any unused investigational drug is disposed of appropriately.

FDA also has the authority to "disqualify" an investigator if they deliberately fail to comply with regulatory requirements or submit false information to the sponsor or to FDA. A disqualified investigator is not eligible to conduct any trials of an FDA-regulated product.

FDA Oversight of Marketed Drugs

FDA and sponsors continue to monitor the safety of drugs and biologics after they have been approved ("licensed" in the case of biologics) and become available for clinical use, and they do so until the agent is potentially no longer approved. This responsibility is an essential function of the agency, given that after approval much larger and more diverse patient populations are exposed to the drug and are often exposed for longer periods than during clinical testing. FDA has a number of mechanisms to collect data on safety—for example, collection of adverse event reports and medication error reports through FDA's MedWatch system or through the use of FDA's Sentinel system. Drug manufacturers are required to report safety information, whereas healthcare professionals and consumers may report safety concerns and experiences, either directly to FDA or to the drug manufacturer, for further evaluation. FDA may also communicate any emergent concerns to sponsors, where they are addressed through review of available data and possibly through the implementation of additional activities (e.g., subsequent research, modifications of manufacturing processes).

Should FDA identify a serious safety issue for a marketed drug, such as the identification of a novel drug–drug interaction, the agency has several ways to take regulatory action. Identification of a serious safety concern will almost always lead to modification of the drug label, which guides clinician prescribing practices. In certain cases, a risk evaluation and mitigation strategy (REMS) may be required to help reduce the occurrence and/or severity of the safety risk identified (Food and Drug Administration Amendments Act of 2007). An REMS may require any of several interventions, ranging from specific training for drug prescribers to ongoing monitoring (e.g., through regular lab tests and clinical assessments) of patients taking the drug. REMS are not limited to the post-marketing setting and may be put in place concurrent with approval of the drug. In exceptional circumstances, FDA may require that the drug be taken off the market.

Studies Requiring or Not Requiring an IND

Studies Requiring an IND

INDs are required for any study of an investigational drug that has never been approved for use in the United States. Additionally, given that FDA drug approvals are limited to specific indications, sponsors may also need to obtain an IND, or amend an existing IND, for certain trials with an approved drug for different (new) populations, dosing, or routes of administration.

Studies Not Requiring an IND

In general, an IND is not required for studies evaluating a marketed drug in a manner consistent with its labeling. Specifically, an IND is *not needed* to conduct a clinical investigation with an approved drug—that is, one that is already marketed in the United States, when *all* of the following apply:

- The investigation is not intended to be reported to FDA in support of a new indication or a significant change in the labeling of the drug.
- In the case of a prescription drug, the investigation is not intended to support a significant change in the advertising for the drug.
- The investigation does not involve a route of administration, dose, patient population, or other factor that significantly increases the risk (or decreases the acceptability of the risk) associated with the use of the drug product.

Importantly, an IND is not required if the drug is administered in the course of medical practice at provider discretion, even if the drug is being given to treat a condition outside of its indicated use ("off-label" use; FDA, 2013).

IRB Involvement in the IND Process

IRBs play an important role throughout the IND process, where they serve to ensure, both in advance of a trial and through periodic review, that appropriate steps are being taken to protect the rights and welfare of human research subjects.

Sponsors and investigators must ensure IRB involvement in the initial and ongoing review of clinical trials, which includes review of research protocols (or protocol changes) and other trial materials to ensure appropriate human research subjects protections, review of investigator qualifications, and review of the adequacy of the trial site. In addition, IRBs may assist investigators or sponsor-investigators in determining whether an IND is necessary for a proposed trial.

IRB review is expected, at least annually, for any ongoing investigation(s) under an IND. As part of its review, the IRB should consider any adverse events (AEs) that may affect the risks presented to human research subjects. In general, an AE should be reported to the IRB as an unanticipated problem only if it is unexpected, serious, and possibly related to the study drug, as determined by the sponsor (FDA, 2009, 2012). If the sponsor makes such a determination, it must report the serious AE to FDA and to all investigators. Investigators, in turn, are responsible for sharing this information with the IRB. Other

SPONSOR AND INVESTIGATOR RESPONSIBILITIES UNDER AN IND

As part of the IND, the sponsor and investigator(s) responsible for conducting the trial(s) commit to different roles and responsibilities associated with human subject protections and data integrity needs.

A sponsor is the party that takes responsibility for and initiates the IND, and the sponsor is responsible for oversight and monitoring of the clinical trial(s) conducted under the IND. The sponsor communicates with FDA and ensures that both FDA and investigators are promptly informed of any significant adverse events or risks associated with the drug that emerge during the course of a trial. Sponsors ultimately have the responsibility to ensure that the trial is conducted in a manner that protects human research subjects and the integrity of the data.

An investigator is an individual who conducts the trial and/or is the person responsible for leading the research team at a particular trial site. Investigators' responsibilities include ensuring appropriate conduct of the trial(s) to: protect the rights, safety, and welfare of the human research subjects participating at their trial site; control the drug(s) under investigation; and meet certain record keeping, retention, and reporting requirements, including reporting safety data to the sponsor. Investigators are also responsible for assuring IRB review of the trial protocol and any protocol changes, and for communicating to the IRB and sponsor any unanticipated problems or protocol deviations involving risk to human research subjects or others.

A sponsor-investigator is an individual who both initiates and conducts a clinical trial and is responsible for both sponsor and investigator responsibilities associated with an IND (FDA, 2015).

unanticipated problems may arise that are not related to the drug, such as breaches of privacy; these should also be reported to the IRB.

Generally, investigators communicate with the IRBs, but FDA will notify the IRB directly if an FDA inspection of the trial site results in any violation, such as a "warning letter" for trial conduct problems or a notice of disqualification proceedings for an investigator or institution (FDA, 2010).

🔗 8-6

FDA regulations require IRBs to follow written procedures for conducting initial and continuing review of research and reporting findings and actions to the investigator and institution; determining which projects require review more often than annually; and ensuring prompt reporting to the IRB of changes in research activity and IRB review, as well as approval of changes, except where necessary to eliminate apparent immediate hazards to the human research subjects. Written procedures are also required for ensuring prompt reporting to the IRB, appropriate institutional officials, and FDA regarding (1) any unanticipated problems involving risks to human subjects or others, (2) any instance of serious or continuing noncompliance with these regulations or the requirements or determinations of the IRB, or (3) any suspension or termination of IRB approval (**21 CFR 56.108 (a)** and **(b)**; FDA, 2018b). FDA requirements for IRB activities can be found in **21 CFR Part 50**, **56**, and **312**; additional information about IRB responsibilities can be found on FDA's website (www.fda.gov).

🔗 2-3
🔗 7-2

🔗 7-1

🔗 7-3
🔗 7-6

Additional Considerations for Drug Development and Review

Biological Products (Biologics)

Drugs are generally small molecules, designed and produced using synthetic chemistry techniques, that can be precisely characterized in terms of chemical structure. In contrast, biological products are usually larger molecules with chemical structures that are more difficult to characterize. For example, FDA oversees the U.S. blood supply, which comprises a far more complex set of molecules, including whole cells. Other biologics, such as vaccines and monoclonal antibodies, are produced in biological systems (e.g., cell culture). In addition, interest has surged recently regarding development of cellular and gene therapies, which are highly complex and novel biological products. That said, most biologics meet the definition of a "drug," making them subject to premarket approval requirements, and, for clinical trials of unapproved biological products, IND requirements apply.

Clinical research on biologics performed under an IND is subject to the same requirements for human research subjects protections and data quality standards as clinical research on drugs. In addition, given that biological products are generally derived from living systems, a robust manufacturing process is critical to ensure batch-to-batch consistency. For a vaccine to be licensed, for example, the sponsor must submit a BLA, which requires that the proposed manufacturing facility be inspected and approved by FDA as a precondition for licensure.

Combination Products

Sponsors may propose to test a product(s) that combines a small molecule drug, a device, and/or a biologic. Examples of combination products include a monoclonal antibody combined with a therapeutic drug (biological product/small molecule drug) or a prefilled drug delivery system (device/drug). When reviewing combination products, FDA assigns to one center (Center for Drug Evaluation and Research [CDER], Center for Devices and Radiological Health [CDRH], or Center for Biologics Evaluation and Research [CBER]) primary jurisdiction over the product's review and regulation. Because combination products are subject to different regulations, research oversight and regulatory evaluation can be complex, depending on the product(s) being proposed for study. The submission of combination products may increase in the future, as emerging technologies and methodologies reduce boundaries between product types.

Looking Forward

FDA recognizes that new technological and methodological tools are continuously being designed to accelerate and improve drug development, and the agency actively considers how these types of tools affect the IND and/or regulatory review process.

For example, the research community has developed innovative trial design strategies to facilitate and accelerate drug development. One example of an innovative trial design is an adaptive trial, which allows for prespecified planned modification(s) to a trial, such as refining the sample size or excluding particular treatments or treatment doses, based on an interim evaluation of data. These types of trials may be more flexible than traditional clinical trials and may be more cost and time efficient, for example, by requiring fewer human research subjects (Pallmann et al., 2018). In 2019, FDA launched the Complex Innovative Trial Design (CID) pilot program to facilitate and advance the use of innovative and complex trial designs for drug development. Sponsors participating in this program will have additional opportunities to meet with FDA to receive agency input on trial design and analyses.

Additionally, FDA is exploring the use of "decentralized" clinical trials (DCTs) to support evidence for drug safety and effectiveness. DCTs adhere to the general principles and processes of traditional clinical trials but use a variety of technological tools, such as telemedicine and digital health technologies, to conduct trial activities at point-of-care locations, such as the participant's home or healthcare provider's office, rather than at a traditional study site. DCTs may provide certain advantages over traditional clinical trials, such as allowing for faster subject recruitment, increasing the diversity of individuals recruited for a study, and/or improving subjects retention.

FDA is also considering specific issues as outlined in the 21st Century Cures Act, a law enacted in 2016 designed to accelerate medical product development and to faster and more efficiently bring new medical innovations to the patients who need them. Under the Cures Act, FDA has been tasked to evaluate if and how real-world data (RWD), defined as data relating to patient health status and/or delivery of health care that is routinely collected from a variety of sources (e.g., electronic health records, insurance claims and billing activities, product and disease registries, and mobile devices) can generate real-world evidence (RWE). In this context, RWE is defined as clinical evidence regarding the usage and potential benefits or risks of a medical analysis derived from analysis of RWD to help support the approval of a new indication for marketed products or to satisfy post-approval study requirements. The use of such data may accelerate approval of new indications for approved drugs based on studies that differ from traditional trials—for example, through collection of RWD for endpoints or use of digital health technologies. In 2018, FDA published a draft framework outlining the agency's proposed program to evaluate the potential of RWE to inform FDA's product approval determinations

(FDA, 2018c). The RWE program is multifaceted, including demonstration projects, internal education and external stakeholder engagement efforts, and guidance documents to assist drug developers interested in using RWD or RWE to support a labeling claim. The agency views this program as a part of its continued efforts to explore the utility of a variety of data sources to support the drug development process.

Conclusion

The goals of the IND process—to protect human research subjects and develop evidence that can be used to support a finding of drug safety and effectiveness—remain constant, but continual advances in our understanding of human biology, coupled with the development of new technologies to assess, treat, and prevent human disease, requires FDA to continue to evolve and refine approaches for the review and oversight of drug development. FDA is actively engaged in efforts to provide regulatory guidance on how the use of emerging research technologies, research methodologies, and study designs may affect clinical research being conducted under an IND and to help ensure that such tools are successfully incorporated into the drug development and review process. FDA's decision making is informed by sponsors, investigators, IRB members, IRB administrative staff, and the general public.

Acknowledgments

We would like to thank FDA's Office of Good Clinical Practice, Dr. John Concato, David Joy, Stefanie Kraus, J. Paul Phillips, Dr. Robert Temple, Julia Tierney, and Sarah Walinsky for providing their review and input into different sections of this chapter. We would especially like to thank Rosemarie Purcell for her help in drafting the chapter.

Resources

21st Century Cures Act. Public Law 114-255, enacted December 13, 2016. www.gpo.gov/fdsys/pkg/PLAW-114publ255/pdf/PLAW-114publ255.pdf

Code of Federal Regulations, Title 21, Chapter 1–Food and Drug Administration, DHHS, Part 312–Investigational New Drug Application (2019). www.accessdata.fda.gov/scripts/cdrh/cfdocs/cfcfr/CFRsearch.cfm?CFRPart=312

Code of Federal Regulations, Title 21, Chapter 1–Food and Drug Administration, DHHS, Part 314–Applications for FDA Approval to Market a New Drug (2019). www.accessdata.fda.gov/scripts/cdrh/cfdocs/cfcfr/CFRsearch.cfm?CFRPart=314

Federal Food, Drug, and Cosmetic Act (FD&C Act). Public Law 75-717, enacted June 25, 1938. https://catalog.archives.gov/id/299847

References

DiMasi, J. A., Grabowski, H. G., & Hansen, R. W. (2016). Innovation in the pharmaceutical industry: New estimates of R&D costs. *Journal of Health Economics, 47,* 20–33.

Food and Drug Administration Amendments Act of 2007. Public Law 110-85, enacted September 27, 2007. www.congress.gov/110/plaws/publ8/PLAW-110publ8.pdf

Food and Drug Administration (FDA). (2009). *Guidance for clinical investigators, sponsors, and IRBs, adverse event reporting to IRBs—improving human subject protection.* www.fda.gov/media/72267/download

Food and Drug Administration (FDA). (2010). *Information sheet guidance for IRBs, clinical investigators, and sponsors, FDA inspections of clinical investigators.* www.fda.gov/media/75185/download

Food and Drug Administration (FDA). (2012). *Guidance for industry and investigators, safety reporting requirements for INDs and BA/BE studies.* www.fda.gov/media/79394/download

Food and Drug Administration (FDA). (2013). *Guidance for clinical investigators, sponsors, and IRBs, investigational new drug applications (INDs)—determining whether human research studies can be conducted without an IND.* www.fda.gov/media/79386/download

Food and Drug Administration (FDA). (2014). *Guidance for industry, expedited programs for serious conditions–drugs and biologics.* www.fda.gov/media/86377/download

Food and Drug Administration (FDA). (2015). *Guidance for industry, investigational new drug applications prepared and submitted by sponsor-investigators.* www.fda.gov/media/92604/download

Food and Drug Administration (FDA). (2018a). *Step 3: Clinical research.* www.fda.gov/patients/drug-development-process/step-3-clinical-research

Food and Drug Administration (FDA). (2018b). *Guidance for institutions and IRBs, institutional review board written procedures.* www.fda.gov/media/99271/download

Food and Drug Administration (FDA). (2018c). *Framework for FDA's real-world evidence program.* www.fda.gov/media/120060/download

Kaitin, K. I. (2010). Deconstructing the drug development process: The new face of innovation. *Clinical Pharmacology and Therapeutics, 83*(3), 356–361.

Moore, T. J., Zhang, H., Anderson, G., & Alexander, G. C. (2018). Estimated costs of pivotal trials for novel therapeutic agents approved by the US Food and Drug Administration, 2015–2016. *JAMA Internal Medicine, 178*(11), 1451–1457.

Pallmann, P., Bedding, A. W., Choodari-Oskooei, B., Dimairo, M., Flight, L., Hampson, L. V., Holmes, J., Mander, A. P., Odondi, L., Sydes, M. R., Villar, S. S., Wason, J., Weir, C. J., Wheeler, G. M., Yap, C., & Jaki, T. (2018). Adaptive designs in clinical trials: Why use them, and how to run and report them. *BMC Medicine, 16*(1), 29.

Woodcock, J., & Marks, P. (2019). *Delivering promising new medicines without sacrificing safety and efficacy.* www.fda.gov/news-events/fda-voices-perspectives-fda-leadership-and-experts/delivering-promising-new-medicines-without-sacrificing-safety-and-efficacy

Research Involving Medical Devices: IRB Review and the FDA's IDE Process

Laverne Estanol
Erica Heath

Abstract

IRB administrators reviewing research involving medical devices should have a working knowledge of the ways new devices arrive on the market, including the classification system for medical devices, the definition of an investigational device, and the complexities of the Food and Drug Administration (FDA) investigational device exemption (IDE) process. This chapter describes the major components of the device regulations that distinguish them from the drug regulations, identifies issues raised in clinical investigations of devices, and discusses the critical and central role that IRBs play in the regulation of medical devices.

Background and History

Although charms and talismans to prevent or cure disease have been used from ancient times, there was rarely more than anecdotal proof as to their safety or their efficacy. The Pure Food and Drug Act of 1906 did not cover medical devices (Pure Food and Drug Act, 1906). The 1938 Food, Drug, and Cosmetic (FD&C) Act gave the U.S. Food and Drug Administration (FDA) jurisdiction over medical devices for the first time but was essentially confined to preventing the sale of products that it believed were adulterated or misbranded, and enforcement was limited (FD&C Act, 1938). There was gradual recognition that the existing law provided an inadequate framework for regulating the rapidly expanding variety of medical devices (Merrill, 1994).

In 1969, the Department of Health, Education, and Welfare (now the Department of Health and Human Services) appointed the Cooper Committee to study the nature and scope of future device legislation. After finding at least 10,000 injuries and 751 fatalities attributable to "therapeutic devices" over 10 years, the Cooper Committee proposed a system whereby existing devices would be assigned to one of three classes; based on these classes, FDA regulatory authority would range from premarket approval (PMA) to simple policing for faulty manufacture or mislabeling (Department of Health, Education and Welfare, 1970). The recommendations of the Cooper Commission were ultimately translated into the Medical Device Amendments (MDA) of 1976 to the Federal Food, Drug, and Cosmetic Act, regulations were issued in 1980, and the FDA's Center for Devices and Radiological Health (CDRH) was created in 1982 (MDA, 1976). Subsequent to the FD&C Act, new legislation, including the Safe Medical Devices Act (1990), the Food and Drug Administration Modernization Act (1997), the Medical Device User Fee and Modernization Act (2002), and the 21st Century Cures Act (2016), have augmented FDA authority and streamlined its operations regarding medical devices.

⊘ 11-2
This chapter describes the major components of the device regulations that distinguish them from the <u>drug regulations</u>, identifies issues raised in clinical investigations of devices, and discusses the critical and central role that IRBs play in the regulation of medical devices.

What Is a Medical Device?

A medical device, as defined by the FD&C Act **21 U.S.C. § 321(h)**, is as follows:

> an instrument, apparatus, implement, machine, contrivance, implant, in vitro reagent, or other similar or related article, including a component part, or accessory which is:
>
> 1. recognized in the official National Formulary, or the United States Pharmacopoeia, or any supplement to them,
> 2. intended for use in the diagnosis of disease or other conditions, or in the cure, mitigation, treatment, or prevention of disease, in man or other animals, or
> 3. intended to affect the structure or any function of the body of man or other animals, and
>
> which does not achieve its primary intended purposes through chemical action within or on the body of man or other animals and which is not dependent upon being metabolized for the achievement of its primary intended purposes.

The category of medical devices is very broad, ranging from crutches, to magnetic resonance imaging (MRI), to in vitro diagnostics. Medical devices include not only hardware but also the software running it; also included are smartphone applications, mobile medical devices, and, perhaps in the not too distant future, artificial intelligence.

Critical to the definition of a medical device is its intended use. According to the definition given earlier, if a device is "intended for use in the diagnosis of disease or other conditions, or in the cure, mitigation, treatment, or prevention of disease . . . or intended to affect the structure or any function of the body," it is likely to be a medical device and thus be regulated by FDA **[21 U.S.C. 321(h)]** (**Table 11.3-1**).

Table 11.3-1 Possible Device Uses and Regulation

Device Used in Study	Nonmedical Device (not FDA regulated)	Medical Device (FDA regulated)
Wrist monitor to measure heart rate	For runners	For diagnosis of disease
Copper bracelet	For feeling more robust (wellness)	For symptoms of arthritis
Genetic test kit	For ancestry	For diagnosis or prediction of disease
Laboratory test	For use in a research laboratory	For diagnostic study

From the point of view of the IRB, only devices classified as medical devices require application of FDA regulations at **21 CFR 50** and **56**.

Classification of Medical Devices [21 CFR 860.3]

The MDA of 1976 established a classification system that codified all novel devices into one of three classes: class I, class II, or class III (MDA, 1976). The classes were not intended to be solely a risk classification schema; they were also intended to designate the level of regulation required to establish that the devices in that class are "safe and effective" (MDA, 1976). Each class requires an increasing amount of regulatory control in order to maintain this assurance of safety and effectiveness and to meet the requirements for entering the market.

Class I (low risk of illness or injury) devices are items such as "elastic bandages, examination gloves, hand-held surgical instruments" (FDA, 2018a); their manufacture and marketing are only subject to *general controls*, which include registration, device listing, premarket notification, and good manufacturing practice requirements. Most class I devices are exempt from premarket review, and manufacturers need not submit an application to FDA prior to marketing.

Class II (moderate risk) includes items such as "powered wheelchairs, infusion pumps, surgical drapes" (FDA, 2018a). In addition to general controls, class II devices require *special controls* in order to mitigate risk. Special controls are usually device-specific and may include special labeling requirements, mandatory performance standards, and postmarket surveillance. Some class II devices are exempt from premarket review.

Class III devices (high risk) include devices that are life supporting or life sustaining, or which present a high or potentially unreasonable risk of illness or injury to a patient. Examples of such devices are "heart valves, silicone gel-filled breast implants, implanted cerebellar stimulators" (FDA, 2018a). All class III devices require general controls, and instead of special controls, most also require premarket FDA approval (see Premarket Approval section).

New devices that are not class I or II are automatically designated as class III unless the manufacturer files a request for reclassification [**FD&C Act §513(f)(2)**]. Magnetic resonance imaging (MRI) entered the market as a completely new class III device and was later reclassified to class II. Safety studies are often required in order to justify reclassification.

LIMITATIONS OF THE SUBSTANTIAL EQUIVALENCE STANDARD

During the first 10 years following enactment of the MDA, over 80% of class III devices entering the market did so on the basis of showing substantial equivalence (510(k)) to devices on the market before the MDA (Institute of Medicine, 2011).

There has been significant debate regarding whether the 510(k) process is sufficiently protective of users of medical devices. The 510(k) process finds that new devices are substantially equivalent to a predicate device. Since all predicate devices were on the market before the 1976 MDA, they have themselves never been systematically assessed to determine their safety and effectiveness.

The negative consequences of this equivalence to a device that has never been systematically assessed to determine its safety and effectiveness is illustrated by the case of the metal-on-metal DePuy ASR XL total hip replacement. By claiming "substantial equivalence" to 95 different previously marketed devices, including devices in use prior to 1976, it cleared without any clinical evaluation in 2008. The ASR XL was recalled two years later, at which time 100,000 devices had already been implanted with a 49% failure rate (Ardaugh et al., 2013).

Routes to Market [21 CFR 814]

In general, the route a medical device takes to market correlates with the class of the device; however, some deviations occur.

As noted previously, most (but not all) class I devices and some class II devices are exempt from premarket review, and manufacturers need not submit an application to FDA prior to marketing. Other devices proceed to market via a number of mechanisms; the three most relevant are discussed here. Importantly, note the difference between device *clearance* (via **FD&C Act §510(k)**) and device *approval* (via PMA and the humanitarian device exemption (HDE)).

- *Substantial Equivalence*
  Section 510(k) of the FD&C Act allows a sponsor to claim to FDA that their device is "substantially equivalent" to a device that was on the market as of 1976 (a "predicate device") **[FD&C Act §513(i)(1)(A)]**. If the 510(k) claim is accepted by FDA, it is *cleared* (not approved) and can join the device already on the market without any demonstration of safety or efficacy. Most class II devices enter the market via the 510(k) pathway.

- *Premarket Approval (PMA)*

  ⊘ 11-2

  PMA is roughly the device equivalent of the new drug application (NDA). In contrast to a 510(k), PMAs generally require some clinical data to determine safety and efficacy before FDA will approve the device **[21 CFR 814 subpart C]**. As will be discussed later, all clinical investigations of investigational devices (unless exempt) must have an IDE before the clinical study is initiated **[21 CFR 812 subpart B]**. Most class III devices use the PMA route; however, some class III devices may be cleared via the 510(k) process.

- *Humanitarian Use Device* **[21 CFR 814.100]**:

  ⊘ 11-5

  Similar to an orphan drug, the humanitarian use device (HUD) designation is for a device designed to treat a disease or condition that affects fewer than 8,000 people in the United States per year. The HUD designation allows market approval "notwithstanding the absence of reasonable assurance of effectiveness that would otherwise be required . . ." **[21 CFR 814.100(b)(2)]**.

Clinical Investigations Involving Medical Devices

21 CFR 812.3(g) defines an investigational device as "a device, including a transitional device, that is the object of an investigation." The concept of "object" is important. Many devices used in studies are not the object of those studies. Some basic science studies and studies in physiology, kinesiology, and physical education use medical devices, but the object of the study is some

physical question rather than the safety or effectiveness of the device; therefore, the device is not considered an investigational device.

Consider the following four scenarios:

1. A marketed device is used to measure what it is designed to measure, within a physiology, drug, or exercise study.
2. A marketed device is used per indication in a clinic, and the doctor is reviewing their records regarding the device's effects or costs.
3. An approved device is being studied for further clarity on its efficacy.
4. An inventor is tinkering with several iterations of their approved device in order to improve the sensitivity, and they are using it in the lab on a small number of human subjects.

All four studies are human subjects research and therefore require IRB review and approval under the Common Rule or institutional requirements. Whether the study is also subject to **21 CFR parts 50**, **56**, and **812** depends on whether the device is the *object of the study*. In examples 1 and 2, the device is not the object, and therefore the study is likely not subject to **21 CFR parts 50**, **56**, or **812**. In examples 3 and 4 the device is the object of the study; therefore, the device is an investigational device, and the research is subject to **21 CFR parts 50**, **56**, and **812**.

Use of an investigational device in a clinical investigation requires an IDE, either abbreviated or full, unless that investigation is exempt from the requirement per **21 CFR 812.2(c)**.

Exempt from IDE

21 CFR 812.2(c) describes categories of investigations that are exempt from the requirement of an IDE. The most common (and most relevant to IRBs) are the following:

- A device that FDA has determined to be "substantially equivalent to a device in commercial distribution" before 1976 (that is, 510(k) devices) and that is used or investigated according to its labeling **[21 CFR 812.2(c)(2)]**.
- Diagnostic devices, if the testing of the device meets four requirements: "(i) Is noninvasive, (ii) Does not require an invasive sampling procedure that presents significant risk, (iii) does not by design or intention introduce energy into a subject, and (iv) is not used as a diagnostic procedure without confirmation of the diagnosis by another, medically established product or procedure" **[21 CFR 812.2(c)(3)]**.
- A device undergoing "consumer preference testing, testing of a modification, or testing of a combination of two or more devices in commercial distribution, if the testing is not for the purpose of determining safety or effectiveness and does not put subjects at risk" **[21 CFR 812.2(c)(4)]**. Note that these investigations may also be exempt from IRB review under **21 CFR 56.104(d)**.

It is important to stress that investigations that are exempt from the requirement for an IDE are still subject to FDA regulations regarding human subject protections **21 CFR 50** and **56**.

Abbreviated or Full IDE

Research use of an investigational device that is not exempt as described earlier requires an IDE. It is the responsibility of the sponsor (usually the manufacturer) of the device to obtain the IDE. The sponsor requirements for obtaining

---

SIGNIFICANT RISK DEVICE

Significant risk device is defined in **21 CFR 812.3(m)** as "an investigational device that:

1. Is intended as an implant and presents a potential for serious risk to the health, safety, or welfare of a subject;
2. Is purported or represented to be for a use in supporting or sustaining human life and presents a potential for serious risk to the health, safety, or welfare of a subject;
3. Is for a use of substantial importance in diagnosing, curing, mitigating, or treating disease, or otherwise preventing impairment of human health and presents a potential for serious risk to the health, safety, or welfare of a subject; or
4. otherwise presents a potential for serious risk to the health, safety, or welfare of a subject."

---

an IDE are extensive; they are described in **21 CFR 812** and are not largely relevant to the IRB (FDA, 2018b).

Under certain circumstances, the sponsor may seek an abbreviated IDE. Responsibilities under an abbreviated IDE are described in **21 CFR 812.2(b)**. These are largely limited to labeling, advertising, monitoring, and record-keeping, as well as meeting the more general investigator obligations to obtain local IRB approval of the study. In an abbreviated IDE, no specific notification or approval from FDA is required; in effect, the IRB acts as a surrogate for FDA.

The critical determining factor regarding whether an abbreviated IDE is appropriate is whether the device is a "significant risk device" (See box, Significant Risk Device). In essence, a significant risk device is one that poses a serious risk to the health, safety, or welfare of a subject.

In order for a sponsor to seek an abbreviated IDE, they must "[obtain] IRB approval of the investigation after presenting the reviewing IRB with a brief explanation of why the device is not a significant risk device" [**21 CFR 812.2(a) (ii)**].

The sponsor designates whether they believe the device is of significant risk (SR) versus nonsignificant risk (NSR) and may provide documents to support their contention. However, the full <u>convened IRB</u> makes the final determination of whether the device is SR or NSR.

✎ 5-7

The IRB's decision regarding SR versus NSR can be complicated. As noted previously, it hinges on the definition of SR device in **21 CFR 812.3(m)**. That regulation focuses primarily on whether *the device* presents a potential for serious risk to the health, safety, or welfare of a subject. However, FDA guidance discusses the risks of "the device study" (FDA, 2006). This encompasses a much broader realm of risks, up to and including risks from clinical care. A reasonable middle-road approach might be for the IRB to consider the risks of the device as it is used *in the context* of the study. This encompasses a measurable set of risks related to the device as altered by the situation of that study. A device could be found to have different risks in different studies or populations, and the determination is not transferable between studies.

It is also important to note that the NSR/SR decision regarding a device (required by **21 CFR 812**) is not the same as the minimal risk/greater than minimal risk IRB determinations required by **21 CFR 56**, although in most cases they align.

If the IRB determines that a device is NSR, then the clinical investigation can proceed, and no report to FDA is required until the data are submitted (i.e., an abbreviated IDE). If the IRB determines that the device is SR, then the sponsor must seek an IDE from FDA. In the case of a multisite study involving more than one IRB, if any IRB determines the device is SR, then an IDE is needed.

Note that FDA may subsequently decide that an NSR determination by the IRB (and sponsor) was incorrect. In that circumstance, FDA may require the study to stop and the sponsor to obtain an IDE

Resources

When considering clinical trials involving medical devices, administrators should be conscious of the myriad FDA guidance documents. FDA provides an up-to-date list of guidance documents on its website that can be browsed by topic or found using a guidance document search function (FDA, 2020). Many FDA guidance documents target sponsors, describing information required for clearance or approval or the kinds of data that are required. Very few guidance documents are specifically targeted to IRBs; however, familiarity with the guidance documents used by sponsors and researchers can assist the IRB in making its required determinations under FDA regulations.

References

21st Century Cures Act. (2016). Pub. L. 114–255, 130 Stat. 1033. www.congress.gov/114 /plaws/publ255/PLAW-114publ255.pdf

Ardaugh, B. M., Graves, S. E., & Redberg, R. F. (2013). The 510(k) ancestry of a metal-on-metal hip implant. *New England Journal of Medicine, 368*(2), 97–100.

Department of Health, Education and Welfare. (1970). *Medical devices: A legislative plan.* https:// books.google.com/books/about/Medical_Devices.html?id=3CwHRAAACAAJ

Federal Food, Drug, and Cosmetic Act (FD&C Act). (1938). Pub. L. 75-717, 52 Stat. 1040.

Food and Drug Administration (FDA). (2006). *Information sheet guidance for IRBs, clinical investigators, and sponsors: Significant risk and nonsignificant risk medical device studies.* www.fda.gov /media/75459/download

Food and Drug Administration (FDA). (2018a). *Regulatory controls.* www.fda.gov/medical-devices /overview-device-regulation/regulatory-controls

Food and Drug Administration (FDA). (2018b). *IDE responsibilities.* www.fda.gov/medical-devices /investigational-device-exemption-ide/ide-responsibilities

Food and Drug Administration (FDA). (2020). *Search for FDA guidance documents.* www.fda.gov /regulatory-information/search-fda-guidance-documents

Food and Drug Administration Modernization Act. (1997). Pub. L. 105–115, 111 Stat. 2296 (1997).

Institute of Medicine. (2011). *Medical devices and the public's health: The FDA 510(k) clearance process at 35 years.* National Academies Press.

Medical Device Amendments Act (MDA). (1976). Pub. L. 94-295, 90 Stat. 539 (1976).

Medical Device User Fee and Modernization Act. (2002). Pub. L. 107-250, 116 Stat. 1588 (2002).

Merrill, R. A. (1994). Regulation of drugs and devices: An evolution. *Health Affairs, 13*(3), 47–69.

Pure Food and Drug Act. (1906). Pub. L. 59-384; p. 768–772.

Safe Medical Devices Act. (1990). Pub. L. 101-629, 104 Stat. 4511 (1990).

Emergency Use, Expanded Access, and Right to Try

Richard Klein

Marjorie A. Speers

Abstract

Food and Drug Administration (FDA) regulations have, for decades, allowed patients with serious or life-threatening illnesses to access investigational products (drugs, biologics, and medical devices) for the purpose of treatment when FDA-approved treatments are not available or not working and the patients are not eligible or able to participate in a clinical trial. These uses of investigational products, called expanded access, are regulated and require the IRB to be involved in the oversight of the usage. More recent federal law, called "Right to Try," permits the use of investigational drugs and biologics by patients for the purpose of treatment for life-threatening diseases and conditions, similar to the traditional FDA pathway but without the involvement of FDA or an IRB. This chapter describes emergency use, nonemergency cases of expanded access, and the Right to Try Act; responsibilities of IRBs; and what IRBs can do to streamline the process that ensures and facilitates responsible review in a time-sensitive situation.

Introduction

The FDA has jurisdiction under the Federal Food, Drug, and Cosmetic Act to regulate drug development in the United States (FDA, 2018). Only products deemed to be safe and effective and that offer a positive risk/benefit ratio are approved for marketing in the United States, making them widely available and usually paid for by third-party insurers.

Prior to marketing, investigational products must be tested in clinical trials to determine whether they are safe and effective for their intended use. FDA does not regulate research, but it does regulate medical products, including those in development.

Sometimes, patients exhaust the approved therapeutic options or are intolerant of the marketed medical products. Some of these patients cannot wait for a promising new drug, biologic, or medical device to be fully tested and approved for marketing. They may choose to participate in a clinical trial that will help determine whether the product works as intended and whether its potential benefits outweigh any harms associated with the product. Although clinical trials are designed and intended to benefit future patients by determining whether a new product is safe and effective, some patients might directly benefit by participating in a trial. Not all patients, however, are able to participate in such trials for a variety of reasons. For example, they might not meet the inclusion criteria for a trial or live too far away from the clinical trial sites.

FDA provides an option that permits some of these patients to access investigational products outside of a clinical trial; this option is called expanded access. Patients who have an immediately life-threatening disease or condition (defined as "a stage of disease in which there is reasonable likelihood that death will occur within a matter of months or in which premature death is likely without early treatment") or a serious disease or condition (defined as "a disease or condition associated with morbidity that has substantial impact on day-to-day functioning") are eligible for this FDA program (FDA, 2017a). Short-lived and self-limiting morbidity is usually not a sufficient condition to meet the requirements of this program; however, the morbidity need not be irreversible, provided it is persistent or recurrent (FDA, 2017a).

Whether a disease or condition is serious is a matter of clinical judgment and is based on its impact on factors such as survival, day-to-day functioning, or the likelihood that the disease will progress from a less severe condition to a more serious one if left untreated.

Other terms commonly applied to the treatment use of an investigational product outside of clinical trials include *preapproval access*, *managed access programs*, and *compassionate use*.

Under appropriate circumstances, if a manufacturer is able and willing to provide the investigational product for the patient, expanded access can provide a regulatory pathway to allow a company to provide access to their investigational agent (unapproved drug, biologic, or medical device) outside of controlled clinical trials for the purpose of treatment. Hereafter, this pathway is referred to as expanded access.

Categories and Tiers of Expanded Access

Expanded access is the use of an investigational drug, biologic, or medical device to treat a patient with a serious disease or condition when there is no comparable or satisfactory alternative treatment available to treat the patient. The purpose of the use is to treat a patient, and the intent is to provide direct benefit to the patient. The regulations governing expanded access for drugs and biologics are found at 21 CFR 312 subpart I and for medical devices at 21 CFR 812.35 and 812.36.

There are two categories of expanded access for an individual patient, based on urgency, for use of drugs, biologics, or medical devices: emergency and nonemergency.

Emergency use is for "a situation that requires a patient to be treated before a written submission can be made" (FDA, 2017a). This is generally an acute medical emergency (such as stroke or heart attack), where time to treatment is critical (e.g., within hours or a day), and no comparable or satisfactory alternative therapy option is available.

Emergency use requires informed consent from the patient, unless "[i]nformed consent cannot be obtained from the subject because of an inability to communicate with, or obtain legally effective consent from, the subject . . . [and] [t]ime is not sufficient to obtain consent from the subject's legal representative" [21 CFR 50.23(a)]. No prospective IRB review is required; however, institutional policies may require consultation with the IRB chair prior to use of the product. FDA regulations require that the IRB be informed of the emergency use within 5 business days. Emergency use applies only to an individual patient [21 CFR 312.310]. Any subsequent use of the test article at the institution is subject to IRB review under 21 CFR 56.104. However, FDA acknowledges that it would be inappropriate to deny emergency treatment to a second individual if the only obstacle is that the IRB has not had sufficient time to convene a meeting to review the issue.

All other individual patient access requests are considered nonemergency. FDA regulations provide for three tiers of nonemergency expanded access, based on the number of patients being treated under a protocol:

1. Nonemergency individual patient investigational new drugs (INDs), as the name implies, are used to treat just one patient with a drug or biologic. Usually, the patient's physician holds the IND and serves as the sponsor/ investigator. This means that the physician will administer the treatment and be responsible for oversight of the patient, as well as securing IRB review of the treatment plan and informed consent document that will be used with the patient. The physician is also responsible for reporting adverse reactions that may be associated with the investigational drug or biologic and submitting a final summary of the treatment use to FDA. Note that in some cases, the product manufacturer may hold the individual patient IND, and when this happens the product manufacturer is responsible for the same obligations as the physician/investigator. The IRB is responsible for reviewing and concurring with the expanded access request prior to the treatment use. In cases of individual patient INDs, the chair or designee may review and concur in lieu of a full board review.

   🔗 11-2

   Individual patient use involving a medical device is called compassionate use. This can be used for devices with or without an investigational device exemption (IDE). The responsibilities of the physician are the same as those for uses involving drugs or biologics. Likewise, the IRB is responsible to review and concur with the expanded access request before the medical device may be used. A product manufacturer (commercial sponsor) may also initiate an individual patient IDE and be the IDE holder of record.

   🔗 11-3

2. An intermediate-size patient population IND allows for the consolidation of several individual patient INDs into a single new IND or when a number of patients are to be treated with an investigational drug or biologic for the same indication. This can significantly reduce paperwork, as additional patients may be treated without having to submit a request for a new IND for each patient.

   As the number of patients to be treated with the investigational drug or biologic increases, less detail is likely to be known about each patient (e.g., overall health status, organ function, and concomitant drugs) at the time the IND application is submitted. FDA usually permits these group INDs to proceed (i.e., be approved) only when there is sufficient safety data to warrant the increased number of patients being exposed to the product.

   There is no set numerical parameter for this type of IND. It is meant to be a practical way to treat a group of patients at the same and/or at different geographic or institutional locations. Additional physicians can be added under the IND by submission to FDA of an IND amendment.

The intermediate-size patient population IND may be requested by an individual physician; by an institution (such as a medical center); by a third party, such as an advocacy organization (if it has a licensed physician making the request); or by the commercial manufacturer.

Most expanded access uses under this type of IND are for products under development; that is, in any phase prior to market approval (e.g., in trials, in data analysis, or application for approval in review at FDA). However, FDA regulations allow access even when a product is not currently in clinical trials. Under certain circumstances, FDA may allow access to drugs that are no longer being developed or products that are for extremely rare diseases when there are too few patients to enroll in a trial.

Intermediate-size patient population expanded access use **[21 CFR 312.315]** may be used under several different types of situations:

- When it is likely the product would be used by, and benefit, a number of patients who have no other treatment options and cannot participate in an ongoing clinical trial.
- In place of multiple single patient uses of an investigational product that is not otherwise available (because it is no longer being developed or has not been approved).
- When a FDA dictated risk evaluation and mitigation strategy (REMS) restricts use of the product to a specific indication, but patients with other conditions might potentially benefit from access to the product.
- To provide broader access to a promising therapeutic product to a limited, defined number of patients under the auspices of an advocacy organization.
- To allow access to treatment with an approved drug or biologic that is no longer marketed or if there is a shortage of product and there is available an unapproved source of the drug (such as from a foreign manufacturer).

Investigational medical devices may also be used under a group IDE called small group access. The product manufacturer or the physician must submit a request to FDA. This option may be used when there is an existing IDE or when there is no existing IDE (FDA, 2019).

3. Widespread treatment access may be afforded to patients through a treatment IND or treatment IDE when a product is being actively developed by a product manufacturer (commercial sponsor), there is enough safety data to justify broader access, and there is sufficient evidence of effectiveness in treating the disease. Usually, these expanded access uses are based on data generated during phase 3 trials or on analyses of the data after the trials are completed. Treatment INDs or IDEs often act as a bridge between the time studies are completed and the product is approved for marketing. In diseases such as HIV/AIDS and cancer, tens of thousands of patients were treated under treatment INDs before the product was approved for marketing. Only a commercial sponsor that is actively developing the product can apply for a treatment IND or IDE (FDA, 2019).

Commercial sponsors may also choose to amend an existing IND or IDE for any of the three tiers of expanded access. These are called, respectively, single patient protocols, intermediate-size patient population protocols or small group access protocols, and treatment protocols (in contrast to single patient INDs or compassionate use IDEs, intermediate-size patient population INDs or small group IDEs, and treatment INDs or treatment IDEs, as described earlier).

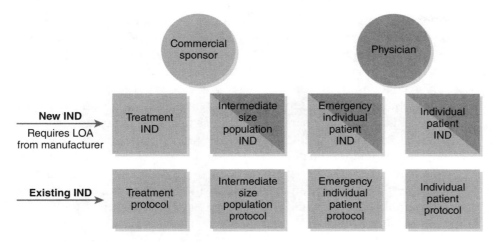

Figure 11.4-1 Summary of the types of expanded access uses and which entity may submit each type of application to FDA.

Individual physicians and institutions cannot apply to amend an existing IND or IDE to provide treatment access unless they are the holder of the existing IND or IDE.

As an example, **Figure 11.4-1** shows the kinds of INDs and protocols that may be used to provide access outside of the clinical trial setting and who may initiate the treatment when the expanded access use involves a drug or biologic.

According to **21 CFR 312.305(a)**, for all expanded access requests, FDA must determine that:

1. The patients or patients to be treated have a serious or immediately life-threatening illness or condition, and there is no comparable or satisfactory alternative therapy to diagnose, monitor, or treat the disease or condition;
2. The potential patient benefit justifies the potential risks of the treatment use and those potential risks are not unreasonable in the context of the disease or condition to be treated; and
3. Providing the investigational product for the requested use will not interfere with the initiation, conduct, or completion of clinical investigations that could support marketing approval of the expanded access use or otherwise compromise the potential development of the expanded access use.

Because FDA regulates investigational products regardless of purpose—research or treatment—expanded access through any of these mechanisms requires IRB review according to **21 CFR 56** and informed consent according to **21 CFR 50**.

Right to Try Legislation

In 2014, Colorado became the first state to pass a right to try law that allows terminally ill patients to bypass FDA for access to investigational products in development that have completed phase 1 testing. As of June 2019, 40 additional states have passed right to try laws that permit physicians to request, from a drug manufacturer, treatment access within their state to investigational drugs that have completed a phase 1 trial, without FDA involvement.

These laws vary from state to state, in terms of definitions, coverage, and eligibilities. For example, some states (e.g., Virginia) require two physicians to certify that a patient has a life-threatening disease. Others (e.g., Tennessee) require that the informed consent specify that parties providing access to an investigational drug cannot be held liable for negative outcomes. There are states that deny access to hospice care for patients who pursue right to try treatment access. Some require IRB involvement, and some do not. Importantly, none of these laws requires companies to provide their investigational drugs to patients outside of clinical trials or insurance companies to cover their use.

A federal Right to Try Bill (the Trickett Wendler, Frank Mongiello, Jordan McLinn, and Matthew Bellina Right to Try Act of 2017) was signed into law in May 2018 but (as of 2019) has not yet been enacted through regulation, nor has FDA published guidance on how the law will be implemented (Right to Try Act, 2017). Although the state laws still exist, it is presumed that the federal law preempts them.

There are notable differences between the expanded access regulations found in **21 CFR 312** and **812** and the federal Right to Try law. The right to try pathway is available solely to individual patients who wish to try an investigational drug or biologic. The right to try pathway is limited to treatment access for individual patients. It is not intended or designed to treat cohorts of patients (as are the intermediate-size patient population IND and treatment IND regulations under the traditional expanded access rules). It does not apply to investigational medical devices. Phase 1 trials must have been completed and the investigational product must be in active development for a marketing application. These two requirements are more restrictive than those for the expanded access pathway (Right to Try Act, 2017).

As noted previously, the expanded access pathway requires the physician/sponsor to submit an IND application with FDA, review and approval by an IRB (or concurrence by the chair or the chair's designee for the individual patient IND), informed consent of the patient that conforms to the requirements of **21 CFR 50**, and reporting of <u>adverse events</u>.

⊘ 7-3

In contrast, in the right to try pathway there is no requirement to submit an application for an IND to FDA and no requirement for IRB review and approval. Institutions, however, may still require IRB review under their own policies and can require the elements of informed consent described in FDA regulations. The Right to Try Act requires the treating physician to obtain informed consent from the patient, but it does not mandate any specific content, as required under **21 CFR 50**.

As with FDA's expanded access regulations, companies are under no legal obligation to provide access to their investigational agents under the Right to Try legislation.

The federal law, like many state laws, limits liability of physicians and product manufacturers, but it does not address liability of IRBs (Right to Try Act, 2017).

What IRBs Can Do to Facilitate the Expanded Access Approval Process

An IRB can be approached at any time to review an expanded access request from a physician to treat a single patient. Whether the request is for an emergency or nonemergency use, there is little time for an IRB to figure out how to handle the request. Thus, an IRB should anticipate receiving a request and have policies and procedures in place for when the situation arises. The IRB is a component in the expanded access process. Other entities within an institution that are likely to be involved are the general counsel; the research pharmacy or the pharmacy where investigational products are stored; the contracting or sponsored programs office, because some institutions and product manufacturers require contracts to transport product; or the office for regulatory affairs, compliance, or quality assurance. Policies about the use of FDA's expanded access program or the right to try pathway are institutional decisions and generally do not rest solely with the IRB.

Policies and Procedures

The first step in developing <u>policies and procedures</u> for handling requests from investigators/physicians and patients to use the expanded access pathways described earlier is for your organization to decide the scope of use of these pathways. The IRB should work with appropriate institutional offices, such as the general counsel or research office to make the following policy decisions:

    🔗 2-3

1. Will the institution permit the use of investigational products through FDA's expanded access program to treat patients? If so, policies and procedures should be developed for emergency and nonemergency uses, because the regulatory requirements are different depending on the urgency of the use and for drugs and biologics, as a group, and medical devices because there are different regulatory requirements depending on the type of investigational product.

2. Will the institution permit the use of investigational drugs and biologics under the federal Right to Try law? And if so, will the institution require IRB review and approval? The federal law does not require IRB review and approval, but an institution may impose additional stipulations to those in the federal law. Does your state have a right to try law, and if so, does it contain additional requirements to the federal law? Do the additional requirements affect the IRB? Are there any inconsistencies between the federal law and your state law?

    If your institution decides not to allow the use of the right to try pathway, it should be stated in institutional policy and included in the IRB policy.

3. Will the institution permit the use of an investigational drug, biologic, or medical device in an emergency situation? If so, the IRB should develop procedures for review of these uses. Procedures should require the physician to report the use to the IRB "…within 5 business days, to submit to FDA a written request for the use within 15 business days of the use, and to comply with the regulatory requirements to obtain informed consent." The regulations at **21 CFR 56.104** do not describe what an IRB must do when it is informed of an emergency use IND or IDE. The IRB should confirm by obtaining the documentation from FDA that the expanded access use was, in fact, an emergency and that the requirements for informed consent as specified in the regulations were met. Policies and procedures should include that any subsequent use of the test article at the institution is subject to IRB review prior to its use. IRBs should make clear to physicians that emergencies are generally considered one-time events and that if they anticipate subsequent uses, to seek prospective IRB approval of a protocol for these uses (see sidebar, Emergency Use).

4. Will the institution permit the use of an investigational drug, biologic, or medical device in a nonemergency situation? If so, develop IRB procedures for drugs and biologics and for medical devices. As shown in Figure 11.4-1, physicians or institutions may be the holder of the IND or IDE for single

EMERGENCY USE

As defined in **21 CFR 56.102(d)**, "[e]mergency use means the use of a test article on a human subject in a life-threatening situation in which no standard acceptable treatment is available, and in which there is not sufficient time to obtain IRB approval." In expanded access situations, emergency use means that the physician does not have enough time to put together the paperwork to apply to FDA before the use of the investigational product must occur. FDA makes the determination that the use is an emergency, *not* the IRB or physician. Most expanded access uses are not emergencies, although time may be precious in terms of treating the patient.

patient uses or for intermediate-size patient population INDs or small group access IDEs. In this case, just clarifying and using terminology consistently will assist IRB members and staff, physicians, and other institutional parties. For example, "single patient" or "individual" is used to describe an expanded access IND, whereas FDA uses the term "compassionate use" for an expanded access IDE for a single patient (FDA, 2019).

Because most expanded access uses involving one patient are time sensitive—the patient is seeking treatment with investigational product outside of a clinical trial and for an immediately life-threatening condition or a serious disease or condition that has substantial impact on day-to-day functioning—the IRB can best serve the patient and treating physician by having streamlined IRB procedures to ensure a quick turnaround time in review and a process whereby expanded access requests are brought to the immediate attention of the IRB and do not get lost in the general IRB flow of business.

The IRB can modify its standard procedures and practices in several ways to facilitate the review process for expanded access uses:

- Inform physicians that they should notify the IRB office when they anticipate having an expanded access request.
  - This could occur at the time the physician submits a request to the product manufacturer or to FDA. This early notification would permit the IRB office to work with the physician to understand the medical condition of the patient and circumstances for the expanded access use and to inform the physician of what will be required in the IRB submission. For individual patient INDs, the IRB office should ensure that the chair or designee, depending on the type of investigational product, is available to review the request when it arrives in the IRB office.
- Request the minimum amount of information necessary for the IRB to review and approve the expanded access request. The objective is to reduce the number of forms or descriptions of the proposed treatment to reduce administrative burden for the physician.
  - For investigational drugs or biologics, it may be sufficient to limit information submitted to FDA Form 3926 (FDA, 2017b), the investigator's brochure (or another source describing risks and potential benefits), FDA documentation for issuance of the IND, and draft informed consent document.
  - For investigational devices, it may be adequate to request a treatment plan that contains the same type of information that is required in FDA Form 3926 (which may only be used for drug and biologic INDs).
- 3-2 • Permit an <u>IRB chair</u> (or their designee for drugs and biologics only) to review and concur with the expanded access request. An IRB chair may determine that full board review is needed. FDA guidance on the manner or criteria for review (or the meaning of "concurrence" as opposed to "approval") is lacking. However, it seems prudent to consider at least the following:
  - Confirm the medical evaluation of the patient's condition. The reviewer must be able to confirm or deny the claim that there is no comparable or satisfactory alternative available, including already approved therapies or other clinical trials for which the patient might be eligible.

- Ensure that informed consent or appropriate permissions will be obtained and documented. Consent documents should meet the requirements listed in **21 CFR 50.25**, using plain language that is specifically aimed at "patients" who expect direct benefit, as opposed to "subjects" for whom direct benefit may not be expected.
- Review documentation that FDA has made its determinations regarding safety and effectiveness, and assure that there is a valid IND or IDE number.
- Review the treatment plan to determine that it makes adequate provision for ensuring the safety of the patient, including adequate monitoring (timing and type of tests/exams, etc.) and appropriate plans for collecting and reporting the data, that the physician is qualified to administer the treatment, and that the treatment facility is adequately equipped.

Additional issues that IRBs should address in their policies and procedures include the following:

- The physician will determine a proposed length of treatment. The IRB may approve the expanded access use for up to 1 year. Sometimes, treatments extend beyond 1 year. At the end of the 1-year period, <u>continuing review</u> is required.   🔗 7-2
- Sometimes, a second course of the treatment is required or there is a change to the treatment use. Changes to treatment use should be reported to the IRB and reviewed by the IRB as modifications to the treatment plan.
- <u>Adverse events</u> related to the treatment may also occur, and if so, they should be reported by the physician to the IRB in addition to the product manufacturer and FDA.   🔗 7-3
- The physician is required to provide a summary report to FDA at the end of the treatment use. Consider asking for a copy of this report to close out the treatment use when it ends.
- All IRB considerations and deliberations related to a treatment use of an investigational agent should be documented and added to the IRB files.

Intermediate-Size Patient Population INDs and Small Group Access IDEs

FDA regulations permit expanded access uses for multiple patients; these are called intermediate-size patient population INDs for drugs and biologics and small group access IDEs for medical devices (FDA, 2019).

In these cases, the IRB must review a treatment protocol. The convened IRB must review the protocol according to the regulatory criteria for approval at **21 CFR 56.111**.

In these cases, the IRB should consider whether there is enough safety data to determine whether the risks are reasonable in relation to the potential benefits. In expanded access uses involving only one patient, the IRB makes a determination about risk and benefit for a specific patient based on the medical evaluation of that patient. When multiple patients will be treated under the expanded access use, the individual patients are not necessarily known, and therefore the determination about risk and potential benefit is made theoretically rather than concretely for specific patients.

When the convened IRB reviews these types of expanded access requests, the IRB must apply the <u>regulatory approval criteria</u> that were designed for   🔗 5-4
evaluating clinical investigations to a treatment use. For example, an IRB should ensure that the <u>informed consent</u> from the patient will be obtained and   🔗 Section 6

documented and that the informed consent documentation refers to a treatment use and not research; that the physician's treatment plan makes adequate provisions for ensuring the safety of the patient, including monitoring and appropriate plans for collecting and reporting data; that <u>Health Insurance Portability and Accountability Act (HIPAA)</u> requirements will be followed to ensure confidentiality of the medical record; and that the treating physician will follow standard medical practice to protect the privacy interests of the patient.

🔗 11-6

Treatment INDs and IDEs

This third type of expanded access is only available to product manufacturers. It is not necessary for IRBs to have procedures to specifically address these types of expanded access uses unless they review expanded access protocols for commercial sponsors. Commercial sponsors generally use a central IRB for this type of broad access, but local institutions may have policies that require their own IRB review. These types of protocols are reviewed similarly to intermediate-size patient population IND protocols or small group access IDEs.

Dissemination of Policies and Procedures

The IRB should include policies and procedures in educational materials for investigators who are physicians and for IRB members. One of the major challenges in using expanded access is that physicians and IRB members are sometimes unfamiliar with the terminology and the regulatory requirements. IRBs can provide a valuable service, particularly to physicians, by disseminating their policies and procedures related to expanded access.

Resources

Code of Federal Regulations. (2019). Food and Drug Administration 21 CFR 312. Subpart I. www.accessdata.fda.gov/scripts/cdrh/cfdocs/cfcfr/CFRSearch.cfm?CFRPart=312&showFR=1&subpartNode=21:5.0.1.1.3.9

Code of Federal Regulations. (2019). Food and Drug Administration 21 CFR 812. www.accessdata.fda.gov/scripts/cdrh/cfdocs/cfcfr/CFRsearch.cfm?CFRPart=812

Code of Federal Regulations. (2019). Food and Drug Administration 21 CFR 312.310(d). www.accessdata.fda.gov/scripts/cdrh/cfdocs/cfcfr/CFRSearch.cfm?fr=312.310

Code of Federal Regulations. (2019). Food and Drug Administration 21 CFR 312.305. www.accessdata.fda.gov/scripts/cdrh/cfdocs/cfcfr/CFRSearch.cfm?fr=312.305

References

Food and Drug Administration (FDA). (2017a). *Expanded access to investigational drugs for treatment use—questions and answers.* www.fda.gov/media/85675/download

Food and Drug Administration (FDA). (2017b). *Individual patient expanded access applications: Form FDA 3926.* www.fda.gov/regulatory-information/search-fda-guidance-documents/individual-patient-expanded-access-applications-form-fda-3926

Food and Drug Administration (FDA). (2018). Federal Food, Drug, and Cosmetic Act (FD&C Act): FD&C Act Reference information. www.fda.gov/regulatory-information/laws-enforced-fda/federal-food-drug-and-cosmetic-act-fdc-act

Food and Drug Administration (FDA). (2019). *Expanded access for medical devices.* www.fda.gov/medical-devices/device-advice-investigational-device-exemption-ide/expanded-access-medical-devices

Trickett Wendler, Frank Mongiello, Jordan McLinn, and Matthew Bellina Right to Try Act of 2017 (Right to Try Act). (2017). Public Law 115-176. 115th Congress. www.congress.gov/bill/115th-congress/senate-bill/204/text

Humanitarian Use Devices

Tracey Craddock

Abstract

A humanitarian use device (HUD) is a device used to treat or diagnose diseases or conditions that occur infrequently, as defined in the Code of Federal Regulations under **21 CFR 814.3(n)** (amended in December 2016 when the 21st Century Cures Act was signed into law; Code of Federal Regulations, 2004). The regulations require a convened IRB to perform the initial review of a protocol using an HUD and to apply the same approval criteria as it does for any FDA-regulated product, even though use of the HUD under the humanitarian device exemption (HDE) is not considered research. The IRB is not required to make a significant risk or nonsignificant risk determination when the device is used as approved by the Food and Drug Administration (FDA) under the HDE for clinical care. Although even when the device is approved for marketing, physicians using an HUD are still required to report serious injuries, deaths, and malfunctions to the HDE holder, FDA, and the IRB as soon as they become aware that the device may have caused or contributed to a death or serious injury.

Introduction

Humanitarian device exemption provides a pathway for manufacturers to develop devices that will benefit small patient populations. HDEs are analogous to orphan drugs under FDA regulations, and both fall under the FDA's Office of Orphan Products Development. The HUD program is relatively young. It was begun in 1990 under the Safe Medical Devices Act (SMD Act, 1990), and it provides a route for marketing devices that would benefit patients with rare conditions or diseases. It was subsequently amended by the 21st Century Cures Act in 2016 (21st Century Cures Act, 2016).

An HUD is a medical device intended to benefit patients in the treatment or diagnosis of a disease or condition that affects or is manifested in not more than 8,000 individuals in the United States per year (21st Century Cures Act, 2016, Section 3052).

An HDE is a marketing application for an HUD (Federal FD&C Act, Section 520(m)) (FDA, 2019a). An HDE is exempt from the effectiveness requirements

APPROPRIATE LOCAL COMMITTEE

"FDA interprets the statutory term "appropriate local committee" to mean a standing committee for the facility that has expertise and experience in reviewing and making treatment decisions for clinical care particularly in applying innovative medical device technologies to clinical care. As such, a standing committee for the facility that includes physicians with experience in the treatment of rare diseases or conditions would be considered an appropriate local committee" (FDA, 2019c). It is recommended the committee include a high-level medical professional or faculty member (FDA, 2019c).

of Section 514 (Performance Standards) and Section 515 (Premarket Approval) of the FD&C Act when used in accordance with FDA-approved indication(s) and is subject to certain profit and use restrictions (FDA, 2018a).

HDE holders are permitted to charge and recoup the costs of research and development, manufacturing, and distribution of the device; under limited conditions, they may also be sold for profit (Pediatric Medical Device Safety and Improvement Act of 2007).

An HUD is a legally marketed device, and its use within its approved indication does not constitute a clinical investigation. However, IRB or appropriate local committee approval is required before an HUD can be used at a facility for clinical care, with the exception of emergency use (discussed later). References to IRB in this chapter denote an IRB or appropriate local committee (see sidebar, Appropriate Local Committee).

The IRB of record for the institution where the device is being used must apply the same approval criteria at **21 CFR 56.111** when it performs an initial review of an HUD as it does for any other FDA-regulated product. FDA approval of the HDE is based on safety and probable benefit and does not provide assurance of effectiveness. Reviewers should consider the following:

1. If the risks are minimized by using procedures that do not unnecessarily expose patients to risk, and if the risks are reasonable in relation to the device being used and its probable benefit.
2. Whether there are adequate provisions to protect the privacy of the patients and the confidentiality of any data being collected.
3. If the device is being used within the scope of the FDA HDE approval order.
4. Whether the patient (or legally authorized representative [LAR]) is given sufficient opportunity to consent to the use of the device for their disease/condition.
5. If consent is applicable, if it is being appropriately documented, and contains the necessary information (discussed later).
6. If no written consent is being required, whether the patient or LAR is being provided with the patient brochure or labeling information for the device.

The IRB should also confirm that there are adequate provisions for monitoring to ensure safety. Physicians should have a clear understanding of their requirements to report any unanticipated device effects and to whom they should be reported.

🔗 5-7   The convened IRB is required under the regulations at **21 CFR 56.108** to initially review the HUD submission. In order to evaluate the risks, probable benefits, and required unanticipated device effects, it is recommended that the following materials be reviewed:

- A copy of the FDA HDE approval order.
- A description of the device.
- Device labeling.
- Any patient information packet or brochure that may be available for the HUD.
- The proposed use, patient population, screening procedures, and overall treatment plan as well as required unanticipated device reporting criteria. The IRB application forms would include all of this information

If the IRB requires a consent form, it should ensure the form is consistent with the HDE-approved labeling and provide sufficient information in lay language for the patient or legally authorized representative to make a decision regarding the use. The consent should be clear that HDE effectiveness has not been demonstrated, it is an HUD, and it is approved by FDA to either treat or diagnose the specific disease or condition. The consent form does not need to contain all the required elements of a research consent form when being used to treat patients under the approved HDE. The consent form should make no reference to research, and a Health Insurance Portability and Accountability Act (HIPAA) authorization for research would not be required. There may be instances when a consent form would be impractical and burdensome to obtain for every patient on the off chance that an HUD may need to be used.

The IRB does not have to make a determination of significant risk (SR) or nonsignificant risk (NSR) when it reviews an HUD to treat or diagnose patients.

The IRB is not required to approve each individual use of an HUD. The IRB may choose to limit the use based on certain factors or reporting requirements to the IRB as it deems appropriate. The IRB may use the FDA expedited review procedure for continuing review **[21 CFR 56.110]**, because the use of the HUD under the approved HDE is not considered research. The IRB of record may have their own policy and procedure for continuing review of an HUD. Whether the IRB decides to perform the continuing review by the <u>convened</u> or the <u>expedited procedure</u>, there should be substantive review of the risk/benefit information, as well as any medical device reports (MDRs) and/or sponsor's annual reports to FDA (FDA, 2019b).

🔗 5-7

🔗 5-5

An IRB is not required to perform any type of post-approval monitoring of patient records for those who have received an HUD, nor are they required to monitor the number of devices distributed each year. The HDE holder is responsible for monitoring the number of devices used and distributed throughout the year. Justification of device charges should not be asked for by the IRB. FDA has already reviewed the HDE-holder financial information.

The collection of safety and efficacy data about the HUD or the use of the HUD outside its FDA-approved indication constitutes a clinical investigation and is subject to **21 CFR Part 56, 21 CFR Part 50**, and the additional safeguards under **21 CFR 50, subpart D** for children (FDA, 2019b). It is required that a clinical investigation of an HUD be reviewed, approved, and supervised only by an IRB. A standing "appropriate local committee" as defined by FDA would not meet the criteria.

If safety and efficacy data is collected about an HUD and it is being used within its approved indication, the device is exempt from the FDA <u>IDE requirements under</u> **21 CFR Part 812**, and no SR or NSR determination needs to be made by the IRB. If the HUD is being used outside its approved indication, the IRB must apply the IDE rules at **21 CFR 812**. Most sponsors would have obtained an FDA-approved IDE before initiating such a study. If there is no IDE, then the IRB would need to make the SR or NSR determination described under **21 CFR 812.66**. The IRB must review and approve the application prior to any use of the device, and informed consent is required when the use is for research outside of the approved indication(s) (FDA, 2019b).

🔗 11-3

A physician in an emergency situation may use an HUD within its approved indication(s) prior to IRB review, only if approval cannot be obtained in time to prevent serious harm or death to the patient. The physician is obligated to report that use within 5 days to the IRB. This report must be provided in writing and include the patient information, reason for the use, and the date the HUD was used (FDA, 2019b).

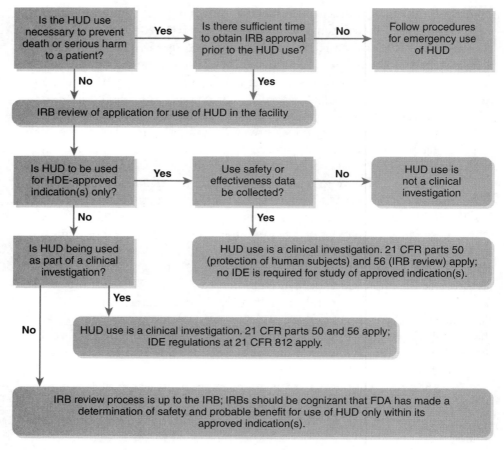

Figure 11.5-1 Decision tree.

If an IRB has reviewed and approved the use of an HUD at an institution, a physician may use it outside of its approved indication(s) in an emergency, or if there is no alternative device for the patient's condition. However, the institution should have a policy for reporting such uses to the IRB, or at least for addressing this in the initial convened IRB approval letter as one of its reporting requirements. The physician should also notify the HDE holder of its use and any <u>adverse events</u> that occur. Serious adverse events and deaths must be reported to FDA and the IRB using the Medical Device Reporting (MDR) system at **21 CFR 803** (FDA, 2019b).

7-3

The FDA's Center for Devices and Radiological Health (CDRH) has a listing of approved HDEs on their website. This listing can be used by the IRB to verify the HDE number, device name, manufacturer, and, most importantly, the FDA-approved indication for use of the HUD (FDA, 2018b, 2019b).

The decision tree in **Figure 11.5-1** can be helpful for IRBs in determining appropriate regulations and processes for the oversight of HUDs.

References

Code of Federal Regulations. (2004). Title 21, Volume 8. 21 CFR 814 Subpart H: Humanitarian Use Devices. www.fda.gov/industry/humanitarian-use-device-laws-regulations-and-guidances/current-regulations-21cfr-814-subpart-h-humanitarian-use-devices

Food and Drug Administration (FDA). (2018a). *Humanitarian device exemption.* www.fda.gov/medical-devices/premarket-submissions/humanitarian-device-exemption

Food and Drug Administration (FDA). (2018b). *Humanitarian use devices and humanitarian device exemption.* www.fda.gov/science-research/pediatrics/humanitarian-use-devices-and-humanitarian-device-exemption

Food and Drug Administration (FDA). (2019a). Humanitarian Device Exemption. www.fda.gov/medical-devices/premarket-submissions/humanitarian-device-exemption

Food and Drug Administration (FDA). (2019b). *Listing of CDRH humanitarian device exemptions.* www.fda.gov/medical-devices/hde-approvals/listing-cdrh-humanitarian-device-exemptions

Food and Drug Administration (FDA). (2019c). *Humanitarian Device Exemption (HDE) Program Guidance for Industry and Food and Drug Administration Staff.* www.fda.gov/media/74307/download

Pediatric Medical Device Safety and Improvement Act of 2007. www.congress.gov/bill/110th-congress/senate-bill/830

Safe Medical Devices Act of 1990 (SDM Act). (1990). Public Law 101-629. www.congress.gov/bill/101st-congress/house-bill/3095

21st Century Cures Act. (2016). Public Law 114-255. Subtitle F—Medical Device Innovations, Sec. 3052 Humanitarian device exemption. www.congress.gov/114/plaws/publ255/PLAW-114publ255.pdf

HIPAA and Research

Mark Barnes

Lawrence H. Muhlbaier

David Peloquin

Abstract

This chapter describes the evolution of the privacy regulations issued under the Health Insurance Portability and Accountability Act of 1996 (HIPAA) and their impact on research in the medical environment. It focuses on the Privacy Rule and includes a discussion of similarities to and differences from the Common Rule. HIPAA imposes several responsibilities on IRBs and privacy boards. A basic understanding of HIPAA is therefore essential for IRB and privacy board members and administrators.

Introduction

The Health Insurance Portability and Accountability Act of (HIPAA) 1996, originally known as the Kassebaum-Kennedy Act of 1996, had two main goals: to make health insurance *portable* and to increase *accountability* in Medicare billing (Department of Health and Human Services [DHHS], 2013a). Health insurance portability enables employees who change jobs to obtain health insurance at a new job without being penalized for preexisting conditions. Accountability efforts sought to address fraud and waste in Medicare billing.

Another section of HIPAA, concerning *administrative simplification*, mandated standards for the secure storage and transmission of healthcare information in electronic form. The Department of Health and Human Services (DHHS) wrote two new regulations: the Standards for Privacy of Individually Identifiable Health Information (the Privacy Rule) and the Security Standards for the Protection of Electronic Protected Health Information (the Security Rule) (see sidebar, Privacy and Security Rules). These rules apply to covered entities (CEs) and their business associates and are codified at 45 CFR Parts 160–164. It is important to note that, as stringent as these rules appear, large amounts of health information are still unprotected by HIPAA (e.g., health information held by many researchers, research sponsors, tumor registries, cash-only healthcare providers), although these types of information are often protected by state health privacy laws. The Privacy and Security Rules have the

PRIVACY AND SECURITY RULES

HIPAA required the Secretary of DHHS to issue privacy regulations implementing this section of HIPAA if Congress did not enact privacy legislation within 3 years of the passage of HIPAA. Because Congress failed to enact privacy legislation during the prescribed time period, DHHS wrote the Privacy Rule and the Security Rule.

The Privacy Rule became effective in April 2003 and the Security Rule in April 2005. DHHS issued substantial modifications to the Privacy and Security Rules in January 2013 through the so-called Omnibus Rule in response to the 2009 Health Information Technology for Economic and Clinical Health (HITECH) Act, and DHHS made additional changes to the Privacy Rule in February 2014 with respect to the treatment of laboratory test results alongside corresponding changes to the Clinical Laboratory Improvement Amendments of 1988 (CLIA) regulations (78 FR 5,566 (2013); 79 FR 7,290 (2014)).

same intent as protections of confidentiality provided under the Common Rule, but they are much more specific. Although the Privacy Rule has received more attention, both the Privacy Rule and Security Rule have led to significant changes in the environment of healthcare research.

According to a strict reading of the HIPAA Privacy Rule and Security Rule [45 CFR Parts 160–164], there is little that an IRB or privacy board must do to be in compliance. The primary requirements are to address waivers or alterations of authorization and to review combined consent and authorization forms. Central or independent IRBs typically limit their involvement with HIPAA to the fulfillment of these two requirements. Institution-based IRBs, however, often become more involved with HIPAA compliance, because anything at the institution that relates to both HIPAA and research is often assigned to the IRB for oversight, whereas many "privacy officers" who oversee the HIPAA compliance program within an institution are often unfamiliar with the nuances of how HIPAA applies to research, as opposed to clinical, activities. This chapter addresses the broader HIPAA topics that often fall within the purview of institution-based IRBs.

This chapter will cover the elements of an authorization in the context of the Common Rule. That is followed by a discussion of other areas that do not require individual authorization and other areas of HIPAA that affect research.

Definition of Protected Health Information and Research

Protected health information (PHI) is, simply, individually identifiable health information held by a CE. A CE is a healthcare provider who conducts certain types of electronic standard transactions, which relate primarily to third-party payer reimbursement, as well as health plans and healthcare clearinghouses. The term "individually identifiable health information" is defined in pertinent part as information that "[r]elates to the past, present, or future physical or mental health or condition of an individual; the provision of health care to an individual; or the past, present, or future payment for the provision of health care to an individual; and [t]hat identifies that individual; or [w]ith respect to which there is a reasonable basis to believe the information can be used to identify the individual" [45 CFR 160.103]. Notably, the definition does not refer to *patients* but rather uses the term *individual*, which means that the rule applies to information about nonpatients as well. Similarly, *identifiable* has taken on a much broader scope than it does under the Common Rule, largely because of the power and availability of computers and nonmedical databases that could be linked to the PHI. For more about identifiability, see the section Deidentified Data later in this chapter. The term *research* is given the same definition under HIPAA as it is under the Common Rule, i.e., "a systematic investigation, including research development, testing, and evaluation, designed to develop or contribute to generalizable knowledge" [45 CFR 46.102(I)].

HIPAA requires that each use or disclosure (i.e., the release, transfer, or provision of access to information outside the entity holding the information) of PHI by a CE is prohibited unless such use or disclosure is permitted by the Privacy Rule. The Privacy Rule permits a CE to use and disclose PHI for treatment, payment, and healthcare operation purposes without the explicit permission of the individual to whom the PHI relates. Use or disclosure of PHI for research, in contrast, requires a separate pathway under the Privacy Rule. The Privacy Rule permits PHI to be used and disclosed for research purposes pursuant to an individual's authorization or pursuant to certain other research-specific provisions. Each of these provisions is discussed next.

Authorization

Authorization is written permission from an individual allowing a CE to use or disclose specified PHI for a particular purpose (for example, for research). The technical requirements for authorizations have been well documented (National Institutes of Health [NIH], 2004a, 2004b). Many of the requirements are similar to or are a restatement of the requirements of <u>consent</u> under the Common Rule (see box, Features of a Valid Authorization).

🔗 Section 6

FEATURES OF A VALID AUTHORIZATION

To be valid, a HIPAA authorization must include the following:

Core Elements **[45 CFR 164.508(c)(1)]**:
  i. A description of the information to be used or disclosed that identifies the information in a specific and meaningful fashion.
  ii. The name or other specific identification of the person(s), or class of persons, authorized to make the requested use or disclosure.
  iii. The name or other specific identification of the person(s), or class of persons, to whom the covered entity may make the requested use or disclosure.
  iv. A description of each purpose of the requested use or disclosure. The statement "at the request of the individual" is a sufficient description of the purpose when an individual initiates the authorization and does not, or elects not to, provide a statement of the purpose.
  v. An expiration date or an expiration event that relates to the individual or the purpose of the use or disclosure. The statement "end of the research study," "none," or similar language is sufficient if the authorization is for a use or disclosure of protected health information for research, including for the creation and maintenance of a research database or research repository.
  vi. Signature of the individual and date. If the authorization is signed by a personal representative of the individual, a description of such representative's authority to act for the individual must also be provided.

Required Statements **[45 CFR 164.508(c)(2)]** (paraphrased here):
  ■ A statement that the individual may revoke the authorization in writing, and instructions on how to exercise such right
  ■ A statement that treatment, payment, enrollment, or eligibility for benefits may not be conditioned on obtaining the authorization if such conditioning is prohibited by the Privacy Rule, or, if conditioning is permitted, a statement about the consequences of refusing to sign the authorization [Note: conditioning may be permitted for research-related treatment]
  ■ A statement about the potential for the PHI to be redisclosed by the recipient and no longer protected by the Privacy Rule

Some key or misinterpreted requirements of authorizations are described as follows:

a. *To whom the PHI will be disclosed*

The authorization must list the "name or other specific identification of the person(s), or class of persons, to whom the covered entity may make the requested use or disclosure" **[45 CFR 164.508(c)(1)(iii)]**. The researchers and the IRB should consider which parties may receive PHI during the course of the study and therefore should be listed in the authorization. The Privacy Rule helpfully provides that the authorization may list "categories" of recipients as opposed to identifying each recipient by name. At this point it is fairly well accepted that the sponsor should be listed by name (but including in most cases a generic reference to any corporate successors or entities that purchase rights to the product under study) whereas the contract research organization (CRO) and its contractors should be described in a general fashion. In addition, the authorization should typically list the Office for Human Research Protections (OHRP), National Institutes of Health (NIH), or the Food and Drug Administration (FDA), as appropriate. Although these offices can all review the records without authorization, listing them will preclude the need for disclosure tracking and serve to inform the subjects more fully.

b. *Redisclosures not protected*

Another technical requirement of the authorization is that it must contain a caution that once PHI has been released to a non-CE pursuant to an authorization, that PHI is no longer protected by HIPAA and may be redisclosed by the recipient to other parties without restriction under HIPAA. For example, if PHI is disclosed to a sponsor or CRO, neither of which are generally CEs, such PHI may no longer be protected by HIPAA and may be subject to redisclosure.

c. *Combined versus separate authorizations*

The Privacy Rule allows an authorization for research to be combined with another authorization and/or with a consent for research. Choosing between a combined or separate authorization is an institutional decision. The argument for separation is that it makes both documents simpler, and the separate authorization does not require review by the IRB. The argument for combining is that there is significant overlap in content, and thus, combining reduces potential inconsistencies and avoids the situation of having one document signed but not the other. Notably, certain state laws, such as California's Confidentiality of Medical Information Act (Cal. Civil Code §56.11), require that the authorization be presented as a separate document, and thus institutions should consider applicable state laws when deciding whether to use a combined or separate authorization.

d. *Authorizations for future research*

An authorization must describe each "purpose" of the uses or disclosures of PHI permitted under the authorization. Under the initial issuance of the Privacy Rule, DHHS interpreted the requirement that the authorization describe the "purpose" of the disclosure to mean that an authorization had to be specific to one research study. In response to concerns raised by the research community, particularly by the DHHS Secretary's Advisory Committee on Human Research Protections (SACHRP), that such a requirement was inconsistent with the Common Rule's practice of allowing consent for future research, DHHS revised its interpretation of the Privacy Rule in the 2013 Omnibus Rule to permit a CE to obtain an authorization for future research. Such an authorization must describe the future research with enough specificity that it is "reasonable" for the individual to expect that their PHI will be used and disclosed for such future research project. Allowing authorizations for future research has been helpful for tissue banks and other research repositories that are housed within CEs by permitting one authorization that can be used for multiple future research projects.

The Omnibus Rule also made an important change to the Privacy Rule's treatment of "compound authorizations," i.e., authorizations that are combined with other documents. The Privacy Rule generally prohibits a CE from conditioning the treatment of an individual on that individual's signing a HIPAA authorization. The Privacy Rule contains an exception to this general prohibition that permits a CE to condition research-related treatment on the individual's signing of an authorization. Under the initial issuance of the Privacy Rule, a CE could not use a "compound authorization" that consisted of a conditioned authorization combined with an unconditioned authorization. For example, a researcher who was part of a CE could not combine in a single form an authorization to use and disclose PHI as part of a clinical trial (known as the "conditioned" authorization, since the individual's receipt of treatment as part of the clinical trial is "conditioned" on the individual's signing the authorization), with an optional authorization to permit PHI collected in the clinical trial to be used and disclosed as part of a tissue bank (known as the "unconditioned" authorization, since the individual's receipt of treatment as part of the clinical trial is not "conditioned" on the individual's signing the authorization). The Omnibus Rule revised the Privacy Rule to permit the combining of a "conditioned" and "unconditioned" research authorization into a single "compound" authorization, provided that the authorization clearly distinguishes between the conditioned and unconditioned components of the research, and the "unconditioned" authorization is presented as an "opt-in," such as through presenting the individual the opportunity to check a box or provide a separate signature to indicate their agreement to the "unconditioned" authorization.

In sum, the Omnibus Rule's revisions to the Privacy Rule to permit a CE to obtain an authorization for future research and to combine "conditioned" and "unconditioned" authorizations into a single form have increased flexibility for tissue repositories, databanks, sponsors, and researchers conducting secondary research by allowing them to combine in a single form an authorization for the present research study with an optional authorization for future research. The future research must be described with enough specificity that it is "reasonable" for the individual to expect that their PHI will be used and disclosed for such future research project.

e. *Limiting a research subject's access to PHI during a research study*

In addition to protecting the privacy of an individual's health information, the Privacy Rule provides individuals with certain rights to obtain copies of their health information (DHHS, 2020). The information that must be disclosed to the individual is called a *designated record set* (DRS). As relevant for most research, the DRS consists of medical records and billing records about individuals maintained by or for a CE healthcare provider and other records that are used, in whole or in part, by a CE to make decisions about individuals. Accordingly, if PHI generated during a research study is stored in a CE's DRS, the individual generally would have a right to obtain such information. Research information that is generated specifically for the research (e.g., lab tests performed specifically for a study) may not be part of the DRS, if that information is not part of the medical record and is not otherwise used to make decisions about the individual.

To protect the integrity of research, such as to maintain the blind in a blinded clinical trial, a researcher may require, as a condition of participating in the research, that a subject suspend this right to access PHI in their designated record set, at least until the research is completed. A subject may subsequently change their mind, but they then may no longer continue in the research.

One area that has received much attention in recent years regarding the DRS and research involves the return of laboratory test results to research subjects. Amendments to the CLIA regulations and the HIPAA Privacy Rule in 2014 state that even results generated in a laboratory subject to CLIA, or exempt from CLIA, are subject to an individual's right of access to PHI (DHHS 2014). This change has been challenging to the research community because laboratory testing performed for research purposes is often performed in research laboratories not certified under CLIA. Such laboratories are prohibited under CLIA from returning individual patient-level results that could be used in diagnosis or treatment. If, however, results generated by such laboratories are part of the DRS, the patient has a right to obtain such results under HIPAA. This can put researchers in a difficult position because returning patient-specific results from a non–CLIA-certified research laboratory is a violation of CLIA, but refusing to return such results can be a violation of the Privacy Rule. Researchers should therefore review carefully at the outset of a research study the CLIA status of laboratories used during the study and whether research results generated at such laboratories could be considered part of the DRS. The researcher can then work with their institution's legal counsel or privacy officer to develop a

🔗 12-1   return of results plan consistent with regulatory requirements.

Waiver of or Alteration to Authorization

Continuing with the avenues to allowable disclosure and use of PHI for research purposes, an IRB or privacy board is permitted to grant a waiver or alteration of authorization to researchers if the research satisfies certain criteria [45 CFR 164.512(i)(1)(i)]. The criteria for waiver or alteration of authoriza-

🔗 6-4   tion are similar to those for the waiver of consent under the Common Rule. The criteria refer to minimal risk to the privacy of the individual rather than minimal risk of all aspects of the study [45 CFR 164.512(i)(2)(ii)(A)]. The HIPAA waiver policy has some more explicit statements about the protections of the PHI, but they follow the Common Rule's intent to minimize risk and require that the research could not practicably be conducted without the waiver of authorization, similar to how the Common Rule requires that the research could not practicably be conducted without the waiver of consent. To obtain a waiver of authorization, the researcher must additionally show that the research could not practicably be conducted without access to and use of PHI, in other words, why the research could not be conducted with deidentified information [45 CFR 164.512(i)(2)(ii)(C)]. This is similar to the requirement in the Common Rule for a waiver of informed consent that the researcher demonstrate that the research could not be conducted without the use of *identifiable* information or biospecimens.

Research that would have a <u>waiver of documentation</u> of consent under the Common Rule can be addressed under HIPAA as an alteration to the authorization. For example, if the only link of a subject to the study is their signature on a consent form, then it can be considered impracticable to the study's completion to obtain a signed authorization as such a requirement might prevent study completion.

🔗 6-5

Notice of Review Preparatory to Research

PHI may be disclosed or used within the context of a notice of review preparatory to research (RPR). The RPR potentially allows researchers to identify, without specific authorization, persons possibly eligible for the study. The use or disclosure of PHI under the notice of RPR has several requirements (NIH, 2004b):

- The use or disclosure is sought solely to review PHI as necessary to prepare the research protocol or other similar preparatory purposes.
- No PHI will be removed from the covered entity during the review.
- The PHI that the researcher seeks to use or access is necessary for the research purposes.

The notice of RPR is a notice to the CE; approval is not required, although most hospital and large clinic CEs maintain internal policies that require preapproval by a privacy officer or research official before an RPR can be undertaken. Notice of RPR should be documented, and someone needs to verify that the required elements are included. Having a form to submit to the CE (likely represented for this purpose by the institution-based IRB, medical records office, or compliance office) makes it easier for both the researcher and the reviewer.

The notice of RPR is subject to the minimum necessary requirement of the Privacy Rule. The "minimum necessary requirement" limits "the use or disclosure of, and requests for, protected health information to the minimum necessary to accomplish the intended purpose" (NIH, 2003). Accordingly, having the researcher specify the data needed for the review would support the CE in the event of an audit of the minimum necessary requirement.

According to 2017 guidance issued by DHHS, CEs can provide researchers with access to PHI through remote access connectivity to conduct RPR provided that such access does not permit the researcher to download, print, or otherwise retain the PHI, and the connection complies with the requirements of the Security Rule (DHHS, 2017a).

Prescreening

The Common Rule, as revised in 2018, permits subject prescreening activities to take place without the subject's consent or an IRB's waiver of consent if the activities are described in a research proposal submitted to and approved by an IRB [45 CFR 46.116(g)].

In accordance with the Privacy Rule, the identification of potential subjects is accomplished with either a notice of RPR or a waiver of authorization. The waiver of authorization is easy to obtain if a researcher is also applying for a waiver of consent. If the prescreening activity does not involve recording any "individual private information" or fits within the Common Rule's exception from informed consent for prescreening activities, a notice of RPR is a direct and easy way to address prescreening.

The act of contacting the individual to seek their authorization can be seen as part of the CE's operations. Thus, the researcher can identify the potential subjects with the notice of RPR and then contact the potential subjects to seek authorization (because the CE is always permitted to disclose PHI back to the individual who is the subject of such PHI). If, however, the researcher is not part of the CE, the researcher must first obtain a waiver of authorization or become a business associate of the CE in order to contact potential subjects.

Decedent Research

Unlike the Common Rule, which applies only to research involving living individuals, HIPAA continues to protect PHI for 50 years after an individual's death. Fortunately, decedent research can be done with a notice to the CE meeting these requirements [45 CFR 164.512(i)(1)(iii)]:

a. Representation that the use or disclosure sought is solely for research on the protected health information of decedents;
b. Documentation, at the request of the covered entity, of the death of such individuals; and
c. Representation that the protected health information for which use or disclosure is sought is necessary for the research purposes.

Like the RPR, decedent research is also subject to the minimum necessary requirement of HIPAA, and thus, asking the researcher to specify the information needed will remind them that they can work only with information pertinent to their question.

Deidentified Data

Another method to use or disclose PHI without authorization is to deidentify the data. A CE is able to deidentify PHI without the patient's authorization because deidentification is considered a "healthcare operation" of the CE. Deidentified data are not subject to the Privacy Rule. In addition, deidentified data are not subject to the minimum necessary criteria, and under most state privacy laws, deidentified data are not protected or the use of them restricted.

Data can be deidentified in either of two ways:

1. Eighteen specific identifiers relating to the individual, the individual's household members, relatives, or employer must be removed. In addition, the CE can have no actual knowledge that the information can be used alone or in combination with other information to identify the individual (DHHS, 2015; 45 CFR 164.514(b)(2)).
2. A person with appropriate knowledge of and experience in generally accepted statistical and scientific principles and methods for rendering information not individually identifiable determines that the risk of reidentification is very small. That person must also document the methods and results of the analysis leading to that determination (DHHS, 2015; 45 CFR 164.514(b)(1)).

The deidentified data can have a reidentification code, but that code cannot be derived from any information about the individual (for example, generated from the individual's SSN or birth date) (DHHS, 2015).

Because dates are an identifier under the Privacy Rule, deidentification is problematic in many research studies. CEs may want to consider "precomputing" the durations of potential interest; (that is, instead of stating that event X occurred on date A, and event Y occurred on date B, stating event Y occurred *n* days after event X).

Limited Data Set With Data Use Agreement

Yet another method to use or disclose PHI for research purposes absent the authorization of the individual is to use a limited data set (LDS) with a data use agreement (DUA) [45 CFR 164.514(e)].

An LDS is PHI from which all of the 18 identifiers required for deidentification have been removed with the exception of dates and certain geocoding (ZIP codes or ZIP+4 codes are allowed, but the specific street address is not allowed). This is typically all that a researcher would want. Before permitting a researcher within the CE to use an LDS for research purposes or disclosing an LDS to an external researcher, the CE must enter a DUA with the recipient researcher or their institution (see sidebar, Data Use Agreements).

Unlike the deidentified data set, the LDS/DUA is still considered PHI and is subject to the minimum necessary requirements of the Privacy Rule. To the IRB, the practical import of this difference is that the researcher should specify the information they will be using under the LDS/DUA. This means that an LDS/DUA should broadly cover the domains of interest to the researcher (e.g., "laboratory values" instead of "LDL cholesterol") and not include irrelevant domains (charge data with no cost-related question).

Some LDS/DUAs are also received from non-CEs (particularly, some NIH public use files). Notably, an LDS/DUA is often considered not to include identifiable private information for purposes of the Common Rule, and thus research involving only an LDS is often declared *not to be research involving human subjects* and not further subject to Common Rule oversight.

Note that while many of the case report forms sent to research sponsors during a clinical trial have the identifiers limited to those that are permitted in an LDS, the CE typically does not enter into a DUA with the research sponsor because the individual has provided their authorization for disclosure of PHI, thus eliminating the need for the DUA.

HIPAA Breach Notification Rule

The HITECH Act mandated privacy and security incident evaluation and breach reporting of uses and disclosure of PHI not permitted by the Privacy Rule (HITECH, 2009). The IRB rarely has PHI that could give rise to a breach, but a CE's researchers do. The institutional compliance office (privacy officer) is generally involved in developing specific steps for the reporting of an incident, its evaluation, mitigation, and corrective actions. As necessary, the privacy officer will coordinate notification of individuals, the public, and the DHHS Office for Civil Rights.

DATA USE AGREEMENTS

The Privacy Rule sets forth specific requirements for DUAs, including that the DUA establish the permitted uses and disclosures of the LDS and that the DUA provide that the recipient of the LDS will "(1) Not use or further disclose the information other than as permitted by the data use agreement or as otherwise required by law, (2) Use appropriate safeguards to prevent use or disclosure of the information other than as provided for by the data use agreement, (3) Report to the covered entity any use or disclosure of the information not provided for by its data use agreement of which it becomes aware; (4) Ensure that any agents to whom it provides the limited data set agree to the same restrictions and conditions that apply to the limited data set recipient with respect to such information; and (5) Not identify the information or contact the individuals" whose information is contained in the LDS [45 CFR 164.514(2)(4)(ii)(c)].

Under HIPAA's Breach Notification Rule, "an impermissible use or disclosure of PHI is presumed to be a breach" unless there is a low probability that the PHI "has been compromised based on a risk assessment of at least the following factors" (DHHS, 2013b):

1. The nature and extent of the PHI involved, including the types of identifiers and the likelihood of reidentification
2. The unauthorized person who used the PHI or to whom the disclosure was made
3. Whether the PHI was actually acquired or viewed
4. The extent to which the risk to the PHI has been mitigated

In recent years, there have been well-publicized breaches of PHI by researchers, and thus it is important that institutions educate researchers regarding the proper use, disclosure, and safeguarding of PHI.

FDA Guidance and International Council on Harmonisation Implications

⚙ 8-2   FDA does not require IRBs to review authorizations. The <u>International Council on Harmonisation (ICH)</u>, in contrast, requires that IRBs review everything that is given to subjects and that is related to research, including the authorization. Therefore, if the organization applies ICH guidance to all of its research, then the authorizations would need to be reviewed by the IRB.

Centers for Disease Control and Prevention Guidance

Most Centers for Disease Control and Prevention (CDC) activities are in the areas of public health. The Privacy Rule contains a provision permitting the use and disclosure of PHI for public health activities [45 CFR 164.512(b)]. CDC guidance on the Privacy Rule includes a few statements related to research (CDC, 2003). Of interest to those who have lived with the OHRP interpretation of the Common Rule for many years is that CDC defines a project as practice (or nonresearch) if a project activity is primarily practice (and, implied, secondarily research), and most OHRP guidance defines a project as research if any portion is research (CDC, 2003).

Business Associate Contracts and Research

Business associate contracts (BACs) between a CE and an external party are typically required before a CE discloses PHI to the external party for activities related to payment, healthcare operations, or certain activities defined in the Privacy Rule as giving rise to a business associate relationship, such as legal or accounting services. Because "research" is not considered a "payment" or "healthcare operation" activity under the Privacy Rule, disclosures of PHI to external parties for research purposes typically do not require the CE to enter a BAC with the researcher or other person performing activities that are essential to the research. In the context of a research study, a BAC is typically only required if a person or entity outside the CE receives PHI to perform a "healthcare operation" activity in connection with the research study, such as obtaining authorizations from prospective research subjects and/or creating a limited or deidentified data set for use in the research.

2018 Common Rule Exemption for Activities Subject to HIPAA

Many research activities fall under the jurisdiction of both the Common Rule and HIPAA, thus requiring researchers to comply with both sets of regulations. The 2018 Common Rule attempted to reduce this overlapping jurisdiction for certain secondary research by introducing a new <u>exemption category</u> for "secondary research" subject to HIPAA **[45 CFR 46.104(d)(4)(iii)]**, sometimes referred to as the "HIPAA Exemption." The Common Rule specifies that "secondary research" is research using identifiable private information that was collected in the course of another primary or initial activity. The new exemption category applies to secondary research performed by a researcher whose use of the information is subject to the Privacy Rule, which can include researchers who are part of a CE or a business associate. Thus, for example, under the 2018 Common Rule, in a retrospective medical record review study occurring within a CE, the researcher requires permission under HIPAA for use and disclosure of PHI as part of the research, such as a waiver of authorization, but under the new exemption they would be "exempt" from the requirements of the Common Rule, meaning that the research would not be subject to IRB oversight and they would not need to obtain a waiver of informed consent. This exemption is likely to increase the extent to which researchers must be familiar with HIPAA requirements, because much secondary research by CEs and their researchers will no longer be subject to IRB oversight but may instead face increased oversight by an institution's compliance function in charge of HIPAA compliance, such as the Privacy Officer. SACHRP has issued guidance addressing this exemption in more detail (DHHS, 2017b).

⊘ 5-3

HIPAA Security Rule and Research

The HIPAA Security Rule, under 45 CFR 160–164, applies to systems within a CE that contain electronic PHI (DHHS, 2017c). An LDS/DUA is still considered PHI and is subject to the Security Rule; similarly, other research activities are subject to the Security Rule to the extent they are done within a CE. It is arguable that PHI obtained with an individual authorization is subject to the Security Rule while still in the possession of a CE. The Security Rule under HIPAA is much more specific about what must be done than the general statements of security seen under the Common Rule (DHHS, 2017c). Researchers and IRBs at CEs need to be aware of this requirement to ensure proper safeguarding of PHI.

Conclusion

Although HIPAA has little official, direct impact on an IRB's functioning, many of the HIPAA requirements of the CE related to research are assigned to institution-based IRBs. This chapter highlights the areas of concern for research and research oversight and offers some practical suggestions to meet these concerns. Identifying a proper basis for the use and disclosure of PHI is an important activity for both researchers within a CE and researchers who draw PHI out of a CE. This requirement of HIPAA has caused changes to the research process, e.g., adding authorizations to research consent forms. Other areas add to the administrative workload of the IRB and researchers but have not caused wholesale changes to the research process.

References

Centers for Disease Control and Prevention (CDC). (2003). HIPAA Privacy Rule and public health: Guidance from CDC and the U.S. Department of Health and Human Services. *Morbidity and Mortality Weekly Report, 52*, 1–12. www.cdc.gov/mmwr/preview/mmwrhtml/m2e411a1.htm

Department of Health and Human Services (DHHS). (2013a). *Office for Civil Rights: Summary of the Health Insurance Portability and Accountability Act.* www.hhs.gov/hipaa/for-professionals/privacy/laws-regulations/index.html

Department of Health and Human Services (DHHS). (2013b). *Breach Notification Rule.* www.hhs.gov/hipaa/for-professionals/breach-notification/index.html

Department of Health and Human Services (DHHS). (2014). *CLIA Program and HIPAA Privacy Rule; Patients' Access to Test Reports.* www.govinfo.gov/content/pkg/FR-2014-02-06/pdf/2014-02280.pdf

Department of Health and Human Services (DHHS). (2015). *Guidance regarding methods for de-identification of protected health information in accordance with the Health Insurance Portability and Accountability Act (HIPAA) Privacy Rule.* www.hhs.gov/hipaa/for-professionals/privacy/special-topics/de-identification/index.html#standard

Department of Health and Human Services (DHHS). (2017a). *21st Century Cures Act Guidance: Remote access to PHI for activities preparatory to research.* www.hhs.gov/sites/default/files/remote-access-research-12-15-17.pdf

Department of Health and Human Services (DHHS). (2017b). *Secretary's Advisory Committee on Human Research Protections. Attachment B – Recommendations on the interpretation and application of §__.104(d)(4) the "HIPAA Exemption."* www.hhs.gov/ohrp/sachrp-committee/recommendations/attachment-b-december-12-2017/index.html

Department of Health and Human Services (DHHS). (2017c). *The Security Rule.* www.hhs.gov/hipaa/for-professionals/security/index.html

Department of Health and Human Services (DHHS). (2020). *Individuals' right under HIPAA to access their health information [45 CFR § 164.524].* www.hhs.gov/hipaa/for-professionals/privacy/guidance/access/index.html

Health Information Technology for Economic and Clinical Health (HITECH) Act of 2009. (2009). Pub. L. No. 111-5, 123 Stat. 226. www.healthit.gov/sites/default/files/hitech_act_excerpt_from_arra_with_index.pdf

National Institutes of Health (NIH). (2003). *Minimum necessary requirement.* www.hhs.gov/hipaa/for-professionals/privacy/guidance/minimum-necessary-requirement/index.html

National Institutes of Health (NIH). (2004a). *Protecting personal health information in research: Understanding the HIPAA Privacy Rule.* http://privacyruleandresearch.nih.gov/pr_02.asp

National Institutes of Health (NIH). (2004b). *Clinical research and the HIPAA Privacy Rule.* http://privacyruleandresearch.nih.gov/clin_research.asp

Planned Emergency Research

Neal W. Dickert
Robert Silbergleit

Abstract

Many medical conditions, such as cardiac arrest, traumatic injury, and seizure, develop quickly and require emergency treatment. The conduct of clinical trials to evaluate existing and novel therapies for these highly mortal and morbid conditions is essential to advancing care. However, conducting clinical trials in emergency settings, where clinical decision making and treatment must happen very quickly and informed consent is often impracticable, is logistically and ethically complex. In recognition of the need for research and the complexity of the emergency setting, particularly regarding informed consent, federal regulations at 21 CFR 50.24 allow an exception from informed consent (EFIC) for some of this type of research. Important clinical trials have been facilitated by the EFIC regulations, and many researchers and IRBs have gained substantial experience working within them. This chapter will briefly describe the EFIC regulations and their origins and discuss several specific elements of emergency research that pose challenges for IRBs.

EFIC Regulations and Their Origin

Prior to 1996, there were no specific provisions to allow the conduct of clinical trials in the emergency setting without prospective informed consent. Researchers and IRBs relied on concepts such as "deferred consent" and provisions related to emergency use of research interventions in permitting the conduct of trials in which prospective consent was not possible. However, neither Food and Drug Administration (FDA) regulations nor the Common Rule specifically permitted a waiver of consent for clinical trials presenting more than minimal risks to subjects (Biros et al., 1996, 1998). In recognition of the lack of explicit regulatory justification for these studies, the Office of Protection for Research Risks declared in 1993 that research in emergency settings that presented more than minimal risk to subjects would not be permitted in the absence of prospective consent (Ellis, 1993).

In 1996, FDA issued regulations [21 CFR 50. 24] to explicitly permit an exception from informed consent for emergency research in specific settings under certain strict criteria (FDA, 2013). The Department of Health and Human Services (DHHS) endorsed the same requirements in the Common Rule through issuance of a secretarial letter without an explicit regulatory change (see box, Key Provisions for Exception from Informed Consent for Research in Emergency Settings). The EFIC regulations include several unique requirements. Regarding the study itself, the most notable requirements are that the condition must be life-threatening, that treatment with the test article must be delivered in a defined (generally very early) therapeutic window, that existing therapy must be considered unsatisfactory or unproven, and that the research presents a possibility for direct benefit. Regarding consent, researchers must demonstrate that prospective consent is not practicable within the necessary therapeutic window and that the study could not be conducted with individuals for whom prospective consent could be obtained. Finally, the regulations require that researchers conduct (and IRBs review) a process of community consultation prior to conducting the study and public disclosure of the study's conduct.

KEY PROVISIONS FOR EXCEPTION FROM INFORMED CONSENT FOR EMERGENCY RESEARCH [21 CFR 50.24]

(a) The IRB responsible for the review, approval, and continuing review of the clinical investigation described in this section may approve that investigation without requiring that informed consent of all research subjects be obtained if the IRB (with the concurrence of a licensed physician who is a member of or consultant to the IRB and who is not otherwise participating in the clinical investigation) finds and documents each of the following:

1. The human subjects are in a life-threatening situation, available treatments are unproven or unsatisfactory, and the collection of valid scientific evidence, which may include evidence obtained through randomized placebo-controlled investigations, is necessary to determine the safety and effectiveness of particular interventions.
2. Obtaining informed consent is not feasible because:
   i. The subjects will not be able to give their informed consent as a result of their medical condition;
   ii. The intervention under investigation must be administered before consent from the subjects' legally authorized representatives is feasible; and
   iii. There is no reasonable way to identify prospectively the individuals likely to become eligible for participation in the clinical investigation.
3. Participation in the research holds out the prospect of direct benefit to the subjects because:
   i. Subjects are facing a life-threatening situation that necessitates intervention;
   ii. Appropriate animal and other preclinical studies have been conducted, and the information derived from those studies and related evidence support the potential for the intervention to provide a direct benefit to the individual subjects; and
   iii. Risks associated with the investigation are reasonable in relation to what is known about the medical condition of the potential class of subjects, the risks and benefits of standard therapy, if any, and what is known about the risks and benefits of the proposed intervention or activity.
4. The clinical investigation could not practicably be carried out without the waiver.
5. The proposed investigational plan defines the length of the potential therapeutic window based on scientific evidence, and the investigator has committed to attempting to contact a legally authorized representative for each subject within that window of time and, if feasible, to asking the legally authorized representative contacted for consent within that window rather than proceeding without consent. The investigator will summarize efforts made to contact legally authorized representatives and make this information available to the IRB at the time of continuing review.
6. The IRB has reviewed and approved informed consent procedures and an informed consent document consistent with 50.25. These procedures and the informed consent document are to be used with subjects or their legally authorized representatives in situations where use of such procedures and documents is feasible. The IRB has reviewed and approved procedures and information to be used when providing an opportunity for a family member to object to a subject's participation in the clinical investigation consistent with paragraph (a)(7)(v) of this section.

7. Additional protections of the rights and welfare of the subjects will be provided, including, at least:
    i.   Consultation (including, where appropriate, consultation carried out by the IRB) with representatives of the communities in which the clinical investigation will be conducted and from which the subjects will be drawn;
    ii. Public disclosure to the communities in which the clinical investigation will be conducted and from which the subjects will be drawn, prior to initiation of the clinical investigation, of plans for the investigation and its risks and expected benefits;
    iii. Public disclosure of sufficient information following completion of the clinical investigation to apprise the community and researchers of the study, including the demographic characteristics of the research population, and its results;
    iv. Establishment of an independent data monitoring committee to exercise oversight of the clinical investigation; and
    v.   If obtaining informed consent is not feasible and a legally authorized representative is not reasonably available, the investigator has committed, if feasible, to attempting to contact within the therapeutic window the subject's family member who is not a legally authorized representative, and asking whether he or she objects to the subject's participation in the clinical investigation. The investigator will summarize efforts made to contact family members and make this information available to the IRB at the time of continuing review.

(b) The IRB is responsible for ensuring that procedures are in place to inform, at the earliest feasible opportunity, each subject, or if the subject remains incapacitated, a legally authorized representative of the subject, or if such a representative is not reasonably available, a family member, of the subject's inclusion in the clinical investigation, the details of the investigation and other information contained in the informed consent document. The IRB shall also ensure that there is a procedure to inform the subject, or if the subject remains incapacitated, a legally authorized representative of the subject, or if such a representative is not reasonably available, a family member, that he or she may discontinue the subject's participation at any time without penalty or loss of benefits to which the subject is otherwise entitled. If a legally authorized representative or family member is told about the clinical investigation and the subject's condition improves, the subject is also to be informed as soon as feasible. If a subject is entered into a clinical investigation with waived consent and the subject dies before a legally authorized representative or family member can be contacted, information about the clinical investigation is to be provided to the subject's legally authorized representative or family member, if feasible.

The most widely discussed elements of the EFIC regulations have been the requirements for community consultation and public disclosure. These processes are not required by regulation for any other kind of study, although they have been used in several other research contexts. Although the requirements for <u>community engagement</u> have been the focus of much discussion, challenges operationalizing the EFIC regulations are not limited to these provisions.

   🔗 12-9

What Studies Qualify for EFIC?

The defining feature of EFIC research is the absence of prospective consent, but the EFIC regulations contain specific criteria related to the study itself. Some of these criteria have proven challenging for IRBs and researchers to interpret.

Life-threatening situation: In an attempt to avoid EFIC studies' being conducted in medical contexts that are not serious, the regulations restrict EFIC to circumstances in which subjects "have a life-threatening medical condition that necessitates urgent intervention" (FDA, 2013). Importantly, this does not mean that all studies conducted under EFIC must be designed to improve mortality. The FDA-issued guidance document, for example, clarifies that morbidity endpoints are acceptable in the context of trials that address treatment for conditions that are, themselves, life-threatening (FDA, 2013). For example, trials of time to seizure resolution in status epilepticus have been approved under the EFIC regulations (Silbergleit et al., 2012). Notably, there have been questions raised regarding the value of the "life-threatening" requirement, because there can be a need for research to improve care for important, non-life-threatening conditions. From an ethical perspective, it is not clear why those studies should not be permitted if other criteria are met (Dickert & Sugarman, 2018).

Available treatments are unproven or unsatisfactory: In an attempt to restrict waivers of consent to instances where there is a strong need for improvement in therapy, the EFIC regulations require that available treatment for the condition under study be unproven or unsatisfactory. There are broad definitions within FDA guidance for both of these terms, and deciding what constitutes unproven or unsatisfactory has at times been a source of substantial controversy (FDA, 2013). Competing accounts of the extent to which blood transfusion is "unsatisfactory" defined much of the debate about the controversial PolyHeme trial in treatment of hemorrhagic shock (Dickert & Sugarman, 2007; Kipnis et al., 2006). Ultimately, an overly restrictive account of what constitutes "unproven or unsatisfactory" results in prohibition of studies that represent important potential improvements to care, whereas a permissive account might only prevent approval of redundant "me too" trials of agents with no potential benefit over existing therapy. As a consequence of difficulty operationalizing this standard, this provision has relatively little effect in practice, especially because the EFIC regulations also incorporate strict risk/benefit assessments that more effectively account for the risks and benefits of the proposed study in relation to standard treatment.

Study design and population are not restricted: It is important to recognize that the EFIC regulations do not specify the types of study designs that are approvable. Placebo-controlled trials, active comparison trials, noninferiority trials, and even trials testing removal of a standard therapy can be approvable under this mechanism, provided other criteria are met. Similarly, EFIC studies are permitted in <u>pediatric</u> populations, assuming other criteria are met and the studies address an important problem in the pediatric population (Nelson, 2006).

9-6

Consent-Related Provisions

Consent is not practicable within the "therapeutic window": In order to approve a study under the EFIC regulations, an IRB must determine that prospective consent from a patient or legally authorized representative is not practicable within the therapeutic window in which the treatment or test article must be provided. If the scientific and regulatory goals of a study can be met by a trial conducted in a population where prospective consent can be obtained, the EFIC mechanism cannot be used. While this requirement seems straightforward, there are subtleties that must be recognized.

First, approval of a trial under EFIC does not mean that there are no attempts to involve patients or legally authorized representatives (LARs) in the enrollment decision, and it does not mean that all patients are enrolled under EFIC. The regulations require that a consent process be in place when an appropriate decision maker is available. As a result, many EFIC studies have enrolled a large number of patients under prospective consent. In the ProTECT III trial in traumatic brain injury, for example, prospective consent was obtained for 30% of enrolled subjects (Wright et al., 2014). This was anticipated at the time of EFIC application, and the justification for EFIC was not that *no* subjects would be enrollable under prospective consent but rather that an insufficient number (and nonrepresentative sample) of subjects would be enrollable under prospective consent within the time frame in which the study intervention was likely to be effective. Other studies, such as the IMMEDIATE trial of suspected acute coronary syndrome, have utilized an assent process upfront (Selker et al., 2012). In that case, the study was being conducted in the prehospital setting. Informed consent was not considered practicable, but most subjects could communicate with paramedics before enrollment in the trial. The assent strategy was utilized as a mechanism for allowing people to opt out of enrollment in a situation where full consent was not considered practicable but some level of meaningful involvement was possible.

Second, a closely related challenge is determining practicability for <u>informed consent</u>. This determination can be difficult for IRBs in several respects. Although the concept of informed consent is well defined, the level of understanding on the part of subjects that is necessary to satisfy criteria for informed consent can be hard to define, especially in the acute setting. A different way in which the practicability criterion may be challenging to apply relates to the length of the therapeutic window. Although a condition such as cardiac arrest requires immediate treatment with absolutely no delay, treatment for traumatic brain injury may have a longer window. While allowing a longer time for obtaining consent may minimize the need for EFIC enrollment, it may compromise the extent to which the treatment being studied is effective and thus compromise the ability to detect its therapeutic value. Guidance on EFIC acknowledges that the therapeutic window is rarely discrete; it often lacks clearly identifiable thresholds. The guidance thus allows researchers to define a scientific rationale for the therapeutic window that makes sense for the trial and intervention under review (FDA, 2013).

⊘ Section 6

Consent must be obtained as soon as practicable: After EFIC enrollment, notification that the enrollment occurred must be provided, and consent to continue in the trial must be pursued as soon as practicable with either the subject or LAR. IRBs have a responsibility for reviewing the plan for this process, but it is important to recognize that the process may accomplish different ends in different studies. When a trial involves a one-time administration of a drug or performance of a procedure, follow-up consent for continued participation is often limited to consent for continued data collection and use. In contrast, if a trial involves a treatment that is delivered over a longer time frame or incorporates additional testing or other procedures, the follow-up consent process may determine whether a subject continues to be exposed to an intervention or assessments of varying invasiveness. In the latter case, there may be more urgency, for example, to identify an LAR than there is in the former case. Importantly, "consent to continue" is distinct from the term "deferred consent." The latter is sometimes used in the literature and regulation outside the United States to refer to retroactive consent given after the fact for an earlier enrollment. Use of this term is discouraged in this case, because it is a misnomer. One may acknowledge and even agree with, but cannot provide consent for, treatment that has been previously administered (Beauchamp, 1980; Levine, 1995).

Opting out and opportunities to object: Many EFIC trials, in conjunction with community engagement activities, provide individuals with a mechanism to opt out of enrollment in advance. Some studies have developed registries of individuals who would not want to be included; more commonly, wristbands or other mechanisms are used. It is important to recognize that opt-out options are not formally required by the EFIC regulations, but they are often incorporated. Available data suggest that very few individuals pursue mechanisms to avoid inclusion in trials and that few individuals who are enrolled in EFIC trials, or in the general public, have heard about the trial prior to enrollment (Dickert et al., 2015; Jacoby et al., 2008; Silbergleit et al., 2012). However, opt-out mechanisms do represent a good faith effort on the part of researchers to allow people to avoid unwanted enrollment in advance.

One important consideration for the IRB to consider is the feasibility of proposed opt-out mechanisms. Wearable opt-out notifications such as medical alert tags or bracelets are easy to distribute and allow individuals to easily change their minds over time, but they may be a nuisance for individuals wearing them. Registries, on the other hand, may be more attractive and less burdensome to potential subjects, but checking a registry prior to EFIC enrollment is often not practical because of time constraints and difficulty verifying identities in the emergency setting. Furthermore, such registries, by definition, collect and maintain personal identifying information or protected health information from individuals who are not research subjects, which is often not desirable to those wishing to opt out of research enrollment.

In contrast to opt-out procedures, the regulations do specify that researchers should attempt to locate a family member within the therapeutic window to offer an "opportunity to object" to enrollment if there is not an appropriate LAR available [21 CFR 50.24(a)(6)]. This requirement has received relatively little attention, and it is unknown what range of approaches to operationalizing it have been employed across EFIC trials. Moreover, there is substantial ambiguity about who should be offered an opportunity to object on behalf of an incapacitated patient. Whether people contacted over the telephone, for example, or distant family members or other acquaintances who may be present should be engaged in this process, and what level of information needs to be communicated for an objection to be valid, remain unsettled questions that are not clearly addressed in the regulations or guidance document (Biros et al., 2015; Vorholt & Dickert, 2019).

Community Consultation and Public Disclosure

As mentioned previously, there is no other type of research for which community consultation and public disclosure are required by regulation. Thus it is not surprising that these two requirements within the EFIC regulations have been the focus of more discussion in the literature than any other aspect of EFIC research and have likely presented the greatest challenge for IRBs and researchers in conducting and reviewing EFIC studies. While the following discussion will focus on areas of uncertainty and challenge for IRBs, several aspects of the community consultation and public disclosure requirements are clear and important, as described in the regulations and formal guidance document (FDA, 2013). First, IRBs must review the researchers' plans for community consultation and public disclosure, and they must review the results of community consultation prior to approval of an EFIC study. Second, the regulations and guidance document do not specify that any particular type of community consultation, and public disclosure must be carried out. These determinations are left to the researchers and the IRB. Third, community consultation should not be conflated with "community consent." It is intended to be an opportunity to discuss a study with and solicit opinions from the relevant community and not a formal approval process that substitutes for individual consent (analogous in some ways to a comment period in governmental rule making). Finally, community consultation and public disclosure have distinct purposes. As elaborated in the FDA guidance document, community consultation is a discussion or "two-way" interaction that is designed to elicit feedback and inform the researchers and the IRB about relevant views and values in the community (FDA, 2013).

🔗 12-9

The principal function of public disclosure is notification; it is a "one-way" process to inform the community about the study and promote transparency. There are activities that may serve both functions, but it is important for IRBs to recognize that the consultation and disclosure processes serve distinct purposes.

Who Should Be Included in Community Consultation?

The EFIC regulations specify that consultation should be conducted with "representatives of the communities in which the clinical investigation will be conducted and from which the subjects will be drawn" [21 CFR 50.24(a)(7)(i)]. This has been interpreted, in practice and within the FDA guidance document, as requiring the involvement of representatives from the geographic area (geographic community) and from groups of individuals affected by the condition under study or at particular risk for the condition under study (condition community; FDA, 2013). As a result, distinct practices of consultation have emerged. Many efforts to consult the "geographic community" have focused on representing (often statistically) the general population in the region where a study will be conducted. Efforts to consult the "condition community," on the other hand, are often more focused and involve advocacy groups, support groups, and direct recruitment of patients and family members to discussions.

In designing and reviewing community consultation, it is important to recognize that neither the regulations nor guidance document specifies that these two "types of community" are necessarily distinct. They also do not require quantitative representation of a general public or, for that matter, involvement of the general public at all. Local health providers, for example, are specifically mentioned in the FDA guidance document as potentially valuable participants from the "community in which the research will be conducted" but clearly do not represent the general public (FDA, 2013). Moreover, within the guidance document, all examples of specific populations to include focus on populations with some connection to the condition under study or increased risk for the condition (i.e., increased chance of being included; FDA, 2013). Coupled with evidence that patients and surrogates of EFIC trials also find involvement of individuals with greater connection to the condition or healthcare providers more meaningful, there is a strong argument for focusing consultation efforts on groups with connections to the condition or the study and not on the geographically defined general public (Fehr et al., 2017; Fordyce et al., 2017). At a practical level, there can also be real challenges to engaging in substantive discussion about an EFIC study with members of the general public. This is especially the case when researchers use tools such as telephone or electronic surveys as a method of assessing the views of large numbers of people. These methods tend to be highly scripted and minimally interactive, and they typically use mostly closed-ended questions (Lewis, 2009; Lo, 2006).

How Should Community Consultation Be Executed?

A wide variety of methods for community consultation have emerged. They range both in the number of people involved and the nature of the discussion. On one end of the spectrum, in-depth interviews with key stakeholders may be conducted; on the other, random-digit-dialed surveys or other highly quantitative tools may be used. These methods provide different combinations of depth and breadth of discussion, and they entail different requirements in terms of monetary and staff resources. One observation in recent years has been that feedback from more quantitative efforts has been relatively constant across studies and geographic locations, suggesting that these efforts tend to assess more general background attitudes toward research. While these efforts may have provided novel insights at the outset of the EFIC era, it is unclear how much they contribute at this stage (Fehr et al., 2015). In addition, having a research team interact in a more substantive way with members of key "communities" through attending community meetings, focus groups, interviews, and other more interactive conversations allows researchers to more directly understand the impact of the proposed study on potential subjects and have more extended discussion about any elements of a study that prompt concern. In general, quality of interaction is more important than quantity (Lewis, 2009). Moreover, more interactive community consultation allows researchers to have a face-to-face interaction with would-be subjects in lieu of the moral exchange that would otherwise be an important but intangible aspect of a consent conversation.

An important trend is that social media have become increasingly used to facilitate community consultation and public disclosure for EFIC studies (Stephens et al., 2016). In most cases, social media serve more of a disclosure function. Interactions tend to be predominantly one way (via ads), and feedback seems to be relatively limited. However, social media may serve a consultative function to some extent, depending on what platform is used and the effort, time, and volume of interaction that researchers pursue. The diversity of community, or lack thereof, on any given social media platform should be considered (Chretien, 2013).

What Should IRBs Do with Negative Feedback During Consultation?

As articulated earlier, the regulations and FDA guidance document are clear that community consultation is not the same as "community consent." It is not a formal approval process nor is it intended to replace individual consent, and the primary goals are to show respect for patients and communities and to solicit input from relevant stakeholders about a particular study. That said, it is intended to help the IRB in reviewing a proposed trial, and it is a foregone conclusion that some participants in any consultation process will not support the study, just as no clinical trial would ever expect 100% enrollment. Because IRBs must review data (surveys and more qualitative descriptions of feedback) from community consultation efforts, they are often confronted with decisions about what to do with objections or lack of support identified during community consultation. There are questions in the literature about what level of dissent should indicate that the ethical justification for an EFIC study is undermined, and there are no accepted standards, although it is commonly the case that roughly 70% of individuals are supportive of personal enrollment in any particular EFIC trial (Baker & Merz, 2018; Fehr et al., 2015). Similar or slightly higher rates of acceptance of enrollment have been observed among EFIC trial enrollees (Dickert et al., 2015). Interestingly, this rate of acceptance tends to mirror general views of randomization in other contexts as well and likely indicates general, background attitudes toward research (Meyer et al., 2019). Although IRBs have to pay attention to unusually high rates of disagreement with a proposed trial, it is more important for IRBs to be informed of and consider specific concerns that are expressed about a study and to evaluate whether there are potential alterations that can be designed to accommodate those concerns.

How Should IRBs Assess Adequacy of Public Disclosure?

Because IRBs are tasked with evaluating public disclosure plans, they must assess whether these plans are adequate. Public disclosure activities may involve traditional media (print, radio, television), social media, billboards, or other community announcements. There is a general consensus, reflected in the guidance, that efforts should be broad and should attempt penetration of communities that are likely to be affected by or enrolled in the proposed study (FDA, 2013). However, it is also widely recognized that community awareness of any particular study is likely to be low despite extensive efforts by researchers. This is reflected by the very low number of enrollees in EFIC trials who, when assessed, have heard of the study in which they were enrolled prior to their own enrollment (Scicluna et al., 2020). The more meaningful goal of public disclosure is thus one of transparency and fostering trust with the public, rather than making actual enrollees aware of the study, for example, so that they can opt out if they wish to do so.

Additional Considerations

Central IRB Review

The requirement for <u>single IRB</u> review in NIH-funded multisite clinical trials, and similar requirements in the 2018 Common Rule, present new challenges to the implementation of EFIC. The review of community consultation results is a quintessentially local task that a central IRB may be less equipped to perform than the IRB at each site. For example, a local IRB has greater opportunity to send representatives to participate or observe local community consultation events. Also, as compared to a central IRB, a local IRB may have insight into aspects of the community served by the site, into local medical practice variation or local statutes or regulations, or into previous experiences with the site investigator team. On the other hand, central IRB review may have advantages in reviewing EFIC trials. Use of a central IRB potentially allows reviews of these trials to be concentrated in a smaller number of boards that are experienced with these regulations. This is important, because many local IRBs are unfamiliar and uncomfortable with conducting these reviews. Indeed, not having a standard operating procedure for implementation of **21 CFR 50.24** is the most common EFIC-related finding in warning letters issued to local IRB by FDA. By reducing variability in application of the regulations, a central IRB inherently provides a more consistent and equitable standard of review. Additionally, because a central IRB can compare community consultation results across diverse sites, it may be better able to identify patterns, expectations, and outliers in findings resulting from community consultation (Goldkind et al., 2014).

Central IRBs will have to identify best practices for reviewing EFIC trial applications to leverage the potential advantages and minimize the limitations of centralized review. There is not yet sufficient experience or operational data available to inform such best practices, but reasonable approaches being developed or implemented include: populating specialized boards with content and regulatory expertise in emergency research, procedures to allow sites to communicate to the central IRB what they know about the people in their communities and other site-specific information, use of standardized EFIC plans that balance predefined expectations with sufficient adaptability to trial site circumstances, and standardized collection and reporting of community consultation

⚲ Section 4

activities and findings as well as public disclosure activities. Ideally, sharing and discussion of systematic empirical evaluation of developing processes will promote increasingly effective and efficient central IRB review of planned emergency research using EFIC.

Non-EFIC Emergency Research

EFIC for emergency research is an important mechanism, but it is only applicable to a narrow range of clinical trials that would not otherwise be possible under FDA regulations or the Common Rule. Many emergency care clinical trials do not require or qualify for EFIC. Researchers, FDA, or an IRB may all determine that asking for consent of the subject or from a surrogate may be practicable, that the condition being studied is not sufficiently life-threatening, or that some other condition of the EFIC regulations has not been met. Discussion of the challenges and variations of planned emergency care research that does not qualify for EFIC is mostly beyond the scope of this chapter, but a few observations are warranted.

Even when an informed consent is practicable, the emergency setting typically has many potential barriers to the process. Trial enrollment decisions in a medical emergency usually need to be made quickly and with limited or incomplete clinical information. Patients are often in pain or under other physiological stress. Both patients and surrogate decision makers are likely to be scared, overwhelmed, distracted, or otherwise emotionally impaired. Research consents may be intertwined with clinical consent processes, causing confusion. Informed consent processes for clinical trials facing these challenges need to be innovative and sensitive to the emergency setting (Dickert et al., 2019). An expedited, or staged consent process may be considered that optimizes the most important and required regulatory components of consent but defers extra information and downstream decision making for subsequent research activities when it may be appropriate to do so (Dickert et al., 2016).

Emergency care research in which informed consent is not practicable but that does not meet all criteria for EFIC is potentially challenging from a regulatory perspective. If the research tests an intervention involving no more than minimal risk, it may be possible to <u>waive or alter elements of informed consent</u> on that basis. Opinion varies widely among IRB professionals as to how broadly minimal risk waivers can be interpreted in the emergency setting. Research that is strictly observational, for example, often clearly presents no more than minimal risk. Clinical trials involving interventions in acute settings, in contrast, are more complicated. Depending on one's interpretation, some randomized interventions could engender no more than minimal risk. For example, <u>standard care studies</u> may systematically allocate subjects to two or more variants of practice that are consistent with the range and distribution of care that would be experienced by patients outside of the trial. In such a trial, the risks to the patient related to the practice variation are similar regardless of whether or not the patient participates in the trial (Wendler et al., 2017). Unfortunately, clinical trials involving situations and settings where informed consent is not practicable, but in which the trial cannot be broadly interpreted to meet either the criteria for EFIC or the minimal risk waiver (if low risk), may not be approvable by an IRB in the current regulatory environment, even if these trials address questions vital to emergency care or public health. Regulatory changes or guidance adopting broader interpretations of existing regulations could help to close this gap in emergency care research. In the absence of these changes, attention to the development and implementation of consent processes that are

🖉 6-4

🖉 10-8

as sensitive to the emergency context as possible represents an important focus, as is recognition on the part of IRB members that consent processes may serve more limited functions in the emergency setting than they do in less stressful contexts (Dickert et al., 2016).

Distributive Justice

Additional concerns about EFIC research are related to distributive justice. One recent review of EFIC trials, for example, found that minority enrollment in EFIC trials may exceed the rate of the study condition in the overall population (Feldman et al., 2018). This concern has salience, especially in the context of historical research abuses. However, there are important contextualizing factors. First, *underenrollment* of minorities is a major problem in most other clinical trial contexts and also raises important distributive justice concerns in terms of ensuring quality care and access to benefits of research among minority populations. In this respect, EFIC may be helpful by ensuring representation. Second, it is likely the case that the driver of perceived overenrollment is not EFIC itself but rather where EFIC studies are performed. Limited available data, for example, suggest that the demographics of EFIC enrollees does tend to match the demographic patterns of the condition under study in the sites where the study is being conducted (Sugarman et al., 2009). Patterns of over-representation may thus reflect the fact that EFIC studies, like other emergency research studies, tend to be conducted in urban academic centers rather than indicating anything about the selectivity of the EFIC enrollment process. An important implication may be that there are reasons to pursue a greater diversity of research sites. These findings also underscore the importance of effective communication with communities about the reasons for EFIC studies and a rigorous process of review and engagement.

Conclusion

The EFIC regulations passed in 1996 offer a comprehensive structure for the review and conduct of key clinical trials in emergency settings. IRBs and researchers have gained substantial experience implementing these regulations since their passage. However, active questions remain. Some of the key challenges highlighted here include how best to implement community consultation and public disclosure requirements, how to approach opportunities to object to inclusion, how to utilize a central IRB process while attending to local context, and how to approach types of research that are important but fall outside the boundaries of current regulatory categories. Ongoing dialogue and evaluation related to each of these challenges will help to continue to refine approaches and facilitate important clinical trials, while respecting critically ill patients.

References

Baker, F. X., & Merz, J. F. (2018). What gives them the right? Legal privilege and waivers of consent for research. *Clinical Trials, 15*(6), 579–586.

Beauchamp, T. L. (1980). The ambiguities of "deferred consent." *IRB, 2*(7), 6–9.

Biros, M. H., Dickert, N. W., Wright, D. W., Scicluna, V. M., Harney, D., Silbergleit, R., Denninghoff, K., & Pentz, R. D. (2015). Balancing ethical goals in challenging individual participant scenarios occurring in a trial conducted with exception from informed consent. *Academic Emergency Medicine, 22*(3), 340–346.

Biros, M. H., Lewis, R. J., Olson, C. M., Runge, J., Cummins, R. O., & Fost, N. (1996). Informed consent in emergency research: Consensus statement from the Coalition Conference of Acute Resuscitation and Critical Care Researchers. *JAMA, 273*(16), 1283–1287.

Biros, M. H., Runge, J., & Lewis, R. J. (1998). Emergency medicine and the development of the FDA's final rule on informed consent and waiver of informed consent in emergency research circumstances. *Academic Emergency Medicine, 1998*(5), 359–368.

Chretien, K. C. (2013). Social media and community engagement in trials using exception from informed consent. *Circulation, 128*(3), 206–208.

Dickert, N. W., Brown, J., Cairns, C. B., Eaves-Leanos, A., Goldkind, S. F., Kim, S. Y., Nichol, G., O'Conor, K. J., Scott, J. D., Sinert, R., Wendler, D., Wright, D. W., & Silbergleit, R. (2016). Confronting ethical and regulatory challenges of emergency care research with conscious patients. *Annals of Emergency Medicine, 67*(4), 538–545.

Dickert, N. W., Scicluna, V. M., Adeoye, O., Angiolillo, D. J., Blankenship, J. C., Devireddy, C. M., Frankel, M. R., Goldkind, S. F., Kumar, G., Ko, Y. A., Mitchell, A. R., Nogueria, R. G., Parker, R. M., Patel, M. R., Riedford, M., Silbergleit, R., Speight, C. D., Spokoyny, I., Weinfurt, K. P., & Pentz, R. D. (2019). Emergency consent: Patients' and surrogates' perspectives on consent for clinical trials in acute stroke and myocardial infarction. *Journal of the American Heart Association, 8*(2), e010905. https://doi.org/10.1161/JAHA.118.010905

Dickert, N. W., Scicluna, V. M., Baren, J. M., Biros, M. H., Fleischman, R. J., Govindarajan, P. R., Jones, E. B., Pancioli, A. M., Wright, D. W., & Pentz, R. D. (2015). Patients' perspectives of enrollment in research without consent: The patients' experiences in emergency research-progesterone for the treatment of traumatic brain injury study. *Critical Care Medicine, 43*(3), 603–612.

Dickert, N. W., & Sugarman, J. (2007). Getting the ethics right regarding research in the emergency setting: Lessons from the PolyHeme Study. *Kennedy Institute of Ethics Journal, 17*(2), 153–169.

Dickert, N. W., & Sugarman, J. (2018). Ethics and regulatory barriers to research in emergency settings. *Annals of Emergency Medicine, 72*(4), 386–388.

Ellis, G. B. (1993). *Informed consent, legally effective and prospectively obtained* [OPRR Letter]. www.hhs.gov/ohrp/regulations-and-policy/guidance/legally-effective-and-prospectively-obtained/index.html

Fehr, A. E., Pentz, R. D., & Dickert, N. W. (2015). Learning from experience: A systematic review of community consultation acceptance data. *Annals of Emergency Medicine, 65*(2), 162–171, e163.

Fehr, A. E., Scicluna, V. M., Pentz, R. D., Haggins, A. N., & Dickert, N. W. (2017). Patient and surrogate views of community consultation for emergency research. *Academic Emergency Medicine, 24*(11), 1410–1414.

Feldman, W. B., Hey, S. P., & Kesselheim, A. S. (2018). A systematic review of the Food and Drug Administration's "exception from informed consent" pathway. *Health Affairs (Millwood), 37*(10), 1605–1614.

Food and Drug Administration (FDA). (2013). *Guidance for institutional review boards, clinical investigators, and sponsors: Exception from informed consent requirements for emergency research.* www.fda.gov/downloads/RegulatoryInformation/Guidances/UCM249673.pdf

Fordyce, C. B., Roe, M. T., & Dickert, N. W. (2017). Maximizing value and minimizing barriers: Patient-centered community consultation for research in emergency settings. *Clinical Trials, 14*(1), 88–93.

Goldkind, S. F., Brosch, L. R., Biros, M., Silbergleit, R. S., & Sopko, G. (2014). Centralized IRB models for emergency care research. *IRB, 36*(2), 1–9.

Jacoby, L. H., Young, B., & Watt, J. (2008). Public disclosure in research with exception from informed consent: The use of survey methods to assess its effectiveness. *Journal of Empirical Research on Human Research Ethics, 3*(1), 79–87.

Kipnis, K., King, N. M. P., & Nelson, R. M. (2006). An open letter to IRBs considering Northfield Laboratories' PolyHeme trial. *American Journal of Bioethics, 6*(3), 18–21.

Levine, R. J. (1995). Research in emergency situations: The role of deferred consent. *JAMA, 273*(16), 1300–1302.

Lewis, R. J. (2009). Community consultation by randomly reaching out to the community. *Annals of Emergency Medicine, 53*(3), 351–353.

Lo, B. (2006). Strengthening community consultation in critical care and emergency research. *Critical Care Medicine, 34*(8), 2236–2238.

Meyer, M. N., Heck, P. R., Holtzman, G. S., Anderson, S. M., Cai, W., Watts, D. J., & Chabris, C. F. (2019). Objecting to experiments that compare two unobjectionable policies or treatments. *Proceedings of the National Academy of Sciences, 116*(22), 10723–10728.

Nelson, R. M. (2006). Challenges in the conduct of emergency research in children: A workshop report. *American Journal of Bioethics, 6*(6), W1–9.

Scicluna, V. M., Biros, M., Harney, D. K., Jones, E. B., Mitchell, A. R., Pentz, R. D., Silbergleit, R., Speight, C. D., Wright, D. W., & Dickert, N. W. (2020). Patient and surrogate post-enrollment perspectives on research using the exception from informed consent: An integrated survey. *Annals of Emergency Medicine, 76*(3), 343–349. https://doi.org/10.1016/j.annemergmed.2020.03.017

Selker, H. P., Beshansky, J. R., Sheehan, P. R., Massaro, J. M., Griffith, J. L., D'Agostino, R. B., Ruthazer, R., Atkins, J. M., Sayah, A. J., Levy, M. K., Richards, M. E., Aufderheide, T. P., Braude, D. A., Pirrallo, R. G., Doyle, D. D., Frascone, R. J., Kosiak, D. J., Leaming, J. M., Van Gelder, C. M., Walter, G. P., ..., Udelson, J. E. (2012). Out-of-hospital administration of intravenous glucose-insulin-potassium in patients with suspected acute coronary syndromes: The IMMEDIATE randomized controlled trial. *JAMA, 307*(18), 1925–1933.

Silbergleit, R., Biros, M. H., Harney, D., Dickert, N., Baren, J., & NETT Investigators. (2012). Implementation of the exception from informed consent regulations in a large multicenter emergency clinical trials network: The RAMPART experience. *Academic Emergency Medicine, 19*(4), 448–454.

Silbergleit, R., Durkalski, V., Lowenstein, D., Conwit, R., Pancioli, A., Palesch, Y., & Barsan, W. (2012). Intramuscular versus intravenous therapy for prehospital status epilepticus. *New England Journal of Medicine, 366*(7), 591–600.

Stephens, S. W., Williams, C., Gray, R., Kerby, J. D., Wang, H. E., & Bosarge, P. L. (2016). Using social media for community consultation and public disclosure in exception from informed consent trials. *Journal of Trauma and Acute Care Surgery, 80*(6), 1005–1009.

Sugarman, J., Sitlani, C., Andrusiek, D., Aufderheide, T., Bulger, E. M., Davis, D. P., Hoyt, D. B., Idris, A., Kerby, J. D., Powell, J., Schmidt, T., Slutsky, A. S., Sopko, G., Stephens, S., Williams, C., Nichol, G., & Resuscitation Outcomes Consortium Investigators. (2009). Is the enrollment of racial and ethnic minorities in research in the emergency setting equitable? *Resuscitation, 80*(6), 644–649.

Vorholt, V., & Dickert, N. W. (2019). Uninformed refusals: Objections to enrollment in clinical trials conducted under an exception from informed consent for emergency research. *Journal of Medical Ethics, 45*(1), 18–21.

Wendler, D., Dickert, N. W., Silbergleit, R., Kim, S. Y., & Brown, J. (2017). Targeted consent for research on standard of care interventions in the emergency setting. *Critical Care Medicine, 45*(1), e105–e110.

Wright, D. W., Yeatts, S. D., Silbergleit, R., Palesch, Y. Y., Hertzberg, V. S., Frankel, M., Goldstein, F. C., Caveney, A. F., Howlett-Smith, H., Bengelink, E. M., Manley, G. T., Merck, L. H., Janis, L. S., Barsan, W. G., & NETT Investigators. (2014). Very early administration of progesterone for acute traumatic brain injury. *New England Journal of Medicine, 371*(26), 2457–2466.

Overview of Select Common Rule Agency Requirements

C. Karen Jeans

Molly M. Klote

Peter Marshall

Daniel K. Nelson

Elizabeth White

Abstract

Every year, the federal government funds and conducts tens of thousands of human subjects research studies within the United States and internationally. As of this writing, 19 federal agencies have agreed to follow the 2018 Common Rule (published January 2017, amended January 2018, effective July 2018), and another (the Department of Justice) intends to do so. Each signatory to the 2018 Common Rule codifies it with an exact duplicate of the wording in **45 CFR 46 subpart A**. To reflect each agency's unique role in government, each agency may write additional agency-specific regulations or policies to define how the agency implements the 2018 Common Rule, the **45 CFR 46 subparts B, C, D,** and **E**, and the Food and Drug Administration (FDA) regulations. In addition, all of the federal agencies presented in this chapter are part of the executive branch and are therefore subject to the Privacy Act, which adds additional restrictions on the release of identifiable information. Additional federal laws may be applicable to the support or conduct of human subjects research studies by federal agencies, unless the federal law excludes a specific federal agency.

Department of Defense

The mission of the Department of Defense (DoD) is to provide the military forces needed to deter war and to protect the security of our country. The DoD Office for Human Research Protections (DOHRP) resides in the office of the

Under Secretary of Defense for Research and Engineering. As the chief technology officer for the DoD, the Under Secretary's mission is to foster globally leading research, ensuring technological advantage for the U.S. warfighter, and the well-being of warfighters, their families, and the public.

DOHRP's vision is to ensure DoD research involving human subjects (HSR) is overseen by irreproachable DoD institutional programs that are constantly safeguarding the welfare of subjects, their data, and their rights, as well as supporting subjects' understanding that their participation is voluntary and not coerced. The mission of every institution within the DoD is to ensure a culture of ethics beyond compliance with federal laws and DoD policies that incorporates best practices in informed consent; protects subjects' privacy, data, and well-being; and respects their desires for how their data is used.

DOHRP Oversight

DOHRP implements the Common Rule at **Part 219 of Title 32, Code of Federal Regulations (CFR)** under the authority: **5 U.S.C. 301, 42 U.S.C. 300v–1(b)**, as well as through DoD Instruction 3216.02, *Protection of Human Subjects and Adherence to Ethical Standards in DoD-Conducted and Supported Research*, by delegation from the Secretary of Defense.

DOHRP oversees DoD human subjects research via the DoD Components' Offices of Human Research Protections (COHRP); COHRPs submit to DOHRP component management plans (CMPs) and policies for their human research protections programs (HRPPs), which oversee their institutions. With an approved CMP and HRPP, DoD components receive authority to issue DoD Federal Assurances and approve institutional HRPPs.

Through the use of templates developed with the COHRPs, DOHRP has been more vigorously standardizing HSR oversight and guidance for research, not just for HSR documentation and processes but also for related documentation, e.g., data use agreements, privacy documentation, and access to electronic health records.

Unique DoD Requirements for HSR

    a. Extramural DoD-supported HSR must receive a Human Research Protection Official (HRPO) written determination before the HSR outlined in the funding instrument may begin. Contracts for DoD-supported research must contain the Defense Federal Acquisition Regulation Supplement (DFARS) clause in its entirety in accordance with **Section 252.235-7004 of Title 48, CFR**. Non-contract funding instruments, e.g., grants, must also define the responsibilities of the non-DoD institution.

    b. Research involving pregnant women, fetuses, or neonates as human subjects must comply with **subpart B** of **45 CFR 46**, with the following modifications:

        1. For purposes of applying this section, the phrase "biomedical knowledge" in **subpart B** of **45 CFR 46**, is replaced with "generalizable knowledge," so that pregnant women are given the ability to decide whether they would like to participate in research.

        2. The applicability of **subpart B** of **45 CFR 46** is limited to research involving:

            a. Pregnant women as human subjects involved in HSR that is more than minimal risk and includes interventions or invasive procedures involving the woman or the fetus; or

            b. Fetuses or neonates as human subjects.

   c. Research involving a detainee, as defined in DoD Directive 2310.01E, or a prisoner of war as a human subject is prohibited.

   d. Research involving large-scale genomic data collected from DoD personnel is subject to component security review and DOHRP approval. The disclosure of DoD personnel's genomic data may pose a risk to national security; accordingly, such research requires administrative, technical, and physical safeguards commensurate with risk, both during and after the conduct of research.

   e. COHRP review of the ethical, legal, and social implications of select research, development, testing, and evaluation involving emerging technologies must be completed prior to the start of such research. A DoD Manual 3216.02 will be issued to further outline the process and goals.

   f. COHRPs have the authority to determine appropriate redactions when posting informed consent forms pursuant to **32 CFR 219** as presented by DoD institutions under their purview. Further guidance on this policy will be issued.

   g. Supervisors, or those in the chain of command, must not be present at any recruitment sessions, or during the consent process for DoD personnel; supervisors are separately approached about their participation in the study.

   h. Use of a single institutional review board (IRB) in accordance with **32 CFR 219.114** is required; however, if the DoD institution feels there needs to be an exception, their COHRP may determine and document that use of a single IRB is not appropriate for the particular context of the proposed HSR. Further guidance on this policy will be issued.

      🔗 Section 4

   i. "Broad consent," as defined in **32 CFR 219**, is permitted in DoD-supported research. The use of broad consent in DoD-conducted research is pursuant to DOHRP guidance and with component notification to DOHRP director.

      🔗 6-9

Department of Veterans Affairs

The mission of the Department of Veterans Affairs (VA) is to fulfill President Lincoln's promise "To care for him who shall have borne the battle, and for his widow, and his orphan" by serving and honoring the men and women who are America's veterans. VA is divided into three subdivisions, which are called administrations. The three administrations are the National Cemetery Administration, the Veterans Benefits Administration, and the Veterans Health Administration (VHA). The VHA is the largest of the three administrations within VA. VHA is the largest integrated healthcare system in the United States, providing care at 1,255 healthcare facilities, including 170 VA medical centers and 1,074 outpatient sites of varying complexity (VHA outpatient clinics). In fiscal year 2018, more than 9 million veterans were enrolled in the VA healthcare system. VHA is one of the nation's largest providers of graduate medical education and a major contributor to medical and scientific research. About 70% of all U.S. physicians have received at least some of their training at VA hospitals.

    For more than 90 years, the Veterans Affairs Research and Development program has been improving the lives of veterans and all Americans through healthcare discovery and innovation. In fiscal year 2019, VHA funded more than $500 million in intramural research grants. The VHA does not fund extramural research. VHA also received more than $500 million in extramural research grants in fiscal year 2019 and conducts multiple studies funded by industry or other organizations, including thousands of clinical trials. VHA is actively involved in multiple partnerships with individuals and organizations that are interested in advancing the health and health care of our nation's veterans.

VA Research's fundamental mission is to advance the health care of veterans. The strategic plan focuses on conducting research that best addresses this mission and ensures that research professionalism and protection of veterans' rights are top priorities. VHA conducts more than 20,000 human subjects research projects at the 108 VA medical centers that are involved in research. These human subjects research projects involve a wide variety of methods and populations, including numerous studies involving big data, because the entire VHA has one integrated medical record system for all of its medical centers. VA does minimal interventional or noninterventional research involving neonates or children. As the number of women who are veterans increases, VA is undertaking increasing numbers of studies focusing on women's health issues. VA maintains national policies that restrict some types of human research studies. For example, VA does not permit greater than minimal risk research involving children. VA also has restrictions, but not prohibitions, on inclusion of nonveterans in VA studies, because VA's research is veteran-centered. When it is to the benefit of the veteran population (e.g., caregiver studies), VA policy will allow nonveterans in VA studies.

The Office of Research Oversight (ORO) is the primary office responsible for research compliance and compliance policy within VHA. The primary office responsible for the peer-review awarding and management of VA's intramural research program and all other VHA national research policy development is the Office of Research and Development (ORD). The VHA Office of Research Protections, Policy, and Education (ORPP&E) is a program office within ORD that is directly responsible for VA policies involving human subjects research and all educational activities to support VHA's research community, including its researchers, research staff, and research offices within VA medical centers and outpatient clinics. ORPP&E houses the VA Central IRB (CIRB), established in 2008 as the first central IRB for use by VA. As of July 2019, the VA CIRB has IRB oversight for more than 245 multisite studies ranging from 2 to 67 sites. VA medical centers conducting nonexempt human subjects research may use the IRB of a VA medical center, an IRB of a university with a medical or dental school, or another federal agency's IRB. Any change in IRB arrangements for any of the VA medical centers must be approved by ORD and ORO prior to the change being implemented. There are 59 additional individual VA IRBs at various VA medical centers around the country, and the remaining VA medical centers either rely on another VA IRB or an affiliate IRB for review. VHA codified the 2018 Common Rule at **38 CFR Part 16**.

VA has numerous other national VA research policies that define the implementation of the 2018 Common Rule and the oversight of research. Some of these national policies include: VHA Directive 1200.05, Requirements for the Protection of Human Subjects in Research; VHA Directive 1200.01, The Research and Development Committee (R&DC); VHA Handbook 1058.01, Research Compliance Reporting Requirements; and VHA Handbook 1108.04, Investigational Drugs and Supplies.

VA has a few unique restrictions on the release of certain types of data as required by **38 CFR 7332**; e.g., drug abuse, alcoholism or alcohol abuse, infection with human immunodeficiency virus, or sickle cell anemia. VHA must obtain a patient's written consent before VA may disclose the protected information unless authorized by the statute.

Each VA medical center director (MCD) must define in the institution's human subjects research protection plan its implementation of VHA policies. They have the option to make local policies more restrictive but not less restrictive. Topics where MCDs vary their policy include, but are not limited to, the following: research with pregnant women, research with children, research with nonveterans, and research with neonates. Non-VA researchers are encouraged to engage the VHA facility or facilities with which they are interested in partnering to learn about any unique restrictions the VHA facility or facilities may have.

Whether serving as the reviewing IRB or not, the VHA institution plays a major role in VHA research review that is codified in the research and development committee. This review is required for all VA research to assess the impact of the research on the facility and to address any institutional issues requiring resolution prior to initiation of the research at the VA facility, including a confirmation that all privacy and information security issues are identified and adequately addressed by the research team. The assistant chief of staff for research and development at the facility is required by VA national research policy to issue an initiation letter to VA researchers; this ensures that all required committee reviews have occurred before the research can begin.

Environmental Protection Agency

The mission of the U.S. Environmental Protection Agency (EPA) is to protect human health and the environment. EPA conducts and supports a wide variety of research involving human subjects in support of this mission, ranging from simple surveys and focus groups to population-based epidemiology studies, controlled exposure research, and interventional trials. Typical examples include projects that examine health status in relation to traffic on nearby roadways, consequences of harmful algal blooms, physiological mechanisms through which summer temperatures and ozone interact to impact the cardiovascular system, fecal contamination at public beaches, environmental concerns of tribal communities, potentially protective effects of fish oil in mitigating the body's response to air pollutants, and web-based applications that track adverse health effects of wildfires.

EPA's version of the Common Rule is codified at **40 CFR 26, subpart A** (EPA, 2013). Beyond the Common Rule, EPA has promulgated additional regulations that provide enhanced protections for human research conducted or supported by the EPA or certain types of third-party research. These agency-specific requirements were added as subparts in 2006 in response to a congressional mandate (Menikoff, 2005; Resnik, 2007; Schonfeld et al., 2017), incorporating guidance from a National Academy of Sciences report on "Intentional Human Dosing Studies for EPA Regulatory Purposes: Scientific and Ethical Issues" (National Research Council, 2004), and were subsequently amended in 2013. The additional subparts are intended to coordinate with subpart A but are generally more restrictive in some aspects that are unique to EPA-related research. In 2019, EPA rule making is under way to harmonize selected subparts with the 2018 Common Rule, incorporating changes that would otherwise create confusion or discrepancies. The EPA-specific regulations are found under **40 CFR 26, subparts B-Q**, summarized as follows:

- *Subpart B*: Categorically prohibits intentional exposure research (defined as the study of a substance in which the exposure would not have occurred but for the research) in children, pregnant women, or nursing women.
- *Subpart C*: Allows for observational research (defined as studies that do not involve intentional exposure) in pregnant women and fetuses, applying the additional protections of **45 CFR 46, subpart B** (i.e., Department of Health and Human Services [DHHS] regulations). There is no allowance, however, for "research not otherwise approvable," as found in **45 CFR 46.207**.

9-4

- *Subpart D*: Allows for observational research (per previous) in children, applying the protections of **45 CFR 46, subpart D**. There is no allowance, however, for research with greater than minimal risk but no direct benefit **[45 CFR 46.406]** or "research not otherwise approvable" **[45 CFR 46.407]**.

9-6

- *Subpart K*: Regulates third-party research involving intentional exposure to pesticides in nonpregnant, nonnursing adults, which is being submitted to EPA for regulatory purposes. This subpart reproduced many elements of the Common Rule **[subpart A]**, excepting those that would not apply to this type of research.
- *Subpart L*: Prohibits third-party research involving intentional exposure in children and pregnant or nursing women, consistent with **subpart B** for EPA-conducted or -supported research.
- *Subpart M*: Sets requirements for submission of information documenting ethical conduct of completed research.
- *Subpart O*: Establishes administrative actions for noncompliance.
- *Subpart P*: Establishes the Human Studies Review Board (HSRB) for review of proposed and completed third-party research involving intentional exposure.
- *Subpart Q*: Sets standards for assessing whether to rely on results of human research in EPA actions.

In addition to these regulatory subparts, EPA also follows EPA Policy Order 1000.17A (adopted 2011, revised 2016), which defines roles and responsibilities for internal review, including the Human Subjects Research Review Official (HSRRO). This Policy Order also establishes procedures and guidance for implementing regulatory requirements under **40 CFR 26** (EPA, 2016).

U.S. DEPARTMENT OF JUSTICE OFFICE OF JUSTICE PROGRAMS

The Office of Justice Programs (OJP), a component of the U.S. Department of Justice (DOJ), provides federal leadership, grants, training, technical assistance, and other resources to improve the nation's capacity to prevent and reduce crime, assist victims, and enhance the rule of law by strengthening the criminal and juvenile justice systems. OJP offices and bureaus include the: National Institute of Justice, Bureau of Justice Statistics, Bureau of Justice Assistance, Office of Juvenile Justice and Delinquency Prevention, Office for Victims of Crime, and Office of Sex Offender Sentencing, Monitoring, Apprehending, Registering, and Tracking.

OJP awards (grants, cooperative agreements, contracts, interagency agreements) that involve research with human subjects are subject to the DOJ regulations for human subject protections. Unlike the other agencies summarized in this chapter, DOJ has not signed on to the 2018 revisions of the Common Rule. DOJ does, however, follow the pre-2018 requirements as codified at **28 CFR Part 46** – Protection of Human Subjects. IRBs reviewing OJP-funded research projects must use **28 CFR Part 46** (pre-2018 Common Rule) and cite this specific regulation and its sections, as applicable, in their determination letters.

Cheryl Crawford Watson

Separate from **28 CFR Part 46**, and applicable only to research awards funded by OJP, are a confidentiality statute **[34 U.S.C. 10231(a)]** and confidentiality regulation **[28 CFR Part 22]**, which afford protections on the use of identifiable data collected using OJP funds. Identifiable data can only be used for research and statistical purposes. It cannot be used for other purposes without subject consent. By federal statute, identifiable data is immune from legal process, and cannot, without the consent of the person furnishing such information, be admitted as evidence or used for any purpose in any action, suit, or other judicial, legislative, or administrative proceedings. **28 CFR Part 22** requires the submission of a privacy certificate by OJP research awardees whenever personally identifiable information is collected as part of a research project. Once approved by the funding agency, the privacy certificate protects the data; there are statutory penalties for noncompliance.

Both regulations **[28 CFR Part 46**; **28 CFR Part 22]** follow the funding stream. If OJP research funds are transferred to another federal, state, or local agency; university; or professional organization; compliance with these regulations is required.

For more guidance and information on these regulations that apply to OJP-funded research involving human subjects and the collection of identifiable data, see https://nij.ojp.gov/funding/human-subjects-and-privacy-protection

Other Federal Agencies

Whereas this chapter contains detailed information in about DoD, VA, EPA, and OJP, there are also other non-DHHS federal agencies that fund and/or conduct human subjects research, such as the Department of Education, the Department of Energy, and the National Science Foundation. For further information about these programs, see the human subjects protection program websites for each of these agencies:

- Department of Education: www2.ed.gov/about/offices/list/ocfo/humansub.html
- Department of Energy: https://science.osti.gov/ber/human-subjects
- National Science Foundation: www.nsf.gov/bfa/dias/policy/human.jsp

Table 11.8-1 Federal Agency Considerations

Topic Area	Department of Defense	Department of Veterans Affairs	Environmental Protection Agency
Assurances	DoD issues DoD assurances and accepts Federalwide Assurance to DHHS. Federalwide assurances are required for DHHS-sponsored human subject research.	In addition to a Federalwide Assurance issued by OHRP, VA (ORO) issues a VA addendum based on internal agency requirements.	EPA accepts Federalwide Assurance to DHHS.
Research/clinical trials		Multisite trials are encouraged.	
Informed consent	In most cases, DoD requires that DoD is listed as an entity that could access research records. Broad consent is permitted in DoD-supported research. The use of broad consent in DoD-conducted research is pursuant to DOHRP guidance and with component notification to DOHRP director.	VA allows for waivers and alterations of informed consent in accordance with the common rule and FDA regulations. VA does not allow broad consent at this printing.	

(continues)

Table 11.8-1 Federal Agency Considerations   (*continued*)

Topic Area	Department of Defense	Department of Veterans Affairs	Environmental Protection Agency
Age of majority	Service academy students, service members, and all reserve component and National Guard members in a federal duty status are considered for purposes of research to be adults.	State law	EPA subparts define "child" as less than 18 years.
Legally authorized representatives (LARs)/capacity	Certain research must be intended to benefit subjects who are unable to provide their own consent **[10 U.S.C. 980]**; **10 U.S.C. 980** is scheduled to be changed in 2020.	In studies with LARs, a HIPAA authorization (separate from the consent form) must be signed by the personal representative (VA Form 10-0493)	
Mental health		No specific VA policy	
Children		Limited applicability to VA mission. No greater than minimal risk research involving children permitted in VA research. All children's research activities require additional approval by VA medical center director.	Intentional exposure studies are prohibited with children.
Pregnant women	DoD-supported research does not fall under subpart B for pregnant women, unless research is more than minimal risk and includes interventions or invasive procedures to the woman or the fetus. The phrase "biomedical knowledge" in **subpart B** of **45 CFR 46** is replaced with "generalizable knowledge" so that pregnant women are given the ability to decide to participate in research.	Additional approval by the CRADO* is required for interventional or invasive monitoring studies.	Intentional exposure studies are prohibited with pregnant or nursing women.
Fetuses or neonates of uncertain viability	Fetal research covered under sections 289g–289g-2 of Title 42, U.S.C., requires DoD component and DOHRP approval.	Limited applicability to VA mission	EPA regulations do not allow intentional exposure of pregnant women. By extension, this prohibition would also apply to fetuses.

Special populations	IRBs must assess risks of research participation to DoD personnel's ability to continue in their duty status.
	   Military and civilian supervisors, officers, and others in the chain of command are prohibited from influencing their subordinates' decision to join research.
	   Supervisors or those in the chain of command of DoD personnel must not be present at any recruitment sessions or during the consent process for DoD personnel.
	   Supervisors are separately approached about whether they would like to participate in the study.
		Trainees are considered a special population, and special considerations are given to ensure that no undue influence exists in their decisions to participate in research.	

Topic Area	Department of Defense	Department of Veterans Affairs	Environmental Protection Agency
	Compensation to DoD personnel for participation in research while on duty is prohibited with some exceptions.		
Wards		Limited applicability to VA mission	
Prisoners	Research involving a detainee as a human subject is prohibited unless research involves investigational new drug or investigational device provisions of **Title 21, CFR**, when the purpose is for diagnosis or treatment of a medical condition in a patient and only when the same product may be available to service members consistent with established medical practice. Actions authorizing or requiring any action by an official of DHHS about any requirements of subparts B–D shall be under the authority of the DOHRP.	CRADO approval is required.	
Embryonic/stem cell research	Fetal research covered under sections 289g–289g-2 of **Title 42, U.S.C.**, requires DoD component and DOHRP approval.	All research activities involving embryonic or stem cells require additional approved by VA medical center director. Use of human stem cells in VA research is governed by the policy set by NIH for recipients of NIH research funding. At this printing, VHA has a prohibition against human embryonic stem cell research.	
Gene transfer		No specific VA policy	
Fetal tissue research	Fetal research covered under sections 289g–289g-2 of **Title 42, U.S.C.**, requires DoD component and DOHRP approval.	At the release of this text, VHA has a prohibition against fetal tissue research.	
Radiation	See previous	Safety review	
Gene transfer/ genomics	DoD security reviews must be conducted before research involving large-scale genomic data collected from DoD personnel may begin, along with DOHRP approval.	No VA-specific policy	
Use of investigational drugs/devices/ supplements		VA follows FDA regulations but does not permit planned emergency research **[21 CFR 50.24]**.	

(continues)

Table 11.8-1 Federal Agency Considerations *(continued)*

Topic Area	Department of Defense	Department of Veterans Affairs	Environmental Protection Agency
Privacy/HIPAA	Applies Privacy Act of 1974 and E-Government Act of 2002 in addition to HIPAA	Applies Privacy Act of 1974 and E-Government Act of 2002 in addition to HIPAA. Additional privacy authority required to allow private individually identifiable information from human subjects to be disclosed outside of VA for research purposes; an IRB or privacy board–approved waiver of HIPAA authorization is not sufficient. Combined consent and HIPAA authorization is encouraged for most research.	
Communicable disease reporting		VA complies with local, state, and federal laws.	
Insurance/ payment requirements		VA is self-insured as a government agency.	
IRBs	Single IRBs encouraged	Single IRB encouraged when allowed by information security requirements; commercial IRBs currently prohibited by policy at this time; however, policy changes are anticipated to allow commercial IRB use.	
Other policies		When nonveterans are considered as a subject population for VA research studies, an additional approval by the R&DC* is required.	Pesticide studies require additional review by EPA Human Subjects Review Board.
Research-related injury (RRI)	Subjects injured in DoD-conducted research may obtain care for the injury at a DoD medical treatment facility on a space-available basis; the costs of care may be billed to the subjects' insurance company.	VA will pay for RRI for veterans enrolled in VA-conducted research that has been approved by an R&DC. Arrangements must be made for RRI care if nonveterans are enrolled.	Controlled exposure studies have a designated amount for medical care of injury.
Internal agency reviews	DoD supported, non-DoD institution–conducted research requires prior approval by human research protection official.	All studies require approval by the R&DC and a study initiation letter from the facility ACOS (R&D).* All research conducted by VA is subject to ORO oversight. Onsite research compliance officers oversee local research programs.	Human studies conducted or supported by EPA require approval by human subjects research review official, in addition to IRB.

*CRADO, chief research and development officer; R&DC, research and development committee; ACOS (R&D) assistant chief of staff (research and development).

Acknowledgment

Stephanie A. Bruce contributed to this chapter.

Resources

Department of Defense (DoD). (2011). *Protection of human subjects and adherence to ethical standards in DoD-supported research*. Department of Defense Instruction 3216.02. www.esd.whs.mil/Portals/54/Documents/DD/issuances/dodi/321602p.pdf

Department of Defense (DoD). (2019). Code of Federal Regulations 32 CFR Part 219 – Protection of human subjects. www.ecfr.gov/cgi-bin/text-idx?tpl=/ecfrbrowse/Title32/32cfr219_main_02.tpl

Department of Veterans Affairs (VA). (2018). *Consent for release of medical records*. www.federalregister.gov/documents/2018/01/19/2018-00758/consent-for-release-of-va-medical-records

Department of Veterans Affairs (VA). (2019a). Code of Federal Regulations 38 CFR 16 – Protection of human subjects. https://ecfr.io/Title-38/cfr16_main

Department of Veterans Affairs (VA). (2019b). *VHA Directive 1200.05 – Requirements for the protections of human subjects in research*. www.va.gov/vhapublications/ViewPublication.asp?pub_ID=8171

References

Annual VHA Site Classifications Summary. (2019). FY18Q4 Site Records Reclassified for October 1, 2018.

Environmental Protection Agency (EPA). (2013). Code of Federal Regulations 40 CFR Part 26 – Protection of human subjects. www.law.cornell.edu/cfr/text/40/part-26

Environmental Protection Agency (EPA). (2016). *Policy and procedures on protection of human subjects in EPA conducted or supported research* (Order 1000.17A). www.epa.gov/sites/production/files/2016-06/documents/2016_policy_order_revision_6-10-16.pdf

Menikoff, J. (2005). Of babies, bugs, and bombast: A look behind the crash-and-burn of the CHEERS pesticide study. *Medical Research Law and Policy Report, 4*(14), 586–590.

National Research Council. (2004). *Intentional human dosing studies for EPA regulatory purposes: Scientific and ethical issues*. National Academies Press.

Resnik, D. B. (2007). The new EPA regulations for protecting human subjects: Haste makes waste. *Hastings Center Report, 37*(1), 17–21.

Schonfeld, T., Gormley, M., & Nelson, D. K. (2017). Dollars and deadlines: Rule reforms in short time frames. *American Journal of Bioethics, 17*(7), 62–64.

Special Topics

Return of Results, Secondary Findings

Sara Chandros Hull

Laura Lyman Rodriguez

Abstract

This chapter will explore topics relevant to how IRBs should consider the return of individual research results to research subjects, particularly secondary findings that are not directly a target of the primary study. Because secondary genomic findings are a useful illustration of broadly applicable issues for IRBs to consider, and because genome sequence analysis is an increasingly common element in a broad range of research, genomic data are used as the framework for the chapter's discussion of challenges, needs, and principles to be deliberated in considering return of research results. The intent herein is to provide IRBs with a resource to support deliberations about returning secondary genomic and other research data, including emerging bioethical scholarship on the key issues and relevant regulations, guidance, and best practices.

Introduction

Questions about the return of individualized research-related findings require researchers to think beyond aggregate data summaries and traditional published reports of their research findings. To what extent are researchers obligated to return information that may be of value to individuals who participate in their studies? Such questions have been debated in the context of many types of data and study designs, but inconsistencies in the terminology used to describe the expansive range of potential research findings are confusing and have made it difficult for IRBs and researchers to develop consistent approaches. For example, the terms "incidental" and "secondary" are often used interchangeably in the literature and guidance. In 2013, the Presidential Commission for the Study of Bioethical Issues (PCSBI) established a detailed taxonomy of research findings that distinguishes between findings that are actively sought and those that are not, as well as those that can be anticipated and those that cannot (**Table 12.1-1**).

Table 12.1-1 PCSBI's Classification of Individualized Results of Medical Tests

Type of Result Discovered	Description	Example
Primary finding	Practitioner aims to discover A, and result is relevant to A	In a child with unknown vaccine history, a test done to determine a child's immunity status before the chickenpox vaccine is administered
Incidental finding: anticipatable	Practitioner aims to discover A but learns B, a result known to be associated with the test or procedure at the time it takes place	Discovering misattributed paternity when assessing a living kidney donor and potential recipient who believe they are biologically related
Incidental finding: unanticipatable	Practitioner aims to discover A but learns C, a result not known to be associated with the test or procedure at the time it takes place	When a direct-to-consumer (DTC) genetic testing company identifies a health risk based on a newly discovered genetic association not knowable at the time a previous sample was submitted
Secondary finding	Practitioner aims to discover A, and also actively seeks D per expert recommendation	The American College of Medical Genetics (ACMG) recommends that laboratories conducting large-scale genetic sequencing for any clinical purpose should look for variants underlying 24 phenotypic traits
Discovery finding	Practitioner aims to discover A through Z by employing a test or procedure designed to detect a broad array of results	A "wellness scan," a whole-body computed tomography (CT) scan, intended to discover any abnormal finding throughout the body

Gutman, A., Wagner, J. W., Allen, A. L., Arras, J., Atkinson, B. F., Farahany, N. A., Grady, C., Hauser, S. L., Kucherlapati, R. S., Michael, N. L., Sulmasy, D. P. (2013). Anticipate and communicate: Ethical management of incidental and secondary findings in the clinical, research and direct-to-consumer contexts. *Presidential Commission for the Study of Bioethical Issues*. https://bioethicsarchive.georgetown.edu/pcsbi/sites/default/files/FINALAnticipateCommunicate_PCSBI_0.pdf

These definitions helpfully inform deliberations about whether and how to return various kinds of results from research in a variety of distinct circumstances. Although medical test results in any category have the potential to be clinically useful, subjects may be more knowledgeable and have different expectations regarding "primary" results from research about a disease that runs in their family, for example, than they do about "incidental" or "secondary" results regarding unfamiliar medical conditions. A subject who enrolled in a longitudinal research protocol with hopes of learning more about their chronic disease is in a different situation from a healthy volunteer who is not expecting any personal health information to be discovered in the course of one-time research participation. PCSBI suggests that all categories of individualized health-related research results should be anticipated by IRBs and researchers and that subject expectations should be managed accordingly. However, incidental and secondary results that are outside of the research focus may raise additional challenges because of their ancillary and unrelated nature. Such results prompt the need for contingency plans that may fall outside of what a researcher is familiar with paying attention to, requiring specialized knowledge both to interpret data and to respond appropriately to findings that fall outside of the researcher's area of clinical expertise.

Following the lead of Darnell et al. (2016), who draw upon the PCSBI taxonomy, we will refer primarily to "secondary findings" in the rest of this chapter, defined as "findings that are anticipated and can be actively sought with a given procedure . . . but are not the primary target of the research evaluation" (Darnell et al., 2016). Secondary findings are salient to a broad range of data types (**Table 12.1-2**). However, given the current rapid evolution of genomic

Table 12.1-2 Common Examples of Secondary Research Findings

Type	Examples
Genetic/genomic	"Discovery of non-paternity determined by genetic testing of parents" (https://irb.research.chop.edu/incidental-findings).
	"[S]ome incidental [sic] findings [that] would likely have medical benefit for the patients and families of patients undergoing clinical sequencing" (Kalia et al., 2017) (e.g., hypertrophic cardiomyopathy, malignant hyperthermia susceptibility).
Imaging	"[O]ften arise when using imaging technologies, such as computed tomography (CT) scans, because a certain organ is the intended focus of the scan but other structures also appear in the field. A CT scan of the colon might show a mass on an adjacent kidney, for example." (Gutman et al., 2013).
	"[F]inding an indication of lung cancer in an X-ray done to look for tuberculosis for research exclusion criteria, finding a brain aneurysm during an MRI conducted for brain mapping purposes" (Department of Health and Human Services [DHHS, 2017a]).
Biomarkers/observational data	"[W]hen testing biological specimens for study purposes or while ascertaining a prospective participant's eligibility to enroll in a study ... [a] researcher could discover that a participant has elevated blood sugar, possibly indicating diabetes, or notice irregularly shaped red blood cells that could indicate sickle cell carrier status" (Gutman et al., 2013).
Behavioral/social	"Discovery that a subject may be suicidal from the results of a quality of life survey" (https://irb.research.chop.edu/incidental-findings).

technology and associated guidance on how to deploy the technology, we have selected genomic research as a secondary findings case study for this chapter. The state of genomic science illustrates the complexities that IRBs should consider in evolving fields where it can be difficult to parse which elements of a protocol represent research versus established clinical knowledge, a subtlety that is paramount for research subjects to understand. The capacities and scale of secondary genomic research findings prompt the need for urgent attention to consistent deliberative approaches, fair practices across different populations and contexts, and the development of centralized resources. Additionally, many principles relevant to the context of genomic study designs will be applicable to other types of clinically relevant research findings. It is important to note that it is not our intent to conflate the attention given herein with a presumption that genomic data are exceptional, deterministic, or (in general) more or less significant than other data types (Rodriguez & Galloway, 2017).

Return of Secondary Genomic Findings: Where We Are

Sophisticated and affordable genome sequencing tools are being utilized in research protocols with increasing frequency to help identify the genetic bases of human disease and behavior (Green et al., 2011). The deployment of these tools across biomedical and behavioral research is generating massive amounts of data about individual research subjects (both new and the assimilation of existing data) that go beyond the primary aims of the study. This reality prompts challenging questions about how best to manage the volume of information (Solomon et al., 2012). Do investigators have obligations to disclose unrelated genomic research findings to subjects? If so, what kinds of findings and under what circumstances? What obligations (or prohibitions) apply to family members who share a DNA connection to the subject? How should researchers manage subjects' expectations about such research-related findings? In the absence of clear regulations and professional guidance to address these questions, IRBs will be faced with deliberating about the best approaches in the context of the specific genomic research protocols they review.

There have been significant disagreements in the bioethics literature about the appropriate management of secondary genomic research findings, including over the basic question of whether results should routinely or rarely be disclosed (see Summer 2008 issue of the *Journal of Law, Medicine, and Ethics*). Emerging empirical research suggests that subjects generally wish to receive their individual results (Bollinger et al., 2012; Facio et al., 2013), and IRB chairs, members, and professionals also generally support return of at least some kinds of research results (Beskow & O'Rourke, 2015; Gliwa et al., 2016). Yet there appears to be a disconnect between practices and preferences among researchers themselves, with only a minority of researchers (40%) in one survey reporting they were either already returning a subset of secondary genomic findings or planning to do so in the future, whereas 95% agreed that secondary genomic findings ought to be returned to subjects (Klitzman et al., 2013).

Best practices in 2020 encourage the return of results that are "actionable," in that they provide potential benefits to the subjects, such as treatments or preventive measures for significant clinical conditions (Fabsitz et al., 2010; Jarvik et al., 2014; National Bioethics Advisory Commission, 1999). The American College of Medical Genetics and Genomics (ACMG) has argued that in the context of clinical care, there is an affirmative obligation to provide patients with genome sequencing results related to 59 specific genes that meet a carefully defined threshold of clinical significance (Kalia et al., 2017). This suggests the emergence of consensus regarding secondary genomic findings in the realm of clinical practice. Interpreting these recommendations in the research context remains challenging, however, and approaches to managing secondary genomic research findings are thus highly variable across institutions and studies (Gutman et al., 2013; Jarvik et al., 2014; Klitzman et al., 2013).

Researchers and IRBs continue to struggle with the appropriate management of secondary genomic findings for many reasons (see box, Challenges to Considering Return of Secondary Genomic Findings). The uncertainty and variation in practice within the research community are problematic for decision making at the level of institutions and IRBs. Operationally, it often falls to IRBs to make determinations about secondary research findings on a protocol-by-protocol basis, and some have suggested that the IRB is indeed the appropriate body to do so (Beskow & O'Rourke, 2015; Darnell et al., 2016).

CHALLENGES TO CONSIDERING RETURN OF SECONDARY GENOMIC FINDINGS

- Debate over the boundaries between clinical care and research
- If and how to solicit subject preferences
- How to assess risks and benefits of disclosure
- The need for subject education to understand the information
- Limited institutional resources and mechanisms to support identification and return of genomic results

A 2016 national survey of 796 IRB professionals found that most IRBs are actively dealing with secondary genomic research findings; three-quarters of respondents indicated some experience thinking through these issues but a lack of consensus about how to address them (Gliwa et al., 2016). Respondents in this study felt that researchers have some obligation to disclose findings to subjects: the majority (65%) indicated that there was "sometimes" an obligation to disclose findings, 13% "always," and another 13% "rarely". Only 2% believed there was never an obligation, and 7% did not know. For those who felt that there was some obligation, views about the ethical principles supporting that obligation were variable; the principles of "duty to warn" (84%), "respect for autonomy" (80%), and "beneficence" (79%) were most commonly cited by respondents (Gliwa et al., 2016).

These findings suggest that the lack of agreement among IRB professionals might stem from terminological confusion or the shifting of beliefs about the scope of an obligation to disclose secondary research findings according to the underlying ethical principle(s) put forward (Eckstein et al., 2014).

The purpose of the discussion that follows is to provide IRBs with a resource to support deliberations concerning secondary genomic research findings, a sense of the evolving bioethical scholarship, and information on emerging regulations, guidance, and best practices. As the costs to analyze secondary genetic variants continue to drop (Darnell et al., 2016) and empirical research demonstrates that the bioethics community's long-standing concerns about the psychosocial harms associated with genetic results have been largely "unfounded, exaggerated, or at least misdirected" (Parens & Appelbaum, 2019), we are shifting toward an emerging consensus that favors disclosure in many circumstances. Although decisions about management of secondary findings are ultimately the responsibility of research institutions (National Academies of Sciences, Engineering, and Medicine [NASEM], 2018), and institutions are starting to develop centralized policies and resources to support investigators, IRBs will continue to be tasked with assessing plans on a protocol-by-protocol basis (Darnell et al., 2016).

Glossary of Terms

Working definitions of terminology commonly used to describe the quality and usefulness of secondary genomic research findings can be found in the sidebar, Characteristics of Genetic Tests. These terms are relevant to both regulatory frameworks and policy decisions regarding what kinds of research results ought to be disclosed to participants.

Regulatory Framework

No regulations or laws directly address the return of secondary genomic research findings (Gutman et al., 2013), which leaves many decisions about how best to manage such findings to the discretion of research teams, institutions, and IRBs. However, IRBs should be aware of the federal regulations that touch upon relevant aspects of returning secondary findings, especially because many of them are also relevant to primary genomic findings.

CHARACTERISTICS OF GENETIC TESTS

- *Analytical validity*: Refers to how well the test predicts the presence or absence of a particular gene or genetic change. Can the test consistently and accurately detect whether a specific genetic variant is present or absent?
- *Clinical validity*: Refers to how well the genetic variant(s) being analyzed is related to the presence, absence, or risk of a specific disease. Has having a specific genetic variant been conclusively shown to increase the risk or likelihood of having a disease or eventually developing a disease?
- *Clinical utility (and/or actionability)*: Refers to whether the test can provide information about diagnosis, treatment, management, or prevention of a disease that will be helpful to patients and their providers. Will use of the test lead to improved health outcomes?
- *Personal utility*: Refers to test information that can reasonably be used for decisions, actions, or self-understanding that are personal in nature. It can be indirectly related to health and disease, but is distinguished from clinical utility because it does not affect clinical management or lead to improved health outcomes.

Excerpted from National Human Genome Research Institute (NHGRI). (2018). *Regulation of genetic tests*. www.genome.gov/about-genomics/policy-issues/Regulation-of-Genetic-Tests; Bunnik, E. M., Janssens, A. C. J., & Schermer, M. H. (2015). Personal utility in genomic testing: Is there such a thing? *Journal of Medical Ethics, 41*(4), 322–326.

The Common Rule makes explicit a requirement for consent forms to include a statement regarding whether, and the conditions under which, clinically relevant research findings will be disclosed to subjects [**45 CFR 46.116(c)(8)**]. This provision neither focuses exclusively on the genomic research context nor is prescriptive about whether there is an affirmative obligation by researchers to disclose such findings. The Common Rule requires IRBs to ensure that appropriate language has been included in consent forms to inform subjects either that they might receive secondary findings in the future or that they will not, but IRBs retain discretion to make tailored decisions on the appropriateness of the plan regarding management of research findings on a protocol-by-protocol basis.

⊘ 5-3

There are more explicit requirements regarding the handling of research findings connected to the Common Rule's <u>exempt</u> category for secondary research involving the use of identifiable private information or biospecimens. This provision, which must conform to the Common Rule requirements for

⊘ 6-9 ⊘ 5-6

<u>broad consent</u> and <u>limited IRB review</u>, requires that investigators *cannot* include the return of individual research findings to subjects in the study plan [**45 CFR 46.104(d)(8)(iv)**]. It is not yet clear how many research institutions and teams will adopt these broad consent and limited IRB review provisions that permit this exempt category to be considered.

⊘ 11-6

The <u>Health Insurance Portability and Accountability Act (HIPAA)</u> Privacy Rule grants individuals a right to access certain aspects of their medical information from covered entities upon request [**45 CFR 164.524**]. Similarly, the Privacy Act affords people the right to request personal data about themselves from federal government agencies, including their medical information (DHHS, 2020). Accordingly, subjects who are enrolled in research studies conducted at either HIPAA-covered entities or government research facilities may be able to receive their secondary genomic research findings irrespective of study design.

The Clinical Laboratory Improvement Act of 1988 (CLIA) establishes, among other things, quality standards for the analytic validity of laboratory testing involving human biological specimens and applies to research if individual-level information is to be reported (Medicare Learning Network, 2018). Because many research labs are not CLIA certified, this has the effect of limiting the research results that can be returned to a subject or to a healthcare provider for health-related uses, defined as ". . .providing information for the diagnosis, prevention, or treatment of any disease or impairment of, or the assessment of the health of, human beings" [**42 U.S.C. 263 a(a)**]. CLIA standards do not address clinical validity or clinical utility/actionability, nor do they address how results that are returned should be explained.

There is some disagreement between legal and ethical analyses of whether research findings generated in non–CLIA-certified laboratories could be returned to subjects. The U.S. Centers for Medicare and Medicaid Services (CMS) has stated clearly that the regulations apply to "laboratories that examine materials derived from the human body for the purpose of providing information for the diagnosis, prevention, or treatment of any disease or impairment of, or the assessment of the health of, human beings" (Medicare Learning Network, 2018). However, legal scholarship in the area has countered that releasing research results to subjects is protected under freedom of speech rights, so the issue remains controversial (Evans, 2014).

Interestingly, the CMS interpretation sets up the potential for HIPAA Privacy Act and CLIA requirements to come into conflict. Under HIPAA's right of access to health data, for example, laboratories within a covered entity that are not CLIA-certified must return identifiable test records if requested by the individual, whereas CMS holds that results must have been generated in a CLIA-certified lab. Although a joint revision to the CLIA and HIPAA regulations was issued in 2017, confusion remained for the community (DHHS, 2017b). Among the recommendations included in the National Academies of Sciences, Engineering, and Medicine's 2018 report on returning individual research results is a call for the development of a "quality management system" for research laboratories (NASEM, 2018). The recommendation's intent is to promote responsible return of individual-level research results and address the regulatory gap by creating an external process for assessing test quality and accuracy in non–CLIA-certified laboratories (NASEM, 2018). Given the regulatory uncertainty, many institutions and research programs that intend to include return of individual research results among their study designs opt to pursue CLIA certification. This involves significant cost and ongoing staff time commitments, so it may not be feasible for all research labs.

The Food and Drug Administration (FDA) also has relevant regulatory purview in genomics research when individual-level genomic research findings are returned to subjects, their providers, or placed in medical records. Although the agency has traditionally exercised enforcement discretion over laboratory-developed tests (LDTs) used for clinical purposes, this is not the case when this type of "medical device" (a category that includes next-generation genome sequencing protocols) is used in research (Donigan, 2017).[1] In those cases, FDA has indicated that such protocols fall under the <u>investigational device exemption (IDE)</u> procedures. Therefore, IRBs should follow their standard procedures to assess the need for, and any parameters appropriate to attach to, an IDE, which includes assessing the risk level (significant risk or nonsignificant risk) associated with the return of genome sequence findings and developing mitigation or reporting expectations where appropriate. As with any IDE consideration, FDA may be consulted for studies where there is not clarity about a risk level determination for a particular protocol. However, the mechanism and role for the IRB in making IDE risk determinations and for overseeing any IDEs issued is the same as in any other research area (e.g., clinical trials involving novel devices). For more information on IDE considerations in genomics research, the National Human Genome Research Institute (NHGRI) has provided points to consider regarding the IDE regulations (NHGRI, 2017). Additional resources on this topic are also available from a 2016 joint FDA-NHGRI workshop (NHGRI, 2016) as well as a policy session at the 2017 American Society of Human Genetics Meeting (Wagner, 2017).

🔗 11-3

IRBs also should consider if any state laws might bear on the return of research results at their institutions. At present, many states that do address the return of research results do so through stipulations regarding consent form content (Doerr et al., 2019). Some large NIH-funded research programs, such as H3Africa, the Undiagnosed Diseases Network, and the *All of Us* research program, have established policies for the return of secondary genomic research findings, and they may represent helpful models for other projects to consider (*All of Us*, 2018; Matimba et al., 2018; Undiagnosed Diseases Network, 2019).

---

1 Note that because Sanger DNA sequencing technology predates the 1976 Medical Device Amendments to the Food, Drug, and Cosmetic Act, FDA considers it to be a "medically established" test, and its use to generate, or in some cases confirm, DNA sequence-based research results may not require an IDE.

Legal scholars have suggested there is a small possibility that researchers could face legal liability under the law for failing to disclose secondary research findings, although no court has specifically addressed the issue of a researcher's legal obligation to do so (Clayton & McGuire, 2012; Pike et al., 2014). An analysis of medical malpractice cases involving "genomic medicine" claims brought through 2016 concluded that while there was a small increase in the frequency of cases brought each year, there did not appear to be a major trend growing in the area (Marchant & Lindor, 2018). Pike and colleagues argue that minimizing legal liability requires researchers, first, to choose from a morally justifiable set of options, avoiding the use of subjective terms such as "clinically relevant" that lack specificity and then to set reasonable expectations among research subjects about the findings that they should expect to receive via the consent process (Pike et al., 2014). Although these concerns regarding legal liability are not equivalent to an analysis of the ethical underpinnings of a researcher's obligations to research subjects, the ethical debate benefits from an awareness of the potential legal ramifications of different avenues of handling secondary genomic research findings. IRBs often find themselves in a position of balancing legally defined research requirements with the ethical goals that have inspired them. Working through an internally consistent and defensible approach to a given return of research results plan that is then transparently described to research subjects in the consent process may help reduce concerns about liability for failure to return results.

Determining What to Return

Given the vast quantities of personal information generated by genome sequencing, it would be impractical to return all possible research findings to subjects in a meaningful way. Most proposals suggest a threshold for identifying findings that are most likely to be beneficial to subjects. The ACMG policy statement on secondary findings represents an effort to reach consensus on genes with medically actionable variants based on current evidence. ACMG acknowledged that their recommended list, which is intended to be applied to clinical sequencing, is only a starting point that will require ongoing refinement based on emerging evidence. ACMG, together with the Association of Molecular Pathology, also published a scoring process for interpreting evidence to classify variant associations with diseases across five categories from "pathogenic" to "benign" (Richards et al., 2015). One study addressing uptake of this scoring system found that its adoption across the globe was high among those labs responding to a survey (Niehaus et al., 2019). Some research programs that investigate the frequency of secondary findings and outcomes associated with disclosing them have developed project-specific lists of variants for disclosure to research subjects (Ceyhan-Birsoy et al., 2019; Schwartz et al., 2018). It is also worth noting that although some research subjects are interested in receiving results that are of significant personal utility (Kohler et al., 2017), few have argued for a default obligation to do so in the research context (Evans, 2014).

Although the ACMG policy statement regarding clinical DNA sequencing could set the default for similar approaches to be followed in research scenarios, the organization has explicitly stated that they discourage application of their statement beyond the clinical context (ACMG Board of Directors, 2019). To date, research guidelines have tended be more circumspect about establishing an affirmative obligation to look for a predetermined list of findings (Gutman et al., 2013; Jarvik et al., 2014). However, as the use of genome sequencing in translational research contributes to the blurring of the line between research and clinical care, more recent research guidelines have followed the ACMG lead and point to an emerging need for a process to identify, validate, and communicate high-impact variants from genomics research with the potential to provide substantial clinical benefit for subjects (Darnell et al., 2016).

It should also be kept in mind that actionability depends on contextual factors that go beyond the characteristics of the genomic tests. Factors such as a subject's age (Ceyhan-Birsoy et al., 2019), prior diagnoses, and medical status may influence how useful a particular finding is to individual subjects. Some proposals have attempted to identify attributes of research protocols and study populations that could modify the obligation to disclose research findings to subjects (**Figure 12.1-1**). For example, a subject who is anonymous to a researcher and has never met them may have less of a claim to results than a subject in a longitudinal protocol who has had regular contact with a researcher. Furthermore, some have posited that there is a different expectation for reciprocity from subjects in longitudinal studies, and the return of research results has been put forward as one way to provide this (Precision Medicine Initiative Working Group, 2015).

The continuously evolving evidence base for genomic variant interpretation raises questions about the scope of researchers' responsibility to recontact individuals with any new information (Bombard et al., 2019). IRBs should work with investigators to ensure that their plan for managing secondary genomic research findings anticipates the length of their commitment to return results, as well as whether genomic research data will be reinterpreted and any updates conveyed over time.

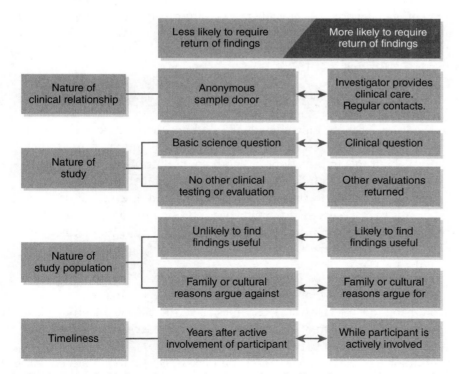

Figure 12.1-1 Guidelines for returning secondary findings in genomic research.

Reproduced from Darnell, A. J., Austin, H., Bluemke, D. A., Cannon, R. O., 3rd, Fischbeck, K., Gahl, W., Goldman, D., Grady, C., Greene, M. H., Holland, S. M., Hull, S. C., Porter, F. D., Resnik, D., Rubinstein, W. S., & Biesecker, L. G. (2016). A clinical service to support the return of secondary genomic findings in human research. *American Journal of Human Genetics, 98*(3), 435–441.

Consent and Managing Participant Expectations

There has been considerable experience with a range of approaches to informed consent for genomics research to date (Pereira et al., 2016). Although genetic literacy among potential research participants is an enduring challenge, a well-designed informed consent process can improve knowledge about both the benefits and limitations of genome sequencing (Kaphingst et al., 2012). Robust online resources with sample consent language and points to consider are available for IRBs (see NHGRI, 2019). In addition, there is a Common Rule requirement to post consent forms on a publicly available federal website, which will be informative about the range of consent language options that IRBs have considered [45 CFR 46.116(h)].

Various approaches to obtaining informed consent prospectively for the potential return of secondary genomic research findings have been proposed. Most have suggested that subjects be given the option to decide whether they wish to receive medically actionable findings (Jarvik, 2014; National Bioethics Advisory Commission, 1999), whereas others have recommended that willingness to receive such findings is a condition of study participation with limited opportunity to opt out (Appelbaum et al., 2014). This question of whether consent forms should give subjects the ability to choose (i.e., to opt in or out of receiving secondary findings) has occupied significant real estate in the bioethics literature. Would it be more appropriate for subjects simply to be informed that they will receive any clinically actionable findings within a defined range? Opt-in/opt-out preferences are typically recorded directly on the consent form via a checkbox or initials distinct from the signature page. Offering this choice reflects the long-standing presumption that subjects have a "right not to know" their genetic information, a notion that does not carry over to other categories of clinically relevant information routinely disclosed to patients and research participants. Critics of the "right not to know" (RNTK) argue that opting out of receiving clinically actionable results should be a rare occurrence (Berkman, 2016):

> For high impact genetic information, I think that it is a mistake to actively solicit preferences. We should inform patients that there is a default set of high impact incidental findings that will be sought and returned. In the rare case that someone independently requests to not learn about this information, in-depth counseling should be provided to ensure that they fully understand the choice being made, but ultimately the decision should be honored if not knowing consistently remains their clearly stated preference. For high impact genetic information, any deviation from regular disclosure should be a clearly defined exception, rather than the basis for a broadly applied conception of the RNTK.

In addition to these arguments, some data suggest that checkboxes can be confusing to subjects, who sometimes leave the choices blank or fill them out inconsistently, which makes tracking and future decision making based on those notations difficult to manage (Chen et al., 2005).

Additional research is needed on complex aspects of the informed consent process regarding the return of genomic research results. For example, managing subject expectations around negative findings and the "false negative" problem is a substantial issue. It is challenging to explain to subjects that the absence of a confirmed "positive" genome sequence result does not mean that no pathogenic variants are present (Sapp et al., 2018). Nor does it make clear that population-level risks remain relevant to them and standard health screening or preventive strategies should be followed. Therefore, consent forms should explain in advance what the absence of a finding does and does not mean, that the interpretation of test results may change over time ("negative for now"), and that especially if patients have a family history for disease, they should still follow the usual recommendations for clinical testing outside of the research setting (Darnell et al., 2016).

Widespread use of <u>previously collected biospecimens</u> in genomics research raises yet another set of challenging questions regarding the adequacy of prior consent. It can be difficult to interpret older consent forms that were written before best practices prompted researchers to address the return of research findings with subjects. Even more challenging are consent forms that stated explicitly that results will not be returned. When a researcher identifies a secondary finding that meets the threshold for return, but it is unclear whether the consent form adequately addressed the issue, they should consult with their IRBs to determine whether disclosure of the result is appropriate (Pereira et al., 2016). An IRB may determine that the previous consent was sufficient or that consent can be <u>waived</u> if they feel benefits of disclosing a research finding outweigh the potential risk to the autonomy of a subject who did not expect to receive such a result. When the consent form states clearly that results would not be returned, however, it may be difficult for an IRB to permit a researcher to make the disclosure (Wolf et al., 2012).

🔗 10-10, 12-3

🔗 6-4

Beyond the topics discussed in this chapter, there are several other important areas of developing practice and scholarship involving the return of secondary genomic research results. For further reading in these areas, see the Resources section.

Conclusion

In summary, the return of secondary genomic research findings is an area experiencing a rapid evolution in knowledge and community practices. The adoption of consistent oversight expectations in the form of regulations or policy, or even best practices and standards, that IRBs might rely upon has yet to happen, especially in the research context. This reality highlights the likelihood that IRBs and institutions will need to consider the appropriate framework for how to proceed on this topic on a case-by-case basis for now. However, NASEM's 2018 recommendations on returning individual research results call on stakeholders in the research enterprise (including researchers, IRBs, institutions, and research sponsors) to promote and support robust attention to the resources, process, and transparency with which any return of results plan is implemented (NASEM, 2018). Returning individual research results can be a beneficial element of a study's design, as it may demonstrate respect for subjects, inform a subject's future health choices, and contribute to the development of increased subject trust and engagement. For these possible outcomes to be realized, deliberate consideration of the complex issues discussed in this chapter must be undertaken up front and at relevant intervals in the course of the research.

Resources

Access of Individuals to Protected Health Information (45 CFR 164.524)

- Department of Health and Human Services. (2011). *Access of individuals to protected health information.* www.govinfo.gov/content/pkg/CFR-2011 -title45-vol1/pdf/CFR-2011-title45-vol1-sec164-524.pdf

Considerations in Pediatric Research

- Ceyan-Birsoy, O., Michini, K., Lego, M. S., Yu, T. W., Agrawal, P. B., Parad, R. B., Holm, I. A., McGuire, A., Green, R. C., Beggs, A. H., & Rehm, H. L. (2017). A curated gene list for reporting results of newborn genomic sequencing. *Genetics in Medicine, 19*(7), 809–818.
- McCullough, L. B., Brothers, K. B., Chung, W. K., Joffe, S., Koenig, B. A., Wilfond, B., & Yu, J. H. (2015). Clinical Sequencing Exploratory Research (CSER) Consortium Pediatrics Working Group: Professionally responsible disclosure of genomic sequencing results in pediatric practice. *Pediatrics, 136*(4), e974–e982.
- Wong, C. S., Kogon, A. J., Warady, B. A., Furth, S. L., Lantos, J. D., & Wilfond, B. S. (2019). Ethical and policy considerations for genomic testing in pediatric research: The path toward disclosing individual research results. *American Journal of Kidney Disease, 73*(6), 837–845.

International Context

- Sullivan, H. K., & Berkman, B. E. (2018). Incidental findings in low-resource settings. *Hastings Center Report, 48*(3), 20–28.
- Knoppers, B. M., Zawati, M. H., & Sénécal, K. (2015). Return of genetic testing results in the era of whole-genome sequencing. *National Review Genetics, 16*, 553–559.
- Thorogood, A., Dalpé, G., & Knoppers, B. M. (2019) Return of individual genomic research results: Are laws and policies keeping step? *European Journal of Human Genetics, 27*, 535–546.

Alternative Informed Consent Platforms for Enhancing Literacy

- Schmidlen, T., Schwartz, M., DiLoreto, K., Kirchner, H. L., & Sturm, A. C. (2019). Patient assessment of chatbots for the scalable delivery of genetic counseling. *Journal of Genetic Counseling, 28*(6), 1166–1177.
- Perrenoud, B., Velonaki, V. S., Bodenmann, P., & Ramelet, A. S. (2015). The effectiveness of health literacy interventions on the informed consent process of health care users: A systematic review protocol. *JBI Database of Systemic Reviews and Implementation Reports, 13*(100), 82–94.

References

ACMG Board of Directors. (2019). The use of ACMG secondary findings recommendations for general population screening: A policy statement of the American College of Medical Genetics and Genomics (ACMG). *Genetics in Medicine, 21*(7), 1467–1468.

All of Us Research Program. (2018). *Protocol v1 Summary.* https://allofus.nih.gov/sites/default /files/all_of_us_protocol_v1_summary.pdf

Appelbaum, P. S., Parens, E., Waldman, C. R., Klitzman, R., Fyer, A., Martinez, J., Price, W. N., 2nd, Chung, W. K. (2014). Models of consent to return of incidental findings in genomic research. *Hastings Center Report, 44*(4), 22–32.

Berkman, B. E. (2016). Refuting the right not to know. *Journal of Health Care Law and Policy, 19,* 1.

Beskow, L. M., & O'Rourke, P. P. (2015). Return of genetic research results to participants and families: IRB perspectives and roles. *Journal of Law, Medicine & Ethics, 43*(3), 502–513.

Bollinger, J. M., Scott, J., Dvoskin, R., & Kaufman, D. (2012). Public preferences regarding the return of individual genetic research results: Findings from a qualitative focus group study. *Genetics in Medicine, 14*(4), 451.

Bombard, Y., Brothers, K. B., Fitzgerald-Butt, S., Nanibaa'A, G., Jamal, L., James, C. A., Jarvik, G. P., McCormick, J. B., Nelson, T. N., Ormond, K. E., Rehm, H. L., Richer, J., Souzeau, E., Vassy, J. L., Wagner, J. K., & Levy, H. P. (2019). The responsibility to recontact research participants after reinterpretation of genetic and genomic research results. *American Journal of Human Genetics, 104*(4), 578–595.

Bunnik, E. M., Janssens, A. C. J., & Schermer, M. H. (2015). Personal utility in genomic testing: Is there such a thing? *Journal of Medical Ethics, 41*(4), 322–326.

Ceyhan-Birsoy, O., Murry, J. B., Machini, K., Lebo, M. S., Timothy, W. Y., Fayer, S., Genetti, C. A., Schwartz, T. S., Agrawal, P. B., Parad, R. B., Holm, I. A., McGuire, A. L., Green, R. C., Rehm, H. L., Beggs, A. H., & BabySeq Project Team. (2019). Interpretation of genomic sequencing results in healthy and ill newborns: Results from the BabySeq project. *American Journal of Human Genetics, 104*(1), 76–93.

Chen, D. T., Rosenstein, D. L., Muthappan, P., Hilsenbeck, S. G., Miller, F. G., Emanuel, E. J., & Wendler, D. (2005). Research with stored biological samples: What do research participants want? *Archives of Internal Medicine, 165*(6), 652–655.

Clayton, E. W., & McGuire, A. L. (2012). The legal risks of returning results of genomics research. *Genetics in Medicine,14*(4), 473.

Darnell, A. J., Austin, H., Bluemke, D. A., Cannon, R. O., 3rd, Fischbeck, K., Gahl, W., Goldman, D., Grady, C., Greene, M. H., Holland, S. M., Hull, S. C., Porter, F. D., Resnik, D., Rubinstein, W. S., & Biesecker, L. G. (2016). A clinical service to support the return of secondary genomic findings in human research. *American Journal of Human Genetics, 98*(3), 435–441.

Department of Health and Human Services (DHHS). (2017a). *Attachment F - Recommendations on reporting incidental findings. SACHRP recommendations approved May 26, 2017. Sharing study data and results: Return of incidental findings.* www.hhs.gov/ohrp/sachrp-committee/recommendations/attachment-f-august-2-2017/index.html

Department of Health and Human Services (DHHS). (2017b). *HHS strengthens patients' right to access lab test reports.* www.hhs.gov/hipaa/for-professionals/special-topics/clia/index.html

Department of Health and Human Services (DHHS). (2020). *The Privacy Act.* www.hhs.gov/foia/privacy/index.html

Doerr, M., Grayson, S., Suver, C., Wilbanks, J., & Wagner, J. (2019). Implementing a universal informed consent process for the All of Us Research Program. *Journal of the Pacific Symposium on Biocomputing, 24,* 427–438.

Donigan, K. (2017). *The intersection of genomics research and the IDE regulation.* www.ashg.org/wp-content/uploads/2020/06/Slides-2017-ASHG-Policy-Luncheon-Donigan.pdf

Eckstein, L., Garrett, J. R., & Berkman, B. E. (2014). A framework for analyzing the ethics of disclosing genetic research findings. *Journal of Law, Medicine & Ethics, 42*(2), 190–207.

Evans, B. J. (2014). The First Amendment right to speak about the human genome. *University of Pennsylvania Journal of Constitutional Law, 16*(3), 549–636.

Fabsitz, R. R., McGuire, A., Sharp, R. R., Puggal, M., Beskow, L. M., Biesecker, L. G., Bookman, E., Burke, W., Burchard, E. G., Church, G., Clayton, E. W., Eckfeldt, J. H., Fernandez, C. V., Fisher, R., Fullerton, S. M., Gabriel, S., Gachupin, F., James, C., Jarvik, G. P., … , Burke, G. L. (2010). Ethical and practical guidelines for reporting genetic research results to study participants: Updated guidelines from a National Heart, Lung, and Blood Institute working group. *Circulation: Cardiovascular Genetics, 3*(6), 574–580.

Facio, F. M., Eidem, H., Fisher, T., Brooks, S., Linn, A., Kaphingst, K. A., Biesecker, L. G., Biesecker, B. B. (2013). Intentions to receive individual results from whole-genome sequencing among participants in the ClinSeq study. *European Journal of Human Genetics, 21*(3), 261–265.

Gliwa, C., Yurkiewicz, I. R., Lehmann, L. S., Hull, S. C., Jones, N., & Berkman, B. E. (2016). Institutional review board perspectives on obligations to disclose genetic incidental findings to research participants. *Genetics in Medicine, 18*(7), 705.

Green, E. D., Guyer, M. S., & National Human Genome Research Institute. (2011). Charting a course for genomic medicine from base pairs to bedside. *Nature, 470*(7333), 204.

Gutman, A., Wagner, J. W., Allen, A. L., Arras, J., Atkinson, B. F., Farahany, N. A., Grady, C., Hauser, S. L., Kucherlapati, R. S., Michael, N. L., Sulmasy, D. P. (2013). Anticipate and communicate: Ethical management of incidental and secondary findings in the clinical, research and direct-to-consumer contexts. *Presidential Commission for the Study of Bioethical Issues.* https://bioethicsarchive.georgetown.edu/pcsbi/sites/default/files/FINALAnticipateCommunicate_PCSBI_0.pdf

Jarvik, G. P., Amendola, L. M., Berg, J. S., Brothers, K., Clayton, E. W., Chung, W., Evans, B. J., Evans, J. P., Fullerton, S. M., Gallego, C. J., Garrison, N. A., Gray, S. W., Holm, I. A., Kullo, I. J., Lehmann, L. S., McCarty, C., Prows, C. A., Rehm, H. L., Sharp, R. R., Salama, J., … , Burke, W. (2014). Return of genomic results to research participants: The floor, the ceiling, and the choices in between. *American Journal of Human Genetics, 94*(6), 818–826.

Kalia, S. S., Adelman, K., Bale, S. J., Chung, W. K., Eng, C., Evans, J. P., Herman, G. E., Hufnagel, S. B., Klein, T. E., Korf, B. R., McKelvey, K. D., Ormond, K. E., Richards, C. S., Vlangos, C. N., Watson, M., Martin, C. L., & Miller, D. T. (2017). Recommendations for reporting of secondary findings in clinical exome and genome sequencing, 2016 update (ACMG SF v2. 0), A policy statement of the American College of Medical Genetics and Genomics. *Genetics in Medicine, 19*(2), 249–255.

Kaphingst, K. A., Facio, F. M., Cheng, M. R., Brooks, S., Eidem, H., Linn, A., Biesecker, B. B., & Biesecker, L. G. (2012). Effects of informed consent for individual genome sequencing on relevant knowledge. *Clinical Genetics, 82*(5), 408–415.

Klitzman, R., Appelbaum, P. S., Fyer, A., Martinez, J., Buquez, B., Wynn, J., Waldman, C. R., Phelan, J., Parens, E., & Chung, W. K. (2013). Researchers' views on return of incidental genomic research results: Qualitative and quantitative findings. *Genetics in Medicine, 15*(11), 888–895.

Kohler, J. N., Turbitt, E., & Biesecker, B. B. (2017). Personal utility in genomic testing: a systematic literature review. *European Journal of Human Genetics, 25*(6), 662.

Marchant, G. E., & Lindor, R. A. (2018). Genomic malpractice: An emerging tide or gentle ripple? *Food and Drug Law Journal, 73*(1), 1.

Matimba, A., de Vries, J., Tindana, P., Littler, K., Madden, E., Nembaware, V., … , Marshall, P. (2018). *H3Africa Guideline for the return of individual genetic research findings.* https://h3africa .org/wp-content/uploads/2018/05/H3Africa%20Feedback%20of%20Individual%20Genetic %20Results%20Policy.pdf

Medicare Learning Network. (2018). *CLIA program and Medicare laboratory services.* www.cms .gov/Outreach-and-Education/Medicare-Learning-Network-MLN/MLNProducts/Downloads /CLIABrochure.pdf

National Academies of Sciences, Engineering, and Medicine (NASEM). (2018). *Returning individual research results to participants: Guidance for a new research paradigm.* The National Academies Press. www.nap.edu/catalog/25094/returning-individual-research-results-to-participants-guidance -for-a-new

National Bioethics Advisory Commission. (1999). *Research involving human biological materials: Ethical issues and policy guidance.* https://bioethicsarchive.georgetown.edu/nbac/hbm.pdf

National Human Genome Research Institute (NHGRI). (2016). *Investigational Device Exemptions (IDEs) and genomics workshop.* www.genome.gov/Multimedia/Slides/IDEWorkshop/IDE _Workshop_meeting_report.pdf

National Human Genome Research Institute (NHGRI). (2017). *Points to consider regarding the Food and Drug Administration's investigational device exemption regulations in the context of genomics research.* www.genome.gov/Pages/PolicyEthics/IDE/FDA_IDE_Points_to_Consider .pdf

National Human Genome Research Institute (NHGRI). (2018). *Regulation of genetic tests.* www .genome.gov/about-genomics/policy-issues/Regulation-of-Genetic-Tests

National Human Genome Research Institute (NHGRI). (2019). *The informed consent resource.* www.genome.gov/about-genomics/policy-issues/Informed-Consent#resource

Niehaus, A., Azzariti, D. R., Harrison, S. M., DiStefano, M. T., Hemphill, S. E., Senol-Cosar, O., & Rehm, H. L. (2019). A survey assessing adoption of the ACMG-AMP guidelines for interpreting sequence variants and identification of areas for continued improvement. *Genetics in Medicine, 21*(8),1699–1701.

Parens, E., & Appelbaum, P. S. (2019). On what we have learned and still need to learn about the psychosocial impacts of genetic testing. *Hastings Center Report, 49*, S2–S9.

Pereira, S., Robinson, J. O., & McGuire, A. L. (2016). Return of individual genomic research results: What do consent forms tell participants? *European Journal of Human Genetics, 24*(11), 1524.

Pike, E. R., Rothenberg, K. H., & Berkman, B. E. (2014). Finding fault? Exploring legal duties to return incidental findings in genomic research. *Georgetown Law Journal, 102*, 795.

Precision Medicine Initiative Working Group. (2015). *The Precision Medicine Initiative Cohort Program – Building a research foundation for 21st century medicine.* www.nih.gov/sites/default/files /research-training/initiatives/pmi/pmi-working-group-report-20150917-2.pdf

Richards, S., Aziz, N., Bale, S., Bick, D., Das, S., Gastier-Foster, J., Grody, W. W., Hegde, M., Lyon, E., Spector, E., Voelkerding, K., Rehm, H. L., & ACMG Laboratory Quality Assurance Committee. (2015). Standards and guidelines for the interpretation of sequence variants: A joint consensus recommendation of the American College of Medical Genetics and Genomics and the Association for Molecular Pathology. *Genetics in Medicine, 17*(5), 405–424.

Rodriguez, L. L., & Galloway, E. (2017). Bringing genomics to medicine: Ethical, policy, and social considerations. In *Genomic and precision medicine* (pp. 283–297). Elsevier.

Sapp, J. C., Johnston, J. J., Driscoll, K., Heidlebaugh, A. R., Sagardia, A. M., Dogbe, D. N., Umstead, K. L., Turbitt, E., Alevizos, I., Baron, J., Bönnemann, C., Brooks, B., Donkervoort, S., Jee, Y. H., Linehan, W. M., McMahon, F. J., Moss, J., Mullikin, J. C., Nielsen, D., Pelayo, E., . . . , Biesecker, L. G. (2018). Evaluation of recipients of positive and negative secondary findings evaluations in a hybrid CLIA-research sequencing pilot. *American Journal of Human Genetics, 103*(3), 358–366.

Schwartz, M. L., McCormick, C. Z., Lazzeri, A. L., D'Andra, M. L., Hallquist, M. L., Manickam, K., Buchanan, A. H., Rahm, A. K., Giovanni, M. A., Frisbie, L., Flansburg, C. N., Davis, F. D., Sturm, A. C., Nicastro, C., Lebo, M. S., Mason-Suares, H., Mahanta, L. M., Carey, D. J., Williams, J. L., Williams, M. S., . . . , Murray, M. F. (2018). A model for genome-first care: Returning secondary genomic findings to participants and their healthcare providers in a large research cohort. *American Journal of Human Genetics, 103*(3), 328–337.

Solomon, B. D., Hadley, D. W., Pineda-Alvarez, D. E., Kamat, A., Teer, J. K., Cherukuri, P. F., Hansen, N. F., Cruz, P., Young, A. C., Berkman, B. E., Chandrasekharappa, S. C., & Mullikin, J. C. (2012). Incidental medical information in whole-exome sequencing. *Pediatrics, 129*(6), e1605–e1611.

Undiagnosed Diseases Network. (2019). *Undiagnosed Diseases Network manual of operations.* https://undiagnosed.hms.harvard.edu/wp-content/uploads/2019/01/UDN-Manual-of-Operations_January-2019.pdf

Wagner, C., (2017). *What you need to know about FDA oversight of genomics research.* ASHG News, November 17. www.ashg.org/publications-news/ashg-news/fda-oversight-genomics-research/

Wolf, S. M., Crock, B. N., Van Ness, B., Lawrenz, F., Kahn, J. P., Beskow, L. M., Cho, M. K., Christman, M. F., Green, R. C., Hall, R., Illes, J., Keane, M., Knoppers, B. M., Koenig, B. A., Kohane, I. S., Leroy, B., Maschke, K. J., McGeveran, W., Ossorio, P., Parker, L. S., . . . , Wolf, W. A. (2012). Managing incidental findings and research results in genomic research involving biobanks and archived data sets. *Genetics in Medicine, 14*(4), 361.

Payment of Research Subjects

Joseph S. Brown

Emily A. Largent

Abstract

The purpose of this chapter is to address offers of payment made to subjects in exchange for their research participation. Although the practice of offering payment to subjects is common and generally acceptable, it remains contentious due to the general lack of regulatory guidance and ethical consensus regarding the practice. This chapter will briefly review the ethical arguments and extant empiric data pertaining to the practice of paying subjects, highlight relevant federal regulations and guidance documents, offer a framework for ethical payment, and address some challenges frequently encountered in practice.

Introduction

The practice of offering payment to research subjects is widespread and long-standing. Nevertheless, offers of payment made in exchange for research participation remain one of the more contentious ethical problems facing many IRBs (Largent et al., 2012). Although concerns over this practice have existed for many years, there is little regulatory guidance and limited ethical consensus to inform IRB policy. This chapter will briefly review the ethical arguments and extant empiric data pertaining to the practice of paying subjects, highlight relevant federal regulations and guidance documents, offer a framework for ethical payment, and address some challenges frequently encountered in practice.

Ethical Arguments

A number of ethical arguments are made about offers of payment to research subjects; four of the most common are considered here.

First, offers of payment to subjects have been described as coercive, unduly influential, or both, and therefore potentially problematic in terms of satisfying the ethical requirement for valid informed consent. The *Belmont Report* explains

🔗 1-1

that "[c]oercion occurs when an overt threat of harm is intentionally presented by one person to another in order to obtain compliance. Undue influence, by contrast, occurs through an offer of an excessive, unwarranted, inappropriate or improper reward or other overture in order to obtain compliance" (National Commission, 1979). Note the sharp conceptual distinction drawn between coercion and undue influence.

An open question in the ethics literature is whether genuine offers, rather than threats, can ever be coercive (McGregor, 2005). Macklin, for example, has explained that the "reason for holding that it is ethically inappropriate to pay patients to be research subjects is that [offers of payment are] likely to be coercive" (Macklin, 1981). Many ethicists have, however, reached a contrary conclusion and assert that genuine offers cannot be coercive. While threats reduce the choices available to an individual (e.g., "do this or be harmed"), genuine offers meaningfully expand an individual's choice set and, therefore, by definition do not coerce (Wertheimer & Miller, 2008). Wertheimer and Miller, champions of this view, are emphatic that the "claim that the offer of financial payments can actually constitute a coercive offer in a manner that undermines informed consent is both false and incoherent, because *genuine offers cannot coerce*" (Wertheimer & Miller, 2014). Following this line of thinking, concerns about offers of payment being "coercive" are misplaced.

COERCION VERSUS UNDUE INFLUENCE

- *Coercion* occurs when an overt threat of harm (e.g., of a violation of rights or a failure to satisfy an obligation to them) is intentionally presented by one person to a second person in order to obtain compliance, in situations where the second person has no reasonable alternative but to comply. For example, it would be coercive for a physician-investigator to condition continued medical treatment on an individual's participation in their research project.
- *Undue influence* occurs through an offer of excessive reward or other overture that results in bad judgment, specifically, a choice that is unreasonably against the offeree's self-defined values and interests. For example, if an investigator offers $10,000 to participate in a Phase 1 study of a novel therapeutic, some subjects may make an unreasonable decision to participate; if so, they are unduly influenced by the offer.

Of course, offers of payment may shape subjects' decision making. Indeed, they are typically offered for just that reason. It is, therefore, essential to differentiate an offer that is a *mere* influence—one that encourages offerees to do something that is reasonable but that they might otherwise choose not to do—from an *undue* influence—one that causes some offerees to participate in research that is unreasonably against their interests. Unlike undue influence, mere influence is not an ethical (or regulatory) concern.

Although it is conceptually straightforward to distinguish mere influence from undue influence, there is general agreement in the bioethics literature that determinations of undue influence are in practice difficult because they are highly contextual. For example, Emanuel and colleagues suggest that "local traditions and economic conditions will influence when financial payments may constitute undue inducements" (Emanuel et al., 2000). Wertheimer and Miller emphasize that the "distinction between an unproblematic . . . inducement and an undue inducement is not a feature of the inducement itself. It is a function of the relation between the inducement and the subject's response to it" (Wertheimer & Miller, 2014). And Grant and Sugarman have written that "[u]nder certain conditions, incentives are implicated in problems of manipulation in the form of undue influence" (Grant & Sugarman, 2004). Stated otherwise, there is no bright line that separates mere inducements from undue ones.

An ethical and practical concern, then, is how IRBs are to discharge their duty to minimize undue influence when it is so hard to identify undue influence in practice. Some have argued that concerns of undue inducement are heightened in studies with greater than minimal risk (Wong & Bernstein, 2011). The primary concern with undue influence is that subjects might be improperly persuaded to assume research-related risks; when risks are relatively low, concerns of undue influence may be mitigated. Others have argued that IRB review may reduce or even eliminate concerns about undue influence (Emanuel, 2005; Largent & Lynch, 2017a). IRB approval is, by regulation, conditioned on a threshold determination that a study has a favorable risk/benefit ratio, and IRBs are directed to make this assessment without weighing any proposed offer of payment to research subjects as a benefit. If an IRB determines that research participation is reasonable for the target study population (at any level of risk), then there should be little concern that an offer of payment will problematically cause subjects to do something *un*reasonable.

A second ethical argument is that it is desirable to recruit altruistically motivated individuals to participate in research studies, and offers of payment undermine this. Jansen observed, "Those who seek to justify clinical research often point to the possibility that participants . . . have altruistic motives for participating" (Jansen, 2009). A minority of commentators believe that altruism should be the *sole* motivation for research participation (Chambers, 2001). For them, this may be a threshold concern as to whether payment should be offered at all. Most commentators, however, have focused on the conditions under which offers of payment can be ethical, suggesting that research participation does not have to be exclusively or even primarily altruistically motivated. The ethical principle of autonomy might be invoked to allow an informed, reasoning person to decide for themselves what value they place on money and what risks they are willing to undertake in exchange for that value.

Another argument is that payment of research subjects may result in "unjust inducement"—that is, the disproportionate participation of economically disadvantaged individuals in research. If so, offers of payment in exchange for research participation would appear to contravene the principle of justice, which requires a fair distribution of the burdens of research. At the same time, however, there is concern that underpayment also might result in unfairness by inadequately remunerating subjects for their contributions to research. Moreover, in the absence of payment, some individuals may encounter financial barriers to participation in studies that offer a prospect of direct benefit (Largent & Lynch, 2018). For example, empirical research has found that lower-income patients are more likely than higher-income patients to worry about how to pay for participation in research and are less likely to participate in cancer clinical trials (Unger et al., 2013). Just as the burdens of research participation should be spread out, justice demands that the benefits be shared widely as well.

A fourth argument against paying research subjects is that payment dehumanizes the subject. It has been said, for example, that "[p]ayment to patients to serve as research subjects is an ethically unacceptable commodification of research practice" (Macklin, 1989). Wartofsky asserted that "payment for participation in research amounts to selling the services of one's body, often at some significant risk" (Wartofsky, 1976). Individuals concerned with commodification find it improper to offer money for certain goods or services, even if the validity of the consent is not in doubt. Again, this may be a threshold concern for some as to whether payment can be offered at all (Largent & Lynch, 2017b). In response, others have pointed out that payment for unskilled, physical labor is not fundamentally unethical: a person's services, capacities, and capabilities are commodities that are regularly exchanged for wages. It should, Lynch has suggested, be "no more worrisome to commodify a person's labor as a research subject than to commodify a person's labor in other contexts, which happens all the time" (Lynch, 2014).

Empirical Data

Data support the notion that payment is an important motivator for subjects, although it is not the only one (Stunkel & Grady, 2011). Increasing evidence also suggests that some individuals encounter significant financial barriers to participating in research and that offers of payment can facilitate their enrollment (Nipp et al., 2016; Unger et al., 2013).

Various studies have sought to understand the effect of payment on subjects' appreciation of research-related risks. Cryder and colleagues found that while higher offers of payment increased willingness to participate in research, these offers also increased perceived risk and the time spent reviewing information about research-related risks (Cryder et al., 2010). Similarly, Slomka and colleagues found that while individuals taking part in HIV prevention studies saw money as a necessary incentive to attract research subjects, some felt large financial incentives might raise subjects' awareness of risks when considering whether or not to participate (Slomka et al., 2007). Halpern and colleagues found no evidence that higher payments altered patients' comprehension of research-related risks, although higher payment increased willingness to participate in a hypothetical trial (Halpern et al., 2004). Bentley and Thacker (2004) determined that higher levels of payment increase willingness to participate but found no association between monetary payment and perceived risk. Finally, an online vignette-based survey revealed that while larger incentives induced greater overall participation, "respondents do not appear to exchange higher incentives for greater risks" (Singer & Couper, 2008). Although more data are needed, collectively these studies do not indicate that higher payment necessarily or even frequently leads to decreased understanding of the risks of research participation. Given subjects' often incomplete or inaccurate perception of risk, however, one might find greater willingness to participate as compensation increases to be a concern, even in the absence of a direct connection between compensation and risk perception.

Empirical evidence does suggest that higher payments may prompt research subjects to lie, deceive, or otherwise conceal information from researchers. For example, some individuals interviewed by Slomka and colleagues "believed that if a large amount of money was offered, individuals would be more likely to provide false information to investigators and 'say anything' to obtain the money" (Slomka et al., 2007). A 2004 study "showed that higher levels of monetary payment may influence subjects' behaviors regarding concealing information about restricted activities," which may in turn distort study results (Bentley & Thacker, 2004). A survey of individuals who had participated in at least two studies in the past year found high rates of self-reported deceptive behavior related to trial eligibility, with significant correlation between deception and monetary reward (Devine et al., 2013). Lynch and colleagues (2019) conducted a randomized survey experiment and found that offers of payment to participate in an online survey were associated with substantial deception by subjects about study eligibility, but higher payments were not associated with higher rates of deception. If it occurs, payment-induced deception—like all deception—may have serious consequences for subject safety and the validity of research results. These effects can often be minimized by using objective measures for eligibility screening and, when possible, relying on objective tests or other methods to reduce deception in the course of the study. Of course, many important measures are inherently subjective (e.g., depression screens, pain scales, etc.). In cases where reliance on subjective measures is unavoidable and concern about deception persists, researchers and IRBs might consider modifying payments.

Regulations and Guidelines

Neither the Common Rule [45 CFR 46] nor the Food and Drug Administration (FDA) [21 CFR 50, 56] regulations offer specific limitations on payment of research subjects. To a considerable extent, then, IRBs—crucial gatekeepers of the research enterprise—are left to their own devices to determine when payment in exchange for research participation is acceptable.

The Common Rule requires IRBs to ensure that researchers "shall seek [informed] consent only under circumstances that provide the prospective subject . . . sufficient opportunity to consider whether or not to participate and that minimize the possibility of coercion or undue influence" [45 CFR 46.116]. The regulations do not specifically address offers of payment. The Office for Human Research Protections (OHRP), the office within DHHS that provides clarification and guidance on ethical and regulatory issues in human subjects research, acknowledges that "[p]aying research subjects in exchange for their participation is a common and, in general, acceptable practice" (DHHS, 2019a). However, this OHRP guidance cautions that "difficult questions must be addressed by the IRB," such as how much payment subjects should receive and whether any aspect of the proposed payment will be an undue influence (DHHS, 2019a). Furthermore, OHRP notes the contextual nature of undue influence and warns that there is a "lack of clear-cut standards on the boundaries of inappropriate and appropriate forms of influence" (DHHS, 2019b).

FDA, like OHRP, describes payment as common and generally acceptable and also "recognizes that payment for participation may raise difficult questions that should be addressed by the IRB" (FDA, 2018). Among other things, FDA advises IRBs to "review both the amount of payment and the proposed method and timing of disbursement to assure that neither are coercive or present undue influence" (FDA, 2018). FDA further clarified that it "does not consider reimbursement for travel expenses to and from the clinical trial site and associated costs such as airfare, parking, and lodging to raise issues regarding undue influence" (FDA, 2018).

Importantly, both OHRP and FDA take the position—widespread in the research ethics community—that payment should not be considered a benefit that offsets study risks. Stated otherwise, payment can permissibly serve many functions (discussed later), but it cannot be viewed as a benefit when assessing whether the risks of participation are reasonable in comparison to the benefits or when deciding whether or not to approve research. If payment was viewed as a benefit, it could problematically allow even very risky research to proceed so long as the "price" was right.

Most international codes provide no firm guidance on payment to subjects. The International Council for Harmonisation (ICH) does not address the issue at all, and the 2013 revision of the World Medical Association Declaration of

Helsinki says only that "[t]he protocol should include information regarding . . . incentives for subjects" and be submitted for consideration and approval to an IRB (World Medical Association, 2018). Only the Council for International Organizations of Medical Sciences (CIOMS) in collaboration with the World Health Organization (WHO) provides more definitive guidance (CIOMS, 2016). Guideline 13 of the *International Ethical Guidelines for Health-Related Research Involving Humans*, "Reimbursement and Compensation for Research Participants," states that subjects

> should be reasonably reimbursed for costs directly incurred during the research, such as travel costs, and compensated reasonably for their inconvenience and time spent. Compensation can be monetary or non-monetary. . . . Compensation must not be so large as to induce potential participants to consent to participate in the research against their better judgment ("undue inducement"). A local research ethics committee must approve reimbursement and compensation for research participants. (CIOMS, 2016)

The commentary accompanying Guideline 13 asserts that subjects "should not have to pay for making a contribution to the social good of research" and therefore encourages reimbursement of expenses (CIOMS, 2016). It goes on to suggest that "[t]he amount of compensation should be proportional to the time spent for research purposes and for travel to the research site. This amount should be calculated using the minimum hourly wage in the region or country as a reference value" (CIOMS, 2016). The commentary argues that the obligation to reimburse and compensate subjects arises even when a study holds the potential of direct benefits for subjects.

A Framework for Ethical Payment

Gelinas and colleagues have advanced an ethical framework to assist investigators in designing and IRBs in evaluating offers of payment to research subjects. According to this framework, there are three primary functions of payment—to reimburse, to compensate, and to incentivize—each supported by distinct ethical underpinnings (Gelinas et al., 2018a). Categorizing payments according to the proposed categories can give both investigators and IRBs a better understanding of the rationale for the total amount of payment offered, thus easing evaluation.

PRIMARY FUNCTIONS OF PAYMENT

- Offers of *reimbursement* seek to restore subjects to their financial baseline by refunding reasonable out-of-pocket expenses incurred as a result of participation in research. For example, a subject might be reimbursed for the cost of taking a taxi to their study visit.
- Offers of *compensation* serve to acknowledge the time and effort subjects contribute to research, as well as the research-related burdens they agree to undertake. For example, a subject might be paid $15 for the hour it takes to complete a research interview.
- *Incentives* are offers of payment beyond what is needed either to reimburse or to compensate subjects. For example, a subject might be offered $100 as a completion bonus.

Reimbursement

Offers of reimbursement seek to restore subjects to their financial baseline by refunding reasonable out-of-pocket expenses incurred as a result of research participation—such as transportation, lodging, or childcare. As discussed previously, subjects ideally will not have to pay out-of-pocket to contribute to socially valuable research, even when their participation holds the prospect of direct medical benefit for them. Gelinas and colleagues suggest that reimbursement should be the default expectation, but allow that the default may be overridden by study-specific considerations, such as budget (Gelinas et al., 2018a). However, if investigators choose not to reimburse participants for research-related expenses, they should explain their reasoning to the IRB and also recognize that this will create financial barriers to participation for some individuals. Because reimbursement is not a net benefit to subjects, it does not raise concerns about undue influence.

Subjects may incur different out-of-pocket expenses and therefore need different amounts to be restored to their financial baseline. For example, subjects who live farther from the study site often have higher out-of-pocket expenses related to travel and lodging than those who live closer (Nipp et al., 2015). Differential payments to reimburse subjects who incur differential out-of-pocket costs raise few ethical concerns because they reflect an equality-based approach: everyone gets the particular costs they incur covered (Persad et al., 2019). As a result, many IRBs currently allow this type of differentiation for reasonable research-related expenses. However, fairness may also be satisfied by reimbursing all participants the same amount. For instance, researchers could offer a standard flat payment to offset subjects' out-of-pocket expenses for transportation to and from the study site.

Compensation

Offers of compensation serve to acknowledge the time and effort subjects contribute to research, as well as the research-related burdens they agree to undertake. When offered, compensation seeks to situate payment for research participation within the context of payment for similarly burdensome activities undertaken outside the research setting, such as work. Compensation rates should be the same for all subjects and reflect the general value of the time required to participate and the burdens assumed by subjects; compensation rates should not be based on subjects' earning potential outside of research. This is similar to Dickert and Grady's influential "wage-payment model," which is premised on the idea that participation in research is unskilled labor that requires little training and some risk and can be compensated with a fairly low standardized hourly wage (Dickert & Grady, 1999). Like reimbursement, offers of compensation should be the ethical default, as treating participants fairly and avoiding exploitation requires adequately recompensing them for their efforts, but there may be overriding considerations in a particular study. If a compensation rate is fair, it should not raise concerns about undue influence.

Differential compensation of subjects participating in the same study can be acceptable when some subjects commit more time or assume greater burdens than others (Koen et al., 2008). For example, some subjects may have more study visits or undergo more research-related interventions. Differential compensation is also appropriate when there are differences in fair local wages between study sites; in these circumstances, although payments differ in amount, they should not meaningfully differ in value (Persad et al., 2019).

Incentives

Incentives are offers of payment beyond what is needed either to reimburse or to compensate subjects. Incentives are the most controversial category of payments, but they should be understood to have an ethical dimension: Many studies do not meet recruitment targets and, as a result, are underpowered or terminate early (Gelinas et al., 2018a). Incentives aim to increase recruitment and retention by making research participation relatively more attractive to subjects and by increasing subjects' willingness to accept research uncertainty and reasonable research-related risks. They are one solution to the problem of unsuccessful trial accrual.

Nevertheless, incentives are discretionary and potentially problematic because they could introduce the possibility of undue influence. As we noted earlier, although subjects do not change (i.e., lower) their perception of the level of risk as inducements increase, their willingness to participate increases. This does not necessarily mean that incentives unduly influence participants; they may simply be a mere influence. We acknowledge, however, that it is possible that incentives might unduly influence participants in at least some circumstances. As noted previously, undue influence is highly contextual and can be difficult to assess, but IRBs can minimize the risk of undue influence by carefully weighing the risks and benefits of a study and ensuring that participation is reasonable for the target study population. In cases where the harms and burdens might be highly subjective or in which subjects might be particularly vulnerable, incentives might be limited or eliminated.

Timing of Payment

FDA clearly requires prorating payments based on the duration of subjects' participation in research. The FDA information sheet on subject payment states that "[a]ny credit for payment should accrue as the study progresses and not be contingent upon the subject completing the entire study" (FDA, 2018). Prorated payment should be made regardless of whether the subjects' withdrawal was voluntary or involuntary. Protocols submitted to the IRB should clearly define the scheme for payment of subjects who withdraw from a study, and this scheme should be described in the consent documents.

FDA does, however, allow for the use of "a small proportion [of payment] as an incentive for completion of the study" (FDA, 2018). A completion bonus is an incentive payment offered to research subjects on the condition that they remain in the study until they reach a prespecified study endpoint, such as completion of planned study therapy, progression of disease, or a toxicity event requiring removal from the study. At these endpoints, subjects' accumulated data is the most valuable to investigators.

Although the practical appeal of offering completion bonuses to subjects is clear, such bonuses remain ethically controversial due to concern that they may cause subjects to not exercise their right to withdraw from research. In order to assuage these concerns, it is appropriate to restrict the bonus amount so that, although it remains an incentive to reach a prespecified study endpoint, it is not so disproportionate to the amount of money a subject might make in the course of the study itself that it becomes likely to unduly influence their judgment (Largent & Lynch, 2019). Furthermore, the consent process should make clear the basic terms under which the completion bonus will become an entitlement and also differentiate reimbursement and compensation payments from completion bonuses so that subjects do not feel that they must continue participation or risk receiving no payment or less than the payment to which they are entitled.

Payment to Minors

The American Academy of Pediatrics (AAP) describes payment as "a common practice for research studies that involve both children and adults" (Shaddy & Denne, 2010). Consistent with this claim, Weise and colleagues (2002) found that the majority (66%) of IRBs allow payment of children who participate in research, although the specifics vary widely. Borzekowski and colleagues (2003) found that 55% of studies involving adolescent subjects offered payment in exchange for participation.

The ethical concerns raised when offering payment to human subjects are magnified when those subjects are minors. Children and adolescents may be prone to overvaluing a financial reward, depending on their age and maturity; at the same time, children and younger adolescents often have limited capability to understand the risks and burdens of research participation and, therefore, may be limited in their ability to make an adequate assessment of risks and benefits. If payment directly to the child is concerning, payment to a parent or guardian is also ethically problematic. In pediatric research, enrollment decisions are frequently made by adults on a child's behalf. Offers of payment in these contexts can raise concerns that the parent or guardian may benefit financially without having to directly assume the burdens and risks of participation and may make a decision inconsistent with the child's best interests.

Yet, if handled thoughtfully, payment to minors can be ethically justified. Wendler and colleagues (2002) have suggested that reimbursement can be directed to the parents, who may incur out-of-pocket expenses such as mileage and parking. Compensation can be directed to the minor, who bears research-related burdens. Even in this context, small incentive payments may be acceptable. The AAP notes, in fact, that "[i]ncentive payments may be essential to the recruitment and retention of pediatric study subjects" (Shaddy and Denne, 2010).

Parallel ethical concerns and strategies may be identified when payment is offered to a surrogate giving consent on behalf of an adult who lacks decision-making capacity, for example, as may occur in Alzheimer's disease research (Largent et al., 2018).

🔗 9-7

Payment in Kind

Ethical concerns may be heightened when offering payment to certain populations. As discussed earlier, children may overvalue money. Populations with substance use disorders may use payments to purchase alcohol or other substances (e.g., drugs), resulting in self-harm and investigator complicity (Festinger & Dugosh, 2012). Some have raised concerns that subjects of low socioeconomic status, including the homeless, may be particularly vulnerable because of their economic situation. For this reason, these populations are sometimes offered payments "in kind"—that is, an item of a value that is appropriate for the study but is not money.

🔗 9-8, 9-9

We find payment in kind to be ethically problematic (Schonfeld et al., 2003). One reason for this is that there is presently little evidence to support the necessity or utility of this approach (Anderson & McNair, 2018). Furthermore, despite attempts at equalization, a payment in kind is almost without exception of lesser value than cash payment. Constraints on the use of payments in kind paternalistically restrict the autonomy of subjects, as they should have the right to spend money earned through their participation in research as they see fit. Thus, offering payment in kind to some populations and not others seems inequitable.

Advertising Payment

Recruitment is considered the start of the informed consent process; thus, advertisements are subject to IRB review. OHRP and FDA briefly address the issue of disclosing information about payment in recruitment materials. FDA states, "Advertisements may state that subjects will be paid, but should not emphasize the payment or the amount to be paid, by such means as larger or bold type" (FDA, 1998). OHRP's guidance on the topic states that "IRBs . . . should carefully review the information to be disclosed to potential subjects to ensure that the [financial or nonfinancial] incentives and how they will be provided are clearly described" (DHHS, 2019b). Regulatory guidance is, therefore, best interpreted as permitting information about payment, including the payment amount offered, to be disclosed on recruitment materials (Gelinas et al., 2018b).

Wright and Robertson (2014) reviewed policies regarding advertising payment at 100 institutions and found significant variation in their content. Most implicitly or explicitly permitted disclosures of the amount of payment. A minority of institutions, however, discouraged or forbade such disclosures, whereas some encouraged or mandated them. The vagueness present in regulatory guidance likely explains the variability in polices at the IRB level.

IRB Responsibilities

It is essential that IRBs develop guidelines to judge the appropriateness of offers of payment made to research subjects. Few institutions have payment-specific policies, and there is significant variability in the quality and content of those policies that exist (Dickert et al., 2002). At a minimum, guidelines developed by IRBs should require that payment is not of a nature that interferes with the ability of potential subjects to give informed consent. Offers of reimbursement and compensation do not raise issues of undue influence. Incentives might, but IRBs can minimize this possibility by ensuring that participation is reasonable for the target study population without considering payment as a benefit to offset risks; in some situations, it may be desirable to limit or eliminate incentives. IRB guidelines should also stress the need for prorating reimbursement and compensation and defining the limited situations under which such proration is not needed. Additionally, guidelines should address issues related to offering completion bonuses, advertising payment, and remunerating minors.

References

Anderson, E., & McNair, L. (2018). Ethical issues in research involving participants with opioid use disorder. *Therapeutic Innovation and Regulatory Science, 52*(3), 280–284.

Bentley, J. P., & Thacker, P. G. (2004). The influence of risk and monetary payment on the research participation decision making process. *Journal of Medical Ethics, 30*(3), 293–298.

Borzekowski, D. L., Rickert, V. I., Ipp, L., & Fortenberry, J. D. (2003). At what price? The current state of subject payment in adolescent research. *Journal of Adolescent Health, 33*(5), 378–384.

Chambers, T. (2001). Participation as commodity, participation as gift. *American Journal of Bioethics, 1*(2), 48.

Council for International Organizations of Medical Sciences in collaboration with the World Health Organization (CIOMS). (2016). *International ethical guidelines for health-related research involving humans.* https://cioms.ch/wp-content/uploads/2017/01/WEB-CIOMS-EthicalGuidelines .pdf

Cryder, C. E., London, A. J., Volpp, K. G., & Loewenstein, G. (2010). Informative inducement: Study payment as a signal of risk. *Social Science and Medicine, 70*(3), 455–464.

Department of Health and Human Services (DHHS). (2019a). *Informed consent FAQs: When does compensating subjects undermine informed consent or parental permission?* www.hhs.gov/ohrp /regulations-and-policy/guidance/faq/informed-consent/index.html

Department of Health and Human Services (DHHS). (2019b). *Informed consent FAQs: What does it mean to minimize the possibility of coercion or undue influence?* www.hhs.gov/ohrp/regulations -and-policy/guidance/faq/informed-consent/index.html

Devine, E. G., Waters, M. E., Putnam, M., Surprise, C., O'Malley, K., Richambault, C., Fishman, R. L., Knapp, C. M., Patterson, E. H., Sarid-Segal, O., Streeter, C., Colanari, L., & Ciraulo, D. A. (2013). Concealment and fabrication by experienced research subjects. *Clinical Trials, 10*(6), 935–948.

Dickert, N., Emanuel, E., & Grady, C. (2002). Paying research subjects: An analysis of current policies. *Annals of Internal Medicine, 136*(5), 368–373.

Dickert, N., & Grady, C. (1999). What's the price of a research subject? Approaches to payment for research participation. *New England Journal of Medicine, 341*(3), 198–203.

Emanuel, E. J. (2005). Undue inducement: Nonsense on stilts? *American Journal of Bioethics, 5*(5), 9–13.

Emanuel, E. J., Wendler, D., & Grady, C. (2000). What makes clinical research ethical? *JAMA, 283*(20), 2701–2711.

Festinger, D. S., & Dugosh, K. L. (2012). Paying substance abusers in research studies: Where does the money go? *American Journal of Drug and Alcohol Abuse, 38*(1), 43–48.

Food and Drug Administration (FDA). (1998). *Information sheet: Recruiting study subjects.* www .fda.gov/regulatory-information/search-fda-guidance-documents/recruiting-study-subjects

Food and Drug Administration (FDA). (2018). *Information sheet: Payment and reimbursement to research subjects.* www.fda.gov/regulatory-information/search-fda-guidance-documents /payment-and-reimbursement-research-subjects

Gelinas, L., Largent, E. A., Cohen, I. G., Kornetsky, S., Bierer, B. E., & Fernandez Lynch, H. (2018a). A framework for ethical payment to research participants. *New England Journal of Medicine, 378*(8), 766–771.

Gelinas, L., Lynch, H. F., Largent, E. A., Shachar, C., Cohen, I. G., & Bierer, B. E. (2018b). Truth in advertising: Disclosure of participant payment in research recruitment materials. *Therapeutic Innovation and Regulatory Science, 52*(3), 268–274.

Grant, R. W., & Sugarman, J. (2004). Ethics in human subjects research: Do incentives matter? *Journal of Medicine and Philosophy, 29*(6), 717–738.

Halpern, S. D., Karlawish, J. H., Casarett, D., Berlin, J. A., & Asch, D. A. (2004). Empirical assessment of whether moderate payments are undue or unjust inducements for participation in clinical trials. *Archives of Internal Medicine, 164*(7), 801–803.

Jansen, L. A. (2009). The ethics of altruism in clinical research. *Hastings Center Report, 39*(4), 26–36.

Koen, J., Slack, C., Barsdorf, N., & Essack, Z. (2008). Payment of trial participants can be ethically sound: Moving past a flat rate. *South African Medical Journal, 98*(12), 926–929.

Largent, E. A., Grady, C., Miller, F. G., & Wertheimer, A. (2012). Money, coercion, and undue inducement: A survey of attitudes about payments to research participants. *IRB, 34*(1), 1.

Largent, E. A., Karlawish, J., & Grill, J. D. (2018). Study partners: Essential collaborators in discovering treatments for Alzheimer's disease. *Alzheimer's Research and Therapy, 10*(1), 101.

Largent, E. A., & Lynch, H. F. (2017a). Paying research participants: The outsized influence of "undue influence." *IRB, 39*(4), 1.

Largent, E. A., & Lynch, H. F. (2017b). Paying research participants: Regulatory uncertainty, conceptual confusion, and a path forward. *Yale Journal of Health Policy Law Ethics, 17*(1), 61–142.

Largent, E. A., & Lynch, H. F. (2018). Addressing financial barriers to enrollment in clinical trials. *JAMA Oncology, 4*(7), 913–914.

Largent, E. A., & Lynch, H. F. (2019). Making the case for completion bonuses in clinical trials. *Clinical Trials, 16*(2), 176–182.

Lynch, H. F. (2014). Human research subjects as human research workers. *Yale Journal of Health Policy Law Ethics, 14*, 122–193.

Lynch, H. F., Joffe, S., Thirumurthy, H., Xie, D., & Largent, E. A. (2019). Association between financial incentives and participant deception about study eligibility. *JAMA Network Open, 2*(1), e187355–e187355.

Macklin, R. (1981). "Due" and "undue" inducements: On paying money to research subjects. *IRB: Ethics and Human Research, 3*(5), 1–6.

Macklin, R. (1989). The paradoxical case of payment as benefit to research subjects. *IRB: Ethics and Human Research, 11*(6), 1–3.

McGregor, J. (2005). "Undue inducement" as coercive offers. *American Journal of Bioethics, 5*(5), 24–25.

National Commission for the Protection of Human Subjects of Biomedical and Behavioral Research. (1979). *The Belmont Report: Ethical principles and guidelines for the protection of human subjects in biomedical and behavioral research.* www.hhs.gov/ohrp/regulations-and-policy/belmont-report/index.html

Nipp, R. D., Lee, H., Powell, E., Birrer, N. E., Poles, E., Finkelstein, D., Winkfield, K., Percac-Lima, S., Chabner, B., & Moy, B. (2016). Financial burden of cancer clinical trial participation and the impact of a cancer care equity program. *Oncologist, 21*(4), 467–474.

Nipp, R. D., Powell, E., Chabner, B., & Moy, B. (2015). Recognizing the financial burden of cancer patients in clinical trials. *Oncologist, 20*(6), 572–575.

Persad, G., Lynch, H. F., & Largent, E. (2019). Differential payment to research participants in the same study: An ethical analysis. *Journal of Medical Ethics, 45*, 318–322.

Schonfeld, T. L., Brown, J. S., Weniger, M., & Gordon, B. (2003). Research involving the homeless: Arguments against payment-in-kind (PinK). *IRB: Ethics and Human Research, 25*(5), 17–20.

Shaddy, R. E., & Denne, S. C. (2010). Guidelines for the ethical conduct of studies to evaluate drugs in pediatric populations. *Pediatrics, 125*(4), 850–860.

Singer, E., & Couper, M. P. (2008). Do incentives exert undue influence on survey participation? Experimental evidence. *Journal of Empirical Research on Human Research Ethics, 3*(3), 49–56.

Slomka, J., McCurdy, S., Ratliff, E. A., Timpson, S., & Williams, M. L. (2007). Perceptions of financial payment for research participation among African-American drug users in HIV studies. *Journal of General Internal Medicine, 22*(10), 1403–1409.

Stunkel, L., & Grady, C. (2011). More than the money: A review of the literature examining healthy volunteer motivations. *Contemporary Clinical Trials, 32*(3), 342–352.

Unger, J. M., Hershman, D. L., Albain, K. S., Moinpour, C. M., Petersen, J. A., Burg, K., & Crowley, J. J. (2013). Patient income level and cancer clinical trial participation. *Journal of Clinical Oncology, 31*(5), 536.

Wartofsky, M. (1976). On doing it for money. In *Research involving prisoners: Report and recommendations.* National Commission for the Protection of Human Subjects of Biomedical and Behavioral Research.

Weise, K. L., Smith, M. L., Maschke, K. J., & Copeland, H. L. (2002). National practices regarding payment to research subjects for participating in pediatric research. *Pediatrics, 110*(3), 577–582.

Wendler, D., Rackoff, J. E., Emanuel, E. J., & Grady, C. (2002). The ethics of paying for children's participation in research. *Journal of Pediatrics, 141*(2), 166–171.

Wertheimer, A., & Miller, F. G. (2008). Payment for research participation: A coercive offer? *Journal of Medical Ethics, 34*(5), 389–392.

Wertheimer, A., & Miller, F. G. (2014). There are (STILL) no coercive offers. *Journal of Medical Ethics, 40*(9), 592–593.

Wong, J. C., & Bernstein, M. (2011). Payment of research subjects for more than minimal risk trials is unethical. *American Journal of the Medical Sciences, 342*(4), 294–296.

World Medical Association. (2018). *Declaration of Helsinki – Ethical principles for medical research involving human subjects.* www.wma.net/policies-post/wma-declaration-of-helsinki-ethical-principles-for-medical-research-involving-human-subjects/

Wright, M. S., & Robertson, C. T. (2014). Heterogeneity in IRB policies with regard to disclosures about payment for participation in recruitment materials. *Journal of Law, Medicine and Ethics, 42*(3), 375–382.

Data Repositories, Data Sharing, and Secondary Use

Aaron J. Goldenberg

Suzanne M. Rivera

Abstract

Human research using data can pose ethical challenges and may invoke a variety of regulatory restrictions in order to protect the rights and welfare of the people from whom the information under study was obtained. Repositories of data increasingly are used for research because they make possible the aggregation, storage, management, and sharing of information that can be used to answer both biomedical and social/behavioral research questions. This chapter examines numerous ethical and regulatory considerations regarding data repositories, including challenges associated with stewardship and sharing of data for secondary uses.

Introduction

Biomedical and behavioral research has evolved to increasingly utilize stored information found in healthcare and other research repositories that facilitate access to data from larger numbers of subjects while conserving resources and time. The kinds of information stored within these repositories can represent a wide and diverse set of data types, including genomic sequence data, information from electronic health records, environmental exposures data, and social or behavioral information from a variety of sources.

The organizations and institutions that maintain these data repositories are just as diverse, ranging from healthcare organizations and academic medical centers, to public health departments, free-standing research institutes, and federal agencies. Many healthcare organizations and academic medical centers maintain repositories of patient data, which can be used by researchers and, in many cases, may include access to complete electronic medical records. Frequently, state health departments or other public health agencies also collect personally identifiable information on a variety of health outcomes such as birth defects, infectious diseases, and cancer incidence (see box, Definition: Personally Identifiable Information). Although the primary purpose for such registries is health surveillance, some states allow these collections to be utilized for research under certain circumstances. For example, the Michigan Biotrust for Health, through the Michigan Neonatal Biobank (a statewide newborn screening biobank), allows researchers to link newborn screening blood spots to deidentified health outcome data contained in state public health registries (Michigan Neonatal Biobank, 2017).

DEFINITION : PERSONALLY IDENTIFIABLE INFORMATION

According to the Office of Management and Budget (OMB), *personally identifiable information* is "information that can be used to distinguish or trace an individual's identity, such as their name, social security number, biometric records, etc. alone, or when combined with other personal or identifying information that is linked or linkable to a specific individual, such as date and place of birth, mother's maiden name, etc." (Executive Office of the President, 2007).

⊘ 10-10   Although biobanks and other specimen repositories are utilized extensively for biomedical research purposes, there is an increasing interest in storing and using the data derived from biological specimens for secondary research purposes. This means the data generated from biospecimens can be shared, aggregated, and analyzed without the physical samples having to change hands or the research to be limited by a physical resource. This form

⊘ 10-13   of data sharing and aggregation is especially useful for genomic information, for which there is an increasing number of databases designed to store genetic variants or genomic sequence data and make them available for research purposes. For example, the Database of Genotypes and Phenotypes (dbGaP), maintained by the National Institutes of Health, "archives and distributes" sequence results from federally funded studies aimed at understanding the "interaction between genotype and phenotype in humans" (National Center for Biotechnology Information, n.d.).

The technologies used to maintain these kinds of data repositories also are evolving quickly. Many repositories are utilizing new bioinformatics techniques to secure and manage their data sets. Some also are starting to store genomic information and other kinds of data in cloud-based systems, which facilitate wider access and data sharing, while utilizing new approaches to maintaining data privacy.

The development, maintenance, and use of data repositories for research present a unique set of questions and challenges regarding ethical and regulatory requirements, including when and how informed consent and other human subjects protections may apply to collections of data that technically are not defined as human subjects. This chapter will outline many of the regulatory and ethical considerations for researchers and research institutions engaged in the creation, management, and use of data repositories. Each of the following sections will highlight key questions necessary for determining regulatory and ethical imperatives throughout the "life" of a data repository.

Development of a Data Repository: Decision Points for Regulatory Oversight

The regulatory requirements for research repositories and databases will depend on a number of crucial features related to the origin and purpose of the data to be collected, stored, and shared. The following points for consideration are meant to help make those determinations.

Purpose

Many health-related databases and registries are developed for purposes other than traditional clinical or public health research. Hospital systems frequently maintain a variety of databases related to patient care, billing, and quality assessment or quality improvement (QA/QI). Determining what kinds of activities constitute QA/QI as opposed to research can be challenging, and the current federal regulations at **45 CFR 46** do not provide comprehensive guidance for making those determinations. Additionally, public health institutions, such as state health departments, often have a number of health registries, such as a birth defects or cancer registry, for population health surveillance purposes.

Although databases and registries meant for QA/QI purposes typically are not governed as human subjects research from a regulatory perspective, questions remain about whether and how the data contained in these repositories may in the future be provided to researchers for secondary uses, and whether these collections may be linked with other sources of data to create a more robust collection for research purposes. This is important because the sources of the data may not have provided informed consent for research, so any research uses of the data represent a departure from the use intended at the time of collection. When no identifying information will be attached to the data, such secondary uses can be approved by IRBs with a <u>waiver</u> of consent under certain circumstances.   🔗 6-4

However, data held in repositories often are more valuable when they contain identifiers that permit aggregation with information from other data sources. Therefore, the provision allowing IRBs to waive informed consent for some kinds of secondary uses of deidentified data may not be viewed as especially helpful for most investigators. Although researchers should design studies in such a way as to collect only the minimum information necessary to achieve study goals, it is important that IRBs do not, even in subtle or inadvertent ways, pressure investigators to use deidentified data when an appropriate and rigorous study design requires access to personally identifying information.

Ultimately, research repositories that contain some personal identifiers and health outcome data may have more intrinsic value for translational research, while at the same time posing higher risks for research participants because of potential privacy breaches. IRBs should work with researchers to find the right balance, and ideally optimization, of both security measures and the research utility of their collected resources. Of course, when personally identifying information is distributed from such a repository for research purposes, the IRB will need to consider what information must be included in the informed consent document so that donors will understand all the future potential uses. This is complicated further when repositories are made up of samples and/or data collected without research consent altogether. A number of scenarios regarding the regulatory needs related to different types of repositories are reviewed next.

First, many research databases are developed as clinical or public health repositories but are subsequently or simultaneously open to researchers wishing to use the stored data. In these cases, the secondary research use of clinical data may have been built into the original design of the repository, in which case IRB oversight would have been needed before the establishment of the collection. Alternatively, there may be instances when an institution may wish to open an existing clinical registry for new research purposes, which would trigger new IRB review and oversight at the time of research intent. In cases where no research consent was obtained at the time of the creation of the repository, the burden would be on the investigators to justify not obtaining consent retrospectively, and they would have to request a waiver of consent to use these data for research purposes.

A second scenario is one that involves a collection of data for the purposes of a more traditional clinical study, but where the researchers also wish to store samples and data once the study concludes for future research possibilities. The secondary use of research data may be conducted by the original researchers who collected that data or may involve opening up access to other researchers either inside or outside their institution. Accordingly, the IRB would need to review the secondary use, because it would not be authorized by the approval given for the original clinical study.

Third, some registries are set up primarily for the purposes of future research studies. These prospective research collections typically are not associated with specific clinical or research questions in mind, but rather are created for the purpose of collecting and distributing research data for a variety of future research studies. Such repositories may be established with more narrow research goals, such as the promotion of studies associated with a particular disease or could represent the new federation of existing collections in order to centralize data from patients across a geographic region or health system. Again, the need for IRB review is triggered at the point of establishing an intention to use the data for research purposes.

The regulatory questions are less murky when a repository is created intentionally to collect, store, and distribute data for research purposes. In these cases, it is possible to collect informed consent from the providers of the data (or specimens from which data will be obtained), with the understanding that the information provided will be released to researchers for future unspeci-

6-9

fied studies. Federal regulations permit the use of a so-called broad consent for collection, storage, maintenance, and secondary research use of identifiable private information [45 CFR 46.111(a)(8)(iii)]. Researchers and institutions developing data repositories for research should work with their institution's IRBs on a case-by-case basis to understand what types of oversight, informed consent, and human subjects protections are necessary. At a minimum, an IRB will want to know (and will need to find) that, "when appropriate, there are adequate provisions to protect the privacy of subjects and to maintain the confidentiality of data" [45 CFR 46.111(a)(7)].

As we have established, determining the regulatory requirements for a database or data repository requires acknowledgment of the original purposes for which the collection was designed. In each of the three preceding scenarios, IRB oversight would be necessary. However, informed consent requirements, determinations regarding future use, and constraints on data sharing will vary depending on the origins of the collection.

Identifiability

Another important factor for determining the regulatory needs of a data repository is the degree to which the data stored within the collection are identifiable.

According to the federal regulations, "Identifiable private information is private information for which the identity of the subject is or may readily be ascertained by the investigator or associated with the information" [45 CFR 46.102(e)(5)].

On one end of the spectrum, some clinical and research registries contain personally identifiable data and private health information (PHI). This is crucial given that, for some research questions, the utility of a database is tied directly to the amount of identifiable information available to researchers, allowing for more connection to health outcome data, electronic health records, and possible future contact with subjects. Alternatively, some repositories collect only nonidentifiable health data with no possible connections to health records or PHI. Although the latter may have inherently lower risk of privacy breaches, these repositories have limited research uses. Increasingly, data repositories fall somewhere in the middle of the spectrum, where data is collected with PHI or other identifiable information but is stored either in a deidentified manner or is deidentified prior to access by researchers. In either case, data repositories can be seen as "honest brokers" or stewards who manage access to PHI and maintain privacy standards for their data (Anderson & Edwards, 2010). Nevertheless, there are concerns that, even if PHI is removed, data may be (or become) identifiable by connecting or cross checking data from multiple registries and other publicly available databases. The possibility of future attempts by bad actors to reidentify subjects without permission by combining deidentified data elements from different sources is a source of concern by privacy advocates and others; however, unauthorized and criminal behavior fall outside the purview of the IRB.

🔗 12-4

Additionally, there are growing concerns that genomic sequence data available through registries may make research subjects identifiable. This concern is grounded by the larger question of whether DNA itself might someday be used to identify individual research subjects and thus should be considered a personal identifier. The Common Rule does not define DNA as an identifier per se; however, the regulations require that federal Common Rule departments and agencies reexamine the definitions of what constitutes "identifiable private information" at regular intervals (DHHS, 2018).

Collecting Data for a Research Repository: Informed Consent

Required informed consent processes and necessary elements of informed consent for the collection and research use of data depend largely on the circumstances. For example, when private identifiable data are collected as part of a traditional clinical trial, the informed consent process for the study must include information about whether and how data and samples may be deidentified and whether "the information or biospecimens could be used for future research studies or distributed to another investigator for future research studies without additional informed consent from the subject or their legally authorized representative" [45 CFR 46.116(b)(9)(i)]. For prospective research repositories and, in some cases, registries created originally for nonresearch purposes, the Common Rule also outlines how broad consent may be used as an alternative to a more traditional informed consent process. Broad consent allows participants to consent to a wider range of unspecified future research; however, the informed consent document must include a number of specific elements including "a general description of the types of research that may be conducted with the identifiable private information or identifiable biospecimens" and

🔗 Section 6

🔗 6-9

"a description of the identifiable private information or identifiable biospecimens that might be used in research, whether sharing of identifiable private information or identifiable biospecimens might occur, and the types of institutions or researchers that might conduct research with the identifiable private information or identifiable biospecimens" [**45 CFR 46.116(d)(3)**]. Additionally, the broad consent process must include information on the length of time private information will be stored, a statement that subjects will not be informed about any specific details regarding any research studies their data is used for, and any plans for returning (or not returning) research results to subjects.

Maintaining Data in a Repository: IRB Considerations

In addition to the regulatory requirements regarding the creation of a research repository and the informed consent processes needed to collect or link data, registries also must develop data security procedures and governance structures for the management and maintenance of their data collections. For example, repositories must develop policies regarding privacy and security, standard operating procedures for the storage and use of data, and methods and procedures for data access and sharing. These procedures and approaches must incorporate and account for federal and state policies regarding data use, emergence of new technologies and research methods, challenges for bioinformatics and the management of "big data" collections, as well as evolving societal concerns about the storage and use of PHI. For example, governance models that rely on the geographic location of data are losing relevance as institutions increasingly are creating networks to link and share data across multiple registries and as digital storage and transfer become cheaper and easier.

📎 12-4

In order to meet their obligations to protect subjects' rights and welfare (including privacy and confidentiality considerations), IRBs must equip themselves with the expertise to review and oversee these plans and governance procedures. Although the regulations are not prescriptive about how to accomplish this, there are some obvious steps an IRB can take. One is to add as a voting member or nonvoting consultant someone with meaningful expertise in techniques for digital collection, storage, and transfer of digital information. That could be a staff person from a university or hospital information technology office. It could also be a nonaffiliated IRB member from a technology field. Such an expert would review proposed security procedures and could provide ongoing education of IRB members. Another step an IRB can take is to send a representative to (or review the minutes from) any community oversight board that may be established to oversee repository governance and operations. This can help to assure that the practices of the repository are consistent with the approved protocol. Finally, given that federal guidance for these kinds of oversight is underdeveloped, there is an opportunity for researchers themselves to work closely with their IRBs and other research infrastructures, such as Clinical and Translational Science Awards (CTSAs), at their institutions to collectively develop a set of internal standard operating procedures and best practices.

Sharing and Aggregation of Data for Research

It increasingly will be the case that solving large, complex problems in science requires large, complex sets of data, likely aggregated from more than one source. Put simply, big questions require big data sets to find answers. There are numerous obvious applications in medicine, where healthcare organizations using sophisticated analytical tools can aggregate a variety of data across a wide range of sources to support evidence-based diagnostic and treatment decisions (Raghupathi & Raghupathi, 2014). These sources can include traditional medical records and data derived from biological specimens as well as from diagnostic images, video, and sensor-based wireless devices for in-home monitoring of patients. There also are research applications of big data using personally identifiable information outside of the healthcare realm, such as consumer behavior information used in the academic discipline of economics.

As explained previously, processes for sharing and/or aggregating data from multiple sources can be very challenging, especially because the circumstances under which the data in question originally were collected vary greatly. Institutional policies regarding data ownership and the sharing for research purposes of personally identifying information can be dramatically different (Goldenberg et al., 2015). Some institutions with stewardship over data repositories may choose not to release data for secondary research uses without contacting the donors/sources to ask for study-specific informed consent or deidentifying the data prior to release. Some institutions may restrict outside access to researchers who have a formal relationship with colleagues at the data's "home" institution, such as coinvestigators, whereas others may restrict access to shared data for secondary use within their own institution or health system, limiting all outside access.

In almost all cases of multi-institutional data sharing, negotiation of data use agreements (DUAs) will be necessary, requiring the involvement of legal counsel and introducing the possibility of significant delays. These agreements govern the mechanisms for transfer of data, the conditions under which they can be used, whether they may be re-shared with a third party, and to what extent there may be plans for revenue sharing among the parties if the data uses should result in a commercializable product. It frequently falls to the IRB to ask the investigator to seek a DUA from the relevant authority at their institution, and in some cases the IRB may withhold approval pending execution of the DUA.

Privacy and Confidentiality Considerations

Although the need to consider practical measures for protecting the privacy and confidentiality of study subjects by securing their data was mentioned previously, this section provides a deeper discussion of the ethical dimensions of informational risks as they relate to human research. As early as the first publication of the World Health Organization's Declaration of Helsinki in 1964, it was acknowledged that researchers have a duty to protect the privacy and dignity of research subjects. The framers likely were thinking about potential privacy violations as collateral risks in the context of biomedical studies, where the primary concern would be the possibility of physical harm. However, in some kinds of human research, the only risks to subjects are informational, meaning that the primary concern is whether association of subjects with identifiable information could place them in jeopardy of criminal or civil penalties, deportation, loss of health insurance, social stigma, or some other penalty. In recognition of the changing nature of research and the risks associated with the collection and use of health data, the Declaration of Helsinki has been amended to explicitly include language on the importance of obtaining consent, when

🔗 1-2

possible, for the use of identifiable health data (World Medical Association, 2018).

Where these risks are obvious, researchers and IRBs already have mechanisms for considering both the likelihood and the magnitude of material and dignitary harms (see sidebar, Material and Dignitary Harms). However, new technologies are challenging traditional notions about both what is private and what is personally identifiable. Take, for example, the phenomenon called "digital phenotyping," in which information from our digital behaviors that is collected from online posts, mobile phones, fitness trackers, and other means are aggregated and analyzed in order to gain insight into potential health issues (Warzel, 2019). These data typically are not subject to <u>Health Insurance Portability and Accountability Act (HIPAA)</u> protections, and IRBs are not accustomed to thinking about this kind of information as potentially risky. Add to this the proliferation and evolution of technologies like cloud-based storage and the Internet of Things, and we find ourselves in ethically challenging waters.

⌚ 11-6

It will be critical for IRBs to avail themselves of IT expertise in order to understand the challenges associated with securing data generated and stored in new technologies such as mobile devices and cloud-based storage services and to assess accurately the likelihood and magnitude of informational risks posed by the use of personally identifiable data for research. Because research subjects do not always know when their data are used in research, it is imperative that the regulatory system for protecting subjects' rights and welfare can adapt to the evolving technology landscape for sharing and storing research data.

MATERIAL AND DIGNITARY HARMS

Material harms are the kind that result in objectively measurable negative outcomes like physical injury, loss of job, or deportation.

Dignitary harms result in the tarnishing of reputation or negative feelings such as humiliation and shame.

Research Exceptionalism and Uses of Data Outside the Research Setting

It is worth noting that the federal requirements for protecting personally identifiable data in a research context are more rigorous than the privacy protections routinely encountered in everyday life, such as when using social media, discount shopper cards, mobile apps, and so-called wearables. The ethical issues raised by research using mobile devices and apps are covered in detail in Chapter 12-5. This section will explore the phenomenon of research exceptionalism (Wilson & Hunter, 2010) and how it contributes to confusion about what kinds of data can be used for studies without the explicit permission of the source.

Users of technology have become accustomed to their personal information being collected in exchange for a perceived benefit. For example, users of the search engine Google understand that, to optimize future searches, information about past searches is captured, saved, and analyzed, thus delivering more accurate results to the user. Google also analyzes data from large numbers of searchers to predict flu outbreaks. Although there is a social good in assisting with health surveillance, Google does not explicitly ask for permission to analyze search terms every time a user looks for local pharmacy hours or prices for cold remedies.

Another example is law enforcement. Police can now solve "cold cases" with information collected from consumer DNA tests such as 23 and Me (Guerrini, 2018). In addition, the city of New York maintains a DNA "databank," known as the Local DNA Index System, which contains information about almost 100,000 people, including both those convicted of crimes and people who are only arrested or questioned. This databank has been used by the Brooklyn district attorney's office to solve hundreds of cases (Ransom & Southall, 2019).

Fiske and Houser stated that, "One might well wonder why academic research is more subject to ethical review than that of business enterprises" (Fiske & Houser, 2014). Indeed, unless an activity meets the federal definition of research and is performed at an institution that receives federal funding or otherwise invokes FDA oversight, the regulations governing protection of subjects' rights and welfare simply do not apply (Rothstein, 2015). Ethical paradigms for oversight of human research and the regulations that followed were developed in response to historical abuses and have been promulgated in the context of federal support for research studies. In this regard, the collection and use of data for academic research are treated exceptionally.

Conclusion

Increasingly, researchers are looking toward the use of existing data sets (including data derived from existing biospecimens) to perform research. This is especially true for translational research meant to promote large population-based studies aimed at precision medicine or public health goals. Accordingly, data repositories will continue to grow both in number and size in the coming years, including both registries created expressly for the purpose of research and repositories that aggregate information derived from other, nonresearch sources. Our regulatory apparatus will need to be nimble enough to address the varying needs of these different kinds of registries and protect research subjects' rights and welfare, while accounting for advances in technology, such as AI, cloud computing, and big data analytics. The slow pace of regulatory reform will hinder important advances in science if the ethical, legal, and social concerns raised by using private identifiable data to solve important problems are not addressed. Accordingly, IRB members and staff need to be thoughtful and creative about how to review and oversee protocols for which there may not always be explicit regulatory guidance. This may require expanding IRB membership to acquire specific technical expertise, exercising the existing flexibility to seek consultation from people outside of the board, and increasing opportunities to work collectively with researchers to develop institutional policies and procedures for the creation and maintenance of registries.

References

Anderson, N., & Edwards, K. (2010). Building a chain of trust: Using policy and practice to enhance trustworthy clinical data discovery and sharing. In *ACM International Conference Proceeding Series* (pp. 15–20). ACM International. https://doi.org/10.1145/1920320.1920323.

Department of Health and Human Services (DHHS). (2018). *Revised common rule Q&As.* www.hhs.gov/ohrp/education-and-outreach/revised-common-rule/revised-common-rule-q-and-a/index.html

Executive Office of the President. (2007). *Office of Management and Budget, memorandum for the heads of executive departments and agencies.* www.whitehouse.gov/sites/whitehouse.gov/files/omb/memoranda/2007/m07-16.pdf

Fiske, S. T., & Hauser, R. M. (2014). Protecting human research participants. *Proceedings of the National Academy of Sciences, 111*(38), 13675–13676.

Goldenberg, A. J., Maschke, K. J., Joffe, S., Botkin, J. R., Rothwell, E., Murray, T. H., & Rivera, S. M. (2015). IRB practices and policies regarding the secondary research use of biospecimens. *BMC Medical Ethics, 16*(1), 32.

Guerrini, C. J., Robinson, J. O., Petersen, D., & McGuire, A. L. (2018). Should police have access to genetic genealogy databases? Capturing the Golden State Killer and other criminals using a controversial new forensic technique. *PLoS Biology, 16*(10), e2006906.

Michigan Neonatal Biobank. (2017). *Providing blood specimens to researchers across the world: Our specimens.* https://mnb.wayne.edu/

National Center for Biotechnology Information. (n.d.). *dbGaP.* www.ncbi.nlm.nih.gov/gap/

Raghupathi, W., & Raghupathi, V. (2014). Big data analytics in healthcare: Promise and potential. *Health Information Science and Systems, 2*(1), 3.

Ransom, J., & Southall, A. (2019, August 15). N.Y.P.D. detectives gave a boy, 12, a soda. He landed in a DNA database. *The New York Times.* www.nytimes.com/2019/08/15/nyregion/nypd-dna-database.html

Rothstein, M. A. (2015). Ethical issues in big data health research: Currents in contemporary bioethics. *Journal of Law, Medicine & Ethics, 43*(2), 425–429.

Warzel, C. (2019, August 13). The Privacy Project: The health data you didn't know you were sharing. *The New York Times.* https://static.nytimes.com/email-content/PRIV_16123.html

Wilson, J., & Hunter, D. (2010). Research exceptionalism. *American Journal of Bioethics, 10*(8), 45–54.

World Medical Association. (2018). *Declaration of Helsinki – Ethical principles for medical research involving human subjects.* www.wma.net/policies-post/wma-declaration-of-helsinki-ethical-principles-for-medical-research-involving-human-subjects/

Big Data Research

Laura Odwazny

Abstract

This chapter examines the regulatory and ethical issues related to human subjects research involving "big data," including informed consent, risks to subjects and others, identifiability, privacy and confidentiality, and data security protections. This information will assist IRBs in identifying considerations specific to reviewing and approving big data research in compliance with U.S. federal regulations and strategies for applying appropriate ethical protections to subjects and others.

Research Involving Big Data: An Overview

Big data has been a part of the research landscape for some time now, and although many of the regulatory and ethical issues presented by big data research are not unique, the exponential increase in the volume, use, and potential for such data highlights the importance of providing appropriate protections to the human beings to whom the data pertains (Buchanan, 2016). The term "big data" generally refers to a data set that includes an extremely large volume of information that may be highly varied in type, structure, and complexity and may be transmitted at a fast rate (Laney, 2001).

These big data sets are derived from many sources, and analysis may require nontraditional technological and software techniques. An IRB may be asked to review big data research protocols that collect and combine data from a variety of both traditional and nontraditional sources for research information. This might include existing databases of stored information, such as medical records; state databases of aggregated health claims information, credit card charges, or other information; and information obtained in near real time from user-generated input on social media feeds, clicks on a webpage, or collected through a mobile app that tracks user action or sensor-enabled <u>wearable devices</u>. This data may be directly or indirectly generated by the user or collected and compiled by an algorithm. The data may be intrinsically sensitive,

📎 12-4

such as health information that an individual would wish to be kept confidential, or sensitive only in context or when combined with other data points or sets. Big data often is not identifiable to the living individuals to whom it pertains but may have the potential to become identifiable through matching techniques or technological manipulation.

A 2018 survey of IRB members showed that 47% of the respondents' IRBs reviewed between 1 and 10 big data research protocols annually, 17% reviewed between 20 and 50 protocols, and 34% reviewed more than 50 protocols (Zimmer, 2019). Given this trend, IRBs increasingly will need expertise in both the technical aspects of the conduct of big data research and the regulatory and ethical aspects of the collection, storage, and use of big data for research purposes.

U.S. Federal Regulatory Requirements

Big data research may be subject to U.S. federal regulations, including the Common Rule, Food and Drug Administration (FDA) regulations, and the Health Insurance Portability and Accountability Act (HIPAA) Privacy Rule.

Common Rule

Big data research does not always fit neatly in the Common Rule paradigm; for example, much big data research using data sets that were collected for purposes other than the current research may not be considered to involve "human subjects" if the data is not both individually identifiable and private. If big data research is reviewed under the Common Rule requirements, the reviewing IRB may have difficulty determining that risks to subjects are minimized, given the possibility that information that would not be considered sensitive or identifiable in and of itself may transform into individually identifiable private information through a combination of multiple data sets and by correlating characteristics that may uniquely identify an individual (Odwazny, 2018). This has been shown in many well-publicized "proof of concept" demonstrations in which researchers were able to link supposedly anonymized or deidentified information to an individual, through combination with other data or through technological manipulation. For example, in one recent such demonstration, researchers applied an algorithm to 120,000 anonymized public records and discerned linkages that allowed the researchers to identify participants in confidential legal cases (Chandler, 2019).

How should an IRB consider the possibility of reidentification of the data used in big data research? The uncertain nature of the probability and magnitude of the risks of big data research may inhibit IRBs in concluding that such research presents no more than minimal risk to subjects. The traditional mechanisms used by researchers for protecting subjects, such as obtaining informed consent or deidentifying research information, are not able to completely protect subjects from the informational risks related to big data analytic techniques. Furthermore, if the reviewing IRB does not determine that the research presents ⏺ 6-4 no more than minimal risk to subjects, the Common Rule's general <u>waiver</u> of informed consent cannot apply to the research, and often, big data research cannot feasibly be conducted if informed consent must be obtained (Odwazny, 2018). That said, it is increasingly common for IRBs to be asked to review and approve big data research in accordance with the Common Rule requirements. The following are the most relevant Common Rule requirements as applied to big data research.

Research

The vast majority of big data projects likely will meet the Common Rule definition of "research," as big data analytics by their nature will ordinarily constitute a systematic investigation that is designed to develop or contribute to generalizable knowledge [45 CFR 46.102(l)]. However, the Common Rule excludes certain activities from the definition of research, so if the big data project would qualify for one of these exclusions, the activity need not follow the Common Rule's requirements. In particular, the exception for certain public health surveillance activities that are "conducted, supported, requested, ordered, required, or authorized by a public health authority" and "limited to those necessary to allow a public health authority to identify, monitor, assess, or investigate potential public health signals, onsets of disease outbreaks, or conditions of public health importance (including trends, signals, risk factors, patterns in diseases, or increases in injuries from using consumer products)" may be relevant to certain big data projects [45 CFR 46.102(l)(2)].

✐ 5-1

Human Subjects

Under the Common Rule definition of "human subject," big data research that involves intervening or interacting with living individuals to obtain their data specifically for purposes of the research protocol involves human subjects. If big data research does not involve direct intervention or interaction with living individuals, and only accessing and analyzing information about living individuals that is collected for purposes other than the proposed research, commonly termed "secondary use research," the information must be both "private" and "individually identifiable" for the research to involve human subjects under the Common Rule [45 CFR 46.102(e)].

- *Individually identifiable.* The Common Rule defines "individually identifiable" to mean that the identity of the subject is or may readily be ascertained by the researcher or associated with the information. A data set may be composed of aggregate information, without individual identifiers linking information directly to living individuals. However, as previously noted, reidentification researchers have demonstrated that individuals may be reidentified through a methodology such as triangulation, in which purportedly deidentified data from multiple big data sets are combined, such that the resulting big data set includes sufficient data elements to identify an individual. Although these demonstrations are intriguing (and perhaps alarming), this does not mean that the IRB must presume that all big data sets include individually identifiable information. Rather, the IRB should assess the planned research and the research context on a case-by-case basis.

    In assessing whether information is individually identifiable, an IRB might consider the researcher, including their relationship to the subject (e.g., a researcher who is also the treating physician for subjects with rare diseases who can recognize those subjects from relatively limited information, or a researcher with access to a mechanism for identification [e.g., the Federal Bureau of Investigation fingerprint database]); the potential identifiers or partial identifiers contained in the information; and the likelihood of reidentification of individuals using technological methods such as triangulation (not just whether this theoretically is possible; Odwazny, 2014).

- *Private.* The Common Rule provides that "[p]rivate information includes information about behavior that occurs in a context in which an individual can reasonably expect that no observation or recording is taking place, and information which has been provided for specific purposes by an individual and which the individual can reasonably expect will not be made public" [45 CFR 46.102(e)(4)].

Collecting already generated information that is presumptively public in which an individual has no reasonable expectation of privacy does not involve human subjects for purposes of the Common Rule. An IRB may consider research analyzing publicly accessible information not to involve human subjects for this reason. However, often it is not clear-cut whether information is private or public under the Common Rule definition of "private information." Privacy scholars generally recognize that there is a sliding scale of privacy interests between the concepts of "public" information and "private" information, and that privacy depends on the nature of the information and the context and situation in which the information is available (Zook et al., 2017). An IRB considering what expectations of privacy of the information are "reasonable" might obtain information about the research context, the potential subjects in that context, and review any relevant terms of service or site policy (e.g., for internet sites) or applicable data use agreement (Odwazny, 2014). For example, even if a researcher can access information from a social media site without a special right of access, an IRB might not consider the information as "public" if the site's terms of service indicate that user-posted information may not be used for research purposes. Another example of when an IRB might opt to consider such information "private" is if the context was one in which users freely shared highly sensitive personal information for a specific purpose, such as a support group website designed for people who engage in self-harming behavior. Furthermore, an IRB may wish to take a more protective stance and consider the information as "private" if the information could endanger the individuals to whom it pertained if it were somehow highlighted through the planned research; for example, a study of an online social network for gay individuals in a country in which homosexuality is outlawed.

Exemptions

5-3 For interventional big data research, the Common Rule exemption for "benign behavioral interventions," in conjunction with the collection of information from the subjects, might be applicable to some big data research [45 CFR 46.104(d)(3)]; Department of Health and Human Services [DHHS], 2017). For example, a proposed manipulation of the landing page through which an individual accesses a particular website, in conjunction with the collection of information from the individuals regarding their perception of the utility of the website, might qualify for this exemption. (Note that this exemption is not applicable to DHHS-conducted or -supported research involving children.)

For secondary use research, in which researchers obtain information or biospecimens already collected from an individual for another purpose, several exemptions potentially are applicable, including an exemption that could apply to big data research if the big data obtained is "publicly available" [45 CFR 46.103(d)(4)(i)]. The utility of this exemption when applied to big data research depends on the challenge in determining whether big data is "private" or "public," as previously discussed. Another of these exemptions applies if the researchers record data such that subjects cannot be identified, and the researcher does not contact or reidentify the subjects [45 CFR 46.103(d)(4)(ii)]. The utility of this exemption may be limited, however, because after obtaining, combining, and using data sets, researchers would need to destroy all identifiable information, which may not be desirable or adequate for assuring research integrity. Lastly, an exemption could apply to big data research conducted at an institution regulated under the HIPAA Privacy Rule (DHHS, 2013) if the secondary research use of information would be considered under HIPAA to be research, healthcare operations, or conducted for public health activities and purposes [45 CFR 46.103(d)(4)(iii)]. (Note that these three exemptions may be applied to DHHS-conducted or -supported research involving children.)

🔗 11-6

🔗 9-6

Risks of Big Data Research

Big data research in general primarily presents informational risk from the unauthorized or inappropriate use or disclosure of information in ways that could be harmful to research subjects. For instance, disclosure of a health condition, illegal or illicit activities, or a psychiatric diagnosis might jeopardize the insurability of subjects, harm their reputation within the community, or cause emotional or psychological distress. In general, informational risks are correlated with both the nature of the information and the degree of identifiability of the information.

The Common Rule defines "minimal risk" as meaning that "the probability and magnitude of harm or discomfort anticipated in the research are not greater in and of themselves than those ordinarily encountered in daily life or during the performance of routine physical or psychological examinations or tests" [45 CFR 46.102(j)]. Because the primary risk of big data research is informational, an IRB will need to compare the probability and magnitude of such risk to the probability and magnitude of the risks of daily life or the performance of routine physical or psychological examinations or tests. If an IRB determines, for example, that informational risk presented by the research is not greater in probability or magnitude than a comparable daily life risk, then a comparison of the risks of big data research to the informational risk experienced in daily life may allow the IRB to determine that the big data research presents no more than minimal risk to subjects. Note that, in conducting the minimal risk assessment, the IRB may consider the data privacy protections of the research to mitigate the risks to privacy presented by the research.

Furthermore, the Common Rule specifically provides that the IRB should not consider possible long-range effects of applying knowledge gained in the research, such as the possible effects of the research on public policy, as among those research risks that fall within the purview of the IRB's responsibility [45 CFR 46.111(b)(2)]. Because many of the risks attendant to big data research might attach to specific populations (for example, through stigmatizing generalizations that affect a particular population or community), rather than to individual research subjects, this regulatory provision serves to highlight the limitations of applying the Common Rule as a protection from all of the potential harms stemming from big data research. Organizations and researchers may choose to consider these risks of harm through other mechanisms than IRB review, for example, by considering when it would be appropriate for a researcher to conduct community outreach before initiating big data research that addresses topics sensitive to the particular community.

🔗 12-9

Informed Consent and Waiver

The Common Rule allows an IRB to waive the requirement for informed consent or approve a waiver or alteration of the required elements of informed consent when certain criteria are met [45 CFR 46.116(e), (f)]. In certain circumstances,

🔗 6-4

big data research may not be able to be conducted under the Common Rule unless an IRB waives the requirement for the research subjects' informed consent. The extremely large numbers of subjects involved in big data research often are a consideration, because the cost of seeking and documenting consent from all of the subjects involved in the research might prevent the researcher from being able to conduct the research. Additionally, for secondary research use of already collected data sets, it may be impracticable (or impossible) to contact all of the subjects whose information would be obtained and used for research purposes, and the exclusion of subjects who cannot consent could have a detrimental effect on the research. For example, consider a big data research protocol involving a nearly real-time secondary use of information collected in the emergency room setting. Requiring informed consent from patient-subjects with an acute health condition in an emergency room setting could bias both the study data and the research results, because many individuals will be unable to give consent and, without a legally authorized representative available, would not be enrolled in the study (Bak, 2018).

⊘ 12-3

As the DHHS Secretary's Advisory Committee on Human Research Protections (SACHRP) recognized in assessing whether to waive informed consent for a secondary research use, an IRB may examine the terms and conditions under which the subject's information originally was collected in order to assess the subject's expectations regarding the use of the information. Much big data used for research purposes probably was collected originally in a nonresearch context. However, if the big data originally was collected for research purposes, then the IRB likely would wish to review the original informed consent provided to the subjects. If the original consent did not include any provisions regarding future research uses of the subject's information; if the informed consent's terms were either consistent with, or not inconsistent with, such future research use; or if there was no informed consent gathered at time of original data collection; then the IRB might favorably consider an application for waiver of informed consent. However, an IRB might refuse to approve a waiver of consent if the original consent had expressly promised that the subject's information would not be used for any purpose other than the original research (DHHS, 2015).

⊘ 6-4

Local Context: Other Legal and Policy Requirements

An IRB's assessment of the local context of the big data research should take into account the other laws and policies that may be applicable to big data research, including state, local, or tribal law, or U.S. federal agency policy. Additionally, non-U.S. laws may be applicable to certain big data research, depending on where the research is conducted and to whom the collected big data pertains. Although a detailed discussion of these is outside of the scope of this chapter, the following policies and laws notably may be relevant to big data research:

- The National Institutes of Health (NIH) genomic data sharing policy on the aggregation and use of large-scale genomic research data outlines NIH's expectation that research use of previously collected genomic research data, even if the data are deidentified, is conducted only if a consent for future data use was obtained through the previous collection (NIH, 2014).
- Consistent with the 2013 White House Office of Science and Technology Policy memorandum "Increasing Access to the Results of Federally Funded Scientific Research" (Executive Office of the President, 2013), many federal agencies have established data sharing policies that might be applicable to big data research.

- The European Union (EU) General Data Protection Regulation (GDPR) is relevant to research that uses data of European citizens, regardless of where the research is conducted (EUGDPR, 2018). The GDPR data protection standards apply to any personally identifiable information and generally operate to require the individual's informed consent for such identifiable information to be processed or shared. The GDPR standards also impose certain restrictions on sharing information with entities outside the EU.

Confidentiality Protections

The Common Rule requires that informed consent must include a <u>statement</u> describing the extent, if any, to which confidentiality of records identifying the subject will be maintained **[45 CFR 46.116(b)(5)]**. Much big data research will not involve records that identify the subject, so this regulatory provision may not apply. Notwithstanding this, from an ethical standpoint, it is advisable for researchers to take steps to protect the individuals to whom the big data pertain and the confidentiality of their information (see the box, Assessing Confidentiality Protections).

🔗 6-2

ASSESSING CONFIDENTIALITY PROTECTIONS

In assessing confidentiality protections, the reviewing IRB may wish to consider some or all of the following:

- What methods will be used to transmit the data from the origin to the research site? How secure should the transmission be? Consider whether the data are identifiable, potentially identifiable, or sensitive.
- Will the data be maintained in an individually identifiable form or a deidentified aggregated form? How will the data be stored—in a public or private cloud, server, or other location?
- Will subject information be disclosed pursuant to data sharing and data use agreements required by funding agencies (for example, NIH and National Science Foundation mandates)? Although not required by the Common Rule, consider whether or not to describe such data sharing in the informed consent.
- Will subject information be disclosed due to funding agency access rights and possible mandatory disclosure to regulatory oversight agencies such as Office for Human Research Protections, FDA, or the Office of Research Integrity? Consider describing this in the informed consent.
- Did the researchers provide a data security plan that outlines the data protection measures? Consider whether the planned measures will adequately address, and perhaps mitigate, the informational risks presented by the research.
- What is the likelihood of reidentification? Will aggregated data (anonymized or deidentified) be made public? Consider the likelihood that the research data actually will be used to link to a specific identified individual; also, consider whether the public release of data should be described in the informed consent (Odwazny, 2014, 2018).

IRB Expertise

The Common Rule explicitly allows an IRB to seek expert assistance. <u>Additional</u> <u>expertise</u> might benefit an IRB when reviewing big data research, depending on the specific protocol. For example, if the proposed research involves complex manipulations of several large data sets, the use and combination of public and private data, a novel analytic strategy, or a highly technical data security

🔗 3-1

plan, the IRB might benefit from seeking help from an expert consultant. Data analysts and scientists, information technology and security professionals, or professors in relevant disciplines might be available to assist the IRB in its review.

FDA Regulations

FDA regulations generally require informed consent from human subjects for all clinical investigations. In order to know whether big data research is regulated by FDA, the initial threshold is whether the research involves human subjects who participate in research, either as a recipient of the test article or as a control [21 CFR 56.102(c), (e)]. In its recommendations on big data research, SACHRP recognized that this determination is not always clear (DHHS, 2015). SACHRP recommended that FDA clarify that human beings are not "recipients of a test article" if the purpose of the proposed big data study is to look at records that involve the use of test articles that were given to individuals for the purposes of the primary study, but not originally given to those individuals for the purpose of obtaining data for a later big data study (DHHS, 2015). If FDA views these activities as not involving human subjects, then they do not meet the definition of clinical investigation, and FDA could accept the data as gathered in a context other than that of a clinical investigation. However, if FDA considers these activities to involve human subjects and to be clinical investigations, then the subject's informed consent is necessary unless the IRB may waive consent in this context.

- *Waiver and alteration of informed consent.* The 21st Century Cures Act provided FDA with the authority to permit an exception from informed consent requirements when the proposed clinical testing poses no more than minimal risk to the subject and includes appropriate safeguards to protect the rights, safety, and welfare of the subject. In accordance with guidance issued by FDA in 2017, FDA will follow the pre-2018 Common Rule provisions regarding waiver and alteration of informed consent until FDA promulgates its own regulations (FDA, 2017). (As of the date of this publication, FDA has published a notice of proposed rule making, which, if finalized, would add a general waiver of informed consent provision to the FDA IRB regulations at 21 CFR part 50 (83 FR 57378; Federal Register, 2018)

HIPAA Privacy Rule

⊘ 11-6

The HIPAA Privacy Rule may apply to big data research undertaken by covered entities (DHHS, 2013). If the <u>Privacy Rule</u> applies, the covered entities can only use or share protected health information in limited circumstances for research: (1) if the individuals to whom the data pertains provided informed consent or authorization [45 CFR 164.508], (2) with waiver of consent from an IRB or a privacy board [45 CFR 164.512(i)], or (3) if the research can be considered an activity for which consent or authorization is not needed, such as analysis for management, quality assurance, or quality improvement [45 CFR 164.506(c)(4)]. In general (and unless an exception applies), the researcher or research institution must either track disclosures of each person's data so that the HIPAA-required accounting of disclosures will be maintained, or a covered entity may maintain a list of studies using more than 50 individual records [45 CFR 164.528].

Ethical Considerations: Beyond the Regulatory Requirements

The Common Rule regulatory requirements provide the floor, and not the ceiling, for the appropriate protection of human subjects, so IRBs generally weigh pertinent ethical sensitivities along with the regulatory standards in their review and approval of research. These considerations are especially appropriate in the review of big data research: as noted previously, such research may not be governed by the Common Rule or may present risks that are not required to be evaluated under the Common Rule. An IRB may wish to consider the following points in its review of big data research:

- Many well-publicized examples demonstrate that people care about the use of their information for research purposes, even information voluntarily shared in a public or quasi-public forum. Research that involves only information that might be considered public still might be controversial to conduct. For example, consider the Facebook emotional contagion study (Meyer, 2014).
- Waiver of informed consent for subjects whose information is used in big data research can be a provocative decision point. On one hand, if appropriate data security and information protections are applied to the big data research, an IRB might find that the balance between autonomy and beneficence weighs in favor of facilitating the conduct of the research. On the other hand, an IRB might consider informed consent to be a baseline level of protection for the subjects of big data research and determine that the subjects' autonomy outweighs facilitating the big data research.
- Remember that reasonable IRBs may disagree about these determinations. One IRB may find that the research involves no more than minimal risk through a comparison to the probability and magnitude of the risks of daily life. Another IRB may use routine physiological or psychological tests or examinations as the comparator in the assessment of minimal risk. Or an IRB may be most comfortable considering any big data study to present more than minimal risk of harm, given the lack of certainty regarding the identifiability of the research data.
- The IRB may wish to consider how the researcher will access the data and whether any other agreements or policies operate regarding data use. For example, is the method in compliance with any applicable terms of service or end-user license agreement? Although the Common Rule does not require that researchers abide by terms of service or end-user license agreements, research use of data that contravenes such restrictions may present ethical considerations.
- Big data research may result in generalizations about a particular geographic community or cultural, ethnic, or racial group. As previously noted, although these concerns are outside of the Common Rule requirements, an IRB might wish to consider such possible downstream effects.

🧠 CASE STUDY 1: Social Influence and Political Mobilization

A researcher at your institution has submitted a new protocol for review that proposes to build on an already conducted study that measured online social influence and the strength of online social networks. The previously conducted research was a randomized controlled trial of political mobilization messages delivered to 61 million Facebook users during the U.S. congressional elections. The research found that the messages directly influenced political self-expression, information seeking, and real-world voting behavior of the Facebook users who received them and the users' friends and friends of friends as well. Users were randomly assigned to a "social message" group, an "informational message" group, or a control group. The social message group was shown a statement in their news feed that encourages the user to vote, provides a link to find local polling places, shows a clickable button reading "I Voted," and displays up to six "profile pictures" of the user's Facebook friends who had already clicked the "I Voted" button. The informational message group was provided with the same information but not the faces of friends. The control group did not receive any message (Bond et al., 2012).

The currently proposed research would build on this earlier study by replicating the same messaging among a similar cohort of Facebook users. Additionally, the research proposes to monitor the users' and friends' social media posts with an algorithm that will collect politically related posts and information about the users' and friends' gender and sexual orientation and to use facial recognition software in order to collect information about the race and ethnicity of the users and friends. Through collection of this information, the researcher hopes to determine what group characteristics correlate with increased influence from one's online social network.

1. The researcher has asked for a not human subjects research determination. How might an IRB administrator consider this request?

   Points to consider:

   a. Is the messaging strategy an interaction with living individuals, involving the collection of data about them, such that this portion of the activity meets the definition of human subjects research? The IRB administrator may wish to consider similarly conducted research, such as the Facebook emotional contagion study, and the discussion as to whether the manipulation of the Facebook users' feed in that study was considered a research interaction (Kramer et al., 2014; Meyer, 2014).

   b. Should the proposed collection of Facebook users' and their friends' posts, demographic information, and photos be considered to involve private information or public information? The IRB administrator may wish to consider a number of factors, including that the information may be "scraped" (a technique that involves extracting data from a website and importing the data to another program) from the Facebook pages without any special right of access, that the Facebook users and friends voluntarily disclosed this information in a way accessible to all, and that the Facebook users and friends disclosed this information for the purposes of participating in a social network and not with the knowledge or intention that their information would be used for research purposes or subjected to analytic technologies such as facial recognition.

2. What extra-regulatory considerations might the IRB evaluate?

   Points to consider:

   a. Research that involves "scraping" social media sites for information presents a variety of ethical challenges, including consideration of the users' autonomy interests and whether social media users may have privacy interests in information that could presumptively be considered public. IRBs might come to very different conclusions regarding this decision point, and the reviewing IRB might wish to document their rationale for considering a particular study to involve private vs. public information.

   b. Regarding the methodology used in the research, whereas the prior research used the messaging technology to influence social media users to vote in a U.S. election, which may be considered a social good, the methodology could equally be used to influence social media users to vote for a particular candidate or to spread a particular belief. In reviewing such protocols, the IRB may wish to focus on the particular purpose for which the big data analytics are employed.

CASE STUDY 2: Public Health Data Analytics

In partnership with the city health department and emergency services department, a researcher at your institution in the advanced analytics unit is developing a predictive application related to opioid overdose reports. The research is designed to help the health department more efficiently focus its limited resources on combating opioid-related deaths and opioid addiction, an important public health issue. Using information obtained from records of 911 calls for emergency services (information that is publicly available), these analytics generate a heat map showing opioid overdose hotspots as they develop across the city. The researcher hopes to develop a spatiotemporal model to identify correlations among 350 different factors and spikes in overdose reports across the city. The researcher notes that these same analytic structures were successfully used to identify 31 factors that predict when and where rodent complaints are most likely to occur over the subsequent week (National Academies of Sciences, Engineering, and Medicine, 2016) and hopes to do the same for opioid overdoses. The resulting internet application would inform the city emergency services department, which would station EMTs in certain areas of the city at certain times of the day to enable a rapid emergency response, and the city health department, which will prioritize hotspots for the location of mobile methadone clinics. Furthermore, the researcher intends to conduct a retrospective review of the hospital records of the individuals who experienced the opioid overdose, to collect basic demographic data such as age, sex or gender, race or ethnicity, as well as blood toxicity information, number of days hospitalized, and outcome (discharge or death), in order to assess whether the internet application reduces the numbers of opioid overdose deaths.

1. The researcher has asked for a not human subjects research determination, as this is a public health surveillance project. How might an IRB administrator consider this request?

    Points to consider:
    a. Does this project fall under the <u>exception</u> from the definition of "research" for certain public health surveillance activities **[45 CFR 46.102(l)(2)]**? If some, but not all, of the planned activities fall within the regulatory exception, could the project be divided such that only the activities that do not qualify for the exception are submitted for IRB review?   ✎ 5-1

    b. Looking at only the retrospective review of the hospital records of the individuals who experienced the opioid overdose: (1) Is this a systematic investigation designed to develop or contribute to generalizable knowledge? Consider that the purpose is to evaluate the use of the internet application to assess the effect, if any, on opioid overdose deaths; and (2) if so, will identifiable and private information about the individuals be collected? If the identifiable or private nature of the information is uncertain, what factors should the IRB administrator weigh in coming to a decision? Should the IRB administrator obtain additional information (e.g., how the researcher will be recording the data from the hospital records.). (Note that, if the decision is that the activity is human subjects research, the IRB administrator could further consider whether the research qualifies for <u>exemption</u> under **45 CFR 46.103(d)(4)**.)   ✎ 5-3

2. Alternatively, if the IRB administrator determines that the project involves human subjects research that must be reviewed and approved by the IRB, the researcher asks for a waiver of informed consent. How might an IRB apply the <u>waiver</u> of informed consent criteria?   ✎ 6-4

    Points to consider:
    a. Regarding whether the research involves no more than minimal risk to the subjects, the IRB might consider what possible risks are presented to the individuals involved in the research and whether the IRB could require data security measures to mitigate such risks to subjects.
    b. When considering whether the research could practicably be carried out without the requested waiver, and whether it is appropriate to provide subjects with additional pertinent information after participation, the IRB

might take into account the number of subjects involved and their availability to provide informed consent.

c. In assessing whether the research could practicably be carried out without using information in an identifiable format, the IRB might consider the factors that weigh in favor, or against, the research information being considered "identifiable" and "private."

d. Regarding whether the waiver adversely affects the rights and welfare of the subjects, the IRB might consider whether there are other requirements for informed consent that might apply.

3. What extraregulatory considerations might the IRB evaluate?

Points to consider:

a. Could the results of this activity be stigmatizing to a geographic community? An IRB might wish to consider the possible impacts on a neighborhood identified as an opioid overdose hotspot and whether they might be perceived as positive or negative.

b. Could the results of this activity be stigmatizing to a cultural, racial, or ethnic group? An IRB might wish to consider possible impacts on a group identified as more likely to experience an opioid overdose.

c. If the institution's involvement in this activity could be controversial, the IRB might wish to discuss with the researcher the possibility of consulting with institutional officials to discuss the conduct of the proposed activity.

Conclusion

When applied to big data research that involves human subjects, the current U.S. federal regulatory framework offers protections that help ensure the confidentiality of subjects' information and the appropriate protection of the subjects' autonomy. It is important to recognize that the Common Rule is intended to provide a floor for protections for human research subjects, and thus institutions and IRBs are free to voluntarily impose additional criteria for the conduct of research. Because of the particular challenges in big data research regarding how to assess the potential identifiability of research data and the possible downstream effects of big data research, IRBs may wish to take into account extraregulatory ethical considerations when reviewing big data research.

Resources

Froomkin, A. M. (2019). Big data: Destroyer of informed consent. *Yale Journal of Health Policy, Law, and Ethics.* https://ssrn.com/abstract=3405482

Metcalf, J., & Crawford, K. (2016). Where are human subjects in Big Data research? The emerging ethics divide. *Big Data & Society, 3*(1),1–14.

References

Bak, M. A. R., Blom, M. T., Tan, H. L., & Willems, D. L. (2018). Ethical aspects of sudden cardiac arrest research using observational data: A narrative review. *Critical Care, 22*(1), 212.

Bond, R. M., Fariss, C. J., Jones, J. J., Kramer, A. D., Marlow, C., Settle, J. E., & Fowler, J. H. (2012). A 61-million-person experiment in social influence and political mobilization. *Nature, 489*(7415), 295–298.

Buchanan, E. (2016). Ethics in digital research. In M. Nolden., G. Rebane, & M. Schreiter (Eds.), *The handbook of social practices and digital everyday worlds* (pp. 1–9). Springer.

Chandler, S. (2019, September 2). *Researchers use big data and AI to remove legal confidentiality.* Forbes. www.forbes.com/sites/simonchandler/2019/09/04/researchers-use-big-data-and-ai -to-remove-legal-confidentiality/#64e814b015f6

Department of Health and Human Services (DHHS). (2013). *Office for Civil Rights: Summary of the Health Insurance Portability and Accountability Act.* www.hhs.gov/hipaa/for-professionals /privacy/laws-regulations/index.html

Department of Health and Human Services (DHHS). (2015). *Secretary's Advisory Committee on Human Research Protections (SACHRP). Attachment A: Human subjects research implications of "Big Data" studies.* www.hhs.gov/ohrp/sachrp-committee/recommendations/2015-april-24-attachment -a/index.html

Department of Health and Human Services (DHHS). (2017). *Secretary's Advisory Committee on Human Research Protections (SACHRP). Attachment B: Recommendations on benign behavioral intervention.* www.hhs.gov/ohrp/sachrp-committee/recommendations/attachment-b-august -2-2017.html

European Union General Data Protection Regulation (EUGDPR). (2018). *General Data Protection Regulation.* https://gdpr-info.eu/

Executive Office of the President. (2013). *Increasing access to the results of federally funded scientific research: Office of Science and Technology policy.* www.epa.gov/sites/production/files/2015-01 /documents/ostp_memo_increasing_public_access.pdf

Federal Register. (2018). *Institutional review board waiver or alteration of informed consent for minimal risk clinical investigations.* 83 FR 57378. www.federalregister.gov/documents /2018/11/15/2018-24822/institutional-review-board-waiver-or-alteration-of-informed-consent -for-minimal-risk-clinical

Food and Drug Administration (FDA). (2017). *IRB waiver or alteration of informed consent for clinical investigations involving no more than minimal risk to human subjects: Guidance for sponsors, investigators, and institutional review boards.* www.fda.gov/media/106587/download

Kramer, A. D. I., Guillory, J. E., & Hancock, J. T. (2014). Experimental evidence of massive-scale emotional contagion through social networks. *Proceedings of the National Academy of Sciences, 111*(24), 8788–8790.

Laney, D. (2001). *3D data management: Controlling data volume, velocity and variety. META Group Research Note, 6.* https://blogs.gartner.com/doug-laney/files/2012/01/ad949-3D-Data -Management-Controlling-Data-Volume-Velocity-and-Variety.pdf

Meyer, M. (2014, June 29). *How an IRB could have legitimately approved the Facebook experiment—and why that may be a good thing.* Bill of Health. https://blog.petrieflom.law.harvard .edu/2014/06/29/how-an-irb-could-have-legitimately-approved-the-facebook-experiment -and-why-that-may-be-a-good-thing/

National Academies of Sciences, Engineering, and Medicine (NASEM). (2016). *Big Data and analytics for infectious disease research, operations, and policy: Proceedings of a workshop.* The National Academies Press. https://doi.org/10.17226/23654

National Institutes of Health (NIH). (2014). *NIH genomic data sharing policy.* https://osp.od.nih.gov /scientific-sharing/policies/

Odwazny, L. (2014). *Conducting internet research: Challenges and strategies for IRBs.* HHS Office for Human Research Protection webinar. https://videocast.nih.gov/summary.asp?Live=13932 &bhcp=1.%0d%0d

Odwazny, L. (2018). The tension between societal lapses in protecting the privacy of individuals and the regulatory definition of "minimal risk." In I. G. Cohen, H. Fernandez Lynch, E. Vayena, & U. Gasser (Eds.), *Big Data, health law, and bioethics* (pp. 223–236). Cambridge University Press.

Zimmer, M. (2019). *Empirical research project on how IRBs review big data research.* Office for Human Research Protections 2019 Exploratory Workshop, Privacy & health research in a data-driven world. www.hhs.gov/ohrp/education-and-outreach/exploratory-workshop/2019-workshop /index.html

Zook, M., Barocas, S., Boyd, D., Crawford, K., Keller, E., Gangadharan, S. P., Goodman, A., Hollander, R., Koenig, B. A., Metcalf, J., Narayanan, A., Nelson, A., & Pasquale, F. (2017). Ten simple rules for responsible big data research. *PLOS Computational Biology 13*(3), e1005399. https://doi .org/10.1371/journal.pcbi.1005399

mHealth, Mobile Technologies, and Apps

Megan Doerr

Sara Meeder

Abstract

In this chapter, we define and describe mHealth and the incorporation of mobile technologies and apps for research. We highlight considerations for reviewers when evaluating mHealth studies, addressing parsimonious data collection, reliability of mHealth data, documentation associated with mHealth studies (e.g., terms of service, privacy policies), data breach procedures, third-party access and use of data, and specific notes regarding regulatory compliance and vulnerable populations. Given the potential "black box" nature of mHealth/mobile technologies/apps, researchers themselves may be unaware of the diverse risks associated with their proposals. We strongly recommend that IRBs allot sufficient time for review, engage with experts, and be unafraid to ask questions when reviewing mHealth studies.

Overview

mHealth research utilizes data gathered on or by a mobile technology, solely or in concert with data collected from other sources (Sahin, 2018). These technologies may be purpose built for a specific study or may be commercial products, used as is or customized to the study. Data used in mHealth research may be gathered actively or passively. Active data are generated by subjects' completion of specific research tasks or activities. By contrast, passive data are generated by subjects in the course of their normal life activities, which is then shared with researchers automatically by the subject's device. These data may be generated by subjects interacting with the mobile technology itself or by other technologies and aggregated on the mobile device within an app (**Figure 12.5-1**).

By definition, mobile technologies, or generically, "devices" (note this is not the FDA term of art, which largely focuses on use of technologies in the diagnosis and treatment of disease), used in mHealth research travel with or within the

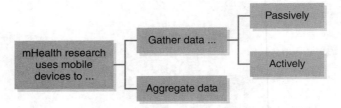

Figure 12.5-1 Defining mHealth research.

DEFINING MHEALTH

mHealth has been a term for over 20 years and has been alternatively referred to as telehealth, digital health, telemedicine, and digital medicine. Each term has slightly different connotations, with definitions evolving over time and varying between organizations. The Healthcare Information and Management Systems Society defined mHealth as involving the use of mobile and wireless technologies in 2012, whereas the FDA refers to the use of mobile devices and apps. The definition of mHealth used for this chapter is the most prevalent in current use and does not differentiate purpose between delivering health care and improving outcomes (Cameron et al., 2017).

research subject. Smartphones, tablets, and wearable sensors are all examples of mobile devices. The world of wearable sensors is continuously expanding, including wearable items like clothing and jewelry; implanted technologies like heart monitors; and ingestible sensors (Chai et al., 2017; Kaisti et al., 2019; Kizakevich et al., 2018), all of which collect data that can be incorporated into mHealth studies. Mobile devices may work in concert with other connected technologies that, while not traveling with or within subjects, may track the movements of the subject or the subject's mobile device. A Bluetooth beacon that transmits signals to a mobile device to allow for collection of data about a subject's location at the same time as the mobile device is collecting accelerometer data would be one example. (Accelerometers detect vibrations to measure acceleration and are frequently built into mHealth devices.)

Two key features of mHealth research are portability and richness of the data being collected. By virtue of their electronic capture and storage, mHealth data are extremely portable. For example, data may be gathered on a watch, aggregated by an app on mobile phone, and uploaded from there to a study database. This portability opens the door to greater opportunity for intentional (malicious) and unintentional (by researchers or third-party vendors) data corruption and siphoning than seen in non-mHealth research endeavors, as data are remotely cached and passed from system to system prior to arriving at the researcher's database.

The true richness of data collected by mobile devices can be surprising to researchers and reviewers alike. For example, many studies of movement disorders use a two-finger tapping activity as a measure of fine motor initiation. Traditionally, the number of taps in a given time period would be the data output of this test. Using a simple smartphone app to administer the test increases the number of primary data outputs from one (the number of taps) to 21 (including number of taps, mean tapping interval, median tapping interval, minimum tapping interval, maximum tapping interval, and 16 others, as shown in **Figure 12.5-2**).

This richness may tell far more about the subject than is needed to accomplish the study's goals. Even the methods chosen by the investigative team for mHealth data collection may impact the risk of participation. For example,

Traditional Capture Measures	mHealth Capture, First-Order Features
Number of taps	Number of taps, Mean tapping interval, Median tapping interval, Minimum tapping interval, Maximum tapping interval, Standard deviation of tapping interval, Kurtosis of tapping interval, Interquartile range of tapping interval, Interquartile range of right button X, Range right button X , Standard deviation right button X, Interquartile range of left button X, Range left button X, Standard deviation left button X, Interquartile range of right button Y, Range right button Y, Standard deviation right button Y, Interquartile range of left button Y, Range left button Y, Standard deviation left button Y, Correlation X and Y, Skew tapping interval, No-button tapping frequency

Figure 12.5-2 Tapping test measures.

Elias Chaibub Neto and Andrew Trister, Sage Bionetworks.

choosing to record GPS coordinates instead of movement vectors (that record a subject's relative movement from a fixed but unknown point) or their nondirectional displacement (a further abstracted description of a subject's relative movement that does not include directional data) may pose additional risks to subjects living in marginalized populations, such as undocumented immigrants, members of the LGBTQ community, and people of color, whose GPS coordinates could be used for tracking and targeting. Furthermore, mHealth data may be used in concert with data from clinical measures, records, social media, educational and criminal justice records, etc., to reveal private information or otherwise put subjects at risk. Each new type of data can introduce added data richness but also new areas requiring scrutiny by IRB reviewers. In our example, if a subject's ZIP code information is merged with movement vector data, subject location may be able to be ascertained nearly as well as through GPS coordinates. Protections afforded by certificates of confidentiality (CoC), or other safeguards provided by Department of Justice and other agencies, may not cover all elements of data collected for mHealth studies. For example, data collected through use of third-party apps may not be included in the protections provided by CoC or other research data protections.

8-3

mHealth research can also suffer from the black box problem: It can be difficult for researchers (and the IRB) to understand the engineering that underlies mHealth tools. For example, apps that are purpose built for research can be open source, meaning that anyone with appropriate knowledge of source code can inspect the source code used to create the app in order to better understand how the app works and how to, potentially, modify it. Apps that are proprietary typically do not allow inspection of source code, so it may not always be possible for a researcher or the IRB to know why the app is behaving the way it does or exactly what data the app is collecting. Whether open source or proprietary, there are generally policies the app developers or distributors put in place about use, modification, and sharing that may dictate whether the apps are suitable for the intended research purpose or whether they can be incorporated with other apps and platforms.

Points of Consideration for IRBs

eConsent

Given their inherent use of devices, mHealth studies frequently employ electronic informed consent (eConsent), either guided by the study team or subject self-navigated. Of particular concern with regard to eConsent use in

6-6

mHealth studies is the collection of data about the subject *prior* to the completion of consent—for example, collecting a prospective subject's time-per-page (as is commonly done by nonresearch apps and websites) as they navigate an eConsent experience. Researchers must be pressed to disclose (and may need to consult with the technical teams that have constructed their eConsent) what, if any, data will be collected prior to subject signature (or equivalent affirmative signal of consent to participate), and provide clear justification for the collection and use of those data. Furthermore, it is important to note that mHealth device documentation (e.g., terms of service, privacy policy, end-user license agreements) may conflict with or undermine terms traditionally set forth within the informed consent process (eConsent or traditional paper consent) for example, regarding data privacy or confidentiality. mHealth device documentation is discussed later in this chapter.

Parsimonious Data Collection

The richness of the data emerging from mobile devices can be intoxicating to researchers. It is important that the IRB recall their mandate to ensure parsimonious (i.e., the minimum necessary) data collection from subjects. Mobile devices' propensity for overcollection of data, for example, automatically identifying and signaling to other connected technologies in their area (Cyr et al., 2019), may pose risks to subjects' privacy and confidentiality. The IRB should consider whether there are ways to mitigate the risk of overcollection, either through changes to study design or through additional protections. This is of particular importance given the potential intimacy of mobile device data (Fuller, 2017; Zook, 2017), as well as the potential for reidentifying individuals

✐ 12-4   whose data are included in <u>aggregated data sets</u>.

During initial study review, researchers and reviewers may not be able to determine the full scope of data collection for the study, because combining data collection streams or using a new device may result in unforeseen data collection. For this reason, the IRB might consider periodic re-review, or approval of a more limited pilot study followed by re-review prior to broad rollout.

Reliability of Data

Researchers may decide to use an existing commercially available app for research purposes, incorporating data collected via a popular fitness tracking app, for example. Researchers may lack a complete understanding of the accuracy and consistency of the data compiled by these apps and the variations that exist between apps and/or a given app when used on different platforms or device models (Brodie et al., 2018). The IRB may play an important role in initiating discussions with researchers about the importance of literature review to assess the accuracy of the readily available mHealth tools for data capture, allowing for better study design from the outset.

Documentation

Documentation for devices and apps is routinely designed for protection of the developer or manufacturer, not for the benefit of the researcher or research subject. It may be helpful for the IRB to think about documentation for mHealth studies in the same way they would think about documenting submission requirements for a traditional drug or device study. IRBs should review all documents related to the devices and apps used in research utilizing mHealth, including terms of use and privacy policies (see box, Necessary Documentation for IRB Review). The IRB should carefully examine all provided documentation to understand what, if any, risks may be posed to subjects by the device or app. Additionally, IRBs should review any documentation provided by the device or app developer/owner regarding permissions for research use, especially those impacting subjects, such as the end-user license agreement (EULA). Documentation may include requirements for arbitration or for sharing of collected data that may not be appropriate for the proposed research or that may affect risk level determination.

NECESSARY DOCUMENTATION FOR IRB REVIEW

Type of Documentation	Areas of Concern/Reason for Review
Privacy policies	Type of data collected, use of data, third-party access, ownership of data in case of sale or dissolution of app/device company
End-user license agreements (EULA)	Exculpatory language
Terms of use	Exculpatory language (e.g., mandatory arbitration clause)
Community reviews	Identified risks
Device manufacturer or software developer specifications	Potential risks or possibility for unintended or undisclosed data collection
Academic literature about device/app, if applicable	Potential risks, ethical or logistical issues associated with device/app

It is the responsibility of researchers to provide all of these documents to the IRB for review. The IRB should ensure that the researcher has included any information that could impact decision making during the consent process and ancillary documents delimiting subjects' rights or protections. Submitted documentation should be the actual documents, not just screenshots or user brochures, although any user-facing documents should be included in the review. Actual documents may contain language about data ownership and access that is not contained in screenshots of promotional material or user brochures, allowing the IRB to more accurately assess potential subject risks. An online search of the device or app should allow the IRB to determine if the appropriate documentation has been submitted.

Additionally, the IRB will need to determine if there are any aspects of the device or app documentation that are not consistent with federal or local research regulations. One important example is the inclusion of exculpatory language, which is defined by OHRP and the FDA as ". . . language that has the general effect of freeing or appearing to free an individual or an entity from malpractice, negligence, blame, fault, or guilt" (FDA, 2011). In the absence of disclosure of such exculpatory language, the researcher and/or institution may be liable for any responsibility disclaimed by the device or app manufacturer in their documentation. It may be possible to negotiate a privacy policy and terms of use specific to a proposed research study or use devices that specifically define and delimit research use within their documentation (e.g., Fitbit 2019a, 2019b). Not all app or device developers will be willing

KEY ITEMS IN MHEALTH PROTOCOL REVIEW

Type of Data Collection	Review Considerations
Measurements of subject motion	Exact geolocation coordinates vs. movement vectors vs. nondirectional displacement
Use of cameras to capture images	Concerns for capture of the subject's full face, inclusion of identifying objects or scenes
Use of microphone to record voice	Inclusion of identifying background sounds
Inclusion of bystanders	In photos, on voice recordings, by sleep measurement devices, etc. (Hausman, 2007; Wagenknecht, 2018)
Open text fields	Be cognizant of documented app-interaction behavior patterns (e.g., texting expecting a response; Doerr et al., 2017); potential for disclosure of identifiable information by subjects
Illicit or criminal behavior	Whether there are mandatory reporting requirements or ethical responsibilities for reporting or intervening

to create research-specific policies. Success in negotiation may depend on the scope of the study (length, number of subjects), the reputation/prestige of the institution undertaking the study, or the nature of the device or app developer. Developers with apps in limited circulation might be willing to negotiate elements of terms of use or privacy policy in the hope that the uptick in research users will help build reputation, whereas long established developers with a wide customer base may be less willing to modify existing policies.

It is important to note that if researchers or IRB reviewers are struggling to understand the documentation associated with a mobile device or app, subjects are sure to be confused as well. If not already required by law (see sidebar, Plain Language and the Law), IRBs should strongly consider requiring researchers to provide plain language translation of key documentation, including privacy policies, terms of use, EULAs, in support of the requirements for transparency and informedness in human subjects research. Plain language translations may require legal review to ensure all key elements of the manufacturer documents are appropriately conveyed.

PLAIN LANGUAGE AND THE LAW

Plain language translation of privacy policies, terms of service, and other end-user license agreements is required under the European Union's General Data Protection Regulation, the California Privacy Protection Act, and likely an increasing number of related regulations.

Data Breach Procedures

Another area of concern involves data breach procedures for the device or app proposed for research use, as well as any other methods of data collection incorporated into the apps or devices, such as an application programming interface (API) that pulls data from a social media platform for the study (Arora, 2014; Clarke & Steele, 2014; Katusiime & Pinkwart, 2019).

The IRB should first identify if researchers have documented breach procedures, especially in studies using purpose-built devices or apps (which may not have undergone documentation procedures as rigorously as commercially available products). If breach procedures are documented, the IRB must evaluate whether the procedures are adequate for the type of data collected. It is important for the IRB to understand who has responsibility for notification of subjects in case of data breach, both in terms of making sure this is clear for subjects and in determining whether the IRB's institution would be responsible for notification or liability in case of breach. Whether there are arbitration requirements in case of data breach should also be considered, in light of the type of data to be collected and the potential risk to subjects.

Third-Party Access and Use

Third-party access is an often overlooked aspect of mHealth studies. The IRB should scrutinize the definition of the investigative team (for example, are the app developers considered part of the investigative team?) and the terms under which parties outside of the investigative team have access to and use of data collected by the device or app. Many commercial products retain a copy of all data collected, regardless of why it was collected. Furthermore, data accessed or collected by third parties (e.g., device manufacturer, app developer) may not be protected by <u>certificates of confidentiality</u> and may be accessible by law enforcement agencies.

🔗 8-3

Closely related are questions of data ownership and right of transfer. Apps purpose built for research may indicate that collected data would be owned by the researcher or research team; commercial products routinely claim ownership of at least a copy of all data collected. The IRB should ask what might happen to subject data when the device or app company changes ownership. Some social media platforms include clauses about deletion of data at the request of the platform, regardless of why the data was collected, which might affect data integrity for studies utilizing this type of data.

No matter who can access or owns the data, subjects must be made aware, in a comprehensible manner, of the limits to their control of what happens to their data.

Data Handling Procedures

Studies should detail data security, including any encryption or authentication procedures (e.g., hashing, a commonly used mechanism for ensuring that data has not been altered in transit), not only for the collection and storage of data but also as it is transferred and verified between devices and databases. Additionally, clear protocols for data access, including any allowable download and use, should be described by researchers within their protocol in advance of data collection.

Regulatory Compliance

FDA The IRB will need to consider FDA's potential for regulatory oversight of mobile devices and/or apps used for research, because researchers may not be aware of these considerations (Barton, 2012; Becker et al., 2014; Cortez et al., 2014). If the product is off-the-shelf, the manufacturer should be responsible for

SOCIAL MEDIA

Although social media is often accessed by mobile devices, research using social media is not *de facto* mHealth research. As examples, the aggregation of social media usage patterns by the iOS Screen Time app could constitute mHealth research, whereas people's browsing patterns while accessing social media from a desktop would not be considered mHealth research. Devices and apps incorporating data collected directly from social media platforms raise third-party access and use concerns unique to each platform. The IRB should keep in mind that if the device or app incorporates data collection from social media platforms, the documentation for those platforms or devices need to be reviewed as well.

assessing whether the FDA has oversight. The FDA considers whether an app, or more particularly the function of an app's software, may be intended for use in the diagnosis, cure, treatment, or prevention of a disease or condition, or for support of a <u>medical device</u>. The rapid evolution of this area of technology means that regulatory guidance may be updated more frequently than in other areas of research under FDA oversight. IRB reviewers should consult the most current FDA guidance and confer with device suppliers to ensure appropriate compliance.

11-3

Geographic region Studies that are not intentionally limited by geographic region may require consideration of national, state/provincial, or other local regulations that could affect mHealth data collection owing to the frequently pan-national nature of electronic data capture, for example, through broadly used social media platforms. Some states and <u>countries</u> have stricter privacy regulations than those at the U.S. federal level, requiring an assessment of whether study design would need to be modified to be in compliance. For example, the European Union's General Data Protection Regulation includes the "right to be forgotten," which allows for data contributors to request that all copies of their electronic data be deleted. Reviewers should ask researchers to explicitly define and justify the geographic region of their data capture and provide plans for regional delimitation. International studies may require in-nation coinvestigators. Within the United States, IRBs should remain abreast of state-level rule making with regard to electronic data privacy protections, for example, the California Privacy Protection Act.

10-9

Certificates of confidentiality Although not unique to mHealth research, the IRB should have a clear understanding of whether their institution will uphold a <u>certificate of confidentiality</u> (CoC) or if the institution will comply with law enforcement requests in spite of the CoC. The degree of protection, or lack thereof, provided by a CoC or similar certificate should be clearly delineated in the study consent form.

8-3

Vulnerable populations Although many concerns with mHealth devices and apps center on confidentiality and sensitivity of data (Fuller, 2017), it is important to consider other types of risk as well. Devices may pose physical risk, depending on their design and the intended research use. There may be special considerations for specific populations, such as <u>vulnerable populations</u>. There may be risks that are not immediately apparent if a commercially available device or app is used in a different population than the one for which it is intended. For example, devices intended for use by adults may pose unintended physical or emotional risk if used in a pediatric population.

Section 9

Children Inclusion of <u>children</u> in research requires a careful assessment of the nature of data collected, whether the data collection method or type might reveal reportable events like child abuse, and whether there are federal, state, or local regulations specific to children regarding data, disclosure, and retention. Research protocols and consents should also be clear about whether children can request deletion of data at age of majority (Dalpé et al., 2019; Schwab-Reese, 2018).

9-6

Persons who are incarcerated The IRB may also need to consider whether mHealth studies have the possibility of inadvertently including <u>persons who are incarcerated</u>, as subjects may become imprisoned over the course of a study or have access to enrollment online while incarcerated, in which case data collection and use requirements for incarcerated individuals may apply.

9-5

Persons with impaired cognition Potential subjects with <u>impaired cognitive ability</u> may be included in mHealth studies as a primary population or

9-7

as part of a broader subject base, requiring consideration of initial and ongoing consent requirements as well as possible risks posed by the nature of the mHealth data collected (Dalpé et al., 2019).

Recommendations

mHealth research can be complex and is constantly changing. Researchers and IRB reviewers should allow additional time for completion of review (Torous & Roberts, 2018). The IRB is likely to have to do research on new technologies or obtain information from the academic literature or online IRB or mHealth forums regarding technologies already in use.

Not all IRBs will have resident experts in mHealth and privacy. Even when experts are available, the IRB should be encouraged to ask questions (even if they seem naïve) regarding areas of subject risk and protection. Researchers are likely to be thinking about how well a device may answer a research question rather than all of the areas of interaction between subject and device that could cause risk.

The mHealth arena is constantly evolving, so it may be necessary to contact experts in the field. Journalists and ethicists who explore the use and misuse of apps, devices, and mHealth may be able to give insight into additional areas of subject protection; alternatively, they may be able to allay fears about some areas of research.

References

Arora, S., Yttri, J., & Nilse, W. (2014). Privacy and security in mobile health (mHealth) research. *Alcohol Research: Current Reviews, 36*(1), 143–151.

Barton, A. J. (2012). The regulation of mobile health applications. *BMC Medicine, 10*(1), 46.

Becker, D., Zhang, J., Heimbach, T., Penland, R. C., Wanke, C., Shimizu, J., & Kulmatycki, K. (2014). Novel orally swallowable IntelliCap(®) device to quantify regional drug absorption in human GI tract using diltiazem as model drug. *AAPS PharmSciTech, 15*(6), 1490–1497.

Brodie, M. A., Pliner, E. M., Ho, A., Li, K., Chen, Z., Gandevia, S. C., & Lord, S. R. (2018). Big data vs accurate data in health research: Large-scale physical activity monitoring, smartphones, wearable devices and risk of unconscious bias. *Medical Hypotheses, 119*, 32–36.

Cameron, J. D., Ramaprasad, A., & Syn, T. (2017). An ontology of and roadmap for mHealth research. *International Journal of Medical Informatics, 100*, 16–25.

Chai, P. R., Carreiro, S., Innes, B. J., Rosen, R. K., O'Cleirigh, C., Mayer, K. H., & Boyer, E. W. (2017). Digital pills to measure opioid ingestion patterns in emergency department patients with acute fracture pain: A pilot study. *Journal of Medical Internet Research, 19*(1), e19.

Clarke, A., & Steele, R. (2014). Local processing to achieve anonymity in a participatory health e-research system. *Procedia: Social and Behavioral Sciences, 147*, 284–292.

Cortez, N. G., Cohen, I. G., & Kesselheim, A. S. (2014). FDA regulation of mobile health technologies. *New England Journal of Medicine, 371*(4), 372–379.

Cyr, B., Horn, W., Miao, D., & Specter, M. (2019). *Security analysis of wearable fitness devices (Fitbit)*. Technical Report. https://api.semanticscholar.org/CorpusID:240133

Dalpé, G., Thorogood, A., & Knoppers, B. M. (2019). A tale of two capacities: Including children and decisionally vulnerable adults in biomedical research. *Frontiers in Genetics, 10*, 289.

Doerr, M., Truong, A. M., Bot, B. M., Wilbanks, J., Suver, C., & Mangravite, L. M. (2017). Formative evaluation of participant experience with mobile eConsent in the app-mediated Parkinson mPower study: A mixed methods study. *JMIR mHealth and uHealth, 5*(2), e14.

FitBit. (2019a). *Research pledge*. https://healthsolutions.fitbit.com/research-pledge/

FitBit. (2019b). *Terms of service*. https://dev.fitbit.com/legal/platform-terms-of-service/

Food and Drug Administration (FDA) (2011). Guidance on Exculpatory Language in Informed Consent. Draft Guidance. www.fda.gov/media/81521/download

Fuller, D., Shareck, M., & Stanley, K. (2017). Ethical implications of location and accelerometer measurement in health research studies with mobile sensing devices. *Social Science & Medicine, 191*, 84–88.

Hausman, D. M. (2007). Third-party risks in research: Should IRBs address them? *IRB: Ethics & Human Research*, 29(3), 1–5.

Kaisti, M., Panula, T., Leppänen, J., Punkkinen, R., Tadi, M. J., Vasankari, T., Jaakkola, S., Kiviniemi, T., Airaksinen, J., Kostiainen, P., Meriheinä, U., Koivisto, T., & Pänkäälä, M. (2019). Clinical assessment of a non-invasive wearable MEMS pressure sensor array for monitoring of arterial pulse waveform, heart rate and detection of atrial fibrillation. *NPJ Digital Medicine*, 2(1), 39.

Katusiime, J., & Pinkwart, N. (2019). A review of privacy and usability issues in mobile health systems: Role of external factors. *Health Informatics Journal*, 25(3), 935–950.

Kizakevich, P. N., Eckhoff, R., Brown, J., Tueller, S. J., Weimer, B., Bell, S., Weeks, A., Hourani, L. L., Spira, J. L., & King, L. A. (2018). PHIT for duty, a mobile application for stress reduction, sleep improvement, and alcohol moderation. *Military Medicine*, 183(Suppl 1), 353–363.

Sahin, C. (2018). Rules of engagement in mobile health: What does mobile health bring to research and theory? *Contemporary Nurse*, 54(4–5), 374–387.

Schwab-Reese, L. M., Hovdestad, W., Tonmyr, L., & Fluke, J. (2018). The potential use of social media and other internet-related data and communications for child maltreatment surveillance and epidemiological research: Scoping review and recommendations. *Child Abuse & Neglect*, 85, 187–201.

Torous, J., & Roberts, L. W. (2018). Assessment of risk associated with digital and smartphone health research: A new challenge for institutional review boards. *Journal of Technology in Behavioral Science*, 3(3), 165–169.

Wagenknecht, S. (2018). Beyond non-/use: The affected bystander and her escalation. *New Media & Society*, 20(7), 2235–2251.

Zook, M., Barocas, S., Boyd, D., Crawford, K., Keller, E., Gangadharan, S. P., Goodman, A., Hollander, R., Koenig, B. A., Metcalf, J., Narayanan, A., Nelson, A., & Pasquale, F. (2017). Ten simple rules for responsible big data research. *PLOS Computational Biology, 13*(3), e1005399. https://doi.org/10.1371/journal.pcbi.1005399

Conflicts of Interest: Researchers

Karen N. Hale
Daniel K. Nelson

Abstract

Conflicts of interest (COIs) are inherent to the conduct of research. Several factors, including historical events, increased funding and competition, and greater involvement of researchers and institutions in commercial endeavors, have moved COI to the forefront as a major concern facing IRBs and the research community. Because COIs can introduce bias that may cause harm, they constitute a risk to be considered and managed. The goals of this chapter are to define COI and provide examples, describe how the research environment has evolved in ways that increase the opportunity for conflicts, review existing regulations and guidelines, and discuss management strategies.

Introduction

COIs are inherent to the conduct of research. This was recognized by the National Commission for the Protection of Human Subjects of Biomedical and Behavioral Research (1978), which wrote that "investigators are always in positions of potential conflict by virtue of their concern with the pursuit of knowledge as well as the welfare of the human subjects of their research." The Commission echoed earlier reports by the National Institutes of Health (NIH) and the U.S. Surgeon General in viewing researchers as poorly situated to reconcile these competing interests on their own and in calling for a shared responsibility that incorporated independent review (e.g., the IRB). The National Bioethics Advisory Commission reiterated this fundamental observation over 20 years later, noting that research "necessarily creates a conflict of interest for investigators" through their use of fellow humans to obtain knowledge (National Bioethics Advisory Commission, 2001). Neither commission held these conflicts to be irreconcilable, nor did they link COIs to character flaws of researchers as individuals or as a class.

Notwithstanding this prior recognition, several factors have converged to propel COIs to the forefront as one of the major concerns facing IRBs and the research community. These factors include increased funding of research, increased competition for that funding, greater involvement of commercial interests, larger payoffs for successful outcomes, more direct participation of researchers and institutions in those rewards, and a shift in the settings where research is performed. Against that background, several events lent credence to the growing concern with COIs in human subjects research. The tragic death of Jesse Gelsinger in a gene transfer study in 1999 prompted a reexamination of many aspects of human subjects research, with particular focus on COI (Agnew, 2000; NIH, 2000a, 2000b). Since then, identification and management of COIs have become part of the expected routine for institutions and IRBs.

1-2

Definitions

Before considering COIs as they relate to research involving human subjects, it is important to establish a working definition. Explaining what is meant by "conflicts of interest" is not straightforward, partly because the topic is emotionally charged and frequently misunderstood (Friedman, 1992; Spece et al., 1996). The core problem to be avoided is bias in judgment; a term is needed to describe situations where the potential for bias is such that decisions may be called into question by others. This is of particular concern in relation to professional roles or obligations to be honest and objective, especially those that come with positions of trust. It is commonly accepted, for example, that judges should recuse themselves from legal cases involving family members, that professors should not be romantically involved with students in their classes, and that the inventor of lab equipment should not be the one making procurement decisions for government or university labs. It is easy to see how these competing interests and "divided loyalties" could influence decisions, yet the same cautionary principle has been difficult to apply to the research setting, where researchers may think that saying a COI exists is calling their personal integrity into question. Acknowledging a COI does not mean that someone acted on their bias or made a wrong decision. As Friedman (1992) explains, "A conflict exists whether or not decisions are affected by the personal interest; a conflict of interest implies only the potential for bias or wrongdoing, not a certainty or likelihood." These misunderstandings about conflicts of interest (as not being synonymous with questions about researcher integrity) may need to be overcome when implementing policies or dealing with individual cases.

With regard to financial relationships, Angell defines COI as "any financial association that would cause an investigator to prefer one outcome . . . to another" (NIH, 2000a). Both Angell and Friedman (1992) argue that terms like "potential" COI are misleading and misused because conflict is a function of the situation and not of the individual's response to that situation. The opportunity need not be acted on for it to represent a COI and a situation worthy of concern.

DEFINITION: CONFLICT OF INTEREST

For the purposes of this chapter, a *conflict of interest* is defined as: a set of conditions in which a researcher's judgment concerning a primary interest (e.g., subject welfare, integrity of research) could be biased by a secondary interest (e.g., personal or financial gain) (Congressional Research Service, 2014; Friedman, 1992; Morin et al., 2002; NIH, 2000a; Spece et al., 1996).

Sources of Conflict of Interest in Research

Although the following discussion largely focuses on financial incentives, it is important to recognize that there are many rewards associated with research that are not directly linked to money (NIH, 2000a, 2000b; Saver, 2012). Admirably, many researchers are driven by the pursuit of knowledge in its purest sense. The altruistic desires to advance scientific frontiers, contribute to society, alleviate suffering, and improve lives are powerful motivators, as are more personal goals that become important to many researchers, including respect of peers, appointments, promotions, tenure, grants, fame, prizes, and the publications that support all of these. Some have argued that these academic pressures present greater conflicts than the prospect for material gain. Anyone who has observed the battles that can be waged over authorship or tenure may be hard pressed to disagree. However, these academic incentives are embedded within the fabric of research. They are widely recognized and broadly shared and, therefore, tend to be viewed with less concern.

More recently, attention has been focused on financial conflict of interest in clinical research, where both the risks and the rewards are potentially the greatest. Examples of such interests include equity holdings in commercial sponsors, consulting fees, royalties, patent rights, and honoraria for serving on advisory boards or for giving lectures. Any of these may be problematic if linked to the sponsor of research or the product under study. Also of concern are scenarios in which faculty may assign students or trainees to work on studies from which the researcher stands to benefit. Even the negotiated budgets to compensate researchers and institutions for conducting research may represent sizable conflicts of interest, depending on how they are structured and how the resulting revenues are handled (Eichenwald & Kolata, 1999).

There is ample evidence that healthcare providers preferentially refer patients to facilities in which they hold a personal financial stake (NIH, 2000a; Spece et al., 1996). Given incentive, researchers might similarly be inclined to enroll as many subjects as possible, push the limits on entry criteria, over-promise the benefits of participation, promote research participation when other alternatives might be preferable, or report positive findings when results are equivocal. At a minimum, without proper management, even the appearance of conflict calls into question the judgment of the researcher and the integrity of the research process. This is no small matter if it jeopardizes the trust and confidence of the public. At its worst, COIs may endanger lives—not only those of the immediate subjects under study, but those of future patients treated on the basis of biased results (Eichenwald & Kolata, 1999; NIH, 2000a). To understand why conditions today create increased opportunities for conflict requires an understanding of how clinical research has evolved.

Evolution of the Clinical Research Enterprise

In the distant past, most biomedical research was funded by the government and conducted in academic centers. The rewards were primarily related to advancement of knowledge. To be sure, advancement of careers and reputations was also a motivator, albeit of a different nature than the current focus on advancement of wealth. Clinical studies tended to be small in scale, observational, investigator-initiated, and relatively inexpensive (NIH, 2000a; Spece et al., 1996).

This picture began to change in the decades after World War II as both federal and industrial funding of research increased. The nature of clinical research also evolved, with large-scale, multicenter, randomized trials providing the safety and efficacy testing that society demanded before new products were brought to market. This growth continued, with investments in U.S. research and development by pharmaceutical companies increasing from approximately $2 billion in 1980 to $90 billion in 2016 (Pharmaceutical Research and Manufacturers of America, 2018). Rapid expansion has also occurred in the international arena. As of 2019, fewer than half of the more than 300,000 clinical studies registered on ClinicalTrials.gov were being conducted in the United States. Of those, only 25% received funding from the U.S. federal government, with 75% supported by industry and other sources (National Library of Medicine, 2019).

During this period, the growth and evolution of managed care also influenced the clinical trial environment at several levels, forcing sponsors to reevaluate every aspect of drug development, including the sites they used to conduct their clinical trials. Academic medical centers were traditionally a locale of choice for conducting clinical trials, owing to their expertise, prestige, and access to large numbers of patients. As pressures mounted, however, sponsors came to view academic centers as "slow, inefficient, expensive, not always top-quality, and sometimes exasperating to work with" (Lightfoot et al., 1998).

Although IRBs are often identified as a bottleneck in this process, other institution-based entities, such as offices for contracts and grants, sponsored programs, legal review, and other peer-review committees, contributed to this perception of a clogged bureaucracy. Faced with a competitive, market-driven environment, sponsors were free to take their business where they pleased, and they did this by actively avoiding academic centers when selecting sites to conduct their trials. Filling the niche were independent sites and private-practice or hospital-based physicians not affiliated with academic centers, perhaps gathered into networks by site management organizations. Contract research organizations (CROs) became a major force, allowing companies to outsource much of the work of managing their trials (Lightfoot et al., 1998).

While managed care exerted pressures on industry, it also created difficulties and opportunities for physicians at an individual level (Eichenwald & Kolata, 1999; Lightfoot et al., 1998). As managed care closed the door on fee-for-service reimbursement on the clinical side, many saw the opportunity to replace lost revenues by conducting industry-sponsored research studies. Although some physicians incorporated research as a supplement to clinical practice, others effectively transferred their focus to conducting clinical trials. Thus was born a new player in this enterprise: the independent for-profit investigative site.

With physicians based outside of academic centers looking to increase their involvement, sponsors were happy to engage this emerging workforce, which came unencumbered with the unwieldy bureaucracies of more traditional sites. The number of private-practice physicians involved in drug studies increased while the proportion of trials conducted in academic medical centers decreased, during a time in which the industry as a whole was enjoying steady growth. From a business perspective, academic centers lost market share (Eichenwald & Kolata, 1999; Kowalczyk, 2000; Lightfoot et al., 1998; Morin et al., 2002).

This migration of clinical trials away from academic medical centers did not go unnoticed by those centers, which faced many of the same financial pressures as community-based practices. In response, many academic centers established clinical trial offices to centralize administrative processes, streamline IRB submissions and contract negotiations, and facilitate interactions with industry sponsors (Lightfoot et al., 1998). Some also formed networks with community-based practices to provide broader access to potential subjects. These efforts had the desired effect, as industry began to return to this traditional base, and academic centers reported increases in revenue from industry grants (Kowalczyk, 2000).

As a backdrop to the economic pressures driving change at corporate, individual, and institutional levels, a change in federal law signaled a shift in the government's approach to the proceeds of research. In 1980, Congress passed the Bayh-Dole Act, which provided universities with incentives to move research results into commercial applications. Before Bayh-Dole, the government retained the intellectual property rights to technology developed through federal support; however, only a tiny fraction of publicly funded technology ever made it to the marketplace. The 1980 legislation allowed academic institutions to retain these intellectual property rights and encouraged institutions to patent new products, license these products to industry, and share resulting royalties with their faculty. This technology transfer paved the way for productive joint ventures between the nonprofit and for-profit sectors. It also, however, paralleled the evolution described previously in creating new and unanticipated opportunities for COIs (NIH, 2000a).

The purpose of the preceding discussion is neither to defend nor criticize the various players in this enterprise but to describe its evolution and current state for readers expected to oversee research conduct. It is undeniable that growth and restructuring are occurring and driven by real-world market forces. Ensuring that this growth can continue in a way that optimizes the safety and well-being of subjects, assures research integrity, and preserves public trust presents challenges for all involved. The government and academic community have helped to confront these challenges in subsequent years by more clearly defining their respective responsibilities in this arena (Association of American Medical Colleges, 2008).

Regulations and Guidance

Reflecting the increased attention to COIs, the October 2000 revision of the Declaration of Helsinki (as well as subsequent revisions in 2004, 2008, and 2013) contained guidance for physician-researchers and IRBs (World Medical Association, 2013). Researchers are instructed to disclose "any possible conflicts of interest" (including institutional affiliations and sources of funding) to independent ethical review committees, to subjects, and in publications resulting from the research. There is no guidance provided, however, as to what constitutes an inappropriate interest from the standpoint of IRB review.

🔗 1-1, 1-2

With regard to U.S. federal regulations governing IRBs, specific requirements are limited to removing IRB members from review of studies in which they have a conflicting interest (e.g., as a researcher [**45 CFR 46.107(d)**; **21 CFR 56.107(e)**]. Beyond that, there is little to guide IRBs in considering researcher COI. (See Chapter 12-7 for a discussion of conflicts of interest at the IRB level.) The requirements for informed consent instruct that "An investigator shall seek consent only under circumstances that . . . minimize the possibility of coercion or undue influence" [**45 CFR 46.116(a)(2)**; **21 CFR 50.20**]. One potential source for such influence is the researchers themselves, if they

🔗 12-7

hold a significant COI in relation to a given study. Similarly, IRBs must determine that risks are minimized, reasonable in relationship to benefits, and disclosed to subjects [**45 CFR 46.111(a)(1) and (2)** and **45 CFR 46.116(b)(2)**; **21 CFR 50.25(a)(2)** and **21 CFR 56.111(a)(1) and (2)**]. COI can be viewed as one such risk. Although federal regulations empower IRBs to act at their discretion, these readings require broad interpretations, and specific guidance is limited (Department of Health and Human Services [DHHS], 2004; NIH, 2000b).

Beginning around 1990, regulations outside the Common Rule began to address researcher COIs (Congressional Research Service, 2014). In July 1995, the Public Health Service (PHS) (which includes NIH) and the National Science Foundation (NSF) issued some of the first guidelines that required disclosure and peer review of any "significant financial interests" held by researchers applying for federal funds (Agnew, 2000; Mervis, 1995). The NIH had first proposed guidelines in 1989 suggesting that conflicts should be prohibited, but these were viewed as overly restrictive by the research community and were withdrawn. The final 1995 regulations gave research institutions discretion in how they would manage conflicts at the local level and stated that they were not required to report details to the government [**42 CFR 50.604** and **42 CFR 50.605**; **45 CFR 94.4** and **45 CFR 94.5**] (DHHS, 2011). The threshold for disclosure was $10,000 in income, $10,000 in equity, or 5% ownership in a company, if these might be affected by the research. Institutions receiving federal funds were charged with establishing and enforcing policies to "manage, reduce, or eliminate" the COI, once disclosed. With much discretion given to institutions, it is not surprising that implementation of these policies led to considerable variability (McCrary et al., 2000).

PHS subsequently revised the 1995 regulations to provide more stringent requirements for disclosure and oversight, i.e., lowering the threshold for disclosures of financial interests from $10,000 to $5,000, requiring institutions to make certain researcher financial interests accessible to the public, reporting financial conflicts of interest to the NIH, and instituting a COI training requirement for researchers [**42 CFR 50.603** and **42 CFR 50.604**; **45 CFR 94.3** and **45 CFR 94.4**] (DHHS, 2011).

In 1998, the Food and Drug Administration (FDA) issued a final rule that required sponsors to certify the absence of financial interests of researchers who conducted their studies or to disclose those interests. Such interests include proprietary interests (e.g., patents, trademarks, copyrights, or licensing agreements); equity interests (e.g., ownership or stock options); compensation affected by the outcome of the study; or payments of $25,000 or more to support researcher activities outside of conducting the study (e.g., equipment, honoraria, or consulting fees) during the time the researcher is carrying out the study and for 1 year following the study's completion. This disclosure is tied to the submission of a marketing application to FDA, and the intent is to protect the integrity of supporting data [**21 CFR 54.1-4**].

Beyond federal regulations, an increasing number of professional organizations have established COI policies to guide their members, including the American Cancer Society (2016), American Society of Transplantation (2014), American Academy of Pediatrics (2010), and the American Society of Gene and Cell Therapy (ASGCT, 2000). The latter, for example, recommended that "investigators and team members directly responsible for patient selection, the informed consent process and/or clinical management in a trial must not have equity, stock options, or comparable arrangements in companies sponsoring the trial" (ASGCT, 2000). Although this policy was originally prompted by problems in gene transfer trials, COIs are by no means limited to this small field, and many other professional groups have adopted equally strong positions to prevent bias in the design, conduct, and reporting of research. Many medical journals follow the recommendations of the International Committee of Medical Journal Editors (2019) for reporting COIs during peer review and publication of scientific work, in order to ensure the credibility of published articles and to maintain the public's trust in the scientific process.

Managing Conflicts of Interest

Disclosure

Disclosure to the Government and Nongovernmental Organizations

Identification of conflicts is an important first step in managing them, and disclosure might occur at one or more levels. As explained, disclosure to the government of researcher conflicts is required by federal agencies (e.g., FDA, PHS, NSF). In the case of grant awards, institutions are expected to manage or eliminate researcher financial COIs, and reporting to the granting agency should include sufficient information to describe the nature and extent of the conflict and the institution's management plan. In the case of marketing applications for new drugs and biologics to FDA, disclosure of researcher financial interests that might affect the reliability of submissions is made through the sponsor. Disclosure occurs at the time of submission to FDA, after the study is completed, and does not apply to practices that might affect subjects (e.g., recruitment incentives). Thus, disclosure to FDA cannot be expected to directly impact the protection of research subjects in a substantive way.

A more recent action aimed at improving disclosure of researcher financial conflicts is "The Physician Payments Sunshine Act" (Section 6002 of the Affordable Care Act implemented by the Centers for Medicare and Medicaid Services [CMS]), requiring applicable manufacturers and group purchasing organizations to disclose payments and "transfers of value," including research-related payments, to physicians and teaching hospitals [42 CFR 403.900, 42 CFR 403.902, 42 CFR 403.904, 42 CFR 403.906] (DHHS, 2013). These disclosures are then publicly posted in a searchable format on the CMS Open Payments website (CMS, 2019). Another disclosure repository (titled "Convey") developed by the Association of American Medical Colleges (AAMC) allows individuals to maintain records of financial interests and disclose them directly to organizations using the system (AAMC, 2018). The goal of these and other efforts to standardize financial disclosure and reporting is to discourage improper relationships without inhibiting productive collaborations that may lead to new discoveries.

Disclosure to the Institution

Disclosure of financial interests to the institution is mandatory for those researchers receiving federal funds, with their institutions given discretion in how they manage any conflicts. Predictably, there is considerable variability in how institutions handle this process. Many institutions have established policies requiring disclosure by all faculty members. However, few institutions initially linked this process to protection of human subjects, as suggested by the fact that none of 235 institutions surveyed in 1999–2000 incorporated disclosure to either IRBs or subjects as a management strategy in their COI policies (McCrary et al., 2000). Several organizations have made efforts to strengthen the link between COI mechanisms and human subjects protections. For example, the Association for the Accreditation of Human Research Protection Programs (AAHRPP) requires institutions it accredits to have policies requiring disclosure and management of researchers' financial interests, and processes must be in place that allow the IRB to have the final authority to decide whether these interests (and their management) allow the study to be approved (AAHRPP, 2018).

🔗 8-7

A complete review of issues that institutions should address in their policies is outside the scope of this chapter and outside the scope of IRB purview, but several sources provide guidance (Congressional Research Service, 2014; DHHS, 2000, 2004; McCrary et al., 2000; National Bioethics Advisory Committee, 2001; NIH, 2000a, 2000b). With regard to the broader goal of protecting all subjects, however, it is important to remember that a majority of industry-sponsored studies are now conducted at sites where there may be no institutional policies. That is, there may be no "institution" beyond the researcher or research team and, therefore, no local oversight.

Disclosure to the IRB

Disclosure to the IRB is increasingly advocated as a routine part of study review. The Office for Human Research Protections (OHRP) has strongly recommended that financial relationships be described when researchers submit IRB applications and that IRBs should take into consideration the funding arrangements between sponsor and researcher institution (DHHS, 2004). Previously, these arrangements tended to be regarded by both researchers and IRBs as "none of our business." For example, a 1999 survey of 200 IRBs that oversee clinical trials found that only 25% reviewed such financial matters (DHHS, 2000). As previously mentioned, AAHRPP requires its accredited organizations to develop processes for the IRB to evaluate and manage researcher financial interests or, if performed by another entity (e.g., COI committee), to inform the IRB of the results of this evaluation, with the IRB having the final authority to decide whether to approve the study (AAHRPP, 2018). Whether it is the IRB or another institutional entity who reviews this information, IRBs should be aware of any financial interests on the part of researchers that have the potential to bias researchers' judgment or actions in areas that affect the rights and welfare of research subjects.

Disclosure to Subjects

🔗 Section 6

Disclosure via the informed consent process is at once the most direct and ethically intuitive route of disclosure and the most difficult to accomplish in a meaningful way (Morin et al., 2002; Weinfurt et al., 2009). At the very least, subjects should be aware that the study is sponsored by outside entities, whether commercial or governmental. The consent form might include a lay definition of what this means (e.g., "researchers/institutions are compensated for the costs of conducting this research"), because sponsorship may not be understood by the public in terms that researchers or IRBs take for granted. IRBs should carefully consider the level of detail (e.g., dollar amounts from study budgets) provided in consent forms. Although there may be a temptation, in the spirit of full disclosure, to suggest language like "your study doctor will receive $7,800 for enrolling you in this study," this begs additional clarification and may only confuse what is already a complicated process. Placing this statement in perspective demands that subjects also understand that (from this seemingly large amount) X goes to pay for the extra MRI scan done for research purposes only, Y goes to hire the study nurse who is attending to their needs, Z goes to institutional overhead, and so on. Thus, dollar amounts may be misleading because they may merely reflect legitimate expenses.

Subjects should certainly be made aware of any COIs on the part of researchers or the institution that might affect their decision to participate and be permitted to decide for themselves whether to participate. On the other hand, IRBs should avoid "passing the buck" to subjects who may not be in a position to fully understand the information provided. If we accept COIs as yet another risk, it is relevant to inform subjects, but disclosure alone is not sufficient and does not obviate the need for IRBs to assess risks (Angell, 2000; Morin et al., 2002; National Bioethics Advisory Committee, 2001; NIH, 2000a).

Managing Beyond Disclosure

Management strategies should be aimed at removing or minimizing COIs. Some have argued that the only acceptable solution is a complete prohibition of interests that could potentially bias the research. These observers suggest banning any institution or researcher from conducting research from which they stand to benefit. Others view that approach as an unattainable, and perhaps even undesirable, goal in the modern environment. They advocate mechanisms to manage the conflict while still permitting what they perceive to be vital relationships to exist. This debate is ongoing and will not be resolved by this chapter (AAMC, 2008; Agnew, 2000; Angell, 2000; Congressional Research Service, 2014; NIH, 2000).

DHHS has, however, issued guidance that provides useful questions to consider (DHHS, 2004). Although IRBs may not be well situated or equipped to directly oversee this management process, they should establish open lines of communication with institutional bodies such as COI committees that can provide this oversight. IRBs should then consider the mechanisms proposed to manage the identified conflict, with a particular eye for aspects that could affect research subjects. This could include removing the conflicted researcher from specific activities such as designing the study, obtaining informed consent, performing procedures, monitoring or reporting adverse events, or analyzing data (Morin et al., 2002). Although excluding researchers from any or all of these aspects of the study may be tantamount to removing them altogether, this remains an option if the IRB or institution determines that a given conflict is unmanageable.

The overarching goal is to ensure that the conflicted individual is not involved in any aspect of research that could be influenced by that conflict. In some cases, the only way to accomplish this goal may be for researchers to divest themselves of their conflicting interest or identify someone else to conduct the research. If the latter approach is taken, the IRB should ensure that the substituted researcher is not subordinate to the conflicted researcher or otherwise situated so that this becomes a meaningless exercise, in which the original researcher still controls the study. The same rationale may be extended to <u>institutional conflicts of interest</u> in a given line of research. If institutional holdings (e.g., major ownership in a start-up company) are such that the integrity of the research can be called into question, it may be preferable to perform the study at a different institution.

Given that even the appearance of impropriety is enough to damage individual careers and institutional reputations, it can truly be said that a cautious approach to these issues is in everyone's mutual interest. IRBs may first need to overcome the perception that managing COIs is reliant on their trust of the

⊘ 12-8

researcher in question. Management should not hinge on anyone's perception of an individual but on an objective assessment of situations in which people have placed themselves. All parties involved in this process should be clear that managing COI has everything to do with the situation and nothing to do with the character or honesty of the individual. Here is another area where proactive education can be helpful, by creating a culture of compliance that promotes self-identification and cooperative resolution of conflicts before they become problems.

Much of the foregoing presumes involvement of an institution, with institution-based mechanisms in place. Managing COIs in the extrainstitutional settings where the majority of clinical trials are now performed presents an even greater challenge for the central IRBs that oversee these sites, for sponsors (who are themselves conflicted, by definition), and for the public at large.

⊘ Section 4

Conclusion and Looking Ahead

Multiple initiatives have had substantial impact on approaches to and management of COI. Several groups, including the Association of American Universities (AAU), AAMC, American Medical Association, NIH, National Bioethics Advisory Commission, OHRP, and Congress have considered financial interests in research (AAMC, 2008; Congressional Research Service, 2014; DHHS, 2004; Morin et al., 2002; NIH, 2005; Steinbrook, 2004). The recommendations and policies from these deliberations have provided guidance in keeping with the modern research environment.

For example, in 2008, the AAU and the AAMC jointly recommended something approaching a "zero tolerance policy" that would prohibit researchers from conducting human subjects research in which they held financial interests, unless there are compelling circumstances (e.g., the conflicted researcher is the only person capable of conducting that research). Other recommendations called for tighter links between COI management and the IRB review process (AAMC, 2008). The same groups have also considered institutional COI, recognizing that arrangements and pressures frequently exist at levels beyond the individual, such that the institutions in which researchers work may be equally conflicted. In the early 2000s, NIH policies in this area came under scrutiny after reports that top-ranking NIH officials were receiving large sums in consulting fees from industry collaborations, including pharmaceutical and biotechnology companies in a position to benefit from NIH decisions and programs (NIH, 2005; Steinbrook, 2004). The appearance of impropriety led to congressional hearings and, in relatively short order, much tighter restrictions on external arrangements by NIH employees. These many initiatives and reports eventually led to the 2011 PHS requirements, which not only provided rules for institutions and researchers receiving federal funds, but also signaled a clear position on COI to the entire research community.

These evolving requirements and events reinforce the notion that, because COIs are common in research and can introduce bias that may cause harm, they continue to be one of the major concerns facing IRBs and the research community. When addressing COIs, IRBs are well advised to stay informed of current requirements and to update their policies as necessary to ensure effective human subjects protections grounded in ethics, regulations, and common sense.

References

Agnew, B. (2000). Bioethics: Financial conflicts get more scrutiny in clinical trials. *Science, 289*(5483), 1266–1267.

American Academy of Pediatrics. (2010). *Policy on conflict of interest and relationships with industry and other organizations.* www.aap.org/en-us/about-the-aap/aap-leadership/Documents/20-IndustryRelations.pdf

American Cancer Society. (2016). *Financial conflict of interest policy for promoting objectivity in research.* www.cancer.org/content/dam/cancer-org/online-documents/en/pdf/policies/financial-conflict-of-interest-policy.pdf

American Society of Gene & Cell Therapy (ASGCT). (2000). *Policy on financial conflict of interest in clinical research.* www.asgt.org/policy/index.html

American Society of Transplantation. (2014). *Conflict of interest policy statement.* www.myast.org/about-ast/who-we-are/bylaws-and-policies/conflict-interest-policy-statement#

Angell, M. (2000). Is academic medicine for sale? *New England Journal of Medicine, 342*(20), 1516–1518.

Association for the Accreditation of Human Research Protection Programs (AAHRPP). (2018). *Evaluation instrument for accreditation. Element I.6.B.* admin.aahrpp.org/Website%20Documents/AAHRPP%20Evaluation%20Instrument%20(2018-05-31)%20published.pdf

Association of American Medical Colleges (AAMC). (2008). *A report of the AAMC-AAU Advisory Committee on Financial Conflicts of Interest in Human Subjects Research. Protecting patients, preserving integrity, advancing health: Accelerating the implementation of COI policies in human subjects research.* www.aamc.org/download/482216/data/protectingpatients.pdf

Association of American Medical Colleges (AAMC). (2018). *Convey global disclosure system.* www.convey.org/?_ga=2.165499900.2138644705.1557755296-1067355313.1556116852

Centers for Medicare and Medicaid Services (CMS). (2019). *Open payments.* www.cms.gov/openpayments/

Congressional Research Service. (2014). *Federal financial conflict of interest rules and biomedical research: A legal overview.* www.everycrsreport.com/reports/R43693.html

Department of Health and Human Services (DHHS). (2000). *Office of Inspector General. Recruiting human subjects: Pressures in industry-sponsored clinical research* (OEI-01-97-00195). oig.hhs.gov/oei/reports/oei-01-97-00195.pdf

Department of Health and Human Services (DHHS). (2004). *Final guidance document: Financial relationships and interests in research involving human subjects: Guidance for human subject protection.* www.hhs.gov/ohrp/regulations-and-policy/guidance/financial-conflict-of-interest/index.html

Department of Health and Human Services (DHHS). (2011). Code of Federal Regulations. 42 CFR Part 50, Subpart F and 45 CFR Part 94. Responsibility of applicants for promoting objectivity in research for which public health service funding is sought and responsible prospective contractors. www.govinfo.gov/content/pkg/FR-2011-08-25/pdf/2011-21633.pdf

Department of Health and Human Services (DHHS). (2013). Code of Federal Regulations. 42 CFR Part 403, Subpart I. Medicare, Medicaid, Children's Health Insurance Programs; Transparency reports and reporting of physician ownership or investment interests. www.govinfo.gov/content/pkg/FR-2013-02-08/pdf/FR-2013-02-08.pdf

Eichenwald, K., & Kolata, G. (1999, May 16). Drug trials hide conflicts for doctors. *The New York Times.* www.nytimes.com/1999/05/16/business/drug-trials-hide-conflicts-for-doctors.html

Friedman, P. J. (1992). The troublesome semantics of conflict of interest. *Ethics and Behavior, 2*(4), 245–251.

International Committee of Medical Journal Editors. (2019). *Conflicts of interest.* icmje.org/recommendations/browse/roles-and-responsibilities/author-responsibilities--conflicts-of-interest.html

Kowalczyk, L. (2000, August 16). Drug trials branch from teaching hospitals: Suburban doctors answer call to help. *The Boston Globe,* p. C01.

Lightfoot, G., Getz, K. A., Harwood, F., Hovde, M., Rauscher, S. M., Reilly, P., & Vogel, J. R. (1998). *Faster time to market.* Association of Clinical Research Professionals. www.acrpnet.org/whitepaper2/white_paper-home.html

McCrary, S. V., Anderson, C. B., Jakovljevic, J., Khan, T., McCullough, L. B., Wray, N. P., & Brody, B. A. (2000). A national survey of policies on disclosure of conflicts of interest in biomedical research. *New England Journal of Medicine, 343*(22), 1621–1625.

Mervis, J. (1995). Conflict of interest: Final rules put universities in charge. *Science, 269*(5222), 294.

Morin, K., Rakatansky, H., Riddick, F. A., Jr, Morse, L. J., O'Bannon, J. M., 3rd, Goldrich, M. S., Ray, P., Weiss, M., Sade, R. M., & Spillman, M. A. (2002). Managing conflicts of interest in the conduct of clinical trials. *JAMA, 287*(1), 78–84.

National Bioethics Advisory Commission. (2001). *Ethical and policy issues in research involving human participants.* U.S. Government Printing Office. bioethics.gov/pubs.html

National Commission for the Protection of Human Subjects of Biomedical and Behavioral Research. (1978). *Report and recommendations: Institutional review boards* (DHEW (OS) 78-0008). Department of Health, Education, and Welfare.

National Institutes of Health (NIH). (2000a). *Transcript of conference on human subject protection and financial conflicts of interest* (Aug. 15–16, 2000). wayback.archive-it.org/3929/20160202182800/http://archive.hhs.gov/ohrp/coi/index.htm

National Institutes of Health (NIH). (2000b). *Financial conflicts of interest and research objectivity: Issues for investigators and institutional review boards.* grants.nih.gov/grants/guide/notice-files/NOT-OD-00-040.html

National Institutes of Health, Office of the Director (NIH). (2005, February 1). NIH announces sweeping ethics reform. *NIH News.* www.nih.gov/news

National Library of Medicine. (2019). *ClinicalTrials.gov.* clinicaltrials.gov/ct2/home

Pharmaceutical Research and Manufacturers of America. (2018). *2018 Biopharmaceutical industry profile.* phrma-docs.phrma.org/industryprofile/2018/pdfs/2018_IndustryProfile_Brochure.pdf

Saver, R. S. (2012). Is it really all about the money? Reconsidering non-financial interests in medical research. *Journal of Law, Medicine & Ethics, 40,* 467–481.

Spece, R. G., Jr., Shimm, D. S., & Buchanan, A. E. (1996). *Conflicts of interest in clinical practice and research.* Oxford University Press.

Steinbrook, R. (2004). Financial conflicts of interest and the NIH. *New England Journal of Medicine, 350*(4), 327–330.

Weinfurt, K. P., Hall, M. A., King, N. M. P., Friedman, J. Y., Schulman, K. A., & Sugarman, J. (2009). Disclosure of financial relationships to participants in clinical trials. *New England Journal of Medicine, 361,* 916–921.

World Medical Association. (2013). *Declaration of Helsinki: Ethical principles for medical research involving human subjects* (last amended 2013). www.wma.net/what-we-do/medical-ethics/declaration-of-helsinki/

Conflicts of Interest: Institutional Review Boards

Ross Hickey
Daniel K. Nelson

Abstract

This chapter discusses conflicts of interest that may influence the objectivity of the IRB. Given their role, IRBs must be mindful to mitigate any bias when conducting their review of studies and must take proactive steps to manage any potential conflicts when they arise. The first part of the chapter discusses commonly encountered conflicts either experienced by individual members or impacting the IRB as an entity. These conflicts include serving as a researcher on the study under review; holding significant financial interest in the study or sponsor; loyalty to colleagues submitting a study for review; pressure to protect or enhance the institution, its reputation, or prestige; potential liability concerns; pressure for speedy reviews; and revenue from study review fees. The second part of the chapter outlines options for managing these conflicts of interest when they arise, particularly in the context of IRB deliberations and voting.

Introduction

Given the central role of IRBs in overseeing the ethical conduct of research involving human subjects, it is critical that they operate free from inappropriate influence. Accordingly, IRB members, chairs, and staff should follow policies and procedures similar to those for researchers in order to eliminate or minimize any conflicts of interest. In this context, a *conflict of interest* can be defined as "any situation or relationship that biases or has the potential to bias the conduct or outcome of IRB review." This chapter reviews conflicts of interest that may be faced by either the IRB as an organizational entity or the individuals that contribute to the IRB's mission.

Possible sources of conflict of interest for IRBs are listed in the sidebar. These might originate or be experienced at individual or institutional levels. None of these scenarios or factors, in and of themselves, may represent unmanageable conflicts. However, any of these could exert inappropriate influence on the IRB and should be considered.

Sources of IRB Conflict of Interest: Individual Level

Research by Members

Perhaps the most widely recognized conflict of interest for IRBs is when research conducted by one of the IRB members comes up for review. The researcher-member has an obvious interest in seeing the research approved for a number of personal and professional reasons. (See Chapter 12-6 for discussion of conflicts of interest facing researchers). This type of conflict is usually apparent, so proper management is largely a procedural matter. However, beyond this direct conflict involving review of members' own research, there are multiple sources for indirect conflict of interest. These may be harder to discern and, therefore, harder to manage.

POSSIBLE SOURCES OF CONFLICT OF INTEREST FOR IRBS

Individual Level

- Member involved in the research under review
- Members or staff hold significant financial interest in study or sponsor
- Loyalty to colleagues submitting for review
- Members closely tied to area of research under review
  - Familiar = too lenient
  - Competitor = too critical
- Possible impact of decisions on member's own work (e.g., policy changes)
- Personal agendas or advocacy positions
- Non-IRB roles of members
  - Grants management or sponsored programs office
  - Legal counsel
  - Risk management

Institutional Level

- Pressure or desire to protect institution
- Concern for institution's reputation or prestige
- Pressure to conform with other members
- Promoting research versus protecting subjects
- Undervaluation of IRB service
- Potential liability
- Institutional or community values
- Pressure for speedy reviews
- Institutional equity or ownership
- Review fees

Members' Financial Interests

One example of these less apparent conflicts is the situation in which an IRB member (or IRB staff member) holds significant equity or other financial interests in the research itself or in the sponsors of research. These might include equity holdings, consulting arrangements, or patent rights—in short, the same types of financial conflicts that researchers might hold. McCrary et al. (2000) showed that, although the majority of academic research institutions have policies governing financial conflicts of interest, these tend to focus on faculty serving as researchers and not as IRB members. The same concerns would apply, however, regarding the objectivity of individuals who stand to gain financially from research they are being asked to review and approve.

Loyalty to Colleagues

Another potential source of conflict is loyalty to colleagues submitting research for IRB review, who may be peers, subordinates, or superiors. IRB members might logically be inclined to support the work of departmental colleagues with whom they interact every day (i.e., more directly than they interact with other IRB members). Beyond mere camaraderie, IRB members may sense a need to promote the work of subordinates or to avoid antagonizing their chief with a critical review. At a practical level, this conflict may be difficult to avoid, because few institutions are large enough to assemble a panel of individuals with sufficient insight who do not also have overlapping interactions with colleagues submitting research.

Members' Areas of Expertise

Selection of IRB members with sufficient expertise to comprehend the complexities of the research under review presents another potential problem. Members whose training or own area of research is closely tied to the studies under review may tend to show more leniency than they might to other areas with which they are less familiar. That is, it may be natural for them to take novel issues or procedures for granted. Conversely, this familiarity might work in the opposite direction if reviewers regard other researchers as competitors or rivals and are thus more critical than they might be otherwise. IRB members in this position might also find themselves with access to proprietary information when reviewing studies, providing tempting insight to ongoing research in their personal area of interest (in essence, a form of "insider trading"). Whether overly lenient or overly critical, neither tendency is conducive to the objective review that the IRB should strive to achieve.

This potential for biased reviews may be something for institutions to consider before establishing "specialty boards" as a means of focusing expertise in a given area. The increased insight that comes with this structure must be viewed as a trade-off for decreased diversity of perspectives.

Impact of Decisions

IRB members might also be mindful of the possible impact of IRB decisions on their own work. For example, an IRB member who does clinical outcome studies may be reluctant to support IRB decisions that strengthen privacy protection, if these lead to policies that restrict their own access to medical records or otherwise impede their ability to conduct research.

Personal Agendas

Personal agendas of IRB members may also interfere with the review process. For example, members of an advocacy group for a given disease or disorder can yield valuable insight as community representatives, but can represent a negative influence if they see their role as promoting a certain agenda, to the detriment of objective, independent review.

Non-IRB Roles

The institutional roles filled by IRB members in their daily work outside the IRB may carry inherent conflicts of interest. For example, the director of the office of sponsored programs, whose primary duties revolve around bringing more research funding into the institution, may not be an appropriate individual to serve on the IRB. The same could be said for any institutional official charged with promoting or supporting the research enterprise, if that obligation might run counter to a critical assessment of studies. Indeed, reliance on individuals with these types of positional conflicts has been cited as an unacceptable situation in federal compliance actions (Department of Health and Human Services [DHHS], 2019). Because of this, the Association for the Accreditation of Human Research Protections (AAHRPP) requires that <u>accredited organizations</u>   🔗 8-7
ensure ethical review is separated from "competing business interests" through its written policies (AAHRPP, 2019, Element II.1.C.).

Another institutional role that may exclude a person from IRB service is that of the in-house counsel. Although legal counsel can be extremely helpful in an advisory capacity, a primary concern for any attorney is effective representation of their client. In this situation their client is the institution and not the human subjects. It can be argued that these goals are not incompatible to the extent that "a happy subject is a happy institution," but care must be exercised to avoid conflicting objectives.

The preceding discussion should not detract from the clear benefit of having IRB members with legal training, which is increasingly important for interpreting and applying regulations, ensuring compliance with state laws, and multiple other functions. Similarly, members with insight on the financing of research or those with roles in some aspect of risk management, can provide valuable input to IRB deliberations. Nevertheless, care should be taken when appointing members who may wear other institutional hats while also serving the IRB.

Sources of IRB Conflicts of Interest: Institutional Level

Protecting the Institution

Although individual IRB members may have an internalized desire to protect the institution, the institution must avoid placing external pressure on the IRB to serve this role. This may be a natural expectation for high-ranking officials (e.g., deans, provosts, presidents), and, although it is not necessarily incompatible with the role of the IRB, protecting the institution should never be confused with the primary role of the IRB to protect human subjects. This separation of roles will be especially important as penalties for noncompliance continue to increase and institutions come to view their IRBs as a chief means of preventing regulatory sanctions.

Enhancing the Institution

In a more positive direction, a related source of conflict could arise from IRB members' innate concerns for their institution's reputation or prestige, to the extent that this is enhanced through an active research portfolio. Once again, this desire is not incompatible with sound IRB review, but should never be an excuse for relaxing standards in the review of research.

Promoting Research

Yet another related concern is the desire on the part of individual IRB members and on the part of the IRB as an agent of the institution to promote research in general. This is a laudable goal but should never be pursued to the extent that it detracts from the IRB's mission to protect the rights and welfare of human subjects.

Undervalued Membership

Undervaluation of service to the IRB is another factor that could translate into a conflict of interest. If members do not believe that their work on the IRB is appreciated or valued by their superiors, they may not believe that they can or should devote the time necessary to do the job well. One national survey of medical school faculty members indicated that only 11% of the respondents served on an IRB in the preceding 3 years. The authors speculated this may be the result of a lack of recognition for the service within the respondents' institutions (Campbell et al., 2003). Department chairs, deans, and other institutional officials should send a clear signal that IRB membership is a necessary and important activity and recognize such service when considering promotions, tenure, and clinical work schedules. Some institutions are going beyond this by purchasing or "protecting" a percentage of faculty effort for IRB service.

Liability

The potential for legal liability is another factor that could influence an IRB's decision making. Although lawsuits implicating the IRB have been few in number, the threat of lawsuit is an ever-present possibility in our litigious society. There is no public record of a successful judgment against an IRB member, but it is difficult to know the details concerning civil cases settled outside of court. Possible sources of lawsuits include not only subjects who have been injured in research, but also researchers who believe their research has been unfairly hindered by an IRB. Most institutions are likely to indemnify IRB members in the performance of their professional duties, acting in good faith on behalf of the institution. This is an area where IRBs should consult with their legal counsel to determine the extent of coverage and representation, as this will vary across institutions.

Institutional or Community Values

Institutional or community values are sources of possible conflict, to the extent these values may be reflected in reviews by individual IRB members or the IRB as a whole. Clearly, there is a regulatory mandate requiring the IRB to be sensitive to community attitudes, but there may be times when these values run counter to the mission of the IRB [45 CFR 46.107(a); 21 CFR 56.107(a)]. For example, some institutions may be particularly sensitive to social or political issues (e.g., abortion) in ways that run counter to regulatory guidance that IRBs should not consider the long-range public policy implications of research under review [45 CFR 46.111(a)(2)]. This separation from institutional values may admittedly be difficult to achieve when beliefs are deeply held.

The mandate for sensitivity to community values highlights the importance of nonaffiliated IRB members. All members must feel their perspective is welcome regardless of how well it aligns with the mission of the institution. There can be an unfortunate perception that these members are expected to be quiet and not ask questions. The pressure to not "stick out" is higher when the composition of the board is mostly from similar backgrounds or disciplines or made up of "experts." This pressure can be subtle, with IRB members not even aware when they are "going along to get along" or engaging in "groupthink" (Saver, 2004). If an IRB member is not reviewing a study independently, but as part of the board collective, the danger increases that the influence from the rest of the committee will bias their objectivity. Community members who have served for many years on an IRB or who possess similar credentials to the researchers or fellow IRB members may run a greater risk of this conformity. Just as a clear signal should be sent that IRB membership is a necessary and important activity for affiliated members, nonaffiliated members should be given tangible evidence that their service is valued.

Pressure for Speed and Lack of Time

IRB members or staff often come under pressure from individual researchers or from the institution for quick turnaround time on review and approval. At larger institutions with high volumes of studies, the typical monthly convened meeting may offer insufficient time to conduct thorough reviews, even when the meeting is several hours long. Although it is in everyone's best interest to establish systems for review that are both effective and efficient, the process should not be hastened to the point that important issues are overlooked.

Institutional Holdings or Interests

Institutions are increasingly entering agreements with industry that may create conflicts of interest for the institution itself. These arrangements might include patent rights for new innovations, spin-off companies, technology licensing, or equity holdings. If an institution will be conducting research in which it bears a direct financial interest, appropriate firewalls should be in place to ensure that the IRB's ethical oversight is not subject to influence from the institution. If the independence of the IRB cannot be assured, it may be preferable to solicit the services of another IRB or to conduct the research at other institutions. (Institutional conflict of interest is addressed in more detail in Chapter 12-8).

Review Fees

Finally, the charging of review fees may create a conflict of interest that biases IRB review. Institutions that compete successfully for federal grant support receive a sizable percentage in the form of indirect costs, which are intended to support a variety of functions necessary to conduct research. Many institutions, perhaps the majority, have begun charging review fees for industry-sponsored studies as a means of generating additional support for the IRB. These fees, ranging from a few hundred to a few thousand dollars, are legitimate sources of revenue for work performed. All parties should be clear, however, that the fees are linked to study submissions and are not contingent on approval by the IRB. It is also highly advisable that the fees be administered through mechanisms separate from the IRB (e.g., sponsored programs office, billing department, or other administrative entities) so that the IRB is not placed in the position of bill collector. Ideally, the IRB should operate in complete ignorance of the billing status of any individual studies.

This also presents a conflict for independent, for-profit IRBs, which may derive their entire revenue from such fees. There is nothing inherently improper in this arrangement, and many independent IRBs conduct credible, ethical review. They are, however, subject to an added element of conflict because they are businesses in their own right. This makes them dependent on the good will and satisfaction of their clients (e.g., pharmaceutical companies or contract research organizations), who are free to take their business elsewhere. This might logically occur if reviews were consistently perceived as being picky, unfavorable, or slow. Thus, independent IRBs may be subject to conflict of interest pressures over and above those facing institution-based IRBs. Conversely, it can be argued that independent IRBs are free from many of the influences discussed previously because they are not subject to institutional expectations and pressures. Each setting has its own set of motivating factors to be considered, and neither is free from conflicts of interest.

Regulatory Requirements and Best Practices

If the IRB is to function in an independent, unbiased manner, it must not be subject to inappropriate pressures. Recognizing this, federal regulations specifically addressed IRB conflict of interest long before researcher conflict of interest became a focus of regulatory guidance. Regulations from both the Department of Health and Human Services (DHHS) and the Food and Drug Administration (FDA) instruct that:

> No IRB may have a member participate in the IRB's initial or continuing review of any project in which the member has a conflicting interest, except to provide information requested by the IRB. **[45 CFR 46.107; 21 CFR 56.107]**

This means that each IRB should have clearly defined mechanisms for identifying conflicts among its members and for excluding conflicted members from a situation where review may be compromised. AAHRPP (2019) standards reinforce this regulatory requirement through Element II.1.D:

> The IRB or EC (Ethics Committee) has and follows written policies and procedures so that members and consultants do not participate in the review of research protocols or plans in which they have a conflict of interest, except to provide information requested by the IRB or EC.

AAHRPP also provides specific guidance on IRB conflict of interest through Tip Sheet 13 on "IRB or EC Member and Consultant Conflict of Interest," which outlines criteria and actions to be included in written policies (AAHRPP, 2013). This guidance identifies many of the sources discussed in this chapter, with an emphasis on financial conflicts of interest, and extends management to family members, as well as the individual IRB member.

Management of IRB Conflicts of Interest

In contrast to the enormous attention paid to researcher conflicts of interest, little attention has been paid to similar conflicts on the part of IRBs. This may be partly because IRBs are not involved directly with the actual conduct of the study and partly because those involved with ethical review are seen as somehow immune to baser instincts. Few authors or policymakers have specifically addressed the conflicts that might be faced by IRBs or the challenges created by conflict resolution (Spece, 1996). Although the IRB functions in a somewhat unique role within an institution, its mandate is analogous to other federally required review boards, such as institutional animal care and use committees and institutional biosafety committees. Experience drawn from developing the policies and procedures for these other committees' members can be instructive in developing similar approaches to managing conflicts of interest for IRB members. In addition, Saver (2004) suggests that IRBs would directly benefit from looking to approaches taken by corporate boards in such areas as institutional level conflicts, time and information constraints, groupthink, potential liability of members, and the need to value board membership service.

As with conflicts for researchers, the first (and perhaps most difficult) task is to recognize that a conflict exists. The written policies of the institution should define what the institution considers an actual conflict and the process that will be taken to identify a conflict for an IRB member. After this potential conflict is identified and acknowledged, steps should be taken as described next to eliminate or minimize its impact.

Member Recusal and Quorum

🔗 3-3   In the setting of a <u>convened meeting</u>, the most obvious solution is that the IRB member in question should physically leave the room (be recused) during consideration of that study. In some circumstances, the IRB may be placed in an untenable position if the physical absence of a conflicted member would force the loss of quorum (the minimum number of members present required by the regulations), thereby halting the meeting. This creates a catch-22 of sorts if the IRB would prefer that any conflicted member leave the room, yet needs that member present in order to meet regulatory requirements for quorum.

Under existing regulations, a majority of IRB members must be present to conduct review at a convened meeting. The minimum membership of an IRB is five, of which three (the minimum quorum for a five-member IRB) must be present [45 CFR 46.108(b), 21 CFR 56.108(c)]. In practice, most IRBs are much larger than this. For example, an IRB with 20 members will require 11 in attendance for a quorum, and will have 10 remaining after temporary recusal of a conflicted member. While it is likely that 10 members will have sufficient expertise to conduct the review, this number does not technically meet the quorum requirement for a 20-member IRB. For institutions with smaller IRBs, the best approach is to ensure that adequate numbers of members will be present so that quorum is never endangered. This can be accomplished through the use of alternates to cover absences, reminders on the days of meetings, and selection of members who will take seriously their commitment to attend. An alternate solution when quorum fails and the approaches discussed earlier are not successful is to seek an IRB where the conflict of interest does not exist, as described previously for conflicts involving institutional holdings.

Regulatory Guidance and Best Practices for Recusal

Regulatory guidance on the question of conflicted members leaving the room is vague and subject to interpretation. As previously noted, the regulations themselves only state that the conflicted member should not "participate" in the review of a given study. In its most recent guidance on this matter, FDA (2019) clarified that:

> The quorum is the count of the number of [voting] members present. If the number present falls below majority, the quorum fails. The regulations only require that a member who is conflicted not participate in the deliberations and voting on a study on which he or she is conflicted. The IRB may decide whether an individual should remain in the room.

This suggests that IRBs have the discretion to keep the conflicted member present but that removing them from the room could endanger quorum, which both FDA and Office for Human Research Protections (OHRP) have cited in the past as a finding of noncompliance.

AAHRPP has taken the position that the IRB members who have a conflict of interest do not count toward quorum (AAHRPP, 2013). In whatever way the recusal of conflicted members is handled, study files and minutes of IRB meetings should reflect the identity of members recused for deliberations or voting. AAHRPP recommends that "policies and procedures for writing IRB or EC minutes [should] indicate that the name of the person with a conflict of interest must be recorded for each applicable vote" (AAHRPP, 2013). Given the increasing attention to detail in minutes, it may be advisable to also note the nature of the member's conflict that led to recusal.

IRB Reporting Structure

Beyond the recusal of researcher-members for deliberations or voting on their own studies, the more systemic forms of conflict may be more difficult to manage, but they are no less important. Attention should be paid to the placement of the IRB within the institution and resulting reporting relationships, as well as to institutional policies that might negate some of the influences already discussed.

🔗 2-1, 2-2

Selection of IRB Members

One of the most effective mechanisms to manage IRB conflict of interest lies in the appointment of a diverse membership (DHHS, 2004). This includes, but is not limited to, recruitment of unaffiliated members not beholden to the host institution [**45 CFR 46.107(c)**; **21 CFR 56.107(d)**]. Consideration of potential conflict of interest should be given when selecting members from inside the institution. Involvement in research gives valuable and necessary insight and should not exclude a potential member from serving on an IRB. However, if circumstances would lead a member to be recused from a majority of studies considered, which might occur in settings where a single researcher or department accounts for a disproportionate amount of the institution's total research portfolio, they may not be a good choice. This creates a dilemma in populating the IRB with sufficient expertise to review studies while simultaneously avoiding conflicts of interest, because the individuals with the greatest insight into scientific aspects of studies under review may also be conflicted. The potential for problems when institutional roles outside of service to the IRB run counter to a primary focus on protecting subjects has already been discussed. This may especially be true in smaller institutions, where individuals may be forced to wear multiple hats.

🔗 3-1

Education

As with every other aspect of human subjects protections, proactive education is another important component of an effective conflict management strategy. Researchers, IRB members and staff, and institutional officials should all be made aware of existing policies and of the potential for conflicts of interest in their own activities. This may be especially relevant for IRB personnel, who may be accustomed to looking for conflicts in the researchers they oversee but not in themselves. The OHRP at DHHS has issued guidance on financial relationships and interests in human subjects research that includes a section on IRB operations and members, providing perhaps the first federal guidance specifically directed at this group of individuals (DHHS, 2004). Along with reiterating the need for education and training activities in this area, this guidance adds financial interests to the conflicts IRB chairs and members should be

🔗 8-5 🔗 8-4

mindful of during the review process. This guidance suggests that IRBs remind their members of policies at the outset of each meeting, providing members with the opportunity to consider any personal conflicts relating to the study they are about to review. They should then follow clear procedures for recusal from deliberations and voting, as previously discussed, and document these actions.

Conclusion

Any conflicts of interest on the part of the IRB undermine the credibility of the process and must be avoided at all costs. Whether a particular influence is real or perceived, originates from within or without, or is felt consciously or subconsciously, IRBs are not immune from conflicts of interest. No one doubts the integrity or motivation of those serving to protect human subjects, but IRB personnel are no more or less human than the researchers they oversee and can only benefit from self-awareness in areas that might impact IRB effectiveness.

References

Association for the Accreditation of Human Research Protection Programs (AAHRPP). (2013). *Tip sheet 13: IRB or EC member and consultant conflict of interest.* admin.aahrpp.org /Website%20Documents/Tip_sheet_13_IRB_or_EC_Member_and_Consultant_Conflict _of_Interest.PDF

Association for the Accreditation of Human Research Protection Programs (AAHRPP). (2019). *Accreditation standards.* www.aahrpp.org/apply/web-document-library/domain-ii-institutional -review-board-or-ethics-committee

Campbell, E. G., Weissman, J. S., Clarridge, B., Yucel, R., Causino, N., & Blumenthal, D. (2003). Characteristics of medical school faculty members serving on institutional review boards: Results of a national survey. *Academic Medicine, 78*(8), 831–836.

Department of Health and Human Services (DHHS). (2004). *Final guidance document: Financial relationships and interests in research involving human subjects: Guidance for human subject protection.* www.hhs.gov/ohrp/regulations-and-policy/guidance/financial-conflict-of-interest/index .html

Department of Health and Human Services (DHHS). (2019). *OHRP determination letters and other correspondence.* www.hhs.gov/ohrp/compliance-and-reporting/determination-letters/index.html

Food and Drug Administration (FDA). (2019). *Information sheet guidance for institutional review boards (IRBs), clinical investigators, and sponsors.* www.fda.gov/science-research/guidance-documents -including-information-sheets-and-notices/information-sheet-guidance-institutional-review -boards-irbs-clinical-investigators-and-sponsors

McCrary, S. V., Anderson, C. B., Jakovljevic, J., Khan, T., McCullough, L. B., Wray, N. P., & Brody, B. A. (2000). A national survey of policies on disclosure of conflicts of interest in biomedical research. *New England Journal of Medicine, 343*(22), 1621–1626.

Saver, R. S. (2004). Medical research oversight from the corporate governance perspective: Comparing institutional review boards and corporate boards. *William & Mary Law Review, 46*(2), 619–730.

Spece, R. G., Jr, Shimm, D. S., & Buchanan, A. E. (1996). *Conflicts of interest in clinical practice and research.* Oxford University Press.

Conflicts of Interest: Institutions

Ross E. McKinney, Jr.
Heather H. Pierce

Abstract

This chapter discusses the unique and significant risks institutional conflicts of interest pose to the institution, to the work of the IRB in protecting research subjects, and to the integrity of research. Institutions and IRBs are familiar with the identification and management of individual researcher conflicts of interest, but when a conflict of interest is created by the interests or investments of the institution itself or its institutional leaders, detailed policies and clear communication across the institution are essential for the identification, evaluation, and management of these situations.

What Is an Institutional Conflict of Interest?

The mechanisms for considering and addressing the conflicts of interest of researchers, IRB members, institutional officials, and institutions differ, but are all rooted in the common understanding that an effective research enterprise seeks to identify conditions that could jeopardize the safety of research subjects or the integrity of the research. An influential 2009 Institute of Medicine report defined a *conflict of interest* as "a set of circumstances that creates a risk that professional judgment or actions regarding a primary interest will be unduly influenced by a secondary interest" (Lo & Field, 2009). In the context of research with human subjects, the focus of both policies and public concern is when the primary interest of conducting ethical research could be compromised by a secondary interest such as personal financial gain or desire to maintain a relationship with a company that has a stake in the outcome of the research.

An *institutional conflict of interest* in research describes one of two situations: (1) when the financial interests of an institution could influence the conduct of the

🔗 2-1   research or the integrity of the <u>human research protections program</u> or (2) when a senior leader of the institution has a personal financial interest that could have an impact on how research taking place at the institution is approved, conducted, or reported. The individuals whose personal interests are considered relevant are identified through an institutional conflict of interest policy and are known as *covered officials*. The justification for considering covered officials' interests as potential conflicts of interest of the institution reflects the concern that high-ranking individuals may hold sufficient authority over the activities of the institution and could influence the decision to engage in a specific research study, the study review process, or the conduct of the research. Even without direct involvement of the senior official in the research or the research review process, it could be perceived that an institution was swayed to conduct certain research because a chief executive was personally invested in the company that funded the research.

DEFINITION: INSTITUTIONAL CONFLICT OF INTEREST

- Financial interests of an institution could influence the conduct of the research or the integrity of the human research protections program; *or*
- A senior leader of the institution has a personal financial interest that could have an impact on how research taking place at the institution is approved, conducted, or reported.

The *financial interests* under consideration when addressing institutional conflicts of interest can include payments, grants, royalties, or gifts received by the institution and equity (private or public) and intellectual property (including patents) held by the institution. In terms of dollar values, there is no fixed threshold over which institutional conflicts of interest automatically become a concern. Institutions set thresholds for conflict of interest review based on the level of risk they see at different levels of investment, and they may or may not have different thresholds for covered officials' interests than for those of the institution itself.

In these policies, private equity is often required to be disclosed and reviewed regardless of the current value of the interest. Private equity holdings in start-up companies are a particular concern. As part of the development process for new drugs, devices, or diagnostics, start-up companies may be created to commercialize the institution's intellectual property through preclinical development, clinical trials, FDA approval, and marketing. In many cases, the institution licenses its intellectual property to the start-up company in exchange for equity in the new venture and the promise of future royalties from patents. Although that equity has no initial short-term value or liquidity, if the idea or eventual product is successful, the company's worth will increase with resulting benefit to the institution, creating powerful incentives for researchers and for the institution to conduct the research and report successful outcomes.

Why Institutional Conflicts of Interest Matter

There are three overarching reasons to be concerned about institutional conflicts of interest: (1) the safety of individuals in a clinical study, (2) the potential for bias in the research, and (3) the reputational risk to the institution if an institutional conflict of interest is identified and publicized after the study.

In terms of safety, the primary concern is that a researcher's judgment could be impaired by the knowledge that the institution that employs the researcher or an institutional leader has a financial interest that could be affected by the conduct or the outcome of the research. A researcher may not put research subjects' interests first if they perceive that an operational or analytical decision could harm the institution's interests or those of an institutional leader. Similarly, there is the concern that an IRB may feel pressure to act in a manner that benefits the institution. For instance, if a company in which the institution has invested or holds equity is looking for clinical sites for early-stage trials of a new drug, that institution's IRB might feel obliged to approve the research, even if there were risks to subjects that would otherwise cause the IRB to reject the proposed research. There is also the perception that an institution might be less diligent in its research oversight if that would be advantageous to the institution's financial position.

⏾ 12-7

Bias on the part of a researcher can manifest in a systematic interpretation of research data that is skewed by an external motivator. In the case of institutional conflict of interest, the worry is that researchers may interpret data in a skewed way if they think a particular interpretation might help their institution or a senior leader on whom the researcher depends for career advancement. Bias can be conscious or unconscious, and although there are instances of research misconduct (falsification or fabrication) to achieve an end, in most cases the bias on the part of the researchers is unconscious. They are unaware that the conflict raised in some cases by financial interests are affecting their judgment. Rationalization of unconsciously biased actions may affect the research results and thus the research integrity or the safety of research subjects. The review of institutional conflicts of interest does not itself identify bias (Lo & Field, 2009). Rather, it serves to identify and mitigate those situations that have the potential to create bias. A bias that might be created through a competing interest can be effectively neutralized by removing the competing interest, rather than trying to define or quantify the specific bias (McKinney & Pierce, 2017).

⏾ 12-6

The reputational risk of institutional conflicts is real and is generally tied to attribution. Clinical research often means some level of risk for the research subjects, but when one or more individuals is harmed through participation in a study, human nature will lead people to question why. If the institution or a significant supervisory person had a financial interest in the outcome of the research, it is highly likely the bad outcome will be attributed to the lack of institutional oversight. This is not to deny that it is possible that oversight issues really did exist, but, regardless of the strength of the institution's *a priori* efforts to prevent harm, it may well be blamed after the fact.

In 1999, in one of the seminal events spurring the development of current conflict of interest programs, Jesse Gelsinger died tragically as a result of his participation in a gene therapy clinical trial at the University of Pennsylvania (Stolberg, 1999). All three of the identified concerns related to institutional conflicts of interest—safety, bias, and institutional reputation—were thrust to the forefront of conflict of interest discussions after the revelations of the institution's financial interest in the outcome of the research. The company that developed the gene transfer protocol was a donor to the University of Pennsylvania's research program and retained rights to develop products based on the outcome of the research. The university and senior leaders in their individual capacity had also invested in the company, which had been founded by the lead researcher (Steinbrook, 2008).

⏾ 1-2

Although the need for principled collaborations and relationships between academic institutions and companies that make drugs and devices has been well recognized, examples of undue influence and financial interests that have led to bias mean that institutions must remain vigilant in assessing the risk of conflicts of interest and the impact that they carry for the institution's reputation (Pizzo et al., 2017). Public awareness of the potential impact of institutional conflicts of interest has increased (Thomas & Ornstein, 2019), leading to renewed discussions at many institutions of whether, for example, the top officials at institutions are permitted to serve on the boards of directors of pharmaceutical or other life sciences companies (Anderson et al., 2014).

Regulations and Guidance

The difficulties in dealing with institutional conflicts of interest are compounded by the fact that there are no federal rules or regulations specifically addressing institutional conflict of interest policies or management.

The U.S. federal rules for identifying and addressing financial conflicts of interest in federally funded research consider only the financial interests of individual researchers. First promulgated in 1995 and revised in 2011, the regulations set forth a process through which institutions conducting research funded by the agencies of the Public Health Service (PHS), including the National Institutes of Health (NIH), must identify and manage conflicts of interest that could affect the research being proposed or undertaken (**42 CFR 50, subpart F**, Responsibility of Applicants for Promoting Objectivity in Research for Which PHS Funding Is Sought; NIH, 2020). Note that the regulations do not require individual researchers to disclose information to the funding agency, but instead rely on the institution to collect and review researchers' disclosures of "significant financial interests." The required identification of conflicts of interest is limited to the researchers who will be responsible for the design, conduct, or reporting of the research and does not apply to the financial interests held by the institution itself or the institution's senior officials.

In 2011, during the rule-making process to revise the PHS conflict of interest regulations, the U.S. Department of Health and Human Services Office of the Inspector General released a report expressing concern that the existing regulations did not include institutional conflicts of interest and urging the NIH to promulgate final regulations that addressed institutional conflicts of interest (DHHS, 2011). Despite this report's conclusions and a similar recommendation from the Institute of Medicine's 2009 report the revised regulations that went into effect in 2012 remained focused solely on the financial interests and conflicts of interest of individual researchers.

Voluntary Recommendations and Standards

In the absence of a federal mandate to have an institutional conflict of interest policy, organizations that conduct or oversee research can look to community standards, model policies, and published best practices to develop their own policies and standards. It is worth noting that one of the requirements of the PHS regulations on individual conflicts of interest is that every funded institution post their conflict of interest policy on a publicly available website. While there is no similar requirement for institutional conflict of interest policies, many research institutions have chosen to make their policies available as well.

A 2008 report by a task force convened by the Association of American Universities and the Association of American Medical Colleges (AAMC) noted that institutional conflicts of interest "are of special concern" in the conduct of human subjects research and renewed an earlier recommendation that all institutions have an institutional conflict of interest policy (AAMC, 2003, 2008). In the report, the task force asserted that when an institutional conflict of interest is identified, a determination as to whether or not the research should be conducted by the institution should be governed by a "rebuttable presumption" that the research *should not* be conducted there. The application of the rebuttable presumption should be a process involving the organization's conflict of interest office (or committee charged with reviewing institutional conflicts of interest) deciding (1) whether there are compelling circumstances that would overcome this presumption and (2) how the conflict should be managed to minimize the risks to the research subjects and the integrity of the research. The report also included an example policy that could be adapted by institutions.

In practice, the policies and procedures employed by institutions that have adopted some form of an institutional conflict of interest policy varies, with some setting forth explicit criteria that must be met before human subjects research may be conducted at the conflicted institution, and some identifying who will make such a determination and leaving the evaluation of the risk and appropriateness of conducting the research up to that reviewing individual or committee.

Accreditation organizations have incorporated the expectation that institutions have an institutional conflict of interest policy. The Association for the Accreditation of Human Research Protection Programs (AAHRPP) includes the following element in its accreditation standards: "The Organization has and follows written policies and procedures to identify, manage, and minimize or eliminate financial conflicts of interest of the Organization that could influence the conduct of the research or the integrity of the Human Research Protection Program" (AAHRPP, 2019). Although AAHRPP requires that institutions have an institutional conflict of interest policy in order to obtain or maintain accreditation of the program, the specifics of that policy—the implementation, degree of stringency, designation of certain positions as covered officials, or definitions of institutional conflict—are not specified.

⊘ 8-7

Prevalence of Institutional Conflict of Interest Policies

Despite the fact that there has been focus on the need to address institutional conflicts of interest since the death of Jesse Gelsinger, many institutions do not have robust policies and processes to identify and address institutional conflict of interest.

A survey of the 100 academic research institutions with the highest research funding in 2010 found that just over a quarter had institutional conflict of interest policies, which were more common in medical schools than in other research institutions (Resnik et al., 2016). The authors suggested that the increased likelihood that a medical school would have such a policy could be attributed to the attention that medical schools had paid to the issue. A previous study, conducted after the recommendations from the Association of American Medical Colleges and the Association of American Universities were published, supports this interpretation (Ehringhaus et al., 2008).

Managing Institutional Conflicts of Interest

The goals of institutional conflict of interest management are to address the three concerns listed earlier in this chapter and focus on (1) protecting research subjects, (2) mitigating bias, and (3) protecting institutional reputation. The fundamental approach is to determine whether the financial risk is significant enough to warrant management and, if it is, what steps to take. Most strategies involve introducing elements of independent or outside review or activities that remove the ability for a conflicted institution to affect the outcome of the ethical review or research outcomes (Resnik, 2019).

For human subjects research, a good approach to take is to identify all the places where institutional oversight might need to be replaced by an unbiased entity. Examples of this approach would be to use an IRB that is not affiliated with the conflicted institution, hire external monitors to evaluate the data as it is being collected to identify any unanticipated results that might pose risks to subjects, or require an independent biostatistician from outside the institution to conduct the data analysis. Forming an external data-safety monitoring board can allow for outside review of the study design, monitoring of its conduct, and evaluation of the publications to be sure they reflect the research in an unbiased way.

🖉 12-6   A common management strategy for <u>individual conflicts of interest</u> is to disclose the researcher's conflicts to potential research subjects through the informed consent document and process. Disclosure should also be used to inform the public about an institution's financial interest in the research and should be a part of publications and other communications about the research. However, disclosure through the informed consent process for subjects is insufficient as a sole management strategy for an identified institutional conflict of interest.

Communication with IRBs

Operationally, the challenge for both the conflict of interest program and for the IRB is to be aware of all relevant situations where the institution has an identified conflict of interest that should be incorporated in the ethical review of proposed human subjects research. Despite the number of institutions that have implemented institutional conflict of interest policies and the increased national attention to problems of institutional conflict of interest, there are few specific published recommendations on how and when information from the conflict of interest operations should be shared with the IRB.

🖉 12-6   In the <u>individual conflict of interest</u> review process, the conflict of interest office, and thus the IRB, relies on a researcher's complete and accurate disclosure of financial interests. Although additional sources of information should be used to verify or supplement these disclosures, it can be assumed that the researcher in question will be personally aware of the existence of each financial interest that may constitute an individual conflict of interest. However, information about an institution's interest in the research would typically not be disclosed by a researcher. Either the researcher would be unaware of the institution's interest in the research or, more likely, the researcher would have no reason to disclose to the institution an interest held by that institution.

For example, if an institution has invested in a start-up company founded by the principal investigator of a proposed clinical trial, both the institution and that investigator should be aware of the potential conflicts of interest at the individual and the institutional levels. However, the investigator may only disclose their own interest in the company, assuming the institutional investment is well known. The fact that institutional resources are committed to the company might not be communicated to the IRB reviewing the proposed research.

In addition to written policies on addressing institutional conflicts of interest, institutions need to build systems and communication channels that will reliably identify relevant institutional interests. This requires regular communication between the institution's technology transfer office, the conflict of interest program, and the IRB, so that any one of the offices that encounters a new and potentially patentable technology alerts the other offices. Designation of which office manages each aspect of the conflict of interest process is important, but the IRB needs the relevant information to understand how the research protocol, conduct, and analysis could impact research subject safety and the consent process.

Conclusion

Institutional conflicts of interest present specific risks and challenges in the protection of human subjects. Although there are no prescribed requirements for an institutional conflict of interest policy, the failure to have such a policy does not relieve the IRB of the need to know when the conduct or reporting of research might be compromised by the investments or financial interests of the institution where the research will be conducted. In assessing the risks to research subjects, an IRB should consider all the ways institutions' interests can impact the ethics of the research: although strong institutional policies and practices can strengthen the human research protection program, the financial interests of the institution and its leaders can threaten the integrity of the research.

References

Anderson, T. S., Dave, S., Good, C. B., & Gellad W. F. (2014). Academic medical center leadership on pharmaceutical company: Boards of directors. *JAMA, 311*(13), 1353–1355.

Association for the Accreditation of Human Research Protection Programs (AAHRPP). (2019). *Domain I accreditation standards.* http://aahrpp.org/apply/web-document-library/domain-i-organization

Association of American Medical Colleges (AAMC). (2003). Task force on financial conflicts of interest in clinical research. Protecting Subjects, Preserving Trust, Promoting Progress II: Principles and Recommendations for Oversight of an Institution's Financial Interests in Human Subjects Research. *Academic Medicine, 78*(2), 237–245.

Association of American Medical Colleges (AAMC). (2008). *Protecting patients, preserving integrity, advancing health: Accelerating the implementation of COI policies in human subjects research.* www.aamc.org/system/files/c/2/482216-protectingpatients.pdf

Department of Health and Human Services (DHHS). (2011). *Office of Inspector General: Institutional conflicts of interest at NIH grantees.* https://oig.hhs.gov/oei/reports/oei-03-09-00480.pdf

Ehringhaus, S. H., Weissman, J. S., Sears, J. L., Goold, S.D., Feibelmann, S., & Campbell, E. G. (2008). Responses of medical schools to institutional conflicts of interest. *JAMA, 299*(6), 665–671.

Lo, B., & Field, M. J. (2009). *Conflict of interest in medical research, education, and practice.* National Academies Press.

McKinney, R. E., & Pierce, H. H. (2017). Strategies for addressing a broader definition of conflicts of interest. *JAMA, 317*(17), 1727–1728.

National Institutes of Health (NIH). (2020). *Financial conflicts of interest.* https://grants.nih.gov/grants/policy/coi/index.htm

Pizzo, P. A., Lawley, T. J., & Rubenstein, A. H. (2017). Role of leaders in fostering meaningful collaborations between academic medical centers and industry while also managing individual and institutional conflicts of interest. *JAMA, 317*(17), 1729–1730.

Resnik, D. B. (2019). Institutional conflicts of interest in academic research. *Science and Engineering Ethics, 25*(6), 1661–1669.

Resnik D. B., Ariansen, J. L., Jamal, J., & Kissling, G. E. (2016). Institutional conflict of interest policies at U.S. academic research institutions. *Academic Medicine, 91*(2), 242–246.

Steinbrook, R. (2008). The Gelsinger case. In E. J. Emanuel, C. Grady, R. A. Crouch, R. Lie, F. Miller, & D. Wendler (Eds.), *The Oxford textbook of clinical research ethics*. Oxford University Press.

Stolberg, S. G. (1999, November 28). The biotech death of Jesse Gelsinger. *New York Times Magazine*. www.nytimes.com/1999/11/28/magazine/the-biotech-death-of-jesse-gelsinger.html

Thomas, K., & Ornstein. C. (2019, January 11). Memorial Sloan Kettering curbs executives' ties to industry after conflict-of-interest scandals. *The New York Times*. www.nytimes.com/2019/04/04/health/memorial-sloan-kettering-conflicts-.html

Patient and Community Engagement

Emily E. Anderson
Ryan Spellecy

Abstract

Patient and community engagement in research has resulted in great strides to improve the health of various communities. Patient and community engagement in research has also been increasing in the past decade, advancing the discussion of what constitutes ethical research and how researchers should best engage with groups outside of academia. For IRBs, this research presents unique ethical and regulatory issues that may be unfamiliar. This chapter will define patient and community engagement in research, highlight the ethical and regulatory issues that an IRB should consider when reviewing this research, and offer suggestions to better equip the IRB in fulfilling its obligation to review and provide oversight for these studies.

Introduction

In the past, researchers have conducted research in and on certain communities and patients without ever truly involving them. There are many lamentable stories of researchers dropping in, conducting their research, and then leaving without ever sharing the results with the community or patient group. This behavior has resulted in certain communities and populations feeling used, underappreciated, and distrustful of researchers. Such feelings exacerbate barriers to leveraging research to improve health disparities faced by these communities and patient groups (Yarborough et al., 2012).

In an attempt to avoid repeating mistakes of the past, and in recognition that ethical research should be done *with* communities and not *to* communities, unique research approaches have been developed. These approaches go by many names, which are listed in the box, Approaches to Patient- and Community-Centered Research. All of these approaches can be broadly understood as efforts to better engage populations that will be affected by the research in question in order to increase transparency, better protect subjects and communities, increase the relevance and benefits of the research, and more generally, respect those communities.

> ## APPROACHES TO PATIENT- AND COMMUNITY-CENTERED RESEARCH
>
> - Community-based participatory research (CBPR) (Israel et al., 1998)
> - Community-engaged research (CEnR) (Michener et al., 2012)
> - Patient-centered (or patient-centered outcomes) research (PCR/PCOR) (Concannon et al., 2014; Sheridan et al., 2017)

This chapter will outline key aspects of research that engages communities that IRBs should consider in reviewing research, establishing policies and procedures, and selecting board members. The phrase "research that engages communities" is used to include a broad range of approaches, methodologies, disciplines, and ideologies. *Communities* refers to groups of people living in the same geographic area or groups of geographically disparate people, including patients with a shared diagnosis, who identify as being part of a particular group. *Community partners* are organizations such as disease-focused education and advocacy groups, neighborhood associations, native tribes, centers that serve LGBTQ youth, school districts, patient groups organized around a disease, health service providers, and others. The term *community partner* can also refer to individuals not formally trained as researchers who are employees or volunteers at such organizations or who are collaborating with researchers without having a specific organizational affiliation.

Researchers use a variety of different strategies to engage communities, and the level of engagement can vary (**Figure 12.9-1**). Common strategies include forming community or patient advisory boards to provide direction on research methods, materials, and dissemination; hiring community partners to recruit research subjects, obtain informed consent, collect data, and/or deliver interventions; or including a community partner as a coinvestigator involved in the development and design of the study (see sidebar, Examples of Community and Patient Engagement in Research). In some cases, research is driven by communities; that is, the research question and design are generated by the community, and the university researcher/research team serves in a consulting rather than leading role.

The concept of "shared ownership" is a common thread across these approaches; that is, shared responsibility for the conduct of the research, shared ownership of the data, and joint decision making about the dissemination of results. Such efforts at engagement aim to ameliorate experiences and perceptions

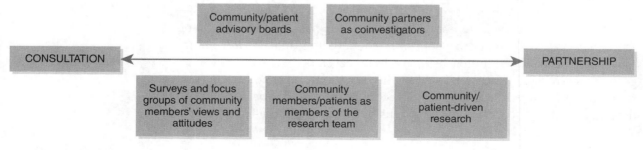

Figure 12.9-1 Types of engagement.

of being used and underappreciated, as well as mistrust, as noted earlier. Engaging communities in research also aims to increase transparency, decrease potential harms, and increase the potential for communities to benefit from research (Clinical and Translational Science Awards Consortium, 2011). Of course, these engagement efforts also carry with them unique ethical and regulatory challenges (Anderson et al., 2012; Mikesell et al., 2013).

Ethical and Regulatory Challenges in Patient and Community Engagement

Determining if a community partner is engaged in research. If a community organization or group is going to be involved in research, then there are certain regulatory considerations, some of which depend upon the federal definition of research "engagement." The federal regulations use the term "engaged" differently from how community-engaged researchers use it: "In general, an institution is considered *engaged* in a particular non-exempt human subjects research project when its employees or agents for the purpose of the research project obtain: 1) data about the subjects of the research through intervention or interaction with them; 2) identifiable private information about the subjects of the research; or 3) the informed consent of human subjects for the research" (Department of Health and Human Services [DHHS], 2008). According to Office for Human Research Protections (OHRP) guidance, before engaging in federally supported, nonexempt human research, an institution must hold or obtain an OHRP-approved <u>Federalwide Assurance (FWA)</u> and certify to the federal funding agency that the research has been reviewed and approved by an IRB designated in the FWA (DHHS, 2008).

🔗 8-1

IRBs must make the final determination as to whether or not a community partner agency is engaged in research, according to the federal definition. Research routinely takes place "in" the community, but the OHRP guidance is concerned with "who" rather than "where." Merely conducting research at a community partner's site does not necessarily mean that agency is engaged in research. If a community partner agency receives federal funds or if employees or volunteers from the organization are considered research personnel, then the agency is considered to be engaged in research.

Patient and community organizations rarely have an FWA or an IRB (although some <u>Native Tribes</u> do have formal IRBs with an FWA). Even completing FWA paperwork can be burdensome for a community partner agency. There are alternatives, such as designating community members on the research team as collaborating individual researchers (either independent or institutional) (Cargill et al., 2016; DHHS, 2017). This may be a preferable option unless a community agency or patient organization is going to frequently engage in research.

🔗 9-10

Regardless of whether or not a partner organization meets the federal definition of engaged or not, the IRB is responsible for confirming that any partner organization has agreed to the terms of the process outlined in the IRB-approved protocol. The researcher should provide the IRB with a letter from the partner organization noting that they have reviewed the research and approve of conducting the research at their site. Specific activities, conditions, and roles should be outlined in this letter to ensure consistency with what is in the protocol.

Determining the role of the community advisory board. Some research studies include CABs (Newman et al., 2011; Strauss et al., 2001). A CAB may be formed specifically for a research project, or a research project may utilize an

EXAMPLES OF COMMUNITY AND PATIENT ENGAGEMENT IN RESEARCH

Scenario 1: A university researcher is collaborating with a community-based service health provider to conduct a survey on those living with chronic obstructive pulmonary disease (COPD). Through a subcontract with the university, health agency employees will identify potential eligible subjects, approach them about the research, obtain informed consent, and collect private, identifiable data.

Scenario 2: A university researcher is collaborating with multiple community-based organizations (CBOs) to develop and test an intervention to address mental health issues in a low-income community. The study will be conducted in three separate phases:

1. Focus groups will be held in the community to assess community practices, interests, and attitudes around mental health.
2. The intervention will be designed, and additional focus groups will be held to ensure community acceptability.
3. The intervention will be pilot tested in a small randomized trial comparing it to a control group.

There will be a community advisory board (CAB) made up of representatives of the various CBOs that will provide input on all project materials and methods, including eligibility criteria, recruitment strategies and flyers, and intervention materials. They will also provide guidance on interpretation and dissemination of study findings. CBOs will assist in recruitment of research subjects in all phases by distributing project materials; interested individuals will call a centralized number staffed by a university employee who will then discuss study eligibility criteria and requirements with them. The intervention will take place at community sites, led by trained mental health professionals employed by the university. CBO employees will not be involved in obtaining informed consent or obtaining or analyzing data.

Scenario 3: A university researcher partners with a national patient advocacy organization to conduct a longitudinal study of individuals living with polycystic kidney disease. Recruitment and data collection will be conducted primarily online; subjects will be mailed a kit to collect saliva samples, which they will return by mail for genetic testing. The advocacy organization executive director is a named coinvestigator on the study.

existing community group as a CAB. CABs can play an important role in ensuring the protection of research subjects and the overall ethical conduct of the research. Although CABs vary in composition and function, their general role is to review research to ensure that it is consistent with the values of the community, protect the interests of the community, and make suggestions regarding research materials and implementation. For example, CABs can be instrumental in improving informed consent documents and other recruitment materials so that they are better understood by potential research subjects. CAB members usually do not have direct contact with research subjects or identifiable data and therefore may not be required to complete standard human research protections training. However, some training on the ethics of human research is recommended, as CABs often provide input on recruitment, informed consent, and data collection processes and materials.

Some studies aim to evaluate the partnership process or effectiveness of the collaboration. This may involve collecting data from CAB members, which may make them research subjects. This does not mean that CAB members are always research subjects, and such evaluation efforts can generally be considered exempt from IRB review and approval.

Determining appropriate human research protections training and providing ongoing support. The IRB or human research protection program (HRPP) is responsible for ensuring that everyone engaged in the conduct of the research has completed appropriate education in the protection of human research subjects (National Institutes of Health [NIH], 2000). It is important to consider that the training generally required for the HRPP's own faculty and employees may be unsuitable for community partners. Some commonly used online research ethics training courses include modules for community-engaged research; there are also stand-alone trainings specifically designed for community partners, who may have limited prior familiarity with research, limited formal education, and specific research responsibilities related to recruitment, informed consent, and data collection (Anderson, 2015; Nebeker, 2015; Solomon et al., 2014a; Solomon et al., 2014b; Solomon & Piechowski, 2011; Yonas et al., 2016).

In addition to initial training in human subjects protections, it is important to provide adequate supervision and ongoing support to those who may experience emotional distress and fatigue associated with recruiting research subjects and gathering data about one's own community (Simon & Mosavel, 2010).

Ensuring appropriate IRB expertise to review research that engages communities. According to **45 CFR 46.107**: "The IRB should be sufficiently qualified through the experience and expertise of its members (professional competence), and the diversity of its members, including race, gender, and cultural backgrounds and sensitivity to such issues as community attitudes, to promote respect for its advice and counsel in safeguarding the rights and welfare of human subjects... The IRB shall therefore include persons knowledgeable in these areas." Given the growth of community engagement in research, in large part driven by both federal (e.g., the NIH, the Centers for Disease Control, and the Patient-Centered Outcomes Research Institute) and private (e.g., the Bill and Melinda Gates Foundation, the Robert Wood Johnson Foundation) research funders, IRBs should include members with the appropriate expertise regarding engagement approaches as well as familiarity with the communities—local and patient—that university researchers frequently engage in their research. Bear in mind that while the regulations require the IRB to include a nonscientist and an unaffiliated member (and these can be the same person), there is no specific regulatory requirement for a "community member." It is, however, certainly advisable to include one or more individuals who meet this definition on the IRB roster (Anderson, 2006).

3-1

For IRBs that frequently review studies that engage communities in research, IRB members and staff should also complete specific training in community-engaged research. For issues related to a specific study, the IRB can avail itself of expert consultation. Just as an IRB might seek advice from a cardiologist if they had specific questions about a heart failure study, it should seek consultation from someone experienced with the community in question if there are study-specific questions, whether that is an individual or the study's CAB.

Considering community-level risks. In the literature and among IRBs, there has been some debate regarding the limitations placed on the IRB when considering risks to communities (Ross et al., 2010a). Specifically, in the context of how IRBs are to evaluate risks posed by a study, the IRB "should not consider possible long-range effects of applying knowledge gained in the research (e.g., the possible effects of the research on public policy) as among those research risks that fall within the purview of its responsibility" [**45 CFR 46.111(a)2**]. Some have interpreted this passage to preclude the IRB from considering the likely potential for long-term harm that may arise from research that engages defined communities, such as negative perceptions or group dissatisfaction that might be generated by the research findings. For example, a hypothetical study seeking to understand literacy levels in a specific community in order to better design interventions might further stigmatize that community by uncovering literacy rates that were lower than initially thought. Another study might investigate a community's views on cancer research, exposing generational differences in perceptions of the value and safety of research, which in turn leads to intergenerational disagreements and discord in the community. As a result of these limits on IRB authority, it is imperative that the IRB have good relations with researchers and community partners. If there are risks that are determined to be outside of the purview of the IRB's deliberations, then community partners, researchers, and CABs can step in to identify and mitigate those risks (Ross et al., 2010b).

Evaluating the potential threats to subject voluntariness of community partners' dual roles. Community research partners may have "dual roles" that may pose risks to the informed consent process and to voluntariness in particular (Anderson et al., 2012; Ross et al., 2010c). An intake coordinator at an Alcohol and Other Drug Abuse (AODA) treatment center routinely involved in research shared the following example: In her role as the intake coordinator, she regularly asks individuals seeking treatment to complete forms providing health histories and other personal information relevant to care planning. She also

Section 6

Case Study: The Havasupai Case and Long-Range Effects

After initially obtaining permission from Havasupai tribal leaders and consent from individual subjects for a diabetes study, researchers from Arizona State University used blood samples from the diabetes study for research on inbreeding in the tribe, schizophrenia, and to further prove the "Bering Strait Theory," which states that Native Americans arrived on the continent by travelling across the Bering strait via a land bridge. All of this additional research was done without the knowledge or consent of the subjects or the tribe leaders, causing harm to the tribe by questioning their cultural identity. As one tribe member stated, using their own blood to contradict their beliefs "hurts the elders who have been telling these stories to their grandchildren" (Harmon, 2010). In the Havasupai case, risks such as stigmatization of a community, intergenerational discord, or harms to a tribe's cultural identity could be considered "possible long-range effects" that the IRB should not consider.

frequently provides information about research to patients. While completion of the health history forms are *required* for admission to the AODA center, research is, of course, optional. However, making sure that this distinction is clear to someone who is desperately seeking treatment for their addiction and is well aware of the limited number of beds for inpatient treatment in the area can pose an ethical challenge. The person seeking inpatient treatment for addiction *must* complete paperwork handed to them by the intake coordinator—when they are acting as the intake coordinator. But when the intake coordinator switches roles and hands a flyer or consent form to the patient, that switch is difficult to understand, threatens the voluntariness of consent, and is exacerbated by the setting.

IRBs should pay special attention to the methods, location, and personnel involved in the process of recruitment and informed consent. In the previous scenario, it might be preferable for someone else to obtain consent, but the reality is that many community partners face staffing limitations and there is simply no one else available. If that is the case, the IRB should work with the researcher and community partner organization to seek solutions to ensure that consent is voluntary and that dual roles are explicit and understood by potential subjects.

Protecting privacy and confidentiality. Dual roles of community service providers also pose risks to privacy and confidentiality. In research that engages communities, community partners may be learning about, and be responsible for, protecting private information about people who are not just research subjects but *people they know in a different context*. Studies may collect sensitive information such as mental health diagnoses, HIV status, income, or participation in illegal or stigmatized behaviors.

For an employee at a community service organization, it might not be unusual in the course of a normal work day to learn of food insecurity from a participant in a preschool program. That employee might regularly place calls to the local food pantry to help the family. However, if that same information about food insecurity is obtained in the course of a focus group conducted for research purposes, making that same call to the food pantry may violate the promise of confidentiality made in the consent form. To that end, the IRB should pay close attention to possible incidental findings (expected or unexpected) and ensure, prior to approval, that plans are in place to meet the requirements of beneficence (both maximizing benefit and minimizing harm) while adhering to research norms about privacy and confidentiality. Specific consent form language should be reviewed carefully to avoid a conflict between breaking promises and protecting subjects from harm.

Conclusion

IRBs should be knowledgeable regarding the specific regulatory and ethical issues that may arise in research that engages communities, and the appropriate solutions to those challenges. However, there is evidence that suggests variation in how IRBs address ethical and regulatory concerns in research that engages communities and that some IRBs may adhere to best practices (Weissman et al., 2018). IRBs should include experts in community-engaged research approaches who are knowledgeable about the communities with which researchers regularly engage. IRBs should seek input from consultants and community advisory boards when appropriate and should work with researchers and community partners to ensure the protection of research subjects.

References

Anderson, E. E. (2006). A qualitative study of non-affiliated, non-scientist institutional review board members. *Accountability in Research, 13*(2), 135–155.

Anderson, E. E. (2015). CIRTification: Training in human research protections for community research partners. *Progress in Community Health Partnerships, 9*(2), 283–288.

Anderson, E. E., Solomon, S., Heitman, E., DuBois, J. M., Fisher, C. B., Kost, R. G., Lawless, M. E., Ramsey, C., Jones, B., Ammerman, A., & Ross, L. F. (2012). Research ethics education for community engaged research: A review and research agenda. *Journal of Empirical Research on Human Research Ethics, 7*(2), 3–19.

Cargill, S. S., DeBruin, D., Eder, M., Heitman, E., Kaberry, J. M., McCormick, J. B., Opp, J., Sharp, R., Strelnick, A. H., Winkler, S. J., Yarborough, M., & Anderson, E. E. (2016). Community-engaged research ethics review: Exploring flexibility in federal regulations. *IRB: Ethics and Human Research, 38*(3), 11–19.

Clinical and Translational Science Awards Consortium Community Engagement Key Function Committee Task Force on the Principles of Community Engagement. (2011). *Principles of community engagement* (2nd ed.). Centers for Disease Control and Prevention, Agency for Toxic Substances and Disease Registry.

Concannon, T. W., Fuster, M., Saunders, T., Patel, K., Wong, J. B., Leslie, L. K., & Lau, J. (2014). A systematic review of stakeholder engagement in comparative effectiveness and patient-centered outcomes research. *Journal of General Internal Medicine, 29*(12), 1692–1701.

Department of Health and Human Services (DHHS). (2008). *Engagement of institutions in human subjects research.* www.hhs.gov/ohrp/regulations-and-policy/guidance/guidance-on-engagement -of-institutions/index.html

Department of Health and Human Services (DHHS). (2017). *Individual investigator agreement.* www.hhs.gov/ohrp/register-irbs-and-obtain-fwas/forms/individual-investigator-agreement /index.html

Harmon, A. (2010, April 21). Indian tribe wins fight to limit research of its DNA. *The New York Times.* www.nytimes.com/2010/04/22/us/22dna.html

Israel, B. A., Schulz, A. J., Parker, E. A., & Becker, A. B. (1998). Review of community based research: Assessing partnership approaches to improve public health. *Annual Review of Public Health, 19*(1), 173–202.

Michener, L., Cook, J., Ahmed, S. M., Yonas, M. A., Coyne-Beasley, T., & Aguilar-Gaxiola, S. (2012). Aligning the goals of community-engaged research: Why and how academic health centers can successfully engage with communities to improve health. *Academic Medicine, 87*(3), 285–291.

Mikesell, L., Bromely, E., & Khodyakov, D. (2013). Ethical community engaged research: A literature review. *American Journal of Public Health, 103*(12), e7–e14.

National Institutes of Health (NIH). (2000). *Required education in the protection of human research participants.* Notice OD-00-039. https://grants.nih.gov/grants/guide/notice-files /NOT-OD-00-039.html

Nebeker, C., Kalichman, M., Talavera, A., & Elder, J. (2015). Training in research ethics and standards for community health workers and promotores engaged in Latino health research. *Hastings Center Report, 45*(4), 20–27.

Newman, S. D., Andrews, J. O., Magwood, G. S., Jenkins, C., Cox, M. J., & Williamson, D. C. (2011). Community advisory boards in community-based participatory research: A synthesis of best processes. *Preventing Chronic Disease, 8*(3), A70.

Ross, L. F., Loup, A., Nelson, R. M., Botkin, J. R., Kost, R., Smith, G. R., & Gehlert, S. (2010a). Human subjects protections in community-engaged research: A research ethics framework. *Journal of Empirical Research on Human Research Ethics, 5*(1), 5–17.

Ross, L. F., Loup, A., Nelson, R. M., Botkin, J. R., Kost, R., Smith, G. R., & Gehlert, S. (2010b). Nine key functions for a human subjects protection program for community-engaged research: Points to consider. *Journal of Empirical Research on Human Research Ethics, 5*(1), 33–47.

Ross, L. F., Loup, A., Nelson, R. M., Botkin, J. R., Kost, R., Smith, G. R., & Gehlert, S. (2010c). The challenges of collaboration for academic and community partners in a research partnership: Points to consider. *Journal of Empirical Research on Human Research Ethics, 5*(1), 19–31.

Sheridan, S., Schrandt, S., Forsythe, L., Hilliard, T. S., & Paez, K. A. (2017). The PCORI engagement rubric: Promising practices for partnering in research. *Annals of Family Medicine, 15*(2), 165–170.

Simon, C., & Mosavel, M. (2010). Community members as recruiters of human subjects: Ethical considerations. *American Journal of Bioethics, 10*(3), 3–11.

Solomon, S., Bullock, S., Calhoun, K., Crosby, L., Eakin, B., Franco, Z., Hardwick, E., Holland, S., Leinberger-Jabari, A., Newton, G., Odell, J., Paberzs, A., & Spellecy, R. (2014a). Piloting a national disseminated, interactive human subjects protection program for community partners: Unexpected lessons learned from the field. *Clinical and Translational Science, 7*(2), 172–176.

Solomon, S., Eakin, B., Kirk, R., Piechowski, P., & Thomas, B. (2014b). Piloting a national disseminated, interactive human subjects protection program for community partners: Design, content, and evaluation. *Clinical and Translational Science, 7*(2), 177–183.

Solomon, S., & Piechowski, P. J. (2011). Developing community partner training: Regulations and relationships. *Journal of Empirical Research on Human Research Ethics, 6*(2), 23–30.

Strauss, R. P., Sengupta, S., Quinn, S. C., Goeppinger, J., Spaulding, C., Kegeles, S. M., & Millett, G. (2001). The role of community advisory boards: Involving communities in the informed consent process. *American Journal of Public Health, 91*(12), 1938–1943.

Weissman, J. S., Campbell, E. G., Cohen, I. G., Fernandez Lynch, H., Largent, E. A., Gupta, A., Rozenblum, R., Abraham, M., Spikes, K., Fagan, M., & Carnie, M. (2018). IRB oversight of patient-centered outcomes research: A national survey of IRB chairpersons. *Journal of Empirical Research in Human Research Ethics, 13*(4), 421–431.

Yarborough, M., Edwards, K., Espinoza, P., Geller, G., Sarwal, A., Sharp, R. R., & Spicer, P. (2012). Relationships hold the key to trustworthy and productive translational science: Recommendations for expanding community engagement in biomedical research. *Clinical and Translational Science, 6*, 310–313.

Yonas, M. A., Jaime, M. C., Barone, J., Valenti, S., Documet, P., Ryan, C. M., & Miller, E. (2016). Community partnered research ethics training in practice: A collaborative approach to certification. *Journal of Empirical Research on Human Research Ethics, 11*(2), 97–105.

Reference Material

Ethical Codes

The Nuremberg Code

Permissible Medical Experiments

The great weight of the evidence before us is to the effect that certain types of medical experiments on human beings, when kept within reasonably well-defined bounds, conform to the ethics of the medical profession generally. The protagonists of the practice of human experimentation justify their views on the basis that such experiments yield results for the good of society that are unprocurable by other methods or means of study. All agree, however, that certain basic principles must be observed in order to satisfy moral, ethical and legal concepts:

1. The voluntary consent of the human subject is absolutely essential.

   This means that the person involved should have legal capacity to give consent; should be so situated as to be able to exercise free power of choice, without the intervention of any element of force, fraud, deceit, duress, over-reaching, or other ulterior form of constraint or coercion; and should have sufficient knowledge and comprehension of the elements of the subject matter involved as to enable him to make an understanding and enlightened decision. This latter element requires that before the acceptance of an affirmative decision by the experimental subject there should be made known to him the nature, duration, and purpose of the experiment; the method and means by which it is to be conducted; all inconveniences and hazards reasonably to be expected; and the effects upon his health or person which may possibly come from his participation in the experiment.

   The duty and responsibility for ascertaining the quality of the consent rests upon each individual who initiates, directs or engages in the experiment. It is a personal duty and responsibility which may not be delegated to another with impunity.

2. The experiment should be such as to yield fruitful results for the good of society, unprocurable by other methods or means of study, and not random and unnecessary in nature.

3. The experiment should be so designed and based on the results of animal experimentation and a knowledge of the natural history of the disease or other problem under study that the anticipated results will justify the performance of the experiment.

4. The experiment should be so conducted as to avoid all unnecessary physical and mental suffering and injury.

5. No experiment should be conducted where there is an *a priori* reason to believe that death or disabling injury will occur; except, perhaps, in those experiments where the experimental physicians also serve as subjects.

6. The degree of risk to be taken should never exceed that determined by the humanitarian importance of the problem to be solved by the experiment.

7. Proper preparations should be made and adequate facilities provided to protect the experimental subject against even remote possibilities of injury, disability, or death.

8. The experiment should be conducted only by scientifically qualified persons. The highest degree of skill and care should be required through all stages of the experiment of those who conduct or engage in the experiment.

9. During the course of the experiment the human subject should be at liberty to bring the experiment to an end if he has reached the physical or mental state where continuation of the experiment seems to him to be impossible.

10. During the course of the experiment the scientist in charge must be prepared to terminate the experiment at any stage, if he has probable cause to believe, in the exercise of the good faith, superior skill and careful judgment required of him that a continuation of the experiment is likely to result in injury, disability, or death to the experimental subject.

Of the ten principles which have been enumerated our judicial concern, of course, is with those requirements which are purely legal in nature—or which at least are so clearly related to matters legal that they assist us in determining criminal culpability and punishment. To go beyond that point would lead us into a field that would be beyond our sphere of competence. However, the point need not be labored. We find from the evidence that in the medical experiments which have been proved, these ten principles were much more frequently honored in their breach than in their observance. Many of the concentration camp inmates who were the victims of these atrocities were citizens of countries other than the German Reich. They were non-German nationals, including Jews and "asocial persons", both prisoners of war and civilians, who had been imprisoned and forced to submit to these tortures and barbarities without so much as a semblance of trial. In every single instance appearing in the record, subjects were used who did not consent to the experiments; indeed, as to some of the experiments, it is not even contended by the defendants that the subjects occupied the status of volunteers. In no case was the experimental subject at liberty of his own free choice to withdraw from any experiment. In many cases experiments were performed by unqualified persons; were conducted at random for no adequate scientific reason, and under revolting physical conditions. All of the experiments were conducted with unnecessary suffering and injury and but very little, if any, precautions were taken to protect or safeguard the human subjects from the possibilities of injury, disability, or death. In every one of the experiments the subjects experienced extreme pain or torture, and in most of them they suffered permanent injury, mutilation, or death, either as a direct result of the experiments or because of lack of adequate follow-up care.

Obviously all of these experiments involving brutalities, tortures, disabling injury, and death were performed in complete disregard of international conventions, the laws and customs of war, the general principles of criminal law as derived from the criminal laws of all civilized nations, and Control Council Law No. 10. Manifestly human experiments under such conditions are contrary to "the principles of the law of nations as they result from the usages established among civilized peoples, from the laws of humanity, and from the dictates of public conscience."

Whether any of the defendants in the dock are guilty of these atrocities is, of course, another question. Under the Anglo-Saxon system of jurisprudence every defendant in a criminal case is presumed to be innocent of an offense charged until the prosecution, by competent, credible proof, has shown his guilt to the exclusion of every reasonable doubt. And this presumption abides with the defendant through each stage of his trial until such degree of proof has been adduced. A "reasonable doubt" as the name implies is one conformable to reason—a doubt which a reasonable man would entertain. Stated differently, it is that state of a case which, after a full and complete comparison and consideration of all the evidence, would leave an unbiased, unprejudiced, reflective person, charged with the responsibility for decision, in the state of mind that he could not say that he felt an abiding conviction amounting to a moral certainty of the truth of the charge.

If any of the defendants are to be found guilty under counts two or three of the indictment it must be because the evidence has shown beyond a reasonable doubt that such defendant, without regard to nationality or the capacity in which he acted, participated as a principal in, accessory to, ordered, abetted, took a consenting part in, or was connected with plans or enterprises involving the commission of at least some of the medical experiments and other atrocities which are the subject matter of these counts. Under no other circumstances may he be convicted.

Before examining the evidence to which we must look in order to determine individual culpability, a brief statement concerning some of the official agencies of the German Government and Nazi Party which will be referred to in this judgment seems desirable.

Nuremberg Code. (1949). *Trials of war criminals before the Nuremberg Military Tribunals under Control Council Law No. 10.* (Vol. 2); 181–182. U.S. Government Printing Office. https://history.nih.gov/display/history/Nuremburg+Code

WMA Declaration of Helsinki – Ethical Principles for Medical Research Involving Human Subjects

Adopted by the 18th WMA General Assembly, Helsinki, Finland, June 1964 and amended by the:

29th WMA General Assembly, Tokyo, Japan, October 1975

35th WMA General Assembly, Venice, Italy, October 1983

41st WMA General Assembly, Hong Kong, September 1989

48th WMA General Assembly, Somerset West, Republic of South Africa, October 1996

52nd WMA General Assembly, Edinburgh, Scotland, October 2000

53rd WMA General Assembly, Washington DC, USA, October 2002 (Note of Clarification added)

55th WMA General Assembly, Tokyo, Japan, October 2004 (Note of Clarification added)

59th WMA General Assembly, Seoul, Republic of Korea, October 2008

64th WMA General Assembly, Fortaleza, Brazil, October 2013

Preamble

1. The World Medical Association (WMA) has developed the Declaration of Helsinki as a statement of ethical principles for medical research involving human subjects, including research on identifiable human material and data.

The Declaration is intended to be read as a whole and each of its constituent paragraphs should be applied with consideration of all other relevant paragraphs.

2. Consistent with the mandate of the WMA, the Declaration is addressed primarily to physicians. The WMA encourages others who are involved in medical research involving human subjects to adopt these principles.

General Principles

3. The Declaration of Geneva of the WMA binds the physician with the words, "The health of my patient will be my first consideration," and the International Code of Medical Ethics declares that, "A physician shall act in the patient's best interest when providing medical care."

4. It is the duty of the physician to promote and safeguard the health, well-being and rights of patients, including those who are involved in medical research. The physician's knowledge and conscience are dedicated to the fulfilment of this duty.

5. Medical progress is based on research that ultimately must include studies involving human subjects.

6. The primary purpose of medical research involving human subjects is to understand the causes, development and effects of diseases and improve preventive, diagnostic and therapeutic interventions (methods, procedures and treatments).

Even the best proven interventions must be evaluated continually through research for their safety, effectiveness, efficiency, accessibility and quality.

7. Medical research is subject to ethical standards that promote and ensure respect for all human subjects and protect their health and rights.

8. While the primary purpose of medical research is to generate new knowledge, this goal can never take precedence over the rights and interests of individual research subjects.

9. It is the duty of physicians who are involved in medical research to protect the life, health, dignity, integrity, right to self-determination, privacy, and confidentiality of personal information of research subjects. The responsibility for the protection of research subjects must always rest with the physician or other health care professionals and never with the research subjects, even though they have given consent.

10. Physicians must consider the ethical, legal and regulatory norms and standards for research involving human subjects in their own countries as well as applicable international norms and standards. No national or international ethical, legal or regulatory requirement should reduce or eliminate any of the protections for research subjects set forth in this Declaration.

11. Medical research should be conducted in a manner that minimises possible harm to the environment.

12. Medical research involving human subjects must be conducted only by individuals with the appropriate ethics and scientific education, training and qualifications. Research on patients or healthy volunteers requires the supervision of a competent and appropriately qualified physician or other health care professional.

13. Groups that are underrepresented in medical research should be provided appropriate access to participation in research.

14. Physicians who combine medical research with medical care should involve their patients in research only to the extent that this is justified by its potential preventive, diagnostic or therapeutic value and if the physician has good reason to believe that participation in the research study will not adversely affect the health of the patients who serve as research subjects.

15. Appropriate compensation and treatment for subjects who are harmed as a result of participating in research must be ensured.

Risks, Burdens and Benefits

16. In medical practice and in medical research, most interventions involve risks and burdens.

Medical research involving human subjects may only be conducted if the importance of the objective outweighs the risks and burdens to the research subjects.

17. All medical research involving human subjects must be preceded by careful assessment of predictable risks and burdens to the individuals and groups involved in the research in comparison with foreseeable benefits to them and to other individuals or groups affected by the condition under investigation.

Measures to minimise the risks must be implemented. The risks must be continuously monitored, assessed and documented by the researcher.

18. Physicians may not be involved in a research study involving human subjects unless they are confident that the risks have been adequately assessed and can be satisfactorily managed.

When the risks are found to outweigh the potential benefits or when there is conclusive proof of definitive outcomes, physicians must assess whether to continue, modify or immediately stop the study.

Vulnerable Groups and Individuals

19. Some groups and individuals are particularly vulnerable and may have an increased likelihood of being wronged or of incurring additional harm.

All vulnerable groups and individuals should receive specifically considered protection.

20. Medical research with a vulnerable group is only justified if the research is responsive to the health needs or priorities of this group and the research cannot be carried out in a non-vulnerable group. In addition, this group should stand to benefit from the knowledge, practices or interventions that result from the research.

Scientific Requirements and Research Protocols

21. Medical research involving human subjects must conform to generally accepted scientific principles, be based on a thorough knowledge of the scientific literature, other relevant sources of information, and adequate laboratory and, as appropriate, animal experimentation. The welfare of animals used for research must be respected.

22. The design and performance of each research study involving human subjects must be clearly described and justified in a research protocol.

The protocol should contain a statement of the ethical considerations involved and should indicate how the principles in this Declaration have been addressed. The protocol should include information regarding funding, sponsors, institutional affiliations, potential conflicts of interest, incentives for subjects and information regarding provisions for treating and/or compensating subjects who are harmed as a consequence of participation in the research study.

In clinical trials, the protocol must also describe appropriate arrangements for post-trial provisions.

Research Ethics Committees

23. The research protocol must be submitted for consideration, comment, guidance and approval to the concerned research ethics committee before the study begins. This committee must be transparent in its functioning, must be independent of the researcher, the sponsor and any other undue influence and must be duly qualified. It must take into consideration the laws and regulations of the country or countries in which the research is to be performed as well as applicable international norms and standards but these must not be allowed to reduce or eliminate any of the protections for research subjects set forth in this Declaration.

The committee must have the right to monitor ongoing studies. The researcher must provide monitoring information to the committee, especially information about any serious adverse events. No amendment to the protocol may be made without consideration and approval by the committee. After the end of the study, the researchers must submit a final report to the committee containing a summary of the study's findings and conclusions.

Privacy and Confidentiality

24. Every precaution must be taken to protect the privacy of research subjects and the confidentiality of their personal information.

Informed Consent

25. Participation by individuals capable of giving informed consent as subjects in medical research must be voluntary. Although it may be appropriate to consult family members or community leaders, no individual capable of giving informed consent may be enrolled in a research study unless he or she freely agrees.

26. In medical research involving human subjects capable of giving informed consent, each potential subject must be adequately informed of the aims, methods, sources of funding, any possible conflicts of interest, institutional affiliations of the researcher, the anticipated benefits and potential risks of the study and the discomfort it may entail, post-study provisions and any other relevant aspects of the study. The potential subject must be informed of the right to refuse to participate in the study or to withdraw consent to participate at any time without reprisal. Special attention should be given to the specific information needs of individual potential subjects as well as to the methods used to deliver the information.

    After ensuring that the potential subject has understood the information, the physician or another appropriately qualified individual must then seek the potential subject's freely-given informed consent, preferably in writing. If the consent cannot be expressed in writing, the non-written consent must be formally documented and witnessed.

    All medical research subjects should be given the option of being informed about the general outcome and results of the study.

27. When seeking informed consent for participation in a research study the physician must be particularly cautious if the potential subject is in a dependent relationship with the physician or may consent under duress. In such situations the informed consent must be sought by an appropriately qualified individual who is completely independent of this relationship.

28. For a potential research subject who is incapable of giving informed consent, the physician must seek informed consent from the legally authorised representative. These individuals must not be included in a research study that has no likelihood of benefit for them unless it is intended to promote the health of the group represented by the potential subject, the research cannot instead be performed with persons capable of providing informed consent, and the research entails only minimal risk and minimal burden.

29. When a potential research subject who is deemed incapable of giving informed consent is able to give assent to decisions about participation in research, the physician must seek that assent in addition to the consent of the legally authorised representative. The potential subject's dissent should be respected.

30. Research involving subjects who are physically or mentally incapable of giving consent, for example, unconscious patients, may be done only if the physical or mental condition that prevents giving informed consent is a necessary characteristic of the research group. In such circumstances the physician must seek informed consent from the legally authorised representative.

If no such representative is available and if the research cannot be delayed, the study may proceed without informed consent provided that the specific reasons for involving subjects with a condition that renders them unable to give informed consent have been stated in the research protocol and the study has been approved by a research ethics committee. Consent to remain in the research must be obtained as soon as possible from the subject or a legally authorised representative.

31. The physician must fully inform the patient which aspects of their care are related to the research. The refusal of a patient to participate in a study or the patient's decision to withdraw from the study must never adversely affect the patient–physician relationship.

32. For medical research using identifiable human material or data, such as research on material or data contained in biobanks or similar repositories, physicians must seek informed consent for its collection, storage and/or reuse. There may be exceptional situations where consent would be impossible or impracticable to obtain for such research. In such situations the research may be done only after consideration and approval of a research ethics committee.

Use of Placebo

33. The benefits, risks, burdens and effectiveness of a new intervention must be tested against those of the best proven intervention(s), except in the following circumstances:

Where no proven intervention exists, the use of placebo, or no intervention, is acceptable; or

Where for compelling and scientifically sound methodological reasons the use of any intervention less effective than the best proven one, the use of placebo, or no intervention is necessary to determine the efficacy or safety of an intervention and the patients who receive any intervention less effective than the best proven one, placebo, or no intervention will not be subject to additional risks of serious or irreversible harm as a result of not receiving the best proven intervention.

Extreme care must be taken to avoid abuse of this option.

Post-Trial Provisions

34. In advance of a clinical trial, sponsors, researchers and host country governments should make provisions for post-trial access for all participants who still need an intervention identified as beneficial in the trial. This information must also be disclosed to participants during the informed consent process.

Research Registration and Publication and Dissemination of Results

35. Every research study involving human subjects must be registered in a publicly accessible database before recruitment of the first subject.

36. Researchers, authors, sponsors, editors and publishers all have ethical obligations with regard to the publication and dissemination of the results of research. Researchers have a duty to make publicly available the results of their research on human subjects and are accountable for the completeness and accuracy of their reports. All parties should adhere to accepted guidelines for ethical reporting. Negative and inconclusive as well as positive results must be published or otherwise made publicly available. Sources of funding, institutional

affiliations and conflicts of interest must be declared in the publication. Reports of research not in accordance with the principles of this Declaration should not be accepted for publication.

Unproven Interventions in Clinical Practice

37. In the treatment of an individual patient, where proven interventions do not exist or other known interventions have been ineffective, the physician, after seeking expert advice, with informed consent from the patient or a legally authorised representative, may use an unproven intervention if in the physician's judgement it offers hope of saving life, re-establishing health or alleviating suffering. This intervention should subsequently be made the object of research, designed to evaluate its safety and efficacy. In all cases, new information must be recorded and, where appropriate, made publicly available.

World Medical Association. (2018). Declaration of Helsinki – Ethical principles for medical research involving human subjects. www.wma.net/policies -post/wma-declaration-of-helsinki-ethical-principles-for-medical-research -involving-human-subjects/

The Belmont Report

Office of the Secretary

Ethical Principles and Guidelines for the Protection of Human Subjects of Research

The National Commission for the Protection of Human Subjects of Biomedical and Behavioral Research

April 18, 1979

AGENCY: Department of Health, Education, and Welfare.

ACTION: Notice of Report for Public Comment.

SUMMARY: On July 12, 1974, the National Research Act (Pub. L. 93-348) was signed into law, thereby creating the National Commission for the Protection of Human Subjects of Biomedical and Behavioral Research. One of the charges to the Commission was to identify the basic ethical principles that should underlie the conduct of biomedical and behavioral research involving human subjects and to develop guidelines which should be followed to assure that such research is conducted in accordance with those principles. In carrying out the above, the Commission was directed to consider: (i) the boundaries between biomedical and behavioral research and the accepted and routine practice of medicine, (ii) the role of assessment of risk-benefit criteria in the determination of the appropriateness of research involving human subjects, (iii) appropriate guidelines for the selection of human subjects for participation in such research and (iv) the nature and definition of informed consent in various research settings.

The Belmont Report attempts to summarize the basic ethical principles identified by the Commission in the course of its deliberations. It is the outgrowth of an intensive four-day period of discussions that were held in February 1976 at the Smithsonian Institution's Belmont Conference Center supplemented by the monthly deliberations of the Commission that were held over a period of nearly four years. It is a statement of basic ethical principles and guidelines that should assist in resolving the ethical problems that surround the conduct of research with human subjects. By publishing the Report in the Federal Register, and providing reprints upon request, the Secretary intends that it may be made readily available to scientists, members of Institutional Review Boards, and Federal employees. The two-volume Appendix, containing the lengthy reports of experts and specialists who assisted the Commission in fulfilling this part of its charge, is available as DHEW Publication No. (OS) 78-0013 and No. (OS) 78-0014, for sale by the Superintendent of Documents, U.S. Government Printing Office, Washington, D.C. 20402.

Unlike most other reports of the Commission, the Belmont Report does not make specific recommendations for administrative action by the Secretary of Health, Education, and Welfare. Rather, the Commission recommended that the Belmont Report be adopted in its entirety, as a statement of the Department's policy. The Department requests public comment on this recommendation.

National Commission for the Protection of Human Subjects of Biomedical and Behavioral Research

Members of the Commission

- Kenneth John Ryan, M.D., Chairman, Chief of Staff, Boston Hospital for Women.

- Joseph V. Brady, Ph.D., Professor of Behavioral Biology, Johns Hopkins University.
- Robert E. Cooke, M.D., President, Medical College of Pennsylvania.
- Dorothy I. Height, President, National Council of Negro Women, Inc.
- Albert R. Jonsen, Ph.D., Associate Professor of Bioethics, University of California at San Francisco.
- Patricia King, J.D., Associate Professor of Law, Georgetown University Law Center.
- Karen Lebacqz, Ph.D., Associate Professor of Christian Ethics, Pacific School of Religion.
- *** David W. Louisell, J.D., Professor of Law, University of California at Berkeley.
- Donald W. Seldin, M.D., Professor and Chairman, Department of Internal Medicine, University of Texas at Dallas.
- *** Eliot Stellar, Ph.D., Provost of the University and Professor of Physiological Psychology, University of Pennsylvania.
- *** Robert H. Turtle, LL.B., Attorney, VomBaur, Coburn, Simmons & Turtle, Washington, D.C.
- *** Deceased.

Ethical Principles & Guidelines for Research Involving Human Subjects

Scientific research has produced substantial social benefits. It has also posed some troubling ethical questions. Public attention was drawn to these questions by reported abuses of human subjects in biomedical experiments, especially during the Second World War. During the Nuremberg War Crime Trials, the Nuremberg code was drafted as a set of standards for judging physicians and scientists who had conducted biomedical experiments on concentration camp prisoners. This code became the prototype of many later codes[1] intended to assure that research involving human subjects would be carried out in an ethical manner.

The codes consist of rules, some general, others specific, that guide the investigators or the reviewers of research in their work. Such rules often are inadequate to cover complex situations; at times they come into conflict, and they are frequently difficult to interpret or apply. Broader ethical principles will provide a basis on which specific rules may be formulated, criticized and interpreted.

Three principles, or general prescriptive judgments, that are relevant to research involving human subjects are identified in this statement. Other principles may also be relevant. These three are comprehensive, however, and are stated at a level of generalization that should assist scientists, subjects, reviewers and interested citizens to understand the ethical issues inherent in research involving human subjects. These principles cannot always be applied so as to resolve beyond dispute particular ethical problems. The objective is to provide an analytical framework that will guide the resolution of ethical problems arising from research involving human subjects.

---

1 Since 1945, various codes for the proper and responsible conduct of human experimentation in medical research have been adopted by different organizations. The best known of these codes are the Nuremberg Code of 1947, the Helsinki Declaration of 1964 (revised in 1975), and the 1971 Guidelines (codified into Federal Regulations in 1974) issued by the U.S. Department of Health, Education, and Welfare. Codes for the conduct of social and behavioral research have also been adopted, the best known being that of the American Psychological Association, published in 1973.

This statement consists of a distinction between research and practice, a discussion of the three basic ethical principles, and remarks about the application of these principles.

Part A: Boundaries Between Practice & Research

A. Boundaries Between Practice and Research

It is important to distinguish between biomedical and behavioral research, on the one hand, and the practice of accepted therapy on the other, in order to know what activities ought to undergo review for the protection of human subjects of research. The distinction between research and practice is blurred partly because both often occur together (as in research designed to evaluate a therapy) and partly because notable departures from standard practice are often called "experimental" when the terms "experimental" and "research" are not carefully defined.

For the most part, the term "practice" refers to interventions that are designed solely to enhance the well-being of an individual patient or client and that have a reasonable expectation of success. The purpose of medical or behavioral practice is to provide diagnosis, preventive treatment or therapy to particular individuals.[2] By contrast, the term "research" designates an activity designed to test an hypothesis, permit conclusions to be drawn, and thereby to develop or contribute to generalizable knowledge (expressed, for example, in theories, principles, and statements of relationships). Research is usually described in a formal protocol that sets forth an objective and a set of procedures designed to reach that objective.

When a clinician departs in a significant way from standard or accepted practice, the innovation does not, in and of itself, constitute research. The fact that a procedure is "experimental," in the sense of new, untested or different, does not automatically place it in the category of research. Radically new procedures of this description should, however, be made the object of formal research at an early stage in order to determine whether they are safe and effective. Thus, it is the responsibility of medical practice committees, for example, to insist that a major innovation be incorporated into a formal research project.[3]

Research and practice may be carried on together when research is designed to evaluate the safety and efficacy of a therapy. This need not cause any confusion regarding whether or not the activity requires review; the general rule is that if there is any element of research in an activity, that activity should undergo review for the protection of human subjects.

---

2 Although practice usually involves interventions designed solely to enhance the well-being of a particular individual, interventions are sometimes applied to one individual for the enhancement of the well-being of another (e.g., blood donation, skin grafts, organ transplants) or an intervention may have the dual purpose of enhancing the well-being of a particular individual, and, at the same time, providing some benefit to others (e.g., vaccination, which protects both the person who is vaccinated and society generally). The fact that some forms of practice have elements other than immediate benefit to the individual receiving an intervention, however, should not confuse the general distinction between research and practice. Even when a procedure applied in practice may benefit some other person, it remains an intervention designed to enhance the well-being of a particular individual or groups of individuals; thus, it is practice and need not be reviewed as research.

3 Because the problems related to social experimentation may differ substantially from those of biomedical and behavioral research, the Commission specifically declines to make any policy determination regarding such research at this time. Rather, the Commission believes that the problem ought to be addressed by one of its successor bodies.

Part B: Basic Ethical Principles

B. Basic Ethical Principles

The expression "basic ethical principle" refers to those general judgments that serve as a basic justification for the many particular ethical prescriptions and evaluations of human actions. Three basic principles, among those generally accepted in our cultural tradition, are particularly relevant to the ethics of research involving human subjects: the principles of respect of persons, beneficence and justice.

1. **Respect for Persons.** Respect for persons incorporates at least two ethical convictions: first, that individuals should be treated as autonomous agents, and second, that persons with diminished autonomy are entitled to protection. The principle of respect for persons thus divides into two separate moral requirements: the requirement to acknowledge autonomy and the requirement to protect those with diminished autonomy.

An autonomous person is an individual capable of deliberation about personal goals and of acting under the direction of such deliberation. To respect autonomy is to give weight to autonomous persons' considered opinions and choices while refraining from obstructing their actions unless they are clearly detrimental to others. To show lack of respect for an autonomous agent is to repudiate that person's considered judgments, to deny an individual the freedom to act on those considered judgments, or to withhold information necessary to make a considered judgment, when there are no compelling reasons to do so.

However, not every human being is capable of self-determination. The capacity for self-determination matures during an individual's life, and some individuals lose this capacity wholly or in part because of illness, mental disability, or circumstances that severely restrict liberty. Respect for the immature and the incapacitated may require protecting them as they mature or while they are incapacitated.

Some persons are in need of extensive protection, even to the point of excluding them from activities which may harm them; other persons require little protection beyond making sure they undertake activities freely and with awareness of possible adverse consequence. The extent of protection afforded should depend upon the risk of harm and the likelihood of benefit. The judgment that any individual lacks autonomy should be periodically reevaluated and will vary in different situations.

In most cases of research involving human subjects, respect for persons demands that subjects enter into the research voluntarily and with adequate information. In some situations, however, application of the principle is not obvious. The involvement of prisoners as subjects of research provides an instructive example. On the one hand, it would seem that the principle of respect for persons requires that prisoners not be deprived of the opportunity to volunteer for research. On the other hand, under prison conditions they may be subtly coerced or unduly influenced to engage in research activities for which they would not otherwise volunteer. Respect for persons would then dictate that prisoners be protected. Whether to allow prisoners to "volunteer" or to "protect" them presents a dilemma. Respecting persons, in most hard cases, is often a matter of balancing competing claims urged by the principle of respect itself.

2. **Beneficence.** Persons are treated in an ethical manner not only by respecting their decisions and protecting them from harm, but also by making efforts to secure their well-being. Such treatment falls under the principle of beneficence. The term "beneficence" is often understood to cover acts of kindness or charity that go beyond strict obligation. In this document, beneficence is understood

in a stronger sense, as an obligation. Two general rules have been formulated as complementary expressions of beneficent actions in this sense: (1) do not harm and (2) maximize possible benefits and minimize possible harms.

The Hippocratic maxim "do no harm" has long been a fundamental principle of medical ethics. Claude Bernard extended it to the realm of research, saying that one should not injure one person regardless of the benefits that might come to others. However, even avoiding harm requires learning what is harmful; and, in the process of obtaining this information, persons may be exposed to risk of harm. Further, the Hippocratic Oath requires physicians to benefit their patients "according to their best judgment." Learning what will in fact benefit may require exposing persons to risk. The problem posed by these imperatives is to decide when it is justifiable to seek certain benefits despite the risks involved, and when the benefits should be foregone because of the risks.

The obligations of beneficence affect both individual investigators and society at large, because they extend both to particular research projects and to the entire enterprise of research. In the case of particular projects, investigators and members of their institutions are obliged to give forethought to the maximization of benefits and the reduction of risk that might occur from the research investigation. In the case of scientific research in general, members of the larger society are obliged to recognize the longer term benefits and risks that may result from the improvement of knowledge and from the development of novel medical, psychotherapeutic, and social procedures.

The principle of beneficence often occupies a well-defined justifying role in many areas of research involving human subjects. An example is found in research involving children. Effective ways of treating childhood diseases and fostering healthy development are benefits that serve to justify research involving children—even when individual research subjects are not direct beneficiaries. Research also makes it possible to avoid the harm that may result from the application of previously accepted routine practices that on closer investigation turn out to be dangerous. But the role of the principle of beneficence is not always so unambiguous. A difficult ethical problem remains, for example, about research that presents more than minimal risk without immediate prospect of direct benefit to the children involved. Some have argued that such research is inadmissible, while others have pointed out that this limit would rule out much research promising great benefit to children in the future. Here again, as with all hard cases, the different claims covered by the principle of beneficence may come into conflict and force difficult choices.

3. Justice. Who ought to receive the benefits of research and bear its burdens? This is a question of justice, in the sense of "fairness in distribution" or "what is deserved." An injustice occurs when some benefit to which a person is entitled is denied without good reason or when some burden is imposed unduly. Another way of conceiving the principle of justice is that equals ought to be treated equally. However, this statement requires explication. Who is equal and who is unequal? What considerations justify departure from equal distribution? Almost all commentators allow that distinctions based on experience, age, deprivation, competence, merit and position do sometimes constitute criteria justifying differential treatment for certain purposes. It is necessary, then, to explain in what respects people should be treated equally. There are several widely accepted formulations of just ways to distribute burdens and benefits. Each formulation mentions some relevant property on the basis of which burdens and benefits should be distributed. These formulations are (1) to each person an equal share, (2) to each person according to individual need,

(3) to each person according to individual effort, (4) to each person according to societal contribution, and (5) to each person according to merit.

Questions of justice have long been associated with social practices such as punishment, taxation and political representation. Until recently these questions have not generally been associated with scientific research. However, they are foreshadowed even in the earliest reflections on the ethics of research involving human subjects. For example, during the 19th and early 20th centuries the burdens of serving as research subjects fell largely upon poor ward patients, while the benefits of improved medical care flowed primarily to private patients. Subsequently, the exploitation of unwilling prisoners as research subjects in Nazi concentration camps was condemned as a particularly flagrant injustice. In this country, in the 1940's, the Tuskegee syphilis study used disadvantaged, rural black men to study the untreated course of a disease that is by no means confined to that population. These subjects were deprived of demonstrably effective treatment in order not to interrupt the project, long after such treatment became generally available.

Against this historical background, it can be seen how conceptions of justice are relevant to research involving human subjects. For example, the selection of research subjects needs to be scrutinized in order to determine whether some classes (e.g., welfare patients, particular racial and ethnic minorities, or persons confined to institutions) are being systematically selected simply because of their easy availability, their compromised position, or their manipulability, rather than for reasons directly related to the problem being studied. Finally, whenever research supported by public funds leads to the development of therapeutic devices and procedures, justice demands both that these not provide advantages only to those who can afford them and that such research should not unduly involve persons from groups unlikely to be among the beneficiaries of subsequent applications of the research.

Part C: Applications

C. Applications

Applications of the general principles to the conduct of research leads to consideration of the following requirements: informed consent, risk/benefit assessment, and the selection of subjects of research.

1. Informed Consent. Respect for persons requires that subjects, to the degree that they are capable, be given the opportunity to choose what shall or shall not happen to them. This opportunity is provided when adequate standards for informed consent are satisfied.

While the importance of informed consent is unquestioned, controversy prevails over the nature and possibility of an informed consent. Nonetheless, there is widespread agreement that the consent process can be analyzed as containing three elements: information, comprehension and voluntariness.

Information. Most codes of research establish specific items for disclosure intended to assure that subjects are given sufficient information. These items generally include: the research procedure, their purposes, risks and anticipated benefits, alternative procedures (where therapy is involved), and a statement offering the subject the opportunity to ask questions and to withdraw at any time from the research. Additional items have been proposed, including how subjects are selected, the person responsible for the research, etc.

However, a simple listing of items does not answer the question of what the standard should be for judging how much and what sort of information should be provided. One standard frequently invoked in medical practice, namely the information commonly provided by practitioners in the field or in the locale, is inadequate since research takes place precisely when a common understanding does not exist. Another standard, currently popular in malpractice law, requires the practitioner to reveal the information that reasonable persons would wish to know in order to make a decision regarding their care. This, too, seems insufficient since the research subject, being in essence a volunteer, may wish to know considerably more about risks gratuitously undertaken than do patients who deliver themselves into the hand of a clinician for needed care. It may be that a standard of "the reasonable volunteer" should be proposed: the extent and nature of information should be such that persons, knowing that the procedure is neither necessary for their care nor perhaps fully understood, can decide whether they wish to participate in the furthering of knowledge. Even when some direct benefit to them is anticipated, the subjects should understand clearly the range of risk and the voluntary nature of participation.

A special problem of consent arises where informing subjects of some pertinent aspect of the research is likely to impair the validity of the research. In many cases, it is sufficient to indicate to subjects that they are being invited to participate in research of which some features will not be revealed until the research is concluded. In all cases of research involving incomplete disclosure, such research is justified only if it is clear that (**1**) incomplete disclosure is truly necessary to accomplish the goals of the research, (**2**) there are no undisclosed risks to subjects that are more than minimal, and (**3**) there is an adequate plan for debriefing subjects, when appropriate, and for dissemination of research results to them. Information about risks should never be withheld for the purpose of eliciting the cooperation of subjects, and truthful answers should always be given to direct questions about the research. Care should be taken to distinguish cases in which disclosure would destroy or invalidate the research from cases in which disclosure would simply inconvenience the investigator.

Comprehension. The manner and context in which information is conveyed is as important as the information itself. For example, presenting information in a disorganized and rapid fashion, allowing too little time for consideration or curtailing opportunities for questioning, all may adversely affect a subject's ability to make an informed choice.

Because the subject's ability to understand is a function of intelligence, rationality, maturity and language, it is necessary to adapt the presentation of the information to the subject's capacities. Investigators are responsible for ascertaining that the subject has comprehended the information. While there is always an obligation to ascertain that the information about risk to subjects is complete and adequately comprehended, when the risks are more serious, that obligation increases. On occasion, it may be suitable to give some oral or written tests of comprehension.

Special provision may need to be made when comprehension is severely limited—for example, by conditions of immaturity or mental disability. Each class of subjects that one might consider as incompetent (e.g., infants and young children, mentally disable patients, the terminally ill and the comatose) should be considered on its own terms. Even for these persons, however, respect requires giving them the opportunity to choose to the extent they are able, whether or not to participate in research. The objections of these subjects to involvement should be honored, unless the research entails providing them a therapy unavailable elsewhere. Respect for persons also requires seeking the permission of other parties in order to protect the subjects from harm. Such persons are thus respected both by acknowledging their own wishes and by the use of third parties to protect them from harm.

The third parties chosen should be those who are most likely to understand the incompetent subject's situation and to act in that person's best interest. The person authorized to act on behalf of the subject should be given an opportunity to observe the research as it proceeds in order to be able to withdraw the subject from the research, if such action appears in the subject's best interest.

Voluntariness. An agreement to participate in research constitutes a valid consent only if voluntarily given. This element of informed consent requires conditions free of coercion and undue influence. Coercion occurs when an overt threat of harm is intentionally presented by one person to another in order to obtain compliance. Undue influence, by contrast, occurs through an offer of an excessive, unwarranted, inappropriate or improper reward or other overture in order to obtain compliance. Also, inducements that would ordinarily be acceptable may become undue influences if the subject is especially vulnerable.

Unjustifiable pressures usually occur when persons in positions of authority or commanding influence—especially where possible sanctions are involved—urge a course of action for a subject. A continuum of such influencing factors exists, however, and it is impossible to state precisely where justifiable persuasion ends and undue influence begins. But undue influence would include actions such as manipulating a person's choice through the controlling influence of a close relative and threatening to withdraw health services to which an individual would otherwise be entitled.

2. Assessment of Risks and Benefits. The assessment of risks and benefits requires a careful arrayal of relevant data, including, in some cases, alternative ways of obtaining the benefits sought in the research. Thus, the assessment presents both an opportunity and a responsibility to gather systematic and comprehensive information about proposed research. For the investigator, it is a means to examine whether the proposed research is properly designed. For a review committee, it is a method for determining whether the risks that will be presented to subjects are justified. For prospective subjects, the assessment will assist the determination whether or not to participate.

The Nature and Scope of Risks and Benefits. The requirement that research be justified on the basis of a favorable risk/benefit assessment bears a close relation to the principle of beneficence, just as the moral requirement that informed consent be obtained is derived primarily from the principle of respect for persons. The term "risk" refers to a possibility that harm may occur. However, when expressions such as "small risk" or "high risk" are used, they usually refer (often ambiguously) both to the chance (probability) of experiencing a harm and the severity (magnitude) of the envisioned harm.

The term "benefit" is used in the research context to refer to something of positive value related to health or welfare. Unlike, "risk," "benefit" is not a term that expresses probabilities. Risk is properly contrasted to probability of benefits, and benefits are properly contrasted with harms rather than risks of harm. Accordingly, so-called risk/benefit assessments are concerned with the probabilities and magnitudes of possible harm and anticipated benefits. Many kinds of possible harms and benefits need to be taken into account. There are, for example, risks of psychological harm, physical harm, legal harm, social harm and economic harm and the corresponding benefits. While the most likely types of harms to research subjects are those of psychological or physical pain or injury, other possible kinds should not be overlooked.

Risks and benefits of research may affect the individual subjects, the families of the individual subjects, and society at large (or special groups of subjects in society). Previous codes and Federal regulations have required that risks to subjects be outweighed by the sum of both the anticipated benefit to the subject, if any, and the anticipated benefit to society in the form of knowledge to be gained from the research. In balancing these different elements, the risks and benefits affecting the immediate research subject will normally carry special weight. On the other hand, interests other than those of the subject may on some occasions be sufficient by themselves to justify the risks involved in the research, so long as the subjects' rights have been protected. Beneficence thus requires that we protect against risk of harm to subjects and also that we be concerned about the loss of the substantial benefits that might be gained from research.

The Systematic Assessment of Risks and Benefits. It is commonly said that benefits and risks must be "balanced" and shown to be "in a favorable ratio." The metaphorical character of these terms draws attention to the difficulty of making precise judgments. Only on rare occasions will quantitative techniques be available for the scrutiny of research protocols. However, the idea of systematic, nonarbitrary analysis of risks and benefits should be emulated insofar as possible. This ideal requires those making decisions about the justifiability of research to be thorough in the accumulation and assessment of information about all aspects of the research, and to consider alternatives systematically. This procedure renders the assessment of research more rigorous and precise, while making communication between review board members and investigators less subject to misinterpretation, misinformation and conflicting judgments. Thus, there should first be a determination of the validity of the presuppositions of the research; then the nature, probability and magnitude of risk should be distinguished with as much clarity as possible. The method of ascertaining risks should be explicit, especially where there is no alternative to the use of such vague categories as small or slight risk. It should also be determined whether an investigator's estimates of the probability of harm or benefits are reasonable, as judged by known facts or other available studies.

Finally, assessment of the justifiability of research should reflect at least the following considerations: **(i)** Brutal or inhumane treatment of human subjects is never morally justified. **(ii)** Risks should be reduced to those necessary to achieve the research objective. It should be determined whether it is in fact necessary to use human subjects at all. Risk can perhaps never be entirely eliminated, but it can often be reduced by careful attention to alternative procedures. **(iii)** When research involves significant risk of serious impairment, review committees should be extraordinarily insistent on the justification of the risk (looking usually to the likelihood of benefit to the subject—or, in some rare cases, to the manifest voluntariness of the participation). **(iv)** When vulnerable populations are involved in research, the appropriateness of involving them should itself be demonstrated. A number of variables go into such judgments, including the nature and degree of risk, the condition of the particular population involved, and the nature and level of the anticipated benefits. **(v)** Relevant risks and benefits must be thoroughly arrayed in documents and procedures used in the informed consent process.

3. Selection of Subjects. Just as the principle of respect for persons finds expression in the requirements for consent, and the principle of beneficence in risk/benefit assessment, the principle of justice gives rise to moral requirements that there be fair procedures and outcomes in the selection of research subjects.

Justice is relevant to the selection of subjects of research at two levels: the social and the individual. Individual justice in the selection of subjects would require that researchers exhibit fairness: thus, they should not offer potentially beneficial research only to some patients who are in their favor or select only "undesirable" persons for risky research. Social justice requires that distinction be drawn between classes of subjects that ought, and ought not, to participate in any particular kind of research, based on the ability of members of that class to bear burdens and on the appropriateness of placing further burdens on already burdened persons. Thus, it can be considered a matter of social justice that there is an order of preference in the selection of classes of subjects (e.g., adults before children) and that some classes of potential subjects (e.g., the institutionalized mentally infirm or prisoners) may be involved as research subjects, if at all, only on certain conditions.

Injustice may appear in the selection of subjects, even if individual subjects are selected fairly by investigators and treated fairly in the course of research. Thus injustice arises from social, racial, sexual and cultural biases institutionalized in society. Thus, even if individual researchers are treating their research subjects fairly, and even if IRBs are taking care to assure that subjects are selected fairly within a particular institution, unjust social patterns may nevertheless appear in the overall distribution of the burdens and benefits of research. Although individual institutions or investigators may not be able to resolve a problem that is pervasive in their social setting, they can consider distributive justice in selecting research subjects.

Some populations, especially institutionalized ones, are already burdened in many ways by their infirmities and environments. When research is proposed that involves risks and does not include a therapeutic component, other less burdened classes of persons should be called upon first to accept these risks of research, except where the research is directly related to the specific conditions of the class involved. Also, even though public funds for research may often flow in the same directions as public funds for health care, it seems unfair that populations dependent on public health care constitute a pool of preferred research subjects if more advantaged populations are likely to be the recipients of the benefits.

One special instance of injustice results from the involvement of vulnerable subjects. Certain groups, such as racial minorities, the economically disadvantaged, the very sick, and the institutionalized may continually be sought as research subjects, owing to their ready availability in settings where research is conducted. Given their dependent status and their frequently compromised capacity for free consent, they should be protected against the danger of being involved in research solely for administrative convenience, or because they are easy to manipulate as a result of their illness or socioeconomic condition.

National Commission for the Protection of Human Subjects of Biomedical and Behavioral Research. (1979). *The Belmont report: Ethical principles and guidelines for the protection of human subjects in biomedical and behavioral research.* www.hhs.gov/ohrp/regulations-and-policy/belmont-report/index.html

Selected U.S. Federal Regulations and Policies

45 CFR 46: DHHS Regulations for the Protection of Human Subjects

CODE OF FEDERAL REGULATIONS

TITLE 45: PUBLIC WELFARE

PART 46—PROTECTION OF HUMAN SUBJECTS

Subpart A—Basic HHS Policy for Protection of Human Research Subjects

§46.101 To what does this policy apply?

(a) Except as detailed in §46.104, this policy applies to all research involving human subjects conducted, supported, or otherwise subject to regulation by any Federal department or agency that takes appropriate administrative action to make the policy applicable to such research. This includes research conducted by Federal civilian employees or military personnel, except that each department or agency head may adopt such procedural modifications as may be appropriate from an administrative standpoint. It also includes research conducted, supported, or otherwise subject to regulation by the Federal Government outside the United States. Institutions that are engaged in research described in this paragraph and institutional review boards (IRBs) reviewing research that is subject to this policy must comply with this policy.

(b) [Reserved]

(c) Department or agency heads retain final judgment as to whether a particular activity is covered by this policy and this judgment shall be exercised consistent with the ethical principles of the Belmont Report.[62]

(d) Department or agency heads may require that specific research activities or classes of research activities conducted, supported, or otherwise subject to regulation by the Federal department or agency but not otherwise covered by this policy comply with some or all of the requirements of this policy.

Subpart A is also known as the Common Rule.

62 The National Commission for the Protection of Human Subjects of Biomedical and Behavioral Research. *Belmont Report*. Washington, DC: U.S. Department of Health and Human Services; 1979.

(e) Compliance with this policy requires compliance with pertinent federal laws or regulations that provide additional protections for human subjects.

(f) This policy does not affect any state or local laws or regulations (including tribal law passed by the official governing body of an American Indian or Alaska Native tribe) that may otherwise be applicable and that provide additional protections for human subjects.

(g) This policy does not affect any foreign laws or regulations that may otherwise be applicable and that provide additional protections to human subjects of research.

(h) When research covered by this policy takes place in foreign countries, procedures normally followed in the foreign countries to protect human subjects may differ from those set forth in this policy. In these circumstances, if a department or agency head determines that the procedures prescribed by the institution afford protections that are at least equivalent to those provided in this policy, the department or agency head may approve the substitution of the foreign procedures in lieu of the procedural requirements provided in this policy. Except when otherwise required by statute, Executive Order, or the department or agency head, notices of these actions as they occur will be published in the FEDERAL REGISTER or will be otherwise published as provided in department or agency procedures.

(i) Unless otherwise required by law, department or agency heads may waive the applicability of some or all of the provisions of this policy to specific research activities or classes of research activities otherwise covered by this policy, provided the alternative procedures to be followed are consistent with the principles of the Belmont Report.[63] Except when otherwise required by statute or Executive Order, the department or agency head shall forward advance notices of these actions to the Office for Human Research Protections, Department of Health and Human Services (HHS), or any successor office, or to the equivalent office within the appropriate Federal department or agency, and shall also publish them in the FEDERAL REGISTER or in such other manner as provided in department or agency procedures. The waiver notice must include a statement that identifies the conditions under which the waiver will be applied and a justification as to why the waiver is appropriate for the research, including how the decision is consistent with the principles of the Belmont Report.

(j) Federal guidance on the requirements of this policy shall be issued only after consultation, for the purpose of harmonization (to the extent appropriate), with other Federal departments and agencies that have adopted this policy, unless such consultation is not feasible.

(k) [Reserved]

(l) Compliance dates and transition provisions:

(1) *Pre-2018 Requirements.* For purposes of this section, the *pre-2018 Requirements* means this subpart as published in the 2016 edition of the Code of Federal Regulations.

(2) *2018 Requirements.* For purposes of this section, the *2018 Requirements* means the Federal Policy for the Protection of Human Subjects requirements contained in this subpart. The general compliance date for the 2018 Requirements is January 21, 2019. The compliance date for §46.114(b) (cooperative research) of the 2018 Requirements is January 20, 2020.

---

63 *Id.*

(3) *Research subject to pre-2018 requirements.* The pre-2018 Requirements shall apply to the following research, unless the research is transitioning to comply with the 2018 Requirements in accordance with paragraph (l)(4) of this section:

(i) Research initially approved by an IRB under the pre-2018 Requirements before January 21, 2019;

(ii) Research for which IRB review was waived pursuant to §46.101(i) of the pre-2018 Requirements before January 21, 2019; and

(iii) Research for which a determination was made that the research was exempt under §46.101(b) of the pre-2018 Requirements before January 21, 2019.

(4) *Transitioning research.* If, on or after July 19, 2018, an institution planning or engaged in research otherwise covered by paragraph (l)(3) of this section determines that such research instead will transition to comply with the 2018 Requirements, the institution or an IRB must document and date such determination.

(i) If the determination to transition is documented between July 19, 2018, and January 20, 2019, the research shall:

(A) Beginning on the date of such documentation through January 20, 2019, comply with the PRE-2018 Requirements, except that the research shall comply with the following:

(*1*) Section 46.102(l) of the 2018 Requirements (definition of research) (instead of §46.102(d) of the pre-2018 Requirements);

(*2*) Section 46.103(d) of the 2018 Requirements (revised certification requirement that eliminates IRB review of application or proposal) (instead of §46.103(f) of the pre-2018 Requirements); and

(*3*) Section 46.109(f)(1)(i) and (iii) of the 2018 Requirements (exceptions to mandated continuing review) (instead of §46.103(b), as related to the requirement for continuing review, and in addition to §46.109, of the pre-2018 Requirements); and

(B) Beginning on January 21, 2019, comply with the 2018 Requirements.

(ii) If the determination to transition is documented on or after January 21, 2019, the research shall, beginning on the date of such documentation, comply with the 2018 Requirements.

(5) *Research subject to 2018 Requirements.* The 2018 Requirements shall apply to the following research:

(i) Research initially approved by an IRB on or after January 21, 2019;

(ii) Research for which IRB review is waived pursuant to paragraph (i) of this section on or after January 21, 2019; and

(iii) Research for which a determination is made that the research is exempt on or after January 21, 2019.

(m) Severability: Any provision of this part held to be invalid or unenforceable by its terms, or as applied to any person or circumstance, shall be construed so as to continue to give maximum effect to the provision permitted by law, unless such holding shall be one of utter invalidity or unenforceability, in which event the provision shall be severable from this part and shall not affect the remainder thereof or the application of the provision to other persons not similarly situated or to other dissimilar circumstances.

[82 FR 7259, 7273, Jan. 19, 2017, as amended at 83 FR 28518, June 19, 2018]

§46.102 Definitions for purposes of this policy.

(a) *Certification* means the official notification by the institution to the supporting Federal department or agency component, in accordance with the requirements of this policy, that a research project or activity involving human subjects has been reviewed and approved by an IRB in accordance with an approved assurance.

(b) *Clinical trial* means a research study in which one or more human subjects are prospectively assigned to one or more interventions (which may include placebo or other control) to evaluate the effects of the interventions on biomedical or behavioral health-related outcomes.

(c) *Department or agency head* means the head of any Federal department or agency, for example, the Secretary of HHS, and any other officer or employee of any Federal department or agency to whom the authority provided by these regulations to the department or agency head has been delegated.

(d) *Federal department or agency* refers to a federal department or agency (the department or agency itself rather than its bureaus, offices or divisions) that takes appropriate administrative action to make this policy applicable to the research involving human subjects it conducts, supports, or otherwise regulates (*e.g.,* the U.S. Department of Health and Human Services, the U.S. Department of Defense, or the Central Intelligence Agency).

(e)(1) *Human subject* means a living individual about whom an investigator (whether professional or student) conducting research:

(i) Obtains information or biospecimens through intervention or interaction with the individual, and uses, studies, or analyzes the information or biospecimens; or

(ii) Obtains, uses, studies, analyzes, or generates identifiable private information or identifiable biospecimens.

(2) *Intervention* includes both physical procedures by which information or biospecimens are gathered (*e.g.,* venipuncture) and manipulations of the subject or the subject's environment that are performed for research purposes.

(3) *Interaction* includes communication or interpersonal contact between investigator and subject.

(4) *Private information* includes information about behavior that occurs in a context in which an individual can reasonably expect that no observation or recording is taking place, and information that has been provided for specific purposes by an individual and that the individual can reasonably expect will not be made public (*e.g.,* a medical record).

(5) *Identifiable private information* is private information for which the identity of the subject is or may readily be ascertained by the investigator or associated with the information.

(6) *An identifiable biospecimen* is a biospecimen for which the identity of the subject is or may readily be ascertained by the investigator or associated with the biospecimen.

(7) Federal departments or agencies implementing this policy shall:

(i) Upon consultation with appropriate experts (including experts in data matching and re-identification), reexamine the meaning of "identifiable private information," as defined in paragraph (e)(5) of this section, and "identifiable biospecimen," as defined in paragraph (e)(6) of this section. This reexamination shall take place within 1 year and regularly thereafter (at least every 4 years). This process will be conducted by collaboration among the Federal departments and agencies implementing this policy. If appropriate and permitted by law, such Federal departments and agencies may alter the interpretation of these terms, including through the use of guidance.

(ii) Upon consultation with appropriate experts, assess whether there are analytic technologies or techniques that should be considered by investigators to generate "identifiable private information," as defined in paragraph (e)(5) of this section, or an "identifiable biospecimen," as defined in paragraph (e)(6) of this section. This assessment shall take place within 1 year and regularly thereafter (at least every 4 years). This process will be conducted by collaboration among the Federal departments and agencies implementing this policy. Any such technologies or techniques will be included on a list of technologies or techniques that produce identifiable private information or identifiable biospecimens. This list will be published in the FEDERAL REGISTER after notice and an opportunity for public comment. The Secretary, HHS, shall maintain the list on a publicly accessible Web site.

(f) *Institution* means any public or private entity, or department or agency (including federal, state, and other agencies).

(g) *IRB* means an institutional review board established in accord with and for the purposes expressed in this policy.

(h) *IRB approval* means the determination of the IRB that the research has been reviewed and may be conducted at an institution within the constraints set forth by the IRB and by other institutional and federal requirements.

(i) *Legally authorized representative* means an individual or judicial or other body authorized under applicable law to consent on behalf of a prospective subject to the subject's participation in the procedure(s) involved in the research. If there is no applicable law addressing this issue, *legally authorized representative* means an individual recognized by institutional policy as acceptable for providing consent in the nonresearch context on behalf of the prospective subject to the subject's participation in the procedure(s) involved in the research.

(j) *Minimal risk* means that the probability and magnitude of harm or discomfort anticipated in the research are not greater in and of themselves than those ordinarily encountered in daily life or during the performance of routine physical or psychological examinations or tests.

(k) *Public health authority* means an agency or authority of the United States, a state, a territory, a political subdivision of a state or territory, an Indian tribe, or a foreign government, or a person or entity acting under a grant of authority from or contract with such public agency, including the employees or agents of such public agency or its contractors or persons or entities to whom it has granted authority, that is responsible for public health matters as part of its official mandate.

(l) *Research* means a systematic investigation, including research development, testing, and evaluation, designed to develop or contribute to generalizable knowledge. Activities that meet this definition constitute research for purposes of this policy, whether or not they are conducted or supported under a program that is considered research for other purposes. For example, some demonstration and service programs may include research activities. For purposes of this part, the following activities are deemed not to be research:

(1) Scholarly and journalistic activities (*e.g.,* oral history, journalism, biography, literary criticism, legal research, and historical scholarship), including the collection and use of information, that focus directly on the specific individuals about whom the information is collected.

(2) Public health surveillance activities, including the collection and testing of information or biospecimens, conducted, supported, requested, ordered, required, or authorized by a public health authority. Such activities are limited to those necessary to allow a public health authority to identify, monitor, assess, or

investigate potential public health signals, onsets of disease outbreaks, or conditions of public health importance (including trends, signals, risk factors, patterns in diseases, or increases in injuries from using consumer products). Such activities include those associated with providing timely situational awareness and priority setting during the course of an event or crisis that threatens public health (including natural or man-made disasters).

(3) Collection and analysis of information, biospecimens, or records by or for a criminal justice agency for activities authorized by law or court order solely for criminal justice or criminal investigative purposes.

(4) Authorized operational activities (as determined by each agency) in support of intelligence, homeland security, defense, or other national security missions.

(m) *Written,* or *in writing,* for purposes of this part, refers to writing on a tangible medium (*e.g.,* paper) or in an electronic format.

§46.103 Assuring compliance with this policy—research conducted or supported by any Federal department or agency.

(a) Each institution engaged in research that is covered by this policy, with the exception of research eligible for exemption under §46.104, and that is conducted or supported by a Federal department or agency, shall provide written assurance satisfactory to the department or agency head that it will comply with the requirements of this policy. In lieu of requiring submission of an assurance, individual department or agency heads shall accept the existence of a current assurance, appropriate for the research in question, on file with the Office for Human Research Protections, HHS, or any successor office, and approved for Federal-wide use by that office. When the existence of an HHS-approved assurance is accepted in lieu of requiring submission of an assurance, reports (except certification) required by this policy to be made to department and agency heads shall also be made to the Office for Human Research Protections, HHS, or any successor office. Federal departments and agencies will conduct or support research covered by this policy only if the institution has provided an assurance that it will comply with the requirements of this policy, as provided in this section, and only if the institution has certified to the department or agency head that the research has been reviewed and approved by an IRB (if such certification is required by §46.103(d)).

(b) The assurance shall be executed by an individual authorized to act for the institution and to assume on behalf of the institution the obligations imposed by this policy and shall be filed in such form and manner as the department or agency head prescribes.

(c) The department or agency head may limit the period during which any assurance shall remain effective or otherwise condition or restrict the assurance.

(d) Certification is required when the research is supported by a Federal department or agency and not otherwise waived under §46.101(i) or exempted under §46.104. For such research, institutions shall certify that each proposed research study covered by the assurance and this section has been reviewed and approved by the IRB. Such certification must be submitted as prescribed by the Federal department or agency component supporting the research. Under no condition shall research covered by this section be initiated prior to receipt of the certification that the research has been reviewed and approved by the IRB.

(e) For nonexempt research involving human subjects covered by this policy (or exempt research for which limited IRB review takes place pursuant to §46.104(d)(2)(iii), (d)(3)(i)(C), or (d)(7) or (8)) that takes place at an institution in which IRB oversight is conducted by an IRB that is not operated by the institution, the institution and the organization operating the IRB shall document the institution's reliance on the IRB for oversight of the research and the responsibilities that each entity will undertake to ensure compliance with the requirements of this policy (*e.g.,* in a written agreement between the institution and the IRB, by implementation of an institution-wide policy directive providing the allocation of responsibilities between the institution and an IRB that is not affiliated with the institution, or as set forth in a research protocol).

(Approved by the Office of Management and Budget under Control Number 0990-0260)

§46.104 Exempt research.

(a) Unless otherwise required by law or by department or agency heads, research activities in which the only involvement of human subjects will be in one or more of the categories in paragraph (d) of this section are exempt from the requirements of this policy, except that such activities must comply with the requirements of this section and as specified in each category.

(b) Use of the exemption categories for research subject to the requirements of subparts B, C, and D: Application of the exemption categories to research subject to the requirements of 45 CFR part 46, subparts B, C, and D, is as follows:

(1) *Subpart B.* Each of the exemptions at this section may be applied to research subject to subpart B if the conditions of the exemption are met.

(2) *Subpart C.* The exemptions at this section do not apply to research subject to subpart C, except for research aimed at involving a broader subject population that only incidentally includes prisoners.

(3) *Subpart D.* The exemptions at paragraphs (d)(1), (4), (5), (6), (7), and (8) of this section may be applied to research subject to subpart D if the conditions of the exemption are met. Paragraphs (d)(2)(i) and (ii) of this section only may apply to research subject to subpart D involving educational tests or the observation of public behavior when the investigator(s) do not participate in the activities being observed. Paragraph (d)(2)(iii) of this section may not be applied to research subject to subpart D.

(c) [Reserved]

(d) Except as described in paragraph (a) of this section, the following categories of human subjects research are exempt from this policy:

(1) Research, conducted in established or commonly accepted educational settings, that specifically involves normal educational practices that are not likely to adversely impact students' opportunity to learn required educational content or the assessment of educators who provide instruction. This includes most research on regular and special education instructional strategies, and research on the effectiveness of or the comparison among instructional techniques, curricula, or classroom management methods.

(2) Research that only includes interactions involving educational tests (cognitive, diagnostic, aptitude, achievement), survey procedures, interview procedures, or observation of public behavior (including visual or auditory recording) if at least one of the following criteria is met:

(i) The information obtained is recorded by the investigator in such a manner that the identity of the human subjects cannot readily be ascertained, directly or through identifiers linked to the subjects;

(ii) Any disclosure of the human subjects' responses outside the research would not reasonably place the subjects at risk of criminal or civil liability or be damaging to the subjects' financial standing, employability, educational advancement, or reputation; or

(iii) The information obtained is recorded by the investigator in such a manner that the identity of the human subjects can readily be ascertained, directly or through identifiers linked to the subjects, and an IRB conducts a limited IRB review to make the determination required by §46.111(a)(7).

(3)(i) Research involving benign behavioral interventions in conjunction with the collection of information from an adult subject through verbal or written responses (including data entry) or audiovisual recording if the subject prospectively agrees to the intervention and information collection and at least one of the following criteria is met:

(A) The information obtained is recorded by the investigator in such a manner that the identity of the human subjects cannot readily be ascertained, directly or through identifiers linked to the subjects;

(B) Any disclosure of the human subjects' responses outside the research would not reasonably place the subjects at risk of criminal or civil liability or be damaging to the subjects' financial standing, employability, educational advancement, or reputation; or

(C) The information obtained is recorded by the investigator in such a manner that the identity of the human subjects can readily be ascertained, directly or through identifiers linked to the subjects, and an IRB conducts a limited IRB review to make the determination required by §46.111(a)(7).

(ii) For the purpose of this provision, benign behavioral interventions are brief in duration, harmless, painless, not physically invasive, not likely to have a significant adverse lasting impact on the subjects, and the investigator has no reason to think the subjects will find the interventions offensive or embarrassing. Provided all such criteria are met, examples of such benign behavioral interventions would include having the subjects play an online game, having them solve puzzles under various noise conditions, or having them decide how to allocate a nominal amount of received cash between themselves and someone else.

(iii) If the research involves deceiving the subjects regarding the nature or purposes of the research, this exemption is not applicable unless the subject authorizes the deception through a prospective agreement to participate in research in circumstances in which the subject is informed that he or she will be unaware of or misled regarding the nature or purposes of the research.

(4) Secondary research for which consent is not required: Secondary research uses of identifiable private information or identifiable biospecimens, if at least one of the following criteria is met:

(i) The identifiable private information or identifiable biospecimens are publicly available;

(ii) Information, which may include information about biospecimens, is recorded by the investigator in such a manner that the identity of the human subjects cannot readily be ascertained directly or through identifiers linked to the subjects, the investigator does not contact the subjects, and the investigator will not re-identify subjects;

(iii) The research involves only information collection and analysis involving the investigator's use of identifiable health information when that use is regulated under 45 CFR parts 160 and 164, subparts A and E, for the purposes of "health care operations" or "research" as those terms are defined at 45 CFR 164.501 or for "public health activities and purposes" as described under 45 CFR 164.512(b); or

(iv) The research is conducted by, or on behalf of, a Federal department or agency using government-generated or government-collected information obtained for nonresearch activities, if the research generates identifiable private information that is or will be maintained on information technology that is subject to and in compliance with section 208(b) of the E-Government Act of 2002, 44 U.S.C. 3501 note, if all of the identifiable private information collected, used, or generated as part of the activity will be maintained in systems of records subject to the Privacy Act of 1974, 5 U.S.C. 552a, and, if applicable, the information used in the research was collected subject to the Paperwork Reduction Act of 1995, 44 U.S.C. 3501 *et seq.*

(5) Research and demonstration projects that are conducted or supported by a Federal department or agency, or otherwise subject to the approval of department or agency heads (or the approval of the heads of bureaus or other subordinate agencies that have been delegated authority to conduct the research and demonstration projects), and that are designed to study, evaluate, improve, or otherwise examine public benefit or service programs, including procedures for obtaining benefits or services under those programs, possible changes in or alternatives to those programs or procedures, or possible changes in methods or levels of payment for benefits or services under those programs. Such projects include, but are not limited to, internal studies by Federal employees, and studies under contracts or consulting arrangements, cooperative agreements, or grants. Exempt projects also include waivers of otherwise mandatory requirements using authorities such as sections 1115 and 1115A of the Social Security Act, as amended.

(i) Each Federal department or agency conducting or supporting the research and demonstration projects must establish, on a publicly accessible Federal Web site or in such other manner as the department or agency head may determine, a list of the research and demonstration projects that the Federal department or agency conducts or supports under this provision. The research or demonstration project must be published on this list prior to commencing the research involving human subjects.

(ii) [Reserved]

(6) Taste and food quality evaluation and consumer acceptance studies:

(i) If wholesome foods without additives are consumed, or

(ii) If a food is consumed that contains a food ingredient at or below the level and for a use found to be safe, or agricultural chemical or environmental contaminant at or below the level found to be safe, by the Food and Drug Administration or approved by the Environmental Protection Agency or the Food Safety and Inspection Service of the U.S. Department of Agriculture.

(7) Storage or maintenance for secondary research for which broad consent is required: Storage or maintenance of identifiable private information or identifiable biospecimens for potential secondary research use if an IRB conducts a limited IRB review and makes the determinations required by §46.111(a)(8).

(8) Secondary research for which broad consent is required: Research involving the use of identifiable private information or identifiable biospecimens for secondary research use, if the following criteria are met:

(i) Broad consent for the storage, maintenance, and secondary research use of the identifiable private information or identifiable biospecimens was obtained in accordance with §46.116(a)(1) through (4), (a)(6), and (d);

(ii) Documentation of informed consent or waiver of documentation of consent was obtained in accordance with §46.117;

(iii) An IRB conducts a limited IRB review and makes the determination required by §46.111(a)(7) and makes the determination that the research to be conducted is within the scope of the broad consent referenced in paragraph (d)(8)(i) of this section; and (iv) The investigator does not include returning individual research results to subjects as part of the study plan. This provision does not prevent an investigator from abiding by any legal requirements to return individual research results.

(Approved by the Office of Management and Budget under Control Number 0990-0260)

§46.105-46.106 [Reserved]

§46.107 IRB membership.

(a) Each IRB shall have at least five members, with varying backgrounds to promote complete and adequate review of research activities commonly conducted by the institution. The IRB shall be sufficiently qualified through the experience and expertise of its members (professional competence), and the diversity of its members, including race, gender, and cultural backgrounds and sensitivity to such issues as community attitudes, to promote respect for its advice and counsel in safeguarding the rights and welfare of human subjects. The IRB shall be able to ascertain the acceptability of proposed research in terms of institutional commitments (including policies and resources) and regulations, applicable law, and standards of professional conduct and practice. The IRB shall therefore include persons knowledgeable in these areas. If an IRB regularly reviews research that involves a category of subjects that is vulnerable to coercion or undue influence, such as children, prisoners, individuals with impaired decision-making capacity, or economically or educationally disadvantaged persons, consideration shall be given to the inclusion of one or more individuals who are knowledgeable about and experienced in working with these categories of subjects.

(b) Each IRB shall include at least one member whose primary concerns are in scientific areas and at least one member whose primary concerns are in nonscientific areas.

(c) Each IRB shall include at least one member who is not otherwise affiliated with the institution and who is not part of the immediate family of a person who is affiliated with the institution.

(d) No IRB may have a member participate in the IRB's initial or continuing review of any project in which the member has a conflicting interest, except to provide information requested by the IRB.

(e) An IRB may, in its discretion, invite individuals with competence in special areas to assist in the review of issues that require expertise beyond or in addition to that available on the IRB. These individuals may not vote with the IRB.

§46.108 IRB functions and operations.

(a) In order to fulfill the requirements of this policy each IRB shall:

(1) Have access to meeting space and sufficient staff to support the IRB's review and recordkeeping duties;

(2) Prepare and maintain a current list of the IRB members identified by name; earned degrees; representative capacity; indications of experience such as board certifications or licenses sufficient to describe each member's chief anticipated contributions to IRB deliberations; and any employment or other relationship between each member and the institution, for example, full-time employee, part-time employee, member of governing panel or board, stockholder, paid or unpaid consultant;

(3) Establish and follow written procedures for:

(i) Conducting its initial and continuing review of research and for reporting its findings and actions to the investigator and the institution;

(ii) Determining which projects require review more often than annually and which projects need verification from sources other than the investigators that no material changes have occurred since previous IRB review; and

(iii) Ensuring prompt reporting to the IRB of proposed changes in a research activity, and for ensuring that investigators will conduct the research activity in accordance with the terms of the IRB approval until any proposed changes have been reviewed and approved by the IRB, except when necessary to eliminate apparent immediate hazards to the subject.

(4) Establish and follow written procedures for ensuring prompt reporting to the IRB; appropriate institutional officials; the department or agency head; and the Office for Human Research Protections, HHS, or any successor office, or the equivalent office within the appropriate Federal department or agency of

(i) Any unanticipated problems involving risks to subjects or others or any serious or continuing noncompliance with this policy or the requirements or determinations of the IRB; and

(ii) Any suspension or termination of IRB approval.

(b) Except when an expedited review procedure is used (as described in §46.110), an IRB must review proposed research at convened meetings at which a majority of the members of the IRB are present, including at least one member whose primary concerns are in nonscientific areas. In order for the research to be approved, it shall receive the approval of a majority of those members present at the meeting.

(Approved by the Office of Management and Budget under Control Number 0990-0260)

§46.109 IRB review of research.

(a) An IRB shall review and have authority to approve, require modifications in (to secure approval), or disapprove all research activities covered by this policy, including exempt research activities under §46.104 for which limited IRB review is a condition of exemption (under §46.104(d)(2)(iii), (d)(3)(i)(C), and (d)(7), and (8)).

(b) An IRB shall require that information given to subjects (or legally authorized representatives, when appropriate) as part of informed consent is in accordance with §46.116. The IRB may require that information, in addition to that specifically mentioned in §46.116, be given to the subjects when in the IRB's judgment the information would meaningfully add to the protection of the rights and welfare of subjects.

(c) An IRB shall require documentation of informed consent or may waive documentation in accordance with §46.117.

(d) An IRB shall notify investigators and the institution in writing of its decision to approve or disapprove the proposed research activity, or of modifications required to secure IRB approval of the research activity. If the IRB decides to disapprove a research activity, it shall include in its written notification a statement of the reasons for its decision and give the investigator an opportunity to respond in person or in writing.

(e) An IRB shall conduct continuing review of research requiring review by the convened IRB at intervals appropriate to the degree of risk, not less than once per year, except as described in §46.109(f).

(f)(1) Unless an IRB determines otherwise, continuing review of research is not required in the following circumstances:

(i) Research eligible for expedited review in accordance with §46.110;

(ii) Research reviewed by the IRB in accordance with the limited IRB review described in §46.104(d)(2)(iii), (d)(3)(i)(C), or (d)(7) or (8);

(iii) Research that has progressed to the point that it involves only one or both of the following, which are part of the IRB-approved study:

(A) Data analysis, including analysis of identifiable private information or identifiable biospecimens, or

(B) Accessing follow-up clinical data from procedures that subjects would undergo as part of clinical care.

(2) [Reserved]

(g) An IRB shall have authority to observe or have a third party observe the consent process and the research.

(Approved by the Office of Management and Budget under Control Number 0990-0260)

§46.110 Expedited review procedures for certain kinds of research involving no more than minimal risk, and for minor changes in approved research.

(a) The Secretary of HHS has established, and published as a Notice in the FEDERAL REGISTER, a list of categories of research that may be reviewed by the IRB through an expedited review procedure. The Secretary will evaluate the list at least every 8 years and amend it, as appropriate, after consultation with other federal departments and agencies and after publication in the FEDERAL REGISTER for public comment. A copy of the list is available from the Office for Human Research Protections, HHS, or any successor office.

(b)(1) An IRB may use the expedited review procedure to review the following:

(i) Some or all of the research appearing on the list described in paragraph (a) of this section, unless the reviewer determines that the study involves more than minimal risk;

(ii) Minor changes in previously approved research during the period for which approval is authorized; or

(iii) Research for which limited IRB review is a condition of exemption under §46.104(d)(2)(iii), (d)(3)(i)(C), and (d)(7) and (8).

(2) Under an expedited review procedure, the review may be carried out by the IRB chairperson or by one or more experienced reviewers designated by the chairperson from among members of the IRB. In reviewing the research, the reviewers may exercise all of the authorities of the IRB except that the reviewers may not disapprove the research. A research activity may be disapproved only after review in accordance with the nonexpedited procedure set forth in §46.108(b).

(c) Each IRB that uses an expedited review procedure shall adopt a method for keeping all members advised of research proposals that have been approved under the procedure.

(d) The department or agency head may restrict, suspend, terminate, or choose not to authorize an institution's or IRB's use of the expedited review procedure.

§46.111 Criteria for IRB approval of research.

(a) In order to approve research covered by this policy the IRB shall determine that all of the following requirements are satisfied:

(1) Risks to subjects are minimized:

(i) By using procedures that are consistent with sound research design and that do not unnecessarily expose subjects to risk, and

(ii) Whenever appropriate, by using procedures already being performed on the subjects for diagnostic or treatment purposes.

(2) Risks to subjects are reasonable in relation to anticipated benefits, if any, to subjects, and the importance of the knowledge that may reasonably be

expected to result. In evaluating risks and benefits, the IRB should consider only those risks and benefits that may result from the research (as distinguished from risks and benefits of therapies subjects would receive even if not participating in the research). The IRB should not consider possible long-range effects of applying knowledge gained in the research (*e.g.,* the possible effects of the research on public policy) as among those research risks that fall within the purview of its responsibility.

(3) Selection of subjects is equitable. In making this assessment the IRB should take into account the purposes of the research and the setting in which the research will be conducted. The IRB should be particularly cognizant of the special problems of research that involves a category of subjects who are vulnerable to coercion or undue influence, such as children, prisoners, individuals with impaired decision-making capacity, or economically or educationally disadvantaged persons.

(4) Informed consent will be sought from each prospective subject or the subject's legally authorized representative, in accordance with, and to the extent required by, §46.116.

(5) Informed consent will be appropriately documented or appropriately waived in accordance with §46.117.

(6) When appropriate, the research plan makes adequate provision for monitoring the data collected to ensure the safety of subjects.

(7) When appropriate, there are adequate provisions to protect the privacy of subjects and to maintain the confidentiality of data.

(i) The Secretary of HHS will, after consultation with the Office of Management and Budget's privacy office and other Federal departments and agencies that have adopted this policy, issue guidance to assist IRBs in assessing what provisions are adequate to protect the privacy of subjects and to maintain the confidentiality of data.

(ii) [Reserved]

(8) For purposes of conducting the limited IRB review required by §46.104(d)(7)), the IRB need not make the determinations at paragraphs (a)(1) through (7) of this section, and shall make the following determinations:

(i) Broad consent for storage, maintenance, and secondary research use of identifiable private information or identifiable biospecimens is obtained in accordance with the requirements of §46.116(a)(1)-(4), (a)(6), and (d);

(ii) Broad consent is appropriately documented or waiver of documentation is appropriate, in accordance with §46.117; and

(iii) If there is a change made for research purposes in the way the identifiable private information or identifiable biospecimens are stored or maintained, there are adequate provisions to protect the privacy of subjects and to maintain the confidentiality of data.

(b) When some or all of the subjects are likely to be vulnerable to coercion or undue influence, such as children, prisoners, individuals with impaired decision-making capacity, or economically or educationally disadvantaged persons, additional safeguards have been included in the study to protect the rights and welfare of these subjects.

§46.112 Review by institution.

Research covered by this policy that has been approved by an IRB may be subject to further appropriate review and approval or disapproval by officials of the institution. However, those officials may not approve the research if it has not been approved by an IRB.

§46.113 Suspension or termination of IRB approval of research.

An IRB shall have authority to suspend or terminate approval of research that is not being conducted in accordance with the IRB's requirements or that has been associated with unexpected serious harm to subjects. Any suspension or termination of approval shall include a statement of the reasons for the IRB's action and shall be reported promptly to the investigator, appropriate institutional officials, and the department or agency head.

(Approved by the Office of Management and Budget under Control Number 0990-0260)

§46.114 Cooperative research.

(a) Cooperative research projects are those projects covered by this policy that involve more than one institution. In the conduct of cooperative research projects, each institution is responsible for safeguarding the rights and welfare of human subjects and for complying with this policy.

(b)(1) Any institution located in the United States that is engaged in cooperative research must rely upon approval by a single IRB for that portion of the research that is conducted in the United States. The reviewing IRB will be identified by the Federal department or agency supporting or conducting the research or proposed by the lead institution subject to the acceptance of the Federal department or agency supporting the research.

(2) The following research is not subject to this provision:

(i) Cooperative research for which more than single IRB review is required by law (including tribal law passed by the official governing body of an American Indian or Alaska Native tribe); or

(ii) Research for which any Federal department or agency supporting or conducting the research determines and documents that the use of a single IRB is not appropriate for the particular context.

(c) For research not subject to paragraph (b) of this section, an institution participating in a cooperative project may enter into a joint review arrangement, rely on the review of another IRB, or make similar arrangements for avoiding duplication of effort.

§46.115 IRB records.

(a) An institution, or when appropriate an IRB, shall prepare and maintain adequate documentation of IRB activities, including the following:

(1) Copies of all research proposals reviewed, scientific evaluations, if any, that accompany the proposals, approved sample consent forms, progress reports submitted by investigators, and reports of injuries to subjects.

(2) Minutes of IRB meetings, which shall be in sufficient detail to show attendance at the meetings; actions taken by the IRB; the vote on these actions including the number of members voting for, against, and abstaining; the basis for requiring changes in or disapproving research; and a written summary of the discussion of controverted issues and their resolution.

(3) Records of continuing review activities, including the rationale for conducting continuing review of research that otherwise would not require continuing review as described in §46.109(f)(1).

(4) Copies of all correspondence between the IRB and the investigators.

(5) A list of IRB members in the same detail as described in §46.108(a)(2).

(6) Written procedures for the IRB in the same detail as described in §46.108(a)(3) and (4).

(7) Statements of significant new findings provided to subjects, as required by §46.116(c)(5).

(8) The rationale for an expedited reviewer's determination under §46.110(b)(1)(i) that research appearing on the expedited review list described in §46.110(a) is more than minimal risk.

(9) Documentation specifying the responsibilities that an institution and an organization operating an IRB each will undertake to ensure compliance with the requirements of this policy, as described in §46.103(e).

(b) The records required by this policy shall be retained for at least 3 years, and records relating to research that is conducted shall be retained for at least 3 years after completion of the research. The institution or IRB may maintain the records in printed form, or electronically. All records shall be accessible for inspection and copying by authorized representatives of the Federal department or agency at reasonable times and in a reasonable manner.

(Approved by the Office of Management and Budget under Control Number 0990-0260)

§46.116 General requirements for informed consent.

(a) *General.* General requirements for informed consent, whether written or oral, are set forth in this paragraph and apply to consent obtained in accordance with the requirements set forth in paragraphs (b) through (d) of this section. Broad consent may be obtained in lieu of informed consent obtained in accordance with paragraphs (b) and (c) of this section only with respect to the storage, maintenance, and secondary research uses of identifiable private information and identifiable biospecimens. Waiver or alteration of consent in research involving public benefit and service programs conducted by or subject to the approval of state or local officials is described in paragraph (e) of this section. General waiver or alteration of informed consent is described in paragraph (f) of this section. Except as provided elsewhere in this policy:

(1) Before involving a human subject in research covered by this policy, an investigator shall obtain the legally effective informed consent of the subject or the subject's legally authorized representative.

(2) An investigator shall seek informed consent only under circumstances that provide the prospective subject or the legally authorized representative sufficient opportunity to discuss and consider whether or not to participate and that minimize the possibility of coercion or undue influence.

(3) The information that is given to the subject or the legally authorized representative shall be in language understandable to the subject or the legally authorized representative.

(4) The prospective subject or the legally authorized representative must be provided with the information that a reasonable person would want to have in order to make an informed decision about whether to participate, and an opportunity to discuss that information.

(5) Except for broad consent obtained in accordance with paragraph (d) of this section:

(i) Informed consent must begin with a concise and focused presentation of the key information that is most likely to assist a prospective subject or legally authorized representative in understanding the reasons why one might or might not want to participate in the research. This part of the informed consent must be organized and presented in a way that facilitates comprehension.

(ii) Informed consent as a whole must present information in sufficient detail relating to the research, and must be organized and presented in a way that does not merely provide lists of isolated facts, but rather facilitates the prospective subject's or legally authorized representative's understanding of the reasons why one might or might not want to participate.

(6) No informed consent may include any exculpatory language through which the subject or the legally authorized representative is made to waive or appear to waive any of the subject's legal rights, or releases or appears to release the investigator, the sponsor, the institution, or its agents from liability for negligence.

(b) *Basic elements of informed consent.* Except as provided in paragraph (d), (e), or (f) of this section, in seeking informed consent the following information shall be provided to each subject or the legally authorized representative:

(1) A statement that the study involves research, an explanation of the purposes of the research and the expected duration of the subject's participation, a description of the procedures to be followed, and identification of any procedures that are experimental;

(2) A description of any reasonably foreseeable risks or discomforts to the subject;

(3) A description of any benefits to the subject or to others that may reasonably be expected from the research;

(4) A disclosure of appropriate alternative procedures or courses of treatment, if any, that might be advantageous to the subject;

(5) A statement describing the extent, if any, to which confidentiality of records identifying the subject will be maintained;

(6) For research involving more than minimal risk, an explanation as to whether any compensation and an explanation as to whether any medical treatments are available if injury occurs and, if so, what they consist of, or where further information may be obtained;

(7) An explanation of whom to contact for answers to pertinent questions about the research and research subjects' rights, and whom to contact in the event of a research-related injury to the subject;

(8) A statement that participation is voluntary, refusal to participate will involve no penalty or loss of benefits to which the subject is otherwise entitled, and the subject may discontinue participation at any time without penalty or loss of benefits to which the subject is otherwise entitled; and

(9) One of the following statements about any research that involves the collection of identifiable private information or identifiable biospecimens:

(i) A statement that identifiers might be removed from the identifiable private information or identifiable biospecimens and that, after such removal, the information or biospecimens could be used for future research studies or distributed to another investigator for future research studies without additional informed consent from the subject or the legally authorized representative, if this might be a possibility; or

(ii) A statement that the subject's information or biospecimens collected as part of the research, even if identifiers are removed, will not be used or distributed for future research studies.

(c) *Additional elements of informed consent.* Except as provided in paragraph (d), (e), or (f) of this section, one or more of the following elements of information, when appropriate, shall also be provided to each subject or the legally authorized representative:

(1) A statement that the particular treatment or procedure may involve risks to the subject (or to the embryo or fetus, if the subject is or may become pregnant) that are currently unforeseeable;

(2) Anticipated circumstances under which the subject's participation may be terminated by the investigator without regard to the subject's or the legally authorized representative's consent;

(3) Any additional costs to the subject that may result from participation in the research;

(4) The consequences of a subject's decision to withdraw from the research and procedures for orderly termination of participation by the subject;

(5) A statement that significant new findings developed during the course of the research that may relate to the subject's willingness to continue participation will be provided to the subject;

(6) The approximate number of subjects involved in the study;

(7) A statement that the subject's biospecimens (even if identifiers are removed) may be used for commercial profit and whether the subject will or will not share in this commercial profit;

(8) A statement regarding whether clinically relevant research results, including individual research results, will be disclosed to subjects, and if so, under what conditions; and

(9) For research involving biospecimens, whether the research will (if known) or might include whole genome sequencing (*i.e.*, sequencing of a human germline or somatic specimen with the intent to generate the genome or exome sequence of that specimen).

(d) *Elements of broad consent for the storage, maintenance, and secondary research use of identifiable private information or identifiable biospecimens.* Broad consent for the storage, maintenance, and secondary research use of identifiable private information or identifiable biospecimens (collected for either research studies other than the proposed research or nonresearch purposes) is permitted as an alternative to the informed consent requirements in paragraphs (b) and (c) of this section. If the subject or the legally authorized representative is asked to provide broad consent, the following shall be provided to each subject or the subject's legally authorized representative:

(1) The information required in paragraphs (b)(2), (b)(3), (b)(5), and (b)(8) and, when appropriate, (c)(7) and (9) of this section;

(2) A general description of the types of research that may be conducted with the identifiable private information or identifiable biospecimens. This description must include sufficient information such that a reasonable person would expect that the broad consent would permit the types of research conducted;

(3) A description of the identifiable private information or identifiable biospecimens that might be used in research, whether sharing of identifiable private information or identifiable biospecimens might occur, and the types of institutions or researchers that might conduct research with the identifiable private information or identifiable biospecimens;

(4) A description of the period of time that the identifiable private information or identifiable biospecimens may be stored and maintained (which period of time could be indefinite), and a description of the period of time that the identifiable private information or identifiable biospecimens may be used for research purposes (which period of time could be indefinite);

(5) Unless the subject or legally authorized representative will be provided details about specific research studies, a statement that they will not be informed of the details of any specific research studies that might be conducted using the subject's identifiable private information or identifiable biospecimens, including the purposes of the research, and that they might have chosen not to consent to some of those specific research studies;

(6) Unless it is known that clinically relevant research results, including individual research results, will be disclosed to the subject in all circumstances, a statement that such results may not be disclosed to the subject; and

(7) An explanation of whom to contact for answers to questions about the subject's rights and about storage and use of the subject's identifiable private

information or identifiable biospecimens, and whom to contact in the event of a research-related harm.

(e) *Waiver or alteration of consent in research involving public benefit and service programs conducted by or subject to the approval of state or local officials*— (1) *Waiver.* An IRB may waive the requirement to obtain informed consent for research under paragraphs (a) through (c) of this section, provided the IRB satisfies the requirements of paragraph (e)(3) of this section. If an individual was asked to provide broad consent for the storage, maintenance, and secondary research use of identifiable private information or identifiable biospecimens in accordance with the requirements at paragraph (d) of this section, and refused to consent, an IRB cannot waive consent for the storage, maintenance, or secondary research use of the identifiable private information or identifiable biospecimens.

(2) *Alteration.* An IRB may approve a consent procedure that omits some, or alters some or all, of the elements of informed consent set forth in paragraphs (b) and (c) of this section provided the IRB satisfies the requirements of paragraph (e)(3) of this section. An IRB may not omit or alter any of the requirements described in paragraph (a) of this section. If a broad consent procedure is used, an IRB may not omit or alter any of the elements required under paragraph (d) of this section.

(3) *Requirements for waiver and alteration.* In order for an IRB to waive or alter consent as described in this subsection, the IRB must find and document that:

(i) The research or demonstration project is to be conducted by or subject to the approval of state or local government officials and is designed to study, evaluate, or otherwise examine:

(A) Public benefit or service programs;

(B) Procedures for obtaining benefits or services under those programs;

(C) Possible changes in or alternatives to those programs or procedures; or

(D) Possible changes in methods or levels of payment for benefits or services under those programs; and

(ii) The research could not practicably be carried out without the waiver or alteration.

(f) *General waiver or alteration of consent*—(1) *Waiver.* An IRB may waive the requirement to obtain informed consent for research under paragraphs (a) through (c) of this section, provided the IRB satisfies the requirements of paragraph (f)(3) of this section. If an individual was asked to provide broad consent for the storage, maintenance, and secondary research use of identifiable private information or identifiable biospecimens in accordance with the requirements at paragraph (d) of this section, and refused to consent, an IRB cannot waive consent for the storage, maintenance, or secondary research use of the identifiable private information or identifiable biospecimens.

(2) *Alteration.* An IRB may approve a consent procedure that omits some, or alters some or all, of the elements of informed consent set forth in paragraphs (b) and (c) of this section provided the IRB satisfies the requirements of paragraph (f)(3) of this section. An IRB may not omit or alter any of the requirements described in paragraph (a) of this section. If a broad consent procedure is used, an IRB may not omit or alter any of the elements required under paragraph (d) of this section.

(3) *Requirements for waiver and alteration.* In order for an IRB to waive or alter consent as described in this subsection, the IRB must find and document that:

(i) The research involves no more than minimal risk to the subjects;

(ii) The research could not practicably be carried out without the requested waiver or alteration;

(iii) If the research involves using identifiable private information or identifiable biospecimens, the research could not practicably be carried out without using such information or biospecimens in an identifiable format;

(iv) The waiver or alteration will not adversely affect the rights and welfare of the subjects; and

(v) Whenever appropriate, the subjects or legally authorized representatives will be provided with additional pertinent information after participation.

(g) *Screening, recruiting, or determining eligibility.* An IRB may approve a research proposal in which an investigator will obtain information or biospecimens for the purpose of screening, recruiting, or determining the eligibility of prospective subjects without the informed consent of the prospective subject or the subject's legally authorized representative, if either of the following conditions are met:

(1) The investigator will obtain information through oral or written communication with the prospective subject or legally authorized representative, or

(2) The investigator will obtain identifiable private information or identifiable biospecimens by accessing records or stored identifiable biospecimens.

(h) *Posting of clinical trial consent form.* (1) For each clinical trial conducted or supported by a Federal department or agency, one IRB-approved informed consent form used to enroll subjects must be posted by the awardee or the Federal department or agency component conducting the trial on a publicly available Federal Web site that will be established as a repository for such informed consent forms.

(2) If the Federal department or agency supporting or conducting the clinical trial determines that certain information should not be made publicly available on a Federal Web site (*e.g.* confidential commercial information), such Federal department or agency may permit or require redactions to the information posted.

(3) The informed consent form must be posted on the Federal Web site after the clinical trial is closed to recruitment, and no later than 60 days after the last study visit by any subject, as required by the protocol.

(i) *Preemption.* The informed consent requirements in this policy are not intended to preempt any applicable Federal, state, or local laws (including tribal laws passed by the official governing body of an American Indian or Alaska Native tribe) that require additional information to be disclosed in order for informed consent to be legally effective.

(j) *Emergency medical care.* Nothing in this policy is intended to limit the authority of a physician to provide emergency medical care, to the extent the physician is permitted to do so under applicable Federal, state, or local law (including tribal law passed by the official governing body of an American Indian or Alaska Native tribe).

(Approved by the Office of Management and Budget under Control Number 0990-0260)

§46.117 Documentation of informed consent.

(a) Except as provided in paragraph (c) of this section, informed consent shall be documented by the use of a written informed consent form approved by the IRB and signed (including in an electronic format) by the subject or the subject's legally authorized representative. A written copy shall be given to the person signing the informed consent form.

(b) Except as provided in paragraph (c) of this section, the informed consent form may be either of the following:

(1) A written informed consent form that meets the requirements of §46.116. The investigator shall give either the subject or the subject's legally

authorized representative adequate opportunity to read the informed consent form before it is signed; alternatively, this form may be read to the subject or the subject's legally authorized representative.

(2) A short form written informed consent form stating that the elements of informed consent required by §46.116 have been presented orally to the subject or the subject's legally authorized representative, and that the key information required by §46.116(a)(5)(i) was presented first to the subject, before other information, if any, was provided. The IRB shall approve a written summary of what is to be said to the subject or the legally authorized representative. When this method is used, there shall be a witness to the oral presentation. Only the short form itself is to be signed by the subject or the subject's legally authorized representative. However, the witness shall sign both the short form and a copy of the summary, and the person actually obtaining consent shall sign a copy of the summary. A copy of the summary shall be given to the subject or the subject's legally authorized representative, in addition to a copy of the short form.

(c)(1) An IRB may waive the requirement for the investigator to obtain a signed informed consent form for some or all subjects if it finds any of the following:

(i) That the only record linking the subject and the research would be the informed consent form and the principal risk would be potential harm resulting from a breach of confidentiality. Each subject (or legally authorized representative) will be asked whether the subject wants documentation linking the subject with the research, and the subject's wishes will govern;

(ii) That the research presents no more than minimal risk of harm to subjects and involves no procedures for which written consent is normally required outside of the research context; or

(iii) If the subjects or legally authorized representatives are members of a distinct cultural group or community in which signing forms is not the norm, that the research presents no more than minimal risk of harm to subjects and provided there is an appropriate alternative mechanism for documenting that informed consent was obtained.

(2) In cases in which the documentation requirement is waived, the IRB may require the investigator to provide subjects or legally authorized representatives with a written statement regarding the research.

(Approved by the Office of Management and Budget under Control Number 0990-0260)

§46.118 Applications and proposals lacking definite plans for involvement of human subjects.

Certain types of applications for grants, cooperative agreements, or contracts are submitted to Federal departments or agencies with the knowledge that subjects may be involved within the period of support, but definite plans would not normally be set forth in the application or proposal. These include activities such as institutional type grants when selection of specific projects is the institution's responsibility; research training grants in which the activities involving subjects remain to be selected; and projects in which human subjects' involvement will depend upon completion of instruments, prior animal studies, or purification of compounds. Except for research waived under §46.101(i) or exempted under §46.104, no human subjects may be involved in any project supported by these awards until the project has been reviewed and approved by the IRB, as provided in this policy, and certification submitted, by the institution, to the Federal department or agency component supporting the research.

§46.119 Research undertaken without the intention of involving human subjects.

Except for research waived under §46.101(i) or exempted under §46.104, in the event research is undertaken without the intention of involving human subjects, but it is later proposed to involve human subjects in the research, the research shall first be reviewed and approved by an IRB, as provided in this policy, a certification submitted by the institution to the Federal department or agency component supporting the research, and final approval given to the proposed change by the Federal department or agency component.

§46.120 Evaluation and disposition of applications and proposals for research to be conducted or supported by a Federal department or agency.

(a) The department or agency head will evaluate all applications and proposals involving human subjects submitted to the Federal department or agency through such officers and employees of the Federal department or agency and such experts and consultants as the department or agency head determines to be appropriate. This evaluation will take into consideration the risks to the subjects, the adequacy of protection against these risks, the potential benefits of the research to the subjects and others, and the importance of the knowledge gained or to be gained.

(b) On the basis of this evaluation, the department or agency head may approve or disapprove the application or proposal, or enter into negotiations to develop an approvable one.

§46.121 [Reserved]

§46.122 Use of Federal funds.

Federal funds administered by a Federal department or agency may not be expended for research involving human subjects unless the requirements of this policy have been satisfied.

§46.123 Early termination of research support: Evaluation of applications and proposals.

(a) The department or agency head may require that Federal department or agency support for any project be terminated or suspended in the manner prescribed in applicable program requirements, when the department or agency head finds an institution has materially failed to comply with the terms of this policy.

(b) In making decisions about supporting or approving applications or proposals covered by this policy the department or agency head may take into account, in addition to all other eligibility requirements and program criteria, factors such as whether the applicant has been subject to a termination or suspension under paragraph (a) of this section and whether the applicant or the person or persons who would direct or has/have directed the scientific and technical aspects of an activity has/have, in the judgment of the department or agency head, materially failed to discharge responsibility for the protection of the rights and welfare of human subjects (whether or not the research was subject to federal regulation).

§46.124 Conditions.

With respect to any research project or any class of research projects the department or agency head of either the conducting or the supporting Federal department or agency may impose additional conditions prior to or at the time of approval when in the judgment of the department or agency head additional conditions are necessary for the protection of human subjects.

Subpart B—Additional Protections for Pregnant Women, Human Fetuses and Neonates Involved in Research

SOURCE: 66 FR 56778, Nov. 13, 2001, unless otherwise noted.

§46.201 To what do these regulations apply?

(a) Except as provided in paragraph (b) of this section, this subpart applies to all research involving pregnant women, human fetuses, neonates of uncertain viability, or nonviable neonates conducted or supported by the Department of Health and Human Services (DHHS). This includes all research conducted in DHHS facilities by any person and all research conducted in any facility by DHHS employees.

(b) The exemptions at §46.101(b)(1) through (6) are applicable to this subpart.

(c) The provisions of §46.101(c) through (i) are applicable to this subpart. Reference to State or local laws in this subpart and in §46.101(f) is intended to include the laws of federally recognized American Indian and Alaska Native Tribal Governments.

(d) The requirements of this subpart are in addition to those imposed under the other subparts of this part.

§46.202 Definitions.

The definitions in §46.102 shall be applicable to this subpart as well. In addition, as used in this subpart:

(a) Dead fetus means a fetus that exhibits neither heartbeat, spontaneous respiratory activity, spontaneous movement of voluntary muscles, nor pulsation of the umbilical cord.

(b) Delivery means complete separation of the fetus from the woman by expulsion or extraction or any other means.

(c) Fetus means the product of conception from implantation until delivery.

(d) Neonate means a newborn.

(e) Nonviable neonate means a neonate after delivery that, although living, is not viable.

(f) Pregnancy encompasses the period of time from implantation until delivery. A woman shall be assumed to be pregnant if she exhibits any of the pertinent presumptive signs of pregnancy, such as missed menses, until the results of a pregnancy test are negative or until delivery.

(g) Secretary means the Secretary of Health and Human Services and any other officer or employee of the Department of Health and Human Services to whom authority has been delegated.

(h) Viable, as it pertains to the neonate, means being able, after delivery, to survive (given the benefit of available medical therapy) to the point of independently maintaining heartbeat and respiration. The Secretary may from time to time, taking into account medical advances, publish in the FEDERAL REGIS-TER guidelines to assist in determining whether a neonate is viable for purposes of this subpart. If a neonate is viable then it may be included in research only to the extent permitted and in accordance with the requirements of subparts A and D of this part.

§46.203 Duties of IRBs in connection with research involving pregnant women, fetuses, and neonates.

In addition to other responsibilities assigned to IRBs under this part, each IRB shall review research covered by this subpart and approve only research which satisfies the conditions of all applicable sections of this subpart and the other subparts of this part.

§46.204 Research involving pregnant women or fetuses.

Pregnant women or fetuses may be involved in research if all of the following conditions are met:

(a) Where scientifically appropriate, preclinical studies, including studies on pregnant animals, and clinical studies, including studies on nonpregnant women, have been conducted and provide data for assessing potential risks to pregnant women and fetuses;

(b) The risk to the fetus is caused solely by interventions or procedures that hold out the prospect of direct benefit for the woman or the fetus; or, if there is no such prospect of benefit, the risk to the fetus is not greater than minimal and the purpose of the research is the development of important biomedical knowledge which cannot be obtained by any other means;

(c) Any risk is the least possible for achieving the objectives of the research;

(d) If the research holds out the prospect of direct benefit to the pregnant woman, the prospect of a direct benefit both to the pregnant woman and the fetus, or no prospect of benefit for the woman nor the fetus when risk to the fetus is not greater than minimal and the purpose of the research is the development of important biomedical knowledge that cannot be obtained by any other means, her consent is obtained in accord with the informed consent provisions of subpart A of this part;

(e) If the research holds out the prospect of direct benefit solely to the fetus then the consent of the pregnant woman and the father is obtained in accord with the informed consent provisions of subpart A of this part, except that the father's consent need not be obtained if he is unable to consent because of unavailability, incompetence, or temporary incapacity or the pregnancy resulted from rape or incest.

(f) Each individual providing consent under paragraph (d) or (e) of this section is fully informed regarding the reasonably foreseeable impact of the research on the fetus or neonate;

(g) For children as defined in §46.402(a) who are pregnant, assent and permission are obtained in accord with the provisions of subpart D of this part;

(h) No inducements, monetary or otherwise, will be offered to terminate a pregnancy;

(i) Individuals engaged in the research will have no part in any decisions as to the timing, method, or procedures used to terminate a pregnancy; and

(j) Individuals engaged in the research will have no part in determining the viability of a neonate.

§46.205 Research involving neonates.

(a) Neonates of uncertain viability and nonviable neonates may be involved in research if all of the following conditions are met:

(1) Where scientifically appropriate, preclinical and clinical studies have been conducted and provide data for assessing potential risks to neonates.

(2) Each individual providing consent under paragraph (b)(2) or (c)(5) of this section is fully informed regarding the reasonably foreseeable impact of the research on the neonate.

(3) Individuals engaged in the research will have no part in determining the viability of a neonate.

(4) The requirements of paragraph (b) or (c) of this section have been met as applicable.

(b) Neonates of uncertain viability. Until it has been ascertained whether or not a neonate is viable, a neonate may not be involved in research covered by this subpart unless the following additional conditions are met:

(1) The IRB determines that:

(i) The research holds out the prospect of enhancing the probability of survival of the neonate to the point of viability, and any risk is the least possible for achieving that objective, or

(ii) The purpose of the research is the development of important biomedical knowledge which cannot be obtained by other means and there will be no added risk to the neonate resulting from the research; and

(2) The legally effective informed consent of either parent of the neonate or, if neither parent is able to consent because of unavailability, incompetence, or temporary incapacity, the legally effective informed consent of either parent's legally authorized representative is obtained in accord with subpart A of this part, except that the consent of the father or his legally authorized representative need not be obtained if the pregnancy resulted from rape or incest.

(c) Nonviable neonates. After delivery nonviable neonate may not be involved in research covered by this subpart unless all of the following additional conditions are met:

(1) Vital functions of the neonate will not be artificially maintained;

(2) The research will not terminate the heartbeat or respiration of the neonate;

(3) There will be no added risk to the neonate resulting from the research;

(4) The purpose of the research is the development of important biomedical knowledge that cannot be obtained by other means; and

(5) The legally effective informed consent of both parents of the neonate is obtained in accord with subpart A of this part, except that the waiver and alteration provisions of §46.116(c) and (d) do not apply. However, if either parent is unable to consent because of unavailability, incompetence, or temporary incapacity, the informed consent of one parent of a nonviable neonate will suffice to meet the requirements of this paragraph (c)(5), except that the consent of the father need not be obtained if the pregnancy resulted from rape or incest. The consent of a legally authorized representative of either or both of the parents of a nonviable neonate will not suffice to meet the requirements of this paragraph (c)(5).

(d) Viable neonates. A neonate, after delivery, that has been determined to be viable may be included in research only to the extent permitted by and in accord with the requirements of subparts A and D of this part.

§46.206 Research involving, after delivery, the placenta, the dead fetus or fetal material.

(a) Research involving, after delivery, the placenta; the dead fetus; macerated fetal material; or cells, tissue, or organs excised from a dead fetus, shall be conducted only in accord with any applicable Federal, State, or local laws and regulations regarding such activities.

(b) If information associated with material described in paragraph (a) of this section is recorded for research purposes in a manner that living individuals can be identified, directly or through identifiers linked to those individuals, those individuals are research subjects and all pertinent subparts of this part are applicable.

§46.207 Research not otherwise approvable which presents an opportunity to understand, prevent, or alleviate a serious problem affecting the health or welfare of pregnant women, fetuses, or neonates.

The Secretary will conduct or fund research that the IRB does not believe meets the requirements of §46.204 or §46.205 only if:

(a) The IRB finds that the research presents a reasonable opportunity to further the understanding, prevention, or alleviation of a serious problem affecting the health or welfare of pregnant women, fetuses or neonates; and

(b) The Secretary, after consultation with a panel of experts in pertinent disciplines (for example: science, medicine, ethics, law) and following opportunity for public review and comment, including a public meeting announced in the FEDERAL REGISTER, has determined either:

(1) That the research in fact satisfies the conditions of §46.204, as applicable; or

(2) The following:

(i) The research presents a reasonable opportunity to further the understanding, prevention, or alleviation of a serious problem affecting the health or welfare of pregnant women, fetuses or neonates;

(ii) The research will be conducted in accord with sound ethical principles; and

(iii) Informed consent will be obtained in accord with the informed consent provisions of subpart A and other applicable subparts of this part.

Subpart C—Additional Protections Pertaining to Biomedical and Behavioral Research Involving Prisoners as Subjects

SOURCE: 43 FR 53655, Nov. 16, 1978, unless otherwise noted.

§46.301 Applicability.

(a) The regulations in this subpart are applicable to all biomedical and behavioral research conducted or supported by the Department of Health and Human Services involving prisoners as subjects.

(b) Nothing in this subpart shall be construed as indicating that compliance with the procedures set forth herein will authorize research involving prisoners as subjects, to the extent such research is limited or barred by applicable State or local law.

(c) The requirements of this subpart are in addition to those imposed under the other subparts of this part.

§46.302 Purpose.

Inasmuch as prisoners may be under constraints because of their incarceration which could affect their ability to make a truly voluntary and uncoerced decision whether or not to participate as subjects in research, it is the purpose of this subpart to provide additional safeguards for the protection of prisoners involved in activities to which this subpart is applicable.

§46.303 Definitions.

As used in this subpart:

(a) *Secretary* means the Secretary of Health and Human Services and any other officer or employee of the Department of Health and Human Services to whom authority has been delegated.

(b) *DHHS* means the Department of Health and Human Services.

(c) *Prisoner* means any individual involuntarily confined or detained in a penal institution. The term is intended to encompass individuals sentenced to such an institution under a criminal or civil statute, individuals detained in other facilities by virtue of statutes or commitment procedures which provide alternatives to criminal prosecution or incarceration in a penal institution, and individuals detained pending arraignment, trial, or sentencing.

(d) *Minimal risk* is the probability and magnitude of physical or psychological harm that is normally encountered in the daily lives, or in the routine medical, dental, or psychological examination of healthy persons.

§46.304 Composition of Institutional Review Boards where prisoners are involved.

In addition to satisfying the requirements in §46.107 of this part, an Institutional Review Board, carrying out responsibilities under this part with respect to research covered by this subpart, shall also meet the following specific requirements:

(a) A majority of the Board (exclusive of prisoner members) shall have no association with the prison(s) involved, apart from their membership on the Board.

(b) At least one member of the Board shall be a prisoner, or a prisoner representative with appropriate background and experience to serve in that capacity, except that where a particular research project is reviewed by more than one Board only one Board need satisfy this requirement.

[43 FR 53655, Nov. 16, 1978, as amended at 46 FR 8386, Jan. 26, 1981]

§46.305 Additional duties of the Institutional Review Boards where prisoners are involved.

(a) In addition to all other responsibilities prescribed for Institutional Review Boards under this part, the Board shall review research covered by this subpart and approve such research only if it finds that:

(1) The research under review represents one of the categories of research permissible under §46.306(a)(2);

(2) Any possible advantages accruing to the prisoner through his or her participation in the research, when compared to the general living conditions, medical care, quality of food, amenities and opportunity for earnings in the prison, are not of such a magnitude that his or her ability to weigh the risks of the research against the value of such advantages in the limited choice environment of the prison is impaired;

(3) The risks involved in the research are commensurate with risks that would be accepted by nonprisoner volunteers;

(4) Procedures for the selection of subjects within the prison are fair to all prisoners and immune from arbitrary intervention by prison authorities or prisoners. Unless the principal investigator provides to the Board justification in writing for following some other procedures, control subjects must be selected randomly from the group of available prisoners who meet the characteristics needed for that particular research project;

(5) The information is presented in language which is understandable to the subject population;

(6) Adequate assurance exists that parole boards will not take into account a prisoner's participation in the research in making decisions regarding parole, and each prisoner is clearly informed in advance that participation in the research will have no effect on his or her parole; and

(7) Where the Board finds there may be a need for follow-up examination or care of participants after the end of their participation, adequate provision has been made for such examination or care, taking into account the varying lengths of individual prisoners' sentences, and for informing participants of this fact.

(b) The Board shall carry out such other duties as may be assigned by the Secretary.

(c) The institution shall certify to the Secretary, in such form and manner as the Secretary may require, that the duties of the Board under this section have been fulfilled.

§46.306 Permitted research involving prisoners.

(a) Biomedical or behavioral research conducted or supported by DHHS may involve prisoners as subjects only if:

(1) The institution responsible for the conduct of the research has certified to the Secretary that the Institutional Review Board has approved the research under §46.305 of this subpart; and

(2) In the judgment of the Secretary the proposed research involves solely the following:

(i) Study of the possible causes, effects, and processes of incarceration, and of criminal behavior, provided that the study presents no more than minimal risk and no more than inconvenience to the subjects;

(ii) Study of prisons as institutional structures or of prisoners as incarcerated persons, provided that the study presents no more than minimal risk and no more than inconvenience to the subjects;

(iii) Research on conditions particularly affecting prisoners as a class (for example, vaccine trials and other research on hepatitis which is much more prevalent in prisons than elsewhere; and research on social and psychological problems such as alcoholism, drug addiction and sexual assaults) provided that the study may proceed only after the Secretary has consulted with appropriate experts including experts in penology medicine and ethics, and published notice, in the FEDERAL REGISTER, of his intent to approve such research; or

(iv) Research on practices, both innovative and accepted, which have the intent and reasonable probability of improving the health or well-being of the subject. In cases in which those studies require the assignment of prisoners in a manner consistent with protocols approved by the IRB to control groups which may not benefit from the research, the study may proceed only after the Secretary has consulted with appropriate experts, including experts in penology medicine and ethics, and published notice, in the FEDERAL REGISTER, of his intent to approve such research.

(b) Except as provided in paragraph (a) of this section, biomedical or behavioral research conducted or supported by DHHS shall not involve prisoners as subjects.

Subpart D—Additional Protections for Children Involved as Subjects in Research

SOURCE: 48 FR 9818, Mar. 8, 1983, unless otherwise noted.

§46.401 To what do these regulations apply?

(a) This subpart applies to all research involving children as subjects, conducted or supported by the Department of Health and Human Services.

(1) This includes research conducted by Department employees, except that each head of an Operating Division of the Department may adopt such nonsubstantive, procedural modifications as may be appropriate from an administrative standpoint.

(2) It also includes research conducted or supported by the Department of Health and Human Services outside the United States, but in appropriate circumstances, the Secretary may, under paragraph (e) of §46.101 of Subpart A, waive the applicability of some or all of the requirements of these regulations for research of this type.

(b) Exemptions at §46.101(b)(1) and (b)(3) through (b)(6) are applicable to this subpart. The exemption at §46.101(b)(2) regarding educational tests is also applicable to this subpart. However, the exemption at §46.101(b)(2) for research involving survey or interview procedures or observations of public behavior does not apply to research covered by this subpart, except for research involving observation of public behavior when the investigator(s) do not participate in the activities being observed.

(c) The exceptions, additions, and provisions for waiver as they appear in paragraphs (c) through (i) of §46.101 of Subpart A are applicable to this subpart.

[48 FR 9818, Mar. 8, 1983; 56 FR 28032, June 18, 1991; 56 FR 29757, June 28, 1991]

§46.402 Definitions.

The definitions in §46.102 of Subpart A shall be applicable to this subpart as well. In addition, as used in this subpart:

(a) *Children* are persons who have not attained the legal age for consent to treatments or procedures involved in the research, under the applicable law of the jurisdiction in which the research will be conducted.

(b) *Assent* means a child's affirmative agreement to participate in research. Mere failure to object should not, absent affirmative agreement, be construed as assent.

(c) *Permission* means the agreement of parent(s) or guardian to the participation of their child or ward in research.

(d) *Parent* means a child's biological or adoptive parent.

(e) *Guardian* means an individual who is authorized under applicable State or local law to consent on behalf of a child to general medical care.

§46.403 IRB duties.

In addition to other responsibilities assigned to IRBs under this part, each IRB shall review research covered by this subpart and approve only research which satisfies the conditions of all applicable sections of this subpart.

§46.404 Research not involving greater than minimal risk.

HHS will conduct or fund research in which the IRB finds that no greater than minimal risk to children is presented, only if the IRB finds that adequate provisions are made for soliciting the assent

§46.405 Research involving greater than minimal risk but presenting the prospect of direct benefit to the individual subjects.

HHS will conduct or fund research in which the IRB finds that more than minimal risk to children is presented by an intervention or procedure that holds out the prospect of direct benefit for the individual subject, or by a monitoring procedure that is likely to contribute to the subject's well-being, only if the IRB finds that:

(a) The risk is justified by the anticipated benefit to the subjects;

(b) The relation of the anticipated benefit to the risk is at least as favorable to the subjects as that presented by available alternative approaches; and

(c) Adequate provisions are made for soliciting the assent of the children and permission of their parents or guardians, as set forth in §46.408.

§46.406 Research involving greater than minimal risk and no prospect of direct benefit to individual subjects, but likely to yield generalizable knowledge about the subject's disorder or condition.

HHS will conduct or fund research in which the IRB finds that more than minimal risk to children is presented by an intervention or procedure that does not hold out the prospect of direct benefit for the individual subject, or by a monitoring procedure which is not likely to contribute to the well-being of the subject, only if the IRB finds that:

(a) The risk represents a minor increase over minimal risk;

(b) The intervention or procedure presents experiences to subjects that are reasonably commensurate with those inherent in their actual or expected medical, dental, psychological, social, or educational situations;

(c) The intervention or procedure is likely to yield generalizable knowledge about the subjects' disorder or condition which is of vital importance for the understanding or amelioration of the subjects' disorder or condition; and

(d) Adequate provisions are made for soliciting assent of the children and permission of their parents or guardians, as set forth in §46.408.

§46.407 Research not otherwise approvable which presents an opportunity to understand, prevent, or alleviate a serious problem affecting the health or welfare of children.

HHS will conduct or fund research that the IRB does not believe meets the requirements of §46.404, §46.405, or §46.406 only if:

(a) The IRB finds that the research presents a reasonable opportunity to further the understanding, prevention, or alleviation of a serious problem affecting the health or welfare of children; and

(b) The Secretary, after consultation with a panel of experts in pertinent disciplines (for example: science, medicine, education, ethics, law) and following opportunity for public review and comment, has determined either:

(1) That the research in fact satisfies the conditions of §46.404, §46.405, or §46.406, as applicable, or

(2) The following:

(i) The research presents a reasonable opportunity to further the understanding, prevention, or alleviation of a serious problem affecting the health or welfare of children;

(ii) The research will be conducted in accordance with sound ethical principles;

(iii) Adequate provisions are made for soliciting the assent of children and the permission of their parents or guardians, as set forth in §46.408.

§46.408 Requirements for permission by parents or guardians and for assent by children.

(a) In addition to the determinations required under other applicable sections of this subpart, the IRB shall determine that adequate provisions are made for soliciting the assent of the children, when in the judgment of the IRB the children are capable of providing assent. In determining whether children are capable of assenting, the IRB shall take into account the ages, maturity, and psychological state of the children involved. This judgment may be made for all children to be involved in research under a particular protocol, or for each child, as the IRB deems appropriate. If the IRB determines that the capability of some or all of the children is so limited that they cannot reasonably be consulted or that the intervention or procedure involved in the research holds out a prospect of direct benefit that is important to the health or well-being of the children and is available only in the context of the research, the assent of the children is not a necessary condition for proceeding with the research. Even where the IRB determines that the subjects are capable of assenting, the IRB may still waive the assent requirement under circumstances in which consent may be waived in accord with §46.116 of Subpart A.

(b) In addition to the determinations required under other applicable sections of this subpart, the IRB shall determine, in accordance with and to the extent that consent is required by §46.116 of Subpart A, that adequate provisions are made for soliciting the permission of each child's parents or guardian. Where parental permission is to be obtained, the IRB may find that the permission of one parent is sufficient for research to be conducted under §46.404 or §46.405. Where research is covered by §§46.406 and 46.407 and permission is to be obtained from parents, both parents must give their permission unless one parent is deceased, unknown, incompetent, or not reasonably available, or when only one parent has legal responsibility for the care and custody of the child.

(c) In addition to the provisions for waiver contained in §46.116 of Subpart A, if the IRB determines that a research protocol is designed for conditions or for a subject population for which parental or guardian permission is not a reasonable requirement to protect the subjects (for example, neglected or abused children), it may waive the consent requirements in Subpart A of this part and paragraph (b) of this section, provided an appropriate mechanism for protecting the children who will participate as subjects in the research is substituted, and provided further that the waiver is not inconsistent with Federal, state or local law. The choice of an appropriate mechanism would depend upon the nature and purpose of the activities described in the protocol, the risk and anticipated benefit to the research subjects, and their age, maturity, status, and condition.

(d) Permission by parents or guardians shall be documented in accordance with and to the extent required by §46.117 of Subpart A.

(e) When the IRB determines that assent is required, it shall also determine whether and how assent must be documented.

§46.409 Wards.

(a) Children who are wards of the state or any other agency, institution, or entity can be included in research approved under §46.406 or §46.407 only if such research is:

(1) Related to their status as wards; or

(2) Conducted in schools, camps, hospitals, institutions, or similar settings in which the majority of children involved as subjects are not wards.

(b) If the research is approved under paragraph (a) of this section, the IRB shall require appointment of an advocate for each child who is a ward, in addition to any other individual acting on behalf of the child as guardian or in loco parentis. One individual may serve as advocate for more than one child. The advocate shall be an individual who has the background and experience to act in, and agrees to act in, the best interests of the child for the duration of the child's participation in the research and who is not associated in any way (except in the role as advocate or member of the IRB) with the research, the investigator(s), or the guardian organization.

Subpart E—Registration of Institutional Review Boards
SOURCE: 74 FR 2405, Jan. 15, 2009, unless otherwise noted.

§46.501 What IRBs must be registered?
Each IRB that is designated by an institution under an assurance of compliance approved for federalwide use by the Office for Human Research Protections (OHRP) under §46.103(a) and that reviews research involving human subjects conducted or supported by the Department of Health and Human Services (HHS) must be registered with HHS. An individual authorized to act on behalf of the institution or organization operating the IRB must submit the registration information.

§46.502 What information must be provided when registering an IRB?
The following information must be provided to HHS when registering an IRB:

(a) The name, mailing address, and street address (if different from the mailing address) of the institution or organization operating the IRB(s); and the name, mailing address, phone number, facsimile number, and electronic mail address of the senior officer or head official of that institution or organization who is responsible for overseeing activities performed by the IRB.

(b) The name, mailing address, phone number, facsimile number, and electronic mail address of the contact person providing the registration information.

(c) The name, if any, assigned to the IRB by the institution or organization, and the IRB's mailing address, street address (if different from the mailing address), phone number, facsimile number, and electronic mail address.

(d) The name, phone number, and electronic mail address of the IRB chairperson.

(e)(1) The approximate numbers of:

(i) All active protocols; and

(ii) Active protocols conducted or supported by HHS.

(2) For purpose of this regulation, an "active protocol" is any protocol for which the IRB conducted an initial review or a continuing review at a convened meeting or under an expedited review procedure during the preceding twelve months.

(f) The approximate number of full-time equivalent positions devoted to the IRB's administrative activities.

§46.503 When must an IRB be registered?
An IRB must be registered before it can be designated under an assurance approved for federalwide use by OHRP under §46.103(a). IRB registration becomes effective when reviewed and accepted by OHRP. The registration will be effective for 3 years.

§46.504 How must an IRB be registered?
Each IRB must be registered electronically through *http://ohrp.cit.nih.gov/efile* unless an institution or organization lacks the ability to register its IRB(s) electronically. If an institution or organization lacks the ability to register an IRB electronically, it must send its IRB registration information in writing to OHRP.

§46.505 When must IRB registration information be renewed or updated?
(a) Each IRB must renew its registration every 3 years.

(b) The registration information for an IRB must be updated within 90 days after changes occur regarding the contact person who provided the IRB registration information or the IRB chairperson. The updated registration information must be submitted in accordance with §46.504.

(c) Any renewal or update that is submitted to, and accepted by, OHRP begins a new 3-year effective period.

(d) An institution's or organization's decision to disband a registered IRB which it is operating also must be reported to OHRP in writing within 30 days after permanent cessation of the IRB's review of HHS-conducted or -supported research.

Federal Register. (2017). Vol. 82, No. 12. 45 CFR 46. www.ecfr.gov/cgi-bin/retrieveECFR?gp=&SID=83cd09e1c0f5c6937cd9d7513160fc3f&pitd=20180719&n=pt45.1.46&r=PART&ty=HTML)

21 CFR 50: FDA Regulations on the Protection of Human Subjects

CODE OF FEDERAL REGULATIONS

TITLE 21–FOOD AND DRUGS

CHAPTER I–FOOD AND DRUG ADMINISTRATION

DEPARTMENT OF HEALTH AND HUMAN SERVICES

SUBCHAPTER A–GENERAL

PART 50 PROTECTION OF HUMAN SUBJECTS

<u>Subpart A–General Provisions</u>

§50.1 Scope.

(a) This part applies to all clinical investigations regulated by the Food and Drug Administration under sections 505(i) and 520(g) of the Federal Food, Drug, and Cosmetic Act, as well as clinical investigations that support applications for research or marketing permits for products regulated by the Food and Drug Administration, including foods, including dietary supplements, that bear a nutrient content claim or a health claim, infant formulas, food and color additives, drugs for human use, medical devices for human use, biological products for human use, and electronic products. Additional specific obligations and commitments of, and standards of conduct for, persons who sponsor or monitor clinical investigations involving particular test articles may also be found in other parts (e.g., parts 312 and 812). Compliance with these parts is intended to protect the rights and safety of subjects involved in investigations filed with the Food and Drug Administration pursuant to sections 403, 406, 409, 412, 413, 502, 503, 505, 510, 513-516, 518-520, 721, and 801 of the Federal Food, Drug, and Cosmetic Act and sections 351 and 354-360F of the Public Health Service Act.

(b) References in this part to regulatory sections of the Code of Federal Regulations are to chapter I of title 21, unless otherwise noted.

[45 FR 36390, May 30, 1980; 46 FR 8979, Jan. 27, 1981, as amended at 63 FR 26697, May 13, 1998; 64 FR 399, Jan. 5, 1999; 66 FR 20597, Apr. 24, 2001]

§50.3 Definitions.

As used in this part:

(a) Act means the Federal Food, Drug, and Cosmetic Act, as amended (secs. 201-902, 52 Stat. 1040 et seq. as amended (21 U.S.C. 321-392)).

(b) Application for research or marketing permit includes:

(1) A color additive petition, described in part 71.

(2) A food additive petition, described in parts 171 and 571.

(3) Data and information about a substance submitted as part of the procedures for establishing that the substance is generally recognized as safe for use that results or may reasonably be expected to result, directly or indirectly, in its becoming a component or otherwise affecting the characteristics of any food, described in 170.30 and 570.30.

(4) Data and information about a food additive submitted as part of the procedures for food additives permitted to be used on an interim basis pending additional study, described in 180.1.

(5) Data and information about a substance submitted as part of the procedures for establishing a tolerance for unavoidable contaminants in food and food-packaging materials, described in section 406 of the act.

(6) An investigational new drug application, described in part 312 of this chapter.

(7) A new drug application, described in part 314.

(8) Data and information about the bioavailability or bioequivalence of drugs for human use submitted as part of the procedures for issuing, amending, or repealing a bioequivalence requirement, described in part 320.

(9) Data and information about an over-the-counter drug for human use submitted as part of the procedures for classifying these drugs as generally recognized as safe and effective and not misbranded, described in part 330.

(10) Data and information about a prescription drug for human use submitted as part of the procedures for classifying these drugs as generally recognized as safe and effective and not misbranded, described in this chapter.

(11) [Reserved]

(12) An application for a biologics license, described in part 601 of this chapter.

(13) Data and information about a biological product submitted as part of the procedures for determining that licensed biological products are safe and effective and not misbranded, described in part 601.

(14) Data and information about an in vitro diagnostic product submitted as part of the procedures for establishing, amending, or repealing a standard for these products, described in part 809.

(15) An Application for an Investigational Device Exemption, described in part 812.

(16) Data and information about a medical device submitted as part of the procedures for classifying these devices, described in section 513.

(17) Data and information about a medical device submitted as part of the procedures for establishing, amending, or repealing a standard for these devices, described in section 514.

(18) An application for premarket approval of a medical device, described in section 515.

(19) A product development protocol for a medical device, described in section 515.

(20) Data and information about an electronic product submitted as part of the procedures for establishing, amending, or repealing a standard for these products, described in section 358 of the Public Health Service Act.

(21) Data and information about an electronic product submitted as part of the procedures for obtaining a variance from any electronic product performance standard, as described in 1010.4.

(22) Data and information about an electronic product submitted as part of the procedures for granting, amending, or extending an exemption from a radiation safety performance standard, as described in 1010.5.

(23) Data and information about a clinical study of an infant formula when submitted as part of an infant formula notification under section 412(c) of the Federal Food, Drug, and Cosmetic Act.

(24) Data and information submitted in a petition for a nutrient content claim, described in 101.69 of this chapter, or for a health claim, described in 101.70 of this chapter.

(25) Data and information from investigations involving children submitted in a new dietary ingredient notification, described in 190.6 of this chapter.

(c) Clinical investigation means any experiment that involves a test article and one or more human subjects and that either is subject to requirements for prior submission to the Food and Drug Administration under section 505(i) or 520(g) of the act, or is not subject to requirements for prior submission to the Food and Drug Administration under these sections of the act, but the results of which are intended to be submitted later to, or held for inspection by, the Food and Drug Administration as part of an application for a research or marketing permit. The term does not include experiments that are subject to the provisions of part 58 of this chapter, regarding nonclinical laboratory studies.

(d) Investigator means an individual who actually conducts a clinical investigation, i.e., under whose immediate direction the test article is administered or dispensed to, or used involving, a subject, or, in the event of an investigation conducted by a team of individuals, is the responsible leader of that team.

(e) Sponsor means a person who initiates a clinical investigation, but who does not actually conduct the investigation, i.e., the test article is administered or dispensed to or used involving, a subject under the immediate direction of another individual. A person other than an individual (e.g., corporation or agency) that uses one or more of its own employees to conduct a clinical investigation it has initiated is considered to be a sponsor (not a sponsor-investigator), and the employees are considered to be investigators.

(f) Sponsor-investigator means an individual who both initiates and actually conducts, alone or with others, a clinical investigation, i.e., under whose immediate direction the test article is administered or dispensed to, or used involving, a subject. The term does not include any person other than an individual, e.g., corporation or agency.

(g) Human subject means an individual who is or becomes a participant in research, either as a recipient of the test article or as a control. A subject may be either a healthy human or a patient.

(h) Institution means any public or private entity or agency (including Federal, State, and other agencies). The word facility as used in section 520(g) of the act is deemed to be synonymous with the term institution for purposes of this part.

(i) Institutional review board (IRB) means any board, committee, or other group formally designated by an institution to review biomedical research involving humans as subjects, to approve the initiation of and conduct periodic review of such research. The term has the same meaning as the phrase institutional review committee as used in section 520(g) of the act.

(j) Test article means any drug (including a biological product for human use), medical device for human use, human food additive, color additive, electronic product, or any other article subject to regulation under the act or under sections 351 and 354-360F of the Public Health Service Act (42 U.S.C. 262 and 263b-263n).

(k) Minimal risk means that the probability and magnitude of harm or discomfort anticipated in the research are not greater in and of themselves than those ordinarily encountered in daily life or during the performance of routine physical or psychological examinations or tests.

(l) Legally authorized representative means an individual or judicial or other body authorized under applicable law to consent on behalf of a prospective subject to the subject's participation in the procedure(s) involved in the research.

(m) Family member means any one of the following legally competent persons: Spouse; parents; children (including adopted children); brothers, sisters, and spouses of brothers and sisters; and any individual related by blood or affinity whose close association with the subject is the equivalent of a family relationship.

(n) Assent means a child's affirmative agreement to participate in a clinical investigation. Mere failure to object should not, absent affirmative agreement, be construed as assent.

(o) Children means persons who have not attained the legal age for consent to treatments or procedures involved in clinical investigations, under the applicable law of the jurisdiction in which the clinical investigation will be conducted.

(p) Parent means a child's biological or adoptive parent.

(q) Ward means a child who is placed in the legal custody of the State or other agency, institution, or entity, consistent with applicable Federal, State, or local law.

(r) Permission means the agreement of parent(s) or guardian to the participation of their child or ward in a clinical investigation.

(s) Guardian means an individual who is authorized under applicable State or local law to consent on behalf of a child to general medical care.

[45 FR 36390, May 30, 1980, as amended at 46 FR 8950, Jan. 27, 1981; 54 FR 9038, Mar. 3, 1989; 56 FR 28028, June 18, 1991; 61 FR 51528, Oct. 2, 1996; 62 FR 39440, July 23, 1997; 64 FR 399, Jan. 5, 1999; 64 FR 56448, Oct. 20, 1999; 66 FR 20597, Apr. 24, 2001; 78 FR 12950, Feb. 26, 2013]

Subpart B–Informed Consent of Human Subjects

§50.20 General requirements for informed consent.

Except as provided in 50.23 and 50.24, no investigator may involve a human being as a subject in research covered by these regulations unless the investigator has obtained the legally effective informed consent of the subject or the subject's legally authorized representative. An investigator shall seek such consent only under circumstances that provide the prospective subject or the representative sufficient opportunity to consider whether or not to participate and that minimize the possibility of coercion or undue influence. The information that is given to the subject or the representative shall be in language understandable to the subject or the representative. No informed consent, whether oral or written, may include any exculpatory language through which the subject or the representative is made to waive or appear to waive any of the subject's legal rights, or releases or appears to release the investigator, the sponsor, the institution, or its agents from liability for negligence.

[46 FR 8951, Jan. 27, 1981, as amended at 64 FR 10942, Mar. 8, 1999]

§50.23 Exception from general requirements.

(a) The obtaining of informed consent shall be deemed feasible unless, before use of the test article (except as provided in paragraph (b) of this section), both the investigator and a physician who is not otherwise participating in the clinical investigation certify in writing all of the following:

(1) The human subject is confronted by a life-threatening situation necessitating the use of the test article.

(2) Informed consent cannot be obtained from the subject because of an inability to communicate with, or obtain legally effective consent from, the subject.

(3) Time is not sufficient to obtain consent from the subject's legal representative.

(4) There is available no alternative method of approved or generally recognized therapy that provides an equal or greater likelihood of saving the life of the subject.

(b) If immediate use of the test article is, in the investigator's opinion, required to preserve the life of the subject, and time is not sufficient to obtain the independent determination required in paragraph (a) of this section in advance of using the test article, the determinations of the clinical investigator shall be made and, within 5 working days after the use of the article, be reviewed and evaluated in writing by a physician who is not participating in the clinical investigation.

(c) The documentation required in paragraph (a) or (b) of this section shall be submitted to the IRB within 5 working days after the use of the test article.

(d)(1) Under 10 U.S.C. 1107(f) the President may waive the prior consent requirement for the administration of an investigational new drug to a member of the armed forces in connection with the member's participation in a particular military operation. The statute specifies that only the President may waive informed consent in this connection and the President may grant such a waiver only if the President determines in writing that obtaining consent: Is not feasible; is contrary to the best interests of the military member; or is not in the interests of national security. The statute further provides that in making a determination to waive prior informed consent on the ground that it is not feasible or the ground that it is contrary to the best interests of the military members involved, the President shall apply the standards and criteria that are set forth in the relevant FDA regulations for a waiver of the prior informed consent requirements of section 505(i)(4) of the Federal Food, Drug, and Cosmetic Act (21 U.S.C. 355(i)(4)). Before such a determination may be made that obtaining informed consent from military personnel prior to the use of an investigational drug (including an antibiotic or biological product) in a specific protocol under an investigational new drug application (IND) sponsored by the Department of Defense (DOD) and limited to specific military personnel involved in a particular military operation is not feasible or is contrary to the best interests of the military members involved the Secretary of Defense must first request such a determination from the President, and certify and document to the President that the following standards and criteria contained in paragraphs (d)(1) through (d)(4) of this section have been met.

(i) The extent and strength of evidence of the safety and effectiveness of the investigational new drug in relation to the medical risk that could be encountered during the military operation supports the drug's administration under an IND.

(ii) The military operation presents a substantial risk that military personnel may be subject to a chemical, biological, nuclear, or other exposure likely to produce death or serious or life-threatening injury or illness.

(iii) There is no available satisfactory alternative therapeutic or preventive treatment in relation to the intended use of the investigational new drug.

(iv) Conditioning use of the investigational new drug on the voluntary participation of each member could significantly risk the safety and health of any individual member who would decline its use, the safety of other military personnel, and the accomplishment of the military mission.

(v) A duly constituted institutional review board (IRB) established and operated in accordance with the requirements of paragraphs (d)(2) and (d)(3) of this section, responsible for review of the study, has reviewed and approved the investigational new drug protocol and the administration of the investigational new drug without informed consent. DOD's request is to include the documentation required by 56.115(a)(2) of this chapter.

(vi) DOD has explained:

(A) The context in which the investigational drug will be administered, e.g., the setting or whether it will be self-administered or it will be administered by a health professional;

(B) The nature of the disease or condition for which the preventive or therapeutic treatment is intended; and

(C) To the extent there are existing data or information available, information on conditions that could alter the effects of the investigational drug.

(vii) DOD's recordkeeping system is capable of tracking and will be used to track the proposed treatment from supplier to the individual recipient.

(viii) Each member involved in the military operation will be given, prior to the administration of the investigational new drug, a specific written information sheet (including information required by 10 U.S.C. 1107(d)) concerning the investigational new drug, the risks and benefits of its use, potential side effects, and other pertinent information about the appropriate use of the product.

(ix) Medical records of members involved in the military operation will accurately document the receipt by members of the notification required by paragraph (d)(1)(viii) of this section.

(x) Medical records of members involved in the military operation will accurately document the receipt by members of any investigational new drugs in accordance with FDA regulations including part 312 of this chapter.

(xi) DOD will provide adequate followup to assess whether there are beneficial or adverse health consequences that result from the use of the investigational product.

(xii) DOD is pursuing drug development, including a time line, and marketing approval with due diligence.

(xiii) FDA has concluded that the investigational new drug protocol may proceed subject to a decision by the President on the informed consent waiver request.

(xiv) DOD will provide training to the appropriate medical personnel and potential recipients on the specific investigational new drug to be administered prior to its use.

(xv) DOD has stated and justified the time period for which the waiver is needed, not to exceed one year, unless separately renewed under these standards and criteria.

(xvi) DOD shall have a continuing obligation to report to the FDA and to the President any changed circumstances relating to these standards and criteria (including the time period referred to in paragraph (d)(1)(xv) of this section) or that otherwise might affect the determination to use an investigational new drug without informed consent.

(xvii) DOD is to provide public notice as soon as practicable and consistent with classification requirements through notice in the Federal Register describing each waiver of informed consent determination, a summary of the most updated scientific information on the products used, and other pertinent information.

(xviii) Use of the investigational drug without informed consent otherwise conforms with applicable law.

(2) The duly constituted institutional review board, described in paragraph (d)(1)(v) of this section, must include at least 3 nonaffiliated members who shall not be employees or officers of the Federal Government (other than for purposes of membership on the IRB) and shall be required to obtain any necessary security clearances. This IRB shall review the proposed IND protocol at a convened meeting at which a majority of the members are present including at least one member whose primary concerns are in nonscientific areas and, if feasible, including a majority of the nonaffiliated members. The information required by 56.115(a)(2) of this chapter is to be provided to the Secretary of Defense for further review.

(3) The duly constituted institutional review board, described in paragraph (d)(1)(v) of this section, must review and approve:

(i) The required information sheet;

(ii) The adequacy of the plan to disseminate information, including distribution of the information sheet to potential recipients, on the investigational product (e.g., in forms other than written);

(iii) The adequacy of the information and plans for its dissemination to health care providers, including potential side effects, contraindications, potential interactions, and other pertinent considerations; and

(iv) An informed consent form as required by part 50 of this chapter, in those circumstances in which DOD determines that informed consent may be obtained from some or all personnel involved.

(4) DOD is to submit to FDA summaries of institutional review board meetings at which the proposed protocol has been reviewed.

(5) Nothing in these criteria or standards is intended to preempt or limit FDA's and DOD's authority or obligations under applicable statutes and regulations.

(e)(1) Obtaining informed consent for investigational in vitro diagnostic devices used to identify chemical, biological, radiological, or nuclear agents will be deemed feasible unless, before use of the test article, both the investigator (e.g., clinical laboratory director or other responsible individual) and a physician who is not otherwise participating in the clinical investigation make the determinations and later certify in writing all of the following:

(i) The human subject is confronted by a life-threatening situation necessitating the use of the investigational in vitro diagnostic device to identify a chemical, biological, radiological, or nuclear agent that would suggest a terrorism event or other public health emergency.

(ii) Informed consent cannot be obtained from the subject because:

(A) There was no reasonable way for the person directing that the specimen be collected to know, at the time the specimen was collected, that there would be a need to use the investigational in vitro diagnostic device on that subject's specimen; and

(B) Time is not sufficient to obtain consent from the subject without risking the life of the subject.

(iii) Time is not sufficient to obtain consent from the subject's legally authorized representative.

(iv) There is no cleared or approved available alternative method of diagnosis, to identify the chemical, biological, radiological, or nuclear agent that provides an equal or greater likelihood of saving the life of the subject.

(2) If use of the investigational device is, in the opinion of the investigator (e.g., clinical laboratory director or other responsible person), required to preserve the life of the subject, and time is not sufficient to obtain the independent determination required in paragraph (e)(1) of this section in advance of using the investigational device, the determinations of the investigator shall be made and, within 5 working days after the use of the device, be reviewed and evaluated in writing by a physician who is not participating in the clinical investigation.

(3) The investigator must submit the written certification of the determinations made by the investigator and an independent physician required in paragraph (e)(1) or (e)(2) of this section to the IRB and FDA within 5 working days after the use of the device.

(4) An investigator must disclose the investigational status of the in vitro diagnostic device and what is known about the performance characteristics of

the device in the report to the subject's health care provider and in any report to public health authorities. The investigator must provide the IRB with the information required in 50.25 (except for the information described in 50.25(a)(8)) and the procedures that will be used to provide this information to each subject or the subject's legally authorized representative at the time the test results are provided to the subject's health care provider and public health authorities.

(5) The IRB is responsible for ensuring the adequacy of the information required in section 50.25 (except for the information described in 50.25(a)(8)) and for ensuring that procedures are in place to provide this information to each subject or the subject's legally authorized representative.

(6) No State or political subdivision of a State may establish or continue in effect any law, rule, regulation or other requirement that informed consent be obtained before an investigational in vitro diagnostic device may be used to identify chemical, biological, radiological, or nuclear agent in suspected terrorism events and other potential public health emergencies that is different from, or in addition to, the requirements of this regulation.

[46 FR 8951, Jan. 27, 1981, as amended at 55 FR 52817, Dec. 21, 1990; 64 FR 399, Jan. 5, 1999; 64 FR 54188, Oct. 5, 1999; 71 FR 32833, June 7, 2006; 76 FR 36993, June 24, 2011]

§50.24 Exception from informed consent requirements for emergency research.

(a) The IRB responsible for the review, approval, and continuing review of the clinical investigation described in this section may approve that investigation without requiring that informed consent of all research subjects be obtained if the IRB (with the concurrence of a licensed physician who is a member of or consultant to the IRB and who is not otherwise participating in the clinical investigation) finds and documents each of the following:

(1) The human subjects are in a life-threatening situation, available treatments are unproven or unsatisfactory, and the collection of valid scientific evidence, which may include evidence obtained through randomized placebo-controlled investigations, is necessary to determine the safety and effectiveness of particular interventions.

(2) Obtaining informed consent is not feasible because:

(i) The subjects will not be able to give their informed consent as a result of their medical condition;

(ii) The intervention under investigation must be administered before consent from the subjects' legally authorized representatives is feasible; and

(iii) There is no reasonable way to identify prospectively the individuals likely to become eligible for participation in the clinical investigation.

(3) Participation in the research holds out the prospect of direct benefit to the subjects because:

(i) Subjects are facing a life-threatening situation that necessitates intervention;

(ii) Appropriate animal and other preclinical studies have been conducted, and the information derived from those studies and related evidence support the potential for the intervention to provide a direct benefit to the individual subjects; and

(iii) Risks associated with the investigation are reasonable in relation to what is known about the medical condition of the potential class of subjects, the risks and benefits of standard therapy, if any, and what is known about the risks and benefits of the proposed intervention or activity.

(4) The clinical investigation could not practicably be carried out without the waiver.

(5) The proposed investigational plan defines the length of the potential therapeutic window based on scientific evidence, and the investigator has committed to attempting to contact a legally authorized representative for each subject within that window of time and, if feasible, to asking the legally authorized representative contacted for consent within that window rather than proceeding without consent. The investigator will summarize efforts made to contact legally authorized representatives and make this information available to the IRB at the time of continuing review.

(6) The IRB has reviewed and approved informed consent procedures and an informed consent document consistent with 50.25. These procedures and the informed consent document are to be used with subjects or their legally authorized representatives in situations where use of such procedures and documents is feasible. The IRB has reviewed and approved procedures and information to be used when providing an opportunity for a family member to object to a subject's participation in the clinical investigation consistent with paragraph (a)(7)(v) of this section.

(7) Additional protections of the rights and welfare of the subjects will be provided, including, at least:

(i) Consultation (including, where appropriate, consultation carried out by the IRB) with representatives of the communities in which the clinical investigation will be conducted and from which the subjects will be drawn;

(ii) Public disclosure to the communities in which the clinical investigation will be conducted and from which the subjects will be drawn, prior to initiation of the clinical investigation, of plans for the investigation and its risks and expected benefits;

(iii) Public disclosure of sufficient information following completion of the clinical investigation to apprise the community and researchers of the study, including the demographic characteristics of the research population, and its results;

(iv) Establishment of an independent data monitoring committee to exercise oversight of the clinical investigation; and

(v) If obtaining informed consent is not feasible and a legally authorized representative is not reasonably available, the investigator has committed, if feasible, to attempting to contact within the therapeutic window the subject's family member who is not a legally authorized representative, and asking whether he or she objects to the subject's participation in the clinical investigation. The investigator will summarize efforts made to contact family members and make this information available to the IRB at the time of continuing review.

(b) The IRB is responsible for ensuring that procedures are in place to inform, at the earliest feasible opportunity, each subject, or if the subject remains incapacitated, a legally authorized representative of the subject, or if such a representative is not reasonably available, a family member, of the subject's inclusion in the clinical investigation, the details of the investigation and other information contained in the informed consent document. The IRB shall also ensure that there is a procedure to inform the subject, or if the subject remains incapacitated, a legally authorized representative of the subject, or if such a representative is not reasonably available, a family member, that he or she may discontinue the subject's participation at any time without penalty or loss of benefits to which the subject is otherwise entitled. If a legally authorized representative or family member is told about the clinical investigation and the subject's condition improves, the subject is also to be informed as soon as feasible. If a subject is entered into a clinical investigation with waived consent and the subject dies before a legally authorized representative or family member can be contacted, information about the clinical investigation is to be provided to the subject's legally authorized representative or family member, if feasible.

(c) The IRB determinations required by paragraph (a) of this section and the documentation required by paragraph (e) of this section are to be retained by the IRB for at least 3 years after completion of the clinical investigation, and the records shall be accessible for inspection and copying by FDA in accordance with 56.115(b) of this chapter.

(d) Protocols involving an exception to the informed consent requirement under this section must be performed under a separate investigational new drug application (IND) or investigational device exemption (IDE) that clearly identifies such protocols as protocols that may include subjects who are unable to consent. The submission of those protocols in a separate IND/IDE is required even if an IND for the same drug product or an IDE for the same device already exists. Applications for investigations under this section may not be submitted as amendments under 312.30 or 812.35 of this chapter.

(e) If an IRB determines that it cannot approve a clinical investigation because the investigation does not meet the criteria in the exception provided under paragraph (a) of this section or because of other relevant ethical concerns, the IRB must document its findings and provide these findings promptly in writing to the clinical investigator and to the sponsor of the clinical investigation. The sponsor of the clinical investigation must promptly disclose this information to FDA and to the sponsor's clinical investigators who are participating or are asked to participate in this or a substantially equivalent clinical investigation of the sponsor, and to other IRB's that have been, or are, asked to review this or a substantially equivalent investigation by that sponsor.
[61 FR 51528, Oct. 2, 1996]

§50.25 Elements of informed consent.

(a) Basic elements of informed consent. In seeking informed consent, the following information shall be provided to each subject:

(1) A statement that the study involves research, an explanation of the purposes of the research and the expected duration of the subject's participation, a description of the procedures to be followed, and identification of any procedures which are experimental.

(2) A description of any reasonably foreseeable risks or discomforts to the subject.

(3) A description of any benefits to the subject or to others which may reasonably be expected from the research.

(4) A disclosure of appropriate alternative procedures or courses of treatment, if any, that might be advantageous to the subject.

(5) A statement describing the extent, if any, to which confidentiality of records identifying the subject will be maintained and that notes the possibility that the Food and Drug Administration may inspect the records.

(6) For research involving more than minimal risk, an explanation as to whether any compensation and an explanation as to whether any medical treatments are available if injury occurs and, if so, what they consist of, or where further information may be obtained.

(7) An explanation of whom to contact for answers to pertinent questions about the research and research subjects' rights, and whom to contact in the event of a research-related injury to the subject.

(8) A statement that participation is voluntary, that refusal to participate will involve no penalty or loss of benefits to which the subject is otherwise

entitled, and that the subject may discontinue participation at any time without penalty or loss of benefits to which the subject is otherwise entitled.

(b) Additional elements of informed consent. When appropriate, one or more of the following elements of information shall also be provided to each subject:

(1) A statement that the particular treatment or procedure may involve risks to the subject (or to the embryo or fetus, if the subject is or may become pregnant) which are currently unforeseeable.

(2) Anticipated circumstances under which the subject's participation may be terminated by the investigator without regard to the subject's consent.

(3) Any additional costs to the subject that may result from participation in the research.

(4) The consequences of a subject's decision to withdraw from the research and procedures for orderly termination of participation by the subject.

(5) A statement that significant new findings developed during the course of the research which may relate to the subject's willingness to continue participation will be provided to the subject.

(6) The approximate number of subjects involved in the study.

(c) When seeking informed consent for applicable clinical trials, as defined in 42 U.S.C. 282(j)(1)(A), the following statement shall be provided to each clinical trial subject in informed consent documents and processes. This will notify the clinical trial subject that clinical trial information has been or will be submitted for inclusion in the clinical trial registry databank under paragraph (j) of section 402 of the Public Health Service Act. The statement is: "A description of this clinical trial will be available on http://www.ClinicalTrials.gov, as required by U.S. Law. This Web site will not include information that can identify you. At most, the Web site will include a summary of the results. You can search this Web site at any time."

(d) The informed consent requirements in these regulations are not intended to preempt any applicable Federal, State, or local laws which require additional information to be disclosed for informed consent to be legally effective.

(e) Nothing in these regulations is intended to limit the authority of a physician to provide emergency medical care to the extent the physician is permitted to do so under applicable Federal, State, or local law.

[46 FR 8951, Jan. 27, 1981, as amended at 76 FR 270, Jan. 4, 2011]

§50.27 Documentation of informed consent.

(a) Except as provided in 56.109(c), informed consent shall be documented by the use of a written consent form approved by the IRB and signed and dated by the subject or the subject's legally authorized representative at the time of consent. A copy shall be given to the person signing the form.

(b) Except as provided in 56.109(c), the consent form may be either of the following:

(1) A written consent document that embodies the elements of informed consent required by 50.25. This form may be read to the subject or the subject's legally authorized representative, but, in any event, the investigator shall give either the subject or the representative adequate opportunity to read it before it is signed.

(2) A short form written consent document stating that the elements of informed consent required by 50.25 have been presented orally to the subject or the subject's legally authorized representative. When this method is used, there shall be a witness to the oral presentation. Also, the IRB shall approve a written

summary of what is to be said to the subject or the representative. Only the short form itself is to be signed by the subject or the representative. However, the witness shall sign both the short form and a copy of the summary, and the person actually obtaining the consent shall sign a copy of the summary. A copy of the summary shall be given to the subject or the representative in addition to a copy of the short form.

[46 FR 8951, Jan. 27, 1981, as amended at 61 FR 57280, Nov. 5, 1996]

Subpart C [Reserved]

Subpart D–Additional Safeguards for Children in Clinical Investigations

§50.50 IRB duties.

In addition to other responsibilities assigned to IRBs under this part and part 56 of this chapter, each IRB must review clinical investigations involving children as subjects covered by this subpart D and approve only those clinical investigations that satisfy the criteria described in 50.51, 50.52, or 50.53 and the conditions of all other applicable sections of this subpart D.

§50.51 Clinical investigations not involving greater than minimal risk.

Any clinical investigation within the scope described in 50.1 and 56.101 of this chapter in which no greater than minimal risk to children is presented may involve children as subjects only if the IRB finds that:

(a) No greater than minimal risk to children is presented; and

(b) Adequate provisions are made for soliciting the assent of the children and the permission of their parents or guardians as set forth in 50.55.

[78 FR 12951, Feb. 26, 2013]

§50.52 Clinical investigations involving greater than minimal risk but presenting the prospect of direct benefit to individual subjects.

Any clinical investigation within the scope described in 50.1 and 56.101 of this chapter in which more than minimal risk to children is presented by an intervention or procedure that holds out the prospect of direct benefit for the individual subject, or by a monitoring procedure that is likely to contribute to the subject's well-being, may involve children as subjects only if the IRB finds that:

(a) The risk is justified by the anticipated benefit to the subjects;

(b) The relation of the anticipated benefit to the risk is at least as favorable to the subjects as that presented by available alternative approaches; and

(c) Adequate provisions are made for soliciting the assent of the children and permission of their parents or guardians as set forth in 50.55.

[66 FR 20598, Apr. 24, 2001, as amended at 78 FR 12951, Feb. 26, 2013]

§50.53 Clinical investigations involving greater than minimal risk and no prospect of direct benefit to individual subjects, but likely to yield generalizable knowledge about the subjects' disorder or condition.

Any clinical investigation within the scope described in 50.1 and 56.101 of this chapter in which more than minimal risk to children is presented by an intervention or procedure that does not hold out the prospect of direct benefit for the individual subject, or by a monitoring procedure that is not likely to contribute to the well-being of the subject, may involve children as subjects only if the IRB finds that:

(a) The risk represents a minor increase over minimal risk;

(b) The intervention or procedure presents experiences to subjects that are reasonably commensurate with those inherent in their actual or expected medical, dental, psychological, social, or educational situations;

(c) The intervention or procedure is likely to yield generalizable knowledge about the subjects' disorder or condition that is of vital importance for the understanding or amelioration of the subjects' disorder or condition; and

(d) Adequate provisions are made for soliciting the assent of the children and permission of their parents or guardians as set forth in 50.55.

[66 FR 20598, Apr. 24, 2001, as amended at 78 FR 12951, Feb. 26, 2013]

§50.54 Clinical investigations not otherwise approvable that present an opportunity to understand, prevent, or alleviate a serious problem affecting the health or welfare of children.

If an IRB does not believe that a clinical investigation within the scope described in 50.1 and 56.101 of this chapter and involving children as subjects meets the requirements of 50.51, 50.52, or 50.53, the clinical investigation may proceed only if:

(a) The IRB finds that the clinical investigation presents a reasonable opportunity to further the understanding, prevention, or alleviation of a serious problem affecting the health or welfare of children; and

(b) The Commissioner of Food and Drugs, after consultation with a panel of experts in pertinent disciplines (for example: science, medicine, education, ethics, law) and following opportunity for public review and comment, determines either:

(1) That the clinical investigation in fact satisfies the conditions of 50.51, 50.52, or 50.53, as applicable, or

(2) That the following conditions are met:

(i) The clinical investigation presents a reasonable opportunity to further the understanding, prevention, or alleviation of a serious problem affecting the health or welfare of children;

(ii) The clinical investigation will be conducted in accordance with sound ethical principles; and

(iii) Adequate provisions are made for soliciting the assent of children and the permission of their parents or guardians as set forth in 50.55.

[66 FR 20598, Apr. 24, 2001, as amended at 78 FR 12951, Feb. 26, 2013]

§50.55 Requirements for permission by parents or guardians and for assent by children.

(a) In addition to the determinations required under other applicable sections of this subpart D, the IRB must determine that adequate provisions are made for soliciting the assent of the children when in the judgment of the IRB the children are capable of providing assent.

(b) In determining whether children are capable of providing assent, the IRB must take into account the ages, maturity, and psychological state of the children involved. This judgment may be made for all children to be involved in clinical investigations under a particular protocol, or for each child, as the IRB deems appropriate.

(c) The assent of the children is not a necessary condition for proceeding with the clinical investigation if the IRB determines:

(1) That the capability of some or all of the children is so limited that they cannot reasonably be consulted, or

(2) That the intervention or procedure involved in the clinical investigation holds out a prospect of direct benefit that is important to the health or well-being of the children and is available only in the context of the clinical investigation.

(d) Even where the IRB determines that the subjects are capable of assenting, the IRB may still waive the assent requirement if it finds and documents that:

(1) The clinical investigation involves no more than minimal risk to the subjects;

(2) The waiver will not adversely affect the rights and welfare of the subjects;

(3) The clinical investigation could not practicably be carried out without the waiver; and

(4) Whenever appropriate, the subjects will be provided with additional pertinent inf1ormation after participation.

(e) In addition to the determinations required under other applicable sections of this subpart D, the IRB must determine, in accordance with and to the extent that consent is required under part 50, that the permission of each child's parents or guardian is granted.

(1) Where parental permission is to be obtained, the IRB may find that the permission of one parent is sufficient for clinical investigations to be conducted under 50.51 or 50.52.

(2) Where clinical investigations are covered by 50.53 or 50.54 and permission is to be obtained from parents, both parents must give their permission unless one parent is deceased, unknown, incompetent, or not reasonably available, or when only one parent has legal responsibility for the care and custody of the child.

(f) Permission by parents or guardians must be documented in accordance with and to the extent required by 50.27.

(g) When the IRB determines that assent is required, it must also determine whether and how assent must be documented.

[66 FR 20598, Apr. 24, 2001, as amended at 78 FR 12951, Feb. 26, 2013]

§50.56 Wards.

(a) Children who are wards of the State or any other agency, institution, or entity can be included in clinical investigations approved under 50.53 or 50.54 only if such clinical investigations are:

(1) Related to their status as wards; or

(2) Conducted in schools, camps, hospitals, institutions, or similar settings in which the majority of children involved as subjects are not wards.

(b) If the clinical investigation is approved under paragraph (a) of this section, the IRB must require appointment of an advocate for each child who is a ward.

(1) The advocate will serve in addition to any other individual acting on behalf of the child as guardian or in loco parentis.

(2) One individual may serve as advocate for more than one child.

(3) The advocate must be an individual who has the background and experience to act in, and agrees to act in, the best interest of the child for the duration of the child's participation in the clinical investigation.

(4) The advocate must not be associated in any way (except in the role as advocate or member of the IRB) with the clinical investigation, the investigator(s), or the guardian organization.

Authority: 21 U.S.C 321, 343, 346, 346a, 348, 350a, 350b, 352, 353, 355, 360, 360c-360f, 360h-360j, 371, 379e, 381; 42 U.S.C. 216, 241, 262, 263b-263n.

Source: 45 FR 36390, May 30, 1980, unless otherwise noted.

Food and Drug Administration. (2019). *21 CFR 50 protection of human subjects.* https://www.ecfr.gov/cgi-bin/text-idx?SID=b245bf060d80dbfb2186856ba6f8fcf4&mc=true&node=pt21.1.50&rgn=div5

21 CFR 56: FDA Regulations Governing Institutional Review Boards

CODE OF FEDERAL REGULATIONS

TITLE 21–FOOD AND DRUGS

CHAPTER I–FOOD AND DRUG ADMINISTRATION

DEPARTMENT OF HEALTH AND HUMAN SERVICES

SUBCHAPTER A–GENERAL

PART 56 INSTITUTIONAL REVIEW BOARDS

Subpart A–General Provisions

§56.101 Scope.

(a) This part contains the general standards for the composition, operation, and responsibility of an Institutional Review Board (IRB) that reviews clinical investigations regulated by the Food and Drug Administration under sections 505(i) and 520(g) of the act, as well as clinical investigations that support applications for research or marketing permits for products regulated by the Food and Drug Administration, including foods, including dietary supplements, that bear a nutrient content claim or a health claim, infant formulas, food and color additives, drugs for human use, medical devices for human use, biological products for human use, and electronic products. Compliance with this part is intended to protect the rights and welfare of human subjects involved in such investigations.

(b) References in this part to regulatory sections of the Code of Federal Regulations are to chapter I of title 21, unless otherwise noted.

[46 FR 8975, Jan. 27, 1981, as amended at 64 FR 399, Jan. 5, 1999; 66 FR 20599, Apr. 24, 2001]

§56.102 Definitions.

As used in this part:

(a) Act means the Federal Food, Drug, and Cosmetic Act, as amended (secs. 201-902, 52 Stat. 1040 et seq., as amended (21 U.S.C. 321-392)).

(b) Application for research or marketing permit includes:

(1) A color additive petition, described in part 71.

(2) Data and information regarding a substance submitted as part of the procedures for establishing that a substance is generally recognized as safe for a use which results or may reasonably be expected to result, directly or indirectly, in its becoming a component or otherwise affecting the characteristics of any food, described in 170.35.

(3) A food additive petition, described in part 171.

(4) Data and information regarding a food additive submitted as part of the procedures regarding food additives permitted to be used on an interim basis pending additional study, described in 180.1.

(5) Data and information regarding a substance submitted as part of the procedures for establishing a tolerance for unavoidable contaminants in food and food-packaging materials, described in section 406 of the act.

(6) An investigational new drug application, described in part 312 of this chapter.

(7) A new drug application, described in part 314.

(8) Data and information regarding the bioavailability or bioequivalence of drugs for human use submitted as part of the procedures for issuing, amending, or repealing a bioequivalence requirement, described in part 320.

(9) Data and information regarding an over-the-counter drug for human use submitted as part of the procedures for classifying such drugs as generally recognized as safe and effective and not misbranded, described in part 330.

(10) An application for a biologics license, described in part 601 of this chapter.

(11) Data and information regarding a biological product submitted as part of the procedures for determining that licensed biological products are safe and effective and not misbranded, as described in part 601 of this chapter.

(12) An Application for an Investigational Device Exemption, described in part 812.

(13) Data and information regarding a medical device for human use submitted as part of the procedures for classifying such devices, described in part 860.

(14) Data and information regarding a medical device for human use submitted as part of the procedures for establishing, amending, or repealing a standard for such device, described in part 861.

(15) An application for premarket approval of a medical device for human use, described in section 515 of the act.

(16) A product development protocol for a medical device for human use, described in section 515 of the act.

(17) Data and information regarding an electronic product submitted as part of the procedures for establishing, amending, or repealing a standard for such products, described in section 358 of the Public Health Service Act.

(18) Data and information regarding an electronic product submitted as part of the procedures for obtaining a variance from any electronic product performance standard, as described in 1010.4.

(19) Data and information regarding an electronic product submitted as part of the procedures for granting, amending, or extending an exemption from a radiation safety performance standard, as described in 1010.5.

(20) Data and information regarding an electronic product submitted as part of the procedures for obtaining an exemption from notification of a radiation safety defect or failure of compliance with a radiation safety performance standard, described in subpart D of part 1003.

(21) Data and information about a clinical study of an infant formula when submitted as part of an infant formula notification under section 412(c) of the Federal Food, Drug, and Cosmetic Act.

(22) Data and information submitted in a petition for a nutrient content claim, described in 101.69 of this chapter, and for a health claim, described in 101.70 of this chapter.

(23) Data and information from investigations involving children submitted in a new dietary ingredient notification, described in 190.6 of this chapter.

(c) Clinical investigation means any experiment that involves a test article and one or more human subjects, and that either must meet the requirements for prior submission to the Food and Drug Administration under section 505(i) or 520(g) of the act, or need not meet the requirements for prior submission to the Food and Drug Administration under these sections of the act, but the results of which are intended to be later submitted to, or held for inspection by, the Food and Drug Administration as part of an application for a research or marketing permit. The term does not include experiments that must meet the provisions of part 58, regarding nonclinical laboratory studies. The terms research, clinical research, clinical study, study, and clinical investigation are deemed to be synonymous for purposes of this part.

(d) Emergency use means the use of a test article on a human subject in a life-threatening situation in which no standard acceptable treatment is available, and in which there is not sufficient time to obtain IRB approval.

(e) Human subject means an individual who is or becomes a participant in research, either as a recipient of the test article or as a control. A subject may be either a healthy individual or a patient.

(f) Institution means any public or private entity or agency (including Federal, State, and other agencies). The term facility as used in section 520(g) of the act is deemed to be synonymous with the term institution for purposes of this part.

(g) Institutional Review Board (IRB) means any board, committee, or other group formally designated by an institution to review, to approve the initiation of, and to conduct periodic review of, biomedical research involving human subjects. The primary purpose of such review is to assure the protection of the rights and welfare of the human subjects. The term has the same meaning as the phrase institutional review committee as used in section 520(g) of the act.

(h) Investigator means an individual who actually conducts a clinical investigation (i.e., under whose immediate direction the test article is administered or dispensed to, or used involving, a subject) or, in the event of an investigation conducted by a team of individuals, is the responsible leader of that team.

(i) Minimal risk means that the probability and magnitude of harm or discomfort anticipated in the research are not greater in and of themselves than those ordinarily encountered in daily life or during the performance of routine physical or psychological examinations or tests.

(j) Sponsor means a person or other entity that initiates a clinical investigation, but that does not actually conduct the investigation, i.e., the test article is administered or dispensed to, or used involving, a subject under the immediate direction of another individual. A person other than an individual (e.g., a corporation or agency) that uses one or more of its own employees to conduct an investigation that it has initiated is considered to be a sponsor (not a sponsor-investigator), and the employees are considered to be investigators.

(k) Sponsor-investigator means an individual who both initiates and actually conducts, alone or with others, a clinical investigation, i.e., under whose immediate direction the test article is administered or dispensed to, or used involving, a subject. The term does not include any person other than an individual, e.g., it does not include a corporation or agency. The obligations of a sponsor-investigator under this part include both those of a sponsor and those of an investigator.

(l) Test article means any drug for human use, biological product for human use, medical device for human use, human food additive, color additive, electronic product, or any other article subject to regulation under the act or under sections 351 or 354-360F of the Public Health Service Act.

(m) IRB approval means the determination of the IRB that the clinical investigation has been reviewed and may be conducted at an institution within the constraints set forth by the IRB and by other institutional and Federal requirements.

[46 FR 8975, Jan. 27, 1981, as amended at 54 FR 9038, Mar. 3, 1989; 56 FR 28028, June 18, 1991; 64 FR 399, Jan. 5, 1999; 64 FR 56448, Oct. 20, 1999; 65 FR 52302, Aug. 29, 2000; 66 FR 20599, Apr. 24, 2001; 74 FR 2368, Jan. 15, 2009]

§56.103 Circumstances in which IRB review is required.

(a) Except as provided in 56.104 and 56.105, any clinical investigation which must meet the requirements for prior submission (as required in parts 312, 812, and 813) to the Food and Drug Administration shall not be initiated unless that investigation has been reviewed and approved by, and remains subject to continuing review by, an IRB meeting the requirements of this part.

(b) Except as provided in 56.104 and 56.105, the Food and Drug Administration may decide not to consider in support of an application for a research or marketing permit any data or information that has been derived from a clinical investigation that has not been approved by, and that was not subject to initial and continuing review by, an IRB meeting the requirements of this part. The determination that a clinical investigation may not be considered in support of an application for a research or marketing permit does not, however, relieve the applicant for such a permit of any obligation under any other applicable regulations to submit the results of the investigation to the Food and Drug Administration.

(c) Compliance with these regulations will in no way render inapplicable pertinent Federal, State, or local laws or regulations.
[46 FR 8975, Jan. 27, 1981; 46 FR 14340, Feb. 27, 1981]

§56.104 Exemptions from IRB requirement.

The following categories of clinical investigations are exempt from the requirements of this part for IRB review:

(a) Any investigation which commenced before July 27, 1981 and was subject to requirements for IRB review under FDA regulations before that date, provided that the investigation remains subject to review of an IRB which meets the FDA requirements in effect before July 27, 1981.

(b) Any investigation commenced before July 27, 1981 and was not otherwise subject to requirements for IRB review under Food and Drug Administration regulations before that date.

(c) Emergency use of a test article, provided that such emergency use is reported to the IRB within 5 working days. Any subsequent use of the test article at the institution is subject to IRB review.

(d) Taste and food quality evaluations and consumer acceptance studies, if wholesome foods without additives are consumed or if a food is consumed that contains a food ingredient at or below the level and for a use found to be safe, or agricultural, chemical, or environmental contaminant at or below the level found to be safe, by the Food and Drug Administration or approved by the Environmental Protection Agency or the Food Safety and Inspection Service of the U.S. Department of Agriculture.
[46 FR 8975, Jan. 27, 1981, as amended at 56 FR 28028, June 18, 1991]

§56.105 Waiver of IRB requirement.

On the application of a sponsor or sponsor-investigator, the Food and Drug Administration may waive any of the requirements contained in these regulations, including the requirements for IRB review, for specific research activities or for classes of research activities, otherwise covered by these regulations.

<u>Subpart B–Organization and Personnel</u>

§56.106 Registration.

(a) Who must register? Each IRB in the United States that reviews clinical investigations regulated by FDA under sections 505(i) or 520(g) of the act and each IRB in the United States that reviews clinical investigations that are intended to support applications for research or marketing permits for FDA-regulated products must register at a site maintained by the Department of Health and Human Services (HHS). (A research permit under section 505(i) of the act is usually known as an investigational new drug application (IND), while a research permit under section 520(g) of the act is usually known as an investigational device exemption (IDE).) An individual authorized to act on the IRB's behalf must submit the registration information. All other IRBs may register voluntarily.

(b) What information must an IRB register? Each IRB must provide the following information:

(1) The name, mailing address, and street address (if different from the mailing address) of the institution operating the IRB and the name, mailing address, phone number, facsimile number, and electronic mail address of the senior officer of that institution who is responsible for overseeing activities performed by the IRB;

(2) The IRB's name, mailing address, street address (if different from the mailing address), phone number, facsimile number, and electronic mail address; each IRB chairperson's name, phone number, and electronic mail address; and the name, mailing address, phone number, facsimile number, and electronic mail address of the contact person providing the registration information.

(3) The approximate number of active protocols involving FDA-regulated products reviewed. For purposes of this rule, an "active protocol" is any protocol for which an IRB conducted an initial review or a continuing review at a convened meeting or under an expedited review procedure during the preceding 12 months; and

(4) A description of the types of FDA-regulated products (such as biological products, color additives, food additives, human drugs, or medical devices) involved in the protocols that the IRB reviews.

(c) When must an IRB register? Each IRB must submit an initial registration. The initial registration must occur before the IRB begins to review a clinical investigation described in paragraph (a) of this section. Each IRB must renew its registration every 3 years. IRB registration becomes effective after review and acceptance by HHS.

(d) Where can an IRB register? Each IRB may register electronically through http://ohrp.cit.nih.gov/efile. If an IRB lacks the ability to register electronically, it must send its registration information, in writing, to the Office of Good Clinical Practice, Office of Special Medical Programs, Food and Drug Administration, 10903 New Hampshire Ave., Bldg. 32, Rm. 5129, Silver Spring, MD 20993.

(e) How does an IRB revise its registration information? If an IRB's contact or chair person information changes, the IRB must revise its registration information by submitting any changes in that information within 90 days of the change. An IRB's decision to review new types of FDA-regulated products (such as a decision to review studies pertaining to food additives whereas the IRB previously reviewed studies pertaining to drug products), or to discontinue reviewing clinical investigations regulated by FDA is a change that must be reported within 30 days of the change. An IRB's decision to disband is a change that must be reported within 30 days of permanent cessation of the IRB's review of research. All other information changes may be reported when the IRB renews its registration. The revised information must be sent to FDA either electronically or in writing in accordance with paragraph (d) of this section.

[74 FR 2368, Jan. 15, 2009, as amended at 78 FR 16401, Mar. 15, 2013]

§56.107 IRB membership.

(a) Each IRB shall have at least five members, with varying backgrounds to promote complete and adequate review of research activities commonly conducted by the institution. The IRB shall be sufficiently qualified through the experience and expertise of its members, and the diversity of the members, including consideration of race, gender, cultural backgrounds, and sensitivity to such issues as community attitudes, to promote respect for its advice and counsel in safeguarding the rights and welfare of human subjects. In addition to possessing the professional competence necessary to review the specific research activities, the IRB shall be able to ascertain the acceptability of proposed research in terms of institutional commitments and regulations, applicable law, and standards of professional conduct and practice. * * * The IRB shall therefore include persons knowledgeable in these areas. If an IRB regularly reviews research that involves a vulnerable category of subjects, such as children, prisoners, pregnant women, or handicapped or mentally disabled persons, consideration shall be given to the inclusion of one or more individuals who are knowledgeable about and experienced in working with those subjects.

(b) Every nondiscriminatory effort will be made to ensure that no IRB consists entirely of men or entirely of women, including the institution's consideration of qualified persons of both sexes, so long as no selection is made to the IRB on the basis of gender. No IRB may consist entirely of members of one profession.

(c) Each IRB shall include at least one member whose primary concerns are in the scientific area and at least one member whose primary concerns are in nonscientific areas.

(d) Each IRB shall include at least one member who is not otherwise affiliated with the institution and who is not part of the immediate family of a person who is affiliated with the institution.

(e) No IRB may have a member participate in the IRB's initial or continuing review of any project in which the member has a conflicting interest, except to provide information requested by the IRB.

(f) An IRB may, in its discretion, invite individuals with competence in special areas to assist in the review of complex issues which require expertise beyond or in addition to that available on the IRB. These individuals may not vote with the IRB.
[46 FR 8975, Jan. 27, 1981, as amended at 56 FR 28028, June 18, 1991; 56 FR 29756, June 28, 1991; 78 FR 16401, Mar. 15, 2013]

Subpart C–IRB Functions and Operations

§56.111 Criteria for IRB approval of research.

(a) In order to approve research covered by these regulations the IRB shall determine that all of the following requirements are satisfied:

(1) Risks to subjects are minimized: (i) By using procedures which are consistent with sound research design and which do not unnecessarily expose subjects to risk, and (ii) whenever appropriate, by using procedures already being performed on the subjects for diagnostic or treatment purposes.

(2) Risks to subjects are reasonable in relation to anticipated benefits, if any, to subjects, and the importance of the knowledge that may be expected to result. In evaluating risks and benefits, the IRB should consider only those risks and benefits that may result from the research (as distinguished from risks and benefits of therapies that subjects would receive even if not participating in the research). The IRB should not consider possible long-range effects of applying knowledge gained in the research (for example, the possible effects of

the research on public policy) as among those research risks that fall within the purview of its responsibility.

(3) Selection of subjects is equitable. In making this assessment the IRB should take into account the purposes of the research and the setting in which the research will be conducted and should be particularly cognizant of the special problems of research involving vulnerable populations, such as children, prisoners, pregnant women, handicapped, or mentally disabled persons, or economically or educationally disadvantaged persons.

(4) Informed consent will be sought from each prospective subject or the subject's legally authorized representative, in accordance with and to the extent required by part 50.

(5) Informed consent will be appropriately documented, in accordance with and to the extent required by 50.27.

(6) Where appropriate, the research plan makes adequate provision for monitoring the data collected to ensure the safety of subjects.

(7) Where appropriate, there are adequate provisions to protect the privacy of subjects and to maintain the confidentiality of data.

(b) When some or all of the subjects, such as children, prisoners, pregnant women, handicapped, or mentally disabled persons, or economically or educationally disadvantaged persons, are likely to be vulnerable to coercion or undue influence additional safeguards have been included in the study to protect the rights and welfare of these subjects.

(c) In order to approve research in which some or all of the subjects are children, an IRB must determine that all research is in compliance with part 50, subpart D of this chapter.
[46 FR 8975, Jan. 27, 1981, as amended at 56 FR 28029, June 18, 1991; 66 FR 20599, Apr. 24, 2001]

§56.112 Review by institution.

Research covered by these regulations that has been approved by an IRB may be subject to further appropriate review and approval or disapproval by officials of the institution. However, those officials may not approve the research if it has not been approved by an IRB.

§56.113 Suspension or termination of IRB approval of research.

An IRB shall have authority to suspend or terminate approval of research that is not being conducted in accordance with the IRB's requirements or that has been associated with unexpected serious harm to subjects. Any suspension or termination of approval shall include a statement of the reasons for the IRB's action and shall be reported promptly to the investigator, appropriate institutional officials, and the Food and Drug Administration.

§56.114 Cooperative research.

In complying with these regulations, institutions involved in multi-institutional studies may use joint review, reliance upon the review of another qualified IRB, or similar arrangements aimed at avoidance of duplication of effort.

§56.108 IRB functions and operations.

In order to fulfill the requirements of these regulations, each IRB shall:

(a) Follow written procedures: (1) For conducting its initial and continuing review of research and for reporting its findings and actions to the investigator and the institution; (2) for determining which projects require review more often than annually and which projects need verification from sources other than the investigator that no material changes have occurred since previous IRB review; (3) for ensuring prompt reporting to the IRB of changes in research activity; and (4) for ensuring that changes in approved research, during the period for which IRB approval has already been given, may not be initiated without IRB review and approval except where necessary to eliminate apparent immediate hazards to the human subjects.

(b) Follow written procedures for ensuring prompt reporting to the IRB, appropriate institutional officials, and the Food and Drug Administration of: (1) Any unanticipated problems involving risks to human subjects or others; (2) any instance of serious or continuing noncompliance with these regulations or the requirements or determinations of the IRB; or (3) any suspension or termination of IRB approval.

(c) Except when an expedited review procedure is used (see 56.110), review proposed research at convened meetings at which a majority of the members of the IRB are present, including at least one member whose primary concerns are in nonscientific areas. In order for the research to be approved, it shall receive the approval of a majority of those members present at the meeting.

[46 FR 8975, Jan. 27, 1981, as amended at 56 FR 28028, June 18, 1991; 67 FR 9585, Mar. 4, 2002]

§56.109 IRB review of research.

(a) An IRB shall review and have authority to approve, require modifications in (to secure approval), or disapprove all research activities covered by these regulations.

(b) An IRB shall require that information given to subjects as part of informed consent is in accordance with 50.25. The IRB may require that information, in addition to that specifically mentioned in 50.25, be given to the subjects when in the IRB's judgment the information would meaningfully add to the protection of the rights and welfare of subjects.

(c) An IRB shall require documentation of informed consent in accordance with 50.27 of this chapter, except as follows:

(1) The IRB may, for some or all subjects, waive the requirement that the subject, or the subject's legally authorized representative, sign a written consent form if it finds that the research presents no more than minimal risk of harm to subjects and involves no procedures for which written consent is normally required outside the research context; or

(2) The IRB may, for some or all subjects, find that the requirements in 50.24 of this chapter for an exception from informed consent for emergency research are met.

(d) In cases where the documentation requirement is waived under paragraph (c)(1) of this section, the IRB may require the investigator to provide subjects with a written statement regarding the research.

(e) An IRB shall notify investigators and the institution in writing of its decision to approve or disapprove the proposed research activity, or of modifications required to secure IRB approval of the research activity. If the IRB decides to disapprove a research activity, it shall include in its written notification a statement of the reasons for its decision and give the investigator an opportunity to respond in person or in writing. For investigations involving an exception to informed consent under 50.24 of this chapter, an IRB shall promptly notify in writing the investigator and the sponsor of the research when an IRB determines that it cannot approve the research because it does not meet the criteria in the exception provided under 50.24(a) of this chapter or because of other relevant ethical concerns. The written notification shall include a statement of the reasons for the IRB's determination.

(f) An IRB shall conduct continuing review of research covered by these regulations at intervals appropriate to the degree of risk, but not less than once per year, and shall have authority to observe or have a third party observe the consent process and the research.

(g) An IRB shall provide in writing to the sponsor of research involving an exception to informed consent under 50.24 of this chapter a copy of information that has been publicly disclosed under 50.24(a)(7)(ii) and (a)(7)(iii) of this chapter. The IRB shall provide this information to the sponsor promptly so that the sponsor is aware that such disclosure has occurred. Upon receipt, the sponsor shall provide copies of the information disclosed to FDA.

(h) When some or all of the subjects in a study are children, an IRB must determine that the research study is in compliance with part 50, subpart D of this chapter, at the time of its initial review of the research. When some or all of the subjects in a study that was ongoing on April 30, 2001, are children, an IRB must conduct a review of the research to determine compliance with part 50, subpart D of this chapter, either at the time of continuing review or, at the discretion of the IRB, at an earlier date.

[46 FR 8975, Jan. 27, 1981, as amended at 61 FR 51529, Oct. 2, 1996; 66 FR 20599, Apr. 24, 2001; 78 FR 12951, Feb. 26, 2013]

§56.110 Expedited review procedures for certain kinds of research involving no more than minimal risk, and for minor changes in approved research.

(a) The Food and Drug Administration has established, and published in the Federal Register, a list of categories of research that may be reviewed by the IRB through an expedited review procedure. The list will be amended, as appropriate, through periodic republication in the Federal Register.

(b) An IRB may use the expedited review procedure to review either or both of the following: (1) Some or all of the research appearing on the list and found by the reviewer(s) to involve no more than minimal risk, (2) minor changes in previously approved research during the period (of 1 year or less) for which approval is authorized. Under an expedited review procedure, the review may be carried out by the IRB chairperson or by one or more experienced reviewers designated by the IRB chairperson from among the members of the IRB. In reviewing the research, the reviewers may exercise all of the authorities of the IRB except that the reviewers may not disapprove the research. A research activity may be disapproved only after review in accordance with the nonexpedited review procedure set forth in 56.108(c).

(c) Each IRB which uses an expedited review procedure shall adopt a method for keeping all members advised of research proposals which have been approved under the procedure.

(d) The Food and Drug Administration may restrict, suspend, or terminate an institution's or IRB's use of the expedited review procedure when necessary to protect the rights or welfare of subjects.

[46 FR 8975, Jan. 27, 1981, as amended at 56 FR 28029, June 18, 1991]

Subpart D–Records and Reports

§56.115 IRB records.

(a) An institution, or where appropriate an IRB, shall prepare and maintain adequate documentation of IRB activities, including the following:

(1) Copies of all research proposals reviewed, scientific evaluations, if any, that accompany the proposals, approved sample consent documents, progress reports submitted by investigators, and reports of injuries to subjects.

(2) Minutes of IRB meetings which shall be in sufficient detail to show attendance at the meetings; actions taken by the IRB; the vote on these actions

including the number of members voting for, against, and abstaining; the basis for requiring changes in or disapproving research; and a written summary of the discussion of controverted issues and their resolution.

(3) Records of continuing review activities.

(4) Copies of all correspondence between the IRB and the investigators.

(5) A list of IRB members identified by name; earned degrees; representative capacity; indications of experience such as board certifications, licenses, etc., sufficient to describe each member's chief anticipated contributions to IRB deliberations; and any employment or other relationship between each member and the institution; for example: full-time employee, part-time employee, a member of governing panel or board, stockholder, paid or unpaid consultant.

(6) Written procedures for the IRB as required by 56.108 (a) and (b).

(7) Statements of significant new findings provided to subjects, as required by 50.25.

(b) The records required by this regulation shall be retained for at least 3 years after completion of the research, and the records shall be accessible for inspection and copying by authorized representatives of the Food and Drug Administration at reasonable times and in a reasonable manner.

(c) The Food and Drug Administration may refuse to consider a clinical investigation in support of an application for a research or marketing permit if the institution or the IRB that reviewed the investigation refuses to allow an inspection under this section.

[46 FR 8975, Jan. 27, 1981, as amended at 56 FR 28029, June 18, 1991; 67 FR 9585, Mar. 4, 2002]

Subpart E–Administrative Actions for Noncompliance

§56.120 Lesser administrative actions.

(a) If apparent noncompliance with these regulations in the operation of an IRB is observed by an FDA investigator during an inspection, the inspector will present an oral or written summary of observations to an appropriate representative of the IRB. The Food and Drug Administration may subsequently send a letter describing the noncompliance to the IRB and to the parent institution. The agency will require that the IRB or the parent institution respond to this letter within a time period specified by FDA and describe the corrective actions that will be taken by the IRB, the institution, or both to achieve compliance with these regulations.

(b) On the basis of the IRB's or the institution's response, FDA may schedule a reinspection to confirm the adequacy of corrective actions. In addition, until the IRB or the parent institution takes appropriate corrective action, the Agency may require the IRB to:

(1) Withhold approval of new studies subject to the requirements of this part that are conducted at the institution or reviewed by the IRB;

(2) Direct that no new subjects be added to ongoing studies subject to this part; or

(3) Terminate ongoing studies subject to this part when doing so would not endanger the subjects.

(c) When the apparent noncompliance creates a significant threat to the rights and welfare of human subjects, FDA may notify relevant State and Federal regulatory agencies and other parties with a direct interest in the Agency's action of the deficiencies in the operation of the IRB.

(d) The parent institution is presumed to be responsible for the operation of an IRB, and the Food and Drug Administration will ordinarily direct any administrative action under this subpart against the institution. However, depending on the evidence of responsibility for deficiencies, determined during the investigation, the Food and Drug Administration may restrict its administrative actions to the IRB or to a component of the parent institution determined to be responsible for formal designation of the IRB.

[46 FR 8975, Jan. 27, 1981, as amended at 81 FR 19035, Apr. 4, 2016]

§56.121 Disqualification of an IRB or an institution.

(a) Whenever the IRB or the institution has failed to take adequate steps to correct the noncompliance stated in the letter sent by the agency under 56.120(a), and the Commissioner of Food and Drugs determines that this noncompliance may justify the disqualification of the IRB or of the parent institution, the Commissioner will institute proceedings in accordance with the requirements for a regulatory hearing set forth in part 16.

(b) The Commissioner may disqualify an IRB or the parent institution if the Commissioner determines that:

(1) The IRB has refused or repeatedly failed to comply with any of the regulations set forth in this part, and

(2) The noncompliance adversely affects the rights or welfare of the human subjects in a clinical investigation.

(c) If the Commissioner determines that disqualification is appropriate, the Commissioner will issue an order that explains the basis for the determination and that prescribes any actions to be taken with regard to ongoing clinical research conducted under the review of the IRB. The Food and Drug Administration will send notice of the disqualification to the IRB and the parent institution. Other parties with a direct interest, such as sponsors and clinical investigators, may also be sent a notice of the disqualification. In addition, the agency may elect to publish a notice of its action in the Federal Register.

(d) The Food and Drug Administration will not approve an application for a research permit for a clinical investigation that is to be under the review of a disqualified IRB or that is to be conducted at a disqualified institution, and it may refuse to consider in support of a marketing permit the data from a clinical investigation that was reviewed by a disqualified IRB as conducted at a disqualified institution, unless the IRB or the parent institution is reinstated as provided in 56.123.

§56.122 Public disclosure of information regarding revocation.

A determination that the Food and Drug Administration has disqualified an institution and the administrative record regarding that determination are disclosable to the public under part 20.

§56.123 Reinstatement of an IRB or an institution.

An IRB or an institution may be reinstated if the Commissioner determines, upon an evaluation of a written submission from the IRB or institution that explains the corrective action that the institution or IRB plans to take, that the IRB or institution has provided adequate assurance that it will operate in compliance with the standards set forth in this part. Notification of reinstatement shall be provided to all persons notified under 56.121(c).

§56.124 Actions alternative or additional to disqualification.

Disqualification of an IRB or of an institution is independent of, and neither in lieu of nor a precondition to, other proceedings or actions authorized by the act. The Food and Drug Administration may, at any time, through the Department of Justice institute any appropriate judicial proceedings (civil or criminal) and any other appropriate regulatory action, in addition to or in lieu of, and before, at the time of, or after, disqualification. The agency may also refer pertinent matters to another Federal, State, or local government agency for any action that that agency determines to be appropriate.

Authority: 21 U.S.C. 321, 343, 346, 346a, 348, 350a, 350b, 351, 352, 353, 355, 360, 360c-360f, 360h, 360i, 360j, 360hh-360ss, 371, 379e, 381; 42 U.S.C. 216, 241, 262.

Source: 46 FR 8975, Jan. 27, 1981, unless otherwise noted.

Food and Drug Administration. (1981). *21 CFR 56 Institutional Review Boards.* https://www.ecfr.gov/cgi-bin/text-idx?SID=b245bf060d80dbfb2186856ba6f8fcf 4&mc=true&node=pt21.1.56&rgn=div5

Final NIH Policy on the Use of a Single Institutional Review Board for Multi-Site Research

Purpose

The National Institutes of Health (NIH) Policy on the Use of a Single Institutional Review Board of Record for Multi-Site Research establishes the expectation that all sites participating in multi-site studies involving non-exempt human subjects research funded by the National Institutes of Health (NIH) will use a single Institutional Review Board (sIRB) to conduct the ethical review required by the Department of Health and Human Services regulations for the Protection of Human Subjects at 45 CFR Part 46. This policy, which is consistent with 45 CFR Part 46.114, is intended to enhance and streamline the process of IRB review and reduce inefficiencies so that research can proceed as expeditiously as possible without compromising ethical principles and protections for human research participants.

Scope and Applicability

This policy applies to the domestic sites of NIH-funded multi-site studies where each site will conduct the same protocol involving non-exempt human subjects research, whether supported through grants, cooperative agreements, contracts, or the NIH Intramural Research Program. It does not apply to career development, research training or fellowship awards.

This policy applies to domestic awardees and participating domestic sites. Foreign sites participating in NIH-funded, multi-site studies will not be expected to follow this policy.

Consistent with the Roles and Responsibilities section, applicants/offerors will be expected to include a plan for the use of an sIRB in the applications/proposals they submit to the NIH. The NIH's acceptance of the submitted plan will be incorporated as a term and condition in the Notice of Award or in the Contract Award. This policy also applies to the NIH Intramural Research Program.

Definitions

The **Authorization Agreement**, which is also called a reliance agreement, is the agreement that documents respective authorities, roles, responsibilities, and communication between an institution/organization providing the ethical review and a participating site relying on the sIRB.

A **multi-site study** uses the same protocol to conduct non-exempt human subjects research at more than one site.

Participating site in a multi-site study is a domestic entity that will rely on the sIRB to carry out the site's IRB review of human subjects research for the multi-site study.

sIRB is the selected IRB of record that conducts the ethical review for participating sites of the multi-site study.

Roles and Responsibilities

Applicant/Offeror. In the application/proposal for research funding, the applicant/offeror is expected to submit a plan describing the use of an sIRB that will be selected to serve as the IRB of record for all study sites. The plan should include a statement confirming that participating sites will adhere to the sIRB Policy and describe how communications between sites and sIRB will be handled. If, in delayed-onset research, an sIRB has not yet been identified, applications/proposals should include a statement that awardees will follow this Policy and communicate plans to use a registered IRB of record to the funding NIH Institute/Center prior to initiating a multi-site study. The applicant/offeror may request direct cost funding for the additional costs associated with the establishment and review of the multi-site study by the sIRB, with appropriate justification; all such costs must be reasonable and consistent with cost principles, as described in the NIH Grants Policy Statement and the Federal Acquisition Regulation (FAR) 31.302 (Direct Costs) and FAR 31.203 (Indirect Costs).

Awardees. Awardees are responsible for ensuring that authorization agreements are in place; copies of authorization agreements and other necessary documentation should be maintained in order to document compliance with this policy, as needed. As appropriate, awardees are responsible for ensuring that a mechanism for communication between the sIRB and participating sites is established. Awardees may delegate the tasks associated with these responsibilities.

Funding Institute or Center (IC). Funding ICs are responsible for management and oversight of the award, including communicating with the awardee regarding the implementation of its proposed plan to comply with the sIRB Policy. In the event that questions arise about the awardee's plan, including the IRB that has been selected to serve as the sIRB, the funding IC will work with the awardee to resolve them.

sIRB. The sIRB is responsible for conducting the ethical review of NIH-funded multi-site studies for participating sites. The sIRB will be expected to carry out the regulatory requirements as specified under the HHS regulations at 45 CFR Part 46. In reviewing multi-site research protocols, the sIRB may serve as a Privacy Board, as applicable, to fulfill the requirements of the HIPAA Privacy Rule for use or disclosure of protected health information for research purposes. The sIRB will collaborate with the awardee to establish a mechanism for communication between the sIRB and the participating sites.

Participating Site. All sites participating in a multi-site study are expected to rely on an sIRB to carry out the functions that are required for institutional compliance with IRB review set forth in the HHS regulations at 45 CFR 46. Participating sites are responsible for meeting other regulatory obligations, such as obtaining informed consent, overseeing the implementation of the approved protocol, and reporting unanticipated problems and study progress to the sIRB. Participating sites must communicate relevant information necessary for the sIRB to consider local context issues and state/local regulatory requirements during its deliberations. Participating sites are expected to rely on the sIRB to satisfy the regulatory requirements relevant to the ethical review. Although IRB ethical review at a participating site would be counter to the intent and goal of this policy, the policy does not prohibit any participating site from duplicating the sIRB. However, if this approach is taken, NIH funds may not be used to pay for the cost of the duplicate review.

Exceptions

Exceptions to this policy will be made where review by the proposed sIRB would be prohibited by a federal, tribal, or state law, regulation, or policy. Requests for exceptions that are not based on a legal, regulatory, or policy requirement will be considered if there is a compelling justification for the exception.

The NIH will determine whether to grant an exception following an assessment of the need.

Effective Date

This policy applies to all competing grant applications (new, renewal, revision, or resubmission) with receipt dates on or after May 25, 2017. Ongoing, non-competing awards will not be expected to comply with this policy until the grantee submits a competing renewal application. For contracts, the policy applies to all solicitations issued on or after May 25, 2017. For the intramural program, the policy applies to intramural multi-site studies submitted for initial review after May 25, 2017.

National Institutes of Health. (2016). *Final NIH policy on the use of a single institutional review board for multi-site research.* https://grants.nih.gov/grants/guide/notice-files/NOT-OD-16-094.html

Human Subject Regulations Decision Charts: 2018 Requirements

Chart 13.2-1 Is an Activity Human Subjects Research Covered by 45 CFR Part 46?

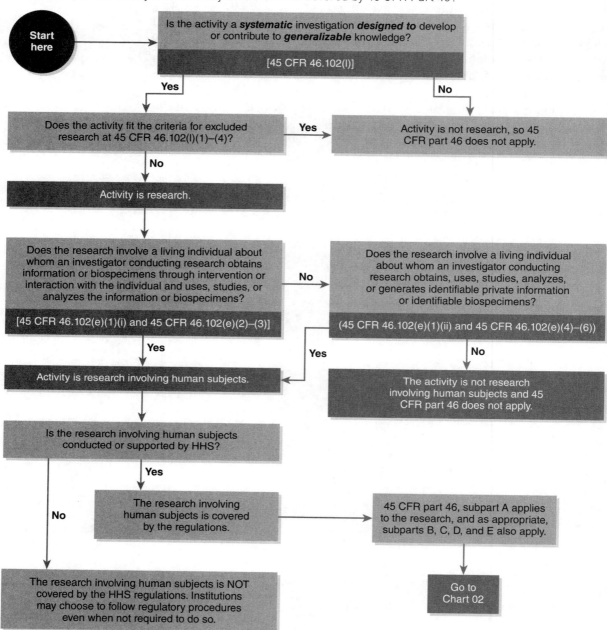

Department of Health and Human Services. (2020). *Human Subject Regulations Decision Charts: 2018 Requirements.* www.hhs.gov/ohrp/regulations-and-policy/decision-charts-2018/index.html

Chart 13.2-2 Is the Research Involving Human Subjects Eligible for Exemption Under 45 CFR 46.104(d)?

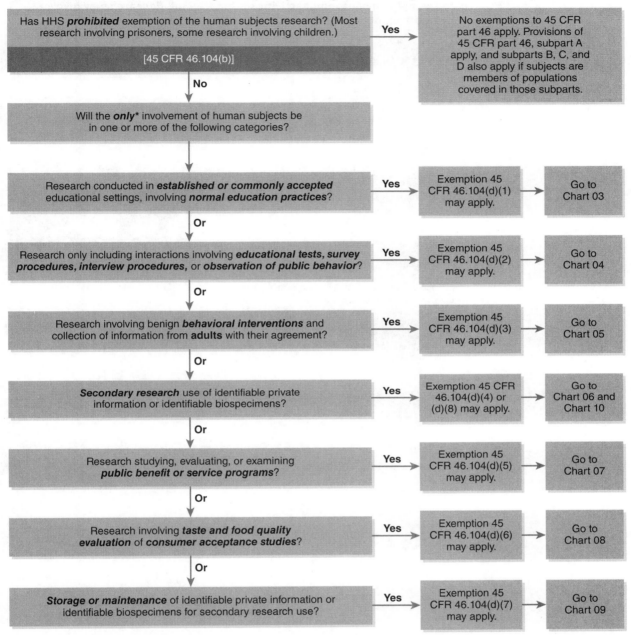

Department of Health and Human Services. (2020). *Human Subject Regulations Decision Charts: 2018 Requirements.* www.hhs.gov/ohrp/regulations-and-policy/decision-charts-2018/index.html

---

* /Only/ means that no nonexempt activities are involved. Research that [includes] both exempt and nonexempt activities is /not/ exempt. Research may involve activities exempt under more than one exemption category.

To be exempt, no nonexempt activities can be involved. Research that includes both exempt and nonexempt activities is not exempt. Research may involve activities exempt under more than one exemption category.

Chart 13.2-3 Does Exemption 45 CFR 46.104(d)(1) for Educational Practices Apply?

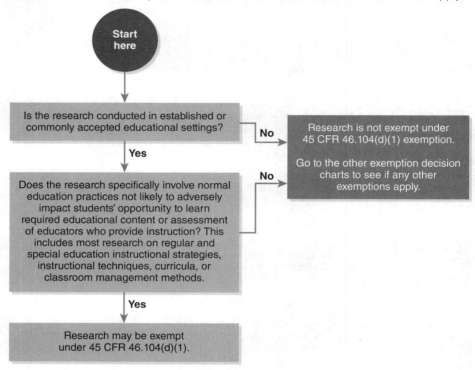

Department of Health and Human Services. (2020). *Human Subject Regulations Decision Charts: 2018 Requirements.* www.hhs.gov/ohrp/regulations-and-policy/decision-charts-2018/index.html

To be exempt, no nonexempt activities can be involved. Research that includes both exempt and nonexempt activities is not exempt. Research may involve activities exempt under more than one exemption category.

Chart 13.2-4 Does Exemption 45 CFR 46.104(d)(2) for Educational Tests, Surveys, Interviews, or Observation of Public Behavior Apply?

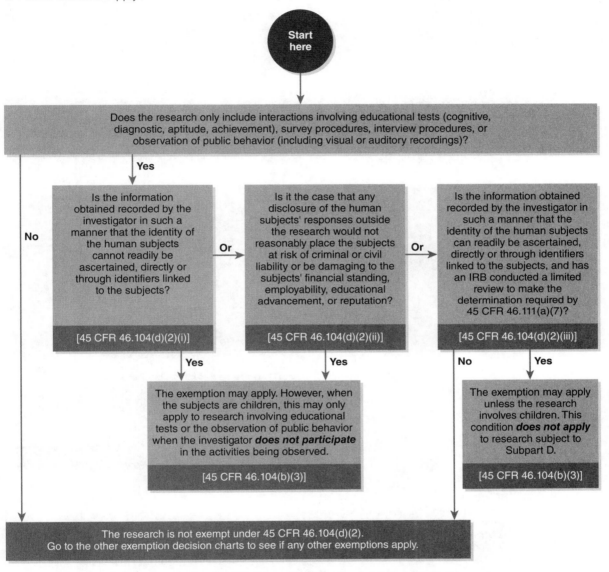

Department of Health and Human Services. (2020). *Human Subject Regulations Decision Charts: 2018 Requirements.* www.hhs.gov/ohrp/regulations-and-policy/decision-charts-2018/index.html

To be exempt, no nonexempt activities can be involved. Research that includes both exempt and nonexempt activities is not exempt. Research may involve activities exempt under more than one exemption category.

Chart 13.2-5 Does Exemption 45 CFR 46.104(d)(3) for Benign Behavioral Interventions Apply?

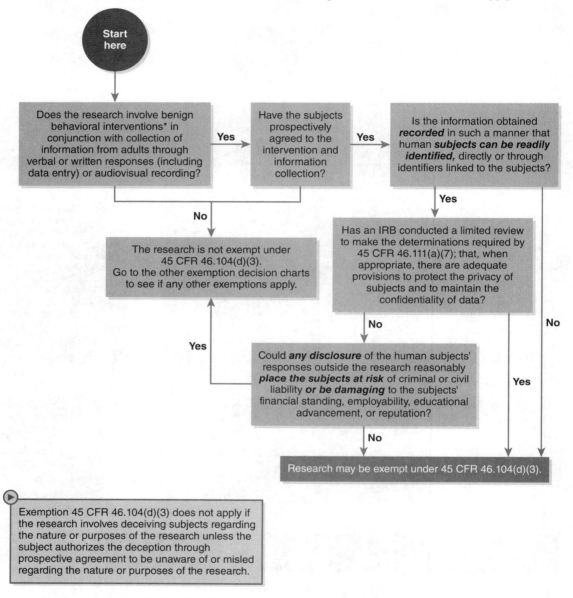

Department of Health and Human Services. (2020). *Human Subject Regulations Decision Charts: 2018 Requirements.* www.hhs.gov/ohrp/regulations-and-policy/decision-charts-2018/index.html

---

* /Benign behavioral interventions/ are brief in duration, harmless, painless, not physically invasive, not likely to have a significant adverse lasting impact on the subjects, and the investigator has no reason to think the subjects will find the interventions offensive or embarrassing.

To be exempt, no nonexempt activities can be involved. Research that includes both exempt and nonexempt activities is not exempt. Research may involve activities exempt under more than one exemption category.

Chart 13.2-6 Does Exemption 45 CFR 46.104(d)(4) for Secondary Research That Does Not Require Consent Apply?

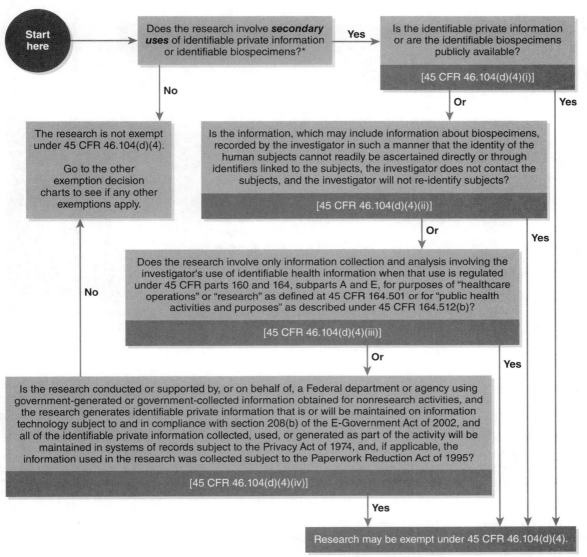

Department of Health and Human Services. (2020). *Human Subject Regulations Decision Charts: 2018 Requirements.* www.hhs.gov/ohrp/regulations-and-policy/decision-charts-2018/index.html

---

* Research use of identifiable private information or identifiable biospecimens collected for either research studies other than the proposed research, or for nonresearch purposes.

To be exempt, no nonexempt activities can be involved. Research that includes both exempt and nonexempt activities is not exempt. Research may involve activities exempt under more than one exemption category.

Chart 13.2-7 Does Exemption 45 CFR 46.104(d)(5) for Public Benefit or Service Programs Apply?

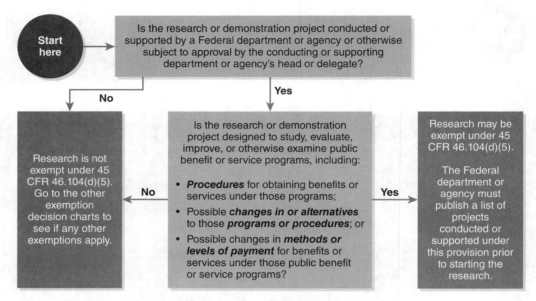

Department of Health and Human Services. (2020). *Human Subject Regulations Decision Charts: 2018 Requirements.* www.hhs.gov/ohrp/regulations-and-policy/decision-charts-2018/index.html

To be exempt, no nonexempt activities can be involved. Research that includes both exempt and nonexempt activities is not exempt. Research may involve activities exempt under more than one exemption category.

Chart 13.2-8 Does Exemption 45 CFR 46.104(d)(6) for Food, Taste, and Acceptance Studies Apply?

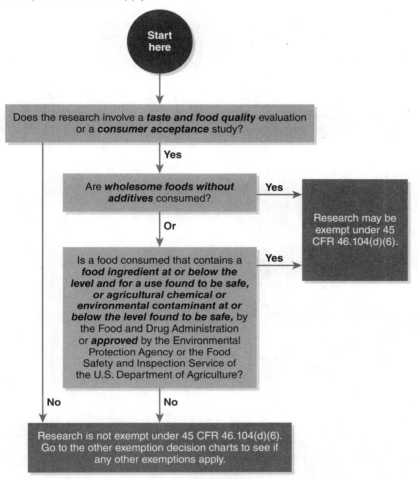

Start here

Does the research involve a *taste and food quality* evaluation or a *consumer acceptance* study?

Yes

Are *wholesome foods without additives* consumed?

Yes

Research may be exempt under 45 CFR 46.104(d)(6).

Or

Is a food consumed that contains a *food ingredient at or below the level and for a use found to be safe, or agricultural chemical or environmental contaminant at or below the level found to be safe,* by the Food and Drug Administration or *approved* by the Environmental Protection Agency or the Food Safety and Inspection Service of the U.S. Department of Agriculture?

Yes

No   No

Research is not exempt under 45 CFR 46.104(d)(6). Go to the other exemption decision charts to see if any other exemptions apply.

Department of Health and Human Services. (2020). *Human Subject Regulations Decision Charts: 2018 Requirements.* www.hhs.gov/ohrp/regulations-and-policy/decision-charts-2018/index.html

To be exempt, no nonexempt activities can be involved. Research that includes both exempt and nonexempt activities is not exempt. Research may involve activities exempt under more than one exemption category.

Chart 13.2-9 Does Exemption 45 CFR 46.104(d)(7), Storage for Secondary Research for Which Broad Consent Is Required, Apply?

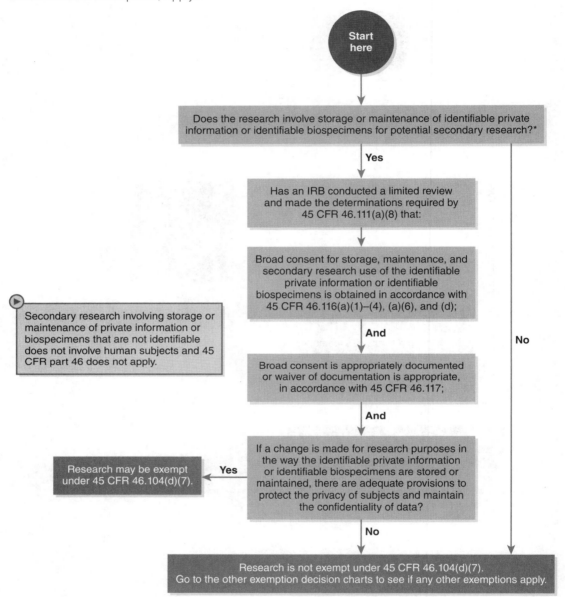

Department of Health and Human Services. (2020). *Human Subject Regulations Decision Charts: 2018 Requirements.* www.hhs.gov/ohrp/regulations-and-policy/decision-charts-2018/index.html

* Research use of identifiable private information or identifiable biospecimens collected for either research studies other than the proposed research, or for nonresearch purposes.

To be exempt, no nonexempt activities can be involved. Research that includes both exempt and nonexempt activities is not exempt. Research may involve activities exempt under more than one exemption category.

Chart 13.2-10 Does Exemption 45 CFR 46.104(d)(8) for Secondary Research for Which Broad Consent Is Required Apply?

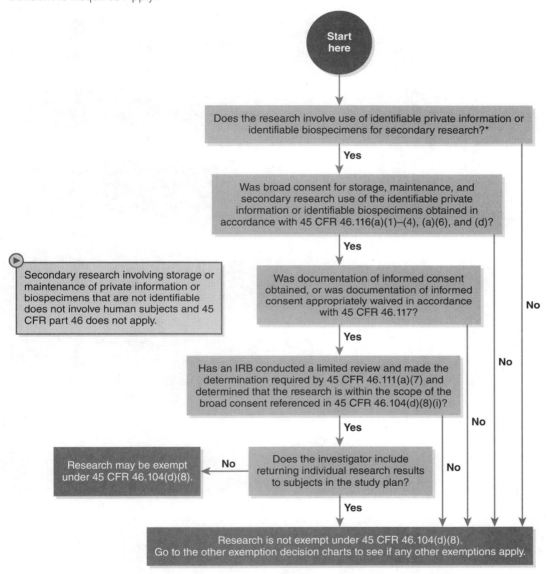

Start here

Does the research involve use of identifiable private information or identifiable biospecimens for secondary research?*

Yes

Was broad consent for storage, maintenance, and secondary research use of the identifiable private information or identifiable biospecimens obtained in accordance with 45 CFR 46.116(a)(1)–(4), (a)(6), and (d)?

Yes

Secondary research involving storage or maintenance of private information or biospecimens that are not identifiable does not involve human subjects and 45 CFR part 46 does not apply.

Was documentation of informed consent obtained, or was documentation of informed consent appropriately waived in accordance with 45 CFR 46.117?

No

Yes

Has an IRB conducted a limited review and made the determination required by 45 CFR 46.111(a)(7) and determined that the research is within the scope of the broad consent referenced in 45 CFR 46.104(d)(8)(i)?

No

Yes

Research may be exempt under 45 CFR 46.104(d)(8).

No

Does the investigator include returning individual research results to subjects in the study plan?

No

Yes

Research is not exempt under 45 CFR 46.104(d)(8).
Go to the other exemption decision charts to see if any other exemptions apply.

Department of Health and Human Services. (2020). *Human Subject Regulations Decision Charts: 2018 Requirements.* www.hhs.gov/ohrp/regulations-and-policy/decision-charts-2018/index.html

---

* Research use of identifiable private information or identifiable biospecimens collected for either research studies other than the proposed research, or for nonresearch purposes.

Chart 13.2-11 Is Continuing Review Required Under 45 CFR 46.109(f)?

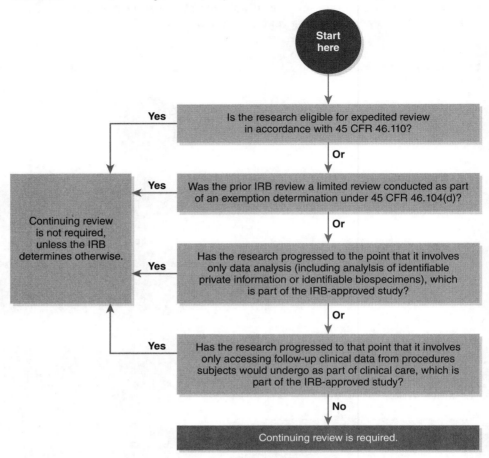

Department of Health and Human Services. (2020). *Human Subject Regulations Decision Charts: 2018 Requirements.* www.hhs.gov/ohrp/regulations-and-policy/decision-charts-2018/index.html

Chart 13.2-12 Waiver or Alteration of Informed Consent in Research Involving Public Benefit and Service Programs Conducted by or Subject to the Approval of State or Local Government Officials [45 CFR 46.116(e)]

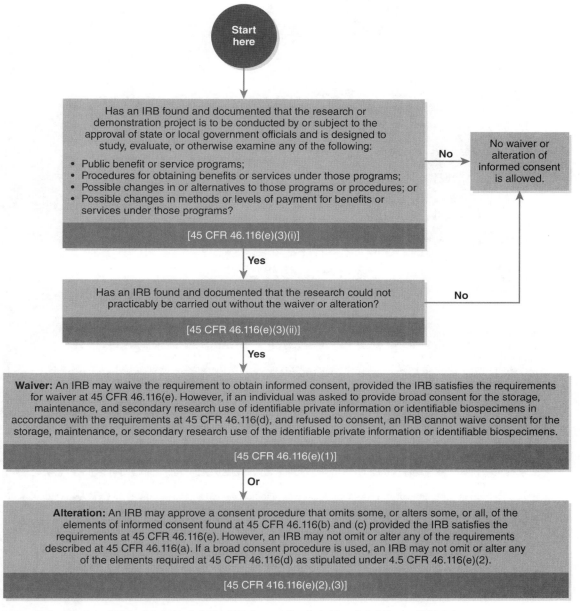

Department of Health and Human Services. (2020). *Human Subject Regulations Decision Charts: 2018 Requirements*. www.hhs.gov/ohrp/regulations-and-policy/decision-charts-2018/index.html

Chart 13.2-13 When Can Informed Consent Be Waived or Altered Under 45 CFR 46.116(f)?

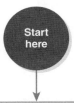

Has an IRB found and documented that **all** of the following conditions have been met?

- The research involves no more than minimal risk to the subjects;
- The research could not practicably be carried out without the requested waiver or alteration;
- If the research involves using identifiable private information or identifiable biospecimens, the research could not practicably be carried out without using such information or biospecimens in an identifiable format;
- The waiver or alteration will not adversely affect the rights and welfare of the subjects; and
- Whenever appropriate, the subjects or legally authorized representatives will be provided with additional pertinent information after participation.

[45 CFR 46.116(f)(3)]

No → No waiver or alteration of informed consent is allowed.

Yes

Waiver: An IRB may waive the requirement to obtain informed consent for research provided the IRB satisfies this requirement. However, if an individual was asked to provide broad consent for the storage, maintenance, and secondary research use of identifiable private information or identifiable biospecimens in accordance with the requirements at 45 CFR 46.116(d), and refused to consent, an IRB cannot waive consent for the storage, maintenance, or secondary research use of the identifiable private information or identifiable biospecimens.

[45 CFR 46.116(f)(1)]

Or

Alteration: An IRB may approve a consent procedure that omits some, or alters some or all, of the elements of informed consent set forth in 45 CFR 46.116(b) and (c) provided the IRB satisfies this requirement. However, an IRB may not omit or alter any of the requirements described at 45 CFR 46.116(a). If a broad consent procedure is used, an IRB may not omit or alter any of the elements required under 45 CFR 46.116(d).

[45 CFR 46.116(f)(2)]

Chart 13.2-14 Can Documentation of Informed Consent Be Waived Under 45 CFR 46.117(c)?

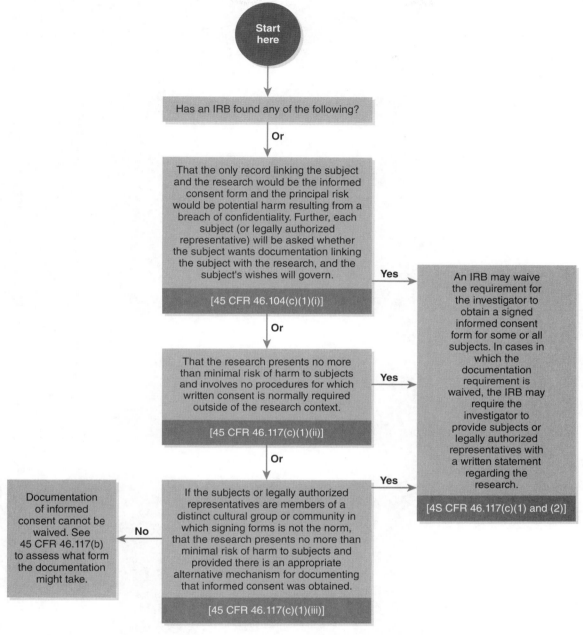

Department of Health and Human Services. (2020). *Human subject regulations decision charts: 2018 requirements.* www.hhs.gov/ohrp/regulations-and-policy/decision-charts-2018/index.html

Adoption of the Common Rule by Participating Agencies

Adoption of the Common Rule

The adoption of the Common Rule by the participating agencies, as modified by agency-specific text, is set forth below.

Department of Homeland Security

List of Subjects in 6 CFR Part 46

Human research subjects, Reporting and record-keeping requirements, Research.

- For the reasons stated in the preamble, the Department of Homeland Security adds 6 CFR part 46, as set forth at the end of the common preamble of this document.

PART 46—PROTECTION OF HUMAN SUBJECTS

Sec. 46.101 To what does this policy apply?

46.102 Definitions for purposes of this policy.

46.103 Assuring compliance with this policy—research conducted or supported by any Federal department or agency.

46.104 Exempt research.

46.105 [Reserved]

46.106 [Reserved]

46.107 IRB membership.

46.108 IRB functions and operations.

46.109 IRB review of research.

46.110 Expedited review procedures for certain kinds of research involving no more than minimal risk, and for minor changes in approved research.

46.111 Criteria for IRB approval of research.

46.112 Review by institution.

46.113 Suspension or termination of IRB approval of research.

Authority: 5 U.S.C. 301; Pub. L. 107–296, sec. 102, 306(c); Pub. L. 108–458, sec. 8306.

Reginald Brothers, Under Secretary for Science and Technology, DHS.

Department of Agriculture

List of Subjects in 7 CFR Part 1c

Human research subjects, Reporting and record-keeping requirements, Research.

- For the reasons stated in the preamble, the Department of Agriculture revises 7 CFR part 1c, as set forth at the end of the common preamble of this document.

PART 1c—PROTECTION OF HUMAN SUBJECTS

1c.121 [Reserved]

1c.122 Use of Federal funds.

1c.123 Early termination of research support: Evaluation of applications and proposals.

1c.124 Conditions.

Authority: 5 U.S.C. 301; 42 U.S.C. 300v–1(b).

Ann M. Bartuska, Acting Under Secretary for Research, Education, and Economics, USDA.

Department of Energy

List of Subjects in 10 CFR Part 745

10 CFR Part 745

Human research subjects, Reporting and record-keeping requirements, Research.

- For the reasons stated in the preamble, the Department of Energy revises 10 CFR part 745, as set forth at the end of the common preamble of this document.

PART 745—PROTECTION OF HUMAN SUBJECTS

Sec. 745.101 To what does this policy apply?

745.102 Definitions for purposes of this policy.

745.103 Assuring compliance with this policy—research conducted or supported by any Federal department or agency.

745.104 Exempt research.

745.105 [Reserved]

745.106 [Reserved]

745.107 IRB membership.

745.108 IRB functions and operations.

745.109 IRB review of research.

745.110 Expedited review procedures for certain kinds of research involving no more than minimal risk, and for minor changes in approved research.

745.111 Criteria for IRB approval of research.

745.112 Review by institution.

745.113 Suspension or termination of IRB approval of research.

745.114 Cooperative research.

745.115 IRB records.

745.116 General requirements for informed consent.

745.117 Documentation of informed consent.

745.118 Applications and proposals lacking definite plans for involvement of human subjects.

745.119 Research undertaken without the intention of involving human subjects.

745.120 Evaluation and disposition of applications and proposals for research to be conducted or supported by a Federal department or agency.

745.121 [Reserved]

745.122 Use of Federal funds.

745.123 Early termination of research support: Evaluation of applications and proposals.

745.124 Conditions.

Authority: 5 U.S.C. 301; 42 U.S.C. 7254; 42 U.S.C. 300v–1(b).

Elizabeth Sherwood-Randall, Deputy Secretary of Energy.

National Aeronautics and Space Administration

List of Subjects in 14 CFR Part 1230

14 CFR Part 1230

Human research subjects, Reporting and record-keeping requirements, Research.

- For the reasons stated in the preamble, the National Aeronautics and Space Administration revises 14 CFR part 1230, as set forth at the end of the common preamble of this document.

PART 1230—PROTECTION OF HUMAN SUBJECTS

Sec.1230.101 To what does this policy apply?

1230.102 Definitions for purposes of this policy.

1230.103 Assuring compliance with this policy—research conducted or supported by any Federal department or agency.

1230.104 Exempt research.

1230.105 [Reserved]

1230.106 [Reserved]

1230.107 IRB membership.

1230.108 IRB functions and operations.

1230.109 IRB review of research.

1230.110 Expedited review procedures for certain kinds of research involving no more than minimal risk, and for minor changes in approved research.

1230.111 Criteria for IRB approval of research.

1230.112 Review by institution.

1230.113 Suspension or termination of IRB approval of research.

1230.114 Cooperative research.

1230.115 IRB records.

1230.116 General requirements for informed consent.

1230.117 Documentation of informed consent.

1230.118 Applications and proposals lacking definite plans for involvement of human subjects.

1230.119 Research undertaken without the intention of involving human subjects.

1230.120 Evaluation and disposition of applications and proposals for research to be conducted or supported by a Federal department or agency.

1230.121 [Reserved]

1230.122 Use of Federal funds.

1230.123 Early termination of research support: Evaluation of applications and proposals.

1230.124 Conditions.

Authority: 5 U.S.C. 301; 42 U.S.C. 300v–1(b).

James D. Polk, Chief Health and Medical Officer, NASA.

Department of Commerce

List of Subjects in 15 CFR Part 27

15 CFR Part 27

Human research subjects, Reporting and record-keeping requirements, Research.

- For the reasons stated in the preamble, the Department of Commerce revises 15 CFR part 27, as set forth at the end of the common preamble of this document.

PART 27—PROTECTION OF HUMAN SUBJECTS

Authority: 5 U.S.C. 301; 42 U.S.C. 300v–1(b).

James Hock, Chief of Staff, Department of Commerce.

Social Security Administration

List of Subjects in 20 CFR Part 431

20 CFR Part 431

Human research subjects, Reporting and record-keeping requirements, Research.

- For the reasons stated in the preamble, the Social Security Administration adds 20 CFR part 431, as set forth at the end of the common preamble of this document.

PART 431—PROTECTION OF HUMAN SUBJECTS

431.110 Expedited review procedures for certain kinds of research involving no more than minimal risk, and for minor changes in approved research.

431.111 Criteria for IRB approval of research.

431.112 Review by institution.

431.113 Suspension or termination of IRB approval of research.

431.114 Cooperative research.

431.115 IRB records.

431.116 General requirements for informed consent.

431.117 Documentation of informed consent.

431.118 Applications and proposals lacking definite plans for involvement of human subjects.

431.119 Research undertaken without the intention of involving human subjects.

431.120 Evaluation and disposition of applications and proposals for research to be conducted or supported by a Federal department or agency.

431.121 [Reserved]

431.122 Use of Federal funds.

431.123 Early termination of research support: Evaluation of applications and proposals.

431.124 Conditions.

Authority: 5 U.S.C. 301; 42 U.S.C. 289(a).

Carolyn W. Colvin, Acting Commissioner of Social Security.

Agency for International Development

List of Subjects in 22 CFR Part 225

22 CFR Part 225

Human research subjects, Reporting and record-keeping requirements, Research.

- For the reasons stated in the preamble, the Agency for International Development revises 22 CFR part 225 as set forth at the end of the common preamble of this document.

PART 225—PROTECTION OF HUMAN SUBJECTS

Sec. 225.101 To what does this policy apply?

225.102 Definitions for purposes of this policy.

225.103 Assuring compliance with this policy—research conducted or supported by any Federal department or agency.

225.104 Exempt research.

225.105 [Reserved]

225.106 [Reserved]

225.107 IRB membership.

225.108 IRB functions and operations.

225.109 IRB review of research.

225.110 Expedited review procedures for certain kinds of research involving no more than minimal risk, and for minor changes in approved research.

225.111 Criteria for IRB approval of research.

225.112 Review by institution.

225.113 Suspension or termination of IRB approval of research.

225.114 Cooperative research.

225.115 IRB records.

225.116 General requirements for informed consent.

225.117 Documentation of informed consent.

225.118 Applications and proposals lacking definite plans for involvement of human subjects.

225.119 Research undertaken without the intention of involving human subjects.

225.120 Evaluation and disposition of applications and proposals for research to be conducted or supported by a Federal department or agency.

225.121 [Reserved]

225.122 Use of Federal funds.

225.123 Early termination of research support: Evaluation of applications and proposals.

225.124 Conditions.

Authority: 5 U.S.C. 301; 42 U.S.C. 300v–1(b), unless otherwise noted.

Irene Koek, Acting Deputy Assistant Administrator for Global Health, U.S. Agency for International Development.

Department of Housing and Urban Development

List of Subjects in 24 CFR Part 60

24 CFR Part 60

Human research subjects, Reporting and record-keeping requirements, Research.

- For the reasons stated in the preamble, the Department of Housing and Urban Development revises 24 CFR part 60 as set forth at the end of the common preamble of this document.

PART 60—PROTECTION OF HUMAN SUBJECTS

Sec. 60.101 To what does this policy apply?

60.102 Definitions for purposes of this policy.

60.103 Assuring compliance with this policy—research conducted or supported by any Federal department or agency.

60.104 Exempt research.

60.105 [Reserved]

60.106 [Reserved]

60.107 IRB membership.

60.108 IRB functions and operations.

60.109 IRB review of research.

60.110 Expedited review procedures for certain kinds of research involving no more than minimal risk, and for minor changes in approved research.

60.111 Criteria for IRB approval of research.

60.112 Review by institution.

60.113 Suspension or termination of IRB approval of research.

60.114 Cooperative research.

60.115 IRB records.

60.116 General requirements for informed consent.

60.117 Documentation of informed consent.

60.118 Applications and proposals lacking definite plans for involvement of human subjects.

60.119 Research undertaken without the intention of involving human subjects.

60.120 Evaluation and disposition of applications and proposals for research to be conducted or supported by a Federal department or agency.

60.121 [Reserved]

60.122 Use of Federal funds.

60.123 Early termination of research support: Evaluation of applications and proposals.

60.124 Conditions.

Authority: 5 U.S.C. 301; 42 U.S.C. 300v–1(b) and 3535(d).

Katherine M. O'Regan, Assistant Secretary for Policy Development and Research, Department of Housing and Urban Development.

Department of Labor

List of Subjects in 29 CFR Part 21

29 CFR Part 21

Human research subjects, Reporting and record-keeping requirements, Research.

- For the reasons stated in the preamble, the Department of Labor adds 29 CFR part 21 as set forth at the end of the common preamble of this document.

PART 21—PROTECTION OF HUMAN SUBJECTS

Sec. 21.101 To what does this policy apply?

21.102 Definitions for purposes of this policy.

21.103 Assuring compliance with this policy—research conducted or supported by any Federal department or agency.

21.104 Exempt research.

21.105 [Reserved]

21.106 [Reserved]

21.107 IRB membership.

21.108 IRB functions and operations.

21.109 IRB review of research.

21.110 Expedited review procedures for certain kinds of research involving no more than minimal risk, and for minor changes in approved research.

21.111 Criteria for IRB approval of research.

21.112 Review by institution.

21.113 Suspension or termination of IRB approval of research.

21.114 Cooperative research.

21.115 IRB records.

21.116 General requirements for informed consent.

21.117 Documentation of informed consent.

21.118 Applications and proposals lacking definite plans for involvement of human subjects.

21.119 Research undertaken without the intention of involving human subjects.

21.120 Evaluation and disposition of applications and proposals for research to be conducted or supported by a Federal department or agency.

21.121 [Reserved]

21.122 Use of Federal funds.

21.123 Early termination of research support: Evaluation of applications and proposals.

21.124 Conditions.

Authority: 5 U.S.C. 301; 29 U.S.C. 551.

Christopher P. Lu, Deputy Secretary of Labor.

Department of Defense

List of Subjects in 32 CFR Part 219

32 CFR Part 219

Human research subjects, Reporting and record-keeping requirements, Research.

- For the reasons stated in the preamble, the Department of Defense revises 32 CFR part 219 as set forth at the end of the common preamble of this document.

PART 219—PROTECTION OF HUMAN SUBJECTS

Sec. 219.101 To what does this policy apply?

219.102 Definitions for purposes of this policy.

219.103 Assuring compliance with this policy—research conducted or supported by any Federal department or agency.

219.104 Exempt research.

219.105 [Reserved]

219.106 [Reserved]

219.107 IRB membership.

219.108 IRB functions and operations.

219.109 IRB review of research.

219.110 Expedited review procedures for certain kinds of research involving no more than minimal risk, and for minor changes in approved research.

219.111 Criteria for IRB approval of research.

219.112 Review by institution.

219.113 Suspension or termination of IRB approval of research.

219.114 Cooperative research.

219.115 IRB records.

219.116 General requirements for informed consent.

219.117 Documentation of informed consent.

219.118 Applications and proposals lacking definite plans for involvement of human subjects.

219.119 Research undertaken without the intention of involving human subjects.

219.120 Evaluation and disposition of applications and proposals for research to be conducted or supported by a Federal department or agency.

219.121 [Reserved]

219.122 Use of Federal funds.

219.123 Early termination of research support: Evaluation of applications and proposals.

219.124 Conditions.

Authority: 5 U.S.C. 301; 42 U.S.C. 300v–1(b).

Stephen P. Welby, Assistant Secretary of Defense (Research and Engineering).

Department of Education

List of Subjects in 34 CFR Part 97

Human research subjects, Reporting and record-keeping requirements, Research.

- For the reasons stated in the preamble, the Department of Education amends 34 CFR part 97 as follows:

PART 97—PROTECTION OF HUMAN SUBJECTS

- 1. The authority citation for part 97 continues to read as follows: Authority: 5 U.S.C. 301; 20 U.S.C. 1221e–3, 3474; 42 U.S.C. 300v–1(b).
- 2. Subpart A is revised as set forth at the end of the common preamble of this document.

Subpart A—Federal Policy for the Protection of Human Subjects (Basic ED Policy for Protection of Human Research Subjects)

Sec. 97.101 To what does this policy apply?

97.102 Definitions for purposes of this policy.

97.103 Assuring compliance with this policy—research conducted or supported by any Federal department or agency.

97.104 Exempt research.

97.105 [Reserved]

97.106 [Reserved]

97.107 IRB membership.

John B. King Jr., Secretary of Education.

Department of Veterans Affairs

List of Subjects in 38 CFR Part 16

38 CFR Part 16

Human research subjects, Reporting and record-keeping requirements, Research.

- For the reasons stated in the preamble, the Department of Veterans Affairs revises 38 CFR part 16 as set forth at the end of the common preamble of this document.

PART 16—PROTECTION OF HUMAN SUBJECTS

16.119 Research undertaken without the intention of involving human subjects.

16.120 Evaluation and disposition of applications and proposals for research to be conducted or supported by a Federal department or agency.

16.121 [Reserved]

16.122 Use of Federal funds.

16.123 Early termination of research support: Evaluation of applications and proposals.

16.124 Conditions.

Authority: 5 U.S.C. 301; 38 U.S.C. 501, 7331, 7334; 42 U.S.C. 300v–1(b).

Gina S. Farrisee, Deputy Chief of Staff, U.S. Department of Veterans Affairs.

Environmental Protection Agency

List of Subjects in 40 CFR Part 26

40 CFR Part 26

Human research subjects, Reporting and record-keeping requirements, Research.

- For the reasons stated in the preamble, the Environmental Protection Agency amends 40 CFR part 26 as follows:

PART 26—PROTECTION OF HUMAN SUBJECTS

- 1. The authority citation for part 26 continues to read as follows:

Authority: 5 U.S.C. 301; 7 U.S.C. 136a(a) and 136w(a)(1); 21 U.S.C. 346a(e)(1)(C); sec. 201, Pub. L. 109–54, 119 Stat. 531; and 42 U.S.C. 300v–1(b).

- 2. Subpart A is revised as set forth at the end of the common preamble of this document.

Subpart A—Basic EPA Policy for Protection of Subjects in Human Research Conducted or Supported by EPA

Sec. 26.101 To what does this policy apply?

26.102 Definitions for purposes of this policy.

26.103 Assuring compliance with this policy—research conducted or supported by any Federal department or agency.

26.104 Exempt research.

26.105 [Reserved]

26.106 [Reserved]

26.107 IRB membership.

26.108 IRB functions and operations.

26.109 IRB review of research.

26.110 Expedited review procedures for certain kinds of research involving no more than minimal risk, and for minor changes in approved research.

26.111 Criteria for IRB approval of research.

26.112 Review by institution.

26.113 Suspension or termination of IRB approval of research.

26.114 Cooperative research.

26.115 IRB records.

26.116 General requirements for informed consent.

26.117 Documentation of informed consent.

26.118 Applications and proposals lacking definite plans for involvement of human subjects.

26.119 Research undertaken without the intention of involving human subjects.

26.120 Evaluation and disposition of applications and proposals for research to be conducted or supported by a Federal department or agency.

26.121 [Reserved]

26.122 Use of Federal funds.

26.123 Early termination of research support: Evaluation of applications and proposals.

26.124 Conditions.

A. Stanley Meiburg, Acting Deputy Administrator, Environmental Protection Agency.

Department of Health and Human Services

List of Subjects in 45 CFR Part 46

45 CFR Part 46

Human research subjects, Reporting and record-keeping requirements, Research.

- For the reasons stated in the preamble, the Department of Health and Human Services amends 45 CFR part 46 as follows:

PART 46—PROTECTION OF HUMAN SUBJECTS

- 1. The authority citation for part 46 is revised to read as follows:

    Authority: 5 U.S.C. 301; 42 U.S.C. 289(a); 42 U.S.C. 300v–1(b).

- 2. Subpart A is revised as set forth at the end of the common preamble of this document.

Subpart A—Basic HHS Policy for Protection of Human Research Subjects

Sec. 46.101 To what does this policy apply?

46.102 Definitions for purposes of this policy.

46.103 Assuring compliance with this policy—research conducted or supported by any Federal department or agency.

46.104 Exempt research.

46.105 [Reserved]

46.106 [Reserved]

46.107 IRB membership.

46.108 IRB functions and operations.

46.109 IRB review of research.

46.110 Expedited review procedures for certain kinds of research involving no more than minimal risk, and for minor changes in approved research.

46.111 Criteria for IRB approval of research.

46.112 Review by institution.

46.113 Suspension or termination of IRB approval of research.

46.114 Cooperative research.

46.115 IRB records.

46.116 General requirements for informed consent.

46.117 Documentation of informed consent.

46.118 Applications and proposals lacking definite plans for involvement of human subjects.

46.119 Research undertaken without the intention of involving human subjects.

46.120 Evaluation and disposition of applications and proposals for research to be conducted or supported by a Federal department or agency.

46.121 [Reserved]

46.122 Use of Federal funds.

46.123 Early termination of research support: Evaluation of applications and proposals.

46.124 Conditions.

Sylvia M. Burwell, Secretary, HHS.

National Science Foundation

List of Subjects in 45 CFR Part 690
45 CFR Part 690
Human research subjects, Reporting and record-keeping requirements, Research.

- For the reasons stated in the preamble, the National Science Foundation revises 45 CFR part 690 as set forth at the end of the common preamble of this document.

PART 690—PROTECTION OF HUMAN SUBJECTS
Sec. 690.101 To what does this policy apply?
690.102 Definitions for purposes of this policy.
690.103 Assuring compliance with this policy—research conducted or supported by any Federal department or agency.
690.104 Exempt research.
690.105 [Reserved]
690.106 [Reserved]
690.107 IRB membership.
690.108 IRB functions and operations.
690.109 IRB review of research.
690.110 Expedited review procedures for certain kinds of research involving no more than minimal risk, and for minor changes in approved research.
690.111 Criteria for IRB approval of research.
690.112 Review by institution.
690.113 Suspension or termination of IRB approval of research.
690.114 Cooperative research.
690.115 IRB records.
690.116 General requirements for informed consent.
690.117 Documentation of informed consent.
690.118 Applications and proposals lacking definite plans for involvement of human subjects.
690.119 Research undertaken without the intention of involving human subjects.
690.120 Evaluation and disposition of applications and proposals for research to be conducted or supported by a Federal department or agency.
690.121 [Reserved]
690.122 Use of Federal funds.
690.123 Early termination of research support: Evaluation of applications and proposals.
690.124 Conditions.
Authority: 5 U.S.C. 301; 42 U.S.C. 300v–1(b).
Lawrence Rudolph, General Counsel, National Science Foundation.

Department of Transportation

List of Subjects in 49 CFR Part 11
49 CFR Part 11
Human research subjects, Reporting and record-keeping requirements, Research.

- For the reasons stated in the preamble, the Department of Transportation revises 49 CFR part 11 as set forth at the end of the common preamble of this document.

PART 11—PROTECTION OF HUMAN SUBJECTS

Sec. 11.101 To what does this policy apply?

11.102 Definitions for purposes of this policy.

11.103 Assuring compliance with this policy—research conducted or supported by any Federal department or agency.

11.104 Exempt research.

11.105 [Reserved]

11.106 [Reserved]

11.107 IRB membership.

11.108 IRB functions and operations.

11.109 IRB review of research.

11.110 Expedited review procedures for certain kinds of research involving no more than minimal risk, and for minor changes in approved research.

11.111 Criteria for IRB approval of research.

11.112 Review by institution.

11.113 Suspension or termination of IRB approval of research.

11.114 Cooperative research.

11.115 IRB records.

11.116 General requirements for informed consent.

11.117 Documentation of informed consent.

11.118 Applications and proposals lacking definite plans for involvement of human subjects.

11.119 Research undertaken without the intention of involving human subjects.

11.120 Evaluation and disposition of applications and proposals for research to be conducted or supported by a Federal department or agency.

11.121 [Reserved]

11.122 Use of Federal funds.

11.123 Early termination of research support: Evaluation of applications and proposals.

11.124 Conditions.

Authority: 5 U.S.C. 301; 42 U.S.C. 300v–1(b).

Anthony R. Foxx, Secretary of Transportation.

Federal Register. (2017). Vol. 82, No. 12. 45 CFR 46 and Preamble (pp. 7269–7274). www.govinfo.gov/content/pkg/FR-2017-01-19/pdf/2017-01058.pdf

Index

Note: Locators followed by 'f' and 't' refers to figures and tables.